CARDIOVASCULAR MAGNETIC RESONANCE

A Companion to BRAUNWALD'S HEART DISEASE

CARDIOVASCULAR MAGNETIC RESONANCE

A Companion to **BRAUNWALD'S HEART DISEASE**

EDITION 4

RAYMOND J. KIM, MD
Director, Duke Cardiovascular Magnetic Resonance Center
Professor, Medicine and Radiology
Duke University Medical Center
Durham, North Carolina

ELSEVIER

Elsevier
1818 Market Street, Suite 3323
Philadelphia, PA 19103-2899

CARDIOVASCULAR MAGNETIC RESONANCE: A COMPANION
TO BRAUNWALD'S HEART DISEASE, FOURTH EDITION ISBN: 978-0-443-12497-6

Senior Content Strategist: Melanie Tucker
Senior Content Development Specialist: Garima Malhotra
Publishing Services Manager: Deepthi Unni
Senior Project Manager: Nayagi Anandan
Design Direction: Renee Duenow

Printed in India by Thomson Press India Private Ltd,
18/35, Delhi-Mathura Road, Faridabad-121007, Haryana

Last digit is the print number: 9 8 7 6 5 4 3 2 1

To my family—the blessings of my life.

R.J.K.

Contributors

Amna Abdel-Gadir, BSc (Hons), MBBS, MRCP, MD(Res)
Cardiology Registrar
Barts Heart Centre
Barts Health NHS Trust
London, United Kingdom

Aiden Abidov, MD, PhD
Professor of Medicine
Radiology and Emergency Medicine
Medicine
Wayne State University School of Medicine
Detroit, Michigan
Section Chief
Cardiology
Medicine
John D. Dingell VA Medical Center
Detroit, Michigan

Fawaz Alenezi, MD, MSC, FACC, FAHA, FASE
Associate Professor of Medicine
Medicine
Duke University
Durham, North Carolina

Andrew E. Arai, MD, FAHA, MSCMR
Cardiologist
Cardiology
University of Utah Health
University of Utah Hospital
Salt Lake City, Utah

Nay Aung, MBBS, MRCP, PhD
Clinical Senior Lecturer
William Harvey Research Institute
Queen Mary University of London
London, United Kingdom
Consultant Cardiologist
Cardiology
Barts Heart Centre
Barts Health NHS Trust
London, United Kingdom

Robert S. Balaban, PHD
Emeritus Scientist
Systems Biology Center
NHLBI
Bethesda, Maryland

Liisa L. Bergmann, MD, MBA
Cardiothoracic Radiology Division Chief,
Associate Professor
Radiology
Medical College of Wisconsin
Milwaukee, Wisconsin

David A. Bluemke, MD, PhD, MsB
Professor
Radiology
University of Wisconsin School of Medicine and Public Health
Madison, Wisconsin

Nadine K. Boehm, MD
Senior Physician
Radiology
Kanstonsspital Graubuenden
Chur, Switzerland

Rene M. Botnar, PhD
Professor
Institute for Biological and Medical Engineering
Pontificia Universidad de Chile
Santiago de Chile, Region Metropolitana, Chile
Professor
Biomedical Engineering and Imaging Sciences
King's College London
London, United Kingdom

Wendy Bottinor, MD, MSCI
Physician
Internal Medicine
VCU
Richmond, Virginia

Adriano Camargo de Castro Carneiro, MD
Medical Coordinator, Division of Cardiovascular MRI and CT
Department of Radiology
Hospital do Coração (HCor)
São Paulo, São Paulo, Brazil
Cardiologist
Emergency Department
Hospital Alemão Oswaldo Cruz
São Paulo, São Paulo, Brazil

Michael J. Campbell, MD, MHA
Professor
Pediatrics
Duke University
Durham, North Carolina

Peter Caravan, PhD
Director
Institute for Innovation in Imaging
Massachusetts General Hospital
Boston, Massachusetts
Professor
Radiology
Harvard Medical School
Boston, Massachusetts
Director of Fundamental Research
Radiology
MassGeneralBrigham
Boston, Massachusetts

Angel Chan, MD, PhD
Assistant Attending
Medicine and Radiology
Memorial Sloan Kettering Cancer Center
New York, New York
Assistant Professor
Medicine
Weill Cornell Medicine – New York Presbyterian Hospital
New York, New York

Enn-Ling Chen, PhD
Assistant Professor of Research
Medicine
Duke University
Durham, North Carolina

Céleste M. Chevalier, MD
Research Faculty
Duke Cardiovascular Magnetic Resonance Center
Duke University Hospital
Durham, North Carolina

Clerio De Azevedo Filho, MD, PhD
Associate Professor
Medicine, Division of Cardiology
Duke University
Durham, North Carolina

Kaoru Dohi, MD, PhD
Professor
Department of Cardiology and Nephrology
Mie University Graduate School of Medicine
Tsu City, Japan

Ingo Eitel, Prof. Dr, MD
Director
Director of Cardiology, Angiology, and Intensive Care Medicine
University Heart Center
Lübeck, Germany

Carlos El-Tallawi, MD, FACC, FASE
Assistant Professor of Cardiology
Department of Cardiology
Houston Methodist Hospital DeBakey Heart and Vascular Center
Houston, Texas

Afshin Farzaneh-Far, MD, PhD
Adjunct Faculty
Cardiology
Duke
Durham, North Carolina
Therapeutic Area Head Cardiology
Solid Biosciences
Boston, Massachusetts

Victor A. Ferrari, MD
Professor
Medicine
Hospital of the University of Pennsylvania
Philadelphia, Pennsylvania
Chair, Penn Cardiovascular Imaging Council
Medicine
Hospital of the University of Pennsylvania
Philadelphia, Pennsylvania

Mark A. Fogel, MD, FACC, FAHA, MSCMR, FNASCI, FAAP
Professor of Pediatrics (Cardiology)/Director of Cardiac MR
Pediatrics and Radiology
Children's Hospital of Philadelphia/Perelman School of Medicine at University of Pennyslvania
Philadelphia, Pennsylvania

Christopher J. François, MD
Radiologist
Radiology
Mayo Clinic
Rochester, Minnesota

Yin Ge, MD
Assistant Professor
Division of Cardiology
University of Toronto
Toronto, Ontario, Canada

John D. Grizzard, MD
Associate Professor
Radiology
VCU Health Systems
Richmond, Virginia

Thomas H. Hauser, MD, MMSc, MPH
Director, Translational Medicine
Cardiovascular and Metabolism
Novartis Biomedical Research
Cambridge, Massachusetts
Lecturer, part-time
Medicine
Harvard Medical School
Boston, Massachusetts
Physician
Cardiovascular Disease
Beth Israel Deaconess Medical Center
Boston, Massachusetts

Chenxi Hu, PhD
Associate Professor
School of Biomedical Engineering
Shanghai Jiao Tong University
Shanghai, China

Gregory W. Hundley, MD
Professor of Medicine/Chief/Director
Cardiology/Internal Medicine
VCU Health Pauley Heart Center
Richmond, Virginia

Masaki Ishida, MD, PhD
Associate Professor
Radiology
Mie University Hospital
Tsu, Mie, Japan

Kelly Jarvis, PhD
Assistant Professor
Radiology
Northwestern University
Chicago, Illinois

Michael Jerosch-Herold, PhD
Associate Professor
Radiology
Harvard Medical School
Boston, Massachusetts
Director of Cardiac Imaging Physics
Radiology
Brigham & Women's Hospital
Boston, Massachusetts

Kim Jiwon, MD
Associate Professor
Department of Medicine (Division of Cardiology)
Weill Cornell Medicine
New York, New York

Jennifer Jordan, PhD, MS, FSCMR
Associate Professor
Department of Biomedical Engineering & Pauley Heart Center
Virginia Commonwealth University
Richmond, Virginia

Robert M. Judd, PhD
Professor Emeritus
Medicine
Duke University
Durham, North Carolina

Yodying Kaolawanich, MD
Associate Professor
Division of Cardiology
Department of Medicine
Faculty of Medicine Siriraj Hospital
Mahidol University
Bangkok Noi, Bangkok, Thailand

Simrat Kaur, MBBS, MD
Cardiology fellow
Cardiovascular Medicine
Cleveland Clinic Foundation
Cleveland, Ohio

Peter Kellman, PhD
Emeritus Staff Scientist
National Heart, Lung, and Blood Institute
National Institutes of Health
Bethesda, Maryland

Han W. Kim, MD
Associate Professor of Medicine
Cardiology
Duke University Medical Center
Durham, North Carolina

Raymond J. Kim, MD
Director, Duke Cardiovascular Magnetic Resonance Center
Professor, Medicine and Radiology
Duke University Medical Center
Durham, North Carolina

Allan L. Klein, MD, FRCP(C), FACC, FAHA, FASE, FESC
Professor of Medicine
Section of Cardiovascular Imaging
Lerner College of Medicine of Case Western University
Cleveland, Ohio
Director
Department of Cardiovascular Medicine/Heart, Vascular and Thoracic Institute
Center for the Diagnosis and Treatment of Pericardial Diseases
Cleveland, Ohio
Past-President
American Society of Echocardiography
Cleveland, Ohio
President
National Board of Echocardiography
Cleveland, Ohio

Igor Klem, MD
Associate Professor of Medicine/Director
Cardiology Consultation and Teaching Service
Duke University Medical Center
Durham, North Carolina

Christopher M. Kramer, M.D.
George A. Beller MD/Lantheus Medical Imaging Distinguished Professor of Cardiovascular Medicine
University of Virginia Health
Charlottesville, Virginia

Raymond Y. Kwong, MD, MPH
Director of Cardiac Magnetic Resonance Imaging
Cardiology
Brigham and Women's Hospital
Chestnut Hill, Massachusetts
Professor of Medicine
Department of Medicine
Harvard Medical School
Boston, Massachusetts

Deborah H. Kwon, MD
Director of Cardiac MRI
Cardiovascular Medicine and Radiology
Heart and Vascular Institute
Cleveland, Ohio
Associate Professor
Medicine
Cleveland Clinic Lerner College of Medicine at Case Western Reserve University
Cleveland, Ohio

David Leslie, PhD
Professor
Digital Environment Research Institute
Queen Mary University of London
London, United Kingdom

Maan Malahfji, MD
Assistant Professor
Department of Cardiology
Houston Methodist Hospital
Houston, Texas

Warren J. Manning, MD
Section Chief, Non-invasive Cardiac Imaging & Testing
Cardiovascular Division
Beth Israel Deaconess Medical Center
Boston, Massachusetts
Professor of Medicine and Radiology
Harvard Medical School
Boston, Massachusetts

Anne M. Valente, MD
Professor
Pediatrics, Medicine
Harvard Medical School
Boston, Massachusetts
Division Chief
Boston Adult Congenital Heart Program
Children's Hospital Boston
Boston, Massachusetts
Staff Cardiologist
Internal Medicine
Division of Cardiology
Brigham and Women's Hospital
Boston, Massachusetts

Michael Markl, PhD
Professor
Radiology
NU
Chicago, Illinois

Manish Motwani, MB ChB, PhD, FSCMR
Consultant
Department of Cardiology
Manchester Heart Institute
Manchester University NHS Foudnation Trust
Manchester, United Kingdom

Eike Nagel, MD, PhD
Director
Institute for Experimental and Translational Cardiovascular Imaging
Goethe University Frankfurt am Main
Frankfurt am Main, Hesse, Germany

Shiro Nakomori, MD, PhD
Senior Lecturer
Cardiology
Mie University Graduate School of Medicine
Tsu, Japan
Staff Scientist
Medicine
Beth Israel Deaconess Medical Center and Harvard Medical School
Boston, Massachusetts

Stefan Neubauer, MD, FRCP, FACC, FMedSci, MSCMR
Professor
Division of Cardiovascular Medicine, Radcliffe Department of Medicine
University of Oxford
Oxford, United Kingdom

Reza Nezafat, PhD
Professor of Medicine
Medicine
Harvard Medical School
Boston, Massachusetts

Christoph A. Nienaber, MD, PhD
Professor
Cardiology, Centre for Aortic Diseases
Guy's and St. Thomas' NHS Foundation Trust
London, United Kingdom

Robin Nijveldt, MD, PhD
Cardiologist
Cardiology
Radboud University Medical Center
Nijmegen, Netherlands

Ankur Pandya, PhD
Associate Professor of Health Decision Science
Health Policy and Management
Harvard T.H. Chan School of Public Health
Boston, Massachusetts

Laura S. Pappas, Dr
Adjunct Lecturer
Cardiovascular Imaging
Institute for Experimental and Translational Cardiovascular Imaging
Frankfurt am Main, Germany

Steffen E. Petersen, MSc MPH MD DPHIL
Professor of Cardiovascular Medicine
William Harvey Research Institute
Queen Mary University of London
London, United Kingdom
Consultant Cardiologist
Barts Heart and Thorax Centre
Barts Health NHS Trust
London, United Kingdom
Interim Director
British Heart Foundation Data Science Centre
Health Data Research UK
London, United Kingdom

Dana C. Peters, PhD
Professor
Radiology and Biomedical Imaging
Yale University
New London, Connecticut

Sven Plein, MD, PhD, FRCP, FESC, FEACVI, MSCMR
Professor of Cardiology
Biomedical Imaging Science Department
University of Leeds
Leeds, United Kingdom

Andrew J. Powell, MD
Chief, Cardiac Imaging Division
Department of Cardiology
Boston Children's Hospital
Boston, Massachusetts
Professor
Department of Pediatrics
Harvard Medical School
Boston, Massachusetts

Oliver J. Rider, BMBCh, DPhil
Professor
Cardiovascular Medicine
University of Oxford
Oxford, United Kingdom

Carlos E. Rochitte, MD, PhD
Associate Professor, Chief-Medical Officer and Director of InCor Reaearch Center, Cardiovascular Magnetic Resonance and Computed Tomography Coordinator
Cardiology
Heart Institute, InCor
University of São Paulo Medical School
São Paulo, Brazil
Cardiovascular Magnetic Resonance and Computed Tomography Director
Cardiology
HCor
São Paulo, Brazil
Cardiovascular MR and CT Senior Leader
Cardiology
Alta Diagnostic Center (DASA Group)
São Paulo, Brazil

Caroline H. Roney, PhD, MRes, MMath
Reader in Computational Medicine
School of Engineering & Materials Science
Queen Mary University of London
London, United Kingdom

Hajime Sakuma, MD, PhD, FAHA
CEO
Department of Radiology
Mie University
Tsu, Japan

Michael Salerno, MD, PhD, MS
Professor
Residence of Medicine and Radiology and Medical Imaging
University of California
San Francisco, California
Hugh and Eila Korpi Distinguished Professor
Cardiology Research
USCF School of Medicine
San Francisco, California
Section Chief of Echocardiography and Cardiac Imaging
Cardiology Division
University of California
San Francisco, California
Director of Multimodality Cardiac Imaging and Advanced Cardiovascular Imaging Fellowship
Cardiology
University of California
San Francisco, California

Michael S. Hansen, PhD
Senior Director
Microsoft Research
Microsoft
Redmond, Washington

Andreas Schuster, MD PhD MBA
Professor of Cardiology
FORUM Cardiology
FORUM Medicine
Rosdorf Göttingen, Germany

Juerg Schwitter, MD
Professor
Department of Cardiovascular Medicine
University Hospital Lausanne, CHUV
Lausanne, Switzerland
Director
Cardiac MR Center of the CHUV
University Hospital Lausanne
Lausanne, Switzerland
Director
Interventional MRI Center of the CHUV
University Hospital Lausanne
Lausannne, Switzerland

Dipan J. Shah, MD
Chief, Division of Cardiovascular Imaging
Cardiology
Houston Methodist Hospital
Houston, Texas

Chetan Shenoy, MBBS, MS
Professor
Cardiovascular Division, Department of Medicine
University of Minnesota
Minneapolis, Minnesota

Orlando P. Simonetti, PhD
Professor
Departments of Radiology and Internal Medicine
The Ohio State University
Columbus, Ohio
John W. Wolfe Professor in Cardiovascular Research

Gregory Slabaugh, PhD
Professor and Director
Digital Environment Research Institute
Queen Mary University of London
London, United Kingdom

Jitka Starekova, MD, Dr. Med
Scientist
Department of Radiology
UW-Madison
Madison, Wisconsin

Cory R. Trankle, MD
Associate Professor
Division of Cardiology, Department of Internal Medicine/Pauley Heart Center
Virginia Commonwealth University
Richmond, Virginia

Ladislav Valkovič, DSc
Associate Professor
OCMR, RDM Cardiovascular Medicine
University of Oxford
Oxford, United Kingdom
Researcher
Department of Imaging Methods
Institute of Measurement Scienec, Slovak Academy of Sciences
Bratislava, Slovakia

Juliet Varghese, PhD
Assistant Professor
Department of Radiology
The Ohio State University
Columbus, Ohio

Pablo Villar-Calle, MD
Clinical Instructor
Cardiology
Weill Cornell Medicine
New York, New York

Jonathan W. Weinsaft, MD
Professor of Medicine (Cardiology)
Medicine
Weill Cornell Medicine
New York, New York

David C. Wendell, PhD
Research Scientist - Senior
Medicine/Cardiology
Duke University
Durham, North Carolina

Mark Westwood, MD, FRCP, FESC
Consultant Cardiologist
Department of Cardiology
London Bridge Hospital
London, United Kingdom

Xun Yuan, MBBS, MMed, PhD
Senior Clinical Fellow
Cardiology
Royal Brompton Hospital
London, United Kingdom
Specialty Doctor in Cardiology
Cardiology
Milton Keynes University Hospital
Milton Keynes, United Kingdom

Robert S. Zhang, MD
Assistant Professor in Medicine
Cardiology
Weill Cornell Medicine
New York City, New York

Foreword

In 1900, Dr. Wilhelm Roentgen received the first Nobel Prize in Physics. His monumental discovery allowed, for the first time, images of the heart in intact patients. Roentgenology, named in honor of its discoverer, ranks high among the greatest advances of modern medicine. The two specialties of imaging sciences and cardiology developed hand in hand during the first half of the 20th century. Imaging progressed with a variety of technologies that included angiography, ultrasound, radionuclide imaging, computed tomography, positron emission tomography, and cardiovascular magnetic resonance (CMR).

Of these, CMR offers a veritable treasure trove of information about the heart and great vessels. It not only provides excellent three-dimensional displays of the structure and function of the cardiac chambers and valves, but is also useful in the assessment of the normal and diseased aorta. The lumina, walls, and obstructive lesions in the major coronary arteries can be visualized, and myocardial perfusion assessed. Myocardial ischemia, necrosis, edema, and fibrosis can be detected and quantified. When combined with the ability to determine myocardial viability and to measure cardiac high-energy phosphate stores noninvasively by CMR spectroscopy, the assessment of patients with ischemic heart disease is greatly enhanced. This noninvasive technique, which does not require ionizing radiation, can reduce the need for coronary angiography, now performed on more than 1.5 million patients each year in the United States alone.

Just as it became necessary for the pioneer cardiologists of the early 20th century to become familiar with cardiac radiology, it is now equally important for their successors to do the same with CMR. Raymond Kim, a distinguished leader of this important technology, and his talented contributors to *Cardiovascular Magnetic Resonance*, have taken an important step toward enabling clinicians and clinical investigators to accomplish this. They deserve the appreciation of cardiovascular specialists, radiologists, and trainees for producing this detailed, authoritative, yet eminently readable book. We are very pleased to welcome this fourth edition of *Cardiovascular Magnetic Resonance* into the family of *Companions to Heart Disease: A Textbook of Cardiovascular Medicine*.

Eugene Braunwald, MD
Robert O. Bonow, MD, MS
Douglas L. Mann, MD
Gordon F. Tomaselli, MD
Deepak L. Bhatt, MD, MPH, MBA
Scott D. Solomon, MD
Peter Libby, MD

Contents

Braunwald's Heart Disease Family of Books

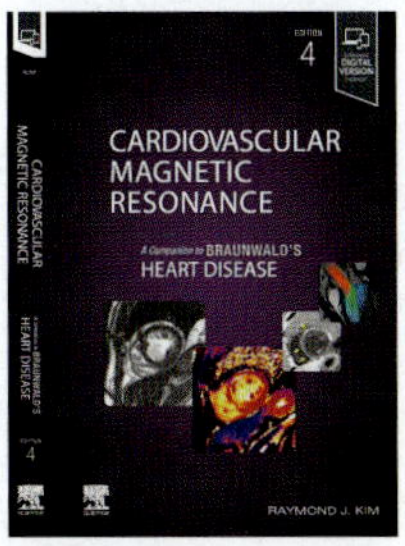

KIM
Cardiovascular Magnetic Resonance

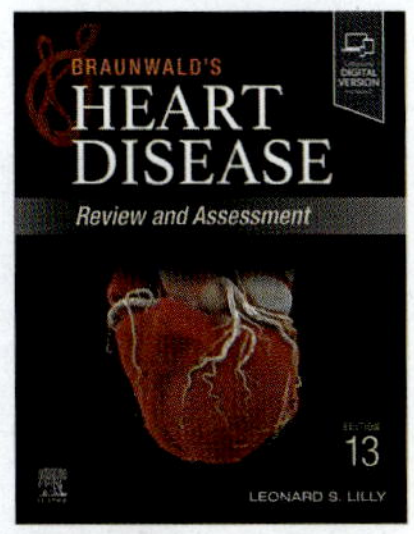

LILLY
Braunwald's Heart Disease Review and Assessment

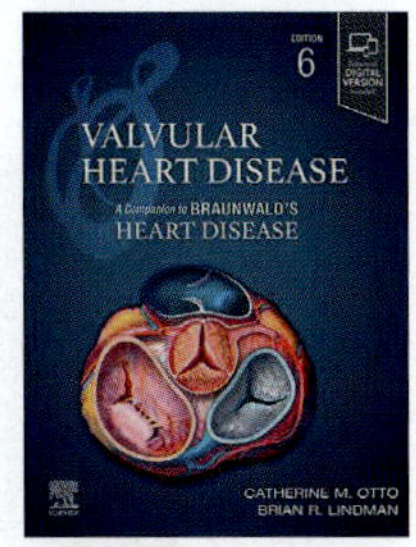

OTTO AND LINDMAN
Valvular Heart Disease

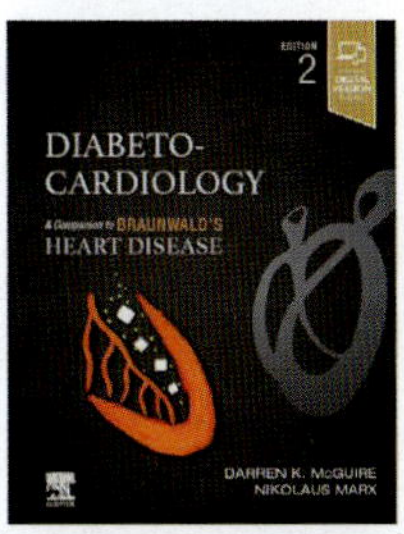

McGUIRE AND MARX
Diabeto-Cardiology

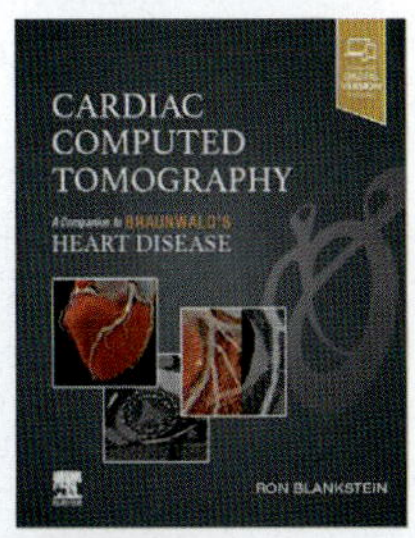

BLANKSTEIN
Computed Cardiac Tomography

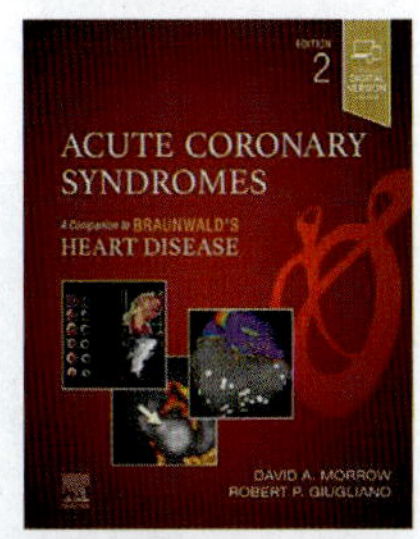

MORROW AND GIUGLIANO
Acute Coronary Syndromes

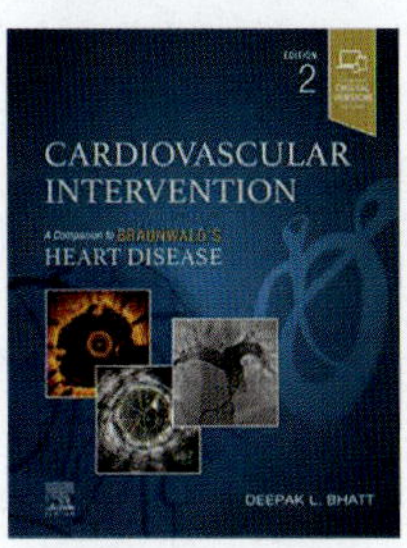

BHATT
Cardiovascular Intervention

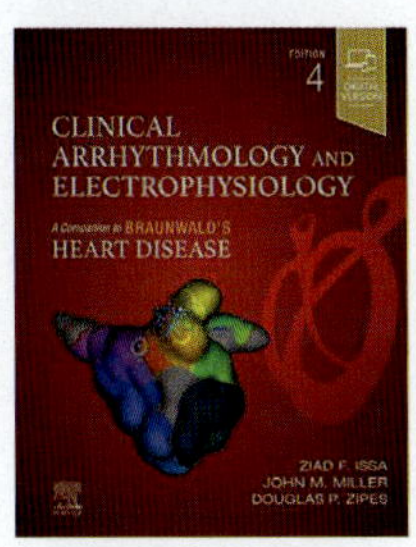

ISSA, MILLER, ZIPES
Clinical Arrhythmology and Electrophysiology

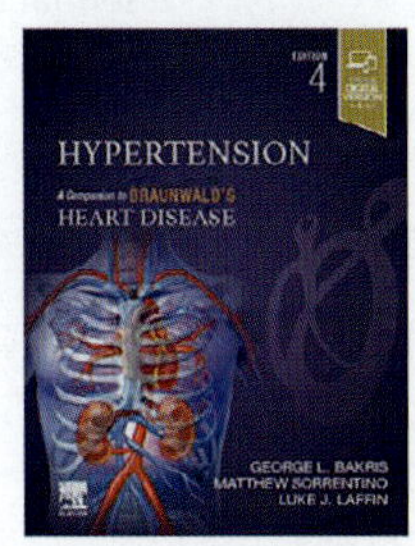

BAKRIS, SORRENTINO, AND LAFFIN
Hypertension

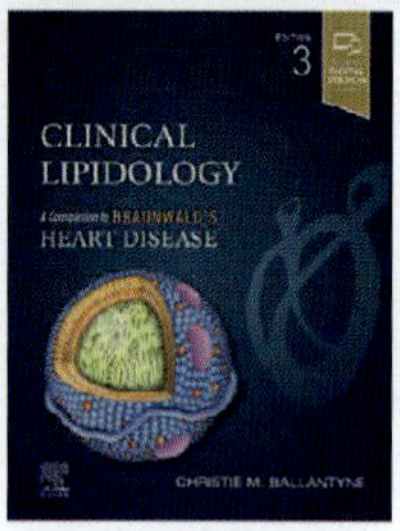

BALLANTYNE
Clinical Lipidology

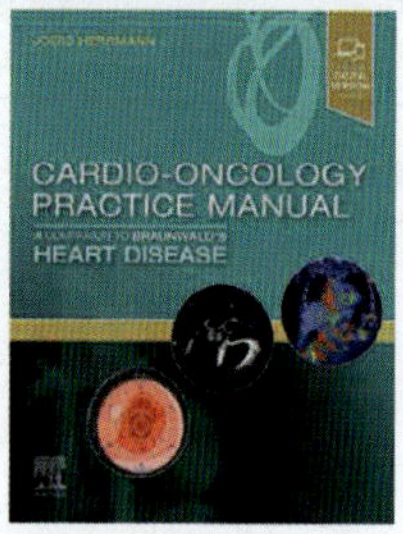

HERRMANN
Cardio-Oncology Practice Manual

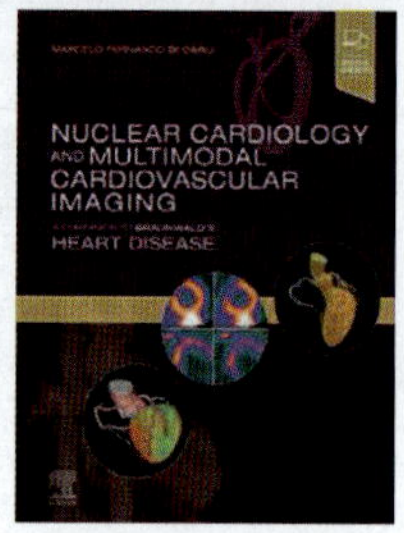

DI CARLI
Nuclear Cardiology and Multimodal Cardiovascular Imaging

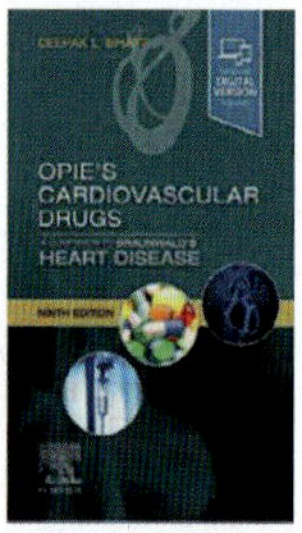

BHATT
Opie's Cardiovascular Drugs

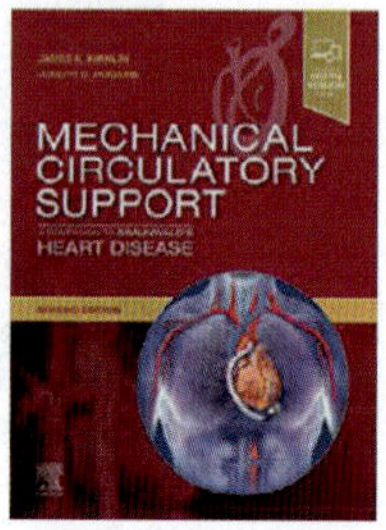

KIRKLIN AND ROGERS
Mechanical Circulatory Support

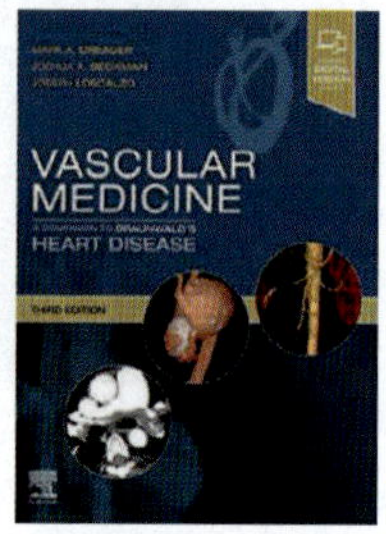

CREAGER
Vascular Medicine

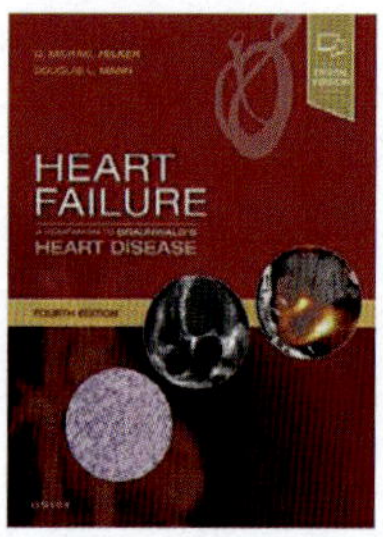

FELKER AND MANN
Heart Failure

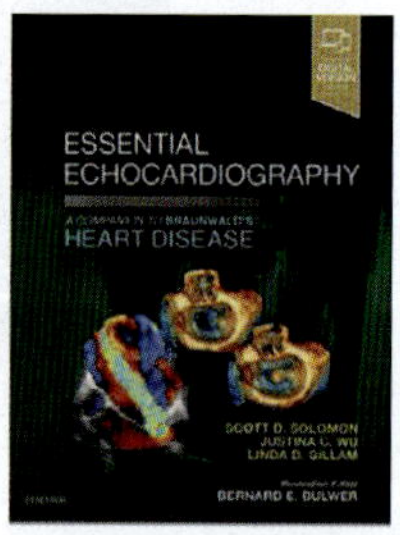

SOLOMON, WU, AND GILLAM
Essential Echocardiography

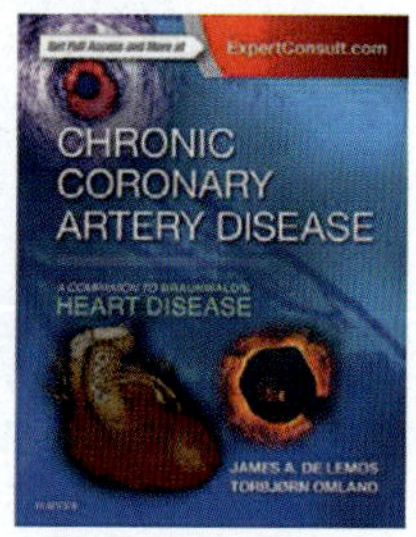

DE LEMOS AND OMLAND
Chronic Coronary Artery Disease

1 Physics, Instrumentation, and Basic Sequences

ROBERT S. BALABAN, CHENXI HU, AND DANA C. PETERS

INTRODUCTION

This introduction to the basic principles of cardiovascular magnetic resonance (CMR) describes the concepts of magnetization, T1, T2, T2*, and image formation, and describes some common magnetic resonance imaging (MRI) pulse sequences and parameters. An overview is presented in Fig. 1.1, but it will require time and rereading to fully appreciate each new concept that together explains MRI.

The human body is composed of mostly water and a lot of fat. The water (H_2O) and fat contain many hydrogen atoms. Hydrogen atoms in turn are made up of a proton (^1H, the hydrogen nucleus) and an electron (Fig. 1.1). Hydrogen protons are in very high concentration in the body, roughly 100 molar (the molarity of ^1H can be estimated as ~[2 moles hydrogen/mole H_2O] × [1 mole H_2O/18 g of tissue] × 1000 g/L[density of the body] ~ 100 mole/L). These hydrogen protons within the body can be imaged through MRI. MRI is possible because hydrogen protons have "spin," and all nuclei with spin interact with magnetic fields. Spin is called the "intrinsic angular momentum," and it is a fundamental property of protons. MRI physics is often called "spin physics" because it describes how the proton spins are used to image the body. In this chapter we will use the term *spin* to indicate the hydrogen proton's spin. MRI images these spins, and in this way it images the tissues in which they are embedded.

MRI uses a main magnetic field called B0. The B0 field in MRI is manufactured to be large (10,000 × stronger than Earth's field), homogeneous, and directed along the tube of the MRI scanner (in the foot-head direction of the patient). While an electric field attracts or repels charged objects, a magnetic field is known to affect magnetic objects by rotating them, using torque, into alignment with the field. In the absence of a magnetic field, spins are randomly oriented (Fig. 1.2A). But if placed in a large homogeneous magnetic field (the scanner), water spins very slightly align in the same orientation of this magnetic field, much like iron filings (Fig. 1.2B), with larger magnetic fields causing greater alignment of the spins. In fact, the bulk magnetization, M_z, is proportional to the strength of the applied field. Unlike iron filings, however, the interaction of the spins with the B_0 field results in the spins rotating around the axis of the magnetic field (Fig. 1.2C). This is why the hydrogen nuclei in MRI are also referred to as spins: they spin (precess) around the B_0 field. The frequency of precession (υ) is a very important property of the spins in a magnetic field and is defined by the Larmor equation:

$$\nu = \frac{\gamma}{2\pi}B \qquad \text{Eq. 1.1}$$

where B is the magnetic field strength experienced by the spin, which is approximately B_0, but includes any variations as described below, υ is the spin's precessional frequency in cycles/s or hertz (Hz), and γ (gamma) is the gyromagnetic ratio, which is a constant related to the mass and charge of the water proton: $\gamma/2\pi = 42.58 \times 10^6$ Hz/Tesla for water protons. The precessional frequency for water protons at 1.5 Tesla (T) (a common CMR field strength) is $\nu = 63.87 \times 10^6$ Hz, or roughly 64 MHz (about the frequency of an FM radio station and one of the reasons the CMR scanner room must be shielded from FM radio waves). According to Eq. (1.1), at 3 T, the precessional frequency is twice this: $\nu = 127.74 \times 10^6$ Hz. The Larmor equation (see Eq. 1.1) looks simple, but it is the basis of both RF excitation and spatial localization.

DETECTION OF THE MAGNETIC RESONANCE IMAGING SIGNAL

Alignment With the Main Magnetic Field

How can the MRI signal from water spins be detected to image the sample? Remember, when a sample (i.e., a patient) is placed in the main magnetic field (i.e., inside the bore of the magnet), the hydrogen spins align with that field (see Fig. 1.2B) and begin to precess at the Larmor frequency. The main magnetic field, B_0, is large and homogeneous and is directed along the Z-axis or longitudinal direction. Since the spins partially align with the B_0 field, they create a net magnetic field along the Z axis (oriented parallel with B_0). However, the spins precess or rotate around the Z axis in a random, incoherent fashion, resulting in no net magnetization in the X-Y plane (also called the transverse plane) (see Fig. 1.2C). Magnetization by the B_0 field (i.e., M_z) is *not* enough to generate a magnetic resonance (MR) signal. The MR signal is measured as the magnetization on the X-Y plane (called M_{xy}). The MR signal is detected by placing a receiver coil (loops of wire tuned to receive signals oscillating at the Larmor frequency) near the subject to detect any spin precession in the X-Y plane. A receiver coil placed to detect the precession of spins in

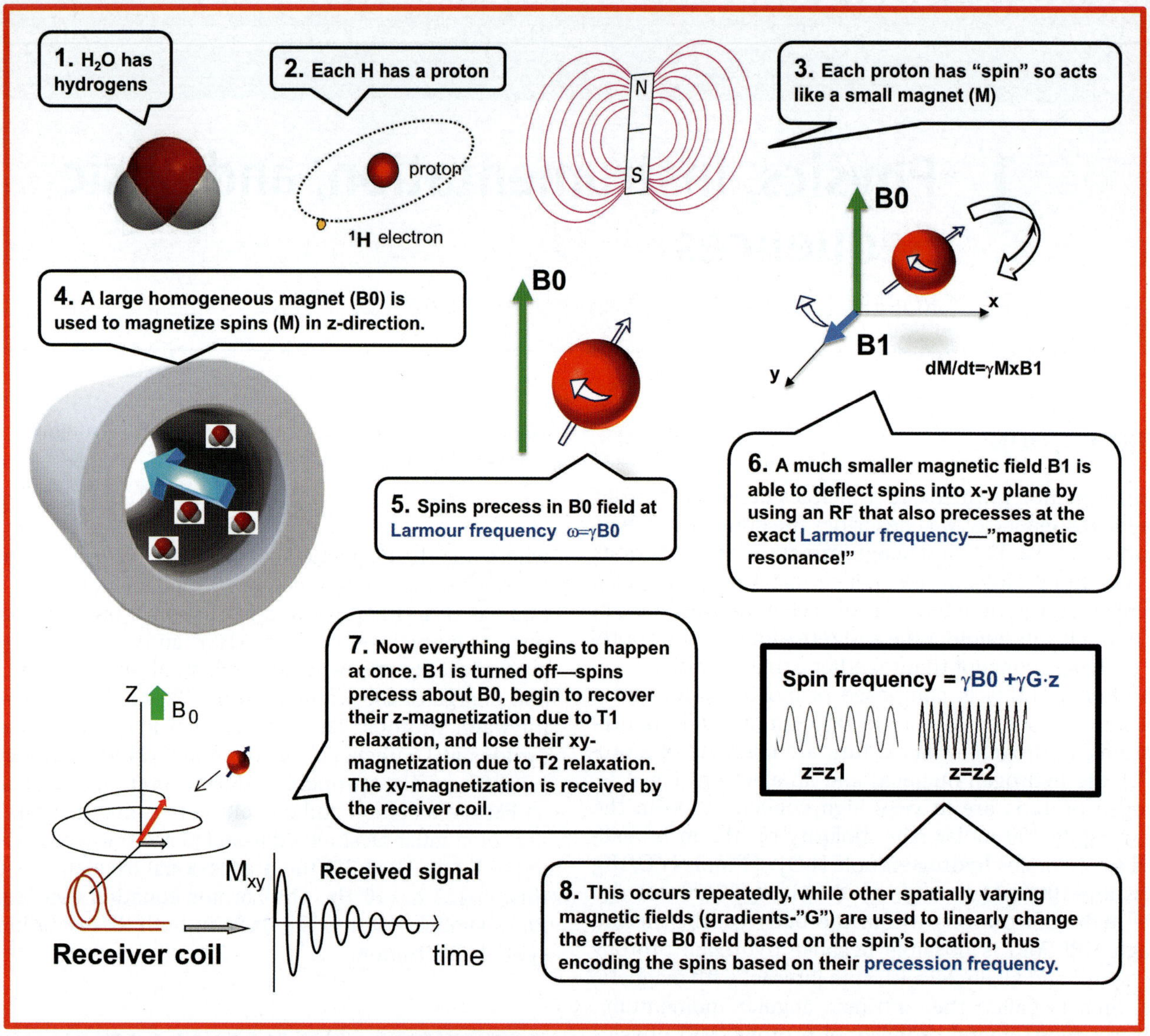

FIG. 1.1 An overview of a magnetic resonance imaging experiment. *RF*, Radiofrequency.

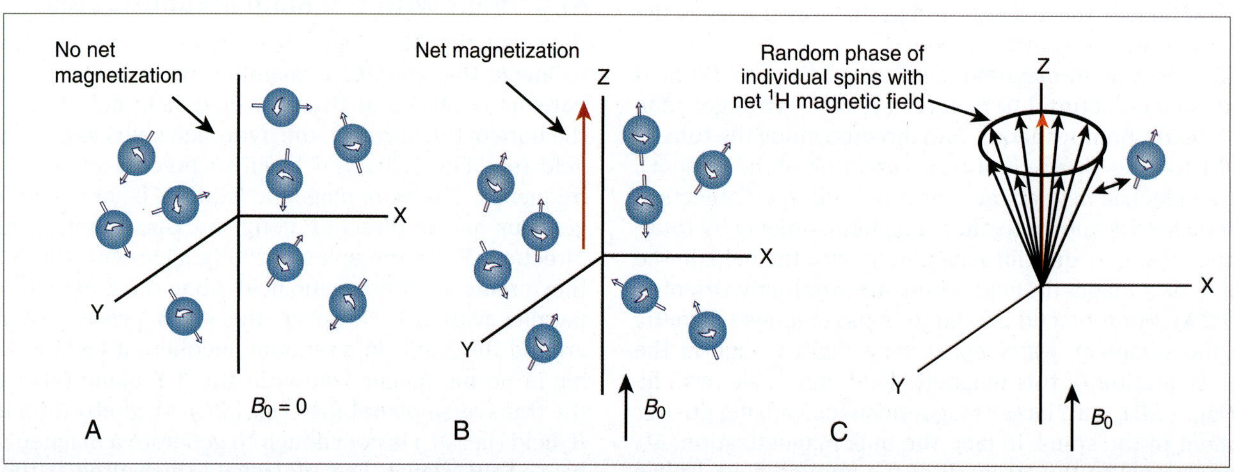

FIG. 1.2 Orientation of molecular spins. (A) With no magnetic field, the spins are oriented randomly, producing no net magnetization. (B) The spins orient with an applied magnetic field (B_0), producing a net magnetic field aligned along B_0. (C) The magnetized spins rotate around the B_0 field (the Z axis) in a random way, resulting in no net magnetization in the X-Y plane.

the X-Y plane will not detect any signal if M_{xy} is zero (see Fig. 1.2C).

Radiofrequency Excitation

To create an MR signal, the water spins must be precessing in a coherent manner in the X-Y plane. To accomplish this task, another (less powerful) magnetic field, with a strength that oscillates at the Larmor frequency (Eq. 1.1), is applied perpendicular to the main magnetic field (Fig. 1.3A). This process is called radiofrequency (RF) excitation, and the field is called an RF pulse or a B_1 field, since it uses a magnetic (B_1) field rotating at a high (radio wave) frequency. The frequency of this perpendicular B_1 field has to precisely match the Larmor frequency of the water to excite the spins in the presence of the stronger B_0 field. (This concept is analogous to exciting a piano string with a tuning fork. Only the string with the same resonant frequency as the tuning fork will efficiently absorb the energy from the fork and resonate. In fact, magnetic *resonance* imaging gets its name from the resonant frequency used for RF excitation.) The excitation field (B_1) has a strength of only a few Gauss compared to the B_0 field, which has a strength of 15,000 Gauss at 1.5 T (1 T = 10,000 Gauss). In addition, the B_1 field is only applied transiently (for milliseconds), long enough to temporarily deflect the spins into the X-Y plane perpendicular to B_0. This effect on the net magnetic field is illustrated in Fig. 1.3A, which shows a B_1 pulse that drives the magnetization completely into the transverse plane (X-Y plane). This is called a 90-degree pulse (or saturation pulse), which refers to the angle through which the initial magnetization *(M_z)* moves relative to the Z axis. However, in practice, the B_1 pulse can be used to flip the magnetization by any angle from 0 to 180 degrees. A small B_1 pulse (<90 degrees) is called an alpha pulse, while a 180-degree pulse is called an inversion pulse. A 180-degree flip is achieved by applying the B_1 field for twice as long or with twice the strength as the 90-degree pulse. The RF pulse is usually directed along the X or Y axis and oscillates at the Larmor frequency, with an amplitude and shape that determine the true flip angle. Once the B_1 field is turned off, the only field affecting the magnetization is the B_0 field. Now, the net magnetization of the water proton spins is in the transverse plane and can be detected as an oscillating signal in the receiver coil (Fig. 1.3B), precessing at the Larmor frequency. This is the signal measured in MRI.

After the RF excitation, the water spins will rotate around the B_0 field on the X-Y plane. Fig. 1.3B shows the signal detected by the receiver coil as the spins precess in the X-Y plane. The signal oscillates at the Larmor frequency and decays in amplitude with time; it is called a free induction decay. The decay in net magnitude in the transverse plane is known as magnetic relaxation. The decay occurs because the spins, having absorbed energy from the transient B_1 field, which is now turned off, return to their original state in equilibrium with the B_0 field, with spins partially aligned along the Z axis (see Fig. 1.2C). This occurs via two extremely important processes called T1 and T2 relaxation. Nature abhors order and seeks to minimize the energy in the system by returning to equilibrium with the main magnetic field, B_0, through T1 and T2 relaxation. T1 and T2 relaxation are the foundations of MRI because they are responsible for MRI's excellent contrast.

T2* and T2 Relaxation: The Effects of Spin Phase

T2 and T2* (T2 star) relaxation describe the randomization of the phase of the spins. After RF excitation, all of the spins

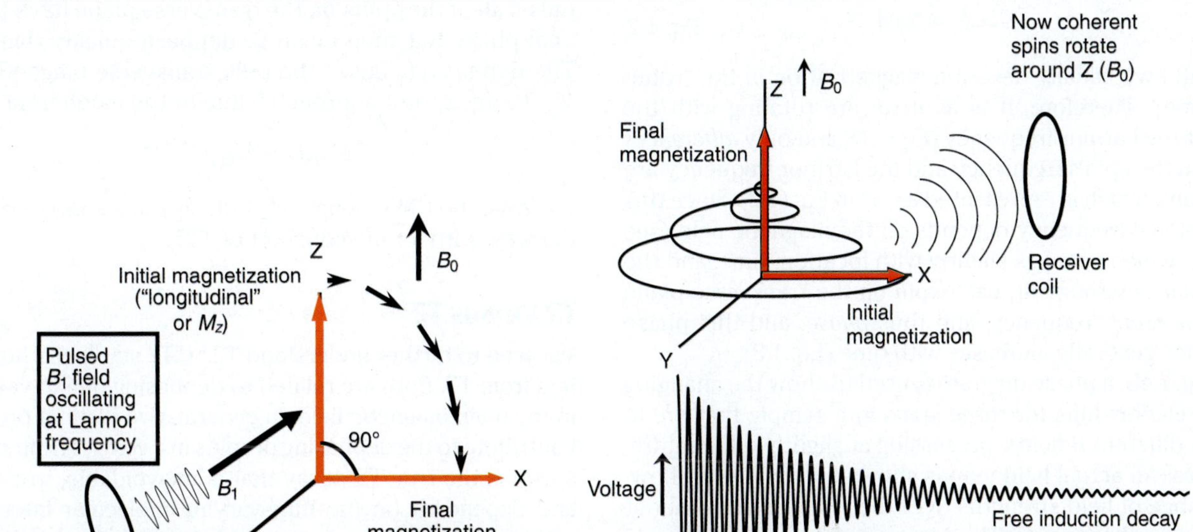

FIG. 1.3 Effects of a perpendicular B_1 magnetic field. (A) The B_1 field oscillating at the Larmor frequency of the spins is absorbed by the spins and causes a rotation around the B_1 field axis (Y axis). A 90-degree RF pulse is shown in which longitudinal magnetization (M_z) becomes transverse magnetization (M_{xy}). (B) Once the B_1 field is removed, the spins continue to rotate around the Z axis at the Larmor frequency, but the signal decays (in the X-Y plane) as equilibrium is reestablished. The result is a coherent oscillating magnetic field that is detected with the coil as the free induction decay (*FID*). The FID is a decaying sinusoidal voltage signal with a frequency equal to the Larmor frequency of the spins. *RF*, Radiofrequency.

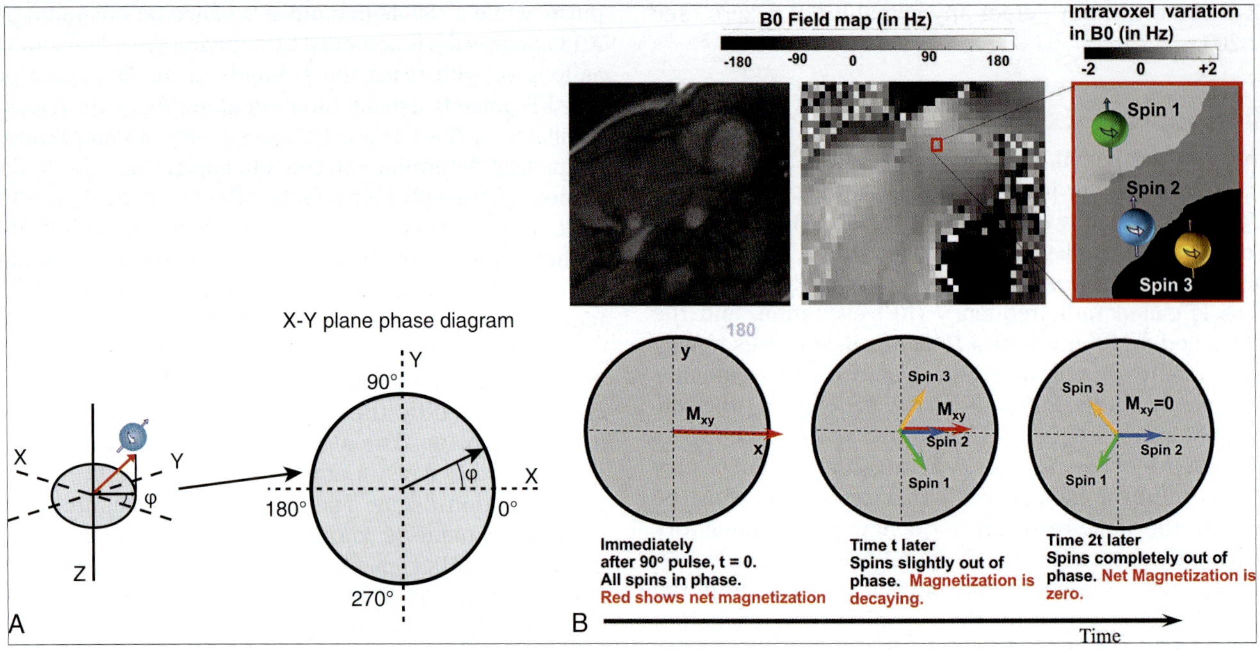

FIG. 1.4 The phase diagram. (A) A phase diagram is a view of the magnetization vectors projected into the X-Y plane. (B) The magnetic field of a sample varies as shown. Spins located in the lower field (spin 1), central field (spin 2), and higher field (spin 3) regions are followed in time after a 90-degree pulse using the phase diagram. The phase diagram presents the phases of the spins relative to spin 2, which is always shown with 0-degree phase. Note that spin 1 lags behind spin 2, while spin 3 is ahead because it has a higher phase velocity. This difference is due to the higher frequency of the spins in the higher magnetic field. This process is called *dephasing*.

precess about the Z axis, with slight differences in the precessional rate, which eventually results in "T2* decay." T2* decay comes from differences in the phase of each spin, so that the net X-Y magnetization, M_{xy}, decays to 0. The phase indicates the direction of the spin in the transverse plane. The phase (ϕ) of a spin in the transverse plane (Fig. 1.4A) depends on its initial phase (ϕ_0), the precessional frequency of that spin, and the time (t) that it has spent in the transverse plane (assuming a constant frequency, ν).

$$\phi = \phi_0 + 2\pi \nu t \qquad \text{Eq. 1.2}$$

In MRI, we usually describe magnetization in the "rotating frame." Therefore, it is as if we are rotating with the spins at the Larmor frequency (Eq. 1.1), and only *differences* between the spin's frequency and the Larmor frequency are important, which is represented as "ν" in Eq. (1.2). Since this precessional frequency depends on the magnetic field (see Eq. 1.1), which changes slightly with location, time, and the molecular environment, each spin on the transverse plane has a different frequency, and thus *phase*, and this phase difference generally increases with time (Eq. 1.2).

In Fig. 1.4B, a phase diagram is used to show the changing phase relationships for three spins in a sample that are in slightly different B fields, precessing at slightly different frequencies. An actual field map is shown for the heart, showing a range of field strengths over the entire heart of about 1 part per million (ppm). This is a map of the "off-resonance" of the spins. However, within any single voxel, there are a quintillion water spins that each precess at a very slightly different frequency depending on the magnetic field experienced (here shown as 2 Hz), but they have an important effect. The B always varies because of imperfections in the main magnetic field and changes in the molecular environment. In the schematic of Fig. 1.4B, the three spins experience different magnetic fields, one higher than B_0, one exactly B_0, and one lower. Therefore, after some time on the X-Y plane, each spin experiences phase accrual until the net magnetization (the sum of all of the spin's magnetization) decreases to 0. This is the process of T2* relaxation.

T2* relaxation can be understood as the characteristic time in which the spins in the X-Y plane become so out of phase that the signal decays (dies out) (Fig. 1.5A). The signal decays because the relative phase of the spins in a single voxel are different. After the initial excitation using a B_1 pulse, all of the spins on the transverse plane have an identical phase but then begin to dephase quickly (Fig. 1.4B). The dephasing causes the bulk transverse magnetization, M_{xy}, to decay and approach 0 due to the incoherent phase.

$$M_{xy}(t) = M_{xy_0} e^{-t/T2*} \qquad \text{Eq. 1.3}$$

Thus, the CMR signal (M_{xy}) decays in a simple exponential way, with a time constant of T2*.

T2 Versus T2*

We need to further understand T2* ("T2 star") and how it differs from T2. Both are related to dephasing due to variability in the main magnetic field. In general, two distinct processes contribute to the dephasing of spins in a voxel. The first mechanism is the true T2 decay that is unavoidable, irreversible, and dependent on the time-varying molecular interactions within a sample. T2 relaxation is also called spin-spin relaxation. It is called this because the mechanism of the relaxation process is through the interaction of spins in the sample with each other at or below the Larmor frequency, making this process dependent on the microscopic motions within the sample. The second process is T2* decay and includes T2 relaxation *and also* relaxation due to *static* inhomogeneity of the main magnetic field (B_0) within the sample. These B_0 field imperfections result from hardware imperfections and

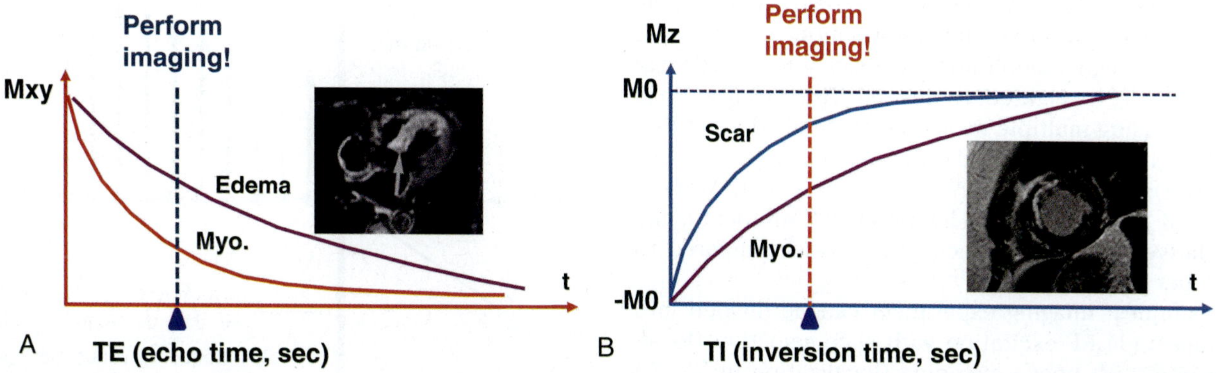

FIG. 1.5 An illustration of T1-weighted and T2-weighted imaging. (A) Edema has a longer T2 relaxation time than normal myocardium due to the increase in water content. Imaging performed at a good echo time (*TE*) can maximize the contrast difference between the two tissues, generating high signals for the edema and low signals for the myocardium. (B) Scar has a faster T1 relaxation than normal myocardium after injection of gadolinium-based contrast agent. Imaging performed at a good inversion time (*TI*) can maximize the contrast difference, ensuring that the myocardium appears dark while the scar appears bright.

TABLE 1.1 T1 and T2 Values.

FIELD STRENGTH	1.5 T		3 T	
Tissue	T1 (ms)[1–3]	T2 (ms)[3]	T1 (ms)[4–6]	T2 (ms)[5,6]
Myocardium	950	55	1150	40
Arterial blood	1550[7]	250	1650[7]	200
Fat	260	110	320	70
Skeletal muscle	1000	45	1400[8]	50[8]

susceptibility-induced B_0 variations due to the influence of the body itself. In the heart, both the lung cavity and the deoxygenated blood in the right heart contribute to B_0 inhomogeneity. B_0 field imperfections also arise from any metallic objects (sternal wires, devices, etc.) near the heart. Both T2 and T2* processes result in a randomization of the spin phases as they precess at different frequencies and a decrease in the net transverse magnetization. However, while T2 relaxation is irreversible, T2* relaxation can be partly reversed since some of it is due to *static* off-resonance. The myocardial T2 relaxation time constant is ~52 ms at 1.5 T (Table 1.1),[9] while myocardial T2* is >20 ms at 1.5 T.[10] *T2* is always less than T2 for all tissues*, because it includes the effects of T2 relaxation, as well as off-resonance effects. Later, we will describe how to obtain only T2 contrast in an image.

T1 Relaxation

T1 relaxation, also known as spin-lattice relaxation, is the release of energy to the environment, or lattice, that results in the reestablishment of the magnetization along the Z axis. Thus, T1 is the time constant by which the longitudinal (or Z) magnetization relaxes to its equilibrium value, M_0. After a 90-degree RF pulse, the Z magnetization, $M_z(t)$, is initially 0 but regrows with a relaxation time of T1 to its equilibrium value (M_0),

$$M_z(t) = M_0(1 - e^{-t/T1}) \quad \text{Eq. 1.4}$$

where t is the time after the 90-degree pulse. Each tissue type has a unique T1, which changes with field strength and in disease.

These basic relaxation processes (T1, T2, and T2*) are key in the generation of *image contrast* as well as in determining the optimal image sequence for gathering information on cardiovascular anatomy, function, and physiology. What is important is that T1, T2, and T2* vary for different tissues, and in disease, thereby providing "contrast" in the CMR image (see Table 1.1). For example, the T1[11] and T2 values are prolonged with increasing water content, as with edema, or myocarditis, which is present in different disease states.[12,13] Overall, myocardial remodeling, or myocyte replacement with connective tissue, also changes the water relaxation properties since the nature of the macromolecules in contact with water are critical for these relaxation processes. T1 is also longer in amyloid cardiomyopathy[14] and Anderson-Fabry disease. In siderotic disease (iron overload), native myocardial T1 is shorter.[15,16] The T1 of normal myocardium can increase during pharmacological stress,[17] while ischemic regions increase less. Finally, most exogenous, intravenously injected CMR contrast agents[18] act by shortening the T1 and T2/T2* of the water spins. As an extremely important example, after contrast agent administration, T1 is shorter in regions of injury where contrast accumulates. Fig. 1.5B shows how this is used to generate contrast between scar and normal myocardium.[19]

By appropriately modifying the imaging sequences, these changes in relaxation properties due to pathology or exogenous contrast agent can be highlighted or even mapped (measured on a pixel-by-pixel basis) in the heart. Before we explain this in more detail, the process of imaging—localizing the T1- or T2-weighted signal to a region—will be explained.

SPATIAL LOCALIZATION

To create a CMR image, the MR signal intensity from the sample (e.g., patient) must be determined in three dimensions (X, Y, and Z). To determine the location of different magnetic spins, the magnetic field (B) is made to vary in strength (linearly) with position (X, Y, and Z) using specialized coils of wire (called "gradient coils") inside the magnet. Although the magnetic field change induced by the gradient is very small, it results in a precessional frequency (υ) that depends on a spin's location in the scanner (as defined by Eq. 1.1). By measuring the number of spins precessing at each location (i.e., at each frequency), an MR image is created,[20] as will be discussed below. For a single image, it is necessary to collect information on X, Y, and Z positions and signal amplitude. This signal amplitude can be T1, T2, or T2* weighted, as desired. This localization is performed using multiple measurements called repetition times (TRs). To localize signal to $Nx \times Ny$ voxels (e.g., a 128 × 128 matrix), approximately $Nx \bullet Ny$ signals (and Ny TRs) are needed. This is actually a limitation of CMR that results in a relatively slow image acquisition rate compared to many other modalities.

The simplest imaging experiment can be divided into four stages: (1) RF excitation with slice selection (localization in Z), (2) phase encoding (localization in Y), (3) gradient and RF rephasing/refocusing, and (4) frequency encoding (localization in X). Each stage is used to encode the MR data with information on the position and the amplitude of the water proton signal. By convention, the Z-position information is encoded in the slice-selection step, the X position is determined in the frequency-encoding/readout step, and the Y position is obtained in the phase-encoding step. In practice, the frequency-encoding (X), phase-encoding (Y), and slice-selection (Z) directions can be rotated in any appropriate direction. MR is tomographic and can create an image of the body along any plane. Indeed, oblique imaging (slicing through a tissue at 45 degrees or any other angle) is possible and common. In this way, CMR differs from other modalities (e.g., computed tomography [CT] or two-dimensional [2D] echocardiography), because CMR can acquire images in any plane.

Magnetic Gradients

Spatial encoding in CMR is performed using magnetic field gradients applied to the main magnetic field: slice-select gradients, phase-encoding gradients, and frequency-encoding gradients. Gradient coils are special coils within the magnet that modify the main magnetic field (B), causing its strength (but not direction) to change slightly in space.

$$B(x, y, z) = B_0 + G_x \cdot x + G_y \cdot y + G_z \cdot z \qquad \text{Eq. 1.5}$$

G_x, G_y, and G_z are called "gradient strengths," and x, y, and z are the spatial coordinates with $x=0$, $y=0$, and $z=0$ at the center of the magnet bore. Eq. (1.5) describes how the main magnetic field strength—which is always directed along the Z axis—varies spatially with x, y, and z. Fig. 1.6 demonstrates the variation of the B field in the presence of an x gradient. In the same way, gradients on the Y or Z axis vary the B field in y or z. Using gradients, the main magnetic field, with which the spins align and around which they precess, varies with spatial position inside the scanner. *Remember, this magnetic field points in the Z direction.* The gradients do not change this direction but slightly increase or decrease its strength spatially. These spatially varying magnetic fields are called gradients because they are added to the main field, B_0, and cause it to vary linearly in space. Of course, since the magnetic field varies with position, the precessional frequency ($\nu[x, y, z]$) and the phase ($\phi[x, y, z, t]$) of the spins also vary with position (see Eqs. (1.1) and (1.3), and Fig. 1.6).

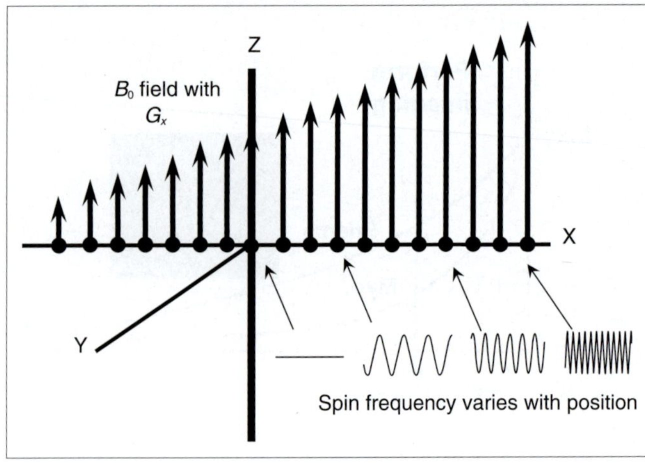

FIG. 1.6 A magnetic field gradient. A gradient is applied along the X axis, causing the B field to vary from less than to greater than B_0 along X. This leads to a linear increase in spin frequency as a function of position along the X direction.

$$\nu = \frac{\gamma}{2\pi} B(x, y, z) = \frac{\gamma}{2\pi}\left(B_0 + G_x \cdot x + G_y \cdot y + G_z \cdot z\right) \text{ Eq. 1.6}$$

The first term, $(\gamma/2\pi) \bullet B_0$, is just the Larmor frequency. In the rotating frame, $\nu = \gamma/2\pi\,(G_x \bullet x + G_y \bullet y + G_z \bullet z)$. Also note that at any time, gradients on the X, Y, and Z axes may be applied together or alone and the amplitudes can be slewed up and down or set to 0.

The phase ($\phi[x, y, z, t]$) of the spins also varies with position. For a constant gradient, $\phi = \gamma B \bullet t = \gamma(G_x \bullet x + G_y \bullet y + G_z \bullet z) \bullet t$ and is related to the gradient strengths, the time (t) that the gradient is on, and the spin's location. Recall that phase accumulation due to precession at the Larmor frequency ($\gamma \bullet B_0 \bullet t$) is omitted, because the phase is described in the rotating frame. For non-constant gradients (e.g., ramped gradients), the phase is proportional to the area of the gradient-time curve (gradient × time):

$$\phi(x, y, z, t) = \gamma[\text{area}(G_x, t) \cdot x + \text{area}(G_y, t) \cdot y + \text{area}(G_z, t) \cdot z] \qquad \text{Eq. 1.7}$$

The idea of gradient "area" is very important. The gradient area is the product of the gradient amplitude (G) and the duration (t) of the gradient. The phase of a spin at any given time is proportional to the total gradient area and the spin's location. Gradients cause the frequency and phase of the spins to depend on location, so that if the frequency and phase of a certain spin can be determined during application of gradients, its position is known.

Slice-Selective Excitation: Position in Z

During slice selection, RF excitation is performed to rotate the spins into the X-Y plane. During excitation, the z spatial localization is determined by only flipping (with the B_1) magnetization from a selected slice of the sample. The magnetization remains unchanged (i.e., aligned with B_0) *except* in that slice. The slice-selection process is illustrated in Fig. 1.7. A linear magnetic field gradient (G_z) is applied to the sample to vary the B_0 field along the slice direction (the Z axis). The magnetic field gradient causes the spins along

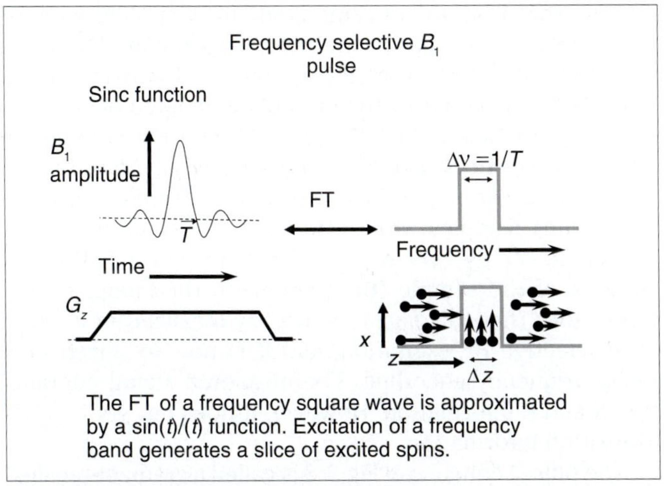

FIG. 1.7 The slice-selective B_1 pulse. The shape of the slice-selective B_1 pulse in time is sin(*t*)/*t*. This is called a "sinc" function. It has the property that it excites a distinct band of frequencies. This is true because the Fourier transform (*FT*) of the sinc B_1 field is a square wave in frequency space. The excitation of a band of frequencies by B_1, used in conjunction with the gradient G_z (similar to Fig. 1.6, but along the Z axis), causes a slice of spins to be placed on the transverse plane.

this axis to have slightly different frequencies, as defined by the Larmor equation:

$$\nu(z) = (G_z \cdot z) \cdot (\gamma/2\pi)$$

The B_1 field is used to excite the spins, but only within a range of precessional frequencies. If only a selected band of frequencies are excited (Δv), then a slice of spins with precessional frequencies in that range (Δz) is placed into the transverse plane, not affecting the rest of the sample. The "slice thickness" can be freely chosen by adjusting the Z gradient. Typical slices range from thin (e.g., 2 mm) slices to thick (e.g., 30 cm) slabs. The slice position can also be freely chosen. Furthermore, if no Z gradient is applied during the slice selection, this is equivalent to an infinite slab thickness, so that all of the spins in the body will be tipped into the transverse plane. This is called a "nonselective" RF pulse and is commonly used in CMR for preparation pulses.

How can the B_1 field, which oscillates at about the Larmor frequency, be used to excite only spins precessing within a range of frequencies? To excite a bandwidth of frequencies, the Z gradient is turned on, and the B_1 strength is modulated in time:

$$B_1(t) = B_{1_0} \cdot \sin(\pi \cdot t/T)/(\pi \cdot t/T) \quad \text{Eq. 1.8}$$

This B_1 shape, sin(*t*)/*t*, is called a "sinc" function and is plotted in Fig. 1.7. This $B_1(t)$ shape excites a well-defined band of frequencies of width $\Delta\nu = 1/T$, centered around the Larmor frequency. Here, a Fourier transform (FT) is used to show how the spins interpret the sin(*t*)/*t* pulse in terms of frequency. If a Z gradient is applied during the sinc RF excitation, then the band of frequencies excited is a "slice" of spins at a certain Z location, with a slice thickness of Δz. Modifications to the sinc pulse are possible to optimize the performance and slice definition of this approach.[21] Wideband pulses can improve slice selection in the presence of devices.[22] Multiband excitations can simultaneously excite two or more slices, which can be used to image multiple slices at once.[23]

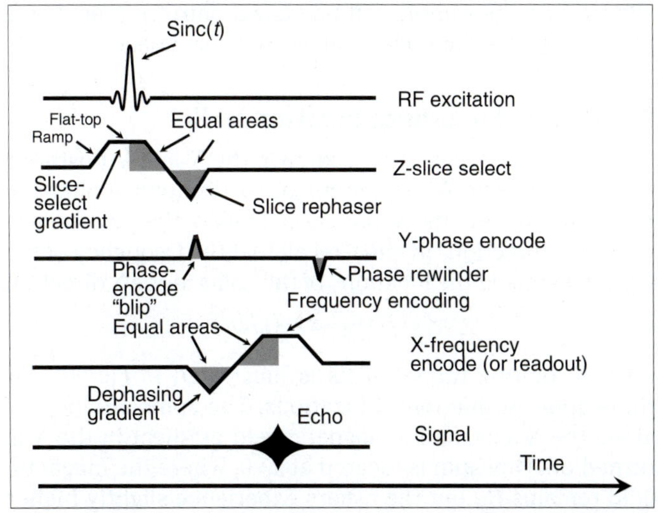

FIG. 1.8 Pulse sequence diagram. In a pulse sequence diagram a timeline is shown for the B_1 pulse, the gradients on each axis, and the signal received. This convention is used in all pulse sequence diagrams. Here the slice-selection process is shown (*see top portion of figure*), in which a Z gradient is used with a sinc B_1 pulse. The frequency encoding is shown on the X axis. The frequency encoding shows a dephasing gradient, and then a flat top, during which time the signal is acquired, as indicated on the last line (*signal*). The phase-encoding gradient "blip" is often applied just prior to frequency encoding. Often after the frequency encoding, the phase-encoding gradient is rephased. During each repeated pulse sequence, only the phase-encoding strength changes. *RF*, Radiofrequency.

Pulse Sequence Diagram

The slice-selection process is summarized in the imaging "pulse sequence diagram" shown in Fig. 1.8. A pulse sequence diagram presents all of the gradients, the B_1 field excitation, and also marks the timing of data collection (i.e., when the receiver coil records the MR signal) on a timeline. In Fig. 1.8, the slice-selection gradient is first increased to a constant level by a ramp. The gradient is maintained while the frequency selective (i.e., slice-selective) B_1 field is applied; note its sinc shape. Subsequently, the slice gradient is ramped down and the rephasing gradient is applied to remove the phase introduced by the slice-select gradient. After performing the slice-select excitation, only a slice of the sample has been placed in the transverse plane and all of the spins are in phase.

The rephasing *Z* gradient shown in Fig. 1.8 is performed so that all of the spins are "in phase" after the slice-selection process. During the 90-degree pulse the spins will dephase depending on where they are in the slice (similar to that seen in Fig. 1.4B), since a magnetic field gradient is applied. Thus, another magnetic field gradient of opposite magnitude must be applied to reverse the dephasing caused by the slice-selection process (shaded regions in Fig. 1.8). The gradient area to rephase the spins is half the slice select area, since the spins reach the transverse plane exactly coincident with the peak of the RF sinc pulse. By applying the gradient in the opposite direction, the spins are forced back to the same phase they were in before application of the slice-select gradient. This small gradient is called a slice-rephasing gradient.

In summary, to selectively excite a slice, a linear magnetic field gradient (G_z) is placed along the axis to be sliced. A sinc B_1 field pulse is applied, and only the predefined slice within the sample will be placed onto the transverse plane for further modification to create an image.

Frequency Encoding: Position in X

While the Z position is now known, the X and Y positions remain unknown. When a gradient (G_x) is applied after the RF excitation in the X direction (called the "frequency-encoding direction" in MRI), recall that the frequency of the spins will reflect the locations of the spins in the X direction

$$\nu(x) = (G_x \cdot x) \cdot (\gamma / 2\pi)$$

(in the rotating frame). This is illustrated in Fig. 1.9 for three spins at different X locations. The spins are located along the X axis, and a magnetic field gradient in the X is turned on. One spin is located at $x = 0$, where the magnetic field remains B_0, but the others experience slightly higher fields. The signal received from each spin depends on its precessional frequency, as shown in Fig. 1.9, with each spin's signal oscillating at a different frequency. The combined signal from all three spins is measured (while G_x is "on") by the receiver coil as the MR signal. The location of each spin can then be determined using an FT, which converts the time oscillating total signal into its frequency (i.e., location) components.

$$\text{FT(signal)} = \int \text{signal}(t) \cdot e^{-2 \cdot \pi \cdot \text{ivt}} \text{dt} \qquad \text{Eq. 1.9}$$

v is related to the X location, as before. Using a frequency-encoding gradient, the MR signal provides a measure of the number of spins precessing at each frequency.

As shown in Fig. 1.8 (bottom two rows), the gradient is applied for a few milliseconds, during which the MR signal is measured. The gradient must remain on for a specific time during frequency encoding to sufficiently record the oscillating signals with high fidelity.

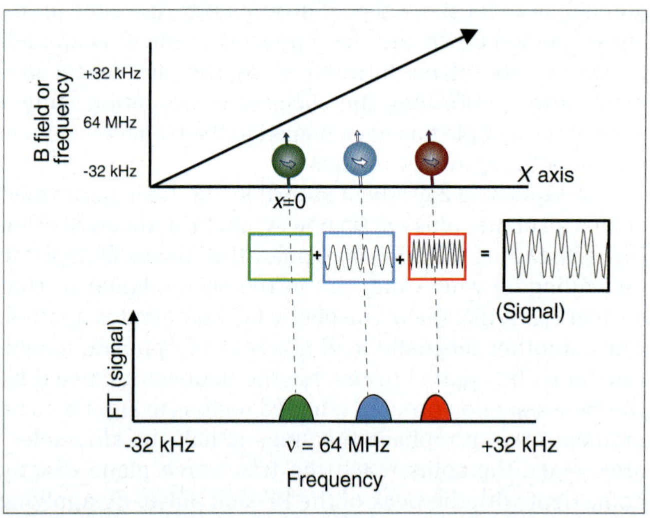

FIG. 1.9 Frequency encoding of position. A frequency-encoding (also called *readout*) gradient is applied on the X axis, causing the *B* field to vary from less than to greater than the main magnetic field. Three spins are shown at different X locations, with different precessional frequencies. The signal from the spins during the application of this gradient is acquired, and its frequency depends on location. The total signal is then *FT* to provide a measurement of the number of spins precessing at each frequency, thereby indicating the X location of each spin.

Note that first a dephasing gradient is applied with an area equal to half that of the readout gradient. The readout gradient is then ramped up and held constant for a period of time, and then the gradient is ramped back down to zero. This time (when G_x is constant) *is the time during which the signal is acquired—the data acquisition.* During this period, the signal is continuously sampled, providing N_x time samples, where the spatial resolution (Δx) is related to N_x, by $\text{FOV}/N_x = \Delta x$. The field of view (FOV) is the size of the sample (the patient) in the imaging field. Remember that this signal is already localized in Z using slice-selective RF excitation, and it is now localized in X using frequency encoding. The measured signal contains this X and Z information. However, it does not yet contain Y-position information.

The pulse sequence of Fig. 1.8 is called a gradient-recalled echo (GRE) or gradient echo since the readout gradient is used to refocus the dephasing gradient applied before it. A rephaser is sometimes applied also, which is similar to a dephaser but is applied after a gradient. A very thoughtful reader may wonder, why are the gradients always "ramped" up and down? The ramps reflect the reality that the magnetic field cannot be changed instantaneously, but rather the change is constrained by the scanner. With current hardware, the gradient coils can be "slewed" to reach their maximum value (currently 4–8 Gauss/cm) within about 100–200 µs. Slew rate is currently constrained by safety concerns related to peripheral nerve stimulation—although continual efforts are underway to utilize higher slew rates safely.[24]

Phase Encoding: Position in Y

Y spatial information is determined through a process called *phase encoding,* which is performed just after the RF pulse (but prior to frequency encoding). The spins can be phase encoded by transiently applying a magnetic field gradient (G_y) along the phase-encoding axis (Y axis by convention) as shown in Fig. 1.8 (labeled a "phase-encoding blip"). This transient gradient or blip imparts a phase to each spin proportional to its area (gradient × time, Eq. 1.7), and to the spin's Y position. A rephaser of the y gradient is commonly applied after frequency encoding to remove any phase accumulations in Y. Importantly, many phase-encoding gradients of progressively increasing areas are required in order to localize a spin in the Y direction, depending on the object size (called an FOV) and the desired spatial resolution (Δy). The number of phase encodings (N_y) is given by the relationship $\text{FOV}/N_y = \Delta y$.

Fig. 1.10 illustrates the phase-encoding process. Consider three spins located at three Y positions, but at any position in X. The Y gradient is "blipped" on, increased for a time (T) to a maximum value (G_y), and then ramped down to 0. The area of the gradient ($G_y \bullet T$) and the spin's Y location determine the phase accumulation (see Eq. 1.7). With no G_y gradient on, all spins precess at the Larmor frequency and have the same phase. If the signal is measured from these spins, it is the bulk signal. The application of a gradient (G_y) for a short time (T) results in a phase that depends on the spin's Y location (and the gradient area). The spins at $y = 0$ accumulate no phase even when gradients are used,

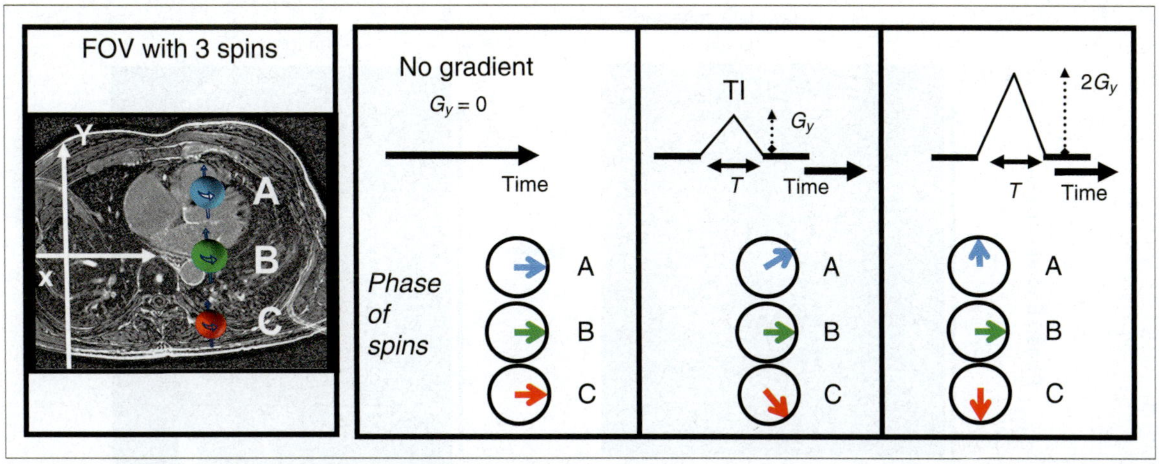

FIG. 1.10 Phase encoding. A Y gradient is transiently applied for a time (*T*) using larger and larger gradient strengths (G_y). Three spins, A, B, and C, located at three different Y locations, respond differently to the phase-encoding gradient. The gradient does not affect the spin at $y=0$ (spin B) because it still precesses at the Larmor frequency. But the gradient causes spin A to precess more slowly and spin C to precess more quickly, resulting in phase differences proportional to the gradient strength (G_y) and the time *t*. These phase differences allow the locations of the spins to be determined. *FOV*, Field of view.

but the other spins accumulate phase depending on their Y location. A larger phase-encoding gradient causes even more phase accumulation at $y \neq 0$. Now, two of the spins are even more "out of phase." The signal measured during each acquisition is dependent on each spin's phase, which in turn is determined by each spin's Y location. With three phase encodings, it is not yet possible to locate the spins in Y, but after collecting the signal from multiple (32 to 512) phase-encoding steps, the signals can be used to determine the Y locations of each spin, using the FT. It is important to realize that for each phase encoding, *an entire frequency encoding must be collected.* When the readout signal is collected during phase encoding, each of the spin's phases is influenced by its position in Y and X. In this way, X and Y spatial information are encoded together. Thus, this slow phase-encoding process provides the last piece of information, the Y-axis position, needed to create the MR image. As noted above, each measurement is called a repetition, and the time to acquire a single measurement is called the TR.

Raw *k*-Space Data and the Fourier Transform (FT)

Fig. 1.8 shows all of the steps of spatial encoding. A separate echo is collected for each phase-encode step. The phase-encode step is most commonly applied immediately after the slice-select process, frequently at the same time as the dephasing gradient for readout occurs (as shown in Fig. 1.8). This is done to minimize the scan time. All of the frequency and phase-encoded raw data are combined to create a *k-space* (Fig. 1.11). The *k*-space in Fig. 1.11 represents the raw data collected at each phase-encoding step. The phase- and frequency-encoding directions are labeled. MR imaging can be understood as acquiring *k*-space data. Each frequency encoding acquires a signal for a full line of *k*-space (k_x) at a single k_y value. Each phase-encoding step moves up along the phase-encoding axis (k_y) to acquire another frequency-encoding line. Once enough *k*-space signal is acquired, this *k*-space signal is converted into an image using a 2D FT. Ideally, the raw *k*-space data contains enough information so that after the 2D FT an image of infinite spatial resolution results. In reality, there are limits on the amount of data that can be collected. The Y resolution of the CMR image is directly related to the number of phase-encoded echoes that are collected ($\Delta y = \text{FOV}_y/N_y$), and therefore infinite spatial resolution would require infinite time to collect. The X resolution is related to the number of frequency-encoding data points acquired ($\Delta x = \text{FOV}_x/N_x$). It is easier to acquire very high resolution in the frequency-encoding direction, and often in CMR spatial resolution in the frequency-encoding direction is higher. In CMR, time is limited due to respiratory and cardiac motions, so the tradeoff between spatial resolution required to observe the structure of interest and scan time is critically important. Schemes to increase the efficiency of collecting *k*-space data (e.g., spiral, radial) will be discussed throughout this book.

PULSE SEQUENCES AND CONTRAST

Spin Echo Imaging

Among the very first pulse sequences used in CMR was the spin echo sequence[25] and, even today, it is routinely used in its accelerated form (fast spin echo). As described earlier, in tissue, T2* causes rapid magnetic relaxation of water protons compared with T2 relaxation. Thus, the decay rate of the M_{xy} signal after an RF pulse excitation is actually a measure of T2*. Since T2* decay is a rapid process, it limits the time that we can detect the MR signal. As noted above, it is possible to circumvent and reverse some of the T2* dephasing, because some of it is caused by fixed B_0 field inhomogeneity. This reversal is accomplished using spin echo imaging. This method uses two B_1 pulses to generate an "echo" (a signal), as outlined in Fig. 1.12 (see lower panel). First, a 90-degree pulse is applied to create M_{xy} magnetization. Due to magnetic field imperfections, the magnetization begins to dephase. Next, a 180-degree B_1 pulse is applied to flip the magnetization by 180 degrees around the X axis. This 180-degree flip is important, because now any slow spins (precessing slower than the Larmor frequency) are "ahead" of fast spins, so that the

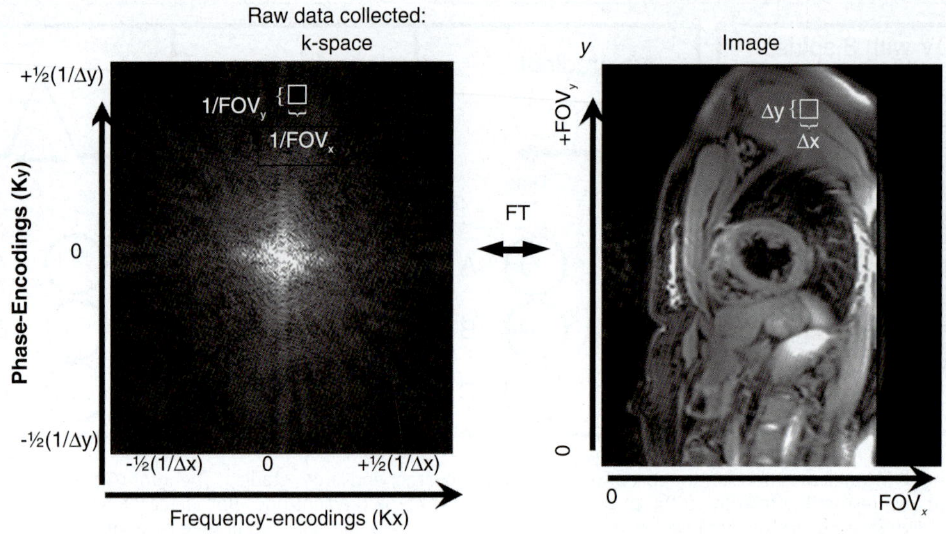

FIG. 1.11 The frequency-encoding data collected during each phase-encoding step is called the *k*-space signal. The *k*-space signal is collected on a grid. The *k*-space signal does not look like an image, but is transformed into an image using the FT. The spacing in *k*-space (Δk_x, Δk_y) determines the field of view (FOV_x, FOV_y) of the image. The width of the *k*-space is related to the pixel size of the image, as shown. Collecting "more" *k*-space reduces the pixel size.

spins now drift back into phase (i.e., "rephase") taking the *same amount of time* to rephase that they were allowed to dephase. This is analogous to two people standing back to back in a field and then walking apart (90-degree pulse) at very different speeds. If at some time later (call it "TE/2"), they turn around (180-degree pulse) and now walk toward each other at that same "individual" pace, they will meet exactly where they had been standing, at exactly twice the time (at time "TE"). This is the nature of the echo that effectively recaptures all of the coherent transverse magnetization that had been destroyed by the B_0 field inhomogeneity in the sample. The spins continue to dephase after reaching the coherent echo due to ongoing field inhomogeneity, just as in the field two people would walk past each other and continue to "dephase." The signal at the time of the spin echo only decays by T2, not T2*.

The spin echo sequence is shown in Fig. 1.12 (upper panel). Note that it is almost identical to the GRE sequence (see Fig. 1.8), except for the 180-degree refocusing pulse. Even in this simple sequence, several factors of its design will change the contrast of the MR image, based on T1 and T2 relaxation. Since a 180-degree refocusing pulse is used in this sequence, the total time that the spins stay in the transverse plane, before the signal is measured, determines the amount of T2 relaxation that will occur (see Eq. 1.2). This time is called the *time to echo* or the *echo time (TE)* and is measured from the center of the RF excitation pulse to the center of the refocused echo during the readout or data acquisition (see Fig. 1.12). Generally, the longer the TE, the more T2 contrast or T2 weighting is generated in the image (see Eq. 1.3).

Another sequence timing parameter that influences the signal amplitude is based on T1 relaxation. The time between each RF excitation pulse (i.e., 90-degree pulse) is the critical factor in this sequence and is the effective TR (see Fig. 1.12). If a shorter TR is used between slice-selective pulses, the spins' Z magnetization will not fully regrow between pulses, which leads to a reduction in the MR signal. This reduction in signal is dependent on the TR and T1 of the sample. Therefore, ***T1 weighting*** *can be achieved using a short TR* combined with a short TE, so that T2 weighting is minimized. ***T2 weighting*** *is achieved with a long TE* and long TR. "*Proton density*" *weighting* (i.e., how many spins are in each location) can be achieved with a short TE and a long TR.

As an example of the importance of TE, the MR water signals from normal (T2 ~52 ms)[9] and acutely infarcted (T2 ~70 ms)[26] regions of the myocardium are shown in Fig. 1.13A. Note that the signals of both tissues decrease with increasing TE, but that the infarcted tissue signal decays more slowly because of its longer T2. This results in a *contrast*, or increased difference, in signal between the normal and the infarcted tissue at prolonged TEs. Inspecting the difference between the signals of the two tissue curves (dotted line), a TE of about 50 ms could be selected to optimize the contrast between these two tissue types. Thus, by simply adjusting the imaging parameters, fundamental information on the heart structure can be obtained. Conversely, pathology may be obscured if the imaging parameters are not ideal.

The impact of TR on signal amplitude is shown in Fig. 1.13B for a spin echo sequence. The effect of TR is illustrated for normal myocardium with a T1 of 950 and abnormal myocardium with a T1 of 1200 ms. Note that the shorter the T1 the more *rapidly* the pulses can be applied and the MR signal still maintained. Also apparent in Fig. 1.13B is that by varying the TR, the contrast or difference between tissues can be altered. Thus, the TR can be used to vary the image contrast based on T1. Note that a TR of 1 s would be optimal in generating the largest difference (or contrast; "dotted" line) between normal and infarcted tissue. Current CMR techniques perform T1 mapping or T1-weighted imaging using inversion recovery, as described in later chapters, to differentiate infarction and normal myocardium.

Fast Spin Echo Imaging

The relatively long TR required for full T1 relaxation is the major reason that the spin echo method is very rarely

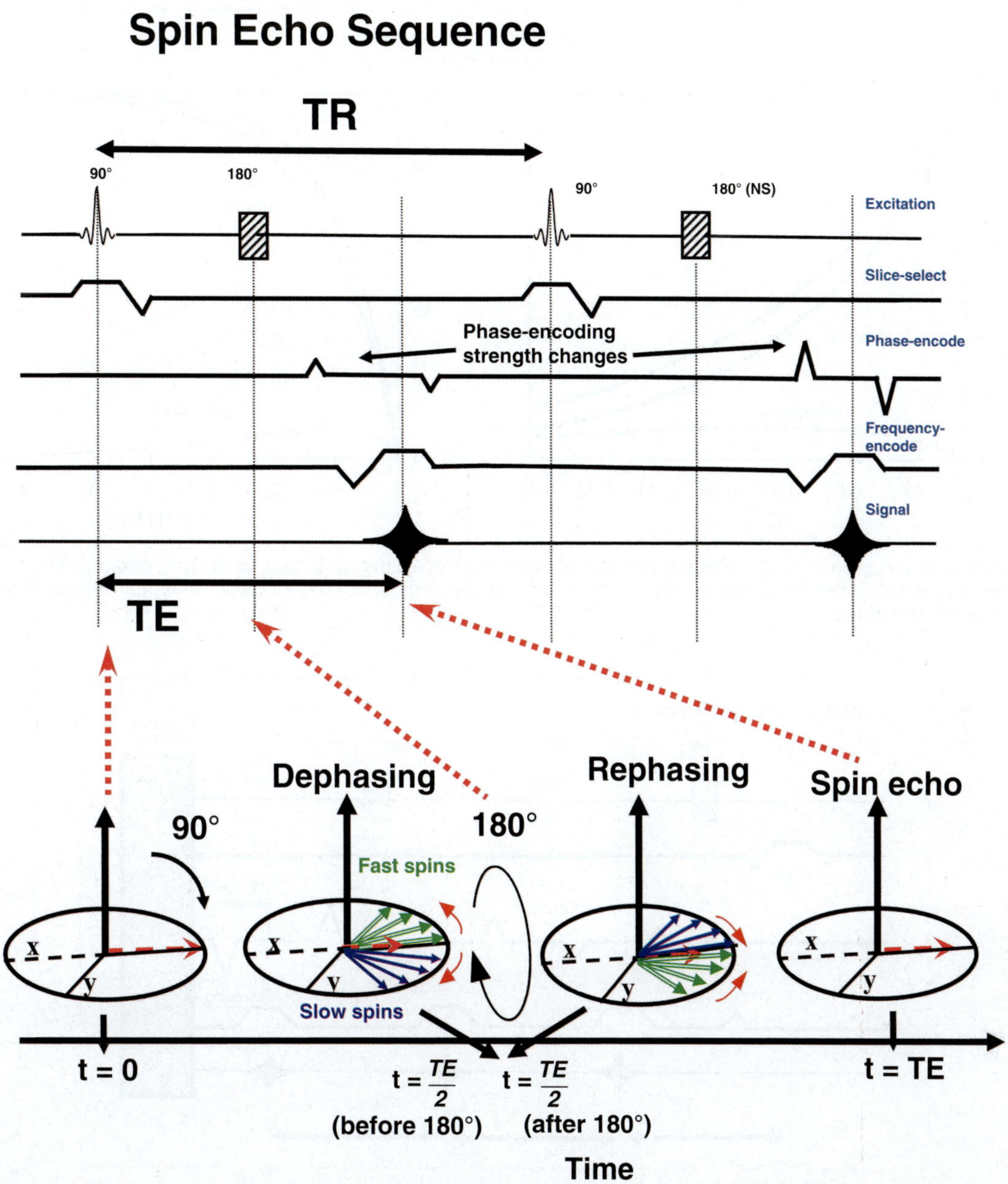

FIG. 1.12 Spin echo: effects of a 180-degree B_1 pulse after a 90-degree B_1 pulse. (*Lower panel*) The spins are first excited by a 90-degree pulse, as in Fig. 1.3. After some time (TE/2), in which dephasing occurs (as in Fig. 1.4B), a 180-degree pulse is applied. By flipping the spins 180 degrees about the X axis, the 180-degree pulse exchanges the phase position of the slower and faster spins so that the faster spins are now lagging the slower spins. The faster spins begin to catch up, and after a time TE/2 is equal to the time of dephasing and the spins are all aligned in the same direction (have the same phase). This process is called "rephasing" or "refocusing" to form a spin echo at time TE. (*Upper Panel*) The pulse sequence diagram for a spin echo pulse sequence. A 90-degree slice-selective excitation is followed by a 180-degree refocusing pulse. Then, phase encoding on the Y and frequency encoding on the X axis are performed. The repetition time *(TR)* and echo time *(TE)* are defined. The diagram shows two TRs. During each repeated TR, everything is the same, except that the phase-encoding strength changes, as shown.

used: scan time (TR • N_y) is too long. To circumvent this problem, one highly useful approach is to use multiple 180-degree refocusing pulses and to collect many echoes during each slice-selective excitation (see Fig. 1.13). This method, called fast spin echo (FSE) or turbo spin echo, is an important technique in CMR.[27] A phase-encoding gradient is applied between each 180-degree pulse, thereby providing multiple phase-encoded steps from a single 90-degree pulse. For CMR, typically 16 to 64 echoes are collected for each slice-selective pulse, thereby reducing the time to collect a spin echo image by 16 to 64 times, respectively. Since large blocks of time are required to collect all of these echoes, this method is usually restricted to relatively motion-free phases of the cardiac cycle, such as diastole. The inherent high signal-to-noise ratio (SNR) of these FSE approaches supports very high spatial resolution images of the heart. In addition, true T2 contrast can be generated by acquiring the central phase-encoding data (which largely controls the image contrast) at a specific time within the echo train. This time is called the effective TE. The longer the time between the initial 90 degrees and the acquisition of central *k*-space (i.e., the longer the effective TE), the more T2 weighting will occur. The FSE technique is very commonly used in CMR to visualize anatomy and measure sizes of cardiac chambers (Fig. 1.14 shows an FSE image). It is usually used with a black-blood

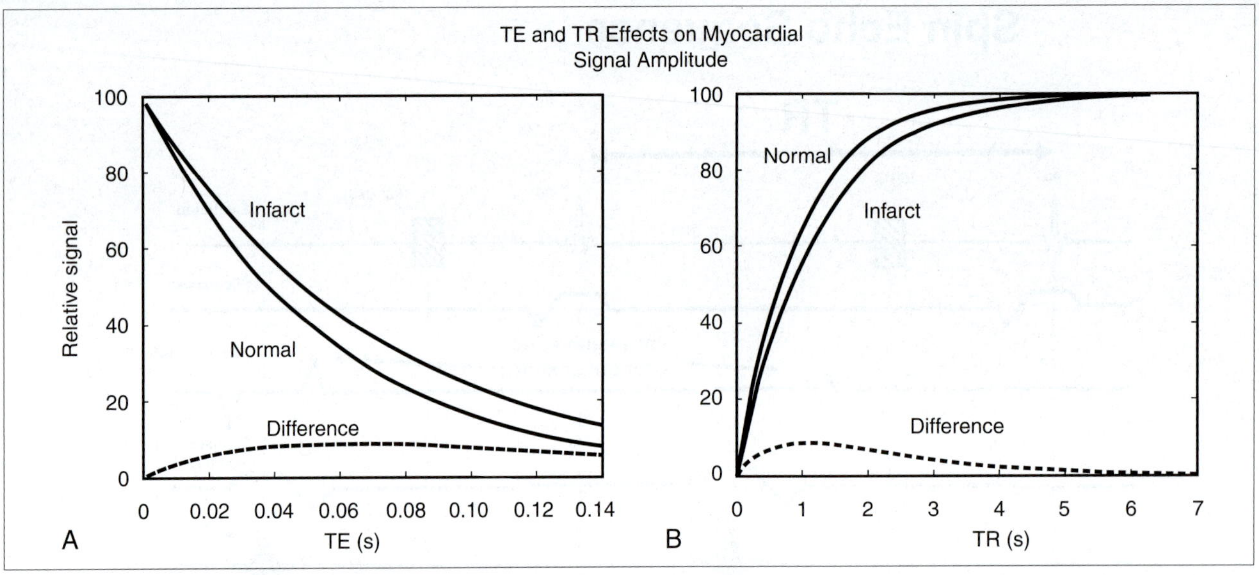

FIG. 1.13 Echo time (*TE*) and repetition time (*TR*) effects on myocardial signal amplitude. Effect of TE (A) and TR (B) on cardiovascular magnetic resonance signal amplitude for normal and infarcted myocardium. Because the T1 and T2 of acutely infarcted myocardium differ from normal myocardium, contrast between these tissues can be created.

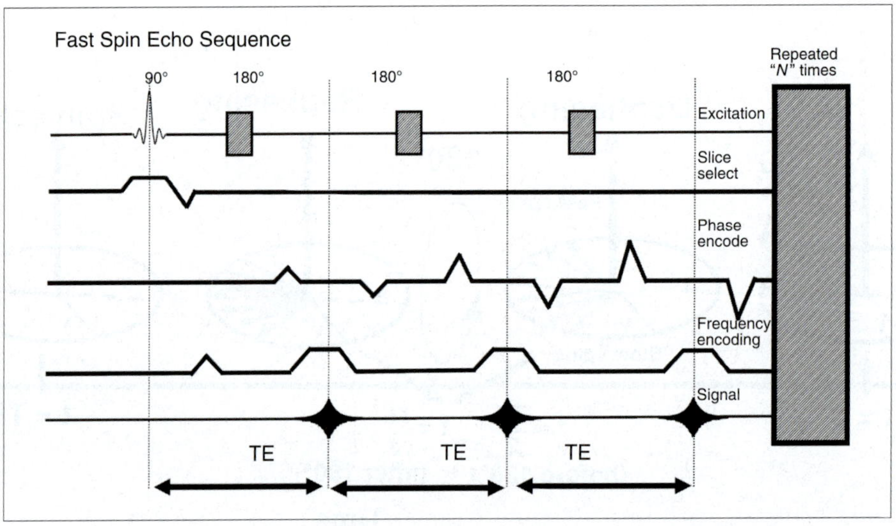

FIG. 1.14 Pulse sequence diagram for fast spin echo imaging. *TE*, Echo time.

preparation pulse, as described below. T2-weighted black-blood FSE has been advocated for identifying edematous tissue associated with acute infarct[27] and for identifying the region at risk.[28,29] In Chapter 4, methods for quantifying myocardial T2 values will be described, which are currently in greater use.

Gradient Echo (GRE) Imaging

GRE imaging, like spin echo, is a fundamental CMR method and enjoys greater use than any other method. For imaging the beating heart and other highly dynamic applications, GRE imaging (also known as FLASH [fast low angle shot], or TFE [turbo field echo])[30] uses very short TRs, providing fast imaging. This sequence was shown in Fig. 1.8, but Fig. 1.15 displays multiple TRs. GRE imaging uses short TRs and lower flip angles. Furthermore, in GRE imaging the 180-degree refocusing pulse is eliminated. The signal on the transverse plane will then decay with T2* instead of T2, but this is acceptable if the TE is very short (TE < 3 ms). As the TR is shortened, the flip angle must be reduced to provide the optimal SNR per unit time. The flip angle provides maximum signal at steady state (i.e., after many slice-selective pulses) and is determined by a tradeoff. A larger flip angle provides more spins on the transverse plane (more signal), but less Z magnetization is preserved, and therefore the following echoes have less signal. A smaller flip angle provides less signal on the transverse plane, but more Z magnetization is preserved for subsequent echoes. The maximum signal at steady state is achieved using the Ernst angle for a given TR and T1:

$$\alpha = \cos^{-1}(e^{-\mathrm{TR}/T1}) \qquad \text{Eq. 1.10}$$

This low flip angle RF pulse is also called an "alpha pulse" and is suitable for short TRs. Short TRs are needed for dynamic imaging. For example, the collection of 32 phase-encode lines in *k*-space, each with a 5-ms TR,

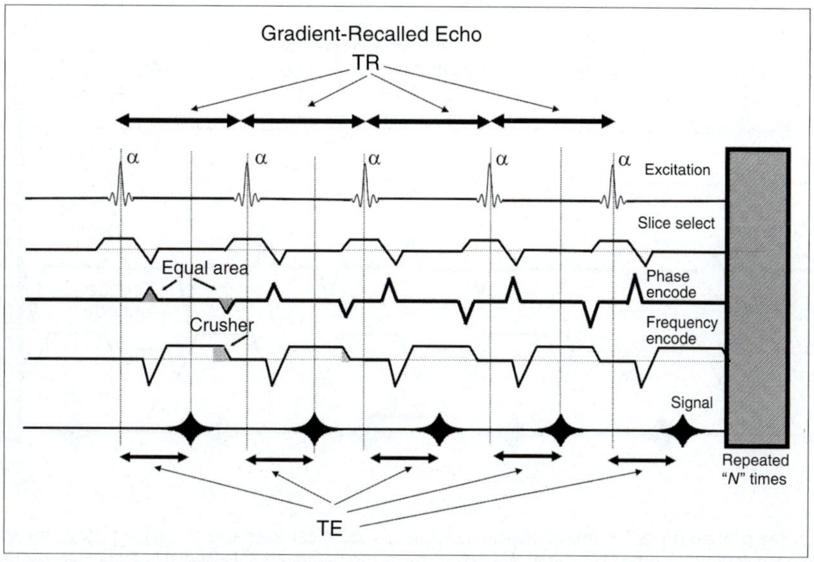

FIG. 1.15 Pulse sequence diagrams for gradient-recalled echo imaging showing multiple repetition times (*TRs*). TRs and echo times (*TE*) are indicated.

requires 160 ms (5 ms × 32 phase-encode lines). This time is sufficiently short that 32 TRs can be acquired in the quiescent diastolic period. Thus, data can be collected rather rapidly using a small excitation pulse rather than the 90-degree pulse. The GRE imaging method uses short TRs, low flip angles (alpha pulses), and no 180-degree refocusing pulse. Note that in GRE imaging (see Figs. 1.8 and 1.15), to keep the phase information intact, rewinding gradients are applied after each acquisition equal and opposite to the phase-encoding gradient. Furthermore, the readout gradient is also rewound, so that on all axes, the spins are in phase after each TR. Usually, an extra gradient is applied at the end of each TR on the X or Z axis, called a "crusher," "killer," or "spoiler" gradient (Fig. 1.15), which dephases any remaining transverse magnetization so that it does not contribute signal during the next phase-encode step (TR). Although the fast GRE images have T2* dephasing, this does not usually reduce image quality, since very short TEs are achievable unless a serious source of magnetic field inhomogeneity (e.g., a metallic implant) is present. Furthermore, the GRE sequence can be used to quantify myocardial T2* (by imaging at multiple TE times), which has revolutionized detection of myocardial iron deposition in diseases such as thalassemia.[10,31,32]

Three-Dimensional Fast Gradient Echo: Magnetic Resonance Angiography

The fast GRE pulse sequence is also used for contrast-enhanced MR angiography, which is the imaging of arteries and veins during the first pass of an exogenous gadolinium contrast agent[33] or in steady state.[34] During the first pass of a gadolinium contrast agent, the blood T1 is reduced to ~30 ms. The Ernst angle equation (see Eq. 1.9) identifies an optimal angle of ~30 degrees for a TR of 5 ms. Because this method is three dimensional (3D), "phase-encoding" in Z (now called "slice encoding") is performed in the slice direction also. Therefore, the scan time is $N_y \cdot N_z \cdot$ TR, where N_z is the number of slice encodings (slices). After the first pass of contrast, the T1 is much higher (~100 ms). However, recent use of iron-based contrast agents (e.g., ferumoxytol)[35–37] in the steady state has demonstrated extraordinary and long-lasting T1-shortening of the blood, which permits high-resolution MR angiography (and T2* is not prohibitively shortened). The acquisition of a 3D fast GRE volume provides high-quality images of vessels (see Chapters 41).

However, without a contrast agent, the SNR of fast GRE imaging can be low, and is mostly generated by spins flowing into the slice or slab. This limitation is partly overcome using balanced steady-state free precession (SSFP).

Balanced Steady-State Free Precession

Directly related to the GRE sequence is the balanced SSFP method (Fig. 1.16). Today, almost all CMR imaging of ventricular function employs this method, and it also is used for anatomical localization, valve visualization, and coronary artery imaging. Balanced SSFP (or bSSFP) was an old technique[38] that was later revived[39] because better scanner hardware allowed for the short TRs (e.g., 2–4 ms) required for balanced SSFP. Balanced SSFP uses a pulse sequence identical to GRE, except for two distinctions. First, after each TR, the spins are rephased on each gradient axis (X, Y, and Z) to zero phase. No crushers, killers, or spoilers are used. This keeps the spins completely in phase (except for dephasing due to magnetic field inhomogeneities) so that the transverse magnetization can be reused in the next TR. For this reason, the sequence is called "balanced." Second, a large flip angle (e.g., 60 degrees) is used, flipping spins around the positive and negative Y axis in alternate TRs. This flip angle alternation scheme reuses the remaining transverse magnetization and mixes it with longitudinal magnetization for increased signal in each TR.

Balanced SSFP provides high SNR of blood and a unique T2/T1 weighting.[40] As stated above, balanced SSFP is highly sensitive to off-resonance, requires short TRs and large flip angles, and is challenging at 3 T, where off-resonance creates artifacts[41] and RF heating concerns (specific

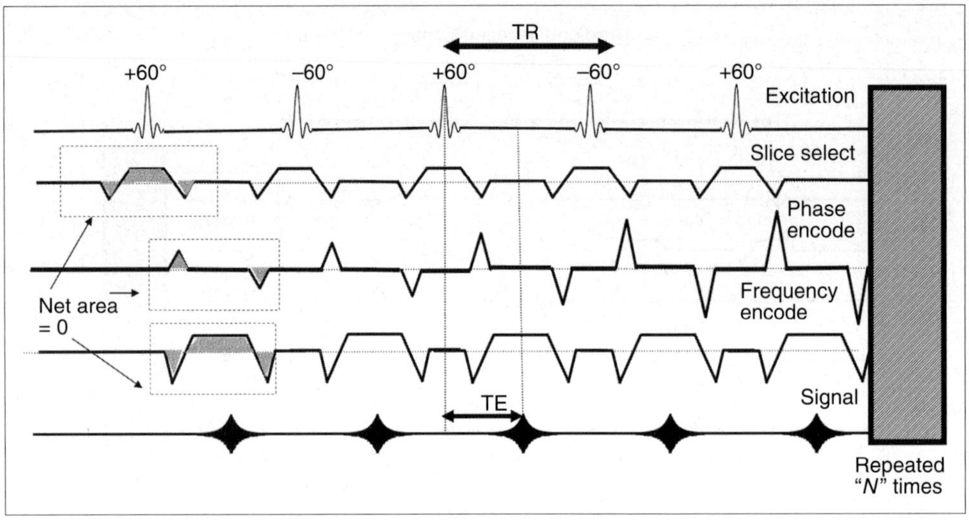

FIG. 1.16 Balanced steady-state free precession (*SSFP*) imaging. The sequence is identical to gradient-recalled echo, except that the flip angle for SSFP is high and its sign is alternated in each repetition time (*TR*). Also, the gradients in the balanced SSFP sequence are fully rephased (*see shaded areas*), so that the net gradient area (summed over the TR) is zero for each gradient axis. *TE*, Echo time.

absorption rate) limit the flip angle. At field strengths lower than 1.5T, it holds tremendous promise.[42]

Echo Planar Imaging, Spiral and Radial

Analogous to reducing scan time, by replacing a spin echo acquisition with a fast spin echo acquisition, the GRE sequence can be accelerated by acquiring a train of gradient-recalled echoes after a single RF pulse. This approach is called multiecho or echo planar imaging (EPI) and was among the first CMR imaging methods described.[43] For anatomy with long T2* tissues (e.g., the head), EPI can result in a complete image collection with a single slice-select pulse and a train of gradient echoes. EPI is the basis for the functional MRI technique widely used in brain mapping. Fig. 1.17 shows an EPI sequence in which, after a single RF excitation, frequency-encoding information at multiple phase-encoding values is acquired. To reduce time between echoes, the readout gradient is rapidly reversed with every phase-encode step, so that MR signals are collected during both the positive and negative lobes of the readout gradient (arrows). This approach is challenging in the heart, where the T2* can be short[16] compared to the brain, but has found early applications in cardiac perfusion[44] and is still used for cardiac diffusion-weighted imaging.[45,46] Because of the acquisition of many phase-encode steps after one RF excitation, the EPI method is fast, but results in poor SNR. EPI (along with spiral and radial, described below) has *k*-space "trajectory" errors that need correction[47–50] and image distortions due to off-resonance. However, these limitations can be overcome by only collecting a few (e.g., 3–9) phase-encode steps per slice-select RF excitation (instead all phase-encode steps) and repeating this process until all of the data have been collected.

Spiral imaging[51,52] is similar to EPI and obtains more image data after a single RF pulse compared to conventional imaging by continuously sampling *k*-space in a spiral pattern,[53,54] and has found applications in flow imaging[55] coronary imaging, myocardial strain imaging,[56] and most recently MR fingerprinting, a method for jointly mapping T1 and T2 and other tissue properties.[57,58] Radial imaging is another trajectory that acquires *k*-space data as radial spokes, analogous to CT. It has been applied to the heart, especially using undersampling of *k*-space for fast imaging.[59–62] Radial imaging was the first imaging method,[20] and its clinical utility has been facilitated by trajectory improvements (e.g., golden angle[63,64]) and recent developments in reconstruction of undersampled MR data using sparsity constraints.[65,66]

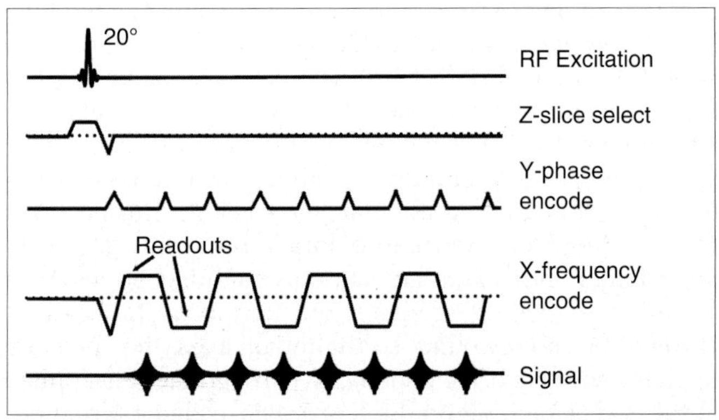

FIG. 1.17 Echo planar imaging (also called *multiecho imaging*), in which a portion of the frequency encodings are collected after each B_1 pulse. Here, eight frequency encodings are collected after a single B_1 excitation pulse (here with a 20-degree flip angle). All of the cardiovascular magnetic resonance data can be acquired after a single excitation, or only a portion. The phase-encoding gradient is blipped with a constant area, which leads to increasing phase encoding, and readouts are acquired using both positive and negative lobes of the frequency-encoding gradient. *RF*, Radiofrequency.

Preparation Pulses

In CMR imaging, preparation pulses are often used to generate contrast by generating M_z magnetization, which is T1 or T2 weighted. Fig. 1.18A shows how preparation pulses are used in CMR. First, a preparation pulse is applied, and then a segment (16–64 lines or more of *k*-space) of the MR data is acquired at a certain time within the cardiac cycle.

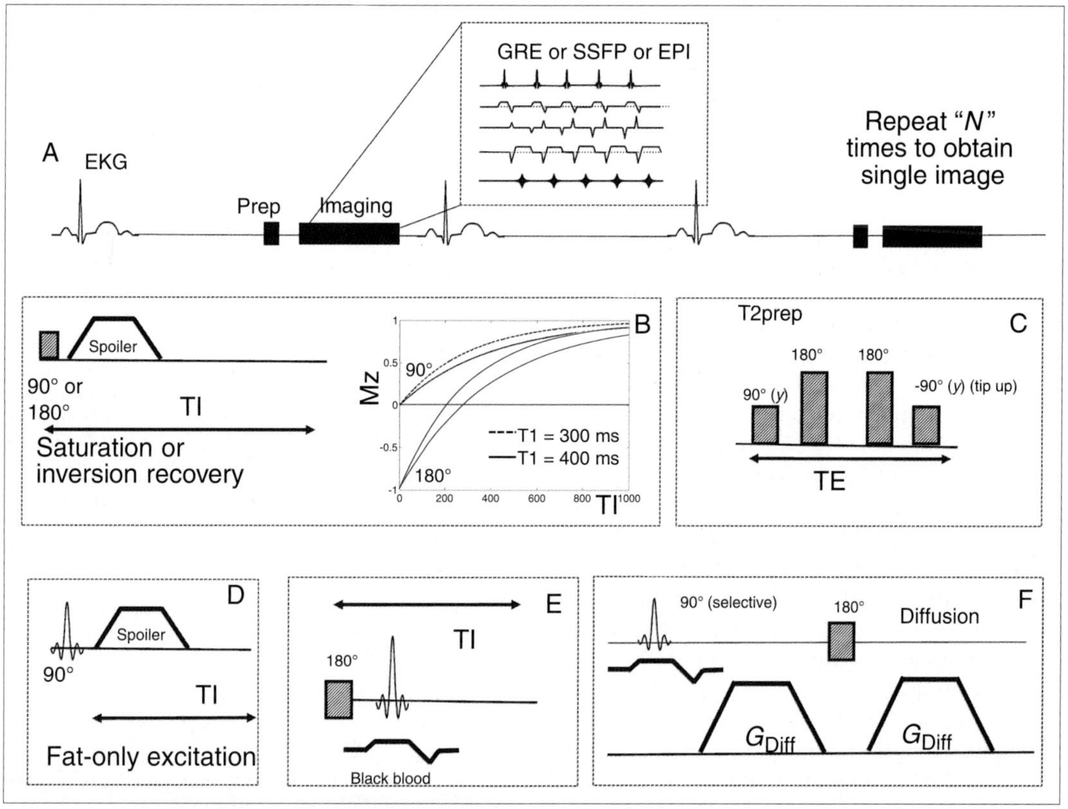

FIG. 1.18 Preparation pulses. (A) A preparation pulse precedes the acquisition of a segment of data (e.g., multiple repetition times [*TRs*] with gradient-recalled echo [*GRE*] or steady-state free precession [*SSFP*]), usually as part of an electrocardiogram (*EKG*)-gated acquisition. All preparations affect the longitudinal magnetization (M_z). (B) A nonselective 180-degree or 90-degree followed by an inversion time (*TI*) pulse generates T1 contrast, because M_z depends on the T1 and the TI time chosen. (C) T2prep uses the method of fast spin echo to refocus magnetization, which is then stored on the M_z axis. This results in Z magnetization, which depends on the T2 of the imaged tissue. (D) Fat saturation is performed by exciting fat with a 90-degree pulse and then crushing the resulting fat M_{xy}. Using a short TI, the M_z of fat is 0 after the saturation pulse, and the fat signal is suppressed. (E) Black-blood preparation inverts all blood and images at a TI when blood M_z magnetization is close to 0. The myocardial signal is unaffected, because a slice of interest is reinverted immediately after the 180 degrees. (F) Diffusion-encoding preparation. *EPI*, Echo planar imaging; *TE*, echo time.

Then, either in the next cardiac cycle or after skipping one or more cycles, another preparation pulse is applied and another segment of data is acquired. Fig. 1.18B–F shows a few important preparation pulses. Fig. 1.18B shows nonselective RF pulses, both a 90-degree "saturation recovery" pulse and a 180-degree "inversion recovery" pulse. These pulses generate T1 weighting, determined by the inversion time choice. A spoiler gradient destroys any M_{xy} magnetization created by the RF pulse. These are commonly used for perfusion and late gadolinium enhancement.[19,67] They are nonselective, so that all spins experience these pulses. Adiabatic RF pulses are often used, which are less susceptible to B_0 inhomogeneity.[68] Eq. (1.4) describes the T1 weighting achieved for a 90-degree saturation pulse.

Fig. 1.18C shows a *T2prep* pulse.[69] This is also nonselective, affecting all of the spins in the magnetic field. A 90-degree excitation is followed by multiple 180-degree refocusing pulses. The signal decays by T2, just like fast spin echo imaging. However, the signal is tipped back to the Z axis with a 90-degree pulse, generating M_z magnetization that is weighted by the T2 of the tissue, with higher M_z for long T2 tissues. Thus, this preparation pulse is called T2prep. It has great importance in T2 mapping.[70]

Very importantly, Fig. 1.18D shows how fat saturation can be achieved using a 90-degree excitation of fat only, which is possible because the Larmor frequency of fat is different from that of water (~210 Hz difference at 1.5 T). After the saturation of fat, a spoiler kills the fat M_{xy}. Imaging then begins, with the fat signal suppressed. Fig. 1.18E shows a double inversion recovery black-blood preparation.[71] This preparation consists of two inversion (180-degree) pulses, which immediately follow each other. The first inversion is a nonselective inversion pulse, which inverts all magnetization. The second inversion is a slice-selective inversion pulse, which reinverts a slice of interest that is centered on the imaging slice but is slightly larger (by a factor of 1.5–2). This preparation is timed so that at the time of acquisition, all blood magnetization has regrown from $-M_z$ to 0 (i.e., is black). Any blood that was reinverted, because it was within the slice of interest, moves out of the imaging slice during systole. Any blood that has flowed into the slice will contribute no signal because it is nulled (see Figs. 1.5A and 1.11 for a black-blood image). Fig. 1.18F shows a "diffusion weighting" preparation. In this technique, the microstructure of the myocardium can be studied. The diffusion of water in the myocardium depends on the myocyte's orientation and therefore fiber structure. The diffusion is measured using preparation pulses: a 90-degree RF saturation pulse to excite the spins, followed by the application of a maximal strength and rather long gradient (~10 ms, on any or multiple axes) to sensitize the signal to microscopic motions (diffusion). This is followed by a 180-degree refocusing pulse and an identical gradient that should rephrase any phase accumulation not due to spin motion. Cardiac diffusion imaging was proposed early on,[72] but is only now gaining acceptance[46] due to lessening concerns about the influences of cardiac and respiratory motion.[73] Many other preparation pulses, such as magnetization transfer,[74] cardiac CEST (chemical exchange saturation transfer),[75,76] and T1rho[77,78] are available for generating contrast.

NEW HARDWARE ADVANCES

For CMR, a B_0 of 1.5 T is most commonly used; however, cardiac imaging at 3 T[79] provides equivalent or improved quality for coronary artery imaging, late gadolinium enhancement, perfusion, and function, and there is progress in CMR at 7 T.[80] It is possible that 5 T might be the field strength of equipoise,[81] balancing between increased SNR and spectral sensitivity provided by 7 T, versus the ease of use (with only minor concerns regarding B1 excitation), quality, and safety (e.g., with respect to specific absorption rate) of 3 T. Recently, 0.55 T has been explored as a potentially important field strength, as it is less expensive to buy, site, and maintain and is thus more accessible, and it has advantages for lung imaging and imaging of devices (including interventional MRI), among other applications.[82,83] Beyond field strength, the number of receiver coil channels has increased from a single surface coil or body coil to 16–32 channels routinely on new systems. Higher gradient strengths of 80 mT/m are now available, which might hold promise for cardiac diffusion imaging.

REFERENCES

1. Dabir D, Child N, Kalra A, et al. Reference values for healthy human myocardium using a T1 mapping methodology: results from the International T1 Multicenter cardiovascular magnetic resonance study. *J Cardiovasc Magn Reson*. 2014;16(1):69. https://doi.org/10.1186/s12968-014-0069-x.
2. Popescu IA, Werys K, Zhang Q, et al. Standardization of T1-mapping in cardiovascular magnetic resonance using clustered structuring for benchmarking normal ranges. *Int J Cardiol*. 2021;326:220–225. https://doi.org/10.1016/j.ijcard.2020.10.041.
3. Messroghli DR, Moon JC, Ferreira VM, et al. Correction to: Clinical recommendations for cardiovascular magnetic resonance mapping of T1, T2, T2* and extracellular volume: a consensus statement by the Society for Cardiovascular Magnetic Resonance (SCMR) endorsed by the European Association for Cardiovascular Imaging (EACVI). *J Cardiovasc Magn Reson*. 2018;20(1):9. https://doi.org/10.1186/s12968-017-0408-9.
4. Roy C, Slimani A, de Meester C, et al. Age and sex corrected normal reference values of T1, T2 T2* and ECV in healthy subjects at 3T CMR. *J Cardiovasc Magn Reson*. 2017;19:72. https://doi.org/10.1186/s12968-017-0371-5.
5. Xu Z, Li W, Wang J, et al. Reference ranges of myocardial T1 and T2 mapping in healthy chinese adults: a multicenter 3t cardiovascular magnetic resonance study. *J Cardiovasc Magn Reson*. 2023;25(1):64. https://doi.org/10.1186/s12968-023-00974-5.
6. von Knobelsdorff-Brenkenhoff F, Prothmann M, Dieringer MA, et al. Myocardial T1 and T2 mapping at 3 T: reference values, influencing factors and implications. *J Cardiovasc Magn Reson*. 2013;15(1):53. https://doi.org/10.1186/1532-429X-15-53.
7. Zhang X, Petersen ET, Ghariq E, et al. In vivo blood t(1) measurements at 1.5 t, 3 t, and 7 t. *Magn Reson Med*. 2013;70(4):1082–1086. https://doi.org/10.1002/mrm.24550.
8. Stanisz GJ, Odrobina EE, Pun J, et al. T1 and T2 relaxation and magnetization transfer in tissue at 3T. *Magn Reson Med*. 2005;54(3):507–512. https://doi.org/10.1002/mrm.20605.
9. Hanson CA, Kamath A, Gottbrecht M, Ibrahim S, Salerno M. T2 relaxation times at cardiac MRI in healthy adults: a systematic review and meta-analysis. *Radiology*. 2020;297(2):344–351. https://doi.org/10.1148/radiol.2020200989.
10. Triadyaksa P, Oudkerk M, Sijens PE. Cardiac T(2) * mapping: techniques and clinical applications. *J Magn Reson Imaging*. 2020;52(5):1340–1351. https://doi.org/10.1002/jmri.27023.
11. Reiter U, Reiter C, Krauter C, Fuchsjager M, Reiter G. Cardiac magnetic resonance T1 mapping. Part 2: diagnostic potential and applications. *Eur J Radiol*. 2018;109:235–247. https://doi.org/10.1016/j.ejrad.2018.10.013.
12. Scholz TD, Martins JB, Skorton DJ. Nmr relaxation times in acute myocardial infarction: relative influence of changes in tissue water and fat content. *Magn Reson Med*. 1992;23(1):89–95. http://www.ncbi.nlm.nih.gov/entrez/query.fcgi?cmd=Retrieve&db=PubMed&dopt=Citation&list_uids=1734185.
13. Kim PK, Hong YJ, Im DJ, et al. Myocardial T1 and T2 mapping: techniques and clinical applications. *Korean J Radiol*. 2017;18(1):113–131. https://doi.org/10.3348/kjr.2017.18.1.113.
14. Karamitsos TD, Piechnik SK, Banypersad SM, et al. Noncontrast T1 mapping for the diagnosis of cardiac amyloidosis. *JACC Cardiovasc Imaging*. 2013;6(4):488–497. https://doi.org/10.1016/j.jcmg.2012.11.013.
15. Alam MH, Auger D, Smith GC, et al. T1 at 1.5T and 3T compared with conventional T2* at 1.5T for cardiac siderosis. *J Cardiovasc Magn Reson*. 2015;17:102. https://doi.org/10.1186/s12968-015-0207-0.
16. Reeder SB, Faranesh AZ, Boxerman JL, McVeigh ER. In vivo measurement of T2* and field inhomogeneity maps in the human heart at 1.5 T. *Magn Reson Med*. 1998;39(6):988–998. http://www.ncbi.nlm.nih.gov/entrez/query.fcgi?cmd=Retrieve&db=PubMed&dopt=Citation&list_uids=9621923.
17. Piechnik SK, Neubauer S, Ferreira VM. State-of-the-art review: stress T1 mapping-technical considerations, pitfalls and emerging clinical applications. *MAGMA*. 2018;31(1):131–141. https://doi.org/10.1007/s10334-017-0649-5.
18. Caravan P, Ellison JJ, McMurry TJ, Lauffer RB. Gadolinium(iii) chelates as mri contrast agents: structure, dynamics, and applications. *Chem Rev*. 1999;99(9):2293–2352. https://doi.org/10.1021/cr980440x.
19. Simonetti OP, Kim RJ, Fieno DS, et al. An improved mr imaging technique for the visualization of myocardial infarction. *Radiology*. 2001;218(1):215–223. http://www.ncbi.nlm.nih.gov/entrez/query.fcgi?cmd=Retrieve&db=PubMed&dopt=Citation&list_uids=11152805.
20. Lauterbur P. Image formation by induced local interactions: examples employing nuclear magnetic resonance. *Nature*. 1973;242:190–191.
21. Conolly S, Glover G, Nishimura D, Macovski A. A reduced power selective adiabatic spin-echo pulse sequence. *Magn Reson Med*. 1991;18(1):28–38. http://www.ncbi.nlm.nih.gov/entrez/query.fcgi?cmd=Retrieve&db=PubMed&dopt=Citation&list_uids=2062239.
22. Singh A, Kawaji K, Goyal N, et al. Feasibility of cardiac magnetic resonance wideband protocol in patients with implantable cardioverter defibrillators and its utility for defining scar. *Am J Cardiol*. 2019;123(8):1329–1335. https://doi.org/10.1016/j.amjcard.2019.01.018.
23. Price AN, Cordero-Grande L, Malik SJ, Hajnal JV. Simultaneous multislice imaging of the heart using multiband balanced ssfp with blipped-caipi. *Magn Reson Med*. 2020;83(6):2185–2196. https://doi.org/10.1002/mrm.28086.
24. Davids M, Dietz P, Ruyters G, et al. Peripheral nerve stimulation informed design of a high-performance asymmetric head gradient coil. *Magn Reson Med*. 2023;90(2):784–801. https://doi.org/10.1002/mrm.29668.
25. Meiboom S, Gill D. Modified spin-echo method for measuring nuclear relaxation times. *Rev Sci Instrum*. 1958;29(8):688–691. https://doi.org/10.1063/1.1716296.
26. Abdel-Aty H, Zagrosek A, Schulz-Menger J, et al. Delayed enhancement and T2-weighted cardiovascular magnetic resonance imaging differentiate acute from chronic myocardial infarction. *Circulation*. 2004;109(20):2411–2416. http://www.ncbi.nlm.nih.gov/entrez/query.fcgi?cmd=Retrieve&db=PubMed&dopt=Citation&list_uids=15123531.
27. Hennig J, Nauerth A, Friedburg H. Rare imaging: a fast imaging method for clinical MR. *Magn Reson Med*. 1986;3(6):823–833. http://www.ncbi.nlm.nih.gov/entrez/query.fcgi?cmd=Retrieve&db=PubMed&dopt=Citation&list_uids=3821461.
28. Aletras AH, Tilak GS, Natanzon A, et al. Retrospective determination of the area at risk for reperfused acute myocardial infarction with T2-weighted cardiac magnetic resonance imaging: histopathological and displacement encoding with stimulated echoes (dense) functional validations. *Circulation*. 2006;113(15):1865–1870. http://www.ncbi.nlm.nih.gov/entrez/query.fcgi?cmd=Retrieve&db=PubMed&dopt=Citation&list_uids=16606793.
29. Ferreira VM, Schulz-Menger J, Holmvang G, et al. Cardiovascular magnetic resonance in nonischemic myocardial inflammation: expert recommendations. *J Am Coll Cardiol*. 2018;72(24):3158–3176. https://doi.org/10.1016/j.jacc.2018.09.072.
30. Haase A, Matthaei D, Hanicke W, Frahm J. Dynamic digital subtraction imaging using fast low-angle shot MR movie sequence. *Radiology*. 1986;160(2):537–541. http://www.ncbi.nlm.nih.gov/entrez/query.fcgi?cmd=Retrieve&db=PubMed&dopt=Citation&list_uids=3523597.
31. Anderson LJ, Holden S, Davis B, et al. Cardiovascular T2-star (T2*) magnetic resonance for the early diagnosis of myocardial iron overload. *Eur Heart J*. 2001;22(23):2171–2179. http://www.ncbi.nlm.nih.gov/entrez/query.fcgi?cmd=Retrieve&db=PubMed&dopt=Citation&list_uids=11913479.
32. Westwood M, Anderson LJ, Firmin DN, et al. A single breath-hold multiecho T2* cardiovascular magnetic resonance technique for diagnosis of myocardial iron overload. *J Magn Reson Imaging*. 2003;18(1):33–39. http://www.ncbi.nlm.nih.gov/entrez/query.fcgi?cmd=Retrieve&db=PubMed&dopt=Citation&list_uids=12815637.
33. Prince MR, Yucel EK, Kaufman JA, Harrison DC, Geller SC. Dynamic gadolinium-enhanced three-dimensional abdominal MR arteriography. *J Magn Reson Imaging*. 1993;3(6):877–881. http://www.ncbi.nlm.nih.gov/entrez/query.fcgi?cmd=Retrieve&db=PubMed&dopt=Citation&list_uids=8280977.

34. Grist TM, Korosec FR, Peters DC, et al. Steady-state and dynamic mr angiography with ms-325: initial experience in humans. *Radiology*. 1998;207(2):539–544. https://doi.org/10.1148/radiology.207.2.9577507.
35. Hope MD, Hope TA, Zhu CC, et al. Vascular imaging with ferumoxytol as a contrast agent. *Am J Roentgenol*. 2015;205(3):W366–W373. https://doi.org/10.2214/Ajr.15.14534.
36. Finn JP, Nguyen KL, Han F, et al. Cardiovascular mri with ferumoxytol. *Clin Radiol*. 2016;71(8):796–806. https://doi.org/10.1016/j.crad.2016.03.020.
37. Yoshida T, Chen JJ, Zhou B, Finn JP, Hu P, Nguyen KL. Ferumoxytol-enhanced 4D multiphase, steady-state imaging with magnetic resonance in congenital heart disease: Ventricular volume and function across 2D and 3D software platforms. *Quant Imaging Med Surg*. 2022;12(9):4377–4389. https://doi.org/10.21037/qims-21-1243.
38. Oppelt A, Graumann R, Barfuss H, Fischer H, Hart W, Shajor W. FISP—a new fast mri sequence. *Electromedica*. 1986;54:15–18.
39. Duerk JL, Lewin JS, Wendt M, Petersilge C. Remember true fisp? A high snr, near 1-second imaging method for T2-like contrast in interventional mri at .2 T. *JMRI-J Magn Reson Imaging*. 1998;8(1):203–208. https://doi.org/10.1002/jmri.1880080134.
40. Scheffler K, Lehnhardt S. Principles and applications of balanced ssfp techniques. *Eur Radiol*. 2003;13(11):2409–2418. http://www.ncbi.nlm.nih.gov/entrez/query.fcgi?cmd=Retrieve&db=PubMed&dopt=Citation&list_uids=12928954.
41. Schar M, Kozerke S, Fischer SE, Boesiger P. Cardiac ssfp imaging at 3 Tesla. *Magn Reson Med*. 2004;51(4):799–806. http://www.ncbi.nlm.nih.gov/entrez/query.fcgi?cmd=Retrieve&db=PubMed&dopt=Citation&list_uids=15065254.
42. Bandettini WP, Shanbhag SM, Mancini C, et al. A comparison of cine CMR imaging at 0.55 T and 1.5 T. *J Cardiovasc Magn Reson*. 2020;22(1):37. https://doi.org/10.1186/s12968-020-00618-y.
43. Mansfield P, Pykett I. Biological and medical imaging by NMR. *J Magn Res*. 1978;29:355–373.
44. Epstein FH, Wolff SD, Arai AE. Segmented k-space fast cardiac imaging using an echo-train readout. *Magn Reson Med*. 1999;41(3):609–613. http://www.ncbi.nlm.nih.gov/entrez/query.fcgi?cmd=Retrieve&db=PubMed&dopt=Citation&list_uids=10204886.
45. Nielles-Vallespin S, Mekkaoui C, Gatehouse P, et al. In vivo diffusion tensor mri of the human heart: reproducibility of breath-hold and navigator-based approaches. *Magn Reson Med*. 2013;70(2):454–465. https://doi.org/10.1002/mrm.24488.
46. Nielles-Vallespin S, Scott A, Ferreira P, Khalique Z, Pennell D, Firmin D. Cardiac diffusion: technique and practical applications. *J Magn Reson Imaging*. 2020;52(2):348–368. https://doi.org/10.1002/jmri.26912.
47. Reeder SB, Atalar E, Faranesh AZ, McVeigh ER. Referenceless interleaved echo-planar imaging. *Magn Reson Med*. 1999;41(1):87–94. http://www.ncbi.nlm.nih.gov/entrez/query.fcgi?cmd=Retrieve&db=PubMed&dopt=Citation&list_uids=10025615.
48. Peters DC, Derbyshire JA, McVeigh ER. Centering the projection reconstruction trajectory: reducing gradient delay errors. *Magn Reson Med*. 2003;50(1):1–6. http://www.ncbi.nlm.nih.gov/entrez/query.fcgi?cmd=Retrieve&db=PubMed&dopt=Citation&list_uids=12815671.
49. Duyn JH, Yang Y, Frank JA, van der Veen JW. Simple correction method for k-space trajectory deviations in MRI. *J Magn Reson*. 1998;132(1):150–153. http://www.ncbi.nlm.nih.gov/entrez/query.fcgi?cmd=Retrieve&db=PubMed&dopt=Citation&list_uids=9615415.
50. Campbell-Washburn AE, Xue H, Lederman RJ, Faranesh AZ, Hansen MS. Real-time distortion correction of spiral and echo planar images using the gradient system impulse response function. *Magn Reson Med*. 2016;75(6):2278–2285. https://doi.org/10.1002/mrm.25788.
51. Ahn CB, Kim JH, Cho ZH. High-speed spiral-scan echo planar NMR imagingl. *IEEE Trans Med Imaging*. 1986;5(1):2–7. https://doi.org/10.1109/TMI.1986.4307732.
52. Meyer CH, Hu BS, Nishimura DG, Macovski A. Fast spiral coronary artery imaging. *Magn Reson Med*. 1992;28(2):202–213. https://doi.org/10.1002/mrm.1910280204.
53. Hardy CJ, Zhao L, Zong X, Saranathan M, Yucel EK. Coronary MR angiography: respiratory motion correction with bacspin. *J Magn Reson Imaging*. 2003;17(2):170–176. http://www.ncbi.nlm.nih.gov/entrez/query.fcgi?cmd=Retrieve&db=PubMed&dopt=Citation&list_uids=12541223.
54. Nayak KS, Pauly JM, Yang PC, Hu BS, Meyer CH, Nishimura DG. Real-time interactive coronary mra. *Magn Reson Med*. 2001;46(3):430–435. http://www.ncbi.nlm.nih.gov/entrez/query.fcgi?cmd=Retrieve&db=PubMed&dopt=Citation&list_uids=11550232.
55. Kowalik GT, Muthurangu V, Khushnood A, Steeden JA. Rapid breath-hold assessment of myocardial velocities using spiral unfold-ed sense tissue phase mapping. *J Magn Reson Imaging*. 2016;44(4):1003–1009. https://doi.org/10.1002/jmri.25218.
56. Zhong X, Spottiswoode BS, Meyer CH, Kramer CM, Epstein FH. Imaging three-dimensional myocardial mechanics using navigator-gated volumetric spiral cine dense MRI. *Magn Reson Med*. 2010;64(4):1089–1097. https://doi.org/10.1002/mrm.22503.
57. Hamilton JI, Jiang Y, Chen Y, et al. Mr fingerprinting for rapid quantification of myocardial t(1), t(2), and proton spin density. *Magn Reson Med*. 2017;77(4):1446–1458. https://doi.org/10.1002/mrm.26216.
58. Rashid I, Cruz G, Seiberlich N, Hamilton JI. Cardiac MR fingerprinting: overview, technical developments, and applications. *J Magn Reson Imaging*. 2023;60(5):1753–1773. https://doi.org/10.1002/jmri.29206.
59. Peters DC, Korosec FR, Grist TM, et al. Undersampled projection reconstruction applied to MR angiography. *Magn Reson Med*. 2000;43(1):91–101. https://doi.org/10.1002/(sici)1522-2594(200001)43:1<91::aid-mrm11>3.0.co;2-4.
60. Barger AV, Block WF, Toropov Y, Grist TM, Mistretta CA. Time-resolved contrast-enhanced imaging with isotropic resolution and broad coverage using an undersampled 3D projection trajectory. *Magn Reson Med*. 2002;48(2):297–305. https://doi.org/10.1002/mrm.10212.
61. Rasche V, de Boer RW, Holz D, Proksa R. Continuous radial data acquisition for dynamic MRI. *Magn Reson Med*. 1995;34(5):754–761. https://doi.org/10.1002/mrm.1910340515.
62. Larson AC, White RD, Laub G, McVeigh ER, Li D, Simonetti OP. Self-gated cardiac cine MRI. *Magn Reson Med*. 2004;51(1):93–102. http://www.ncbi.nlm.nih.gov/entrez/query.fcgi?cmd=Retrieve&db=PubMed&dopt=Citation&list_uids=14705049.
63. Winkelmann S, Schaeffter T, Koehler T, Eggers H, Doessel O. An optimal radial profile order based on the golden ratio for time-resolved mri. *IEEE Trans Med Imaging*. 2007;26(1):68–76. https://doi.org/10.1109/TMI.2006.885337.
64. Wundrak S, Paul J, Ulrici J, et al. Golden ratio sparse mri using tiny golden angles. *Magn Reson Med*. 2016;75(6):2372–2378. https://doi.org/10.1002/mrm.25831.
65. Lustig M, Donoho D, Pauly JM. Sparse MRI: the application of compressed sensing for rapid MR imaging. *Magn Reson Med*. 2007;58(6):1182–1195. http://www.ncbi.nlm.nih.gov/entrez/query.fcgi?cmd=Retrieve&db=PubMed&dopt=Citation&list_uids=17969013.
66. Block KT, Uecker M, Frahm J. Undersampled radial MRI with multiple coils. Iterative image reconstruction using a total variation constraint. *Magn Reson Med*. 2007;57(6):1086–1098. http://www.ncbi.nlm.nih.gov/entrez/query.fcgi?cmd=Retrieve&db=PubMed&dopt=Citation&list_uids=17534903.
67. Kim RJ, Wu E, Rafael A, et al. The use of contrast-enhanced magnetic resonance imaging to identify reversible myocardial dysfunction. *N Engl J Med*. 2000;343(20):1445–1453. http://www.ncbi.nlm.nih.gov/entrez/query.fcgi?cmd=Retrieve&db=PubMed&dopt=Citation&list_uids=11078769.
68. Rashid S, Rapacchi S, Vaseghi M, et al. Improved late gadolinium enhancement mr imaging for patients with implanted cardiac devices. *Radiology*. 2014;270(1):269–274. https://doi.org/10.1148/radiol.13130942.
69. Brittain JH, Olcott EW, Szuba A, et al. Three-dimensional flow-independent peripheral angiography. *Magn Reson Med*. 1997;38(3):343–354. https://doi.org/10.1002/mrm.1910380302.
70. Giri S, Chung YC, Merchant A, et al. T2 quantification for improved detection of myocardial edema. *J Cardiovasc Magn Reson*. 2009;11(1):56. https://doi.org/10.1186/1532-429X-11-56.
71. Simonetti OP, Finn JP, White RD, Laub G, Henry DA. "Black blood" T2-weighted inversion-recovery MR imaging of the heart. *Radiology*. 1996;199(1):49–57. https://doi.org/10.1148/radiology.199.1.8633172.
72. Reese TG, Weisskoff RM, Smith RN, Rosen BR, Dinsmore RE, Wedeen VJ. Imaging myocardial fiber architecture in vivo with magnetic resonance. *Magn Reson Med*. 1995;34(6):786–791. https://doi.org/10.1002/mrm.1910340603.
73. Aliotta E, Wu HH, Ennis DB. Convex optimized diffusion encoding (code) gradient waveforms for minimum echo time and bulk motion-compensated diffusion-weighted mri. *Magn Reson Med*. 2017;77(2):717–729. https://doi.org/10.1002/mrm.26166.
74. Wolff SD, Balaban RS. Magnetization transfer imaging: practical aspects and clinical applications. *Radiology*. 1994;192(3):593–599. https://doi.org/10.1148/radiology.192.3.8058919.
75. Ayala C, Luo H, Godines K, et al. Individually tailored spatial-spectral pulsed cest mri for ratiometric mapping of myocardial energetic species at 3t. *Magn Reson Med*. 2023;90(6):2321–2333. https://doi.org/10.1002/mrm.29801.
76. Ward KM, Aletras AH, Balaban RS. A new class of contrast agents for MRI based on proton chemical exchange dependent saturation transfer (cest). *J Magn Reson*. 2000;143(1):79–87. https://doi.org/10.1006/jmre.1999.1956.
77. Han Y, Liimatainen T, Gorman RC, Witschey WR. Assessing myocardial disease using t(1rho) MRI. *Curr Cardiovasc Imaging Rep*. 2014;7(2):9248. https://doi.org/10.1007/s12410-013-9248-7.
78. Thompson EW, Iyer SK, Solomon MP, et al. Endogenous T1ρ cardiovascular magnetic resonance in hypertrophic cardiomyopathy. *J Cardiovasc Magn Reson*. 2021;23(1):120. https://doi.org/10.1186/s12968-021-00813-5.
79. Graves MJ. 3 T: The good, the bad and the ugly. *Br J Radiol*. 2022;95(1130):20210708. https://doi.org/10.1259/bjr.20210708.
80. Niendorf T, Schulz-Menger J, Paul K, Huelnhagen T, Ferrari VA, Hodge R. High field cardiac magnetic resonance imaging: a case for ultrahigh field cardiac magnetic resonance. *Circ Cardiovasc Imaging*. 2017;10(6). https://doi.org/10.1161/CIRCIMAGING.116.005460.
81. Lin L, Liu PJ, Sun G, et al. Bi-ventricular assessment with cardiovascular magnetic resonance at 5 Tesla: a pilot study. *Front Cardiovasc Med*. 2022;9:913707. https://doi.org/10.3389/fcvm.2022.913707.
82. Campbell-Washburn AE, Ramasawmy R, Restivo MC, et al. Opportunities in interventional and diagnostic imaging by using high-performance low-field-strength MRI. *Radiology*. 2019;293(2):384–393. https://doi.org/10.1148/radiol.2019190452.
83. Varghese J, Jin N, Giese D, et al. Building a comprehensive cardiovascular magnetic resonance exam on a commercial 0.55 T system: A pictorial essay on potential applications. *Front Cardiovasc Med*. 2023;10:1120982. https://doi.org/10.3389/fcvm.2023.1120982.

2 Cardiovascular Magnetic Resonance Contrast Agents

PETER CARAVAN

The vast majority of cardiovascular magnetic resonance (CMR) studies use a gadolinium-based contrast agent (GBCA).[1] The CMR contrast agent typically makes diseased tissue appear brighter (or in some cases darker) than the surrounding tissue. Cardiovascular applications, such as magnetic resonance angiography (MRA), functional imaging of myocardial perfusion, viability with late gadolinium enhancement imaging, and extracellular volume mapping to estimate myocardial fibrosis represent the bulk of CMR scans that use a contrast agent. The first approved contrast agent for magnetic resonance (MR), gadopentetate (Gd-DTPA), appeared in 1988, and several other compounds followed. These first contrast agents were extracellular fluid (ECF) agents. The contrast agent gadobutrol has been approved by the US Food and Drug Administration (FDA) "to assess myocardial perfusion (stress, rest) and late gadolinium enhancement in adult patients with known or suspected coronary artery disease." While other GBCAs do not have this indication, they are frequently used "off-label." In addition to ECF agents, there is also an approved hepatobiliary contrast agent. Another material used in CMR is an iron oxide preparation developed to treat anemia but that is also used off-label as an intravascular agent for steady-state contrast-enhanced MRA. At the clinical development and preclinical stages, there are exciting advancements in nongadolinium contrast agents and molecular imaging agents that can report on molecular markers of inflammation, fibrosis, ischemia, cardiomyocyte function, and magnetically labeled cells.

This chapter focuses first on the general underlying chemistry and biophysics of contrast agents in clinical CMR. The mechanism of action of different classes of contrast agents is described, with examples drawn from CMR applications. Finally, there is a brief survey of novel contrast agents potentially useful for cardiovascular indications that are currently in clinical or preclinical development.

The vast majority of CMR agents in clinical use are small molecules based on chelated gadolinium (Gd). The bulk of this chapter focuses on GBCAs, including their chemistry, biophysics, and applications. Other exogenous compounds have been used to change signal properties in magnetic resonance imaging (MRI; e.g., chelated manganese, fluorine-19, iron particles, hyperpolarized nuclei), and these will be discussed as appropriate to CMR. This chapter assumes that the reader has a basic understanding of CMR vocabulary.

INTRODUCTION TO THE BIOPHYSICS OF MAGNETIC RESONANCE IMAGING

All contrast agents shorten both T1 and T2 relaxation times. However, it is useful to classify CMR contrast agents into two broad groups based on whether the substance increases the transverse relaxation rate (1/T2) by roughly the same amount that it increases the longitudinal relaxation rate (1/T1) or whether 1/T2 is altered to a much greater extent. The first category is referred to as "T1 agents" because, on a percentage basis, these agents alter 1/T1 of tissue more than 1/T2 as a result of endogenous transverse relaxation in tissue. With most pulse sequences, this dominant T1-lowering effect gives rise to *increases* in signal intensity, and thus these agents are referred to as "positive" contrast agents. The T2 agents largely increase the 1/T2 of tissue selectively and cause a *reduction* in signal intensity, and thus they are known as "negative" contrast agents. Paramagnetic gadolinium-based contrast agents are examples of T1 agents, whereas ferromagnetic large iron oxide particles are examples of T2 agents.

There are many mechanisms by which contrast agents shorten T1 and T2. Considerable chemistry and biophysics can be applied to understand or predict these mechanisms. However, in many cases, the effect of these mechanisms can be reduced to a single constant, called "relaxivity." Fig. 2.1 shows the effect and definition of relaxivity.

Fig. 2.1A shows the effect of a typical contrast agent on the relaxation time of two hypothetical tissues, one with T1 = 1200 ms (similar to heart muscle at 1.5 T) and one with T1 = 400 ms. At low concentrations (left side of the graph), it appears that the contrast agent has a larger effect (change in T1) on the tissue with a longer T1. At higher contrast agent concentrations (right side of Fig. 2.1A), both tissues approach approximately the same T1. A simple way to quantify this effect is to consider the rate of relaxation, 1/T1 (sometimes denoted "R1"). In most cases in medical imaging, the contrast agent increases the relaxation rate proportional to the amount of contrast agent:

$$\frac{1}{T1} = \frac{1}{T1_0} + r_1\ [\mathrm{CA}] \qquad \text{Eq. 2.1}$$

where T1 is the observed T1 with contrast agent in the tissue, $T1_0$ is the T1 before addition of the contrast agent, [CA] is the concentration of contrast agent, and r_1 is the longitudinal relaxivity, often just "relaxivity." The conventional units for r_1 are $mM^{-1}s^{-1}$ (per millimolar per second, sometimes

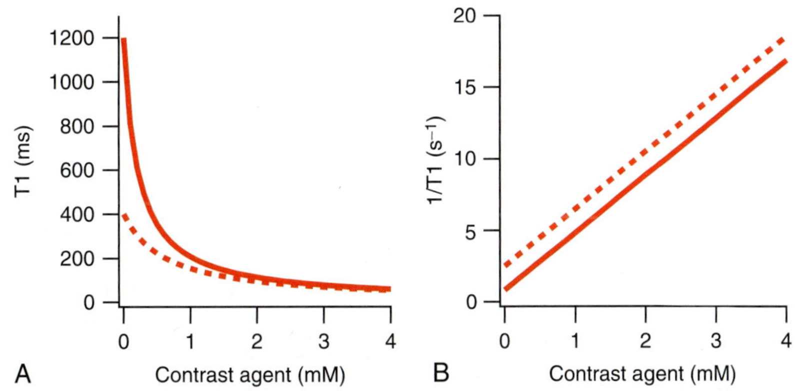

FIG. 2.1 Change in (A) longitudinal relaxation time (T1) and (B) longitudinal relaxation rate (1/T1) for typical myocardial tissue (*solid line*, T1 = 1200 ms at 1.5 T) and short T1 tissue (*dashed line*, T1 = 400 ms).

L•mol^{-1}s^{-1}). Thus, the slope of 1/T1 as a function of contrast agent concentration (Fig. 2.1B) shows the relaxivity, in this case, 4 mM^{-1}s^{-1}. Fig. 2.1B shows that the effect of the contrast agent on the relaxation rate is independent of the initial T1 of the tissue; that is, in terms of relaxation rate, the contrast agent has the same effect, regardless of initial T1. Transverse, or T2, relaxivity is defined in an analogous way:

$$\frac{1}{T1} = \frac{1}{T2_0} + r_2\ [CA] \qquad \text{Eq. 2.2}$$

For all contrast agents, r_2 is larger than r_1. Relaxivity is dependent on magnetic field strength, temperature, and in some instances protein binding, pH, or even the presence of enzymes.

Contrast agent behavior in vivo is seldom as simple as the pure linear effect relaxation rate shown in Fig. 2.1. Even in the simple case of pure linear relaxation, the effect of the contrast agent on the CMR image is generally nonlinear.[2] In traditional spin echo sequences, nonlinearity can be a result of T1 saturation or T2 signal loss. Once the contrast agent reduces T1 < repetition time (TR)/2, increasing contrast agent concentration will have little effect on increasing the available longitudinal magnetization because the tissue will have nearly fully recovered the magnetization before the next radiofrequency (RF) pulse. Furthermore, because contrast agents affect both T1 and T2 relaxation, at a high enough concentration, the contrast agent will reduce T2 to the order of the echo time (TE), and will then decrease magnetic resonance (MR) image intensity. These effects are seen in Fig. 2.2, where signal intensity is plotted versus contrast agent concentration for T1- and T2-weighted spin echo sequences. Fig. 2.2 was generated assuming a contrast agent relaxivity of 4 mM^{-1}s^{-1}, typical of many commercial ECF gadolinium agents, and tissue relaxation times typical of myocardium at 1.5 T (T1 = 1200 ms, T2 = 50 ms). For the T1-weighted sequence (TE/TR = 15/600) in Fig. 2.2A, signal intensity begins to level out at a contrast agent concentration between 0.5 and 1.0 mM. From Fig. 2.1A, this is the range at which the T1 of the myocardium decreased to approximately 300 ms, or TR/2. At concentrations >1 mM, the T1 effect is saturated, and the only *imaging* effect of the contrast agent is to make T2 shorter and cause signal loss, even on this T1-weighted sequence. Signal is lost because even a T1-weighted sequence has a finite TE, and T2 effects can enter when T2 is short enough.

The signal intensity plateau on the T2-weighted scan (TE/TR = 80/3000), Fig. 2.2B, occurs at a much lower contrast agent concentration. Because TR is so long, the only real effect of the contrast agent is to reduce (rather than increase) signal intensity on this T2-weighted scan. However, this negative contrast can also be medically useful, and certain contrast agents (notably, iron oxide particles) create negative contrast exactly by providing enhanced T2 relaxation, and thus darker images on T2-weighted scans.

Increasing the relaxivity (r_1 or r_2) will have the effect of pushing the simulated curves in Fig. 2.2A to the left, which means that peak signal and subsequent signal loss will occur at *lower* contrast agent concentrations. A more linear response of the signal to contrast agent can be achieved with a fast three-dimensional (3D) spoiled gradient-recalled echo (GRE) sequence. This is seen in Fig. 2.2C, where signal intensity is plotted versus contrast agent concentration using the same tissue relaxation times and relaxivities as in Figs. 2.2A and 2.2B for a typical fast 3D spoiled GRE sequence: TE/TR/flip = 2.2/9.0/40 degrees. The short TR and very short TE ensure that signal intensity increases across the entire concentration range. At high concentrations, the effect of the contrast agent becomes nonlinear, but the signal still increases with increasing contrast agent concentration.

Commercial Contrast Agents and Those in Clinical Development

The addition of paramagnetic materials to reduce relaxation times goes back to the earliest days of MR. In the 1940s, Bloch and colleagues used ferric nitrate to enhance the relaxation rate of water.[3] Exogenous contrast was applied to MRI in 1978 when Lauterbur and associates reported using manganese dichloride to differentiate normal from infarcted myocardium in dogs.[4] Carr and colleagues reported the first use of a gadolinium complex, gadopentetate dimeglumine (Gd-DTPA; Magnevist, Bayer, Berlin, Germany), in patients with brain tumors in 1984.[5] By 1988, Gd-DTPA was FDA-approved for clinical use.

Extracellular Agents

The most common contrast agents used clinically are ECF agents. These all behave in a very similar manner, and are

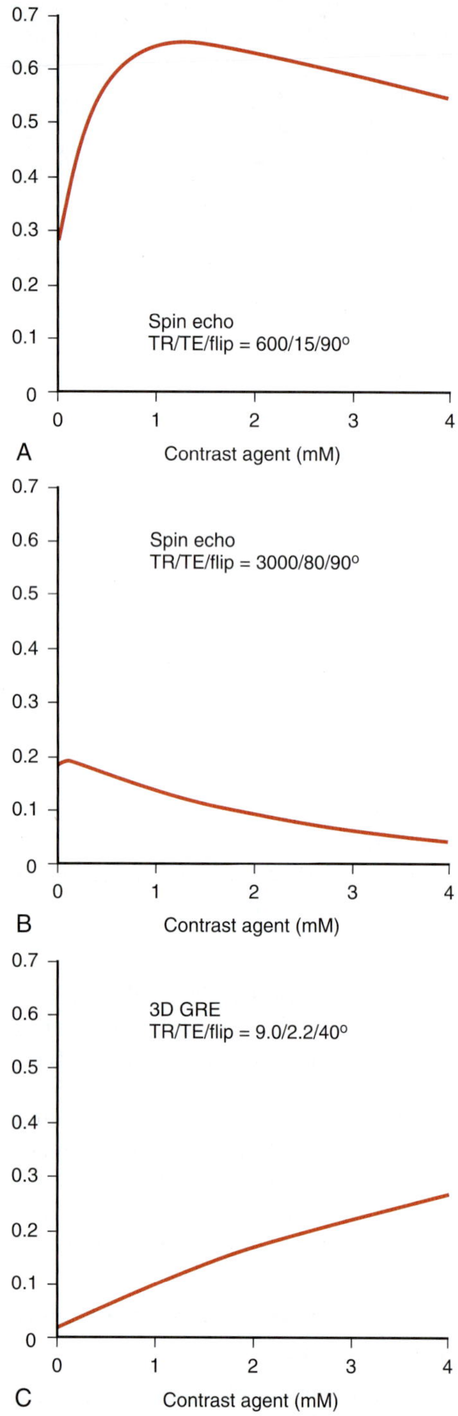

FIG. 2.2 Effect of contrast agent on myocardial image intensity on T1-weighted and T2-weighted spin echo scans. (A) T1-weighted spin echo (repetition time [*TR*] = 600 ms) assumes a patient with a heart rate of 100 beats per minute and shows a linear increase of signal only for contrast agent concentrations <0.5 mM. (B) T2-weighted spin echo images (TR = 3000 ms) show only T2 signal loss effects as a result of contrast agent with no T1 enhancement because of the long TR. (C) Typical short-TR fast spoiled gradient-recalled echo (*GRE*) sequence. The very short echo time (*TE*) and short TR give monotonically increased image intensity across the entire range of contrast agent concentrations typically found in clinical scans.

typically referred to as "gadolinium" or "gado" agents. Fig. 2.3 shows the chemical structures of several approved ECF agents. Chemically, these compounds exhibit three similar features: they all contain Gd, they all contain a 7- or 8-coordinate ligand binding to Gd, and they all contain one or two water molecules bonded to Gd. Nomenclature for contrast agents can be confusing: there is a generic name (e.g., gadoterate), a trade name (e.g., Dotarem, Clariscan), and usually a chemical code name or abbreviation (e.g., Gd-1,4,7,10-tetraazacyclododecane-1,4,7,10-tetraacetic acid or Gd-DOTA). Any of these three names may be used in the scientific literature.

The multidentate ligand is required for safety.[6] The ligand encapsulates the Gd, resulting in a high thermodynamic stability and kinetic inertness with respect to metal loss. This enables the contrast agent to be excreted intact, an important property because these contrast agents tend to be much less toxic than their substituents. For example, the DTPA ligand and gadolinium chloride both have an LD_{50} of 0.5 mmol/kg in rats (LD_{50} = dose that causes death in 50% of the animals), whereas the Gd-DTPA complex has a safety margin that is higher by nearly a factor of 20, with an LD_{50} of 8 mmol/kg for the Gd-DTPA complex.[7]

The Gd ion and coordinated water molecule are essential to providing contrast. The Gd (III) ion has a high magnetic moment and a relatively slow electronic relaxation rate, properties that make it an excellent relaxer of water protons. The proximity of the coordinated water molecule leads to efficient relaxation. The coordinated water molecule is in rapid chemical exchange (10^6 exchanges/s) with solvating water molecules.[8] This rapid exchange leads to a catalytic effect whereby the Gd complex effectively shortens the relaxation times of the bulk solution.

ECF agents have very similar properties, which are summarized in Table 2.1. They are all very hydrophilic complexes with excellent safety profiles and can be formulated at high concentrations. On injection, these ECF agents quickly and freely distribute to the extracellular space. Administration of any of these agents yields similar diagnostic information.

There are some differences among the physical properties. All the approved agents are formulated at concentrations that are hyperosmotic. Osmolality depends on both the concentration and number of species in solution. A charge neutral compound like gadobutrol will have only one species in solution whereas an ionic compound like gadoterate will have equal numbers of the gadoterate complex and meglumine counterion. Thus, the osmolality is higher for ionic complexes formulated at the same concentration as neutral complexes. While there is a known benefit of neutral, lower osmolality contrast agents for x-ray/computed tomography (CT) applications, for CMR the injection volumes are much *smaller* than the volumes used for x-ray angiography or CT angiography. Thus, the overall increase in osmolality after injection of a CMR contrast agent is minimal. Unlike with x-ray contrast, there is no documented safety benefit in using nonionic CMR contrast agents. One benefit of nonionic compounds is the ability to formulate them at high concentration (1 M) without drastically increasing osmolality or viscosity (see Table 2.1).[9] These high-concentration formulations may be useful in fast dynamic studies, such as dynamic MRA or myocardial perfusion. These ECF agents, as with iodinated preparations used for x-ray and CT, are excreted by the kidneys. As a result, clearance is impaired in patients with impaired/reduced renal function (discussed later).

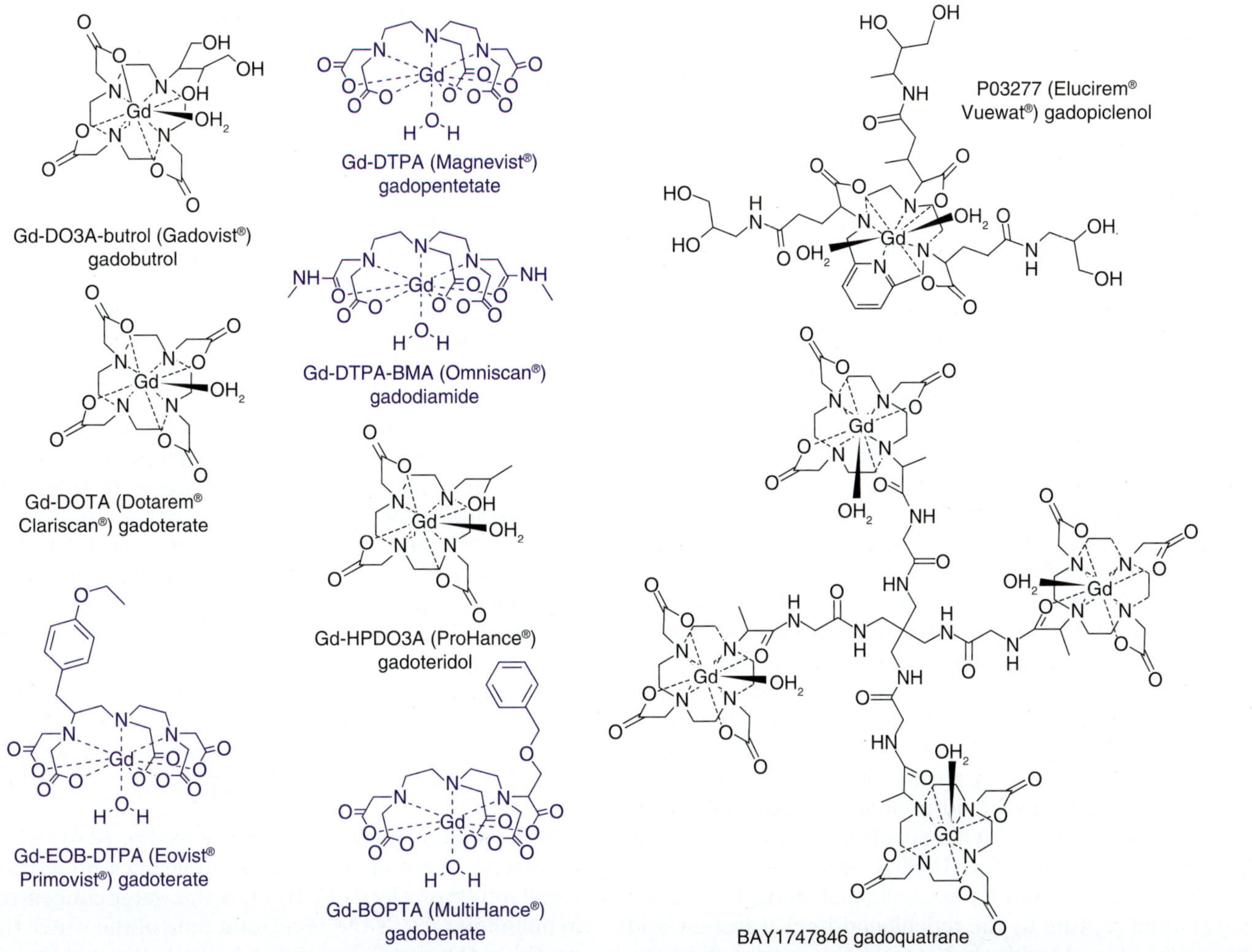

FIG. 2.3 Chemical structures of commercial (United States or Europe) magnetic resonance contrast agents. Macrocyclic agents are shown in *black* and linear agents in *blue*. Gadoquatrane has completed phase 3 clinical trials as of October 2024, but is not yet approved for commercial use.

TABLE 2.1 Approved[a] (October 2024) magnetic resonance imaging contrast agents—formulation properties.

GENERIC NAME	PRODUCT NAME	CHEMICAL ABBREVIATION	CLASS	CONCENTRATION (MOLAR)	APPROVED DOSE (MMOL/KG)	OSMOLALITY (OSMOL/KG)	VISCOSITY (CP)
Gadopentetate	Magnevist	Gd-DTPA	Linear	0.5	0.1	1.96	2.9
Gadoterate	Dotarem Clariscan	Gd-DOTA	Macrocyclic	0.5	0.1	1.35	2.0
Gadodiamide	Omniscan	Gd-DTPA-BMA	Linear	0.5	0.1	0.79	1.4
Gadoteridol	Prohance	Gd-HPDO3A	Macrocyclic	0.5	0.1	0.63	1.3
Gadobutrol	Gadovist	Gd-DO3A-butrol	Macrocyclic	1.0	0.1	1.39	3.7
Gadobenate	Multihance	Gd-BOPTA	Linear	0.5	0.1		
Gadopiclenol	Elucirem Vueway	P03277	Macrocyclic	0.5	0.05	1.11	2.0
Gadoxetate	Eovist Primovist	Gd-EOB-DTPA	Linear		0.025		
Gadoquatrane		BAY 1747846	Macrocyclic	0.3 (in Gd)	0.04	0.294	1.22

[a]As of writing, gadoquatrane had completed clinical trial enrollment but was not yet approved for use.

Blood Pool Agents

Because CMR contrast agents are administered intravenously, they are all potentially capable of imaging the blood lumen. The ECF agents described earlier are used routinely for contrast-enhanced MRA. One potential drawback of using ECF agents for MRA is their pharmacokinetics. ECF agents rapidly leak out of the vascular space into all the interstitial spaces of the body. Angiography with ECF agents is thus typically limited to dynamic/first-pass arterial studies. There has been considerable effort made toward designing specific blood pool agents that are tailored for vascular imaging. The ideal blood pool agent should remain in the vascular compartment and not leak out into the extracellular space. It should be capable of being given as a bolus such that a dynamic arterial image can be obtained. While there was a gadolinium-based MRA agent approved (gadofosveset, Ablavar/Vasovist, MS-325), it is no longer marketed.[10,11] Gadofosveset was a derivative of Gd-DTPA that bound reversibly to serum albumin. Albumin is the most abundant protein in plasma, and its concentration is high enough (600–700 μM) to reversibly bind most of the gadofosveset after injection. Reversible albumin binding serves four purposes: (1) the albumin slows the leakage of the contrast agent out of the intravascular space; (2) the reversible binding still allows a path for excretion—the unbound fraction can be filtered through the kidneys or taken up by hepatocytes; (3) the bound fraction is "hidden" from the liver and kidneys, leading to an extended plasma half-life; and (4) the relaxivity of the contrast agent is increased fourfold to 10-fold on binding to albumin (discussed later).[12,13] Gd-BOPTA (gadobenate; see Fig. 2.3) has weak affinity for albumin (~10% bound), which leads to a modest increase in relaxivity relative to other ECF agents.[14,15] Other approaches to blood pool agents have involved making molecules that were too large to rapidly cross the endothelial wall but were still small enough to be filtered by the kidneys. Gadomer and Vistarem were examples of this approach that advanced to clinical trials but which were ultimately abandoned.[16,17]

Currently, the only blood pool agent available is ferumoxytol (Feraheme), which is an ultrasmall superparamagnetic particle of iron oxide (USPIO). Ferumoxytol particles are very large (10–30 nm), but still small enough to evade substantial capture by the reticuloendothelial system, and have a long blood residency time.[18] Such particles also have strong r_1 relaxivity, especially at lower field strengths. Ferumoxytol (Feraheme) is a carboxymethyldextran-coated USPIO that is approved as an intravenous iron replacement therapy.[19] Ferumoxytol has been used off-label as a blood pool agent and has seen some use in pediatric CMR owing to its long circulating blood half-life, which facilitates high-resolution imaging and obviates the need for timing of boluses.[20,21] Ferumoxytol must be administered as an infusion, and there is an FDA boxed warning about its safety, especially if administered too quickly. Ferumoxytol can also be used to image monocytes and macrophages on delayed phase imaging (next day), as accumulation in the reticuloendothelial system is the ultimate fate of these particles.[22,23] The iron oxide particles are not excreted; the iron is eventually resorbed into the body.

RELAXIVITY

Because their effect is indirect, CMR contrast agents differ from other diagnostic imaging agents. Water and fat are imaged, and it is the action of the contrast agent on the relaxation properties of the water hydrogen nuclei that generates contrast; in x-ray contrast media and nuclear imaging agents, the observed effect is more direct. Because water is present at a very high concentration (55,000 mM) and the contrast agent is typically at a much lower concentration (0.1–1 mM), the contrast agent must act catalytically to relax the water protons for there to be a measurable effect. Relaxivity (r_1 and r_2) thus describes this catalytic efficiency. Some compounds are better magnetic catalysts than others (have higher relaxivity). Moreover, relaxivity is dependent on the external magnetic field, B_0. This section explains these differences and the molecular basis for them. For discrete ions, such as Gd(III) and manganese (Mn[II]), the factors influencing relaxivity are the same; for iron oxide particles, the relaxation mechanism is different and will be treated separately.

Relaxivity can be factored into inner- and outer-sphere terms. "Inner sphere"

$$r_1 = \frac{\Delta(1/T_1)}{[\mathrm{Gd}]} = r_1^{\mathrm{IS}} + r_1^{\mathrm{OS}} \qquad \text{Eq. 2.3}$$

refers to the relaxation enhancement because of the exchangeable waters in the inner sphere. "Outer sphere" refers to relaxivity resulting from water in the second and outer-coordination spheres. This separation is often used because the inner-sphere component is easier to understand from a theoretical framework and the effect of changing specific molecular parameters on relaxivity can be tested. For ECF agents, the inner-sphere and outer-sphere contribution to relaxivity is about the same, whereas for newer, high-relaxivity contrast agents, the inner-sphere component accounts for the majority of overall relaxivity.

$$r_1^{\mathrm{IS}} = \frac{q/[H_2O]}{T_{1m} + \tau_m} \qquad \text{Eq. 2.4}$$

Inner-sphere relaxivity is given by Eq. (2.4), where q represents the number of water molecules bound to the metal ion (typically $q = 1$), $[H_2O]$ is the water concentration in millimolar, T_{1m} is the relaxation time of the water that is bound to the metal ion, and τ_m is the lifetime of the water molecule in the inner sphere. Eq. (2.4) shows that the more sites available for water to bind (q), the more efficient the process. Likewise, the T1 of the bound water (T_{1m}) should be very short. This is indicative of how effectively the metal ion can relax the coordinated water. The lifetime τ_m of the bound water is the inverse of the water exchange rate ($k_{ex} = 1/\tau_m$). If turnover is slow (τ_m is long), then it will not matter how efficiently the bound water is relaxed if this relaxation cannot be transmitted to the bulk water.

Paramagnetic relaxation ($1/T_{1m}$) occurs via a dipolar mechanism. At a magnetic field encountered in medical imaging, $1/T_{1m}$ is shown in Eq. (2.5), where C is a constant,

$$\frac{1}{T_{1m}} = C\frac{S(S+1)}{r_{\mathrm{MH}}^6}\left[\frac{3\tau_c}{1+\omega_H^2\tau_c^2}\right] \qquad \text{Eq. 2.5}$$

S is the spin quantum number, r_{MH} is the metal ion-to-proton distance, τ_c is the correlation time, and ω_H is the hydrogen Larmor frequency.[6] The product $S(S+1)$ is proportional to the magnetic moment. All other factors being equal, the higher the magnetic moment, the more efficient the relaxation. This is why Gd^{3+} ($S = 7/2$) is preferred to copper (Cu^{2+}, $S = 1/2$) because the $S(S+1)$ term is 9 times higher. The dipolar effect depends on the distance between the ion and the hydrogen nucleus (r_{MH}) to the inverse sixth power. The inner-sphere water is critical; it has the shortest metal-to-hydrogen distance of water hydrating the metal complex. The Mn^{2+} ion ($S = 5/2$) has a smaller magnetic moment

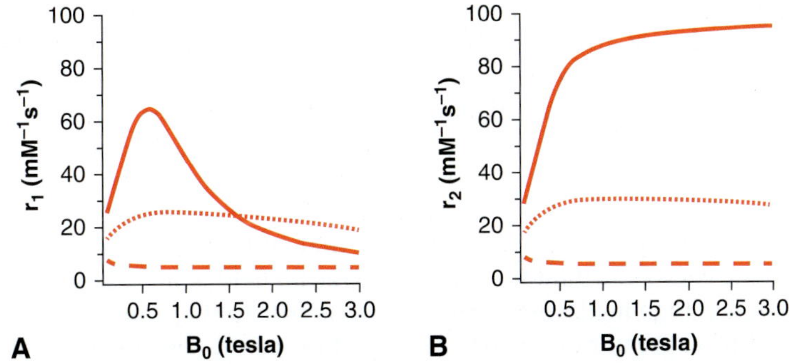

FIG. 2.4 Effect of rotational correlation time on longitudinal (r_1, A) and transverse (r_2, B) relaxivities as a function of field strength. Long correlation time (τ_R = 10 ns, *solid line*), typical of albumin binding, gives high r_1 that decreases with increasing field and high r_2; intermediate correlation time (τ_R = 1 ns, *short dashed line*) shows relaxivity maximum pushed out to a higher field; short correlation time (τ_R = 0.1 ns, *long dashed line*), typical of extracellular fluid agents, shows low, roughly field-independent r_1, r_2. Simulations with other parameters typical of gadolinium-based agents.

than Gd^{3+}, but the distance from the Mn^{2+} to the water hydrogen atom is shorter than for Gd^{3+} complexes, which enables Mn^{2+} complexes to have similar or even higher relaxivity than Gd^{3+} complexes.[24,25]

The correlation time, τ_c, is the time constant that governs the interaction between the electron spin of the ion and the nuclear spin of the hydrogen. Depending on the ion and the field strength, the correlation time is either the time constant for rotational diffusion of the molecule, τ_R, or the electronic T1 of the metal ion, T_{1e}. In the MR experiment, nuclei are excited by applying RF energy at the Larmor frequency. To relax these nuclei, there needs to be a resonant source for energy transfer. A paramagnetic molecule tumbling in solution creates a fluctuating magnetic field. Molecules tumble (undergo rotational diffusion) because of thermal energy; however, because they also collide with each other, there is a distribution of rotational diffusion rates, with a mean rate characterized by $1/\tau_R$. The closer this tumbling rate is to the Larmor frequency, the more efficient the relaxation by the contrast agent.

Small molecules such as gadopentetate tumble very fast, in the gigahertz range (1 GHz = 1000 MHz), but the Larmor frequency for protons at imaging fields is much slower. For example, at 1.5 T, the Larmor frequency is approximately 65 MHz, so relaxation is not as efficient as it could be. Larger molecules, such as proteins, tumble much more slowly. When contrast agents are made to tumble more slowly, relaxivity is increased. One way to increase relaxivity is to bind noncovalently to a protein target where the relaxivity would be increased on binding because the contrast agent would take on the rotational characteristics of the protein. An example of this is with gadobenate, for which the relaxivity measured at 37°C in water at 1.5 T is 4.0, but increases over 50% to 6.3 $mM^{-1}s^{-1}$ when measured in blood plasma under the same conditions.[26] Gadobenate binds weakly to serum albumin, with about 10% bound after administration, but the relaxivity of the albumin-bound form is so high that it raises the measured relaxivity. Increasing the molecular size is another way to increase relaxivity. Gadoquatrane is a tetramer of 4 Gd chelates (Fig. 2.3), and this increased size results in slower motion and higher relaxivity. For example, the relaxivity per Gd^{3+} ion in gadoquatrane is about 3 times higher than that of gadoteridol, which is solely due to the larger size of the gadoquatrane molecule.[27] On a *molecular* basis the relaxivity of gadoquatrane is 4 times higher still because the molecule contains 4 Gd^{3+} ions. A benefit of this high relaxivity is that gadoquatrane can be formulated at isotonic osmolality.

Gadopiclenol has higher relaxivity compared to most GBCAs because of two design features. First, unlike other GBCAs, there are two water molecules, which double the inner-sphere relaxation effect compared to other agents. Equally important are the three "arms" of the molecule that bear OH groups, which serve to slow down the molecular tumbling of the complex and enhance relaxivity further.[28]

Electrons undergoing relaxation in a paramagnetic ion also generate a fluctuating field that can cause nuclear relaxation. It is the faster of the two processes (rotation or electronic relaxation) that define how efficiently the hydrogen is relaxed. For Gd and Mn complexes, electronic relaxation depends on the applied field, and it gets slower as the magnetic field is increased. At low fields (<0.5 T), electronic relaxation governs hydrogen relaxation, whereas at higher fields, rotational diffusion is the dominant mechanism. Gd^{3+} and Mn^{2+} have symmetrical electronic configurations (half-filled *f* and *d* shells, respectively), and as a result, electronic relaxation is relatively slow. Other ions, such as dysprosium (Dy^{3+}), have a higher magnetic moment, but are rather poor relaxors because electronic relaxation is so fast.

Eq. (2.5) also indicates that at higher magnetic fields, the T1 relaxation mechanism becomes less efficient as $\omega_H^2\tau_c^2 > 1$. The magnetic field at which this condition is met is dependent on the magnitude of the correlation time. This is exemplified by gadobenate. The relaxivity of gadobenate is 4.2, 4.0, 4.0, and 4.0 $mM^{-1}s^{-1}$ when measured in water at 0.47, 1.5, 3, and 4.7 T, respectively.[26] The lack of field dependence on relaxivity for gadobenate in water indicates that $\omega_H^2\tau_c^2 < 1$. As mentioned above, the relaxivity of gadobenate is increased in plasma because of transient binding to serum albumin. The albumin binding effect is more pronounced at lower fields and then disperses as $\omega_H^2\tau_c^2$ becomes greater than 1. The relaxivity of gadobenate in plasma is 9.2, 6.3, 5.5, and 5.2 at 0.47, 1.5, 3, and 4.7 T, respectively.[26] Fig. 2.4 further illustrates the effects of correlation time and field strength on relaxivity. In Fig. 2.4, r_1 and r_2 are simulated over a range of fields encountered in CMR for correlation times of 0.1 ns (typical of ECF agents), 1 ns (intermediate motion), and 10 ns (typical of albumin-bound agents). Fig. 2.4 shows that the benefits of very slow rotation are seen at lower field strengths. Note also that r_1 does not go to zero because there is also an outer-sphere component to relaxivity,[12] and the correlation times that govern outer-sphere relaxivity are quite short.[6] Transverse relaxivity is defined by equations similar to Eqs. (2.4) and (2.5), with the exception that there are other mechanisms causing r_2 to increase at high fields.[6,29,30] The r_2 is always greater than r_1, and for very slow-tumbling systems, the r_2/r_1 ratio becomes large at high fields. Electronic and nuclear relaxation is described in greater detail in various reviews and books.[6,8,31]

Fig. 2.4 suggests that slow-tumbling T1 agents become less effective at high fields, but relaxation times for tissue are longer at high fields and the signal-to-noise ratio (SNR) increases with increased field strength (B_0). These factors and the choice of sequence mean that a contrast agent with a lower relaxivity at 3T than at 1.5T may still provide greater contrast at 3T than at 1.5T.

Iron oxide–based contrast agents are not discrete molecules, but crystals of iron oxide (Fe_3O_4) surrounded by a coating. The individual spins of each iron cooperatively, via quantum mechanical interactions, build up to give the crystal a very large total spin, and thus relaxivity is a function of the number of spins. Such a material is called "ferromagnetic," and its magnetism persists outside the external magnetic field. A weaker form of this is superparamagnetism, in which small particles of iron oxides with aligned spins occur in a magnetic field. Because the particles are small (submicron), the magnetic susceptibility effect is smaller than for large crystals of ferrites. Superparamagnets are no longer magnetic outside of the external field.

Iron oxide particles consist of a core of one or more magnetic crystals of Fe_3O_4 embedded in a coating. Because these are materials rather than discrete molecular entities, there is a distribution of sizes. USPIOs have a single crystal core and a submicron diameter. SPIOs have cores containing more than one crystal of Fe_3O_4 and are larger than USPIOs, but are still submicron in size. USPIOs and SPIOs are small enough to form a stable suspension and can be administered intravenously. The difference in particle size determines their pharmacokinetic behavior. There are no inner-sphere water molecules in iron particles, and relaxation of water arises from the water molecules diffusing near the particle. However, the mechanism of outer-sphere relaxation differs from that described earlier. One feature is that the crystals have a net magnetization, and as the external field is increased, this magnetization is increased (as is true for Gd, but the effect is much smaller). The modulation of this net magnetization can cause proton relaxation and have field dependence.[32]

There are some generalities about relaxivity in these particles. For USPIOs, longitudinal relaxivity (r_1) can be quite high, and these can function as effective T1 agents. The r_2/r_1 ratio for USPIOs is significantly larger than for Gd complexes, and r_2 increases with increasing magnetic field. When there is aggregation of crystals, which is the case in SPIOs, r_1 tends to decrease and r_2 increases. Thus, for the particles themselves, as well as for aggregates of particles, the ratio of r_2/r_1 typically increases as the size of the particles or aggregates increases, although the T2 relaxivity as a function of particle size can be quite complicated. The effect of aggregation of crystals is that the aggregate itself can be considered a large, magnetized sphere whose magnetic moment increases with increasing field strength. This gives rise to susceptibility effects, and SPIOs can act as T2* relaxation agents. This has important consequences when considering the effects of contrast agent compartmentalization on imaging (discussed later).

Table 2.2 gives r_1 and r_2 values in plasma at 1.5 and 3T for a range of contrast media. The ECF agents have a slightly lower r_1 at 3T and low r_2/r_1 ratios. Weak albumin binders have higher relaxivities, and slower tumbling Gd compounds, such as gadoquatrane or gadopiclenol (which also benefits from two inner-sphere water molecules), have several-fold higher relaxivities than ECF agents. As Fig. 2.4 suggests, the slow-tumbling compounds also have significantly lower r_1 at 3T than at 1.5T and the r_2/r_1 ratio

TABLE 2.2 Approved[a] (October 2024) magnetic resonance imaging contrast agents—relaxivity properties measured in human plasma.

GENERIC NAME	PRODUCT NAME	CHEMICAL ABBREVIATION	R_1 1.5T ($mM^{-1}S^{-1}$)	R_2 1.5T ($mM^{-1}S^{-1}$)	R_1 3T ($mM^{-1}S^{-1}$)	R_2 3T ($mM^{-1}S^{-1}$)
Gadopentetate	Magnevist	Gd-DTPA	4.1	4.6	3.7	5.2
Gadoterate	Dotarem Clariscan	Gd-DOTA	3.6	4.3	3.5	4.9
Gadodiamide	Omniscan	Gd-DTPA-BMA	4.3	5.2	4.0	5.6
Gadoteridol	Prohance	Gd-HPDO3A	4.1	5.0	3.7	5.7
Gadobenate	Multihance	Gd-BOPTA	6.3	8.7	5.5	11.0
Gadobutrol	Gadovist	Gd-DO3A-butrol	5.2	6.1	5.0	7.1
Gadopiclenol	Elucirem Vueway	P03277	12.8	15.1	11.6	14.7
Gadoxetate	Eovist Primovist	Gd-EOB-DTPA	6.9	8.7	6.2	11.0
Gadoquatrane		BAY 1747846	11.8	NA	10.5	NA
Ferumoxytol	Feraheme		19.0	64.9	9.5	65.2

[a]As of writing, gadoquatrane had completed clinical trial enrollment but was not yet approved for use. Relaxivities taken from Rohrer et al.[26] except gadopiclenol,[28] gadoquatrane,[27] and ferumoxytol.[33]

is increased at 3 T. Ferumoxytol has good T1 relaxivity at 1.5 T, but at 3 T, the transverse relaxivity starts to dominate.

CONTRAST-ENHANCED TISSUE RELAXATION

The extent to which a metal complex influences tissue relaxation rates depends on three factors.

1. The chemical environment encountered by the metal complex. Binding of the agent to macromolecules can cause significant relaxivity enhancement, as was discussed for gadobenate above.
2. Compartmentalization of the metal complex in tissue. Generally, tissue water is compartmentalized into intravascular, interstitial (fluid space between cells and capillaries), and intracellular space, constituting roughly 5%, 15%, and 80% of total water, respectively. Cellular organelles further subdivide the intracellular component. If water exchange between any of these compartments is slow relative to the relaxation rate in the compartment with the longest T_1, multiexponential relaxation may result. This can decrease the effective tissue relaxivity of an agent because not all of the tissue water is encountering the paramagnetic center.
3. The magnetic susceptibility of the contrast agent. The contrast agent causes a microscopic field inhomogeneity on a biologic scale of 10 to 1000 nm rather than on the chemical scale of 0.1 to 1 nm. This results in a reduction in apparent T2 (i.e., in T2*).

The result of the first two effects is that the simple relaxivity equation (Eq. 2.1) is often not valid in a biologic setting; likewise, describing the effects on a CMR pulse sequence with a single tissue relaxivity can be misleading. Care must be taken when trying to estimate the concentration of a contrast agent from signal intensity changes.

The actual relaxivity within a compartment might be affected by the biologic milieu. For some compounds with strong or weak albumin binding (e.g., gadofosveset or gadobenate), local variation in the albumin concentration will affect the amount of contrast agent bound to albumin and thus affect the overall relaxivity. For example, in the plasma space, the albumin concentration is typically high (0.6–0.7 mM) compared with the extracellular space in the normal heart (0.2–0.3 mM).

ECF agents interact very weakly if at all with plasma proteins and membrane structures. Tweedle, Wedeking, and colleagues showed that the relaxivity in blood and soft tissue of gadopentetate and gadoterate is the same as the relaxivity in aqueous solution.[34,35] In extreme settings, the actual relaxivity could vary.[36,37] Except for pathologic situations, most CMR contrast agents in use today are excluded from intact cells. Thus, the contrast agent will be localized to the *extracellular* space. As a result, the simple relaxivity equations do not necessarily hold. For a Gd-based ECF agent in a test tube, it takes approximately 3 μs for water to diffuse between Gd molecules; in the time of a typical imaging repetition time (TR), a given water molecule may interact with thousands or millions of Gd molecules, and all water molecules will interact with approximately the same number of Gd ions.[38] However, if that same ECF agent is compartmentalized solely within the cardiac microvasculature, it takes between 2 and 20 seconds for most of the water in the tissue (85% of it is extravascular) to physically diffuse into the microvasculature; most of the water in the tissue does not have the opportunity to be relaxed by the Gd within the TR of an imaging acquisition, resulting in a lower signal enhancement than that predicted by Eq. (2.1), assuming a uniform distribution of contrast agent throughout the tissue.

To deal with compartmentalization, the concepts of "water exchange" and "exchange time" (τ) between compartments are often used.[39,40] The water exchange rate and the size of the compartments will determine the effect of the contrast agent on the CMR signal. To illustrate this phenomenon, the two limiting causes of exchange will be described.[38,39] In one extreme, water moves so quickly between the biologic compartments that the net effect is as if the contrast agent were uniformly spread throughout the entire tissue. This situation, called "fast exchange," occurs whenever the exchange rate (1/τ) between the compartments is much faster than the difference in relaxation rates between the compartments.[41] This occurs in blood, where red cells have a short water exchange time, on the order of 5 to 10 ms.[42] An intact red blood cell prevents most CMR contrast agents from entering the cell, but as long as the plasma T1 is longer than 20 ms, the two compartments of the blood (plasma + red cells) are in fast exchange and blood behaves, for CMR purposes, as if the contrast agent were spread uniformly throughout the blood. In this case, the effective relaxation rate will be the weighted average of the relaxation in the two compartments. That is, if for compartment *i* the volume fraction is f_i, the initial T1 is $T1_i$, and the concentration of agent is C_i (which could be zero), the entire tissue together will behave as shown:

$$\frac{1}{T1} = f_1\left(\frac{1}{T1_1} + r_1C_1\right) + f_2 \qquad \text{Eq. 2.6}$$

In "slow exchange," the water exchange rate is much slower than the difference in relaxation rates between the compartments. In this case, a single relaxation time, and thus a single relaxivity, is meaningless because the two microscopic compartments will relax with their own relaxation times. Very few biologic compartments show true slow exchange, whereas the intermediate case, when exchange is neither slow nor fast ("intermediate exchange"), occurs very commonly. With intermediate exchange, relaxation behavior appears biexponential, although both the apparent compartment size and the effective T1 of the two compartments will vary from their true biologic size and T1. It is possible to model the signal intensity behavior as a function of contrast agent concentration to estimate water exchange times in vivo. Although characterizing human tissue as having only one or two compartments is an oversimplification, these types of models have proved useful for explaining the effects of biologic water mobility on contrast-enhanced scans.[43]

Biologic compartmentalization also results in susceptibility contrast. The contrast agent causes microscopic field inhomogeneities, sometimes called "mesoscopic" inhomogeneities.[44] Water diffusion causes the protons to dephase from one another because of the different magnetic fields that they experience. Even in the absence of water diffusion, the field inhomogeneity causes intravoxel dephasing and thus signal loss on GRE images because of the different microscopic magnetic fields within the voxel. The strength of the perturbing magnetic field is directly proportional to the contrast agent concentration and its molar magnetic susceptibility (χ). The actual magnitude and even the direction of the magnetic field shifts depend strongly on the size and shape of the biologic compartment in which the contrast agent resides; the size of the susceptibility contrast effect depends on how the water diffuses through the tissue.[44]

NOVEL CONTRAST AGENTS IN DEVELOPMENT

Although the current approved contrast agents are all based on gadolinium, there has been effort in recent years to develop ECF and other agents that utilize an essential element like iron or manganese instead of gadolinium to enhance the signal. This move has been prompted by safety concerns around nephrogenic systemic fibrosis and retention of gadolinium in the brain and body. RVP-001 (Mn-PyC3A, Fig. 2.5) is a small Mn-based chelate designed as a replacement for GBCAs.[45] RVP-001 has a similar relaxivity to GBCAs like gadopentetate and gadoterate and is eliminated unchanged from the body.[45–48] RVP-001 was shown to provide equivalent MR contrast to GBCAs in different animal models. Fig. 2.6 shows CMR applications of RVP-001 in large animal models.[45–49] Fig. 2.6A–C shows that MRA with RVP-001 performed in baboons at 3 T provided equivalent arterial contrast to gadopentetate administered at the same dose. Fig. 2.6D–F shows that RVP-001 provided equivalent delayed enhancement to gadoterate in a pig model of myocardial infarction and that the scar volume measured with RVP-001–enhanced MR was the same as that measured using gadoterate in the same animal. RVP-001 is currently (October 2024) being investigated in clinical trials (NCT05413668 and NCT06322342).

Mangafodipir (MnDPDP, Fig. 2.5) is a manganese-based contrast agent that was approved for liver and pancreas imaging. Mangafodipir acts as a prodrug and releases a free Mn^{2+} ion, which is rapidly taken up by transporters in

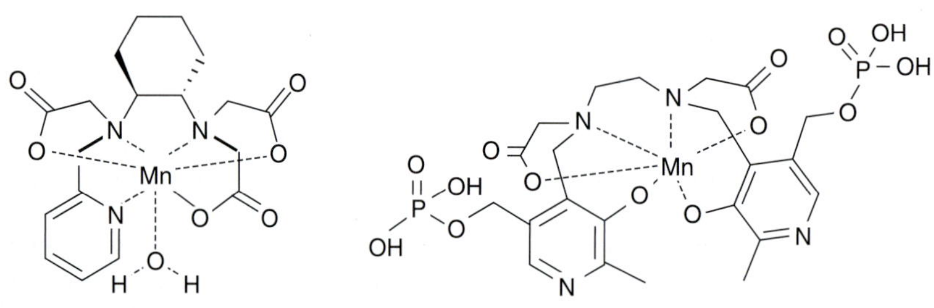

FIG. 2.5 Manganese-based contrast agents RVP-001 (Mn-PyC3A) and mangafodipir (MnDPDP).

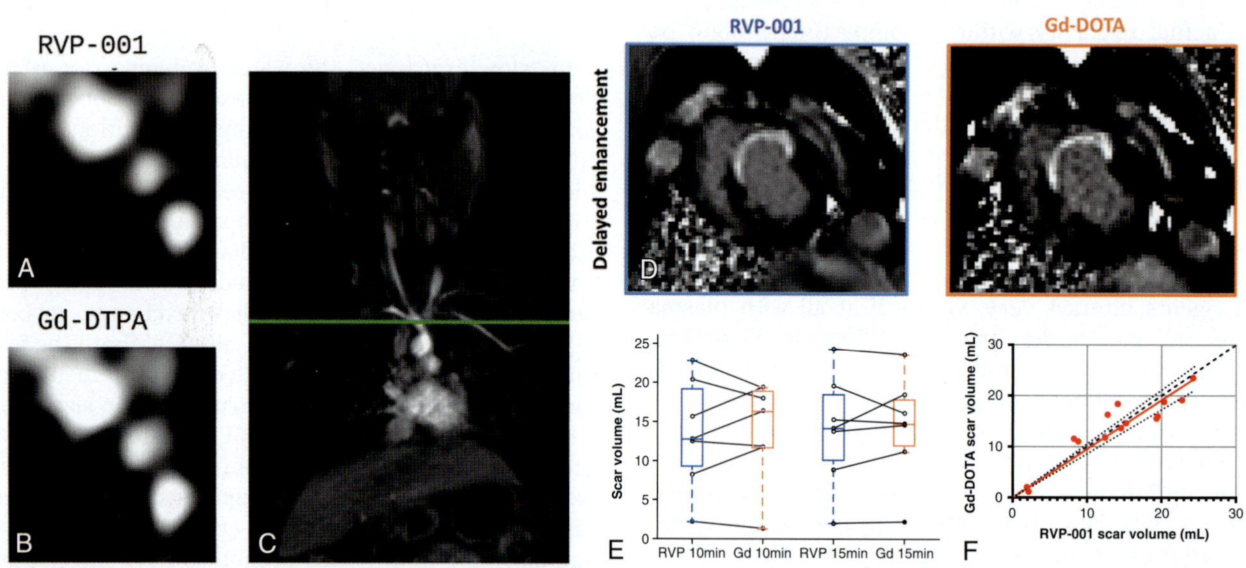

FIG. 2.6 Axial T1-weighted images of branch arteries of the thoracic aorta of baboons acquired 9 seconds after bolus intravenous administration of 0.1 mmol/kg RVP-001 (A) or gadopentetate (Gd-DTPA) (B) show similar enhancement in arterial contrast between the two agents. The *green line* in the coronal image in panel (C) shows the level at which the axial images were acquired. (D) Short-axis, delayed enhancement magnetic resonance (MR) images of the heart of a pig that underwent ischemia reperfusion injury of the left anterior descending coronary artery. Delayed RVP-001 image on left and late gadolinium (gadoterate [Gd-DOTA]) enhanced image on the right. (E) Paired box-and-whisker plots of gross lesion volume, as measured by RVP-001 (*blue*) and Gd-DOTA (*orange*). (F) Correlation plot of the myocardial scar volumes measured by RVP-001–enhanced MR (x axis) and those measured by Gd-DOTA (y axis). The *solid red line* represents linear regression and the *dotted black lines* represent the 95% confidence bands of the regression; identity line is *dashed black line*. (Adapted from Gale EM, Wey HY, Ramsay I, et al. A manganese-based alternative to gadolinium: contrast-enhanced mr angiography, excretion, pharmacokinetics, and metabolism. *Radiology*. 2018;286(3):865–872. Bonner BP, Yurista SR, Coll-Font J, et al. contrast-enhanced cardiac magnetic resonance imaging with a manganese-based alternative to gadolinium for tissue characterization of acute myocardial infarction. *J Am Heart Assoc*. 2023;12(8):e026923.)

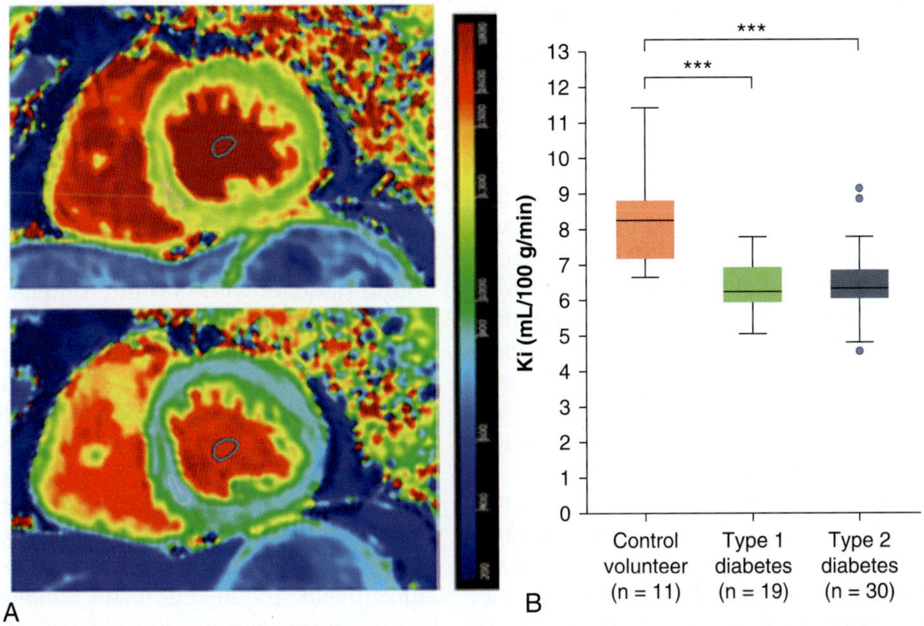

FIG. 2.7 Mangafodipir-enhanced cardiovascular magnetic resonance in type 1 and type 2 diabetes. (A) T1 maps of the myocardium and blood pool in a control and diabetic subject. (B) Kinetic modeling to assess manganese uptake rates (*Ki*) revealed that people with type 1 and type 2 diabetes had lower manganese uptake compared with healthy volunteers. ****P*<.001. (Adapted from Dattani A, Joshi S, Yeo JL, et al. Impaired myocardial calcium uptake in patients with diabetes mellitus: a manganese-enhanced cardiac magnetic resonance study. *JACC Cardiovasc Imaging*. 2023;16(12):1623–1625.)

the liver and pancreas, resulting in strong T1 contrast.[50] The Mn^{2+} ion is also taken up via Ca^{2+} channels on cardiomyocytes and mangafodipir-enhanced CMR has been used to assess cardiac function.[51–53] Mn^{2+} cardiac uptake is determined by both the delivery of Mn^{2+} to the myocardium (blood flow) and the amount that is taken up into the intercellular space via Ca^{2+} channels (function). Kinetic modeling of the signal versus time curve allows quantitative assessment of function using the Mn^{2+} influx constant Ki.[54] Fig. 2.7 shows an example of mangafodipir CMR being applied to patients with type I or type II diabetes.[55] The authors observed striking reductions in myocardial calcium (Mn^{2+}) uptake in people with diabetes who had no prevalent cardiac disease and in the absence of any apparent left ventricular systolic or diastolic dysfunction. While mangafodipir is no longer being marketed by its original sponsor, a new company, IC Targets AS, is working to make mangafodipir commercially available again.

Molecular imaging has been defined as "the in vivo characterization and measurement of biological processes at the cellular and molecular level."[56] Combining the high-resolution anatomic and functional imaging ability of CMR with the specificity of molecular targeting is very appealing, but somewhat limited by the inherent sensitivity limitations of CMR. Examples of molecular CMR contrast agents used for cardiovascular applications are numerous. The vast majority of these agents have only been studied in animal models. A few examples are described here.

An early example of a molecularly targeted contrast agent that advanced into clinical development was EP-2104R, which targeted fibrin, an abundant component of thrombus. EP-2104R was a peptide sequence specific for fibrin that was conjugated to four Gd-DOTA chelates.[57] EP-2104R was shown to positively enhance thrombus visualization in animal models of atherosclerotic plaque rupture and carotid artery thrombus, and in embolic models of thrombus in the coronary arteries, left atrium, lung, and stroke.[58–65] EP-2104R uptake was shown to correlate with fibrin content in a murine model of venous thrombosis.[66] This contrast agent has also been shown to visualize arterial, venous, and cardiac thrombus in human subjects, one of the first examples of clinical translation of a molecular MR probe.[67,68]

Molecular MR imaging requires targets that are highly abundant, like fibrin, typically with micromolar concentrations for detection. Another protein that has been successfully imaged with molecular MR is type I collagen, which is highly abundant in fibrotic tissue. EP-3533 is a type I–specific peptide conjugated to three Gd-DTPA chelates for signal enhancement.[69] This probe has been used to show specific in vivo molecular imaging of fibrosis in a mouse model of healed postinfarction myocardial scarring.[70] Because the extracellular matrix of the heart is very rich in collagen, a similar compound was used to assess myocardial perfusion in a pig model of coronary artery stenosis. Collagen binding served to retain the probe in the myocardial extracellular matrix for extended periods such that a delayed, high-resolution, steady-state image of the heart could be obtained that reflected the initial perfusion of the contrast agent.[71] EP-3533 has also been used to quantify diffuse myocardial and skeletal muscle fibrosis in a mouse model of Duchenne muscular dystrophy.[72] Recently, a peptide-based probe targeting type III collagen was reported and shown to be more selective for the detection of fibrogenesis in a mouse model of myocardial infarction wherein higher uptake was seen at 10 days post myocardial infarction (MI) compared to imaging 21 days postMI. Collagen oxidized by the lysyl oxidase enzyme has been shown to be a marker of fibrogenesis, and recent work has shown that oxidized collagen can be imaged with a molecular MR probe in the myocardium of mice with diffuse fibrosis.[73–77]

An agent that targets elastin has also been developed. Elastin levels are largely increased following injury to load-bearing tissues. Elastin content in injury or healing cardiovascular tissue is a sufficiently abundant biomarker for monitoring tissue remodeling. The elastin-specific magnetic resonance contrast agent Gd-ESMA targets elastin with high affinity and specificity.[78] Gd-ESMA was used to visualize rupture of the aortal elastic lamina and monitor the compensatory increase in elastin content of the dilated vessel over the course of weeks in a mouse model of aortic abdominal aneurysm.[79] Gd-ESMA has also been used to visualize the vascular remodeling process at the site of disrupted plaques in a rabbit model of atherosclerosis.[80] Changing elastin content postmyocardial infarction in both the infarcted and remote myocardium has serially monitored Gd-ESMA out to 3 weeks in a mouse model.[81] In another study, Gd-ESMA was used to quantify intrascar elastin out to 3 weeks following myocardial infarction in a mouse model.[82] Newer peptide-based probes targeting tropoelastin have also been reported as imaging biomarkers of atherosclerotic plaque instability.[83,84]

The preceding examples relied on targeting the contrast agent to a specific protein. Another mechanism to obtain molecular information is to design a probe sensitive to enzymatic activity. Ischemic injury of the myocardium causes timed recruitment of neutrophils and monocytes/macrophages, which produce substantial amounts of local myeloperoxidase (MPO). MPO forms reactive chlorinating species capable of inflicting oxidative stress and altering protein function by covalent modification. A series of Gd-based probes that are activated by MPO have been reported and contain a 5-hydroxytrypamide (5-HT) moiety conjugated to a Gd chelate.[85–87] In the presence of MPO, the 5-HT moiety is oxidized to a radical, which then either spontaneously oligomerizes or binds to matrix proteins, leading to enhanced spin-lattice relaxivity and delayed washout kinetics. These MPO-targeting probes have been used to noninvasively measure inflammatory responses after myocardial ischemia or stroke in murine models[88,89] and vascular inflammation in a murine model of Kawasaki disease and a rabbit model of aneurysm.[88–92] Using MPO knockout and heterozygous mice, differing degrees of contrast enhancement at the site of myocardial infarction could be seen, showing a clear correlation between infarct enhancement and local MPO activity.[89]

USPIOs passively accumulate in macrophages. This property has been exploited to provide negative contrast in macrophage-rich atherosclerotic plaques.[93] For macrophage uptake, imaging is typically performed 24h after administration to allow time for macrophage uptake to occur and also for the blood pool signal to diminish. Ferumoxytol has been shown to detect macrophages in the first 2 weeks following acute MI.[23] This CMR-detected ferumoxytol pattern of cellular inflammation was distinct and different from myocardial edema detected via T2 mapping, which persisted for a much longer period. On the other hand, delayed ferumoxytol CMR could not detect the presence of macrophages in patients with acute myocarditis, which may indicate that there is a threshold of macrophage-associated inflammation that must be reached before ferumoxytol is detectable by CMR.[94]

Iron oxides have also been used to label cells, and the cells then tracked in vivo using CMR.[95,96] Visualization of mesenchymal stem cells engrafted into the myocardium of a pig has been demonstrated at 1.5T.[97,98] Injection sites containing $>10^5$ cells could be detected in vivo.[97] MR tracking of USPIO-labeled, bone marrow–derived autologous mesenchymal stem cells (MSCs) after intramyocardial injection in patients with chronic ischemic heart disease was reported in a small cohort of patients. The treatment was safe, and cells were detectable at injection sites up to 14 days after transplantation.[99] Care must be taken in interpreting MRI data to track USPIO-labeled stem cells because the local presence of USPIO will void the MRI signal, regardless of cell viability. A recent study using MRI and histology to track the fate of USPIO-labeled mesenchymal stem cells implanted into infarcted myocardium provides a cautionary example. Four weeks after implantation of the labeled cells, the injection site remained hypointense but histologic analysis revealed very few viable stem cells. The USPIOs had accumulated in macrophages that infiltrated the injection site.[100]

Gadolinium-, manganese-, and iron oxide–based compounds all act as contrast agents. That is, they change the contrast in a proton MR image by changing the relaxation time of water in regions where the compound accumulates. These contrast agents are detected indirectly by their effect on the water proton MR signal. Water is detected because water is the most abundant source of protons in the body and MRI is a rather insensitive technique. It is possible to detect a probe directly, but actions must be taken to address the issue of sensitivity.

After hydrogen, the fluorine ^{19}F atom is the next most sensitive stable isotope for detection by MRI. Perfluorocarbons are inert polymers that have been used as blood substitutes. There are numerous examples of MRI applications involving perfluorocarbon nanoemulsions to deliver the very high concentration of ^{19}F atoms needed for detection by MRI. Perfluorocarbon nanoemulsions have been used to label cells for the purpose of cell tracking studies, and this technology has been applied to humans.[101–103]

Perfluorocarbon emulsions can also be derivatized with targeting vectors (e.g., peptides, antibodies) that result in binding of the emulsion to a molecular target; numerous examples have been reported.[104–110] Different perfluorocarbons can be used to form the emulsion, and these different perfluorocarbons have different ^{19}F chemical shifts.[111] Designing perfluorocarbon-based probes with differing chemical shifts offers the potential for multiplexing. An example of this is summarized in Fig. 2.8. The authors prepared a perfluorooctyl bromide (PFOB) emulsion derivatized with alpha-2-antiplasmin (α2AP) for targeting Factor 13a, termed $^{\alpha2AP}$PFOB, a perfluoro-1,3,5-trimethylcyclohexane (PFCH) emulsion derivatized with a peptide specific to fibrin, termed ^{fbn}PFCH, and a perfluorocrown ether emulsion (PFCE) that targeted cardiovascular inflammation.[112] The authors developed a multichemical shift-selective imaging sequence to specifically detect each probe based on its chemical shift (Fig. 2.8A). They showed that $^{\alpha2AP}$PFOB specifically labeled only newly formed

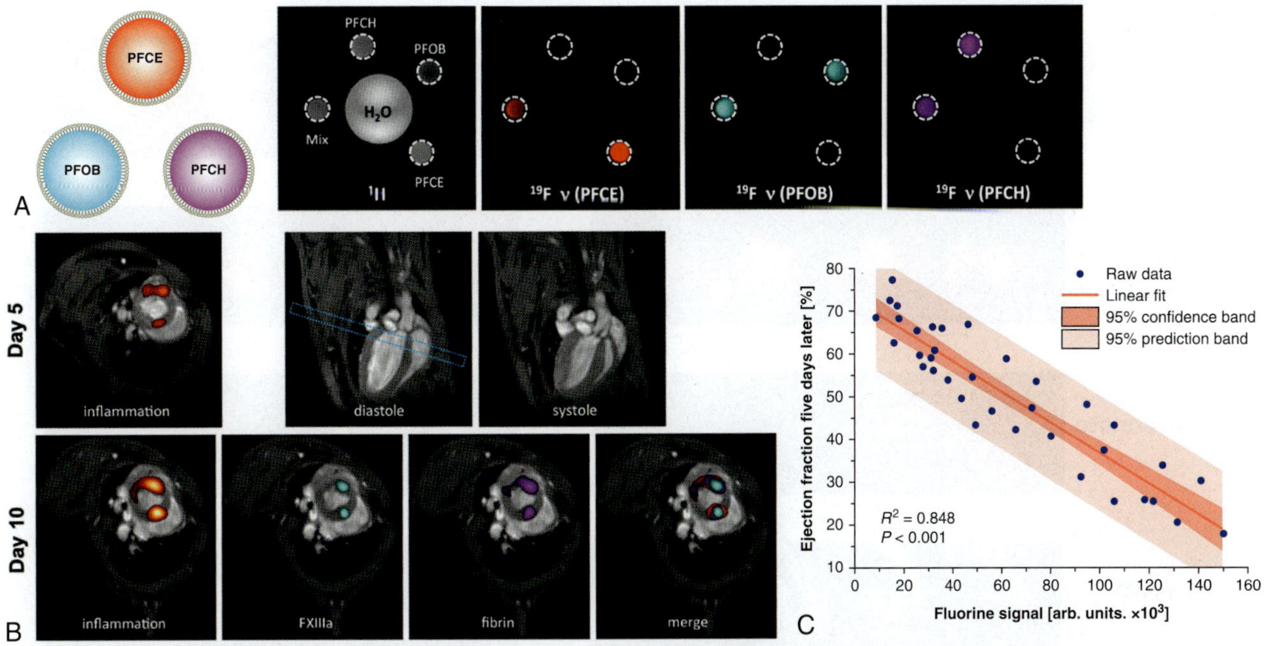

FIG. 2.8 (A) ^{19}F multichemical shift selective imaging of perfluorocrown ether emulsion (PFCE), perfluorooctyl bromide (PFOB), perfluoro-1,3, 5-trimethylcyclohexane (PFCH), and a mixture of all perfluorocarbons, showing the ability to spectrally discriminate each probe. (B) ^{19}F imaging of inflammation by PFCE (*red*), FXIIIa by PFOB (*cyan*), and fibrin by PFCH (*magenta*) in mice that received a special diet to induce myocardial infarction. (C) Linear correlation between detectable ^{19}F signal at day x and cardiac function at day x+5. (Adapted from Flogel U, Temme S, Jacoby C, et al. Multi-targeted (1)H/(19)F MRI unmasks specific danger patterns for emerging cardiovascular disorders. *Nat Commun*. 2021;12(1):5847.)

thrombi, while ^{fbn}PFCH bound to both newly formed and aged thrombi. They intravenously administered a mixture of PFCE/$^{\alpha 2AP}$PFOB/^{fbn}PFCH probes to a diet-induced mouse model of spontaneous myocardial infarction. As shown in Fig. 2.8B, at day 5 the only probe accumulating in the myocardium was the inflammation probe PFCE; upregulation of Factor 13a and fibrin occurred at day 10 as detected by $^{\alpha 2AP}$PFOB and ^{fbn}PFCH, respectively. Linear regression analysis showed that the in vivo ^{19}F signal linearly correlated with the change in cardiac function assessed 5 days after imaging (Fig. 2.8C), indicating that the multiplexed ^{19}F signal quantification can be used to predict further functional impairment.

Another way to overcome the poor sensitivity of direct detection probes is to use hyperpolarization. The lack of sensitivity in CMR stems from the very small degree of polarization among the nuclear spins. In a magnetic field there is a net magnetization, but it is small, and approximately 0.0006% of the spins are polarized. A technique called "spin exchange" uses a high-powered laser (also called "optical pumping") to increase the polarization by four to five orders of magnitude (hyperpolarization).[113] Other methods like parahydrogen hydrogenation are also being developed for this purpose.[113] Isotopes with long T1 values can be hyperpolarized and used as contrast agents. The long T1 is necessary to maintain the contrast medium in a hyperpolarized state long enough to obtain an image before the spins relax back to the equilibrium value.

For CMR, most work has been performed with hyperpolarized carbon C-13, most frequently with [1–^{13}C]-pyruvate, which can be produced on commercial devices.[114] Pyruvate is metabolized rapidly, and in addition to its distribution, one can also image the conversion of pyruvate to its metabolites alanine, lactate, and bicarbonate.[113] Rapid dynamic imaging enables the estimation of metabolic flux, and the ratios of metabolites formed provide information on the dominant metabolic pathway.[113] In the heart, the relative contribution of glucose oxidation and fatty acid oxidation to energy production are measured by pyruvate conversion to [1–^{13}C]-bicarbonate, which is catalyzed by pyruvate dehydrogenase, and conversion to [1–^{13}C]-lactate, which is catalyzed by lactate dehydrogenase. The difference between these two metabolic pathways can be nicely shown by chemical shift imaging of subjects who have fasted versus those who have been recently fed (Fig. 2.9). ^{13}C-bicarbonate, reflecting pyruvate dehydrogenase activity, was very low in the fasting state, and primarily localized to left ventricular (LV) myocardium in the fed state. Patient CMR imaging studies have shown decreased myocardial pyruvate dehydrogenase activity in patients who have received the cardiotoxin doxorubicin as part of cancer treatment.[116] In patients with type 2 diabetes, there is reduced pyruvate dehydrogenase activity and increased lactate dehydrogenase activity in the myocardium compared to healthy controls.[117] In addition to [1–^{13}C]-pyruvate, there have also been human studies performed with [2–^{13}C]-pyruvate and [^{13}C]-urea.[118,119]

A major benefit of hyperpolarized contrast media is the excellent sensitivity with no background (high SNR). Challenges include the distribution and availability of hyperpolarization equipment and imaging hardware compatibility for imaging nonhydrogen nuclei (not available on all clinical scanners). Because of the short times involved from hyperpolarization to administration, the hyperpolarized material must be prepared onsite. However, there are commercial polarizers available.

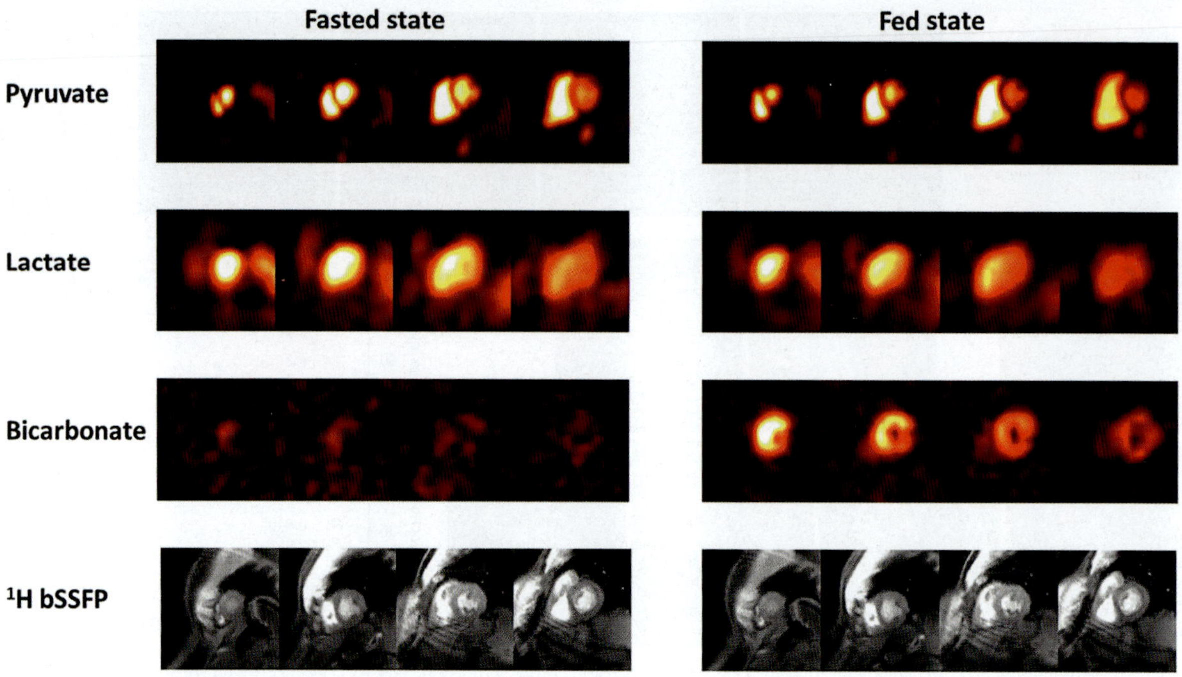

FIG. 2.9 Representative ^{13}C images of pyruvate, lactate, and bicarbonate in fasted and fed states with corresponding ^{1}H short-axis balanced steady state free procession (bSSFP) images in a healthy volunteer. The ^{13}C metabolite images (*raw*) are scaled identically across experiments and slices within each metabolite and clearly show the alteration in pyruvate metabolism within the heart. (Taken from Larson PEZ, Tang S, Liu X, et al. Regional quantification of cardiac metabolism with hyperpolarized [1-(13)C]-pyruvate CMR evaluated in an oral glucose challenge. *J Cardiovasc Magn Reson*. 2023;25(1):77.[115])

SAFETY

The safety of CMR contrast agents, which themselves offer no direct therapeutic benefit, is always a question of appropriate medical concern. Gd-based chelates were initially considered among the safest injectable compounds in medical use, with a specific reputation for superior safety in patients with renal dysfunction (compared with iodinated preparations used in fluoroscopy and CT). This view has changed with the apparent link between Gd contrast and nephrogenic systemic fibrosis (NSF).

A very rare but potentially devastating condition affecting patients with acute or chronic kidney disease, NSF has an estimated prevalence of >10% among patients receiving Gd who are on hemodialysis.[120,121] Although presenting primarily with skin thickening, tethering, hyperpigmentation, and disabling joint flexion contractures, patients with NSF can also have multiorgan/systemic fibrosis, leading to organ dysfunction and even death.[122,123] The universal feature of NSF is Gd administration and acute or chronic kidney disease, most commonly with an estimated glomerular filtration rate of <30 mL/min/1.73 m^2.[123–126] However, NSF-like symptoms have also been reported in patients with apparently normal renal function.[127,128] Gd has been shown to be present in skin biopsy specimens of patients with NSF,[129–132] and also in internal organs.[133] The prevailing hypothesis is that acute or chronic kidney disease results in prolonged exposure to the contrast agent, providing opportunity for the Gd to dissociate from its chelator, and this dissociated Gd is believed to be responsible for the toxic response.[121] The least stable and least kinetically inert (to Gd dissociation) contrast agent, gadodiamide, is the agent that has been most frequently associated with NSF,[134] but other Gd compounds also pose a risk.[10] All commercially available GBCAs now carry an FDA boxed warning about the risk of gadolinium (Gd) in renally impaired patients.[135]

Although ECF agents are similar in terms of their imaging efficacy, they differ in terms of how well they bind Gd. Metal complexes such as Gd contrast agents are characterized in terms of their thermodynamic stability and kinetic inertness. Stability is a measure of the affinity of a chelator for the metal ion and is expressed as an equilibrium constant for the association of the chelator (ligand) with the metal. Stability constants for approved agents have the order gadoterate > gadoteridol ~ gadobutrol ~ gadobenate ~ gadopentetate > gadodiamide.[6]

Stability constants describe equilibrium values, but do not indicate how quickly equilibrium is reached. In the biologic milieu, protons and other metal ions compete to bind the chelator ligand, whereas there are ions such as phosphate and carbonate that have a high affinity for Gd. Under conditions that favor dissociation of Gd (e.g., low pH), two complexes with comparable stability may have very different rates of dissociation. For example, the macrocyclic complex gadoteridol is a compound that is more kinetically inert to Gd loss than gadopentetate, which has a similar stability constant.[136] Laurent and colleagues measured the rate of Gd loss in the presence of zinc and phosphate under a standard set of conditions for various approved agents.[137] The macrocyclic complexes gadoterate, gadoteridol, and gadobutrol were the most inert with respect to Gd loss. Recent studies with gadopiclenol and gadoquatrane have shown that these agents are also both very inert.[27,28] The compound that released Gd the most rapidly was gadodiamide. These differences in kinetics and thermodynamic stabilities may well translate into safety with regard to patients with chronic kidney disease. For instance, there is a much lower incidence of NSF among patients who received macrocyclic GBCAs, which is likely related to increased kinetic inertness. Today, the linear agents gadodiamide, gadopentetate, and gadoversetamide are no longer available in Europe because regulators removed them from the market for safety reasons. Most radiology practices today use a macrocyclic contrast agent.

A series of studies published since 2013 have raised concerns over long-term Gd retention in the brain, bone, and skin of patients receiving multiple contrast agent-enhanced examinations, including patients with normal renal function. The observation that the dentate nucleus and globus pallidus appear hyperintense in contrast-free, T1-weighted scans of patients having received multiple prior contrast-enhanced scans suggested residual gadolinium accumulation in those regions of the brain.[138,139] Elemental analysis of autopsy specimens collected from patients receiving numerous injections of Gd-based contrast agents confirmed that there was measurable gadolinium in the brain, albeit at low levels.[140,141] The amount of central nervous system (CNS) Gd deposition may depend on the type of contrast agent received. CNS tissue enhancement by residual Gd appears to be greater after receiving multiple injections of Gd contrast with acyclic chelators.[140] This is evidenced by consistently hyperintense dentate nuclei in patients receiving multiple doses of Gd complexes with acyclic chelators, whereas the effect is not observed in patients exclusively receiving Gd complexes with macrocyclic chelators. Nonetheless, postmortem elemental analysis detects nonnegligible Gd levels in CNS tissue of patients receiving only macrocyclic agents, including healthy patients receiving a single dose in their lifetime, and imaging studies demonstrate retained Gd after high doses of macrocytic agents.[142,143] The same study found highly elevated Gd levels in the bone of all patients receiving both acyclic and macrocyclic agents; Gd retention in the skin was also observed.

The speciation of Gd retained in the skin, bone, and CNS remains largely underexplored (chelated vs. unchelated), as do the mechanisms by which Gd is accumulated and the corresponding health risks.[144,145] One study used chromatography coupled with elemental spectroscopy to evaluate Gd speciation in the skin of a patient with healthy kidney function who received 61 contrast-enhanced examinations over the course of 11 years. Speciation analysis revealed skin accumulation of intact gadopentetate and gadobenate as well as still uncharacterized Gd-containing species that likely exist in particulate form or are protein bound.[146] In 2015, the FDA announced a formal investigation into the safety risks of Gd retained in the CNS and subsequently recommended against the use of linear agents and issued a new class warning for all GBCAs. An analysis of data from the multinational multicenter European Society of Cardiovascular Radiology MR/CT Registry collected between January 2013 and October 2019 showed that the use of linear GBCAs in CMR had decreased to less than 1% of all GBCAs used; in other words, the field had completely adopted macrocyclic chelates in Europe.[147]

Regarding other side effects, Kirchin and Runge reviewed the safety record of clinically approved contrast agents as of 2003; gadopentetate, gadoterate, gadobenate, gadodiamide, gadoversetamide, gadobutrol, and gadoteridol appeared indistinguishable with respect to their safety profile.[148] The most common adverse events were headache, nausea, taste perversion, and urticaria (hives). Nearly all adverse events with these agents were transient, mild, and self-limiting. These findings were echoed in a 2018 meta-analysis of nine studies with a combined 716,978 administrations of GBCAs. The overall rate of patients who had immediate allergic-like reactions was 9.2 per 10,000 administrations. Severe immediate allergic-like reactions can occur, but are as rare as 0.52 per 10,000 administrations.[149] Interestingly, gadodiamide had the lowest rate of reactions at 1.5 per 10,000 administrations, which was significantly less than that of linear ionic GBCAs (e.g., gadopentetate) at 8.3 per 10,000 administrations and less than that for nonionic macrocyclic GBCAs at 16 per 10,000 administrations. GBCAs known to be associated with protein binding (e.g., gadobenate) had a higher rate of reactions, at 17 per 10,000 administrations. Prince reported that from 2004 to 2009, the FDA received reports on 40 gadolinium-based contrast agent US deaths unrelated to NSF, with an incidence per million doses of 0.15, 0.19, 0.97, 2.7, and 0.7 for gadodiamide, gadoversetamide, gadopentetate dimeglumine, gadobenate dimeglumine, and gadoteridol, respectively.[150] At the time of writing, very large studies with gadopiclenol have not yet been reported. Gd-based ECF contrast agents have been studied, and most are approved for pediatric use in patients older than 2 years, although there are differences in their approval wording. Gadobutrol and gadoterate are also approved for use in patients younger than 2 years of age in the United States.

The safety profile for current CMR contrast agents of course will not necessarily be the same for future compounds. For all contrast agents, the package insert should always be consulted for the latest safety information.

CONCLUSION

A large number of contrast agents have been approved for MRI in the last 36 years. A significant number of new agents, including gadolinium-free and tissue-specific agents that are potentially relevant for CMR, are currently in development. The behavior of these agents, which is often summarized by a single effectiveness parameter (r_1), is actually quite complex, in terms of both the underlying chemistry and the biophysics in vivo. Although many elements of that complexity remain active areas of research, both for understanding existing agents as well as for creating new agents and new uses for those agents, the relative safety and ease of use of these agents has brought them into routine use in many medical applications. As clinical CMR expands, no doubt the use of these contrast agents will expand as well, but CMR practitioners need to be cognizant of potential moderate-term complications, including NSF in patients with renal dysfunction. The long-term impact of Gd retention in the CNS and elsewhere remains uncertain.

REFERENCES

1. Bruder O, Wagner A, Lombardi M, et al. European cardiovascular magnetic resonance (EuroCMR) registry-multi national results from 57 centers in 15 countries. *J Cardiovasc Magn Reson*. 2013;15(1):9.
2. Norris EC, Schneider G, Clark TJ, et al. Efficacy of whole-blood model of gadolinium-based contrast agent relaxivity in predicting vascular MR signal intensity in vivo. *J Magn Reson Imaging*. 2024;60(2):615–627.
3. Bloch F, Hansen WW, Packard M. The nuclear induction experiment. *Phys Rev*. 1948;70:474–485.
4. Lauterbur PC, Mendonca Dias MH, Rudin AM. Augmentation of tissue water proton spin-lattice relaxation rates by in vivo addition of paramagnetic ions. In: Dutton PO, Leigh J, Scarpa A, eds. *Frontiers of Biological Energetics*. Academic Press; 1978:752–759.
5. Carr DH, Brown J, Bydder GM, et al. Intravenous chelated gadolinium as a contrast agent in NMR imaging of cerebral tumours. *Lancet*. 1984;1(8375):484–486.
6. Caravan P, Ellison JJ, McMurry TJ, Lauffer RB. Gadolinium(III) chelates as MRI contrast agents: structure, dynamics, and applications. *Chem Rev*. 1999;99(9):2293–2352.
7. Gries H. Extracellular MRI contrast agents based on gadolinium. *Top Curr Cehm*. 2002;221:1–24.
8. Wahsner J, Gale EM, Rodriguez-Rodriguez A, Caravan P. Chemistry of MRI contrast agents: current challenges and new frontiers. *Chem Rev*. 2019;119(2):957–1057.
9. Tombach B, Heindel W. Value of 1.0-M gadolinium chelates: review of preclinical and clinical data on gadobutrol. *Eur Radiol*. 2002;12(6):1550–1556.
10. Goyen M, Edelman M, Perreault P, et al. MR angiography of aortoiliac occlusive disease: a phase III study of the safety and effectiveness of the blood-pool contrast agent MS-325. *Radiology*. 2005;236(3):825–833.
11. Rapp JH, Wolff SD, Quinn SF, et al. Aortoiliac occlusive disease in patients with known or suspected peripheral vascular disease: safety and efficacy of gadofosveset-enhanced MR angiography-multicenter comparative phase III study. *Radiology*. 2005;236(1):71–78.
12. Caravan P, Cloutier NJ, Greenfield MT, et al. The interaction of MS-325 with human serum albumin and its effect on proton relaxation rates. *J Am Chem Soc*. 2002;124(12):3152–3162.
13. Lauffer RB, Parmelee DJ, Dunham SU, et al. MS-325: albumin-targeted contrast agent for MR angiography. *Radiology*. 1998;207(2):529–538.
14. de Haen C, La Ferla R, Maggioni F. Gadobenate dimeglumine 0.5 M solution for injection (MultiHance) as contrast agent for magnetic resonance imaging of the liver: mechanistic studies in animals. *J Comput Assist Tomogr*. 1999;23(suppl 1):S169–S179.
15. Vander Elst L, Maton F, Laurent S, et al. A multinuclear MR study of Gd-EOB-DTPA: comprehensive preclinical characterization of an organ specific MRI contrast agent. *Magn Reson Med*. 1997;38(4):604–614.
16. Herborn CU, Watkins DM, Baumann S, et al. Contrast-enhanced magnetic resonance angiography: P792 blood pool agent versus Gd-DOTA in rabbits at 3.0 T versus 1.5 T. *Invest Radiol*. 2007;42(9):622–628.
17. Krombach GA, Higgins CB, Chujo M, Saeed M. Gadomer-enhanced MR imaging in the detection of microvascular obstruction: alleviation with nicorandil therapy. *Radiology*. 2005;236(2):510–518.
18. Li SD, Huang L. Pharmacokinetics and biodistribution of nanoparticles. *Mol Pharm*. 2008;5(4):496–504.
19. Lu M, Cohen MH, Rieves D, Pazdur R. FDA report: Ferumoxytol for intravenous iron therapy in adult patients with chronic kidney disease. *Am J Hematol*. 2010;85(5):315–319.
20. Nguyen KL, Ghosh RM, Griffin LM, et al. Four-dimensional multiphase steady-state MRI with ferumoxytol enhancement: early multicenter feasibility in pediatric congenital heart disease. *Radiology*. 2021;300(1):162–173.
21. Nguyen KL, Yoshida T, Kathuria-Prakash N, et al. Multicenter safety and practice for off-label diagnostic use of ferumoxytol in MRI. *Radiology*. 2019;293(3):554–564.
22. Iv M, Samghabadi P, Holdsworth S, et al. Quantification of macrophages in high-grade gliomas by using ferumoxytol-enhanced MRI: a pilot study. *Radiology*. 2019;290(1):198–206.
23. Stirrat CG, Alam SR, MacGillivray TJ, et al. Ferumoxytol-enhanced magnetic resonance imaging assessing inflammation after myocardial infarction. *Heart*. 2017;103(19):1528–1535.
24. Troughton JS, Greenfield MT, Greenwood JM, et al. Synthesis and evaluation of a high relaxivity manganese(II)-based MRI contrast agent. *Inorg Chem*. 2004;43(20):6313–6323.
25. Caravan P. Divalent manganese complexes as potential replacements for gadolinium-based contrast agents. *Invest Radiol*. 2024;59(2):187–196.
26. Rohrer M, Bauer H, Mintorovitch J, et al. Comparison of magnetic properties of MRI contrast media solutions at different magnetic field strengths. *Invest Radiol*. 2005;40(11):715–724.
27. Lohrke J, Berger M, Frenzel T, et al. Preclinical profile of gadoquatrane: a novel tetrameric, macrocyclic high relaxivity gadolinium-based contrast agent. *Invest Radiol*. 2022;57(10):629–638.
28. Robic C, Port M, Rousseaux O, et al. Physicochemical and pharmacokinetic profiles of gadopiclenol: a new macrocyclic gadolinium chelate with high T1 relaxivity: erratum. *Invest Radiol*. 2019;54(12):810.
29. Laurent S, Elst LV, Muller RN. Superparamagnetic iron oxide nanoparticles for MRI. In: *The Chemistry of Contrast Agents in Medical Magnetic Resonance Imaging*. Wiley Online Library; 2013:427–447.
30. Caravan P, Greenfield MT, Bulte JW. Molecular factors that determine Curie spin relaxation in dysprosium complexes. *Magn Reson Med*. 2001;46(5):917–922.
31. Tóth é, Helm L, Merbach A. Relaxivity of gadolinium(III) complexes: theory and mechanism. In: *The Chemistry of Contrast Agents in Medical Magnetic Resonance Imaging*. Wiley Online Library; 2013:25–81.
32. Jung CW, Jacobs P. Physical and chemical properties of superparamagnetic iron oxide MR contrast agents: ferumoxides, ferumoxtran, ferumoxsil. *Magn Reson Imaging*. 1995;13(5):661–674.
33. Knobloch G, Colgan T, Wiens CN, et al. Relaxivity of ferumoxytol at 1.5 T and 3.0 T. *Invest Radiol*. 2018;53(5):257–263.
34. Wedeking P, Sotak CH, Telser J, et al. Quantitative dependence of MR signal intensity on tissue concentration of Gd(HP-DO3A) in the nephrectomized rat. *Magn Reson Imaging*. 1992;10(1):97–108.
35. Tweedle MF, Wedeking P, Telser J, et al. Dependence of MR signal intensity on Gd tissue concentration over a broad dose range. *Magn Reson Med*. 1991;22(2):191–194; discussion 5-6.
36. Wang Y, Spiller M, Caravan P. Evidence for weak protein binding of commercial extracellular gadolinium contrast agents. *Magn Reson Med*. 2010;63(3):609–616.
37. Stanisz GJ, Henkelman RM. Gd-DTPA relaxivity depends on macromolecular content. *Magn Reson Med*. 2000;44(5):665–667.
38. Donahue KM, Weisskoff RM, Burstein D. Water diffusion and exchange as they influence contrast enhancement. *J Magn Reson Imaging*. 1997;7(1):102–110.
39. Li X, Rooney WD, Springer Jr CS. A unified magnetic resonance imaging pharmacokinetic theory: intravascular and extracellular contrast reagents. *Magn Reson Med*. 2005;54(6):1351–1359.
40. Hazlewood CF, Chang DC, Nichols BL, Woessner DE. Nuclear magnetic resonance transverse relaxation times of water protons in skeletal muscle. *Biophys J*. 1974;14(8):583–606.
41. McLaughlin AC, Leigh JS. Relaxation times in systems with chemical exchange: approximate solutions for the nondilute case. *J Magn Reson*. 1973;9(2):296–304.
42. Wright GA, Hu BS, Macovski A. 1991 I.I. Rabi Award. Estimating oxygen saturation of blood in vivo with MR imaging at 1.5 T. *J Magn Reson Imaging*. 1991;1(3):275–283.
43. Donahue KM, Weisskoff RM, Chesler DA, et al. Improving MR quantification of regional blood volume with intravascular T1 contrast agents: accuracy, precision, and water exchange. *Magn Reson Med*. 1996;36(6):858–867.
44. Sukstanskii AL, Yablonskiy DA. Gaussian approximation in the theory of MR signal formation in the presence of structure-specific magnetic field inhomogeneities. Effects of impermeable susceptibility inclusions. *J Magn Reson*. 2004;167(1):56–67.
45. Gale EM, Atanasova I, Blasi F, et al. A manganese alternative to gadolinium for MRI contrast. *J Am Chem Soc*. 2015;137(49):15548–15557.
46. Erstad DJ, Ramsay IA, Jordan VC, et al. Tumor contrast enhancement and whole-body elimination of the manganese-based magnetic resonance imaging contrast agent Mn-PyC3A. *Invest Radiol*. 2019;54(11):697–703.
47. Gale EM, Wey HY, Ramsay I, et al. A manganese-based alternative to gadolinium: contrast-enhanced MR angiography, excretion, pharmacokinetics, and metabolism. *Radiology*. 2018;286(3):865–872.
48. Zhou IY, Ramsay IA, Ay I, et al. Positron emission tomography-magnetic resonance imaging pharmacokinetics, in vivo biodistribution, and whole-body elimination of Mn-PyC3A. *Invest Radiol*. 2021;56(4):261–270.
49. Bonner BP, Yurista SR, Coll-Font J, et al. Contrast-enhanced cardiac magnetic resonance imaging with a manganese-based alternative to gadolinium for tissue characterization of acute myocardial infarction. *J Am Heart Assoc*. 2023;12(8):e026923.
50. Toft KG, Hustvedt SO, Grant D, et al. Metabolism and pharmacokinetics of MnDPDP in man. *Acta Radiol*. 1997;38(4 Pt 2):677–689.
51. Skjold A, Amundsen BH, Wiseth R, et al. Manganese dipyridoxyl-diphosphate (MnDPDP) as a viability marker in patients with myocardial infarction. *J Magn Reson Imaging*. 2007;26(3):720–727.
52. Skjold A, Kristoffersen A, Vangberg TR, et al. An apparent unidirectional influx constant for manganese as a measure of myocardial calcium channel activity. *J Magn Reson Imaging*. 2006;24(5):1047–1055.
53. Skjold A, Vangberg TR, Kristoffersen A, et al. Relaxation enhancing properties of MnDPDP in human myocardium. *J Magn Reson Imaging*. 2004;20(6):948–952.
54. Spath NB, Singh T, Papanastasiou G, et al. Assessment of stunned and viable myocardium using manganese-enhanced MRI. *Open Heart*. 2021;8(1):e001646.
55. Dattani A, Joshi S, Yeo JL, et al. Impaired myocardial calcium uptake in patients with diabetes mellitus: a manganese-enhanced cardiac magnetic resonance study. *JACC Cardiovasc Imaging*. 2023;16(12):1623–1625.
56. Weissleder R, Mahmood U. Molecular imaging. *Radiology*. 2001;219(2):316–333.
57. Overoye-Chan K, Koerner S, Looby RJ, et al. EP-2104R: a fibrin-specific gadolinium-Based MRI contrast agent for detection of thrombus. *J Am Chem Soc*. 2008;130(18):6025–6039.
58. Uppal R, Ay I, Dai G, et al. Molecular MRI of intracranial thrombus in a rat ischemic stroke model. *Stroke*. 2010;41(6):1271–1277.
59. Spuentrup E, Katoh M, Buecker A, et al. Molecular MR imaging of human thrombi in a swine model of pulmonary embolism using a fibrin-specific contrast agent. *Invest Radiol*. 2007;42(8):586–595.
60. Stracke CP, Katoh M, Wiethoff AJ, et al. Molecular MRI of cerebral venous sinus thrombosis using a new fibrin-specific MR contrast agent. *Stroke*. 2007;38(5):1476–1481.
61. Sirol M, Fuster V, Badimon JJ, et al. Chronic thrombus detection with in vivo magnetic resonance imaging and a fibrin-targeted contrast agent. *Circulation*. 2005;112(11):1594–1600.
62. Spuentrup E, Fausten B, Kinzel S, et al. Molecular magnetic resonance imaging of atrial clots in a swine model. *Circulation*. 2005;112(3):396–399.
63. Spuentrup E, Katoh M, Wiethoff AJ, et al. Molecular magnetic resonance imaging of pulmonary emboli with a fibrin-specific contrast agent. *Am J Respir Crit Care Med*. 2005;172(4):494–500.
64. Spuentrup E, Buecker A, Katoh M, et al. Molecular magnetic resonance imaging of coronary thrombosis and pulmonary emboli with a novel fibrin-targeted contrast agent. *Circulation*. 2005;111(11):1377–1382.
65. Botnar RM, Buecker A, Wiethoff AJ, et al. In vivo magnetic resonance imaging of coronary thrombosis using a fibrin-binding molecular magnetic resonance contrast agent. *Circulation*. 2004;110(11):1463–1466.
66. Andia ME, Saha P, Jenkins J, et al. Fibrin-targeted magnetic resonance imaging allows in vivo quantification of thrombus fibrin content and identifies thrombi amenable for thrombolysis. *Arterioscler Thromb Vasc Biol*. 2014;34(6):1193–1198.
67. Vymazal J, Spuentrup E, Cardenas-Molina G, et al. Thrombus imaging with fibrin-specific gadolinium-based MR contrast agent EP-2104R: results of a phase II clinical study of feasibility. *Invest Radiol*. 2009;44(11):697–704.
68. Spuentrup E, Botnar RM, Wiethoff AJ, et al. MR imaging of thrombi using EP-2104R, a fibrin-specific contrast agent: initial results in patients. *Eur Radiol*. 2008;18(9):1995–2005.
69. Caravan P, Das B, Dumas S, et al. Collagen-targeted MRI contrast agent for molecular imaging of fibrosis. *Angew Chem Int Ed Engl*. 2007;46(43):8171–8173.
70. Helm PA, Caravan P, French BA, et al. Postinfarction myocardial scarring in mice: molecular MR imaging with use of a collagen-targeting contrast agent. *Radiology*. 2008;247(3):788–796.
71. Spuentrup E, Ruhl KM, Botnar RM, et al. Molecular magnetic resonance imaging of myocardial perfusion with EP-3600, a collagen-specific contrast agent: initial feasibility study in a swine model. *Circulation*. 2009;119(13):1768–1775.
72. Murphy AP, Greally E, O'Hogain D, et al. Noninvasive quantification of fibrosis in skeletal and cardiac muscle in mdx mice using EP3533 enhanced magnetic resonance imaging. *Magn Reson Med*. 2019;81(4):2728–2735.
73. Chen HH, Waghorn PA, Wei L, et al. Molecular imaging of oxidized collagen quantifies pulmonary and hepatic fibrogenesis. *JCI Insight*. 2017;2(11).
74. Ma H, Zhou IY, Chen YI, et al. Tailored chemical reactivity probes for systemic imaging of aldehydes in fibroproliferative diseases. *J Am Chem Soc*. 2023;145(38):20825–20836.
75. Moon BF, Zhou IY, Ning Y, et al. Simultaneous positron emission tomography and molecular magnetic resonance imaging of cardiopulmonary fibrosis in a mouse model of left ventricular dysfunction. *J Am Heart Assoc*. 2024;13:e034363.
76. Ning Y, Zhou IY, Roberts Jr JD, et al. Molecular MRI quantification of extracellular aldehyde pairs for early detection of liver fibrogenesis and response to treatment. *Sci Transl Med*. 2022;14(663):eabq6297.
77. Ning Y, Zhou IY, Rotile NJ, et al. Dual hydrazine-equipped turn-on manganese-based probes for magnetic resonance imaging of liver fibrogenesis. *J Am Chem Soc*. 2022;144(36):16553–16558.
78. Makowski MR, Wiethoff AJ, Blume U, et al. Assessment of atherosclerotic plaque burden with an elastin-specific magnetic resonance contrast agent. *Nat Med*. 2011;17(3):383–388.
79. Botnar RM, Wiethoff AJ, Ebersberger U, et al. In vivo assessment of aortic aneurysm wall integrity using elastin-specific molecular magnetic resonance imaging. *Circ Cardiovasc Imaging*. 2014;7(4):679–689.

80. Phinikaridou A, Andia ME, Indermuehle A, et al. Vascular remodeling and plaque vulnerability in a rabbit model of atherosclerosis: comparison of delayed-enhancement MR imaging with an elastin-specific contrast agent and unenhanced black-blood MR imaging. *Radiology*. 2014;271(2):390–399.
81. Protti A, Lavin B, Dong X, et al. Assessment of myocardial remodeling using an elastin/tropoelastin specific agent with high field magnetic resonance imaging (MRI). *J Am Heart Assoc*. 2015;4(8):e001851.
82. Wildgruber M, Bielicki I, Aichler M, et al. Assessment of myocardial infarction and postinfarction scar remodeling with an elastin-specific magnetic resonance agent. *Circ Cardiovasc Imaging*. 2014;7(2):321–329.
83. Phinikaridou A, Lacerda S, Lavin B, et al. Tropoelastin: a novel marker for plaque progression and instability. *Circ Cardiovasc Imaging*. 2018;11(8):e007303.
84. Lavin B, Lacerda S, Andia ME, et al. Tropoelastin: an in vivo imaging marker of dysfunctional matrix turnover during abdominal aortic dilation. *Cardiovasc Res*. 2020;116(5):995–1005.
85. Querol M, Chen JW, Bogdanov Jr AA. A paramagnetic contrast agent with myeloperoxidase-sensing properties. *Org Biomol Chem*. 2006;4(10):1887–1895.
86. Rodriguez-Rodriguez A, Shuvaev S, Rotile N, et al. Peroxidase sensitive amplifiable probe for molecular magnetic resonance imaging of pulmonary inflammation. *ACS Sens*. 2019;4(9):2412–2419.
87. Wang C, Cheng D, Jalali Motlagh N, et al. Highly efficient activatable MRI probe to sense myeloperoxidase activity. *J Med Chem*. 2021;64(9):5874–5885.
88. Breckwoldt MO, Chen JW, Stangenberg L, et al. Tracking the inflammatory response in stroke in vivo by sensing the enzyme myeloperoxidase. *Proc Natl Acad Sci U S A*. 2008;105(47):18584–18589.
89. Nahrendorf M, Sosnovik D, Chen JW, et al. Activatable magnetic resonance imaging agent reports myeloperoxidase activity in healing infarcts and noninvasively detects the antiinflammatory effects of atorvastatin on ischemia-reperfusion injury. *Circulation*. 2008;117(9):1153–1160.
90. DeLeo 3rd MJ, Gounis MJ, Hong B, et al. Carotid artery brain aneurysm model: in vivo molecular enzyme-specific MR imaging of active inflammation in a pilot study. *Radiology*. 2009;252(3):696–703.
91. King RM, Caroff J, Langan ET, et al. In situ decellularization of a large animal saccular aneurysm model: sustained inflammation and active aneurysm wall remodeling. *J Neurointerv Surg*. 2021;13(3):267–271.
92. Su HS, Nahrendorf M, Panizzi P, et al. Vasculitis: molecular imaging by targeting the inflammatory enzyme myeloperoxidase. *Radiology*. 2012;262(1):181–190.
93. Sadat U, Usman A, Gillard JH. Imaging pathobiology of carotid atherosclerosis with ultrasmall superparamagnetic particles of iron oxide: an update. *Curr Opin Cardiol*. 2017;32(4):437–440.
94. Stirrat CG, Alam SR, MacGillivray TJ, et al. Ferumoxytol-enhanced magnetic resonance imaging in acute myocarditis. *Heart*. 2018;104(4):300–305.
95. Bulte JW, Kraitchman DL. Monitoring cell therapy using iron oxide MR contrast agents. *Curr Pharm Biotechnol*. 2004;5(6):567–584.
96. Modo MMJ, Bulte JWM. *Molecular and Cellular MR Imaging*. CRC Press; 2007.
97. Hill JM, Dick AJ, Raman VK, et al. Serial cardiac magnetic resonance imaging of injected mesenchymal stem cells. *Circulation*. 2003;108(8):1009–1014.
98. Kraitchman DL, Heldman AW, Atalar E, et al. In vivo magnetic resonance imaging of mesenchymal stem cells in myocardial infarction. *Circulation*. 2003;107(18):2290–2293.
99. Mathiasen AB, Qayyum AA, Jorgensen E, et al. In vivo MRI tracking of mesenchymal stromal cells labeled with ultrasmall paramagnetic iron oxide particles after intramyocardial transplantation in patients with chronic ischemic heart disease. *Stem Cells Int*. 2019;2019:2754927.
100. Ma N, Cheng H, Lu M, et al. Magnetic resonance imaging with superparamagnetic iron oxide fails to track the long-term fate of mesenchymal stem cells transplanted into heart. *Sci Rep*. 2015;5:9058.
101. Ahrens ET, Helfer BM, O'Hanlon CF, et al. Method for estimation of apoptotic cell fraction of cytotherapy using in vivo fluorine-19 magnetic resonance: pilot study in a patient with head and neck carcinoma receiving tumor-infiltrating lymphocytes labeled with perfluorocarbon nanoemulsion. *J Immunother Cancer*. 2023;11(6):e007015.
102. Ahrens ET, Helfer BM, O'Hanlon CF, Schirda C. Clinical cell therapy imaging using a perfluorocarbon tracer and fluorine-19 MRI. *Magn Reson Med*. 2014;72(6):1696–1701.
103. Chapelin F, Capitini CM, Ahrens ET. Fluorine-19 MRI for detection and quantification of immune cell therapy for cancer. *J Immunother Cancer*. 2018;6(1):105.
104. Croci D, Santalla Méndez R, Temme S, et al. Multispectral fluorine-19 MRI enables longitudinal and noninvasive monitoring of tumor-associated macrophages. *Sci Transl Med*. 2022;14(667):eabo2952.
105. Diou O, Fattal E, Delplace V, et al. RGD decoration of PEGylated polyester nanocapsules of perfluorooctyl bromide for tumor imaging: influence of pre or post-functionalization on capsule morphology. *Eur J Pharm Biopharm*. 2014;87(1):170–177.
106. Matsushita H, Mizukami S, Sugihara F, et al. Multifunctional core–shell silica nanoparticles for highly sensitive (19)F magnetic resonance imaging. *Angew Chem Int Ed Engl*. 2014;53(4):1008–1011.
107. Schmieder AH, Wang K, Zhang H, et al. Characterization of early neovascular response to acute lung ischemia using simultaneous (19)F/(1)H MR molecular imaging. *Angiogenesis*. 2014;17(1):51–60.
108. Schmieder AH, Winter PM, Williams TA, et al. Molecular MR imaging of neovascular progression in the Vx2 tumor with αvβ3-targeted paramagnetic nanoparticles. *Radiology*. 2013;268(2):470–480.
109. Temme S, Grapentin C, Quast C, et al. Noninvasive imaging of early venous thrombosis by 19F magnetic resonance imaging with targeted perfluorocarbon nanoemulsions. *Circulation*. 2015;131(16):1405–1414.
110. Xu X, Zhang R, Liu F, et al. (19)F MRI in orthotopic cancer model via intratracheal administration of α(v)β(3)-targeted perfluorocarbon nanoparticles. *Nanomedicine*. 2018;13(20):2551–2562.
111. van Heeswijk RB, Bauer WR, Bonner F, et al. Cardiovascular molecular imaging with fluorine-19 MRI: the road to the clinic. *Circ Cardiovasc Imaging*. 2023;16(9):e014742.
112. Flogel U, Temme S, Jacoby C, et al. Multi-targeted (1)H/(19)F MRI unmasks specific danger patterns for emerging cardiovascular disorders. *Nat Commun*. 2021;12(1):5847.
113. Larson PEZ, Bernard JML, Bankson JA, et al. Current methods for hyperpolarized [1-(13)C]pyruvate MRI human studies. *Magn Reson Med*. 2024;91(6):2204–2228.
114. Frijia F, Flori A, Giovannetti G, et al. MRI application and challenges of hyperpolarized carbon-13 pyruvate in translational and clinical cardiovascular studies: a literature review. *Diagnostics*. 2024;14(10).
115. Larson PEZ, Tang S, Liu X, et al. Regional quantification of cardiac metabolism with hyperpolarized [1-(13)C]-pyruvate CMR evaluated in an oral glucose challenge. *J Cardiovasc Magn Reson*. 2023;25(1):77.
116. Park JM, Reed GD, Liticker J, et al. Effect of doxorubicin on myocardial bicarbonate production from pyruvate dehydrogenase in women with breast cancer. *Circ Res*. 2020;127(12):1568–1570.
117. Rider OJ, Apps A, Miller J, et al. Noninvasive in vivo assessment of cardiac metabolism in the healthy and diabetic human heart using hyperpolarized (13)C MRI. *Circ Res*. 2020;126(6):725–736.
118. Chen HY, Gordon JW, Dwork N, et al. Probing human heart TCA cycle metabolism and response to glucose load using hyperpolarized [2-(13) C]pyruvate MRS. *NMR Biomed*. 2024;37(3):e5074.
119. Liu X, Tang S, Mu C, et al. Development of specialized magnetic resonance acquisition techniques for human hyperpolarized [(13) C,(15) N(2)]urea + [1-(13) C]pyruvate simultaneous perfusion and metabolic imaging. *Magn Reson Med*. 2022;88(3):1039–1054.
120. Todd DJ, Kagan A, Chibnik LB, Kay J. Cutaneous changes of nephrogenic systemic fibrosis: predictor of early mortality and association with gadolinium exposure. *Arthritis Rheum*. 2007;56(10):3433–3441.
121. Todd DJ, Kay J. Gadolinium-induced fibrosis. *Annu Rev Med*. 2016;67:273–291.
122. Cowper SE. Nephrogenic systemic fibrosis: a review and exploration of the role of gadolinium. *Adv Dermatol*. 2007;23:131–154.
123. Cowper SE, Kuo PH, Bucala R. Nephrogenic systemic fibrosis and gadolinium exposure: association and lessons for idiopathic fibrosing disorders. *Arthritis Rheum*. 2007;56(10):3173–3175.
124. Grobner T. Gadolinium-a specific trigger for the development of nephrogenic fibrosing dermopathy and nephrogenic systemic fibrosis? *Nephrol Dial Transplant*. 2006;21(4):1104–1108.
125. Grobner T, Prischl FC. Gadolinium and nephrogenic systemic fibrosis. *Kidney Int*. 2007;72(3):260–264.
126. Thomsen HS. Nephrogenic systemic fibrosis: a serious late adverse reaction to gadodiamide. *Eur Radiol*. 2006;16(12):2619–2621.
127. Burke LM, Ramalho M, AlObaidy M, et al. Self-reported gadolinium toxicity: a survey of patients with chronic symptoms. *Magn Reson Imaging*. 2016;34(8):1078–1080.
128. Semelka RC, Commander CW, Jay M, et al. Presumed gadolinium toxicity in subjects with normal renal function: a report of 4 cases. *Invest Radiol*. 2016;51(10):661–665.
129. Abraham JL, Thakral C, Skov L, et al. Dermal inorganic gadolinium concentrations: evidence for in vivo transmetallation and long-term persistence in nephrogenic systemic fibrosis. *Br J Dermatol*. 2008;158(2):273–280.
130. High WA, Ayers RA, Chandler J, et al. Gadolinium is detectable within the tissue of patients with nephrogenic systemic fibrosis. *J Am Acad Dermatol*. 2007;56(1):21–26.
131. High WA, Ayers RA, Cowper SE. Gadolinium is quantifiable within the tissue of patients with nephrogenic systemic fibrosis. *J Am Acad Dermatol*. 2007;56(4):710–712.
132. Thakral C, Alhariri J, Abraham JL. Long-term retention of gadolinium in tissues from nephrogenic systemic fibrosis patient after multiple gadolinium-enhanced MRI scans: case report and implications. *Contrast Media Mol Imaging*. 2007;2(4):199–205.
133. Kay J, Bazari H, Avery LL, Koreishi AF. Case records of the Massachusetts general hospital. Case 6-2008. A 46-year-old woman with renal failure and stiffness of the joints and skin. *N Engl J Med*. 2008;358(8):827–838.
134. Rydahl C, Thomsen HS, Marckmann P. High prevalence of nephrogenic systemic fibrosis in chronic renal failure patients exposed to gadodiamide, a gadolinium-containing magnetic resonance contrast agent. *Invest Radiol*. 2008;43(2):141–144.
135. Yang L, Krefting I, Gorovets A, et al. Nephrogenic systemic fibrosis and class labeling of gadolinium-based contrast agents by the food and drug administration. *Radiology*. 2012;265(1):248–253.
136. Frenzel T, Lengsfeld P, Schirmer H, et al. Stability of gadolinium-based magnetic resonance imaging contrast agents in human serum at 37 degrees C. *Invest Radiol*. 2008;43(12):817–828.
137. Laurent S, Elst LV, Muller RN. Comparative study of the physicochemical properties of six clinical low molecular weight gadolinium contrast agents. *Contrast Media Mol Imaging*. 2006;1(3):128–137.
138. Kanda T, ishii K, Kawaguchi H, et al. High signal intensity in the dentate nucleus and globus pallidus on unenhanced T1-weighted MR images: relationship with increasing cumulative dose of a gadolinium-based contrast material. *Radiology*. 2014;270:834–841.
139. Kanda T, Kawaguchi H. Hyperintense dentate nucleas and globus pallidus on unenhanced T1-weighted MR images are associated with gadolinium-based contrast media. *Neuroradiology*. 2013;55:1268–1269.
140. Kanda T, Osawa M, Oba H, et al. High signal intensity in dentate nucleus on unenhanced T1-weighted MR images: association with linear versus macrocyclic gadolinium chelate administration. *Radiology*. 2015;275(3):803–809.
141. McDonald RJ, McDonald JS, Kallmes DF, et al. Intracranial gadolinium deposition after contrast-enhanced MR imaging. *Radiology*. 2015;275(3):772–782.
142. Murata N, Gonzalez-Cuyar LF, Murata K, et al. Macrocyclic and other non-group 1 gadolinium contrast agents deposit low levels of gadolinium in brain and bone tissue: preliminary results from 9 patients with normal renal function. *Invest Radiol*. 2016;51(7):447–453.
143. Murata N, Murata K, Gonzalez-Cuyar LF, Maravilla KR. Gadolinium tissue deposition in brain and bone. *Magn Reson Imaging*. 2016;34(10):1359–1365.
144. Le Fur M, Caravan P. The biological fate of gadolinium-based MRI contrast agents: a call to action for bioinorganic chemists. *Metallomics*. 2019;11(2):240–254.
145. McDonald RJ, Levine D, Weinreb J, et al. Gadolinium retention: a research roadmap from the 2018 NIH/ACR/RSNA workshop on gadolinium chelates. *Radiology*. 2018;289(2):517–534.
146. Roberts DR, Lindhorst SM, Welsh CT, et al. High levels of gadolinium deposition in the skin of a patient with normal renal function. *Invest Radiol*. 2016;51(5):280–289.
147. Uhlig J, Al-Bourini O, Salgado R, et al. Gadolinium-based contrast agents for cardiac MRI: use of linear and macrocyclic agents with associated safety profile from 154 779 European patients. *Radiol: Cardiothorac Imaging*. 2020;2(5):e200102.
148. Kirchin MA, Runge VM. Contrast agents for magnetic resonance imaging: safety update. *Top Magn Reson Imaging*. 2003;14(5):426–435.
149. Behzadi AH, Zhao Y, Farooq Z, Prince MR. Immediate allergic reactions to gadolinium-based contrast agents: a systematic review and meta-analysis. *Radiology*. 2018;286(2):471–482.
150. Prince MR, Zhang H, Zou Z, et al. Incidence of immediate gadolinium contrast media reactions. *AJR Am J Roentgenol*. 2011;196(2):W138–W143.

3 Gating, Motion Correction, and Image Acceleration

ORLANDO P. SIMONETTI AND JULIET VARGHESE

INTRODUCTION

Magnetic resonance imaging (MRI) data acquisition for all applications typically takes on the order of seconds to minutes. This timescale is slow relative to cardiac and respiratory motion, and any motion-induced variability in the acquired k-space data leads to image artifacts if specific measures are not taken to avoid them or correct their effects. A variety of strategies are used to minimize the impact of motion: data acquisition can be synchronized to cardiac and respiratory motion using external or MRI-derived signals for gating and triggering, respiratory motion can be avoided by patient breath-holding, motion effects may be corrected prospectively or retrospectively, and data acquisition can be accelerated to the degree that motion artifacts are reduced or eliminated. The success of cardiovascular magnetic resonance (CMR) in recent years can be largely attributed to significant improvements in image quality and reliability due to advances in gating strategies, motion correction methods, and image acceleration techniques. These innovations have reduced the frequency and severity of motion artifacts and have increased workflow efficiency by reducing overall scan time. This chapter provides a comprehensive overview of these techniques, focusing on important considerations for practitioners.

PART I—SYNCHRONIZATION WITH PHYSIOLOGICAL MOTION

Cardiac Triggering and Gating

Cardiac triggering or gating techniques synchronize image acquisition with the cardiac cycle, enabling high-resolution imaging of the heart and vasculature free of motion artifacts. Cardiac synchronization also supports dynamic cine imaging to evaluate cardiac function and blood flow with high temporal and spatial resolution. While the terms "triggering" and "gating" are often used interchangeably, "triggering" typically refers to prospective initiation of data acquisition based on a physiological signal, for example, the R-wave of the electrocardiogram (ECG). "Gating," on the other hand, generally refers to the process of accepting or rejecting data based on timing relative to physiological motion or the binning of data into multiple motion phases spanning a cyclical motion pattern such as a cardiac or respiratory cycle. Gating as a data acceptance or rejection technique is typically applied prospectively, while the process of binning to resolve distinct motion phases is often termed "retrospective" gating. The basic concepts of "triggering" and "gating" are illustrated in Fig. 3.1.

CARDIAC SYNCHRONIZATION SIGNALS: ECG, PULSE OXIMETER, PILOT TONE, AND SELF-GATING

In cardiac MRI, precise synchronization of data acquisition with the cardiac cycle is critical to avoid motion artifact and accurately depict dynamic contraction and blood flow. Various physiological signals are used to achieve this synchronization, each offering unique advantages for different applications. Here, we provide a brief overview of the key signals employed in cardiac MRI synchronization.

Electrocardiogram

The ECG is the physiological signal most commonly used to synchronize MRI data acquisition with cardiac motion. The ECG R-wave provides a sharp voltage spike that is easily detected and initiates the start of ventricular contraction, a convenient point for the timing of subsequent data acquisition to specific phases of the cardiac cycle, such as end diastole or end systole, or to cover the entire R-to-R interval for dynamic cine and flow imaging. There are some challenges, however; the ECG is susceptible to electromagnetic interference caused by flowing blood in high magnetic fields (the magnetohydrodynamic effect), and MRI gradients and radiofrequency (RF) pulses can lead to signal distortion or dropout that may cause erroneous triggering or missed heartbeats. ECG synchronization requires the placement of ECG electrodes on the chest of the patient, which may cause discomfort or skin irritation and adds time to the exam. Misplacement or poor skin contact can result in an unreliable signal, and patient motion or chest muscle contractions may degrade signal quality, leading to gating inaccuracies. Despite these limitations, ECG synchronization is widely utilized in practice due to its overall simplicity and effectiveness.

Finger Pulse Oximeter

The finger pulse oximeter signal is proportional to peripheral blood oxygen saturation (SpO_2) and is primarily used for monitoring patient well-being during MRI scans. However, it can be used to provide a cardiac timing signal via the pulsatile changes in blood volume in the fingertip and can be used as an alternative or complementary method for cardiac synchronization.

It offers the advantages of being less invasive and easier to apply than ECG electrodes, requiring only a probe to be clipped on a finger; as an optical signal, it is less susceptible

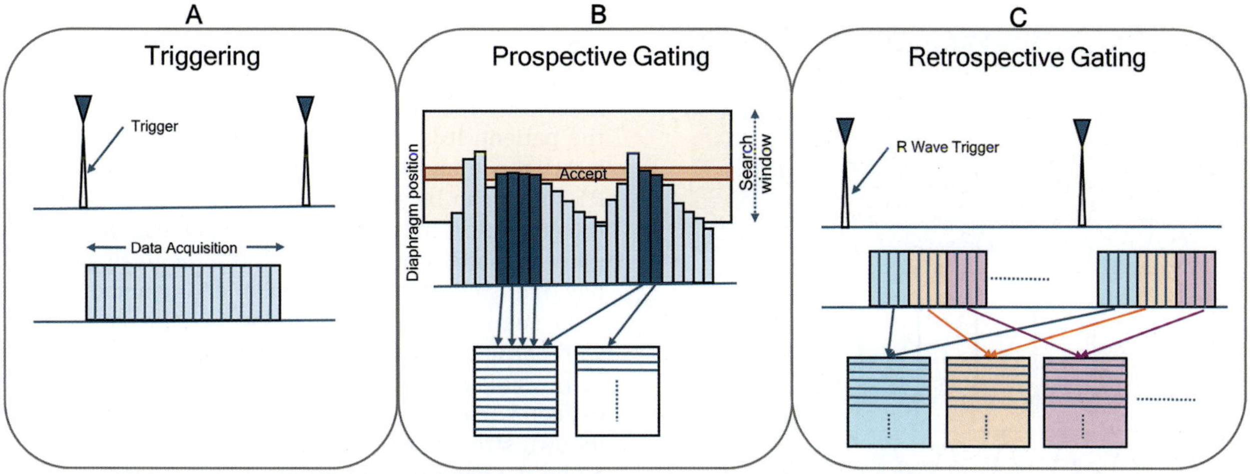

FIG. 3.1 The Basic Concepts of "Triggering" and "Gating." The terms "triggering" and "gating" can apply to synchronization of data acquisition with either cardiac or respiratory motion. Panel A represents the concept of prospective triggering. In this mode, the physiological trigger signal, which can be cardiac or respiratory, initiates data acquisition for a predefined time window. Panel B illustrates the concept of gating as the acceptance or rejection of data based on a gating window; this method is applied only to respiratory motion. In this example, data are only accepted when the position of the lung diaphragm falls within a predetermined window corresponding to end-expiration. Panel C illustrates the concept of gating as binning the acquired data to correspond with different motion states. This is frequently referred to as "retrospective gating" and is commonly applied to cardiac cine imaging, although the same method is sometimes used for respiratory resolved imaging. In this illustration, the timing within the R-R interval is used to determine the bin to which the k-space data will be assigned, with each bin corresponding to a motion state (systole, diastole, etc.) in the cardiac cycle.

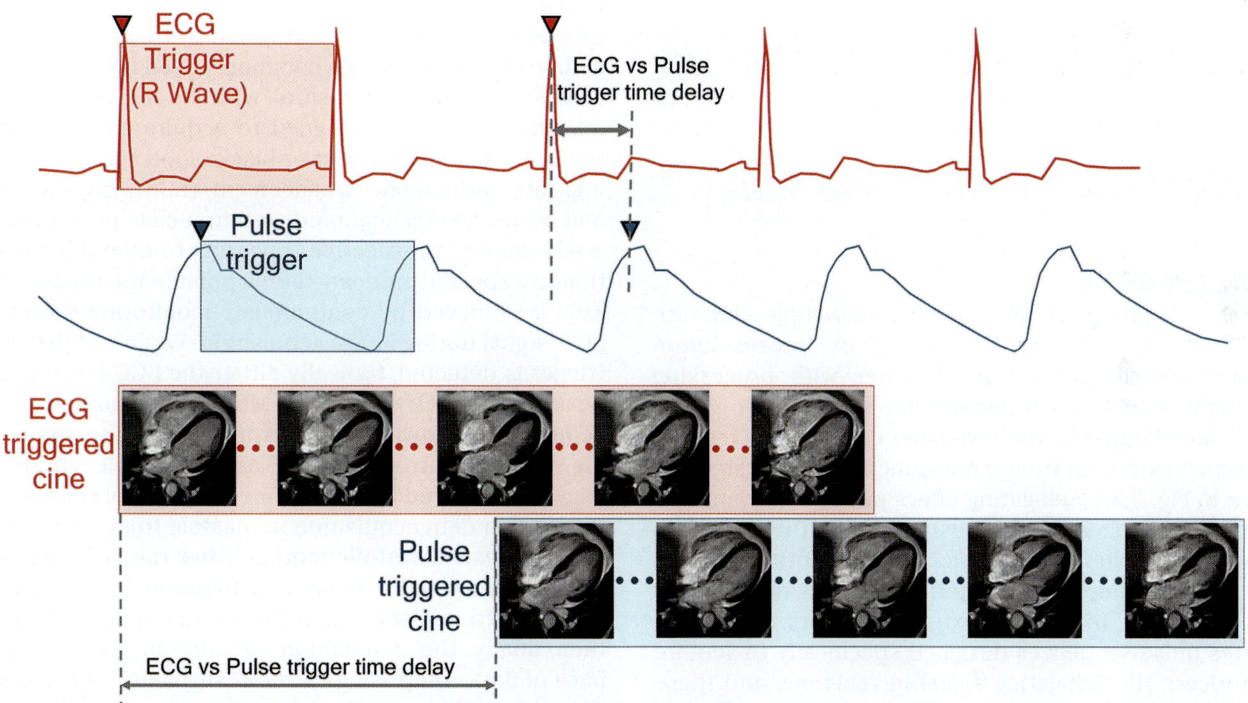

FIG. 3.2 The Timing Difference Between electrocardiogram (ECG) and Finger-Pulse Cardiac Triggering. The ECG and finger pulse oximeter are the physiological signals most commonly used for cardiac synchronization. The R-wave of the ECG is typically used as the trigger and initiates systolic contraction. On the other hand, the peak of the pulse oximeter signal used as a trigger corresponds when the pulse wave of blood flow reaches the finger, typically just after peak systolic contraction. This delay between the R-wave and the peak flow signal must be accounted for when acquiring or analyzing cardiac MRI images. This time shift is evident from the cardiac phase order in the cardiac cine images acquired with ECG versus pulse triggering. The ECG triggered cine progresses through systole to diastole, while the pulse triggered cine progresses through diastole to systole.

to electromagnetic interference than the ECG, especially at higher fields, and SpO_2 provides additional physiological information. Unlike the sharp peak of the ECG R-wave, however, the pulse signal is smoothly varying, and this can lead to timing inconsistencies relative to cardiac motion. Furthermore, the pulse trigger typically reflects the peak blood flow at the fingertip, which lags the R-wave trigger by some 200 to 300 ms, making it difficult or impossible to time data acquisition to end systole. Because this delay is variable from patient to patient, it may be necessary to calibrate sequence timing based on a pulse-triggered cine scan. The trigger timing difference between ECG and pulse is illustrated in Fig. 3.2. Pulse oximeter signal quality may be compromised or even undetectable in patients with poor peripheral circulation and is susceptible to artifacts caused by finger motion.

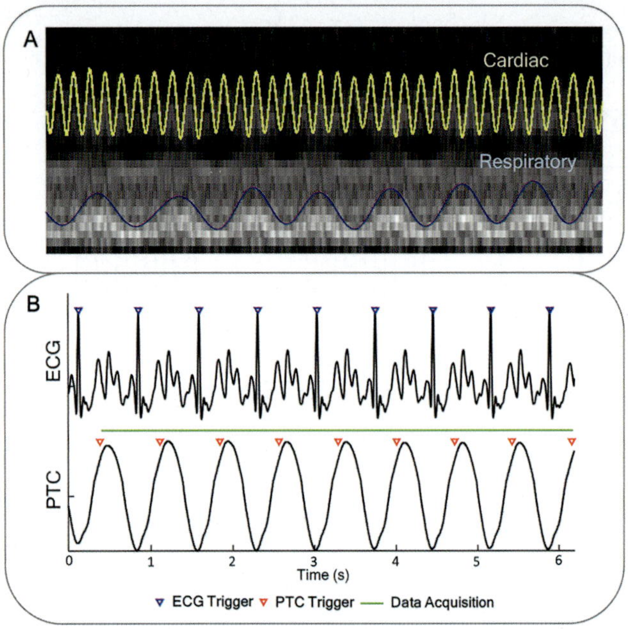

FIG. 3.3 Self-Gating and Pilot-Tone Gating. Panel A shows the temporal profile of the one-dimensional signal extracted from a self-gated acquisition. The cardiac (shown in *yellow*) and respiratory (shown in *blue*) signals extracted from the self-gated profile are overlaid on the image. The data can be binned to different cardiac and respiratory phases based on this information. Panel B shows the timing difference between ECG and pilot-tone cardiac (PTC) triggering. The pilot tone signal reflects cardiac motion. Similar to the pulse oximeter signal, the PT trigger (shown in *red*) typically lags the ECG R-wave (shown in *blue*) by 200 to 300 ms. This temporal lag must be accounted for when setting up data acquisition to correspond with mid-diastole, for example, or when analyzing dynamic cine or flow image series.

Cardiac Self-Gating

Cardiac self-gating[1] is an emerging technique that utilizes a one-dimensional MRI signal, or low-resolution two-dimensional (2D) image, together with processing algorithms to detect cardiac motion and derive a gating signal. An example of the self-gated cardiac and respiratory signal extracted from a one-dimensional MR signal is shown in Fig. 3.3A. Self-gating offers potential advantages in terms of simplicity and robustness in that it eliminates the need for external physiological monitoring devices and is less susceptible to interference and motion artifacts compared to ECG or external sensors. Self-gating requires pulse sequences designed specifically to acquire and process the self-gating signal in real-time, and these techniques are not widely available. Variability in cardiac motion patterns between patients may require customization of gating algorithms for optimal performance.

Pilot Tone

The pilot tone (PT) is a recently introduced technology that is gaining in utility as a motion synchronization signal.[2–4] The PT signal is derived from the transmission of RF energy by a separate generator incorporated into a receiver coil or somewhere inside the magnet bore. The PT frequency is outside of the imaging frequencies, but detectable by the receiver coils. The received signal is modulated by both cardiac and respiratory motion, and signals proportional to both types of motion can be separated out by signal processing. This typically requires some form of calibration prescan. An example of the PT-derived cardiac signal in comparison to the ECG trigger is shown in Fig. 3.3B. The primary advantage of PT gating is that it eliminates the need to place ECG electrodes or other devices on the patient. It is also less susceptible to electromagnetic interference and signal distortion compared to ECG. The PT signal can be sensitive, however, to the positioning of the generator on the patient and may exhibit variability in different patient populations. It is a relatively new technology that is not yet widely available for clinical use.

In summary, synchronization of MRI data acquisition with cardiac motion can be accomplished using a variety of physiological signals, including the ECG, finger pulse oximeter, cardiac self-gating, and PT. Each method has its own strengths and limitations, and the choice of technique depends on factors including scanner capabilities, patient characteristics, and specific imaging requirements. Understanding these factors is critical for ultimately ensuring accurate and reliable image quality devoid of cardiac motion artifact.

CARDIAC SYNCHRONIZATION TECHNIQUES: PROSPECTIVE TRIGGERING AND RETROSPECTIVE GATING

Prospective cardiac triggering and retrospective cardiac gating[5] (Fig. 3.4) are both commonly used in cardiac MRI to synchronize image acquisition with the cardiac cycle. Most imaging techniques designed to acquire static images of the heart, including bright or black-blood anatomical imaging, late gadolinium enhancement (LGE), myocardial T1 and T2 parameter mapping, and first-pass perfusion, generally employ prospective triggering to time data acquisition to a specific predefined time point in the cardiac cycle. This is achieved by continuously monitoring the ECG or SpO_2 signal during image acquisition. When a physiological trigger is detected, typically either the ECG R-wave or the peak of the SpO_2 signal, the MRI scanner initiates image acquisition following predetermined pulse sequence timing. Using ECG-triggered LGE as an example, the R-wave trigger is followed by a predefined trigger delay prescribed to position data acquisition in diastole to avoid rapid systolic and early diastolic motion. After the delay, an inversion recovery pulse is applied followed by an inversion delay set to null the signal from viable myocardium, and then finally the acquisition of multiple phase-encoded lines of data comprising either a "segment"[6] of the k-space data that will be used to form an image, or, in the case of single-shot imaging, all of the data needed to reconstruct an entire image (Fig. 3.4A).

Retrospective cardiac gating,[5] on the other hand, is commonly used for dynamic cine and flow imaging. The goal in these applications is to acquire and reconstruct a multiframe series of images spanning the entire cardiac cycle (R-R interval) with sufficient temporal resolution to evaluate cardiac function and blood flow. Unlike prospective triggering, retrospective or retrogating involves acquiring data continuously throughout the cardiac cycle. The ECG or SpO_2 signal is monitored during data acquisition and used to switch, in real-time, to acquire different k-space lines in each cardiac cycle. During image reconstruction, the k-space data are retrospectively sorted into cardiac

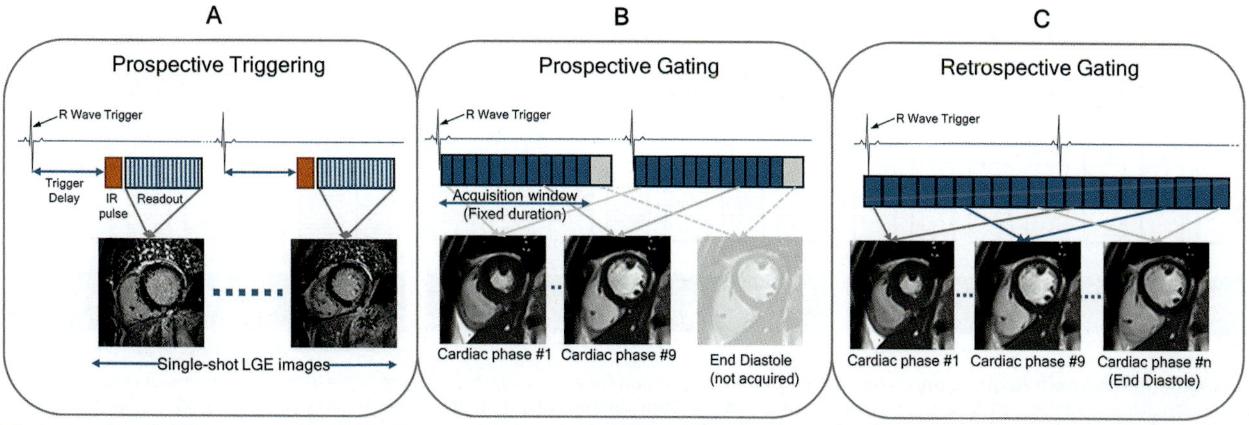

FIG. 3.4 Prospective Triggering, Prospective Gating, and Retrospective Gating. Prospective triggering is commonly used for static imaging, including late gadolinium enhancement (LGE) as shown, single-shot balanced steady state free precession, and turbo spin echo imaging. For prospective triggering illustrated in panel A, the physiological trigger initiates a predefined sequence of gradient and radiofrequency pulses, typically comprising some magnetization preparation followed by data acquisition to generate static pictures with a specific image contrast. In this example of single-shot LGE imaging, inversion recovery magnetization preparation is applied followed by a single-shot image readout. A trigger delay is specified in order to time the image acquisition in diastole. In panel B, the term "prospective gating" typically applies to dynamic cine or flow imaging. In this case, a series of k-space data segments is acquired over a predetermined time window specified to end prior to the next expected cardiac cycle. This method for cine imaging can be useful in patients with arrhythmias as the acquisition window can be set short enough to capture systolic contraction in all or most beats even when the heart rate is variable. However, the end diastolic cardiac phase may not be acquired due to the predetermined scan time being shorter than the cardiac cycle. In panel C, retrospective gating is illustrated. This is the most commonly used synchronization method for cine and flow imaging as it captures the entire cardiac cycle. In this example, k-space segments are acquired continuously over the duration of multiple heartbeats. k-Space data from a given segment across multiple beats are used to fill the k-space corresponding to a specific cardiac phase. This method of cine imaging is useful in patients who have consistent cardiac rhythm and are capable of performing breath-holds.

phases based on the recorded trigger signals (Fig. 3.4C). This allows for flexibility in selecting the desired number of cardiac phases or frames in the resulting cine loop. However, because data are acquired throughout the entire cardiac cycle, retrospective gating may be more susceptible to motion artifacts, particularly if the patient experiences irregular heart rhythms that lead to longer and shorter R-R intervals during acquisition.

The choice between prospective triggering and retrospective gating primarily depends on the imaging application; static images of the heart are generally acquired using prospective triggering and dynamic imaging with retrogating. However, dynamic cine imaging can also be performed with prospective triggering, and this can offer an advantage over retrogating in the presence of arrhythmias. For example, if the R-R interval is widely varying, prospective triggering can be used to acquire a prescribed number of frames covering only the duration of systolic contraction, which tends to be fairly consistent even with arrhythmias (Fig. 3.4B). While diastole will not be depicted with this acquisition strategy, in some instances, systolic contraction may be of most interest, and the variability of diastole with arrhythmia may introduce severe motion artifact. Real-time cine techniques[7,8] are also a viable strategy when severe arrhythmias are encountered; these generally require highly accelerated acquisition/reconstruction techniques to achieve sufficient spatial and temporal resolution.

In summary, prospective cardiac triggering and retrospective cardiac gating are complementary techniques and both are widely used in cardiac MRI to synchronize image acquisition with the cardiac cycle. The choice between the two techniques depends on the clinical scenario and imaging goals.

SEGMENTED K-SPACE VERSUS REAL-TIME AND SINGLE-SHOT ACQUISITION

Data acquisition methods for CMR can generally be divided into segmented k-space or real-time and single-shot scans. Each of these methods has distinct uses and benefits, tailored to meet the requirements of different imaging applications and different patient characteristics.

As the term implies, a segmented k-space scan acquires a subset or "segment" of the k-space data in each cardiac cycle,[9] and data from multiple heartbeats are combined to reconstruct a complete image or series of images (see Fig. 3.5). Segmenting the data acquisition in this fashion, rather than acquiring all of the data for one or more images in a single heartbeat, allows for high spatial and temporal resolution imaging while minimizing motion artifacts. This method relies, however, on the assumption that cardiac motion is periodic and virtually identical in every heartbeat, and that there is no respiratory movement from one beat to the next. Therefore, segmented k-space acquisitions can be challenging in patients with arrhythmias and typically require some form of respiratory motion avoidance (i.e., patient breath-hold or respiratory gating) or respiratory motion compensation. These strategies are discussed in subsequent sections.

In real-time/single-shot acquisition techniques, on the other hand, all of the necessary k-space data for one or more images are acquired within one heartbeat (see Fig. 3.6). Acceleration techniques are used to reduce the total number of k-space lines needed to reconstruct complete images, and compromises in spatial and temporal resolution are made to achieve scan times in the range of tens to a few hundred milliseconds per image. Thus single-shot images can be acquired fast enough to "freeze" respiratory motion and obviate the need for breath-holding or

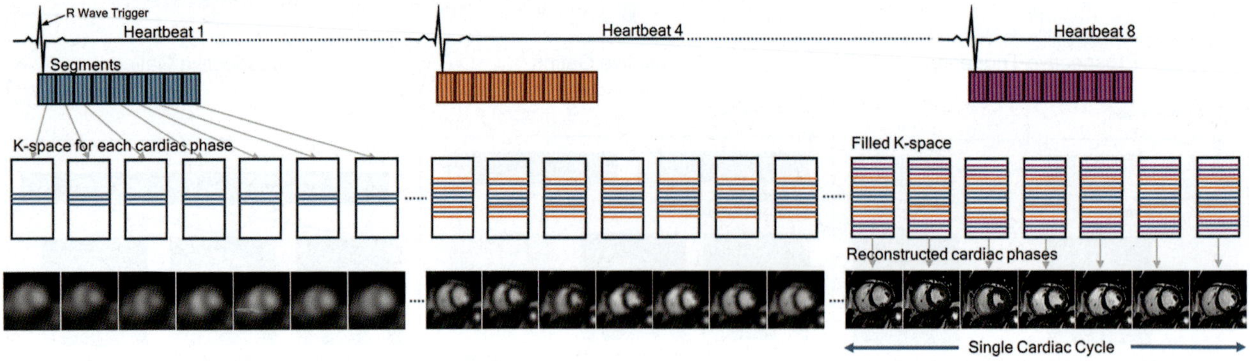

FIG. 3.5 Segmented k-Space Acquisition. A segmented k-space acquisition for a static 2D image or dynamic series such as cine or flow imaging requires data acquisition across multiple heartbeats to represent a single cardiac cycle. In this illustration of the acquisition of a segmented cine, eight heartbeats are required. Once data acquisition is initiated with the detection of an R-wave trigger, several k-space segments are collected within each R-R interval. Based on their timing within the R-R interval, specific k-space segments correspond to a particular cardiac phase. As shown in the illustration, k-space information from a single heartbeat only partially contributes to the cine phases. The k-space for all cardiac phases continues to be filled with each successive heartbeat. Once the entire k-space information is acquired after the eighth heartbeat, the images for all cardiac phases are reconstructed, providing a 2D cine that represents a single complete cardiac cycle.

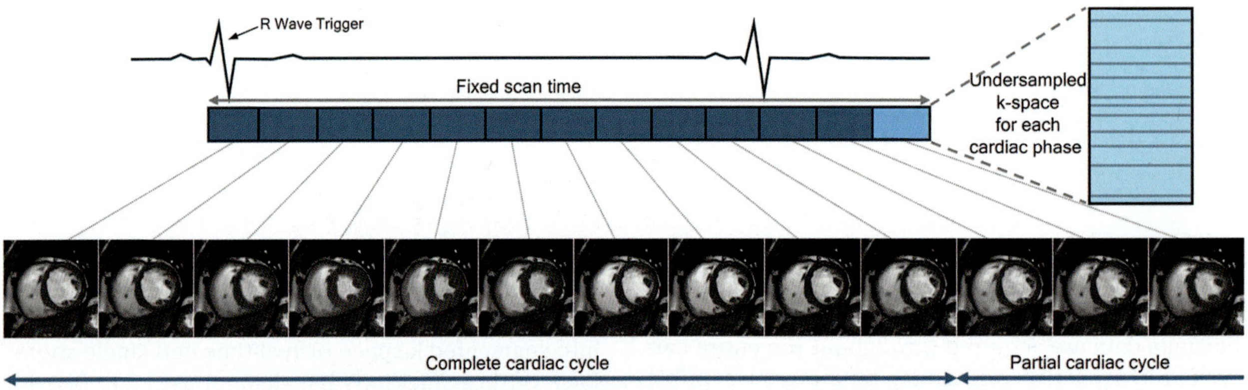

FIG. 3.6 Real-Time/Single-Shot Acquisitions. Real-time images or single-shot images are "snapshot" images, where the entire k-space required for an image is acquired within a single heartbeat. When this concept is extended to cine imaging as illustrated here, data are acquired for a fixed period of time (e.g., 1500 ms) after initiated by a physiological trigger. A set of k-space lines are acquired for every cardiac phase and are reconstructed to provide a complete image. As the scan duration is fixed, more than one cardiac cycle may be acquired and reconstructed—one complete heartbeat and one partial heartbeat are acquired in this example. Real-time cine imaging provides high-speed acquisition by using image acceleration strategies to collect a heavily undersampled and often nonuniformly filled k-space (shown in the illustration) and utilizes image reconstruction methods to recover the missing k-space information. Compared to a segmented cine acquisition, spatial and temporal resolution is usually sacrificed to afford fast real-time imaging.

respiratory gating, and a series of such images can be acquired in rapid succession for real-time cine imaging, analogous to the way dynamic echocardiographic and fluoroscopic scans are performed.

Segmented k-space and real-time/single-shot acquisition strategies are complementary, with situations and applications where one may be advantageous over the other. By dividing up data acquisition over multiple heartbeats, k-space segmentation is particularly useful when high spatial and/or high temporal resolution are required, or if a large amount of data must be acquired such as for high-resolution three-dimensional (3D) anatomy, or four-dimensional (4D) flow imaging. Higher spatial resolution, anatomical coverage, and signal-to-noise ratio (SNR) can be achieved as compared to single-shot techniques by leveraging longer scan times to accumulate data over multiple heartbeats. Similarly, higher temporal resolution can be realized by limiting the number of k-space lines acquired in each beat. For these reasons, segmented k-space is often used for applications where detailed morphological information is needed with high spatial resolution, and where detailed temporal information is required to assess function and flow. However, since data collection spans multiple cardiac cycles and k-space data for individual images are pieced together from different heartbeats, segmented acquisitions are sensitive to heart rate variability and respiratory motion. Longer scan times are required as well, which may be challenging for patients who have difficulty holding their breath and can extend overall exam time, creating challenges for patient comfort and operational efficiency.

While real-time and single-shot scans generally cannot achieve the spatial and temporal resolution of segmented scans, there are applications where this approach is essential to capture dynamic processes in real time (e.g., first-pass perfusion imaging or respiratory cycle dependent flow variations) or preferred when higher spatial or temporal resolution is unnecessary (e.g., "scouting" or slice-planning and imaging for gross morphology). Furthermore, because these techniques are robust against motion artifact, real-time and single-shot imaging have become important clinical tools enabling reliable image quality in patients who have severe arrhythmias or difficulty holding their breath. Scan time is inherently faster than segmented acquisitions, and therefore total exam time can be reduced significantly. The primary disadvantages of real-time/single-shot techniques are lower spatial resolution compared to segmented acquisitions due to the limited time available to collect data, and the potential for blurring if motion is rapid and significant within the longer "temporal footprint" (i.e., poorer temporal resolution) of single-shot data collection. Choosing between these techniques generally involves a trade-off between image quality and practicality in a clinical setting, tailored to the specific diagnostic requirements and patient condition. However, modern approaches to image acceleration based on iterative compressed sensing (CS), and, more recently, the development of deep learning (DL) reconstruction and denoising methods, have narrowed the gap in image quality and spatiotemporal resolution between segmented and real-time/single-shot methods. Based on this evolution, it is likely that real-time/single-shot methods will supplant the use of segmented k-space acquisitions for most CMR applications in the future,[10] except for those requiring large 3D volumes of data.

Respiratory Gating

While patient breath-holding is commonly used in CMR to suspend respiratory motion and thereby avoid motion-induced artifacts,[9] many patients are unable to hold their breath consistently and repeatedly, and the duration of some scans such as high-resolution 3D angiography and 4D flow, exceeds a reasonable breath-hold duration. For these situations, respiratory gating strategies have been developed. Similar to cardiac motion synchronization, a variety of signals can be used to provide a respiratory motion signal or surrogate, including pressure and motion sensors, navigator echoes and images, self-gating, and PT.

RESPIRATORY SYNCHRONIZATION SIGNALS: PRESSURE AND MOTION SENSORS, NAVIGATOR ECHOES, SELF-GATING, PILOT TONE

Pressure and Motion Sensors

Pressure sensors, sometimes called respiratory bellows,[11] can be placed on or around the chest or abdomen of the patient to detect the expansion and contraction associated with breathing. The pressure change is converted into an electrical signal used to synchronize data acquisition with respiration, typically to acquire data at end-expiration when motion is minimal. Respiratory bellows devices have been deployed for many years but require additional setup time and are often not reliable. An important recent innovation involves the use of a separate small RF transmit/receive coil embedded in the patient table.[12] This coil operates outside of the MRI frequency to avoid interaction with the imaging process. Respiratory motion affects the coil loading, causing changes in a small current applied to the coil that can be detected and translated into a respiratory motion signal. Multiple such coils may be embedded in the patient table to effectively detect a respiratory signal whether the patient is positioned head or feet-first into the magnet. The respiratory signal from these devices is automatically detected and displayed without any additional setup and is therefore always available as a means for the technologist to monitor breathing patterns and compliance with breath-hold instructions. However, utilizing this signal for respiratory gating requires pulse sequences specifically designed for this purpose.

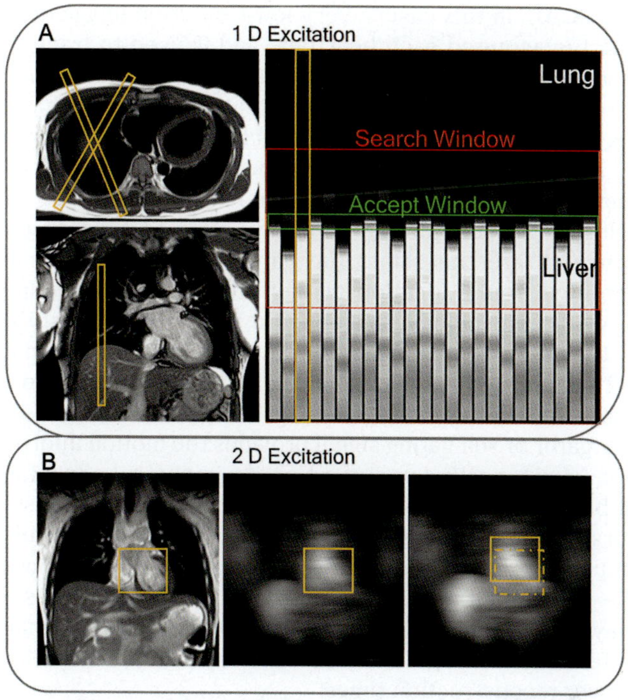

FIG. 3.7 One-Dimensional (1D) and Two-Dimensional (2D) Respiratory Navigator Gating Strategies. Respiratory navigator gating strategies track the respiratory positions to either acquire data or to perform motion correction. In the example shown in panel A, a crossed pair of slice-selective pulses are positioned over the right hemidiaphragm (placement shown in an axial and coronal scout image) to generate 1D navigator echoes. As shown in the image on the right, a predefined search and acceptance window is determined based on an initial brief survey of the individual's respiratory pattern. During the image acquisition, a navigator echo is generated for each heartbeat (a single echo is highlighted by the *yellow box*). The large signal intensity differences between the lung and the liver allow clear detection of the position of the diaphragm. In this example, image data are only accepted at end-expiration heartbeats when the position of the diaphragm falls within the acceptance window. Panel B shows a 2D image-based navigator acquisition. A low-resolution 2D image is acquired within each heartbeat. The position of the heart is tracked with each navigator image, and the information can be used to correct for motion or to resolve the data to different cardiac and respiratory phases. 2D image-based navigators can provide more efficient scan times compared to 1D navigator gating but require more complex data processing.

Respiratory Navigator and Self-Gating

One-dimensional respiratory navigator techniques[13,14] incorporate a navigator-echo readout within the MRI pulse sequence to track the position of the diaphragm at the lung-liver interface (Fig. 3.7A). The navigator echo is acquired each heartbeat, by reading out a single line of MR data from tissue in the path of a "navigator beam", that is oriented in the head-to-foot direction and positioned over the dome of the right hemidiaphragm. This tissue is excited to generate the navigator echo using either a specially designed RF excitation pulse, or the crossing of slice-selective 90- and 180-degree pulse pairs. The received MR signal reflects the head-to-foot movement of the diaphragm during respiration. 2D image-based navigators[15,16] or "iNav" can also be used to track the motion of the heart itself

(Fig. 3.7B). In this case, a very low-resolution image of the heart is acquired each heartbeat and is used to track the translational motion of the heart. Both 1D and 2D navigators can be used for gating of data acquisition that is, accepting or rejecting data in each heartbeat depending on respiratory phase, or for prospective and retrospective motion correction. The distinction between navigator and self-gating techniques is not always clear, and the general concepts are the same. Navigator signals are typically acquired from a location distinct from the imaging plane or volume specifically targeting the motion of interest that is, the diaphragm or the heart, while the self-gating signal[17] is typically derived from a subset of the MRI data used to generate the final image (see Fig. 3.3A). In both cases, the navigator or self-gating signal provides the motion information used for gating or correction. An important advantage of both methods is that they do not require external sensors or other devices; however, they do necessitate pulse sequences designed specifically to acquire and process the navigator or self-gating signals. Complex processing may be required to extract and utilize the motion signals, potentially leading to increased computational load and slower reconstruction times.

Pilot Tone

The same PT technology described previously for cardiac gating (see Fig. 3.3B) can also be utilized for respiratory gating. In fact, the raw PT signal is modulated by both cardiac and respiratory motion, and these can be separated and extracted by signal processing methods.[2]

The PT can provide a continuous real-time respiratory motion signal without the need for placement of an external sensor. However, an additional calibration scan is typically required to reliably suppress interference from RF signals generated as part of the imaging process.[3] Utilization of the PT signal for respiratory gating does require specific signal processing and pulse sequence modifications, and these are only recently becoming available for clinical use.

Choosing the appropriate respiratory motion signal to be used for gating or correction depends on the specific clinical requirements, patient condition, and available MRI technology. It is important that the CMR practitioner understands the strengths and limitations of each method and is able to select the appropriate technique to address various clinical imaging scenarios.

PART II—MOTION CORRECTION

Prospective Motion Correction

Prospective motion correction and slice tracking techniques in cardiac MRI proactively address the root cause of motion artifacts during data acquisition to improve image quality. Prospective motion correction generally applies only to respiratory motion and can potentially eliminate the need for patient breath-holding. This approach involves real-time detection of respiratory movement, typically through the use of 1D[14] or 2D[16] navigators (Fig. 3.7) or a self-gating signal[17] (Fig. 3.3). Prospective motion correction adjusts the imaging parameters (e.g., slice position, orientation, and sometimes the encoding gradients) to track with the respiratory motion of the heart in real time. Specialized hardware (like optical tracking systems) or imaging sequences (such as navigator echoes or self-gating) are used to monitor the position and motion of the heart and chest during the MRI scan. This information is continuously fed back to the MRI system, and based on the real-time motion data, the position and orientation of the imaging plane or volume is adjusted to follow the respiratory motion of the heart. Prospective motion correction can be applied in both single-shot and segmented k-space acquisitions. In the case of single-shot imaging, this can help with the registration of multiple slices acquired for averaging or for alignment of 2D slices for 3D reformatting. In segmented k-space imaging, prospective correction is often used in combination with gating (acceptance/rejection) to apply prospective corrections to slice position only within a narrow gating window. Other techniques[16] rely solely on prospective respiratory motion correction to achieve 100% gating efficiency and provide the convenience of a fixed scan time, which is not the case if acceptance/rejection gating is employed. Prospective respiratory motion correction can obviate the need for patient breath-hold, which is especially beneficial for patients who have difficulty doing so, such as young children, the elderly, or those with advanced cardiovascular disease.

Retrospective Motion Correction

Retrospective motion correction typically does not employ the use of internal or external signals, but rather most commonly is applied to register multiple single-shot images of the same slice acquired during free-breathing for the purpose of averaging to boost SNR[18] or to generate parameter maps such as T1,[19] T2,[20] T2*,[21] and myocardial blood flow[22] (Fig. 3.8). In these applications, the original single-shot images are acquired fast enough to be insensitive to respiratory motion artifacts; retrospective motion correction has no effect on motion artifact in the original images but is instead used to align images to enable further processing. This method is often referred to as MOCO, as an acronym for MOtion COrrection. In the MOCO-LGE technique,[18] multiple single-shot LGE images are acquired during free-breathing, using acceleration techniques to achieve spatial and temporal resolution comparable to segmented breath-hold imaging at the expense of SNR (Fig. 3.8A). Registering these original source images to each other can compensate for in-plane respiratory motion, permitting simple averaging to be used to recover SNR. This method cannot account for through-plane motion, however, and thus some gating or rejection of those original images requiring the greatest amount of motion correction is often employed. This same strategy is commonly utilized to generate myocardial T1 and T2 maps, which requires image registration to fit T1 recovery or T2 decay curves on a pixel-wise basis[20,22] (Fig. 3.8B). The technique is similarly applied to generate myocardial blood flow maps from first-pass perfusion images, where retrospective motion correction is used to align the images dynamically acquired following the bolus injection of contrast agent (Fig. 3.8C).

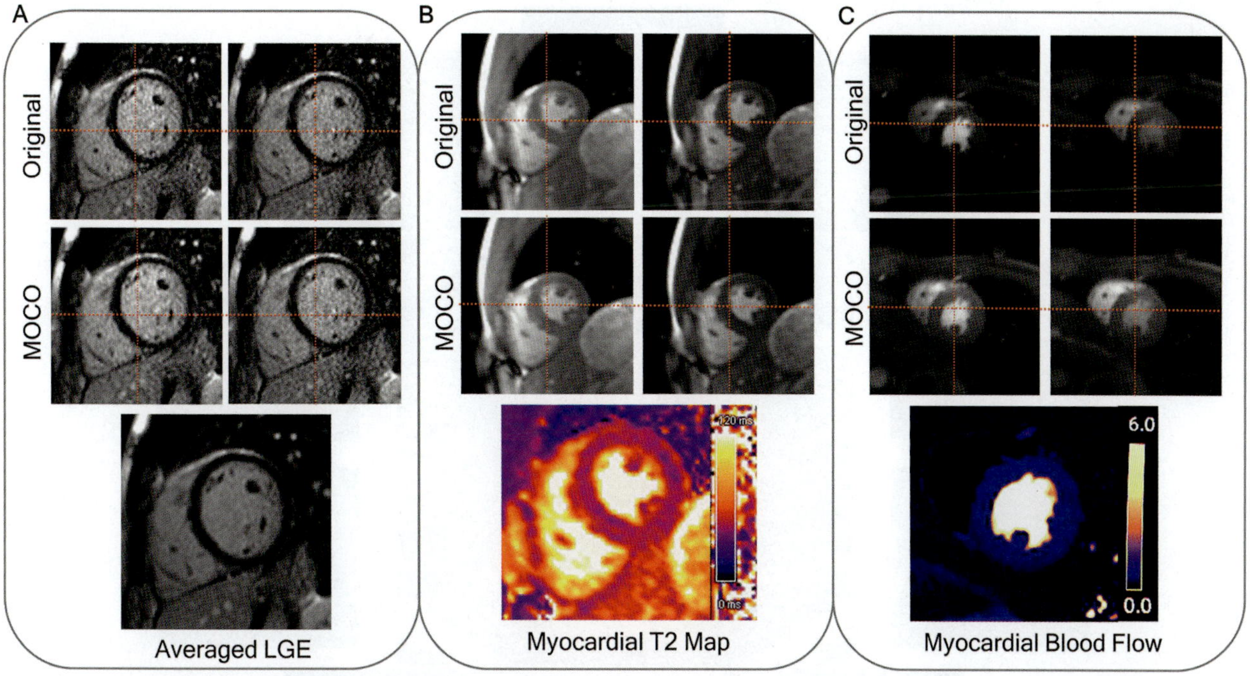

FIG. 3.8 Retrospective Motion Correction Applications. Retrospective motion correction strategies can be applied to register single-shot images for different cardiac magnetic resonance applications. Panel A shows the example of motion-corrected and averaged single-shot late gadolinium enhancement (LGE) imaging. High spatial resolution single-shot LGE images are collected free-breathing across multiple heartbeats (typically eight or more images). A motion correction algorithm is then retrospectively applied to register the individual LGE images. The motion-corrected images are then averaged together to generate an image that has high signal-to-noise ratio compared to the individual single-shot images. Panel B shows the same motion correction algorithm applied to myocardial T2 mapping. Single-shot images collected with different T2 preparation times (typically three images in total) are motion corrected and registered together. A pixel-wise fit is then performed across the images to generate a quantitative T2 map. Panel C shows motion correction applied to register the individual single-shot perfusion images (typically 40 to 60 images in total) acquired during bolus injection of gadolinium-based contrast. The registered images can then be used to derive a quantitative myocardial blood flow map. For simplified illustration, only two of the single-shot source images are shown for each application.

PART III—ACCELERATION TECHNIQUES

While the strategies for motion synchronization and correction outlined in the previous sections can successfully reduce or avoid motion artifact, advanced acceleration methods including parallel imaging (PI), CS, and artificial intelligence (AI) DL-based reconstruction are instrumental in increasing the efficiency and reliability of CMR. Acceleration techniques can be combined with gating to reduce breath-hold times and overall exam times, increasing patient comfort and compliance. Higher acceleration can reduce scan times to the point that high-quality real-time and single-shot imaging is possible, eliminating the need for breath-holding and for cardiac and respiratory synchronization in many applications. This section provides a summary of currently utilized acceleration techniques, along with their comparative advantages and disadvantages.

Parallel Imaging Reconstruction

PI is one of the earliest and most widely adopted methods used to reduce MRI scan times. PI techniques take advantage of the spatial sensitivity profiles of multiple receiver coil arrays to reduce the number of phase-encoding steps required during acquisition, thereby shortening the total scan duration. Each coil element has a unique spatial sensitivity profile, that is, it receives signals from different regions of the body with varying intensities. By combining the data from multiple coils, PI can effectively "fill in" the missing information in undersampled data (Fig. 3.9). The two most commonly used PI methods in cardiac MRI are sensitivity encoding (SENSE)[23] and generalized autocalibrating partially parallel acquisitions (GRAPPA).[24] The SENSE technique directly reconstructs the image by solving an inverse problem that combines data from all coils using their individual sensitivity maps. The coil sensitivity maps are typically obtained through precalibration scans or autocalibration techniques. The SENSE algorithm works by solving a set of linear equations that enforce data consistency based on the coil sensitivities, which allows the reconstruction of undersampled data. GRAPPA operates in k-space (the raw data space). It estimates the missing k-space lines by using data from neighboring acquired lines, with the assumption that the acquired data contains sufficient spatial information. GRAPPA requires a set of calibration data (often acquired at the center of k-space) to estimate the weights needed for interpolation of missing k-lines.

By reducing the number of acquired k-space lines, PI techniques accelerate cardiac MRI scans, reducing motion artifacts and improving patient comfort by minimizing the time required to hold their breath or stay still.[25] Reduction in scan time by acceleration techniques is particularly beneficial for patients who have difficulty holding their breath or for capturing dynamic processes in real-time. PI techniques are widely compatible and are commonly utilized

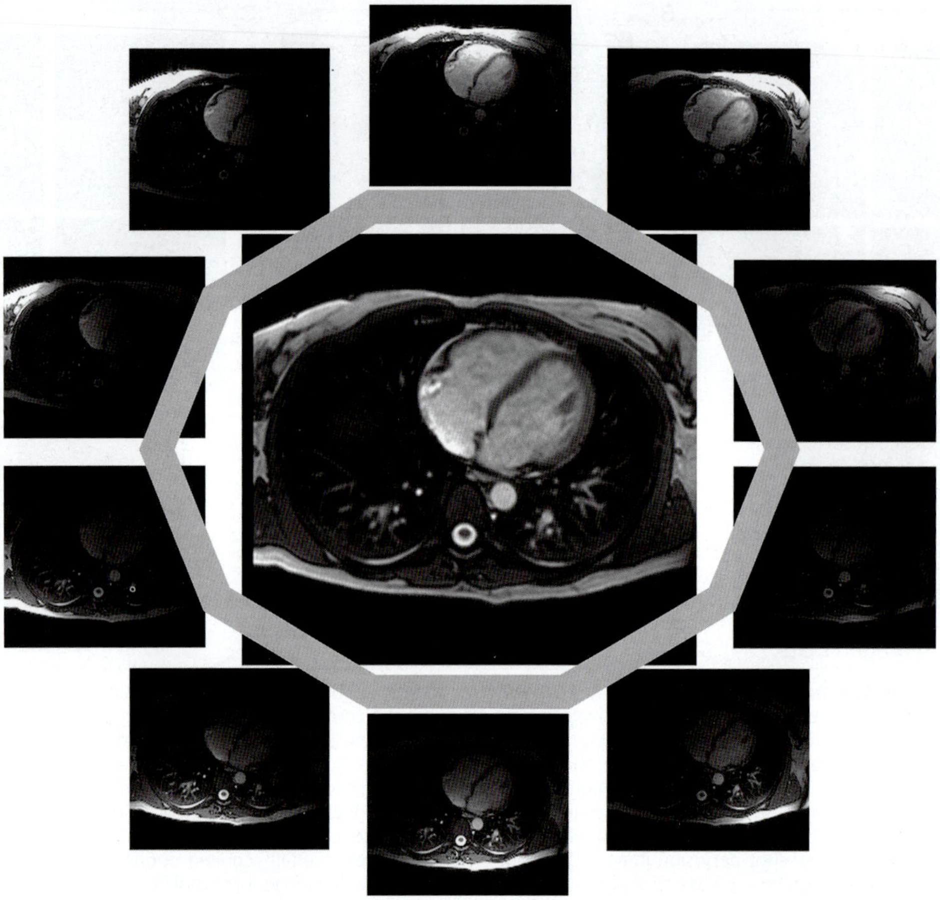

FIG. 3.9 Parallel Imaging. Parallel imaging is an acceleration strategy to reduce the total scan duration. In this example, the central image is an axial single-shot image of the chest acquired using an acceleration rate 2, that is, the k-space is undersampled by a factor of 2. The individual coil images are shown surrounding the reconstructed image, demonstrating the variation in signal intensities based on the proximity of the coil element to the anatomical structure. For simplified illustration, not all coil images are displayed. A generalized autocalibrating partially parallel acquisitions–based reconstruction will interpolate the missing k-space lines to reconstruct the image, while a sensitivity encoding–based reconstruction will utilize the individual coil sensitivity information.

with nearly all cardiac MRI sequences across various clinical applications.

PI techniques, however, are limited in the acceleration rates that can be achieved. Aggressive acceleration factors may amplify noise, degrading image quality, and inaccuracies in coil sensitivity maps can lead to ghosting and blurring artifacts. Coil sensitivity calibration methods must account for coil and patient movement throughout the scan, which present challenges for free-breathing acquisitions. Balancing acceleration with signal-to-noise and artifact considerations is crucial for optimal results, and for most cardiac imaging applications, the acceleration rates are limited to factors of 2 or 3; that is, sampling of one-half to one-third of full k-space data (Fig. 3.10). While PI achieves only modest acceleration rates compared to the more recently developed CS and DL methods, the image quality is highly reliable, and this degree of acceleration has proven sufficient to enable a broad range of robust clinical applications.

Compressed Sensing (CS) Reconstruction

CS is a more recently developed technique used to reconstruct undersampled k-space data that builds on the observation that cardiac MRI data are sparse in some transform domain (e.g., wavelet or temporal Fourier domain).[26] This sparsity means that the raw MRI data can be represented by relatively few nonzero coefficients in the appropriate domain. The key idea behind CS is to exploit this sparsity to reconstruct images from undersampled data using an iterative optimization process.[27] This process enforces both data consistency (i.e., the reconstructed image must closely match the acquired k-space data) and sparsity (i.e., the image should have a compact representation in the chosen transform domain). The reconstruction problem is typically formulated as an optimization problem:

$$\hat{\rho} = argmin_{\rho} \, \|E_{\rho} - s\|_2^2 + \lambda R(\rho)$$

where E is the encoding operator that includes the coil sensitivities and Fourier transform, $\hat{\rho}$ is the image to be reconstructed, $\boldsymbol{s}$ is the acquired k-space data, and $\lambda R(\rho)$ is the regularization term that promotes sparsity. The parameter λ controls the trade-off between data fidelity and regularization.

Instead of uniformly undersampling the k-space lines as is usually done with PI reconstruction methods, CS techniques employ pseudorandomly sampled k-space lines.[28,29] This approach is fundamentally different from traditional MRI sampling strategies and helps in distributing the undersampling aliasing artifacts throughout the field of view as incoherent noise rather than as coherent ghost artifacts. Incoherent

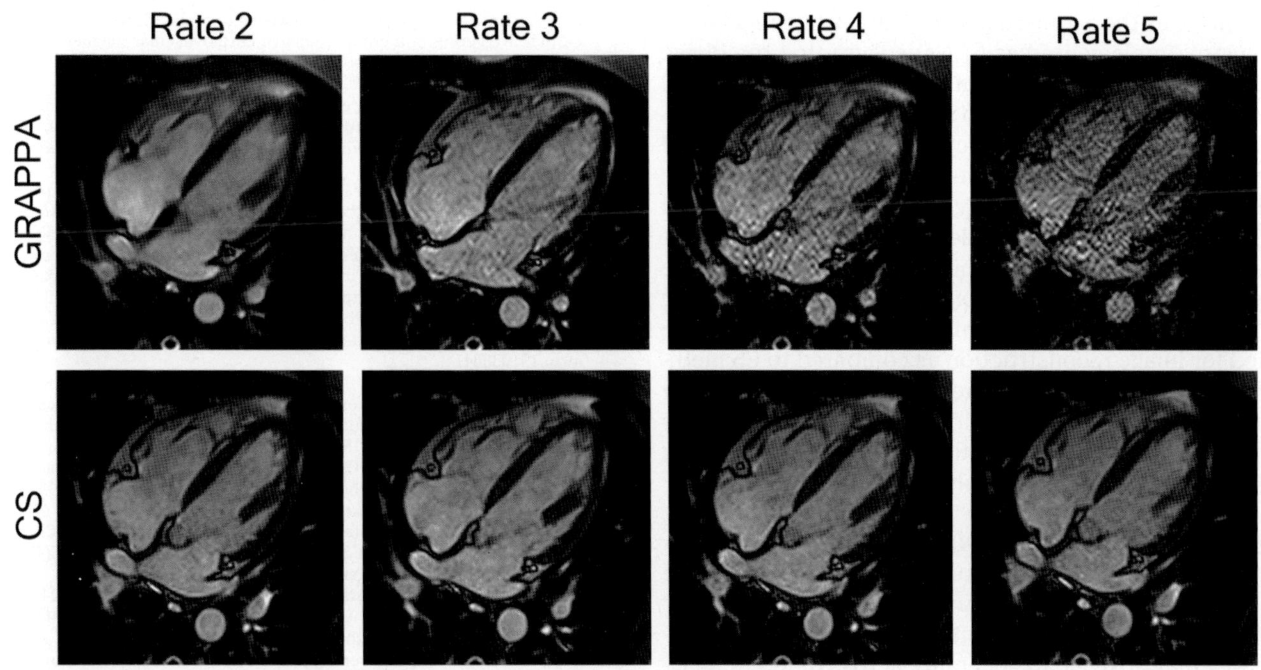

FIG. 3.10 Image Acceleration and Image Quality. An end-diastole cardiac phase of a breath-held segmented cine acquisition in a four-chamber view of the heart is shown for different image acceleration rates. The top row shows images reconstructed with generalized autocalibrating partially parallel acquisitions (GRAPPA)–based acceleration, while the bottom row shows images reconstructed with compressed sensing (CS). As observed, image quality significantly degrades at acceleration rates 4 and 5 for GRAPPA, while image quality is relatively preserved for the CS reconstruction even at rate 5 acceleration.

noise can be more easily minimized during the CS reconstruction process. In practice, CS-based reconstruction involves nonlinear iterative algorithms, such as the split Bregman or FISTA (fast iterative shrinkage-thresholding algorithm), which apply the sparsity-enforcing regularization term and maintain data consistency.[27] These algorithms iteratively minimize the difference between the measured undersampled data and the predicted data from the reconstructed images while ensuring the images remain sparse in the transform domain. By leveraging these principles, CS reconstruction techniques can achieve higher acceleration compared to PI without significant loss in image quality (Fig. 3.10). In practice, CS has been shown to achieve acceleration factors of 5 to 10 times in various cardiac imaging applications, such as dynamic real-time cine imaging and 4D flow imaging.

One disadvantage of CS-based reconstruction is that these are iterative techniques that are computationally demanding, leading to longer reconstruction times that can be disruptive to clinical imaging workflow and decrease efficiency. This problem has largely been solved through programming strategies for computational speed and through the use of powerful GPU-based computers for image reconstruction; however, when applied to a sequence that generates large datasets, such as multidimensional cine and flow, the reconstruction times are still on the order of several minutes. One potential pitfall of CS reconstruction is that the quality of the reconstructed image heavily depends on the chosen sparsity constraint and reconstruction algorithm parameters, which may not be properly tuned for a given imaging scenario. Additionally, CS requires careful tuning of multiple parameters, such as the sparsity basis, regularization weight, and reconstruction algorithm, to achieve high-quality results. If these parameters are not chosen carefully, the reconstructed images may appear overly smooth or artificial. Careful optimization of acquisition and reconstruction parameters is necessary to minimize these effects.

DL Reconstruction

Recent advances in AI, particularly DL, have introduced new opportunities to overcome the limitations of PI and CS reconstruction techniques.[27,30–34] DL-based reconstruction methods leverage large datasets of previously acquired MRI data to learn and model the relationship between undersampled k-space data, or aliased/noisy images reconstructed from undersampled data, and high-quality images reconstructed from fully sampled k-space. Once trained, these models can potentially be applied to new, undersampled datasets to rapidly provide high-quality images from highly undersampled data.

Convolutional neural networks (CNNs) are well suited for analyzing spatial and temporal patterns in image data. In this context, CNNs are trained to learn the mapping between undersampled k-space data and fully sampled images. *End-to-end* CNNs take undersampled images as input and directly output fully reconstructed images. The CNN learns to "denoise" the undersampled data and fill in missing details, effectively performing the role of the traditional iterative reconstruction algorithms used in CS. One notable architecture is the *U-Net*, which is popular for medical imaging tasks due to its ability to capture multiscale features. *Unrolled networks* mimic the iterative optimization algorithms used in CS and PI, but with learned parameters. In these models, the iterative process is "unrolled" into a series of network layers, where each layer corresponds to one step in the iterative algorithm. A data consistency layer enforces that the reconstructed image matches the acquired k-space data, while regularization layers (implemented as CNNs) ensure that the image is sparse or smooth in certain domains. These unrolled networks can be trained end to end, learning both the regularization and data consistency steps needed to go from undersampled k-space to reconstructed images.

DL methods can potentially correct for artifacts and improve image fidelity at acceleration rates beyond what PI- and CS-based methods alone can achieve. Once the model is trained, reconstruction can be very fast, offering near real-time processing, significantly reducing the time needed for image reconstruction as compared to CS methods.[35,36] AI models also have the potential to continuously improve over time with exposure to more data, potentially offering even faster reconstruction speeds and higher image quality as the model evolves.

LIMITATIONS AND CHALLENGES

DL models are often specific to the type of MRI sequence and anatomy on which they were trained, limiting their generalizability across different clinical scenarios; therefore, they may struggle to generalize across different imaging protocols, anatomies, or scanner vendors. Fine-tuning or retraining models on diverse datasets representative of clinical variability can improve generalization performance. AI-based reconstruction models require large amounts of training data to learn robust representations of image structures and artifacts; such data can be difficult to obtain, especially if raw k-space data are needed. Ensuring the quality and diversity of training data is essential to prevent overfitting and improve reconstruction accuracy. Training and deploying AI models for real-time image reconstruction can be computationally demanding, requiring high-performance computing resources. The "black-box" nature of DL models can make it difficult to understand how the model is making its reconstruction decisions, raising potential concerns for clinical applications.

SUMMARY

In summary, the technologies developed for gating, motion correction, and acceleration techniques have significantly improved the efficiency and quality of cardiac MRI. By integrating physiological synchronization with innovative acceleration methods like PI, CS, and DL, we can achieve faster, more reliable imaging with fewer artifacts. These improvements not only enhance image quality, reliability, and workflow efficiency, but also contribute to greater patient comfort and compliance. As DL continues to evolve, it is poised to play a pivotal role in the future of cardiovascular imaging, supporting even higher acceleration rates than currently achievable by PI and CS techniques alone.

REFERENCES

1. Larson AC, White RD, Laub G, McVeigh ER, Li D, Simonetti OP. Self-gated cardiac cine MRI. *Magn Reson Med.* 2004;51(1):93–102. https://doi.org/10.1002/mrm.10664.
2. Chen C, Liu Y, Simonetti OP, et al. Cardiac and respiratory motion extraction for MRI using pilot tone-a patient study. *Int J Cardiovasc Imaging.* 2024;40(1):93–105. https://doi.org/10.1007/s10554-023-02966-z.
3. Pan Y, Varghese J, Tong MS, et al. Two-center validation of Pilot Tone based cardiac triggering of a comprehensive cardiovascular magnetic resonance examination. *Int J Cardiovasc Imaging.* 2024;40(2):261–273. https://doi.org/10.1007/s10554-023-03002-w.
4. Vahle T, Bacher M, Rigie D, et al. Respiratory motion detection and correction for MR using the pilot tone: applications for MR and simultaneous PET/MR examinations. *Invest Radiol.* 2020;55(3):153–159. https://doi.org/10.1097/RLI.0000000000000619.
5. Feinstein JA, Epstein FH, Arai AE, et al. Using cardiac phase to order reconstruction (CAPTOR): a method to improve diastolic images. *J Magn Reson Imaging.* 1997;7(5):794–798. https://doi.org/10.1002/jmri.1880070505.
6. Edelman RR, Wallner B, Singer A, Atkinson DJ, Saini S. Segmented turboFLASH: method for breath-hold MR imaging of the liver with flexible contrast. *Radiology.* 1990;177(2):515–521. https://doi.org/10.1148/radiology.177.2.2171014.
7. Debbins JP, Riederer SJ, Rossman PJ, et al. Cardiac magnetic resonance fluoroscopy. *Magn Reson Med.* 1996;36(4):588–595. https://doi.org/10.1002/mrm.1910360414.
8. Lee VS, Resnick D, Bundy JM, Simonetti OP, Lee P, Weinreb JC. Cardiac function: MR evaluation in one breath hold with real-time true fast imaging with steady-state precession. *Radiology.* 2002;222(3):835–842. https://doi.org/10.1148/radiol.2223011156.
9. Atkinson DJ, Edelman RR. Cineangiography of the heart in a single breath hold with a segmented turboFLASH sequence. *Radiology.* 1991;178(2):357–360. https://doi.org/10.1148/radiology.178.2.1987592.
10. Contijoch F, Rasche V, Seiberlich N, Peters DC. The future of CMR: all-in-one vs. real-time CMR (Part 2). *J Cardiovasc Magn Reson.* 2024;26(1):100998. https://doi.org/10.1016/j.jocmr.2024.100998.
11. Santelli C, Nezafat R, Goddu B, et al. Respiratory bellows revisited for motion compensation: preliminary experience for cardiovascular MR. *Magn Reson Med.* 2011;65(4):1097–1102. https://doi.org/10.1002/mrm.22687.
12. Runge VM, Richter JK, Heverhagen JT. Motion in magnetic resonance: new paradigms for improved clinical diagnosis. *Invest Radiol.* 2019;54(7):383–395. https://doi.org/10.1097/RLI.0000000000000566.
13. Ehman RL, Felmlee JP. Adaptive technique for high-definition MR imaging of moving structures. *Radiology.* 1989;173(1):255–263. https://doi.org/10.1148/radiology.173.1.2781017.
14. Wang Y, Rossman PJ, Grimm RC, Riederer SJ, Ehman RL. Navigator-echo-based real-time respiratory gating and triggering for reduction of respiration effects in three-dimensional coronary MR angiography. *Radiology.* 1996;198(1):55–60. https://doi.org/10.1148/radiology.198.1.8539406.
15. Henningsson M, Botnar RM. Advanced respiratory motion compensation for coronary MR angiography. *Sensors (Basel).* 2013;13(6):6882–6899. https://doi.org/10.3390/s130606882.
16. Henningsson M, Smink J, Razavi R, Botnar RM. Prospective respiratory motion correction for coronary MR angiography using a 2D image navigator. *Magn Reson Med.* 2013;69(2):486–494. https://doi.org/10.1002/mrm.24280.
17. Larson AC, Kellman P, Arai A, et al. Preliminary investigation of respiratory self-gating for free-breathing segmented cine MRI. *Magn Reson Med.* 2005;53(1):159–168. https://doi.org/10.1002/mrm.20331.
18. Kellman P, Larson AC, Hsu LY, et al. Motion-corrected free-breathing delayed enhancement imaging of myocardial infarction. *Magn Reson Med.* 2005;53(1):194–200. https://doi.org/10.1002/mrm.20333.
19. Xue H, Davies RH, Brown LAE, et al. Automated inline analysis of myocardial perfusion MRI with deep learning. *Radiol Artif Intell.* 2020;2(6):e200009. https://doi.org/10.1148/ryai.2020200009.
20. Giri S, Shah S, Xue H, et al. Myocardial T(2) mapping with respiratory navigator and automatic nonrigid motion correction. *Magn Reson Med.* 2012;68(5):1570–1578. https://doi.org/10.1002/mrm.24139.
21. Jin N, da Silveira JS, Jolly MP, et al. Free-breathing myocardial T2* mapping using GRE-EPI and automatic non-rigid motion correction. *J Cardiovasc Magn Reson.* 2015;17:113. https://doi.org/10.1186/s12968-015-0216-z.
22. Xue H, Shah S, Greiser A, et al. Motion correction for myocardial T1 mapping using image registration with synthetic image estimation. *Magn Reson Med.* 2012;67(6):1644–1655. https://doi.org/10.1002/mrm.23153.
23. Pruessmann KP, Weiger M, Scheidegger MB, Boesiger P. SENSE: sensitivity encoding for fast MRI. *Magn Reson Med.* 1999;42(5):952–962.
24. Griswold MA, Jakob PM, Heidemann RM, et al. Generalized autocalibrating partially parallel acquisitions (GRAPPA). *Magn Reson Med.* 2002;47(6):1202–1210. https://doi.org/10.1002/mrm.10171.
25. Deshmane A, Gulani V, Griswold MA, Seiberlich N. Parallel MR imaging. *J Magn Reson Imaging.* 2012;36(1):55–72. https://doi.org/10.1002/jmri.23639.
26. Lustig M, Donoho D, Pauly JM. Sparse MRI: the application of compressed sensing for rapid MR imaging. *Magn Reson Med.* 2007;58(6):1182–1195. https://doi.org/10.1002/mrm.21391.
27. Bustin A, Fuin N, Botnar RM, Prieto C. From compressed-sensing to artificial intelligence-based cardiac MRI reconstruction. *Front Cardiovasc Med.* 2020;7:17. https://doi.org/10.3389/fcvm.2020.00017.
28. Ahmad R, Xue H, Giri S, Ding Y, Craft J, Simonetti OP. Variable density incoherent spatiotemporal acquisition (VISTA) for highly accelerated cardiac MRI. *Magn Reson Med.* 2015;74(5):1266–1278. https://doi.org/10.1002/mrm.25507.
29. Rich A, Gregg M, Jin N, et al. CArtesian sampling with Variable density and Adjustable temporal resolution (CAVA). *Magn Reson Med.* 2020;83(6):2015–2025. https://doi.org/10.1002/mrm.28059.
30. Hammernik K, Klatzer T, Kobler E, et al. Learning a variational network for reconstruction of accelerated MRI data. *Magn Reson Med.* 2018;79(6):3055–3071. https://doi.org/10.1002/mrm.26977.

31. Knoll F, Hammernik K, Zhang C, et al. Deep-learning methods for parallel magnetic resonance imaging reconstruction: a survey of the current approaches, trends, and issues. *IEEE Signal Process Mag.* 2020;37(1):128–140. https://doi.org/10.1109/MSP.2019.2950640.
32. Oscanoa JA, Middione MJ, Alkan C, et al. Deep learning-based reconstruction for cardiac MRI: a review. *Bioengineering (Basel).* 2023;10(3). https://doi.org/10.3390/bioengineering10030334.
33. Vornehm M, Wetzl J, Giese D, et al. CineVN: variational network reconstruction for rapid functional cardiac cine MRI. *Magn Reson Med.* 2024. https://doi.org/10.1002/mrm.30260.
34. Zhu B, Liu JZ, Cauley SF, Rosen BR, Rosen MS. Image reconstruction by domain-transform manifold learning. *Nature.* 2018;555(7697):487–492. https://doi.org/10.1038/nature25988.
35. Jaubert O, Montalt-Tordera J, Knight D, et al. Real-time deep artifact suppression using recurrent U-Nets for low-latency cardiac MRI. *Magn Reson Med.* 2021a;86(4):1904–1916. https://doi.org/10.1002/mrm.28834.
36. Jaubert O, Steeden J, Montalt-Tordera J, Arridge S, Kowalik GT, Muthurangu V. Deep artifact suppression for spiral real-time phase contrast cardiac magnetic resonance imaging in congenital heart disease. *Magn Reson Imaging.* 2021b;83:125–132. https://doi.org/10.1016/j.mri.2021.08.005.

4 Techniques for T1, T2, and Extra-Cellular Volume (ECV) Mapping

PETER KELLMAN AND MICHAEL S. HANSEN

Many disease processes alter the local molecular environment of the myocardium and consequently, the longitudinal (T1) and transverse (T2) relaxation times can change. While such changes may be observed directly as changes in image contrast,[1–6] the tissue processes may be global and diffuse, hampering reliable detection of the disease. Quantitative methods for characterizing myocardial tissue based on parametric mapping of T1 and T2 have been proposed as objective ways of detecting and quantifying both focal and global changes in tissue. In combination with extracellular contrast agent injection, T1 mapping can also provide an estimate of the extracellular volume (ECV).

Native T1 mapping and ECV mapping are currently being explored as diagnostic tools for a wide range of cardiomyopathies; native T1 changes are detectable in both acute and chronic myocardial infarction (MI)[7,8] and may be used to characterize the edematous area at risk.[4,9,10] Elevated native T1 has also been reported in a number of diseases with cardiac involvement including myocarditis,[11] amyloidosis,[12] lupus,[13] and system capillary leakage syndrome,[14] and decreases in native T1 have been associated with Anderson-Fabry disease[15] and high iron content.[16,17] Native T2 mapping is used to detect edema in acute MI and myocarditis[18-20] and to identify the area at risk[4] in acute MI. Application of tissue characterization using parametric mapping for detection of disease is discussed in a following chapter.

This chapter describes state of the art methods for measuring T1, T2, and ECV in the myocardium. Since the purpose of such techniques is quantitative (objective) evaluation of biomarkers and disease, the discussion of the available techniques is framed in terms of accuracy, precision, and general reliability. In parametric mapping it is important to understand errors in quantification and other artifact mechanisms, which may be less familiar than conventional cardiovascular magnetic resonance (CMR) artifact mechanisms. Method imperfections may manifest themselves as subtle changes in measured tissue parameters and artifactual changes may well be correlated with specific patient groups (i.e., they are potential confounders). In particular, estimated parameter values such as T1 may be affected by other variables such as myocardial wall thickness, T2, protocols settings, or scanner adjustments. Although this is not new to magnetic resonance imaging (MRI), in which T1-weighted contrast may have some T2 contrast, these confounding effects may influence the interpretation of parametric maps. Normal values for parameters may depend on the field strength and the specific measurement technique or imaging protocol. Therefore, well-controlled and optimized protocols are key to reproducibility, which is particularly important in applications aiming at detection of subtle fibrosis and preclinical disease, and when normal values need to be established for specific protocols. Limited spatial resolution will lead to errors caused by partial volume effects, particularly between myocardium and adjacent blood pool or fat tissue. Despite limitations, parametric mapping is a powerful tool in the assessment of diffuse myocardial disease.

T1 AND EXTRA-CELLULAR VOLUME MAPPING

Changes in both native T1 and T1 following administration of gadolinium (Gd) contrast agents are considered important biomarkers and multiple methods have been suggested for quantifying myocardial T1 in vivo.[21] In general, methods for measuring myocardial T1 consist of three components: (1) a perturbation of the longitudinal magnetization (i.e., an inversion or saturation), (2) an experiment to sample the relaxation curve as the longitudinal magnetization returns to its original level, and (3) a model used to fit the sampled curve and extract the myocardial T1. This chapter focuses on the technical aspects of key methods and imaging protocols and describes their limitations and the factors that influence their accuracy, precision, and overall reproducibility. The accuracy and precision of these measurements affect the detection and quantification of abnormal myocardial tissue.

Late Gd enhancement (LGE) is currently the primary tool for tissue characterization in CMR since it provides excellent depiction of MI and focal scar and has become an accepted standard for assessing myocardial viability.[22] LGE is also useful for detecting and characterizing fibrosis that is "patchy" in appearance (e.g., as seen in nonischemic cardiomyopathies such hypertrophic cardiomyopathy).[23] Diffuse myocardial fibrosis is, however, more difficult to distinguish using LGE since the myocardial signal intensity may be nearly isointense and may be globally "nulled," thus appearing to be normal tissue.[24] Alternatively, quantitative measurement of myocardial T1 following administration of an extracellular Gd contrast agent has been shown to be sensitive to the increased ECV associated with diffuse myocardial fibrosis. However, a single post-contrast T1 measurement has limitations due to a variety of confounding factors such as Gd clearance rate, time of measurement, injected dose, body composition, and hematocrit.[25,26] These factors cause a significant variation in post-contrast T1 making it difficult to distinguish diseased and normal tissue based on absolute T1 values alone. Pre-contrast T1 varies with water content and may be elevated in cases of diffuse myocardial fibrosis. Pre-contrast T1 also varies significantly with field strength.[27] Direct measurement of ECV was initially developed for quantifying the myocardial extracellular fractional distribution volume[28] and has been proposed as a means for detection and quantification of diffuse myocardial fibrosis.[24,29–34] This approach is based on the change in T1 following administration of an extracellular contrast agent and circumvents the limitation of a single postcontrast T1 measurement in detecting a global change in T1. Myocardial ECV is measured as the percent of tissue comprised of extracellular space, which is a physiologically intuitive unit of measurement and is independent of field strength. ECV has been shown to correlate with collagen volume fraction in some diseases.[29,31]

Brief History of Methods for T1 Mapping in the Heart

Methods for measuring myocardial T1 were initially based on region of interest (ROI) analysis rather than pixel-wise parametric maps. Inversion recovery images at different inversion times were acquired with multiple breath-holds[35] or inversion recovery cine protocols were used as a means of acquiring data in a single breath-hold.[36] These early methods were ROI-based schemes and were not suitable for pixel-wise mapping. Pixel-wise T1-mapping was introduced with the modified Look-Locker inversion recovery (MOLLI) imaging strategy,[37] which propelled the use of T1 mapping in CMR and inspired many new methods. MOLLI is widely used today with some protocol optimization and other adaptations. A shortened breath-hold adaptation with conditional curve fitting (ShMOLLI)[38] was proposed as a means of mitigating heart rate dependence as well as shortening the breath-hold. Further protocol optimization has been aimed at shortening the breath-hold and optimizing precision.[32,39] Motion correction was developed to mitigate respiratory motion for subjects with poor breath-holding[40] and phase-sensitive inversion recovery reconstruction with motion correction further improved image quality.[41] A number of publications analyzed the accuracy of T1 measurements,[37,38,42–45] leading to a better understanding of the influence of various protocol parameters on T1 measurement errors. Saturation recovery methods that were initially developed for T1 measurements during first pass contrast-enhanced perfusion (SAP-T1)[46] have recently been adapted for T1 mapping using saturation recovery single-shot acquisition (SASHA)[47] with a steady-state free precession (SSFP) readout as a means of mitigating the T1 underestimation in MOLLI and reducing the influence of confounding factors such as T2, magnetization transfer (MT), heart rate, and off-resonance. Even more recently, hybrid schemes have been proposed that incorporate both inversion and saturation recovery methods (SAPPHIRE).[48] ECV measurements were initially introduced using ROI-based measurements[28–30] and pixel-wise ECV mapping was

TABLE 4.1 Widely used inversion and saturation recovery methods for T1 mapping in the heart.

Inversion Recovery (IR)	Multiple breath-hold FLASH[35] MOLLI[37] ShMOLLI[38] modified MOLLI Protocols[32,33,44,45]
Saturation recovery (SR)	SAP-T1[46] SASHA[47,51,52] SASHA VFA[53] SMART1[54] mSASHA[55,56]
Combined IR/SR	SAPPHIRE[48]

later introduced.[33,39] Improvements to T1 and ECV mapping are continuously being introduced such as navigated methods for higher resolution 3D[49] or 2D multislices.[50]

This chapter focuses on the basic concepts behind the widely used MOLLI and SASHA acquisition strategies for T1 mapping, followed by a review of factors influencing accuracy and precision. The discussion includes a description of other limitations and a summary of pros and cons of various protocols.

T1 Mapping Methods

The currently used protocols for T1 mapping in the heart (Table 4.1) are based on inversion (IR) or saturation recovery (SR). Images are acquired at multiple time points on the recovery curve, and pixel-wise curve fitting is performed to estimate the relaxation time parameter and produce a pixel map of T1. Images are generally acquired at the same cardiac phase and respiratory position to eliminate tissue motion. Although initial implementation involved multiple breath-holds, current methods generally use single breath-hold protocols with single-shot 2D-imaging. To achieve higher spatial resolution and/or 3D imaging segmentation may be required.

The original scheme known as MOLLI, proposed by Messroghli, et al.,[37] is illustrated in Fig. 4.1. For each inversion, the MOLLI method samples the IR curve at multiple inversion times using single-shot imaging spaced at heartbeat intervals. Multiple inversions are used with different trigger delays in order to acquire measurements at different inversion times to sample the IR curve more finely. Recovery periods are needed between the inversions to ensure that samples from the different inversions are from the same recovery curve (i.e., each inversion starts at the same initial condition). The precision of the T1 map is related to the number and position of samples along the IR curve, and the accuracy of the signal model is also affected by the sampling strategy due to the influence of the readout on the apparent recovery.

The MOLLI method uses an SSFP readout. The readout drives the IR to recover more quickly and reaches a steady state that is less than the equilibrium magnetization (M0). The effect of the readout (Fig. 4.2) is an apparent recovery time referred to as T1*, which is less than the actual longitudinal recovery time, T1, which is the desired tissue

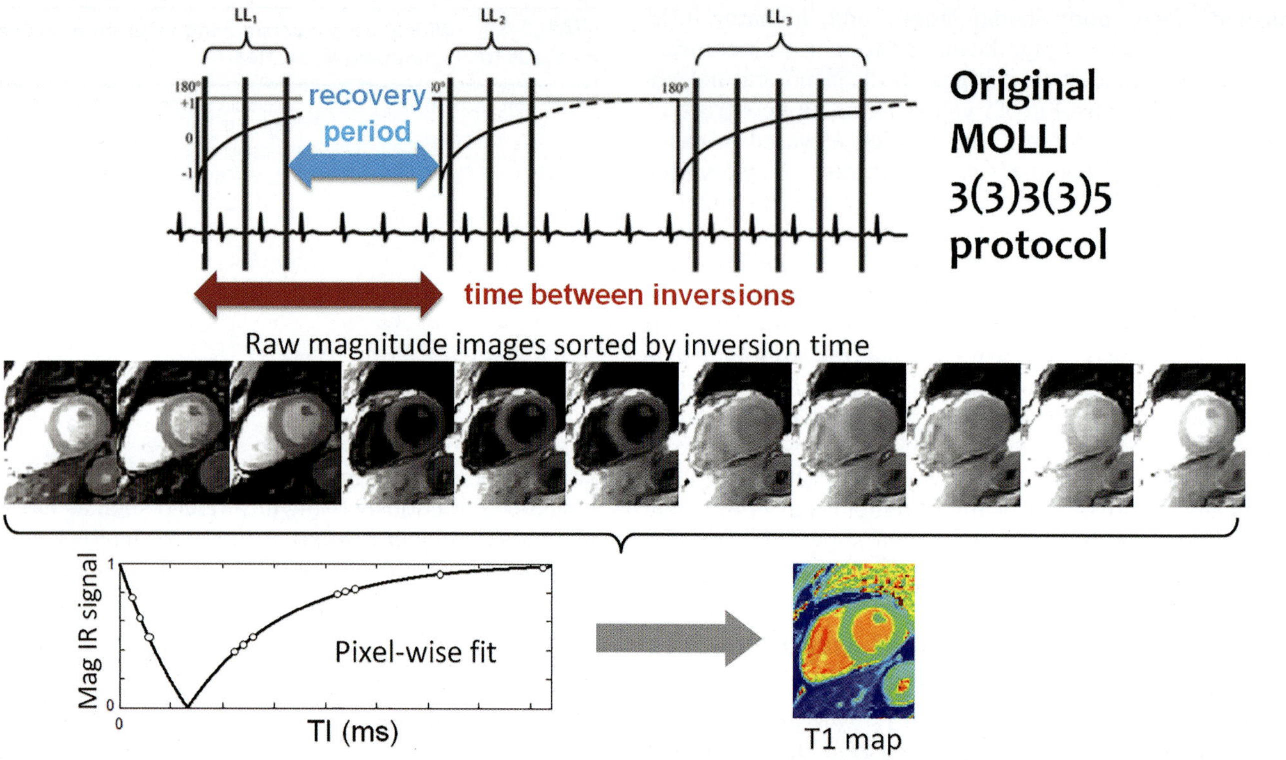

FIG. 4.1 Modified Look-Locker inversion recovery (*MOLLI*) scheme for T1-mapping in the heart.[37] The original protocol employed three inversions with 3, 3, and 5 images acquired in the beats following inversions, and three heartbeat recovery periods between inversions, referred to here as 3(3)3(3)5. All images are acquired at the same delay from the R-wave trigger for middiastolic imaging. Curve fitting is performed on a pixel-wise basis using the actual measured inversion times. *IR*, Inversion recovery; *TI*, inversion time. (Kellman P, Hansen MS. T1-mapping in the heart: accuracy and precision. *J Cardiovasc Magn Reson*. 2014;16:2.)

parameter. As a result of the influence of the readout, the inversion recovery curve follows a 3-parameter exponential signal model, $S(t) = A - B\exp(-t/T1^*)$, where t represents the inversion time and T1* is the apparent T1. The measured values may be fit to the 3-parameter model to estimate A, B, and T1*, which may be used to approximate $T1 \approx T1^*(B/A-1)$. The derivation for the so-called "Look-Locker" correction factor (B/A−1) is based on a continuous readout using fast low-angle shot (FLASH).[57] Despite the fact that the MOLLI uses a gated SSFP readout, the signal model behaves as a 3-parameter model in which the Look-Locker correction is reasonably effective at low-readout excitation flip angles.

The analytic relationship between T1* and T1 for SSFP has been derived for continuous SSFP under somewhat idealized conditions such as an ideal slice profile.[58] Useful analytic derivations for gated SSFP with realistic slice profiles have not been developed due to complexity. Bloch simulations may be used to calculate the error inherent in this approximation[43] and to gain insight into the sensitivity of various protocol parameters and design variables. The influence of various parameters such as T2, heart rate, off-resonance, actual flip angle are referred to as confounders and are discussed later.

A number of modifications (Table 4.2) to the original MOLLI protocol have been proposed to shorten the acquisition duration or to improve accuracy or precision.[32,38,39,44,45] A shorthand nomenclature is used to label these protocols. The notation captures how many inversions (or saturations) are included in the experiment, how many images are acquired after each inversion, and how long the waiting period is between inversions. For example, a 3(3)3(3)5 protocol indicates that there are a total of three inversions; three images are acquired (over three RR intervals) after the first inversion, which is followed by a waiting period of three RR intervals, then three images are acquired followed by another three RR waiting period, and finally a third inversion occurs after which five images are acquired. In an extension of this nomenclature, an "s" can be added to the intervals to indicate that images are acquired for a certain number of seconds and that the waiting period is in seconds; that is, 5s(3s)3s indicates two inversions with an acquisition of images for at least 5s, followed by a recovery of at least 3s, and a second inversion with images acquired for at least 3s. Since the number of ECG-triggered images must be a whole number, the acquisition and recovery periods are rounded to the nearest multiple of the RR period to ensure an adequate duration. In order to avoid acquiring too few images for low heart rates (<60 bpm), the sequence never acquires fewer than the specified number of images (i.e., 5 + 3 = 8 in this example). The recovery period is never less than the specified number of seconds. Acquiring and recovering with a fixed minimum time periods helps gain independence of heart rate.

Saturation recovery (SR) is an alternative to inversion recovery that has gained renewed attention. Despite having a reduced dynamic range, saturation recovery has potential for improved accuracy. SR methods that use a saturation preparation for each measurement have the

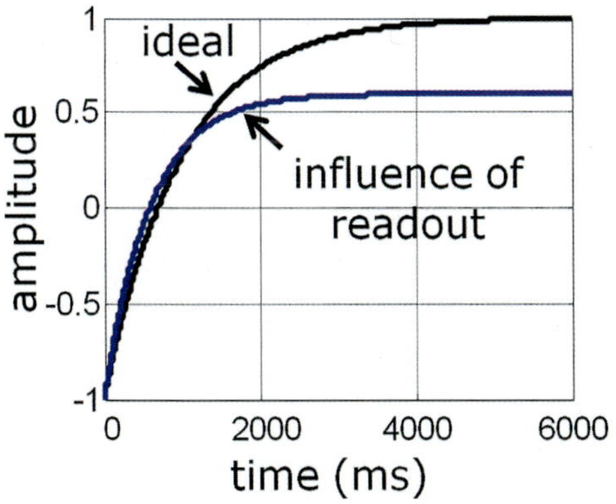

FIG. 4.2 The apparent inversion recovery (T1*) is influenced by the steady-state free precession readout. The effective inversion recovery is fit using a 3-parameter model, and the T1 is estimated using the so-called Look-Locker correction. (Kellman P, Hansen MS. T1-mapping in the heart: accuracy and precision. *J Cardiovasc Magn Reson*. 2014;16:2.)

TABLE 4.2 Reported schemes for modified Look-Locker inversion recover sampling.

MOLLI	3(3)3(3)5	Messrohli et al.[37](original publication)
	3(3)5	Ugander et al.[33] & Salerno, et al. [44]
	5(3)3	Kellman et al.[39]
	4(1)3(1)2	Schelbert, et al.[32]
	2(2)2(2)4	Salerno et al.[44]
	5(3s)3	Kellman et al.[59,60]
	4(1s)3(1s)2	Kellman et al.[59]
	5s(3s)3s	Kellman et al.[45]
	4s(1s)3s(1s)2s	Kellman et al.[45]
ShMOLLI	5(1)1(1)1 (with conditional fitting)	Piechnik et al.[38]

MOLLI, modified Look-Locker inversion recover; *ShMOLLI*, shortened MOLLI.

benefit that each measurement becomes independent of the others. By starting the recovery from a saturated state, the prior history is erased. Recovery periods between successive measurements are not required unless longer saturation recovery times are needed for fitting. The method known as SASHA[47] is diagrammed in Fig. 4.3. The SASHA method using an SSFP readout is very similar to the earlier short acquisition period–T1 (SAP-T1) method,[46] which used a spoiled gradient-recalled echo (GRE) readout.

The SASHA method acquires multiple time points on the SR curve and does a pixel-wise curve fit. In order to acquire a fully recovered image, an image is initially acquired prior to any saturation preparation (i.e., starting from the equilibrium magnetization). Images are acquired on successive heart beats using SR preparations with varying trigger delays. In the original proposed SASHA protocol there are 10 images acquired at saturation delays uniformly spaced over the RR interval plus the initial fully recovered image, which serves as an important anchor point for the curve fit. The order in which the various delays are acquired is not of significant importance for fitting, assuming ideal saturation. Importantly, the SR curve recovers as T1 and is not influenced by the readout so that it is not shortened to an apparent T1* < T1, as in the case of MOLLI. Therefore, no correction is necessary, which eliminates the source of many inaccuracies of the IR-based MOLLI scheme. Since the readout does not lead to an apparent T1*, a higher flip angle readout is possible, which makes up for some of the lost dynamic range in using SR. The higher readout flip angle using SSFP with linear phase-encode ordering does slightly alter the shape of the recovery curve, causing an apparent bias (i.e., curve does not start at 0 for 0 delay). Thus, the otherwise 2-parameter signal model $S(t) = A(1-\exp(-t/T1))$ for SR, assuming ideal saturation, becomes a 3-parameter model: $S(t) = A-B \exp(-t/T1)$. The 3-parameter model also absorbs any imperfection in the saturation efficiency due

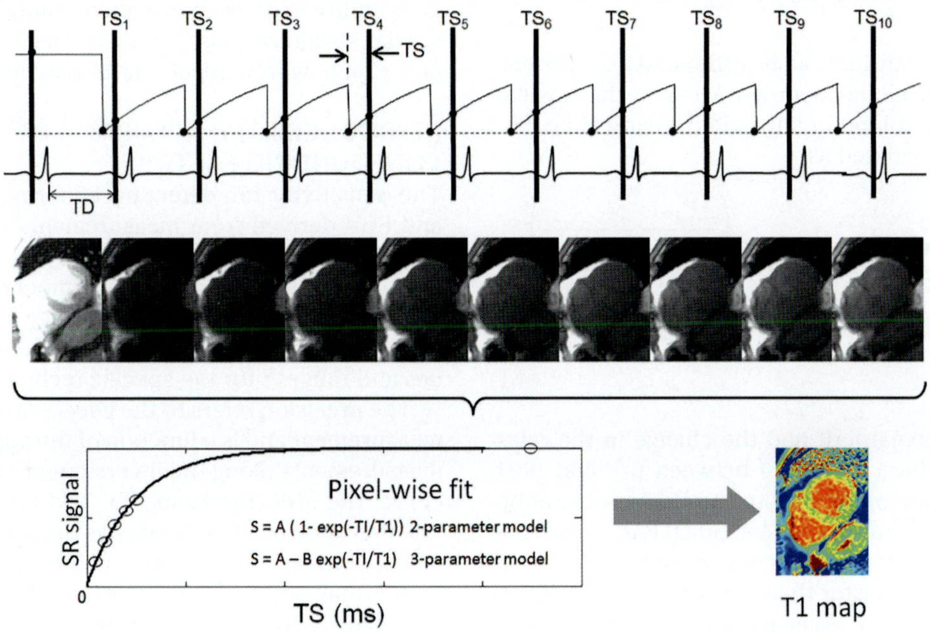

FIG. 4.3 Saturation recovery (*SR*) single-shot acquisition scheme for T1 mapping in the heart.[47] A single image is acquired without saturation and used as the fully recovered measurement followed by a series of saturation recovery images at different saturation recovery times (*TSi*). All images are acquired at the same trigger delay (*TD*) from the R-wave trigger for middiastolic imaging. Curve fitting is performed on a pixel-wise basis. (Kellman P, Hansen MS. T1-mapping in the heart: accuracy and precision. *J Cardiovasc Magn Reson*. 2014;16:2.)

to the RF (radio frequency) saturation pulse. However, the cost of estimating the additional parameter is loss of precision. Therefore, there is a trade-off between accuracy and precision in considering whether to use 2- or 3-parameter fitting. Although a center-out phase-encode order in which the center of k-space is acquired first has the potential to completely remove the influence of the readout, the use of center-out ordering with SSFP is problematic due to artifacts, and the use of center-out FLASH is associated with a significant loss of signal-to-noise ratio (SNR). An improved version of SASHA[53] that uses variable flip angle (VFA) for the SSFP readout minimizes the small bias due to a linear phase-encode order and therefore makes 2-parameter fitting practical with negligible loss in accuracy. The SASHA VFA also has the benefit of improved transition to steady state, which greatly reduces ghost artifacts, particularly due to off-resonant fat, which was an issue with the original implementation.

The SASHA sampling scheme may be altered to acquire longer saturation delay measurements by allowing one or more heartbeat recovery periods between saturations. Measurements strategies that use recovery periods such as SMART1[54] may improve precision for specific ranges of T1 and heart rate but reduce the overall SNR efficiency somewhat. Optimized sampling strategies for SASHA for both 2- and 3-parameter fitting are described in [52] and [51], respectively. Schemes that simply use a MOLLI strategy replaced with SR[61] incur the problems of an apparent T1* without gaining the main benefits of SR. A combined IR/SR approach known as saturation pulse prepared heart rate independent inversion-recovery (SAPPHIRE)[48] has many of the benefits of IR and SR but still retains some of the problems associated with IR. Each method has its strengths and weaknesses in terms of accuracy, precision, and overall reproducibility.

Extra-Cellular Volume Mapping Methods

METHODS

The ECV in the myocardium can be estimated from the concentration of extracellular contrast agent in the myocardium relative to the blood in a dynamic steady state.[28,29,33] The ECV can be calculated as:

$$\mathrm{ECV} = (1-\mathrm{hct})\frac{\Delta R1_{\mathrm{myo}}}{\Delta R1_{\mathrm{blood}}} = (1-\mathrm{hct})\frac{\left(\frac{1}{T1_{\mathrm{myo\ post}}}-\frac{1}{T1_{\mathrm{myo\ pre}}}\right)}{\left(\frac{1}{T1_{\mathrm{blood\ post}}}-\frac{1}{T1_{\mathrm{blood\ pre}}}\right)} \tag{4.1}$$

where hct is the hematocrit and the change in the relaxation rate $\Delta R1$ (where $R1 = 1/T1$) between pre and postcontrast is directly proportional to the Gd concentration: $\Delta R1 = \gamma[\mathrm{Gd}]$ ($\gamma = 4.5\,\mathrm{L\ mmol^{-1}sec^{-1}}$ for Gd-DTPA). A dynamic steady state exists for tissues that have a contrast exchange rate with blood that is faster than the net clearance of contrast from the blood.[28] A dynamic steady state between the plasma and interstitium may be achieved by slow intravenous infusion[24,29] or by imaging 15 minutes after an intravenous bolus administration[32,33] for normally perfused myocardium, although 15 minutes may not be adequate for recently infarcted myocardium.[62] The bolus method is more generally used since it fits well with the clinical workflow and permits conventional late enhancement imaging at the desired dose. The ECV formula (Eq. 4.1) implies that our myocardial ECV measurements include both the intra and extravascular space. The factor (1-hct), which varies between individuals, represents the blood volume of distribution (blood ECV) and converts the equation from a partition coefficient calculation to a myocardial ECV.

Pre- and postcontrast image series are acquired in separate breath-holds, which are typically 15–30 minutes apart. Even small differences in respiratory position or changes in patient position due to movement will cause significant misregistration of the images. Care must be taken that the patient does not move, and coregistration of the pre and postcontrast images must be performed using a nonrigid image registration to mitigate in-plane motion.[40,41] The complete processing workflow may be fully automated[39] to include pre and postcontrast T1 mapping with respiratory motion correction and blood pool segmentation. A prototype ECV mapping tool has been integrated onto a clinical scanner.[63] In-line ECV mapping presumes that the hematocrit has been measured prior to the scan using point-of-care devices. For instances in which the hematocrit has not been measured it is possible to estimate an approximate hematocrit from the value of blood T1 and use this derived hct for a synthetic ECV.[64] In this way, the ECV map may be available immediately following the completion of the postcontrast T1 map regardless of whether hct was measured.

Although detecting global changes that are difficult to see on nonquantitative imaging has been a driver for quantitation, there is also potential value in cases of focal abnormalities in determining whether remote tissue is in fact normal and in measuring border zones. Given adequate precision, the strength of pixel-wise mapping of T1 is its ability to detect small abnormalities and discriminate spatial structures. Fig. 4.4 illustrates T1 and ECV maps in cases ranging from focal scar to patchy to diffuse.

REPRODUCIBILITY: ACCURACY, PRECISION, AND CONFOUNDING FACTORS

The sensitivity for detecting abnormal elevations of T1 and ECV derived from measurements of T1 is fundamentally limited by the reproducibility of T1 estimates. The reproducibility is affected by a number of factors including measurement precision and accuracy as well as biological variability. It is important to establish normal baseline values and ranges[21] for the specific technique and protocol.

The precision refers to the effect of random noise on the measurement and is a function of the number and timing of measurements along the inversion- or saturation-recovery curve, the SNR, the tissue T1, and the method of fitting. The precision of T1 methods has been well characterized,[45] and a pixel-wise map of the standard deviation (SD) due to thermal noise may be generated as a quality map.[59] Example T1 and corresponding SD maps are shown (Fig. 4.5) for a normal subject for four different mapping protocols. This example illustrates several points: (1) normal T1 values vary considerably by method and specific imaging

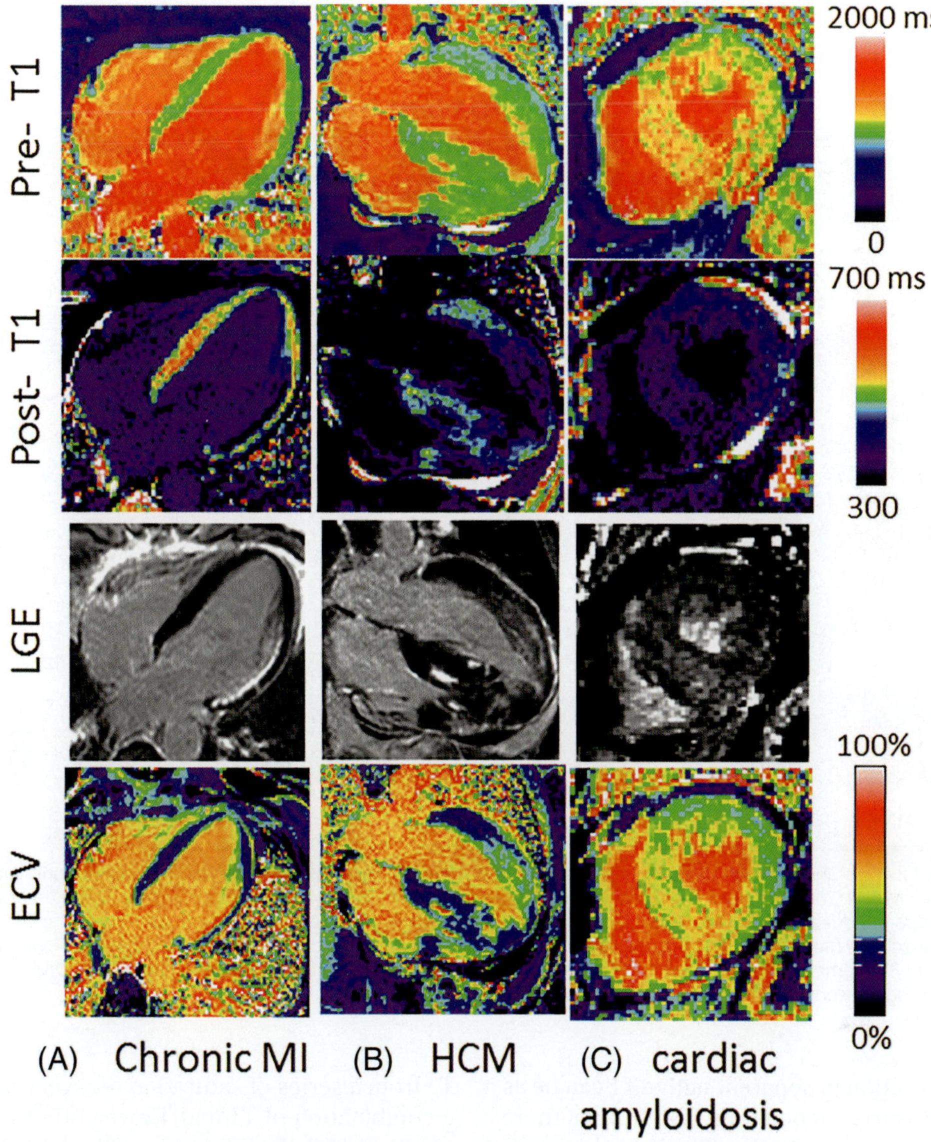

FIG. 4.4 Examples illustrating mapping in cases ranging from focal, patchy, to diffuse disease. Native (precontrast) T1-maps (*top row*), postcontrast T1-maps (*second row*), late gadolinium enhancement (*LGE; third row*), and extracellular volume (*ECV*) maps (*bottom row*) for patients with (A) chronic myocardial infarction (*MI*), (B) hypertrophic cardiomyopathy (*HCM*), and (C) cardiac amyloidosis. (Kellman P, Wilson JR, Xue H, et al. Extracellular volume fraction mapping in the myocardium, part 2: initial clinical experience. *J Cardiovasc Magn Reson*. 2012;14[1]:64.)

protocol, (2) the SD varies across the heart as the SNR varies due to surface coil drop off with distance, and (3) different methods of T1 mapping have different precisions, leading to differing sensitivities.

Other factors that contribute to measurement error and are not random further limit the reproducibility and are highly dependent on the technique and specific protocol. Some of these factors may depend on scanner adjustments such as off-resonance errors[60] due to center frequency adjustment error, inability to shim the volume perfectly, or variation in the actual flip angle due to transmitter field inhomogeneity or flip angle adjustment error. Techniques must be designed to be robust in the presence of such variations since these variables are generally not well controlled. Variations may also relate to the actual tissue composition. For instance, inversion recovery methods using an SSFP readout are dependent on the tissue T2[43,45,47] and MT resulting from the macromolecular content of proteins.[65] Still other variables relating to the patient such as heart rate, heart rate variability, and cardiac or respiratory motion may affect estimates of T1. The accuracy for a given technique may also be influenced by specific protocol parameters such as flip angle, matrix size, repetition rate (TR), and sampling strategy. The sensitivities of the MOLLI (Fig. 4.6) and SASHA (Fig. 4.7) techniques have been calculated based on Bloch simulations for a common protocol with matrix size 256×144, partial Fourier factor 7/8, factor two acceleration, bandwidth 1085 Hz/pixel, TR = 2.8 ms, excitation flip angle (FA) 35 degrees, minimum TI 100 ms, and TI (inversion time) increment 80 ms. These calculations illustrate the dependencies on T2, HR (heart rate), FA (flip angle), and off-resonance, leading to an underestimation of T1. The MOLLI-based methods have the largest sensitivity to adjustments and protocol parameters. For a 25% variation in transmit FA, often seen in practice, the variation in apparent native T1 is 2%. For 100 Hz

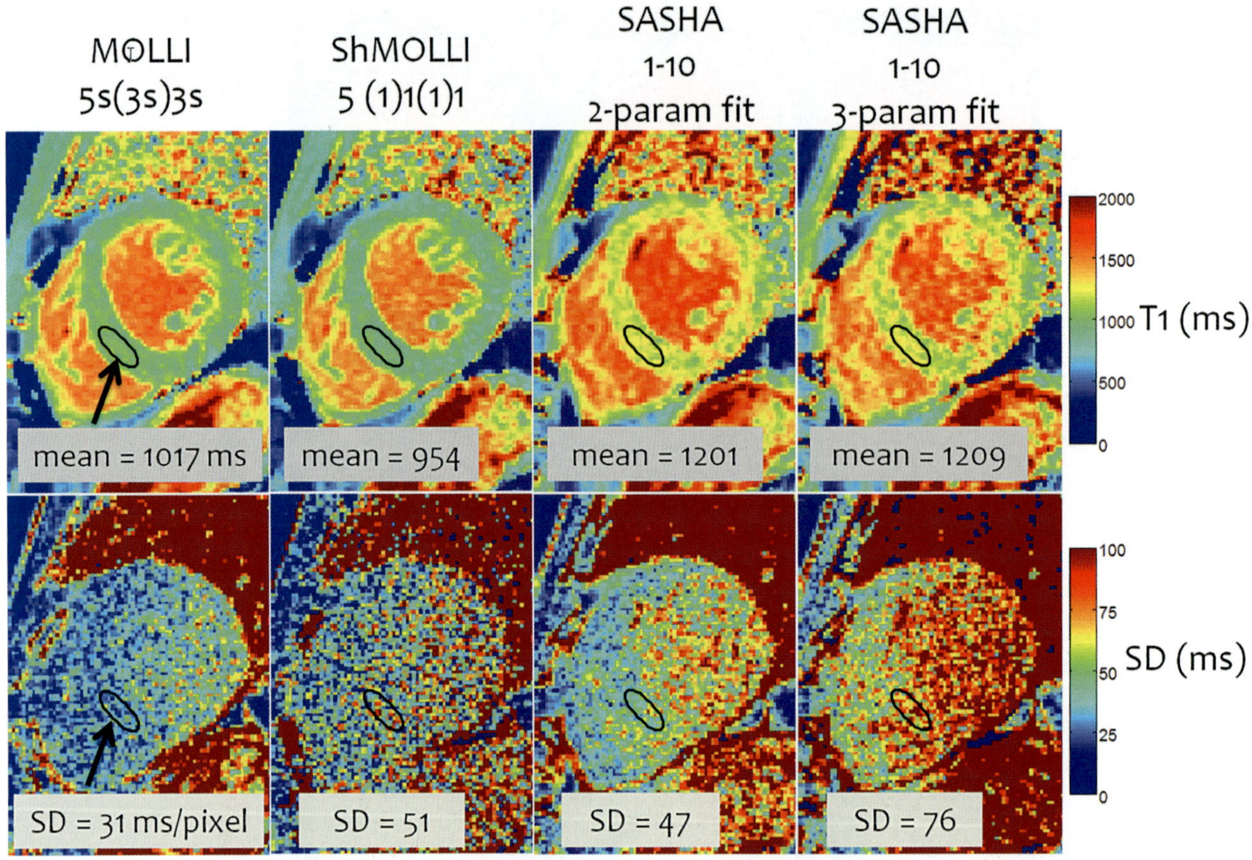

FIG. 4.5 Example in-vivo T1 maps and corresponding pixel-wise standard deviation (*SD*) maps acquired using modified Look-Locker inversion recovery (*MOLLI*) 5s(3s)3s, shortened MOLLI (*ShMOLLI*), and saturation recovery single-shot acquisition (*SASHA*) protocols using 2- and 3-parameter fitting. Variation in SD across the heart is apparent due to variation in the signal-to-noise ratio from surface coil sensitivity roll-off. MOLLI has the best precision but underestimates T1 due to the approximate nature of the Look-Locker correction and due to magnetization transfer. Note that SASHA with 2-parameter fitting has a small T1 underestimation; 3-parameter fitting is more accurate but has significant loss of precision. (Kellman P, Hansen MS. T1-mapping in the heart: accuracy and precision. *J Cardiovasc Magn Reson*. 2014;16:2.)

off-resonance, the variation in apparent native T1 can be as high as 4%. For heart rate variation from 60–120 bpm, there is a 2.5% variation in apparent native T1. Over the range of normal to highly edematous T2 (45 to 90 ms), the native T1 will vary approximately 4%. The SR-based method of SASHA is much less sensitive to these variables. However, the IR methods such as MOLLI achieve a higher precision.[45]

An example of how edematous myocardium may confound the measurement of native T1 (Fig. 4.8) is presented for a subject with acute MI. The edematous region of MI has an elevated value of T2 that is 15 ms greater than remote. The increase in T1 for this MI region is 227 ms above remote as measured using MOLLI, and is elevated 199 ms as measured using SASHA. The difference in T1 elevation (227–199 = 28 ms) is explained in part due to the 15 ms elevation of T2 due to edema as seen in a plot of MOLLI sensitivity to T2 (Fig. 4.6) and due to the different degree of MT between the MI and remote region. The MT will be less in the edematous region due to increased water content, thus the T1 underestimation of MOLLI due to MT will be less, corresponding to an increased T1. The SASHA method is relatively insensitive to both T2 and MT.

To further improve the precision of saturation recovery methods and reduce the confounding between T1 and T2, a multiparametric SASHA method (known as mSASHA) has been developed.[55] This approach jointly estimates T1 and T2 from a series of saturation recovery measurements with a combination of T1 and T2 weightings. By jointly estimating T1 and T2, the influence of T1 on T2 is eliminated. A free-breathing mSASHA protocol was developed[56] that permits longer acquisitions, thus improving the precision of both T1 and T2 compared to breath-hold acquisitions. In this way, the free-breathing mSASHA can achieve precision comparable to the breath-hold inversion recovery approach.

LIMITATIONS AND POTENTIAL PITFALLS

The use of T1 to characterize myocardial tissue is a simplification, or first-order model. The myocardium consists of several compartments such as myocytes, interstitium, and capillaries, each with a different constituent molecular makeup that includes free water and macromolecules. The interactions between the proton spins that contribute to the observed MRI signal are highly complex. Despite the fact that current T1 mapping largely ignores these complexities in measuring a single macroscopic T1, the T1 measurements have been demonstrated to have potential clinical use.

The potential for the quantification of myocardial tissue is to detect small changes due to disease processes or treatment. The desire to measure subtle changes

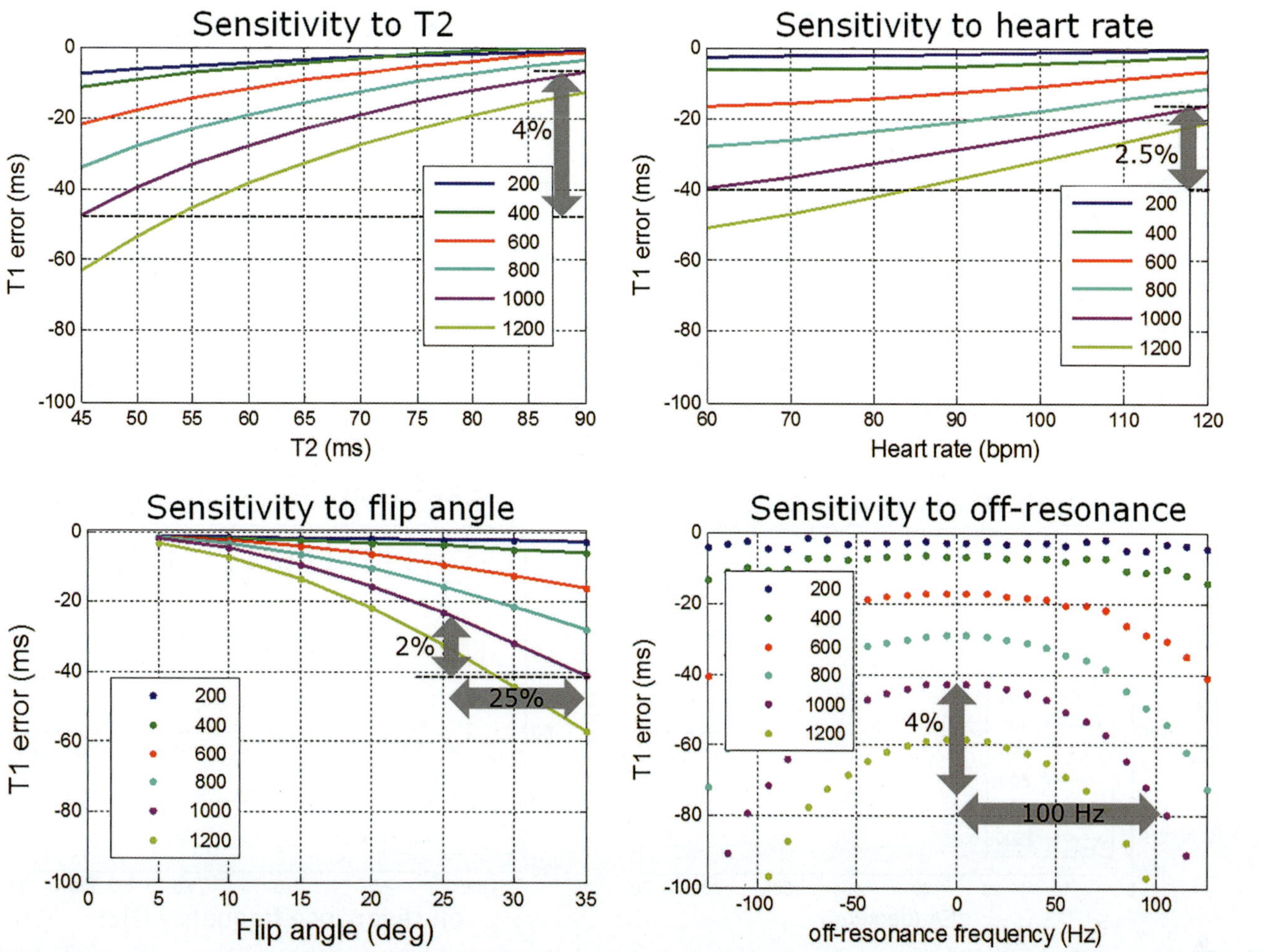

FIG. 4.6 Sensitivity of T1 estimates using modified Look-Locker inversion recovery method to T2, heart rate, flip angle, and off-resonance frequency using 5s(3s)3s sampling scheme. (Kellman P, Hansen MS. T1-mapping in the heart: accuracy and precision. *J Cardiovasc Magn Reson*. 2014;16:2.)

places stringent requirements on the reliability of the measurement. For this reason, there is great emphasis on accuracy, precision, and general reproducibility. In addition to the confounding factors described above, wherein estimates of T1 may be affected by tissue T2, MT, patient heart rate, off-resonance (B_0), or actual flip angle (transmitted B_1), there are other artifact mechanisms that may affect measurement. One of the most important limitations is the partial volume contamination of the myocardium by the adjacent blood pool signal, which is generally greater than the myocardium. Blood pool contamination is due to both limited in-plane spatial resolution as well as through-plane resolution. A voxel in a myocardial region may contain a mixture of myocardium and blood and thus be biased. The degree of bias due to this partial volume between myocardium and blood will depend on proximity to the blood pool as well as effective spatial resolution. With an in-plane image resolution of 1.5–2 mm and thin myocardial walls (<1 cm), there may be only a few (2–5) pixel widths across the myocardial wall. Gibb's ringing can lead to fluctuations of 5% or greater in T1 values even midwall, and errors can be much larger close to the blood-myocardial boundary. For slices in which there is through-plane angulation of the wall, particularly at the apex, there can be additional partial volume effects. Caution must be exercised in making and interpreting measurements for thin walls, particularly when comparing populations with different wall thickness.

Fig. 4.9 illustrates the effect of spatial resolution on native T1 maps for two subjects with different wall thicknesses and heart rates. Subject 1 (left) has a myocardial wall thickness of approximately 10 mm (approx. 6 pixels) in the septum and a heart rate of approximately 55 bpm. A profile plot of T1 across the septal wall shows a ringing of approximately 50 ms (5%) due to Gibb's effect and a smooth transition between the myocardium and adjacent blood pool of approximately 2 pixels. Subject 2 (right) has a thinner myocardial wall (approx. 7 mm) and a higher heart rate. For the higher heart rate (approx. 92 bpm), a slightly reduced matrix size was used to mitigate temporal motion blur, resulting in a myocardial wall thickness corresponding to 3–4 pixels. In this case, the measured T1 (see profile plot) is contaminated by adjacent blood for all but the midwall, thereby compromising the accuracy of measurements. Most clinical image viewers use interpolation to display images when zoomed, thus hiding the true resolution limits that would be apparent when displaying the pixelated image. Depending on the displayed range (window level), the zoomed and interpolated maps often appear to have distinct boundaries, even in situations with significant partial volume contamination.

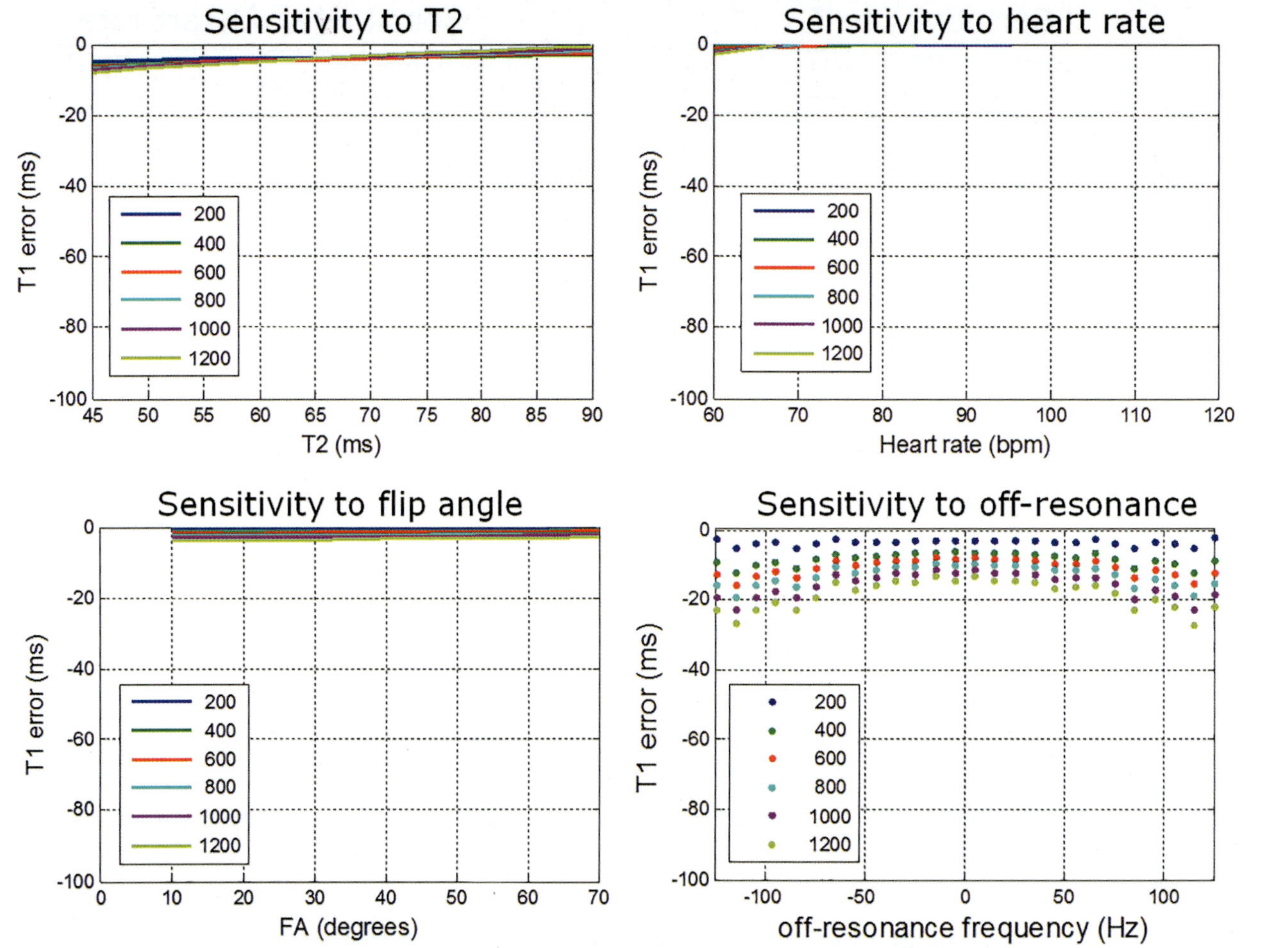

FIG. 4.7 Sensitivity of T1 estimates using saturation recovery single-shot acquisition variable flip angle 2-parameter method to T2, heart rate, flip angle (*FA*), and off-resonance frequency using NS + [(0)1]^9 sampling scheme.

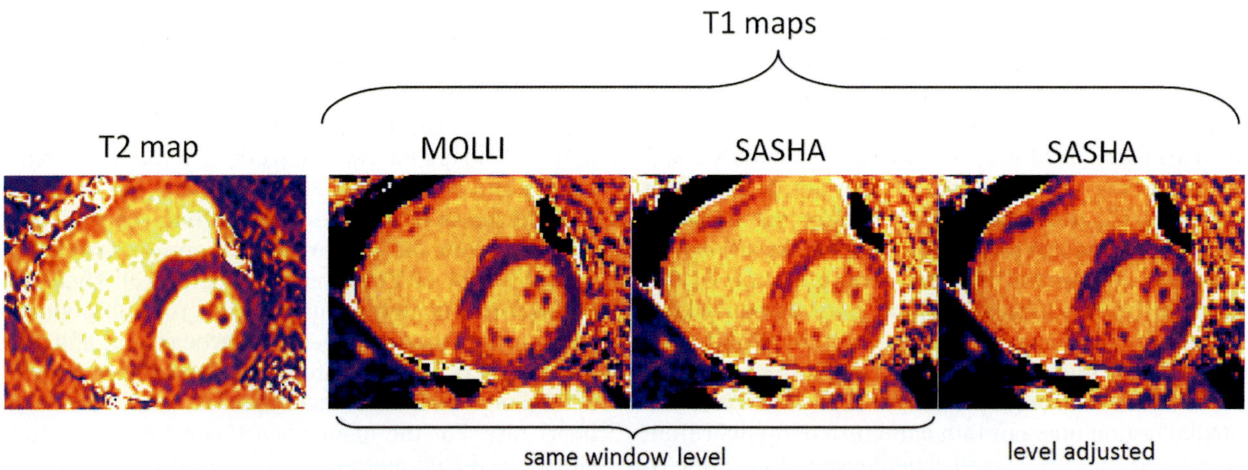

	Edema	Remote	difference
T1 (MOLLI)	1231	1004	227
T1 (SASHA)	1382	1183	199
T2	59	44	15

FIG. 4.8 Example of T1 and T2 maps for subject with edematous acute myocardial infarction. The edematous region is elevated 15 ms above remote, and T1 is elevated 227 ms (using modified Look-Locker inversion recovery [*MOLLI*]) and 199 ms (using saturation recovery single-shot acquisition [*SASHA*]). The greater increase in apparent T1 for MOLLI edema is due to the confounding effects of T2 and magnetization transfer. Note that the baseline values for SASHA are greater than for MOLLI.

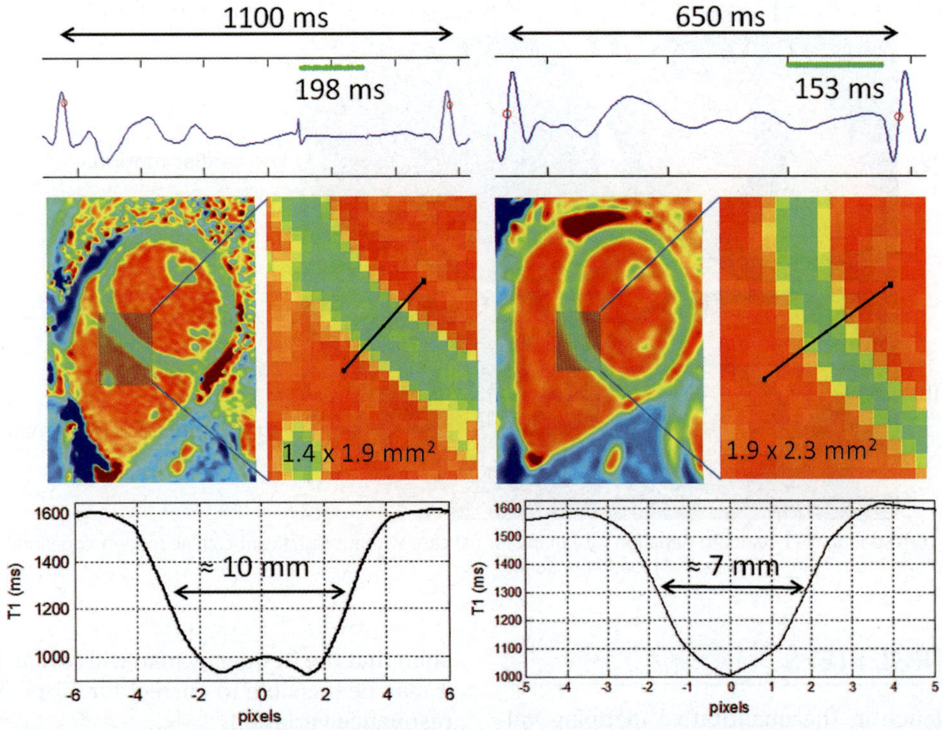

FIG. 4.9 Example of T1 maps in two subjects. (*left*) Subject with heart rate of 58 bpm acquired using a modified Look-Locker inversion recovery protocol with a 256 × 144 matrix and (*right*) subject with heart rate of approximately 90 bpm using a 192 × 120 matrix. Although the interpolated maps are of good quality, the subject with higher heart rate and thinner wall has only about 3.5 pixels across the septum, leading to a degree of partial volume error in region of interest measurements. (Kellman P, Hansen MS. T1-mapping in the heart: accuracy and precision. *J Cardiovasc Magn Reson*. 2014;16:2.)

In addition to limited spatial resolution, there may be additional blurring due to cardiac motion in cases of higher heart rates, variations in RR interval, or imaging during a period of the cardiac cycle in which there is wall motion. The temporal duration of image acquisition can be reduced to mitigate blurring by using higher parallel imaging acceleration, although this may come at the expense of loss in SNR. The partial volume bias due to potential blurring at heart rates is important to consider and is distinct from the previously described heart rate dependence of the MOLLI-type sequences. Finally, imperfect respiratory motion correction may lead to an additional source of blurring.

There are partial volume errors for voxels with a mixture of myocardium and fat.[66] This may occur at tissue boundaries or within the myocardium in the case of lipomatous metaplasia of replacement fibrosis, which is commonly seen in chronic MI or other scarring. The presence of fat leads to a bias in T1 measurement, which may be either a positive or negative bias depending on the specific protocol and off-resonance frequency. T1 biases will be additive or subtractive depending on whether the center frequency corresponds to the myocardium and fat being in phase or out of phase, respectively. Lipomatous metaplasia is prevalent and often difficult to detect at low fat fractions. The influence on T1 at these low fat fractions is significant and is readily misinterpreted. Although this may be mitigated to some extent by means of chemical shift fat suppression (i.e., fat saturation), the fat saturation may also influence the measurement of normal myocardial T1 if there is any significant off-resonance error due to imperfect shim.

Quality maps such as goodness of fit or standard deviation maps[59] may be used for quality control as a means of detecting cases for which there is increased error due to cardiac or respiratory motion when the motion is fairly extreme. However, quality maps do not account for all partial volume errors. Other potentially useful quality metrics are off-resonance field maps and flip angle maps. When ECV is elevated, it may not be clear whether this is due to fibrosis, edema, or both, which may be either diffuse or focal. In such instances, precontrast T1 or T2 maps, in addition to patient history and contextual imaging clues like signs of heart failure, may help to differentiate these mechanisms.

One of the attractive aspects of ECV measurement is that the value represents a quantitative measurement. However, biases in the measurement of pre and postcontrast T1 do not cancel out and methods with different baseline normal values of T1 such as MOLLI and SASHA will yield different baseline normal values of ECV.

The ability to distinguish partial volume border pixels and correctly determine whether pixels are contaminated by partial volume effects or are a true pathophysiology, such as subendocardial or subepicardial fibrosis, is a residual and important issue, as shown in the T1 mapping example. This issue is not only important in terms of the visual readout, but may introduce biases into quantitative measurements, which become particularly significant in the context of more subtle diseases. One approach to reducing bias in measurements is to restrict the measurement to the midwall region, although one must exercise caution for subjects with thin-walled myocardium or patients with thin rims of subendocardial fibrosis.

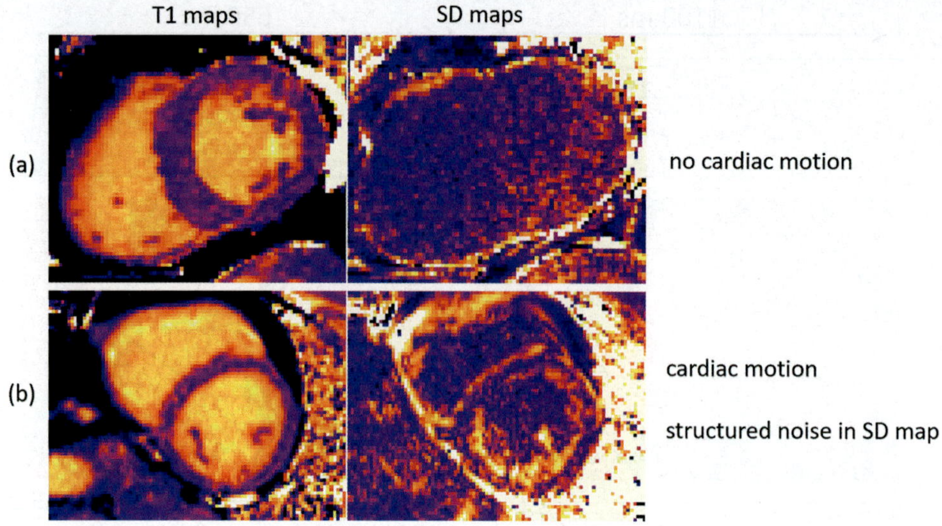

FIG. 4.10 T1 maps and corresponding T1 standard deviation (*SD*) maps for (A) case without significant cardiac motion appearing noise-like, and (B) case with cardiac motion resulting in structure at myocardial blood boundaries.

QUALITY CONTROL STEPS

To improve confidence in the quantitative mapping values, a number of quality control steps may be performed manually: (1) checking for motion correction errors due to breathing or mistriggering, (2) checking for adequate shim, (3) checking that spatial resolution is adequate, (4) checking for the presence of fat, and (5) checking for edema.

Motion correction may have errors that can lead to errors in the quantitative maps. In some implementations, the mapping may provide an error map of SD, as shown in Fig. 4.10. If the SD map has a structured (Fig. 4.10B) rather than noise-like appearance (Fig 4.10A), it is an indication of error due to motion, which may increase the T1 mapping error at that location. For implementations that do not have an SD map, one can load the motion-corrected series of images into a viewer and manually trace endocardial and epicardial contours for one of the inversion recovery images with good contrast and copy these contours to all measurements, as illustrated in Fig. 4.11. In this case, it is possible to assess the quality of image registration, and to be sure all images are acquired at the same cardiac phase.

Poor shimming can lead to off-resonance, which may result in local variation or a global shift in center frequency. If the off-resonance is great enough, the raw images will have dark banding artifacts due to the b-SSFP (steady state free precession) readout. However, there may be significant errors in T1 due to less severe off-resonance that does not lead to banding artifacts and is not readily apparent. Sensitivity to off-resonance is shown in Fig. 4.6 (lower right panel) for inversion recovery T1 mapping such as MOLLI or ShMOLLI. It is recommended to shim locally around the heart, as shown in Fig. 4.12, and use a field map when available for additional quality assurance. Field maps may be a by-product of multiecho Dixon water fat-separated imaging and display the spatial variation in off-resonance frequency. Ideally, the off-resonance would be within +/−50 Hz across the heart. In patients with implantable devices such as pacemakers or implantable cardioverter defibrillators, there may be a substantial gradient in off-resonance in shim that the frequency map will reveal. In some instances, it may be possible to correct for T1 map errors due to off-resonance variation.[67]

One of the largest sources of error in quantitative mapping is partial volume error due to contamination of the myocardial signal from either the adjacent blood pool or adjacent epicardial fat. The degree of partial volume contamination relates to the effective spatial resolution and myocardial wall thickness. The importance of spatial resolution is illustrated in Fig. 4.13. In this case, the septal wall thickness is only 2 pixels, as shown on the left prior to interpolation, and the transition between the myocardium and adjacent blood pool is between 1 and 2 pixels. Fig. 4.14 shows the septal profiles for native T1 maps for a second case for which the acquisition window is varied to illustrate how the duration and timing of the image may affect the spatial blurring due to cardiac motion. In the absence of disease, the myocardial wall will ideally have a constant T1 transmurally, as shown in Fig. 4.14 (top), but small changes in timing can cause blur such that it is not possible to make an error that is not contaminated by the blood signal. Therefore, it is important to use the correct timing during image acquisition. It is most common to trace endo and epicardial contours on interpolated images and use a small erosion factor such as 10% to account for the boundary being somewhat blurred. However, 10% may not be adequate depending on how the original contours are drawn or how blurred the border is. For quality assurance in dealing with partial volume, myocardial profiles are very useful. If profile tools are not available, then the window width may be decreased to be sure that the blood is not within the myocardial region of interest.

In the presence of intramyocardial fat such as lipomatous metaplasia, voxels may contain a mixture of myocytes and white adipose cells. The measurement of T1 for a mixture of "fat" and "water" can lead to erroneous values of T1, even for small values of fat fraction,[66] as illustrated in Fig 4.15. A partial volume mixture of fat and myocardium may lead to myocardial T1 errors that either increase the apparent T1 or decrease the apparent T1 depending on the center frequency and field strength, thereby making T1

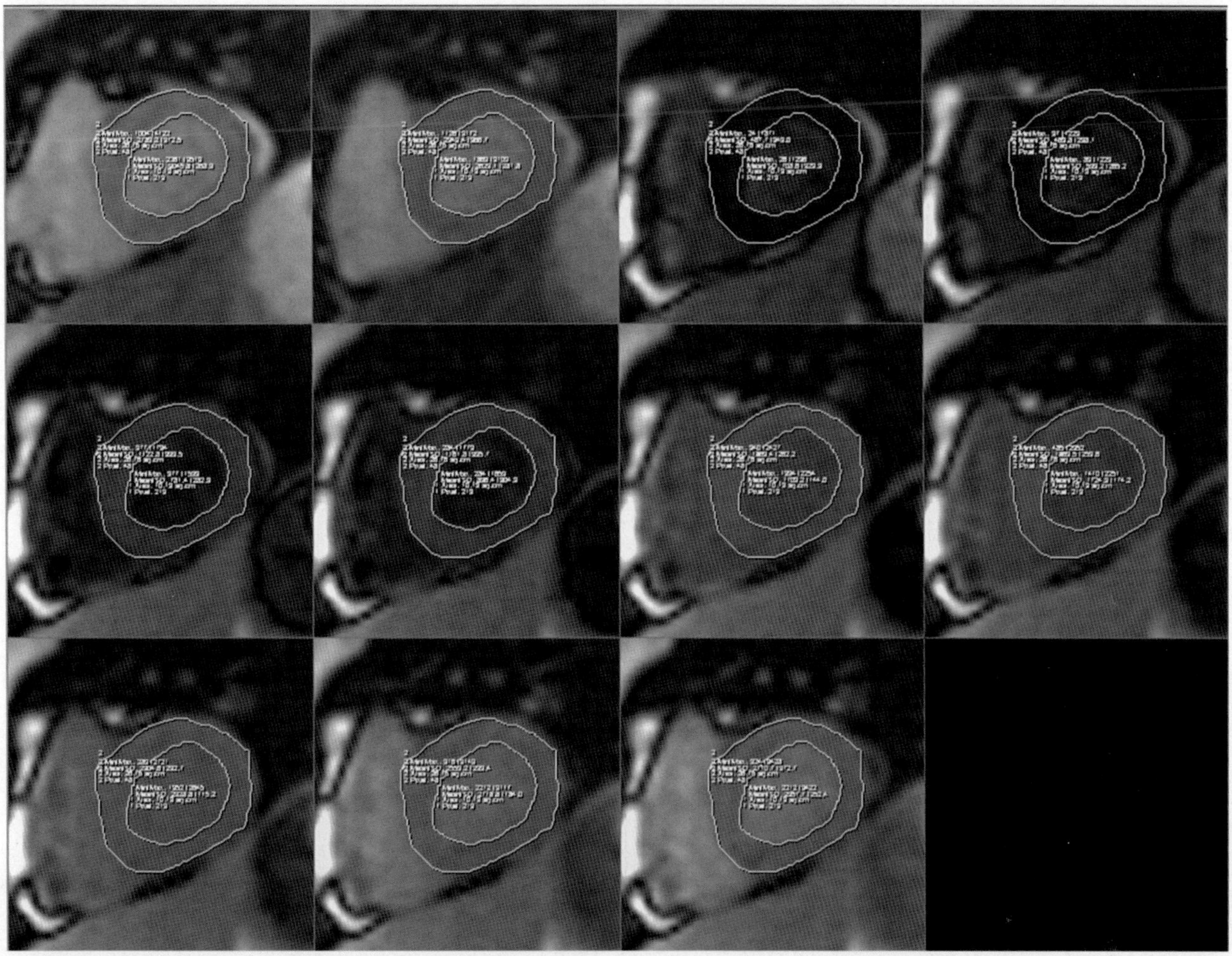

FIG. 4.11 Motion-corrected inversion recovery images may be checked for adequate motion correction by manually tracing endo and epicardial contours and copying for all images to ensure proper image registration.

measurement in the presence of fat unreliable. In this case, it is useful to acquire a water-fat separated image that aids in identifying whether there is fat present and provides the field map of off-resonance. When there is known to be fat, then it is preferable to reacquire with fat saturation when one case ensures the center frequency is well tuned. Fat saturation may lead to T1 errors if not well shimmed; therefore, it is not recommended to use this by default.

The measurement of T1 may also be influenced by T2 when using inversion recovery T1 methods such as MOLLI or ShMOLLI, as shown in Fig. 4.6 (upper left panel). Elevated values of myocardial T2 will further increase the myocardial T1 and may confound the interpretation depending on the application. For this reason, it is recommended to acquire T2 maps in conjunction with T1 maps to aid in interpreting T1 values.

Putting it all together (Fig. 4.16), it is recommended to: (1) perform a local volume shim, (2) acquire a multiecho Dixon water fat image with field map, (3) acquire T1 maps and T2 maps of each slice, (4) ensure good ECG triggering and diastolic timing, (5) reacquire with fat saturation if the presence of intramyocardial fat is detected, (6) check motion-corrected images for adequate image registration, and (7) check spatial resolution to ensure that measurements are not contaminated by adjacent blood or fat tissue.

SUMMARY

There are a number of methods and imaging protocols for T1 mapping in the heart and new methods are emerging. A comparison of several of the widely used protocols is shown in Table 4.3. This assessment of pros and cons, albeit subjective, is meant to capture the key issues that relate to overall reproducibility and affect the ability to detect subtle changes in T1 from normal values. The inherent difficulty of tightly controlling the shim and uniformity of the transmit flip angle in clinical scanners reduces the overall reproducibility of MOLLI-based methods that use inversion recovery and SSFP readout compared to the saturation recovery approach. Limitations such as partial volume effects are common to all of these protocols. In this table, falsely elevated T1 due to partial volume with fat is considered an artifact.

ECV mapping appears promising as a complement to LGE imaging in cases of more homogenously diffuse myocardial disease states that affect the myocardial extracellular space. The ability to display ECV maps in quantitative units that may be interpreted on an absolute scale offers the potential for simplified detection and measurement of the extent of abnormalities affecting the myocardial ECV. There is a continuous spectrum of spatial heterogeneity

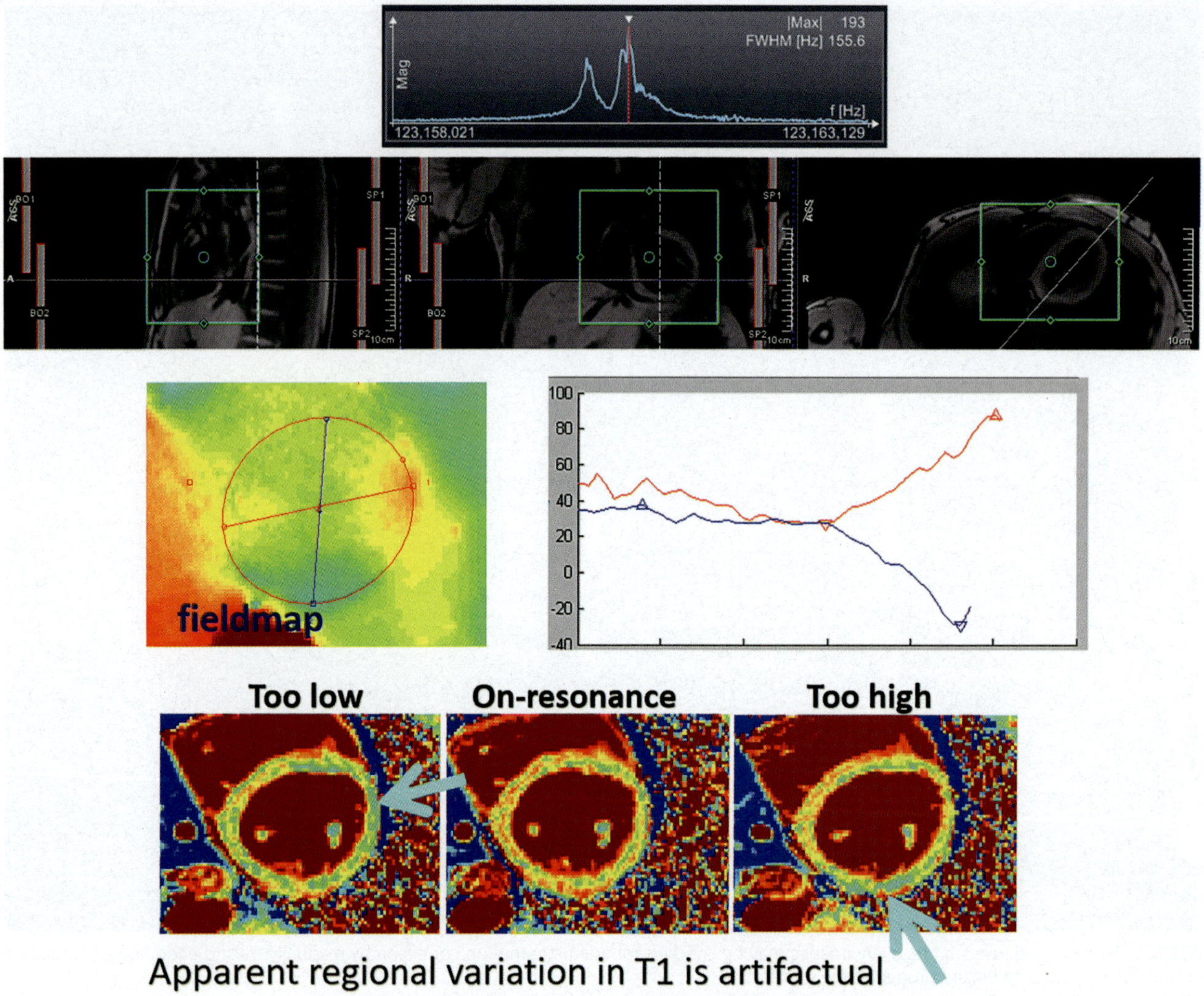

FIG. 4.12 T1 map sensitivity to shim and center frequency adjustment.

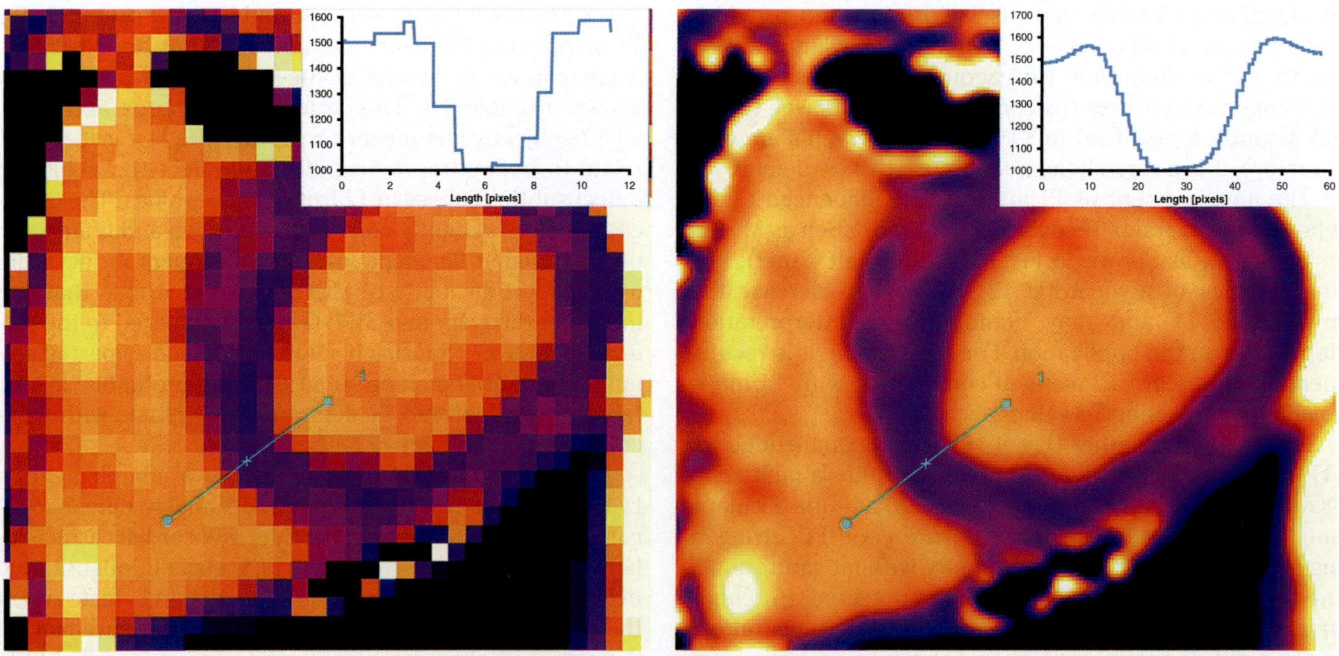

FIG. 4.13 Native T1 maps of heart with septal profile for pixelated map (*left*) and interpolated map (*right*), for case illustrating septal wall thickness of approximately 2 pixels in true acquired resolution.

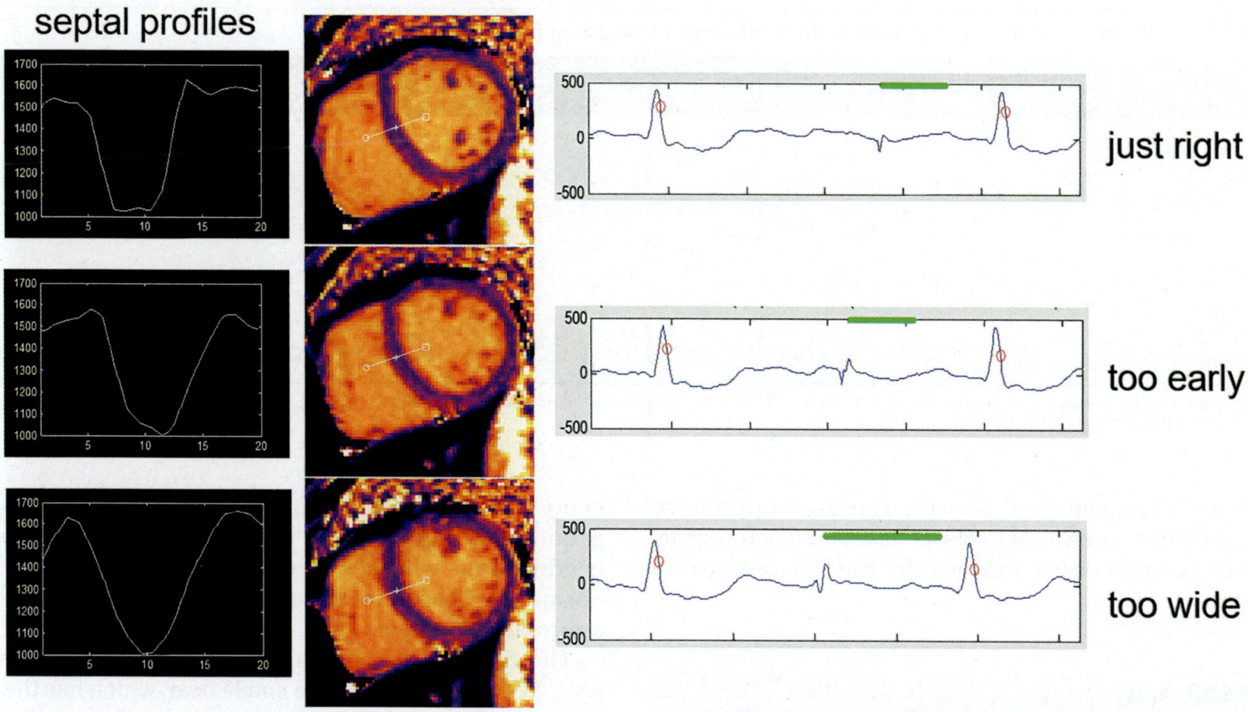

FIG. 4.14 Effect of temporal acquisition window on effective spatial resolution.

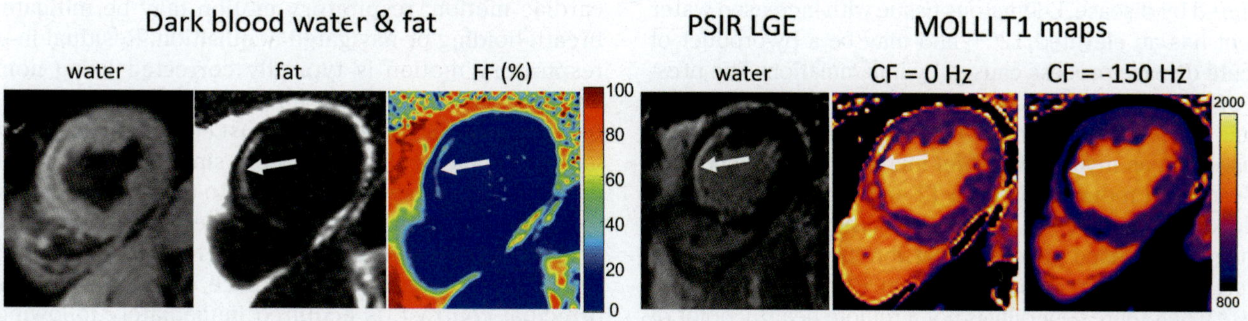

FIG. 4.15 Intramyocardial fat due to lipomatous metaplasia can lead to artifactual T1 estimate in voxels containing a mixture of water and fat, and the apparent T1 become dependent on the off-resonance frequency. *CF*, Center frequency; *FF*, fat fraction; *LGE*, late gadolinium enhancement; *MOLLI*, modified look locker inversion recovery; *PSIR*, phase sensitive inversion recovery.

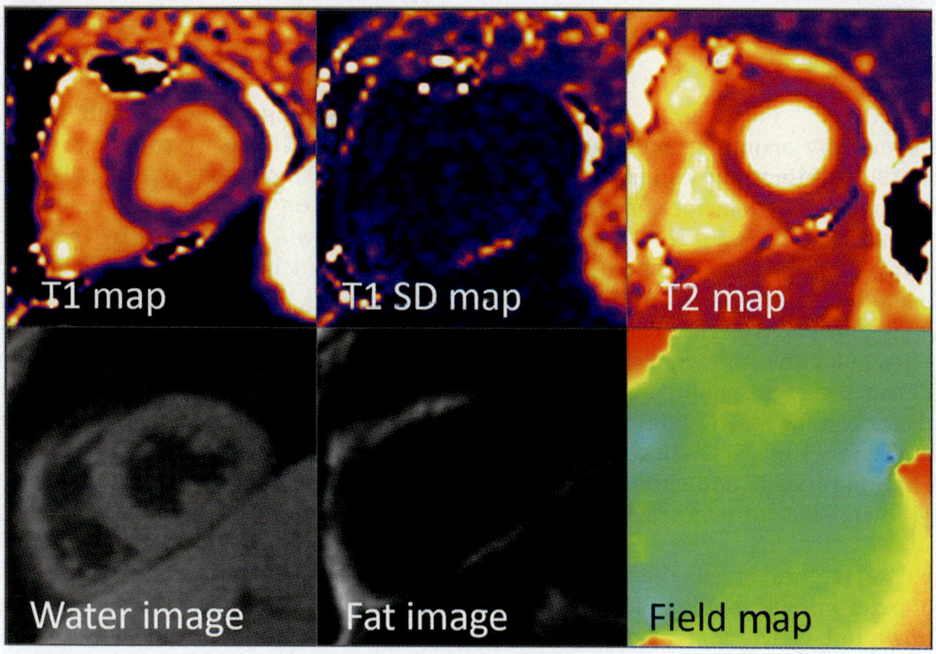

FIG. 4.16 Recommended imaging for performing quality assurance steps in T1 mapping. *SD*, Standard deviation.

TABLE 4.3 Summary of pros and cons of various reported T1 mapping protocols.

	MOLLI 3(3)3(3)5	MOLLI 5S(3S)3S	MOLLI 4S(1S)3S(1S)1S	SHMOLLI	SASHA 2P-FIT	SASHA 3P-FIT	SASHA VFA 2P-FIT	MSASHA
Short breath-hold	–	+	+	+	+	+	+	Free-breathing
HR insensitivity	–	+	+	+	++	++	++	++
Absolute accuracy	–	–	–	–	+	++	+	++
Precision	++	++	++	+	+	–	+	++
Few image artifacts	+	+	+	+	–	–	+	++
Reproducibility	–	+	+	+	–	–	++	++

HR, heart rate; *MOLLI*, modified Look-Locker inversion recovery; *mSASHA*, multiparametric SASHA; *SASHA*, saturation recovery single-shot acquisition; *ShMOLLI*, shortened MOLLI; *VFA*, variable flip angle.

between diffuse and focal fibrosis. The use of pixel-wise mapping offers a new tool to better assess the heterogeneity of myocardial tissue and measure the ECV of diseased regions.

T2 MAPPING

The transverse relaxation time (T2) of myocardial tissue may be altered by disease. Edematous tissue with increased water content has an elevated T2[18,19] and may be a by-product of an acute disease process caused by inflammation. The presence or absence of edema is used to differentiate acute and chronic MI,[1] identify the area at risk,[4] and assess nonischemic disease such as myocarditis.[68] An increased iron concentration leads to a reduction in both T2 and T2*, as seen in iron overload, for example Thalassemia.[17] Although T2-weighted imaging may be used to detect focal abnormalities, it is more challenging to detect global changes in T2 caused by diffuse disease when there generally is not a remote healthy point of reference. T2 mapping provides a means of automatic, quantitative measurement of T2 on a pixel-wise basis, which may be used in the diagnosis of diseases across a spectrum of heterogeneity, from diffuse to focal.

Methods

T2 mapping is performed by acquiring multiple images ($N \geq 2$) with different T2 weightings and estimating the T2 at each pixel by performing a 2-parameter curve fit to the measured signal for each pixel: $S_n(x,y)$. A monoexponential model ($S_n = PD \exp[-TE_n/T2]$) is used, where T2 is the unknown to be estimated, PD is the unknown proton density, and TE_n (known) is the effective echo time of the individual T2-weighted image for the *n*th acquisition ($n = 1,2, \ldots, N$). T2-weighted images may be acquired by a number of methods. Methods for cardiac MRI T2 mapping include: (1) T2-prepared SSFP (T2p-SSFP),[69] (2) multiecho spin echo (MESE),[70] and (3) a hybrid of MESE and either turbo spin echo (TSE)[71,72] or gradient-recalled echo planar imaging (GraSE).[73,74]

The most widely used method at this time is the T2p-SSFP. An example of pixel-wise T2 mapping for a subject with acute MI is shown in Fig. 4.17 for T2p-SSFP. In this example, three T2-weighted images are acquired with echo times of TE = 0, 25, and 55 ms, where the TE = 0 is acquired without any T2 preparation. The anterior MI is edematous with elevated T2 (approx. 72 ms), and the normal myocardium remote from the MI has a T2 of approximately 48 ms.

The single-shot T2-prepared readout approach acquires each T2-weighted image in a single beat, which has the benefit of being robust to cardiac and respiratory motion. ECG gating is used with acquisition in middiastole to minimize cardiac motion; respiratory motion may be mitigated by breath-holding or navigated acquisition. Residual in-plane respiratory motion is typically corrected using nonrigid image registration. Either an SSFP or FLASH readout may be used.[69] An SSFP readout is most commonly used to maximize SNR, particularly at 1.5 T. A single-shot SSFP readout uses a linear phase-encode order to minimize artifacts due to eddy currents. It is possible to use centric phase-encode ordering with a single-shot FLASH readout. By using centric ordering, the center of k-space, which determines the principal contrast, is acquired immediately following the T2 preparation. However, by using linear ordering there is some delay following the T2 preparation and the center of k-space, during which there is T1 regrowth of the magnetization that leads to a T1 dependent bias = $PD(1-\exp(-TS/T1))$, where TS is the time from the end of the preparation to the center of k-space.

With the T2p-SSFP approach, it is necessary to have several heart beats (typically 3 or 4 seconds) between image acquisitions to allow for full magnetization recovery (dependent on T1). If there is insufficient signal recovery, the images will be affected by the preceding image, thus altering the estimated value of T2 and introducing a dependence on T1. Alternately, it has been proposed to use a saturation preparation to reset the initial condition for each heartbeat to a fixed value.[75] In this way, the number of images acquired may be increased since no recovery beats are required, but there is a significant SNR loss due to the incomplete saturation recovery.

The T2 preparation is implemented by tipping the magnetization vector down on the transverse plane for a prescribed duration (TE), followed by tipping the vector back and crushing any residual transverse magnetization. Refocusing pulses are used between the tip-down and tip-up pulses to avoid dephasing due to myocardial motion or blood flow, which can result in artifacts. T2 preparations

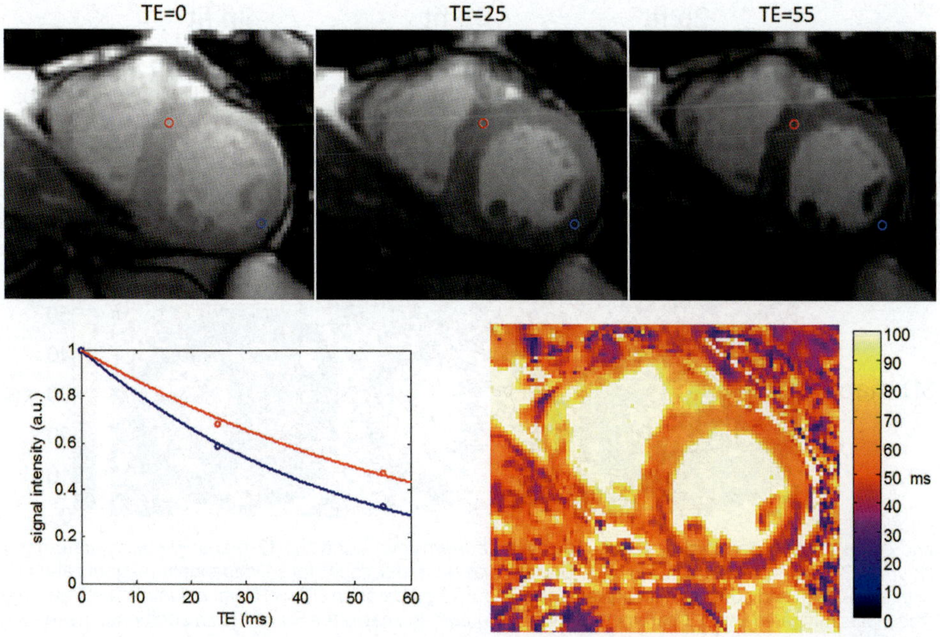

FIG. 4.17 Illustration of T2 mapping approach using T2-prepared steady-state free precession to (A) acquire images at three echo times, (B) perform a monoexponential curve fit to signal intensities at each pixel to estimate T2, and (C) produce a pixel-wise T2 map. *TE*, Echo time.

have been designed that are robust to variations in both B0 (off-resonance) and B1 (effective transmitted FA). These are based on either composite pulses[20,76] or adiabatic RF designs.[77,78] The minimum TE for the T2 preparation is dependent on the duration and number of refocusing pulses. For designs that use several refocusing pulses a short TE is not feasible,[20] and in this case a readout without any T2 preparation is used for an effective TE = 0. A significant error in FA due to inhomogeneity in transmitted B_1+ or a calibration error that results in a reduced signal for the prepared measurements, and not the TE = 0 measurement, may lead to an underestimate of T2. This may be mitigated using a T2 preparation for all measurements and shortening the overall refocusing duration.

The multi echo spin echo (MESE) approach acquires data in a segmented fashion, with multiple echoes with different TEs acquired at each beat for a given phase encode using a spin echo train. This requires a lengthy breath-hold or navigated scan and is included here for completeness of discussion. The MESE is acquired in conjunction with a dark blood preparation to avoid blood flow artifacts, typically double inversion recovery (DIR) applied immediately following the R-wave ECG trigger.

The acquisition of MESE may be accelerated by acquiring multiple phase encodes at each echo time using a hybrid approach such as GraSE,[79,80] which employs a short echo train gradient-recalled echo-planar imaging (EPI) readout between 180 degree refocusing pulses. In this way, 3–7 echoes may be acquired per heartbeat, accelerating the image acquisition for T2 mapping.[73,74] This scheme is also used in conjunction with a DIR dark blood preparation, and may be either breath-held or navigated. An EPI readout is prone to artifacts due to off-resonance or fat chemical shift and is often used in conjunction with chemical-shift fat saturation. To mitigate ghosting artifacts, a linear interleaved phase-encode order is typically used with echo time shifting to ensure a smooth phase transition across k-space for different EPI echoes.

Spin echo methods are highly motion sensitive. DIR dark blood preparations rely on imaging at the same cardiac phase as the DIR preparation, which is difficult to achieve at higher heart rates or in patients with motion during the imaging interval in diastole. Furthermore, the spin echo readout itself is sensitive to motion. It is common for myocardial wall motion to cause signal loss or complete signal drop out.

Reproducibility: Accuracy, Precision, and Confounding Factors

Similar to the discussion of T1 and ECV mapping, many of the same factors and considerations affect reproducibility. These include blood pool contamination due to partial volume effects, dependence on off-resonance and transmitted FA, a confounding influence of T1, and SNR.

With the T2p-SSFP approach, there is a T1 bias due to the magnetization regrowth following the T2 preparation and acquisition of the center of k-space. This signal bias can lead to an overestimation of T2 by 5–10 ms. While in theory, a 3-parameter fit ($S = PD\ \exp[-TE/T2] + b$) may be used to eliminate this confounding bias variable (b), a 3-parameter fit with only a few relatively short TE measurements is very noisy. It has been proposed that the bias term can be directly measured[81] by acquiring an image using a saturation recovery preparation without any T2 preparation, which corresponds to the $TE = \infty$ image. In this way, a 3-parameter fit may be used without incurring a large SNR penalty, thus effectively eliminating this T1 confounder. This is illustrated in Fig. 4.18, which shows the reduced benefit of a 3-parameter fit in reducing the T2 bias and the improvement in SD of the 3-parameter fit using the additional $TE = \infty$ measurement.

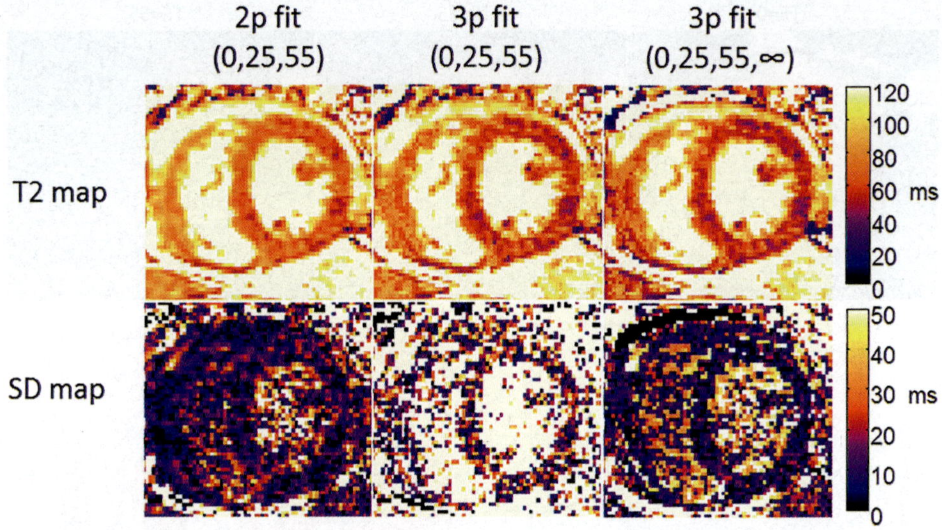

FIG. 4.18 T2 (*top row*) and corresponding standard deviation (*SD*) maps (*bottom row*) using the T2-prepared steady-state free precession method with 2-parameter fitting (*left column*), 3-parameter fitting including a constant bias term to account for T1-dependent magnetization regrowth (*center column*), and 3-parameter fitting with a bias term and additional measurement without T2 preparation (TE = ∞) (*right column*). The 2-parameter fit overestimates the T2 due to the bias term. The bias is mitigated using 3-parameter fitting but greatly increases the SD unless an additional measurement at TE = ∞ is included. *TE*, Echo time; *SD*, standard deviation.

The SSFP readout itself has image contrast dependent on T1 and T2. To a large extent, the image contrast is shared for all of the T2-weighted images and does not affect the fit. However, single-shot imaging is acquired on the approach to steady state and the contrast depends on the initial conditions, which in turn depends on the TE of the T2 preparation. Thus, there is some residual T1 contrast dependent on the readout, which may alter the T2 estimate.

The T2-SSFP measurement is sensitive to off-resonance. The SSFP readout has an off-resonance response that is different for the different T2 preparation echo times (TEs). This leads to an overall dependence of the T2 measurement on the off-resonance frequency. The T2 error has been characterized experimentally[82] for a specific imaging protocol and found to vary significantly for off-resonance > ±150 Hz, and for errors of approximately 5% at ± 100 Hz. The frequency dependence of the T2 preparation also contributes to the response. The off-resonance sensitivity is reduced by using a lower excitation FA. The T2 error is shown in Fig. 4.19, which illustrates off-resonance sensitivity and the FA dependence, as well as on-resonance bias, described above. The composite hard pulse design is wideband, but the adiabatic designs used for greater independence of FA generally have a narrower bandwidth. Thus, care must be taken to ensure the volume is properly shimmed. The T2p-SSFP approach will not work well in the presence of device implants.

Using the GraSE approach, there is also a significant bias.[73] Using a TSE approach, it is difficult to completely eliminate stimulated echo pathways, which may also lead to a T1 dependence in the contrast. This bias is not well characterized, and there are no methods for eliminating the bias.

The precision of the T2 measurement is determined by the SNR, the number of measurements, the actual value of T2, and the specific echo times used. The SD of the T2 estimate due to random noise (Fig. 4.20) was calculated

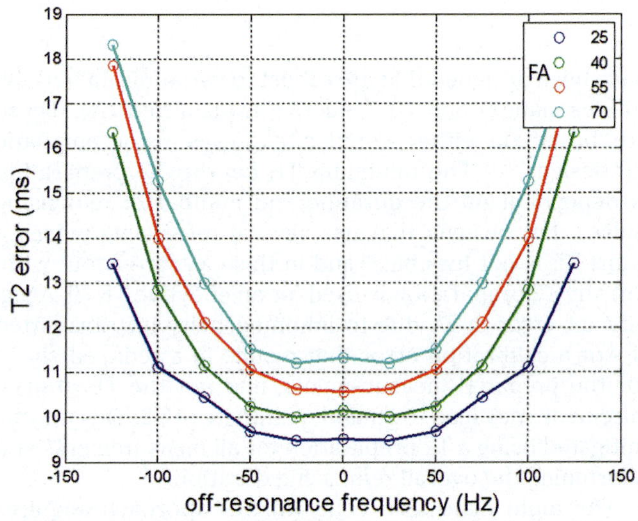

FIG. 4.19 T2 estimates using the T2-prepared steady-state free precession method are sensitive to off-resonance and flip angle (*FA*), with increasing errors at higher FAs. Significant errors are observed for off-resonance greater than ±50 Hz.

analytically for a myocardial T2 of 45 ms at various SNRs for three echo time measurements (solid) and four echo time measurements (dotted). Measurements were equally spaced at 0, $TE_{max}/2$, TE_{max} for 3 TEs and 0, $TE_{max}/3$, $2TE_{max}/3$, and TE_{max} for 4 TEs. These agree well with a numerical simulation performed for a specific T2-SSFP protocol[82] with three measurements constrained to be 0, TE, and 2 TE, where the best TE was found for normal myocardium at T2 = 45 ms to be in the range 30–40 ms (i.e., echo times 0, 30, 60 ms to 0, 40, 80 ms). The SD may be calculated on a pixel-wise fashion in a similar manner as for T1[59] or T2*.[83] An example of T2 and SD maps for the case shown in Fig 4.17 is shown in Fig 4.21. The pixel-wise noise SD for this case is approximately 2.1 ms in a remote region with T2 = 44 ms and the SD is approximately 3.7 ms in the edematous region with elevated T2 = 68 ms.

Limitations and Potential Pitfalls

The dark blood preparation used in spin echo–based techniques such as GraSE help eliminate contamination of myocardial signal due to partial volume effects. However, spin echo readouts and DIR dark blood preparations are highly motion sensitive and prone to signal loss, particularly at higher heart rates. Off-resonance leads to bias errors in SSFP methods and to artifacts in EPI methods; therefore, it is essential to ensure the volume is adequately shimmed.

T1-weighted contrast may confound the T2 measurement due to magnetization regrowth in the case of T2p-SSFP and stimulated echoes in SE methods. Methods have been proposed to mitigate bias in T2p-SSFP,[81] but may not be widely available. This may be avoided by using T2p single-shot FLASH with a centric readout, particularly at 3T where the SNR of FLASH may be adequate. It is also important to avoid T2 mapping after administering Gd contrast to avoid short T1.

Current imaging protocols have been designed for myocardial T2 measurement and are not suitable for accurate measurement of blood T2. The echo times are much shorter than the T2 of the blood, leading to poorly conditioned fitting and sensitivity to blood signal loss due to dephasing at longer echo times.

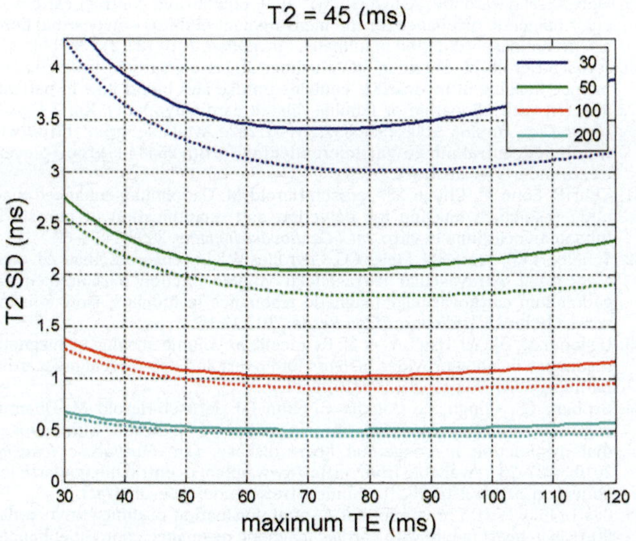

FIG. 4.20 Variation of standard deviation (*SD*) for T2 estimates with equally spaced echo times between 0 and the maximum echo time (TE_{max}) using three measurements (*solid*) and 4 measurements (*dotted*). Baseline normal myocardium T2 = 45 ms is used in this calculation, and SD is fairly insensitive to TE_{max} over a wide range (50–100 ms).

SUMMARY

T2 mapping in the heart using 2D imaging is feasible in a clinical environment and has sufficient accuracy and precision to be of value to answer a number of clinical questions. Absolute baseline values will depend on the field strength, and to some extent on the method. T2p-SSFP is the most widely used method and fairly robust in terms of image quality.

DISCUSSION

Future developments to address the current limitations in quantitative measurement are focused on reduction in partial volume effects, differentiation between edema and fibrosis, establishment of baseline normal values, standardization, and quality control. Quantitative methods of T1, T2, and ECV mapping have been successful in population-based studies. Addressing the remaining issues is key to the reliable application of quantitative methods to the diagnosis of disease in individual patients.

A better understanding of confounding factors such as the effect of T2 on T1 measurement is important for interpretation of measurements. Understanding how scanner adjustments such as off-resonance or flip angle may affect quantitative measurements is important for the reliable detection of subtle disease. Multiparametric measurements may help differentiate between edema and fibrosis and may also play a role in disentangling the coupling in measurements of T1 and T2.

Partial volume contamination by the adjacent blood pool or intramyocardial fat is an important issue in current protocols. Use of higher spatial resolution or 3D imaging help mitigate partial volume to some extent. Suppression of blood or fat may be required to further reduce this contamination; however, these methods may introduce other side effects.

Standardization encompasses methods for acquiring quantitative maps, displays, region-of-interest measurements, and reporting. Visualization of parametric maps is most commonly done by color display. However, there is

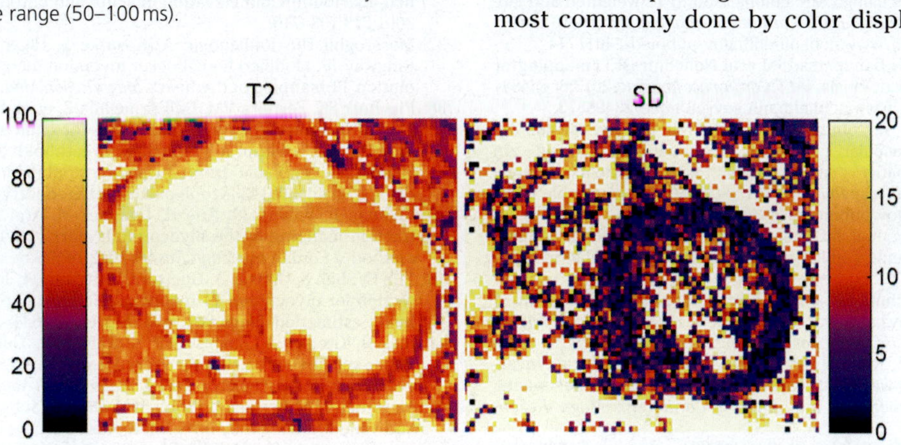

FIG. 4.21 Example T2 and standard deviation (*SD*) maps using T2-prepared steady-state free precession for subject with acute myocardial infarction. SD is increased in edematous region due to elevated T2.

no current consensus on the scale or colormap. The visual display has a significant effect on the classification of normal versus abnormal tissue and on the assessment of the quality of the map. Use of quality control phantoms may also play a role in standardization.[84]

Quantitative mapping has the potential for increasing the objectiveness of CMR and improving the sensitivity for detecting subtle changes in global state due to disease processes. Mapping has come a long way in the past decade, and technical developments continue to improve methods and uncover new and interesting clinical and research applications.

ACKNOWLEDGMENTS

Portions of text and figures have been excerpted and modified from the Journal of Cardiovascular Magnetic Resonance Open Access publication.[39,45]

REFERENCES

1. Abdel-Aty H, Zagrosek A, Schulz-Menger J, et al. Delayed enhancement and T2-weighted cardiovascular magnetic resonance imaging differentiate acute from chronic myocardial infarction. *Circulation*. 2004;109:2411–2416.
2. Bohl S, Wassmuth R, Abdel-Aty H, et al. Delayed enhancement cardiac magnetic resonance imaging reveals typical patterns of myocardial injury in patients with various forms of non-ischemic heart disease. *Int J Cardiovasc Imaging*. 2008;24:597–607.
3. Friedrich MG, Kim HW, Kim RJ. T2-weighted imaging to assess post-infarct myocardium at risk. *JACC Cardiovasc Imaging*. 2011;4:1014–1021.
4. Ugander M, Bagi PS, Oki AJ, et al. Myocardial edema as detected by pre-contrast T1 and T2 CMR delineates area at risk associated with acute myocardial infarction. *JACC Cardiovasc Imaging*. 2012;5:596–603.
5. Zagrosek A, Abdel-Aty H, Boyé P, et al. Cardiac magnetic resonance monitors reversible and irreversible myocardial injury in myocarditis. *JACC Cardiovasc Imaging*. 2009;2:131–138.
6. Kim R, Wu E, Rafael A, Chen E, et al. The use of contrast-enhanced magnetic resonance imaging to identify reversible myocardial dysfunction. *N Engl J Med*. 2000;343:1445–1453.
7. Messroghli DR, Walters K, Plein S, et al. Myocardial T1 mapping: application to patients with acute and chronic myocardial infarction. *Magn Reson Med*. 2007;58:34–40.
8. Messroghli DR, Niendorf T, Schulz-Menger J, Dietz R, Friedrich MG. T1 Mapping in Patients with Acute Myocardial Infarction. *J Cardiovasc Magn Reson*. 2003;5:353–359.
9. Dall'armellina E, Piechnik SK, Ferreira VM, et al. Cardiovascular magnetic resonance by non contrast T1 mapping allows assessment of severity of injury in acute myocardial infarction. *J Cardiovasc Magn Reson [Internet]*. 2012;14(1):15. Available from: http://www.ncbi.nlm.nih.gov/pubmed/22309452.
10. Ferreira VM, Piechnik SK, Armellina ED, et al. Non-contrast T1-mapping detects acute myocardial edema with high diagnostic accuracy: a comparison to T2-weighted cardiovascular magnetic resonance. *J Cardiovasc Magn Reson*. 2012;14:1-12.
11. Ferreira VM, Piechnik SK, Dall'Armellina E, et al. T(1) mapping for the diagnosis of acute myocarditis using CMR: comparison to T2-weighted and late gadolinium enhanced imaging. *JACC Cardiovasc Imaging*. 2013;6(10):1048–1058. Available from: http://www.ncbi.nlm.nih.gov/pubmed/24011774.
12. Karamitsos TD, Piechnik SK, Banypersad SM, et al. Noncontrast T1 mapping for the diagnosis of cardiac amyloidosis. *JACC Cardiovasc Imaging*. 2013;6(4):488–497. Available from: http://www.ncbi.nlm.nih.gov/pubmed/23498672.
13. Puntmann VO, D'Cruz D, Smith Z, et al. Native myocardial T1 mapping by cardiovascular magnetic resonance imaging in subclinical cardiomyopathy in patients with systemic lupus erythematosus. *Circ Cardiovasc Imaging*. 2013;6(2):295–301. Available from: http://www.ncbi.nlm.nih.gov/pubmed/23403334.
14. Ertel A, Pratt D, Kellman P, et al. Increased myocardial extracellular volume in active idiopathic systemic capillary leak syndrome. *J Cardiovasc Magn Reson*. 2015;17(1):76.
15. Sado DM, White SK, Piechnik SK, et al. Identification and assessment of Anderson-Fabry disease by cardiovascular magnetic resonance noncontrast myocardial T1 mapping. *Circ Cardiovasc Imaging*. 2013;6(3):392–398.
16. Pedersen SF, Thrysøe SA, Robich MP, et al. Assessment of intramyocardial hemorrhage by T1-weighted cardiovascular magnetic resonance in reperfused acute myocardial infarction. *J Cardiovasc Magn Reson*. 2012;14(1):1–8.
17. Feng Y, He T, Carpenter JP, et al. In vivo comparison of myocardial T1 with T2 and T2* in thalassaemia major. *J Magn Reson Imaging*. 2013;38(3):588–593. Available from: http://www.ncbi.nlm.nih.gov/pubmed/23371802.
18. Thavendiranathan P, Walls M, Giri S, et al. Improved detection of myocardial involvement in acute inflammatory cardiomyopathies using T2 mapping. *Circ Cardiovasc Imaging*. 2012;5(1):102–110.
19. Verhaert D, Thavendiranathan P, Giri S, et al. Direct T2 quantification of myocardial edema in acute ischemic injury. *JACC Cardiovasc Imaging*. 2011;4(3):269–278. Available from: http://www.pubmedcentral.nih.gov/articlerender.fcgi?artid=4282779&tool=pmcentrez&rendertype=abstract.
20. Giri S, Chung Y-C, Merchant A, et al. T2 quantification for improved detection of myocardial edema. *J Cardiovasc Magn Reson*. 2009;11(1):56.
21. Moon JC, Messroghli DR, Kellman P, et al. Myocardial T1 mapping and extracellular volume quantification: a Society for Cardiovascular Magnetic Resonance (SCMR) and CMR Working Group of the European Society of Cardiology consensus statement. *J Cardiovasc Magn Reson*. 2013;15(1):92.
22. Pennell DJ, Sechtem UP, Higgins CB, et al. Clinical indications for cardiovascular magnetic resonance (CMR): Consensus Panel report. *Eur Heart J*. 2004;25(21):1940–1965.
23. Hunold P, Schlosser T, Vogt FM, et al. Myocardial late enhancement in contrast-enhanced cardiac mri: distinction between infarction and non-infarction-related disease. *AJR Am J Roentgenol*. 2005;184(5):1420–1426.
24. Sado DM, Flett AS, Moon JC. Novel imaging techniques for diffuse myocardial fibrosis. *Future Cardiol*. 2011;7(5):643–650.
25. Gai N, Turkbey EB, Nazarian S, et al. T1 mapping of the gadolinium-enhanced myocardium: adjustment for factors affecting interpatient comparison. *Magn Reson Med*. 2011;65(5):1407–1415.
26. Mewton N, Liu CY, Croisille P, Bluemke D, Lima JAC. Assessment of myocardial fibrosis with cardiovascular magnetic resonance. *J Am Coll Cardiol*. 2011;57(8):891–903. Available from http://www.pubmedcentral.nih.gov/articlerender.fcgi?artid=3081658&tool=pmcentrez&rendertype=abstract.
27. Lee JJ, Liu S, Nacif MS, et al. Myocardial T1 and extracellular volume fraction mapping at 3 tesla. *J Cardiovasc Magn Reson*. 2011;13(1):75.
28. Arheden H, Saeed M, Higgins CB, et al. Measurement of the gadopentetate dimeglumine at echo-planar MR imaging to quantify myocardial infarction : comparison with 99m Tc-DTPA autoradiography in rats. *Radiology*. 1999;311(3):698–708.
29. Flett AS, Hayward MP, Ashworth MT, et al. Equilibrium contrast cardiovascular magnetic resonance for the measurement of diffuse myocardial fibrosis: preliminary validation in humans. *Circulation*. 2010;122(2):138–144.
30. Jerosch-Herold M, Sheridan DC, Kushner JD, et al. Cardiac magnetic resonance imaging of myocardial contrast uptake and blood flow in patients affected with idiopathic or familial dilated cardiomyopathy. *Am J Physiol Heart Circ Physiol*. 2008;295(3):H1234–H1242. Available from: http://www.pubmedcentral.nih.gov/articlerender.fcgi?artid=2544489&tool=pmcentrez&rendertype=abstract.
31. Kehr E, Sono M, Chugh SS, Jerosch-Herold M. Gadolinium-enhanced magnetic resonance imaging for detection and quantification of fibrosis in human myocardium in vitro. *Int J Cardiovasc Imaging*. 2008;24:61–68.
32. Schelbert EB, Testa SM, Meier CG, Ceyrolles WJ, Levenson JE, Blair AJ, et al. Myocardial extravascular extracellular volume fraction measurement by gadolinium cardiovascular magnetic resonance in humans: slow infusion versus bolus. *J Cardiovasc Magn Reson*. 2011;13:16.
33. Ugander M, Oki AJ, Hsu L-Y, et al. Extracellular volume imaging by magnetic resonance imaging provides insights into overt and sub-clinical myocardial pathology. *Eur Heart J*. 2012;33(10):1–11.
34. Broberg CS, Chugh SS, Conklin C, Sahn DJ, Jerosch-Herold M. Quantification of diffuse myocardial fibrosis and its association with myocardial dysfunction in congenital heart disease. *Circ Cardiovasc Imaging*. 2010;3:727–734. Available from: http://www.pubmedcentral.nih.gov/articlerender.fcgi?artid=3048790&tool=pmcentrez&rendertype=abstract.
35. Iles L, Pfluger H, Phrommintikul A, et al. Evaluation of diffuse myocardial fibrosis in heart failure with cardiac magnetic resonance contrast-enhanced T1 mapping. *J Am Coll Cardiol*. 2008;52(19):1574–1580. Available from: http://www.ncbi.nlm.nih.gov/pubmed/19007595.
36. Flacke SJ, Fischer SE, Lorenz CH. Cardiac imaging abbreviations: gadopentetate dimeglumine partition coefficient in human myocardium in vivo: normal distribution and elevation in acute and chronic infarction 1. *Radiology*. 2001;218:703–710.
37. Messroghli DR, Radjenovic A, Kozerke S, Higgins DM, Sivananthan MU, Ridgway JP. Modified Look-Locker inversion recovery (MOLLI) for high-resolution T1 mapping of the heart. *Magn Reson Med*. 2004;52:141–146.
38. Piechnik SK, Ferreira VM, Dall'Armellina E, et al. Shortened Modified Look-Locker Inversion recovery (ShMOLLI) for clinical myocardial T1-mapping at 1.5 and 3 T within a 9 heartbeat breathhold. *J Cardiovasc Magn Reson*. 2010;12:69. Available from: http://www.pubmedcentral.nih.gov/articlerender.fcgi?artid=3001433&tool=pmcentrez&rendertype=abstract.
39. Kellman P, Wilson JR, Xue H, Ugander M, Arai AE. Extracellular volume fraction mapping in the myocardium, part 1: evaluation of an automated method. *J Cardiovasc Magn Reson*. 2012;14:63.
40. Xue H, Shah S, Greiser A, Guetter C, Littmann A, Jolly MP, et al. Motion correction for myocardial T1 mapping using image registration with synthetic image estimation. *Magn Reson Med*. 2012;67:1644–1655.
41. Xue H, Greiser A, Zuehlsdorff S, Jolly M-P, Guehring J, Arai AE, et al. Phase-sensitive inversion recovery for myocardial T1 mapping with motion correction and parametric fitting. *Magn Reson Med*. 2013;69:1408–1420.
42. Messroghli DR, Greiser A, Fröhlich M, Dietz R, Schulz-Menger J. Optimization and validation of a fully-integrated pulse sequence for modified look-locker inversion-recovery (MOLLI) T1 mapping of the heart. *J Magn Reson Imaging*. 2007;26:1081–1086.

43. Gai ND, Stehning C, Nacif M, Bluemke DA. Modified Look-Locker T(1) evaluation using Bloch simulations: Human and phantom validation. *Magn Reson Med.* 2012;69(2):329–336. Available from: http://www.ncbi.nlm.nih.gov/pubmed/22457268.
44. Salerno M, Janardhanan R, Jiji RS, et al. Comparison of methods for determining the partition coefficient of gadolinium in the myocardium using T(1) mapping. *J Magn Reson Imaging.* 2012;38(1):217–224. Available from: http://www.ncbi.nlm.nih.gov/pubmed/23197434.
45. Kellman P, Hansen MS. T1-mapping in the heart: accuracy and precision. *J Cardiovasc Magn Reson.* 2014;16:2.
46. Higgins DM, Ridgway JP, Radjenovic A, Sivananthan UM, Smith MA. T1 measurement using a short acquisition period for quantitative cardiac applications. *Med Phys.* 2005;32:1738. Available from: http://link.aip.org/link/MPHYA6/v32/i6/p1738/s1&Agg=doi.
47. Chow K, Flewitt JA, Green JD, Pagano JJ, Friedrich MG, Thompson RB. Saturation recovery single-shot acquisition (SASHA) for myocardial T(1) mapping. *Magn Reson Med.* 2014;71:2082–2095.
48. Weingärtner S, Akçakaya M, Basha T, et al. Combined saturation/inversion recovery sequences for improved evaluation of scar and diffuse fibrosis in patients with arrhythmia or heart rate variability. *Magn Reson Med.* 2013;71(3):1024–1034.
49. Mehta BB, Chen X, Bilchick KC, Salerno M, Epstein FH. Accelerated and navigator-gated look-locker imaging for cardiac T1 estimation (ANGIE): Development and application to T1 mapping of the right ventricle. *Magn Reson Med.* 2015;73:150–160. Available from: http://www.pubmedcentral.nih.gov/articlerender.fcgi?artid=4128906&tool=pmcentrez&rendertype=abstract.
50. Weingärtner S, Roujol S, Akçakaya M, Basha TA, Nezafat R. Free-breathing multislice native myocardial T 1 mapping using the slice-interleaved T 1 (STONE) sequence. *Magn Reson Med.* 2014;74(1):115–124. https://doi.org/10.1002/mrm.25387.
51. Akcakaya M, Weingartner S, Manning WJ, Nezafat R. Selection of sampling points for saturation recovery based myocardial T1 mapping. *J Cardiovasc Magn Reson.* 2014;73(5):1741–1753. Available from: http://www.jcmr-online.com/content/16/S1/W32.
52. Kellman P, Xue H, Chow K, Spottiswoode BS, Arai AE, Thompson RB. Optimized saturation recovery protocols for T1-mapping in the heart: influence of sampling strategies on precision. *J Cardiovasc Magn Reson.* 2014;16:55.
53. Chow K, Spottiswoode BS, Pagano JJ, Thompson RB. Improved precision in SASHA T1 mapping with a variable flip angle readout. *J Cardiovasc Magn Reson.* 2014;16:M9.
54. Stainsby JA, Slavin GS. Comparing the accuracy and precision of SMART-1Map, SASHA and MOLLI. *J Cardiovasc Magn Reson.* 2014;16(suppl 1):P11. Available from: http://www.jcmr-online.com/content/16/S1/P11.
55. Chow K, Hayes G, Flewitt J, et al. Improved accuracy and precision with three–parameter simultaneous myocardial T1 and T2 mapping using multiparametric SASHA. *Magn Res Med.* 2022:1–17.
56. Kellman P, Xue H, Chow K, et al. Bright-blood and dark-blood phase sensitive inversion recovery late gadolinium enhancement and T1 and T2 maps in a single free-breathing scan: an all-in-one approach. *J Cardiovasc Magn Reson.* 2021;23:1–14. https://doi.org/10.1186/s12968-021-00823-3.
57. Deichmann R, Haase A. Quantification of Tl Values by SNAPSHOT-FLASH NMR Imaging. *J Magn Reson.* 1992;612:608–612.
58. Schmitt P, Griswold M a, Jakob PM, Kotas M, Gulani V, Flentje M, et al. Inversion recovery TrueFISP: quantification of T(1), T(2), and spin density. *Magn Reson Med.* 2004;51:661–667. Available from: http://www.ncbi.nlm.nih.gov/pubmed/15065237.
59. Kellman P, Arai AE, Xue H. T1 and extracellular volume mapping in the heart: estimation of error maps and the influence of noise on precision. *J Cardiovasc Magn Reson.* 2013;15:56.
60. Kellman P, Herzka DA, Arai AE, Hansen MS. Influence of off-resonance in myocardial T1-mapping using SSFP based MOLLI method. *J Cardiovasc Magn Reson.* 2013;15:63.
61. Song T, Stainsby JA, Ho VB, Hood MN, Slavin GS. Flexible cardiac T1 mapping using a modified Look-Locker acquisition with saturation recovery. *Magn Reson Med.* 2012;67:622–627. Available from: http://www.ncbi.nlm.nih.gov/pubmed/22344580.
62. Klein C, Schmal TR, Nekolla SG, Schnackenburg B, Fleck E, Nagel E. Mechanism of late gadolinium enhancement in patients with acute myocardial infarction. *J Cardiovasc Magn Reson.* 2007;9:653–658. Available from: http://www.ncbi.nlm.nih.gov/pubmed/17578720.
63. Spottiswoode BS, Ugander M, Kellman P. Automated inline extracellular volume (ECV) mapping. *J Cardiovasc Magn Reson.* 2015;17:W6. Available from: http://www.jcmr-online.com/content/17/S1/W6.
64. Treibel TA, Fontana M, Maestrini V, et al. Automatic measurement of the myocardial interstitium: synthetic extracellular volume quantification without hematocrit sampling. *JACC Cardiovasc Imaging.* 2016;9:54–63.
65. Robson MD, Piechnik SK, Tunnicliffe EM, Neubauer S. T1 measurements in the human myocardium: The effects of magnetization transfer on the SASHA and MOLLI sequences. *Magn Reson Med.* 2013;670:664–670. Available from: http://www.ncbi.nlm.nih.gov/pubmed/23857710.
66. Kellman P, Bandettini WP, Mancini C, Hammer-Hansen S, Hansen MS, Arai AE. Characterization of myocardial T1-mapping bias caused by intramyocardial fat in inversion recovery and saturation recovery techniques. *J Cardiovasc Magn Reson.* 2015;17:33.
67. Bhuva AN, Treibel TA, Seraphim A, et al. Measurement of T1 mapping in patients with cardiac devices: off-resonance error extends beyond visual artifact but can be quantified and corrected. *Front Cardiovasc Med.* 2021;8:1–9.
68. Bohnen S, Radunski UK, Lund GK, et al. Performance of t1 and t2 mapping cardiovascular magnetic resonance to detect active myocarditis in patients with recent-onset heart failure. *Circ Cardiovasc Imaging.* 2015;8(6):e003073. Available from: http://www.ncbi.nlm.nih.gov/pubmed/26015267.
69. Giri S, Shah S, Xue H, et al. Myocardial T2 mapping with respiratory navigator and automatic nonrigid motion correction. *Magn Reson Med.* 2012;68:1570–1578. Available from: http://www.ncbi.nlm.nih.gov/pubmed/22851292.
70. Baeßler B, Schaarschmidt F, Stehning C, Schnackenburg B, Maintz D, Bunck AC. A systematic evaluation of three different cardiac T2-mapping sequences at 1.5 and 3T in healthy volunteers. *Eur J Radiol.* 2015;84:2161–2170. Available from: http://www.ncbi.nlm.nih.gov/pubmed/26276731.
71. He T, Gatehouse PD, Anderson LJ, et al. Development of a novel optimized breathhold technique for myocardial T2 measurement in thalassemia. *J Magn Reson Imaging.* 2006;24:580–585. Available from: http://www.ncbi.nlm.nih.gov/pubmed/16892203.
72. Krumm P, Martirosian P, Rath D, et al. Signal decay mapping of myocardial edema using dual-contrast fast spin-echo MRI. *J Magn Reson Imaging.* 2015;44(1):186–193. Available from: http://www.ncbi.nlm.nih.gov/pubmed/26717865.
73. Baeßler B, Schaarschmidt F, Stehning C, Schnackenburg B, Maintz D, Bunck AC. Cardiac T2-mapping using a fast gradient echo spin echo sequence - first in vitro and in vivo experience. *J Cardiovasc Magn Reson.* 2015;17:67.
74. Fernández-Jiménez R, Sánchez-González J, Aguero J, et al. Fast T2 gradient-spin-echo (T2-GraSE) mapping for myocardial edema quantification: first in vivo validation in a porcine model of ischemia/reperfusion. *J Cardiovasc Magn Reson.* 2015;17:92. Available from: http://www.pubmedcentral.nih.gov/articlerender.fcgi?artid=4634909&tool=pmcentrez&rendertype=abstract.
75. Ding H, Fernandez-de-Manuel L, Schär M, et al. Three-dimensional whole-heart T2 mapping at 3T. *Magn Reson Med.* 2015;74:803–816. Available from: http://www.ncbi.nlm.nih.gov/pubmed/25242141.
76. Brittain JH, Hu BS, Wright GA, Meyer CH, Macovski A, Nishimura DG. Coronary angiography with magnetization-prepared T2 contrast. *Magn Reson Med.* 1995;33:689–696.
77. Jenista ER, Rehwald WG, Chen E-L, et al. Motion and flow insensitive adiabatic T2 -preparation module for cardiac MR imaging at 3 Tesla. *Magn Reson Med.* 2013;70:1360–1368. Available from: http://www.pubmedcentral.nih.gov-/articlerender.fcgi?artid=3926429&tool=pmcentrez&rendertype=abstract.
78. Nezafat R, Stuber M, Ouwerkerk R, Gharib AM, Desai MY, Pettigrew RI. B1-insensitive T2 preparation for improved coronary magnetic resonance angiography at 3 T. *Magn Reson Med.* 2006;55:858–864. Available from: http://www.ncbi.nlm.nih.gov/pubmed/16538606.
79. Oshio K, Feinberg A. GRASE (Gradient- and spin-echo) imaging: a novel fast MRI technique. *Magn Reson Med.* 1991;20:344–349.
80. Oshio K, Feinberg DA. Single-shot grase imaging without fast gradients. *Magn Reson Med.* 1992;26:355–360.
81. Akçakaya M, Basha TA, Weingärtner S, Roujol S, Berg S, Nezafat R. Improved quantitative myocardial T2 mapping: Impact of the fitting model. *Magn Reson Med.* 2014;74(1):93–105. Available from: http://www.ncbi.nlm.nih.gov/pubmed/25103908.
82. Bano W, Feliciano H, Coristine AJ, Stuber M, van Heeswijk RB. On the accuracy and precision of cardiac magnetic resonance T2 mapping: A high-resolution radial study using adiabatic T2 preparation at 3 T. *Magn Reson Med.* 2016;77(1):159–169. Available from: http://www.ncbi.nlm.nih.gov/pubmed/26762815.
83. Sandino CM, Kellman P, Arai AE, Hansen MS, Xue H. Myocardial T2* mapping: Influence of noise on accuracy and precision. *J Cardiovasc Magn Reson.* 2015;17:7.
84. Captur G, Gatehouse P, Kellman P, et al. A T1 and ECV phantom for global T1 mapping quality assurance: The T1 mapping and ECV standardisation in CMR (T1MES) program. *J Cardiovasc Magn Reson.* 2016;18:571–572.

5 Blood Flow Velocity Assessment

MICHAEL MARKL AND KELLY JARVIS

ACKNOWLEDGMENT

Thanks to Elizabeth Weiss, PhD, for assisting with Fig. 5.11.

INTRODUCTION AND HISTORY OF BLOOD FLOW VELOCITY ASSESSMENT WITH MRI

Flow-sensitive magnetic resonance imaging (MRI) is a widespread noninvasive imaging method for the clinical evaluation of blood flow in cardiovascular disease. Soon after the discovery of nuclear magnetic resonance (NMR) in the late 1940s, Herman Carr and Edwin Purcell observed that the NMR signal was affected by motion.[1] In 1960, Erwin Hahn recorded the motion of seawater with flow-sensitive NMR.[2] After the discovery of MRI in the 1970s, images of flowing blood were produced in the early 1980s.[3–6] Later discoveries combined cardiac gated time-resolved (cine) MRI with velocity encoding to produce time-resolved images of blood flow.[7,8] The term "phase contrast" (PC) refers generally to techniques that encode motion in the MR signal phase. Since the 1980s, PC-MRI has become ubiquitous for the clinical assessment of blood flow and is a feature of all modern MRI systems.[3–5,9,10] Such techniques offer the unique possibility to acquire spatially registered functional information simultaneously with the morphological data within a single examination. Visualization and quantification of blood flow and tissue motion using PC-MRI have been widely used in a number of applications. Characterization of the dynamic components of blood flow and cardiovascular function provides insight into normal and pathological cardiovascular physiology and is a part of imaging protocols in daily clinical routine.

Traditionally, MRI imaging of flow using PC techniques is accomplished using methods that resolve single-directional flow in two spatial dimensions (2D) of an individual slice. More recently, time-resolved three-dimensional (3D) PC-MRI with 3D velocity encoding (four-dimensional [4D] flow MRI) has been introduced that allows for the measurement of blood flow velocities in all three spatial dimensions along the cardiac cycle, providing a time-resolved 3D velocity field.[11] Acquisition of 4D information (4D = 3D + time over the cardiac cycle) enables the visualization of multidirectional flow patterns inside the vessels and eliminates the need for precise plane positioning. Furthermore, by capturing a full volumetric velocity dataset in a single acquisition, areas at any location within the 3D data can be retrospectively analyzed to quantify blood flow and velocities.[12] Over the past decade, there has been increasing interest in the use of 4D flow MRI in a wide range of cardiac and vascular diseases. Since its introduction, 4D flow MRI has undergone extensive development that enabled it to become part of clinical routine in large medical centers.

The purpose of this chapter is to provide an overview of the clinical applications of 2D flow and 4D flow MRI in cardiovascular diseases. This chapter introduces the basics of flow imaging with encoding gradients using the PC principle. A special focus is placed on the relationship between resolution and scan time and how these parameters play a role in the design of flow imaging protocols. The assessment of both 2D and 3D blood flow dynamics with MRI has achieved considerable progress in recent years, and this chapter covers topics such as advanced imaging acceleration techniques for real-time flow imaging and efficient 4D flow MRI. The authors would like to emphasize, however, that this review is by no means complete or exhaustive but is a summary of the methodological development and clinical applications that have accumulated in the literature. For more extensive overviews and additional information of future research directions, the reader is referred to several recently published review articles.[13–16]

2D FLOW IMAGING

2D Flow Imaging Principles

The MRI signal is derived from tissue or blood magnetization (also referred to as spins), which can be characterized by its magnitude (strength of magnetization) and phase (orientation of magnetization). The basic principle of flow encoding is the application of bipolar velocity encoding gradients to encode motion as information in the phase of the blood magnetization and MRI signal phase.[7,8,17–20] To understand flow encoding, it is helpful to consider a simple experiment with an object consisting of two compartments side by side: stationary tissue and a blood vessel as shown in Fig. 5.1. A "bipolar velocity encoding gradient" is applied, consisting of a positive magnetic field gradient, followed a certain time later by an equal but opposite negative magnetic field gradient in the direction of the flow. During the period of the positive gradient, flowing and stationary materials in a particular location will change their orientation (i.e., phase) that depends on their position along the velocity encoding gradient.

At the start of the experiment, the velocity encoding gradient is off; stationary tissue and flowing blood have the same initial magnetization phase. Next, during Time 1, the

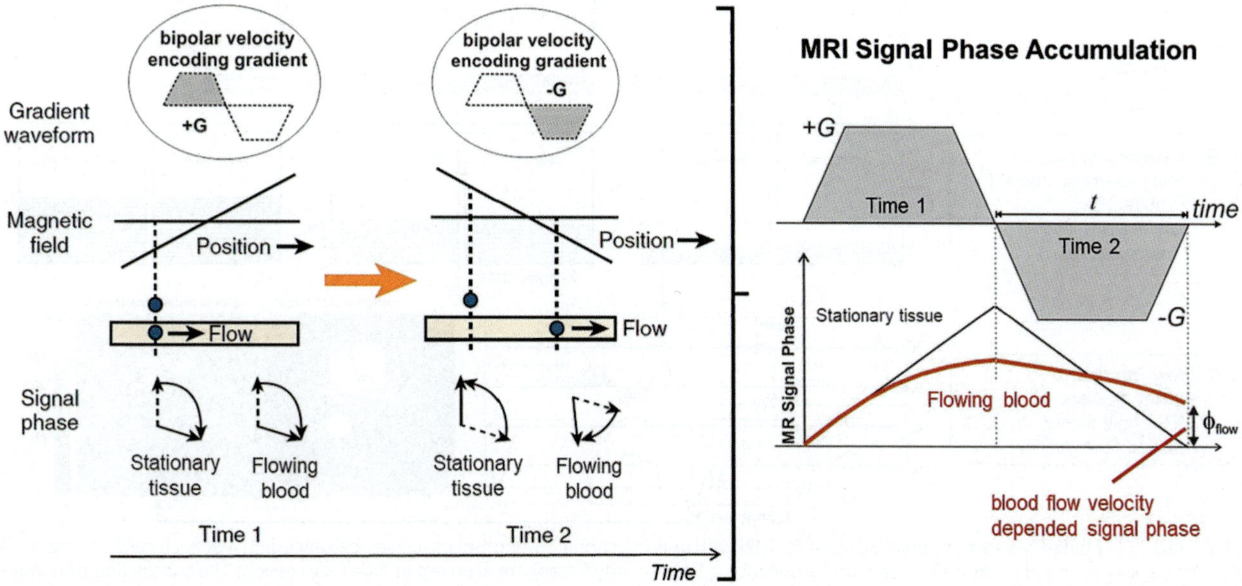

FIG. 5.1 Principles of phase velocity encoding. At Time 1, the positive part of the bipolar velocity encoding gradient is applied that results in an equal accumulation of magnetization phase for both stationary tissue and flowing blood. At Time 2, the equal but opposite part of the bipolar velocity encoding gradient is applied. By this time, the magnetization in the flowing blood has moved to be in a different strength of magnetic field during the gradient application. The result is that although the phase of the stationary tissue magnetization will be returned to zero, the flowing magnetization will accumulate a different phase ϕ_{flow} proportional to the blood flow velocity.

first half of the velocity encoding gradient (+G) is turned on and generates a spatially varying magnetic field, whose amplitude varies linearly with position. Stationary tissue and moving blood experience different magnetic field strengths (constant for stationary spins, changing field along the motion direction for moving blood) and thus accumulate different magnetization phases. Finally, during Time 2, the second half of the velocity encoding gradient (-G, inverted magnetic field) is played out. Stationary tissue magnetization returns to its initial phase (it gained some phase during Time 1 and lost the same phase during the second half). In contrast, flowing blood will continue to accumulate a different phase ϕ_{flow} directly proportional to the blood flow velocity. The relationship between phase ϕ_{flow} and velocity v is

$$\phi_{flow} = \gamma G v t^2$$

where γ is the gyromagnetic ratio, a measure of the magnetic polarizability of hydrogen nuclei, G is the gradient field amplitude, and t is the duration of one half of the bipolar velocity encoding gradient. The gyromagnetic ratio, magnetic field, and duration are known, and the magnetization phase is measured from the MRI signal. As a result, it is possible to compute the blood flow velocity from the measured phase change.

However, the flow-encoded signal phase includes an unknown background phase caused by undesired heterogeneity of the MRI magnetic field. To remove this unwanted contribution to the MRI signal phase, it is necessary to perform two MRI scans (one reference scan followed by a flow-encoded scan). Subtraction of the MRI signal phase of the two scans (i.e., calculation of phase difference) allows for the removal of the unknown background phase and calculation of the final flow velocity images. This approach is generally referred to as PC-MRI, flow-sensitive MRI, or MRI velocity mapping.

Cardiovascular 2D Flow Imaging Techniques

In current clinical practice, the most common type of flow-encoded scan is 2D cine PC-MRI with single-direction velocity encoding to measure time-resolved pulsatile blood flow, most frequently along the through-pane direction. Due to time constraints, standard 2D flow imaging cannot be performed during a single heartbeat and data are acquired over several cardiac cycles. As shown in Fig. 5.2, echocardiographic (ECG) gating is used to synchronize data acquisition with the cardiac cycle, and a segmented pulse sequence scheme is used. For each heartbeat, only a subset (or segment) of all required MRI raw data is measured. The procedure is repeated for several successive heartbeats until the full raw dataset is collected. Time-resolved (cine) images can then be reconstructed from the raw data that depict the pulsatile flow through-plane flow. The selection of the number of lines per segment (N_{Seg}) determines the temporal resolution (time to collect data for a single time frame) and a total scan time of the acquisition. For a typical repetition time (TR) on the order of 5 ms and N_{Seg} = 3–4, measurements can be performed during breath-holding and with temporal resolutions of 30–40 ms.

2D CINE FLOW IMAGES AND FLOW QUANTIFICATION

Fig. 5.3 shows a series of time-resolved phase velocity images with through-plane velocity encoding for a 2D imaging plane location at the thoracic aorta. Following the delineation of vessel contours, flow-time curves across the cardiac cycle can be derived. This approach allows for the calculation of peak systolic velocities, net, forward, regurgitant, and shunt flows in congenital and acquired cardiovascular and heart valve disease. Based on peak velocity measurements, peak and mean pressure gradients

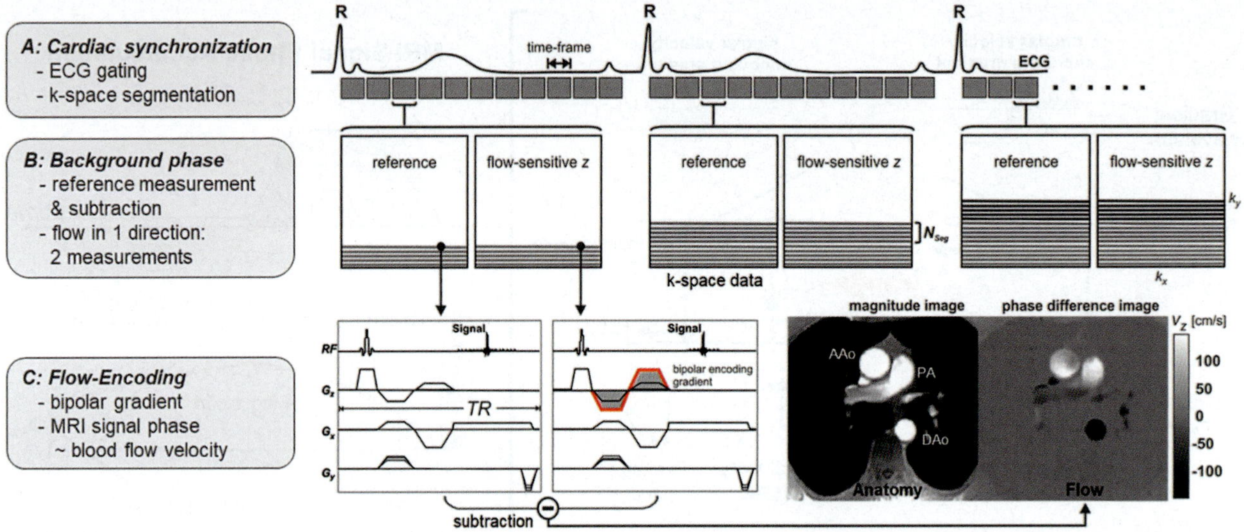

FIG. 5.2 Standard ECG gated two-dimensional (2D) cine PC-MRI with one-directional through-plane (*z*) velocity encoding. For each cardiac time frame (*gray squares*), two velocity encoded scans (reference scan followed by a flow encoded scan) are acquired in direct succession. The subtraction of phase images from both datasets provides phase difference images that contain quantitative blood flow velocities as shown in a 2D slice normal to the ascending (*AAo*) and descending (*DAo*) aorta.

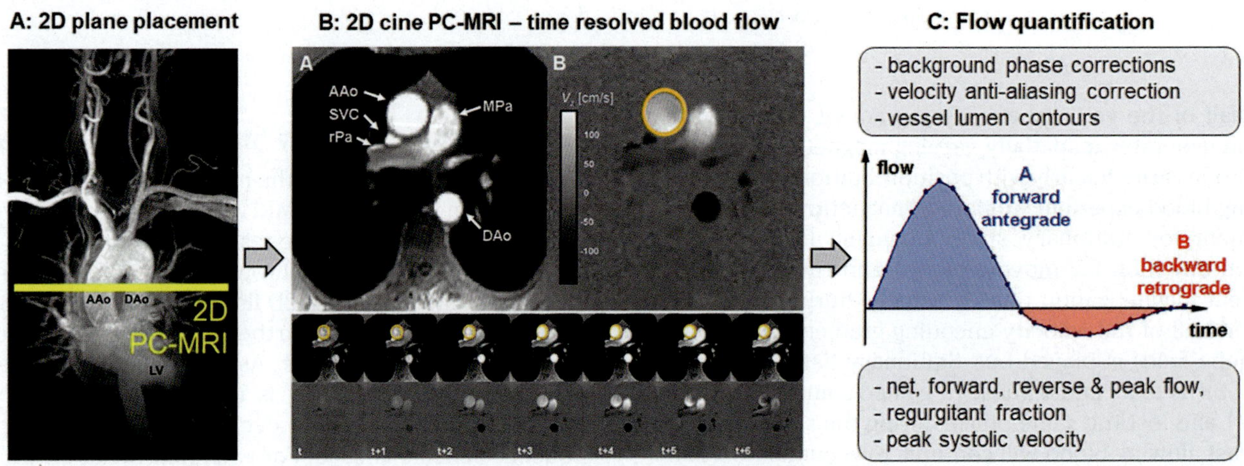

FIG. 5.3 Two-dimensional (*2D*) flow imaging in the aorta. (A) 3D contrast-enhanced MR angiography of the thoracic aorta and placement of the 2D plane for flow imaging in the ascending (*AAo*) and descending aorta (*DAo*) with through-plane flow encoding. (B) Resulting 2D flow images depicting pulsatile flow over the cardiac cycle. Gray scale values correspond to the measured through-plane blood flow velocities in superior/inferior direction. The *bottom row* depicts changes over time during systole and early diastole. (C) Flow analysis can quantify antegrade forward and retrograde flow volumes to regurgitant fraction (B/A × 100). *PA,* pulmonary artery; *LV* left ventricle.

(in mm Hg) can be estimated via the simplified Bernoulli equation pressure gradient = $4v_{peak}^{2}$.[21–23] Under pulsatile flow conditions, the changes in vessel wall position and area over the cardiac cycle typically require adjusting vessel lumen contours for each cardiac time frame.

Cardiac Gating

For cardiac gating of the 2D cine PC-MRI data acquisition, most protocols will provide two alternatives: prospective or retrospective ECG gating. In both techniques, the ECG waveform is continuously analyzed to detect the R-wave and used as the trigger signal to synchronize data acquisition with the cardiac cycle.

- Prospective ECG gating (illustrated in Fig. 5.2): The number of cardiac time frames is determined in advance. Following R-wave detection, the scanner collects the raw data segments for all cardiac time frames prior to the next R-wave. Since the number of cardiac time frames is predetermined, scanning covers only 80%–90% of the heartbeat duration to accommodate possible changes in heart rate. A limitation of this approach is related to the lack of data during late diastole, which can be important for applications such as atrioventricular fluid transport across the mitral or tricuspid valves.
- Retrospective ECG gating: Data are continuously acquired throughout the entire cardiac cycle. To accomplish this task, the continuously acquired MRI raw data are retrospectively interpolated to match the user-selected number of cardiac time frames. It should be noted that the resulting temporal resolution (number of time frames per heartbeat) is different from the true underlying acquired temporal resolution. A limitation of retrospective gating is related to its sensitivity to

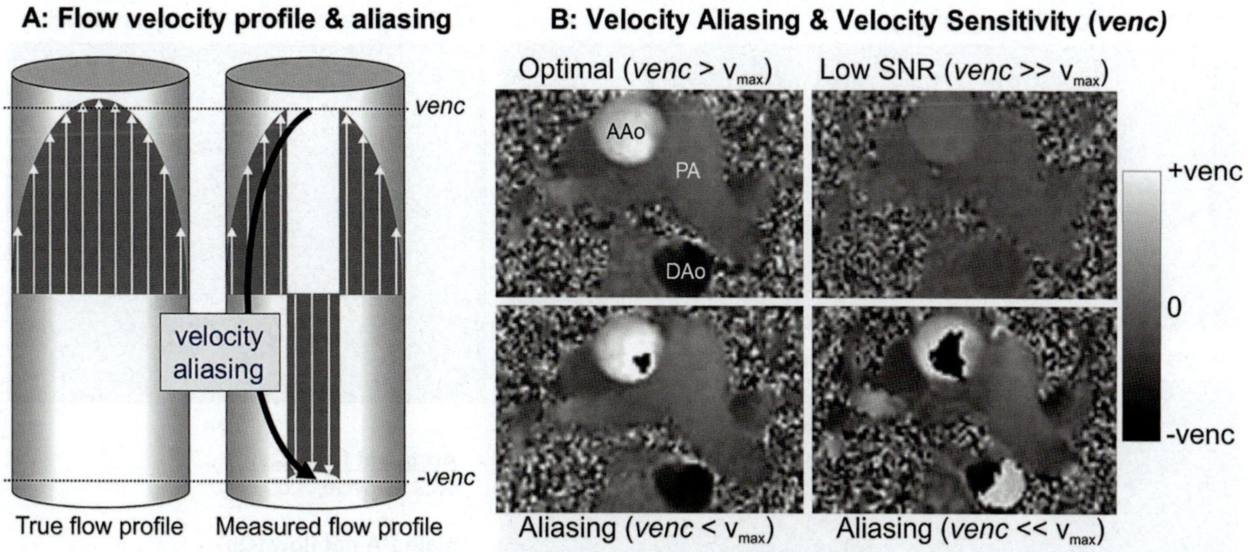

FIG. 5.4 (A) Velocity aliasing for a parabolic flow profile. If the velocity sensitivity venc is smaller compared to the highest occurring flow velocities, aliasing toward inverted velocity values occurs. (B) PC-MRI with through-plane velocity encoding in the ascending and descending aorta. The individual phase difference images show the encoded blood flow velocities during peak systole in the same subject for four different velocity sensitivities (venc).

changes in heart rate, which limits its applications in patients with cardiac arrhythmia.

It should be noted that the cine acquisition for both ECG gating methods is based on a periodic cardiac cycle. The regularity of the heart rate is important to ensure that data are consistently acquired for all time frames and heart beats. To avoid such inaccuracies, arrhythmia rejection algorithms have been introduced in clinical cine PC-MRI protocols.

Spatial and Temporal Resolution and Scan Time

Like most other MRI techniques, different imaging 2D flow imaging protocols can be constructed that are subject to tradeoffs between scan time and spatial and temporal resolution. For example, an increase in spatial resolution will result in an increasing scan time or decreasing temporal resolution. Similarly, an increase in temporal resolution would require longer scan time or decrease in spatial resolution. Typical measurement parameters (spatial resolution: 1.5–2.5 mm, temporal resolution: 30–60 ms, slice thickness: 5–8 mm) permit the acquisition of 2D cine PC-MRI data during a 10- to 20-second breath-hold. In case the patient cannot hold their breath or for pediatric 2D flow imaging application, data can be acquired during free breathing with 3–4 averages to mitigate respiration artifacts. This strategy will allow for application in these patient cohorts but is associated with a 3- to 4-fold scan time increase.

Velocity Sensitivity, Aliasing, and Encoding Directions

An important user-defined parameter in 2D flow imaging is the velocity encoding sensitivity (venc), which represents the maximum blood flow velocity that can be accurately measured without encountering velocity aliasing. As shown in Fig. 5.4, when the maximum blood flow velocity exceeds venc, velocity aliasing can occur, which is typically visible as a sudden change from positive to negative velocity (see Fig. 5.4B). For example, a velocity of 120 cm/s measured with a venc of 100 cm/s will yield a velocity of −80 cm/s in the phase difference image. It is important to note, however, that velocity noise is also directly related to venc. Therefore, selecting a high venc may reduce velocity aliasing but will also increase the level of velocity noise in flow velocity images.[24] As a result, the venc should ideally be selected as high as needed to avoid aliasing but as close as possible to the maximum expected blood flow velocity. If velocity aliasing effects are present, accurate flow quantification may be compromised unless velocity antialiasing correction can be successfully performed. Alternatively, the 2D flow imaging scan may have to be repeated with increased venc to avoid or minimize velocity aliasing.

Most MR systems offer imaging protocols permitting both in-plane and through-plane velocity encoding. In-plane velocity mapping can be performed in one or two directions and is mainly used for visualizing flow patterns within the imaging plane such as jets through stenosed vessels or valves. The velocity encoding direction should be parallel to the direction of the flow in the vessel of interest. An in-plane acquisition of a high-velocity jet can be helpful for planning a subsequent through-plane scan on the jet location with maximum velocities, especially for the assessment of mitral or tricuspid valve regurgitation. Applications that require measurement of stroke volume, stenosis, or regurgitant volumes orient the image orthogonal to the flow encoding direction (through-plane velocity encoding).

Sources of Errors and Artifacts

There are a number of sources of inaccuracies in PC-MRI, which can result in errors in the measured velocities. The major sources of errors include eddy current effects,[25] Maxwell terms,[26] and gradient field distortions.[27] Appropriate correction strategies should thus be applied to ensure

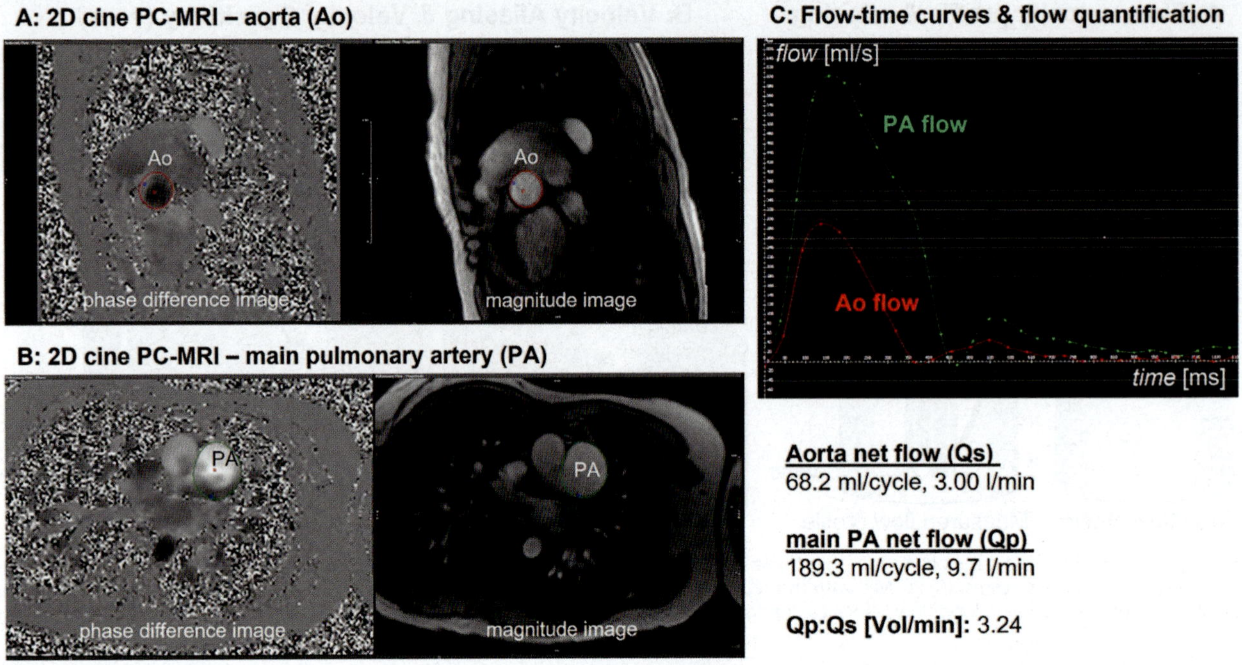

FIG. 5.5 Two-dimensional (*2D*) flow imaging with 2D cine PC-MRI in a 36-year-old patient with anomalous pulmonary venous return. 2D imaging places were positioned in the ascending aorta (A) and main pulmonary artery (B) to derive flow-time curves (C) for the calculation of systemic (Q_S) and pulmonary (Q_P) net flow to quantify the Q_P:Q_S ratio.

accurate flow quantification using PC-MRI data. Correction of these errors typically includes the identification of image regions that contain static tissue in order to estimate the spatial distribution of background phase offsets (using a first- or second-order fit to the static tissue phase difference data). Background phase errors can subsequently be removed by subtraction of the estimated offset from the entire velocity data. An additional factor affecting the accuracy of the flow measurement methods is flow-related signal loss. This is typically the result of highly deranged or turbulent blood flows, which can lead to regional signal loss and may result in an inability to accurately measure the encoded blood flow velocity.

Clinical Applications

Some of the most common indications for 2D cine PC-MRI include applications in patients with heart valve disease (mitral, tricuspid, pulmonary, and aortic valves) to quantify the severity of valve stenosis and/or associated valve insufficiency and regurgitant fraction, aortic coarctation to assess severity and collateral flows, flow shunting in atrial and ventricular septal defects, assessment of flow distribution in complex congenital heart disease (e.g., caval venous, pulmonary, and aortic flow parameters in patients with single ventricle physiology), or assessment of flow jets and peak velocities in patient with pulmonary artery stenosis.

Flow quantification with through-plane velocity encoding can be used to estimate the fraction of regurgitant flow in case of valve defects or to quantify global cardiac function such as stroke volume and cardiac output.[7,28] Typical velocity sensitivities are venc = 150 cm/s for aortic and pulmonary flow measurements. However, it should be noted that in the case of a valve or vessel stenosis, blood flow velocities can reach values of up to 400–600 cm/s. To avoid velocity aliasing, the PC-MRI scan should be repeated using a higher velocity sensitivity venc until the phase aliasing has disappeared to allow for an appropriate flow analysis.

In the presence of pulmonary-systemic shunts, the pulmonary/systemic flow ratio can be determined and used to assess the severity of the disease.[29–31] To quantify the shunt volume, two 2D cine PC-MRI measurements are performed. 2D planes positioned in the ascending aorta and in the pulmonary artery are used to quantify the left and right ventricular stroke volumes Q_S and Q_P, respectively. The ratio Q_P/Q_S represents the direction of shunt and the shunt volume. For $Q_P/Q_S = 1$, no shunt is present, if $Q_P/Q_S >$, 1 a shunt from the aortic circulation to the pulmonary circulation is present and vice versa for $Q_P/Q_S < 1$. Fig. 5.5 illustrates the clinical use of 2D flow imaging for assessing aortic and pulmonary flows in a 36-year-old patient with anomalous pulmonary venous return and an abnormal Q_P:Q_S ratio of 3.2 to 1.

Rapid 2D Flow Imaging Methods and Future Directions

Advances in MRI hardware such as high-field MRI systems for improved signal-to-noise ratio, improved gradient performance, and multichannel receiver coils have enabled parallel imaging with high acceleration factors. These advances have led to promising new applications for flow imaging in patients. Specifically, highly accelerated imaging with spatiotemporal undersampling and compressed sensing/parallel imaging reconstruction can be employed to assess flow with greater flexibility (spatial and temporal resolution) and with short scan times. An emerging and promising technique is real-time flow imaging, which can

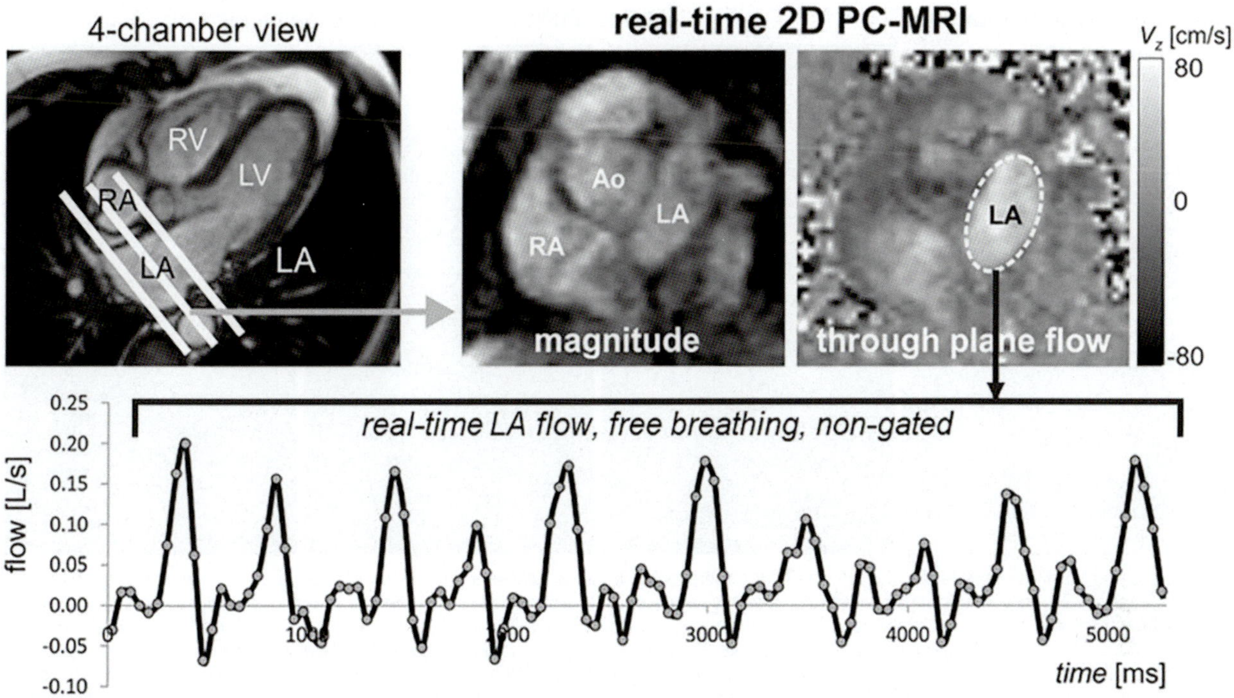

FIG. 5.6 Real-time imaging of flow in the left atrium (*LA*) based on 2D PC with echo planar imaging data readout, shared velocity encoding, and imaging acceleration (temporal resolution per image = 50 ms). Data was acquired without ECG gating and through-plane velocity encoding (total scan time = 10 seconds, venc = 80 cm/s). Data analysis included the calculation of left atrium (*LA*) flow in regions of interest delineating the *LA* boundary. Resulting flow-time curves at mid-atrial short axis level show arrhythmic flow changes over multiple heart beats in a patient with atrial fibrillation.

greatly simplify flow imaging by data acquisition during free breathing and without the need for ECG gating.

Recent advances in MRI data acquisition strategies allow for real-time assessment of beat-to-beat variation in the presence of atrial fibrillation and breathing exercises (such as the Valsalva and Müller maneuvers),[32–34] which cannot easily be performed with standard 2D flow imaging methods. To achieve sufficiently high frame rates needed for real-time flow acquisitions, optimized and accelerated 2D flow imaging pulse sequences have been developed, which combine effective data readout modules (e.g., echo planar imaging) with data undersampling and parallel imaging data reconstruction (e.g., compressed sensing, k-t acceleration in spatial and temporal dimension). In addition, shared velocity encoding[35,36] has been proposed to further improve temporal resolution and is based on the concept of sharing sets of full k-space data between adjacent time frames in order to double the effective frame rate. Based on these developments, 2D real-time flow imaging with through-plane velocity encoding can be performed with temporal update rates on the order of 30–50 ms (see Fig. 5.6).

4D FLOW

The technique of 4D flow MRI builds on 2D PC-MRI by acquiring data in all three velocity encoding directions (Vx, Vy, and Vz) for a prescribed 3D imaging volume.[11,37,38] Anatomical coverage can range from a focused volume (e.g., aortic acquisition in sagittal oblique orientation) to a full coronal acquisition of the whole chest. For an in-depth review and recommendations for clinical applications of 4D flow MRI, the reader is referred to consensus statements that have been published on this technique with details of the acquisition and analysis approach.[12,39]

Data Acquisition

A typical cardiovascular 4D flow MRI sequence takes about 5–15 minutes to acquire data. During this time, heart rate is monitored by an MRI-compatible electrocardiogram to enable either prospective or retrospective cardiac gating. For each time frame of the cardiac cycle, one reference scan and three velocity-encoded scans are captured. Since the data cannot be acquired in a breath-hold, data are acquired during free breathing with the option to use respiratory gating methods to minimize respiration artifacts.[40] In addition to heart rate, the time it takes to acquire 4D flow MRI depends on the scan parameters selected. For example, achieving higher spatial or temporal resolution requires longer scan times. Protocol optimization involves adjusting the scan parameters to give optimal data quality in a reasonable scan time, both for patient comfort and ease of adding the 4D flow MRI sequence to existing protocols. Scan times have been made faster using imaging acceleration techniques such as parallel imaging[41–43] and compressed sensing.[44,45] More recently, imaging acceleration by deep learning has been explored.[46,47] After data capture, image reconstruction results in a large series of images (ranging from 3000 to 10,000), giving time-resolved anatomic (magnitude) and three-directional flow (Vx, Vy, and Vz) images.

Data Analysis Workflow

Similar to 2D flow imaging, the resulting 4D flow MRI data require preprocessing to correct for inaccuracies related

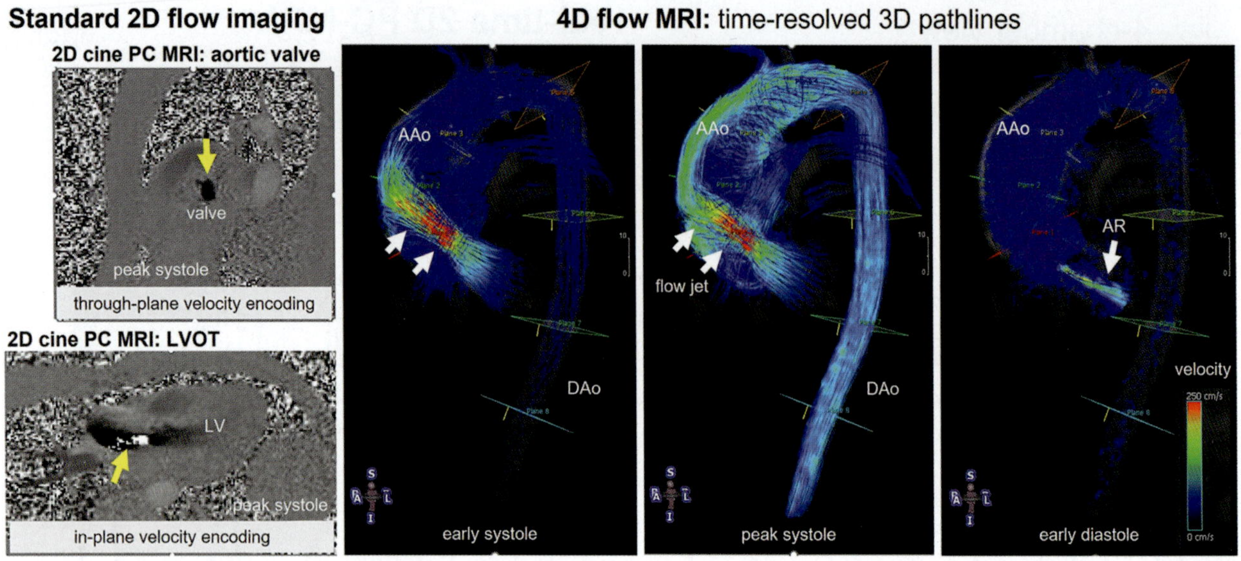

FIG. 5.7 Example of two-dimensional (*2D*) PC-MRI and four-dimensional (*4D*) flow MRI in a patient with bicuspid aortic valve disease and severe aortic valve stenosis. Standard 2D flow imaging at the level of the aortic valve (*top left*, orthogonal to the aorta, through-plane velocity encoding) and in the left ventricular outflow tract (*bottom left*, *LVOT*, in-plane velocity encoding) shows high systolic velocities and velocity aliasing distal to the narrowed aortic valve (*yellow arrows*). Aortic 4D flow MRI has several advantages over 2D flow imaging, including the detailed 3D visualization of aortic flow patterns such as a marked systolic valve flow jet (*white arrows*) and early diastolic aortic regurgitation (*AR*, *white arrow*). In addition, 4D flow MRI allows for retrospective flow quantification using 2D analysis planes at any location along the aorta, while *2D* flow analysis is limited to the location that was selected by the MRI technologist during the MRI exam. Hemodynamic quantification using 2D analysis planes revealed a systolic peak velocity of 4.2 m/s, indicating severe aortic valve stenosis. *AAo,* Ascending aorta; *DAo,* descending aorta.

to phase offset errors (eddy current effects), measurement noise, and velocity aliasing. In a next step, a 3D phase-contrast MR angiogram (PC-MRA) can be calculated from the 4D flow MRI data to depict the cardiovascular geometry.[48] Vessels of interest can be segmented from the 3D PC-MRA data to mask 4D flow data for further analysis inside the vessel of interest. For example, in whole heart analysis, the aorta; the main, left, and right pulmonary arteries; the superior and inferior vena cava; and the left and right atria and ventricles can be depicted by the 3D PC-MRA data and identified for subsequent 3D segmentation. Next, 4D flow MRI postprocessing includes both 3D visualization and quantification of hemodynamics. Figs. 5.7 and 5.8 show examples of the use of 4D flow-derived 3D PC-MRA data for guiding the 3D visualization and analysis of blood flow in patients with aortic disease. While 4D flow data analysis workflow has undergone substantial improvements, including commercially available software solutions by multiple vendors, manual interaction with the data is often still needed. More recently, new deep learning analysis methods have been introduced that have high potential to further simplify and accelerate analysis workflows.[49,50]

3D Blood Flow Visualization and Hemodynamic Quantification

3D visualization of 4D flow MRI data can be performed using approaches such as velocity maximum intensity projections (MIPs) and particle trace streamlines or pathlines. MIPs are used to show intuitive maps of the velocity distribution (see Fig. 5.8), while streamlines and pathlines further depict the flow patterns in three dimensions and over time. Streamlines show the instantaneous trajectory of a virtual particle in the velocity data field for one time frame of the cardiac cycle (Fig. 5.8). Pathlines show the time-resolved trajectory of a virtual particle along the entire cardiac cycle using data from all time frames (see Figs. 5.7 and 5.9).

Hemodynamic quantification of standard 4D flow MRI parameters includes those obtained by 2D PC-MRI, such as net flow, forward flow, reverse flow, regurgitant fraction, and peak velocity. However, in contrast to 2D flow imaging, 4D flow MRI enables the retrospective analysis of those parameters anywhere in the imaging region and at multiple locations. For example, Fig. 5.7 illustrates the analysis of 4D flow MRI in the aorta with the manual placement of several 2D analysis planes along the entire aorta in an orthogonal orientation. For a more automated approach, a 3D vessel centerline can be calculated and 2D analysis planes placed along the centerline without the need for user interaction. Quantification of velocity can be performed by planar analysis (as described above) or by a voxel-wise hemodynamic parameter mapping approach. Peak velocity,[51] obtained by either a planar or voxel-wise method, is an important parameter for characterizing hemodynamics. Analysis of 3D flow jets by 4D flow MRI enables the severity assessment of nearby vessel narrowing or valve stenosis (e.g., higher peak velocity indicates more narrowing or stenosis).

Advanced parameters from 4D flow MRI require additional analysis and are an ongoing area of research. Several candidates have emerged as promising measures for clinical application, and we will highlight a few in this chapter. Aortic wall shear stress (WSS), known for stimulating vessel wall remodeling and degeneration, can be calculated from 4D flow MRI velocity data for the evaluation of pathologies such as acquired and congenital aortic valve disease.[52] Patient-specific WSS heat maps can be computed to indicate elevated regions compared to average WSS maps of healthy age- and sex-matched controls[53,54] (Fig. 5.10). Several studies have shown that WSS has the potential to

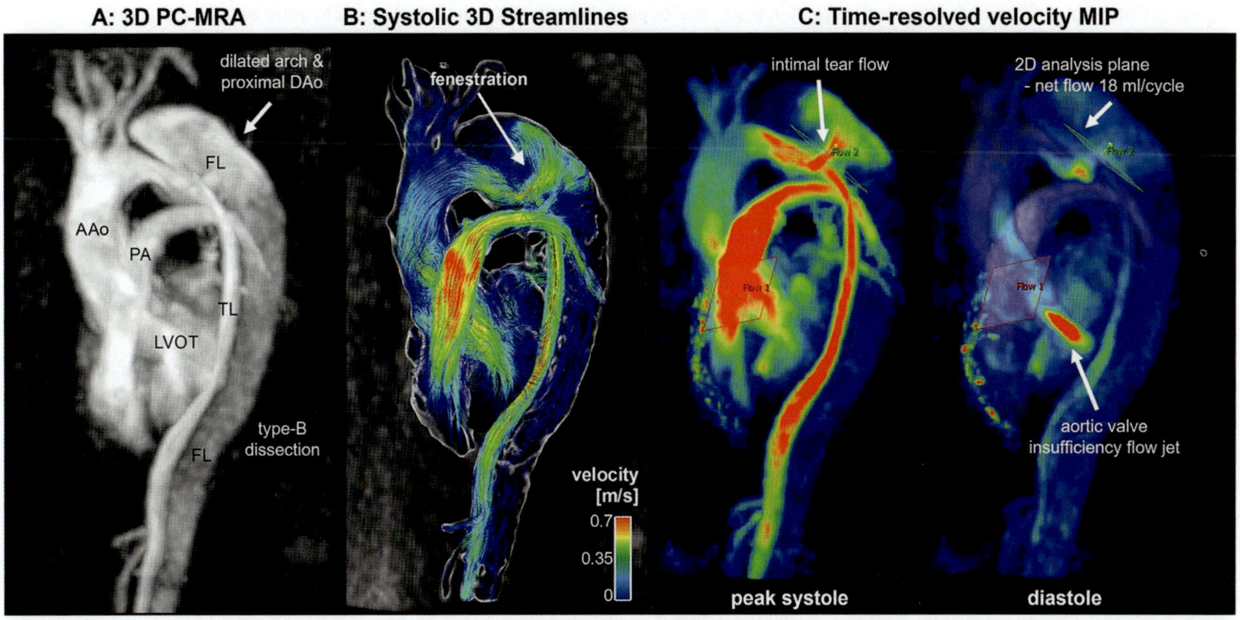

FIG. 5.8 Aortic four-dimensional (*4D*) flow MRI in a patient with type B dissection illustrating the comprehensive anatomic and hemodynamic information that can be derived from a single 4D flow MRI scan. (A) 4D flow-derived three-dimensional (*3D*) PC-MRA data show aortic anatomy and the geometry of the true and false lumen in the aortic arch and descending aorta (*DAo*). (B) Systolic streamlines illustrate 3D flow patterns, including high flow in the true lumen and flow entering the false lumen via a fenestration in the proximal descending aorta. (C) Time-resolved velocity maximum intensity projections (MIPs) provide intuitive maps of the velocity distribution over the cardiac cycle and can be used to identify abnormal flow patterns such as the intimal tear flow and retrograde flow through the insufficient aortic valve. Further, velocity MIPs can guide the optimal placement of two-dimensional (2D) analysis planes, for example, in this case to measure the flow from the true to the false lumen.

help risk stratify patients with bicuspid aortic valve disease, but as with other advanced 4D flow MRI parameters, larger studies are needed to further characterize clinical relationships.[55] Turbulent kinetic energy[56,57] is an advanced 4D flow MRI parameter that can aid in the assessment of aortic stenosis by evaluating the pressure loss in poststenotic flow noninvasively, providing results that are complementary to echo. Turbulent kinetic energy reflects the pressure loss caused by energy dissipation and the hemodynamic significance of the stenosis. Similarly, 4D flow MRI-derived pressure drop assessment based on turbulence production can provide complimentary information to the conventional Bernoulli method.[58] Lastly, pulse wave velocity is a clinical measure of vascular stiffness that can be obtained using various methods, such as tonometry, echo, and MRI. Using 2D PC-MRI or 4D flow MRI enables a more focused measure of pulse wave velocity (PWV) in the thoracic aorta.[59] Recently, larger cross-sectional studies across the aging spectrum have been performed using 4D flow MRI. These studies demonstrated increased aortic PWV with age.[60,61] Assessment of PWV in the regions of the aorta (e.g., ascending and descending) has been explored.[62] However, regional assessment of aortic PWV is limited by temporal resolution of 4D flow MRI, which is typically on the order of 40 ms.

Clinical Application

Over the past decade, 4D flow MRI has become more widely available and supported by the main manufacturers of MRI scanners. In addition, 4D flow MRI analysis tools are now commercially available. This has led to an increased use of this technique both for research studies and in clinical practice at large medical centers across the world.[39]

Aortic diseases, such as bicuspid aortic valve disease[52,63] and aortic dissection,[64,65] present challenges for diagnosis and risk stratification where 4D flow MRI may offer valuable hemodynamic information. The comprehensive evaluation of 3D flow jets and complex flow patterns of these pathologies is a promising application of this technique (see Figs. 5.7 and 5.8).

Valvular heart disease, such as mitral or tricuspid valve regurgitation, is another key area of clinical application.[66,67] Using 4D flow MRI with retrospective valve tracking, the net flow of all four heart valves can be measured in a single scan.[68] Retrospective valve tracking can be performed manually or in an automated fashion.[69] The 4D flow MRI measurements of mitral and tricuspid regurgitant volume have demonstrated potential to be used in place of conventional multiplanar MRI methods.[66]

Congenital heart disease applications for 4D flow MRI include, among other pathologies, the evaluation of complex blood flow in patients with Fontan physiology,[70–73] transposition of the great arteries,[74,75] and tetralogy of Fallot[76–78] (see Fig. 5.11). The flexibility and retrospective nature of this technique lend itself to assessment of these pathologies that may not have standardized vascular geometry or flow patterns for routine evaluation.

Imaging Considerations and Quality Control

Quality control involves setting up the imaging workflow optimally and then performing consistency checks on the resulting data. This includes prescribing the acquired

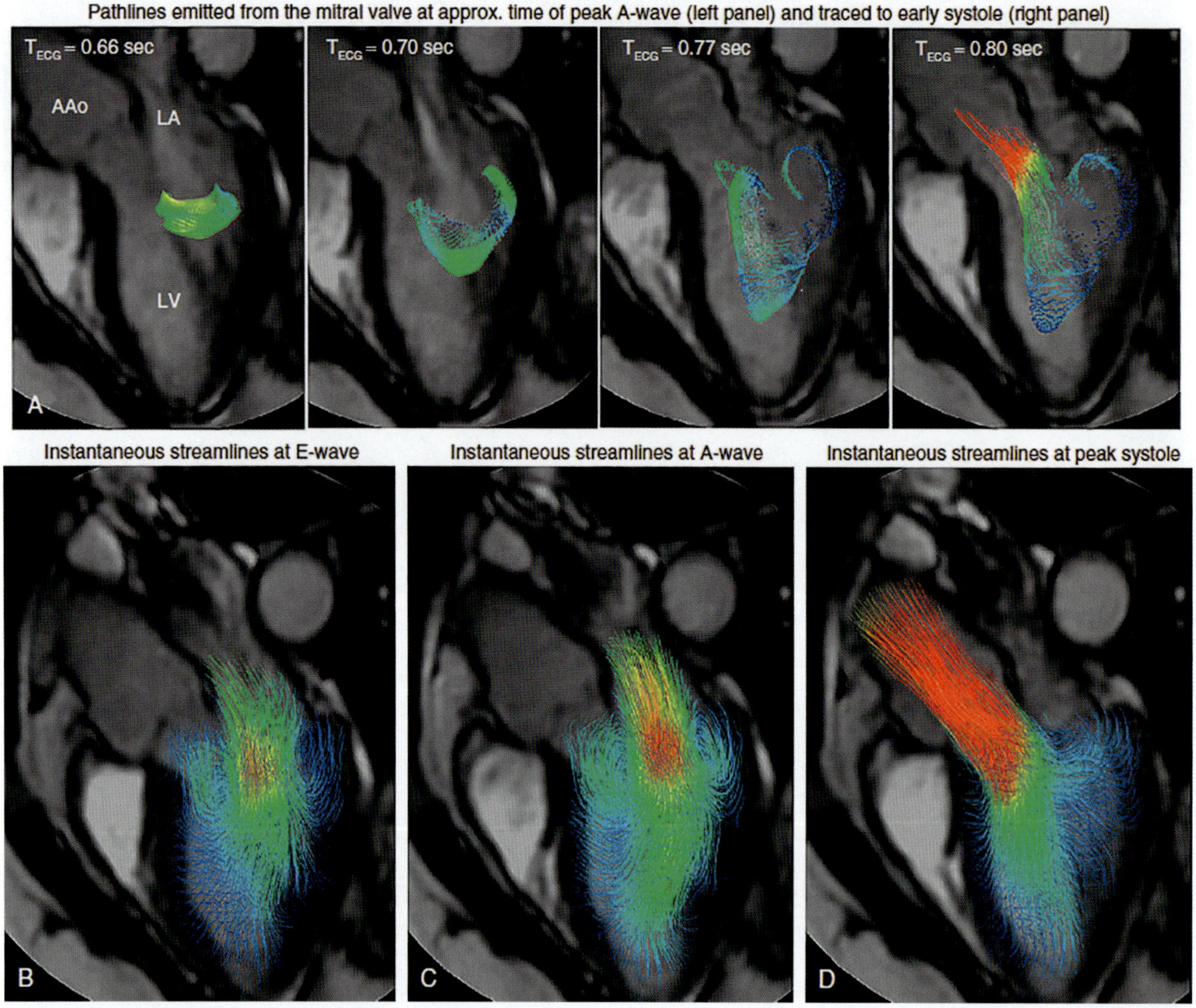

FIG. 5.9 Examples of four-dimensional (4D) flow MRI in the normal heart. Flow visualization is overlaid onto a 2D balanced Steady State Free Precession (bSSF) acquisition in a three-chamber view. Pathlines indicate the flow patterns of pulsatile blood flow over time. (A) Blood through the left ventricle (*LV*) is shown by pathlines emitted from the mitral valve from the time of peak A-wave to early systole. (B–D) Streamlines show parts of the intracardiac velocity field at the time of peak early filling (E-wave), peak late filling (A-wave), and peak systole. *AAo,* Ascending aorta; *LA,* left atrium. (From Dyverfeldt P, Bissell M, Barker AJ, et al. 4D flow cardiovascular magnetic resonance consensus statement. *J Cardiovasc Magn Reson*. 2015;17:72.)

spatial resolution to be isotropic and allow for at least the recommended 5–6 voxels across the vessel diameter.[79] Several protocols can be prepared in advance to optimize the acquisition for different age groups and pathologies. Venc should be set as low as possible (e.g., usually 10% above the maximum expected velocity and not more than 25%) to mitigate velocity noise and optimize dynamic range but not too low as to induce velocity aliasing.[12,80] Typical venc settings are 150 cm/s for the aorta and pulmonary artery and 250 cm/s if stenosis is suspected.[14,39] Previous imaging or an additionally acquired 2D PC-MRI can be a helpful reference when prescribing venc for the individual patient. During acquisition, the ECG leads may need to be adjusted to ensure full capture of heart rhythm and 4D flow MRI data. After data collection, internal flow consistency measures can be used to check the imaging workflow based on the conservation of mass. For example, within the same 4D flow MRI dataset, the following flow measurements should be comparable: main pulmonary artery = left + right pulmonary artery, main pulmonary artery = inferior + superior caval veins, flow across all four heart valves, and so forth. Consistency measures are described in more detail in the recent 4D flow MRI consensus statement.[39] When setting up new 4D flow MRI sequences and analysis workflows, intra- and interobserver studies are helpful to ensure analysis steps are consistent among raters. In addition, test-retest studies (e.g., scanning healthy individuals twice within 1 month) can provide important information on reproducibility. Agreement within 10% is usually considered acceptable.

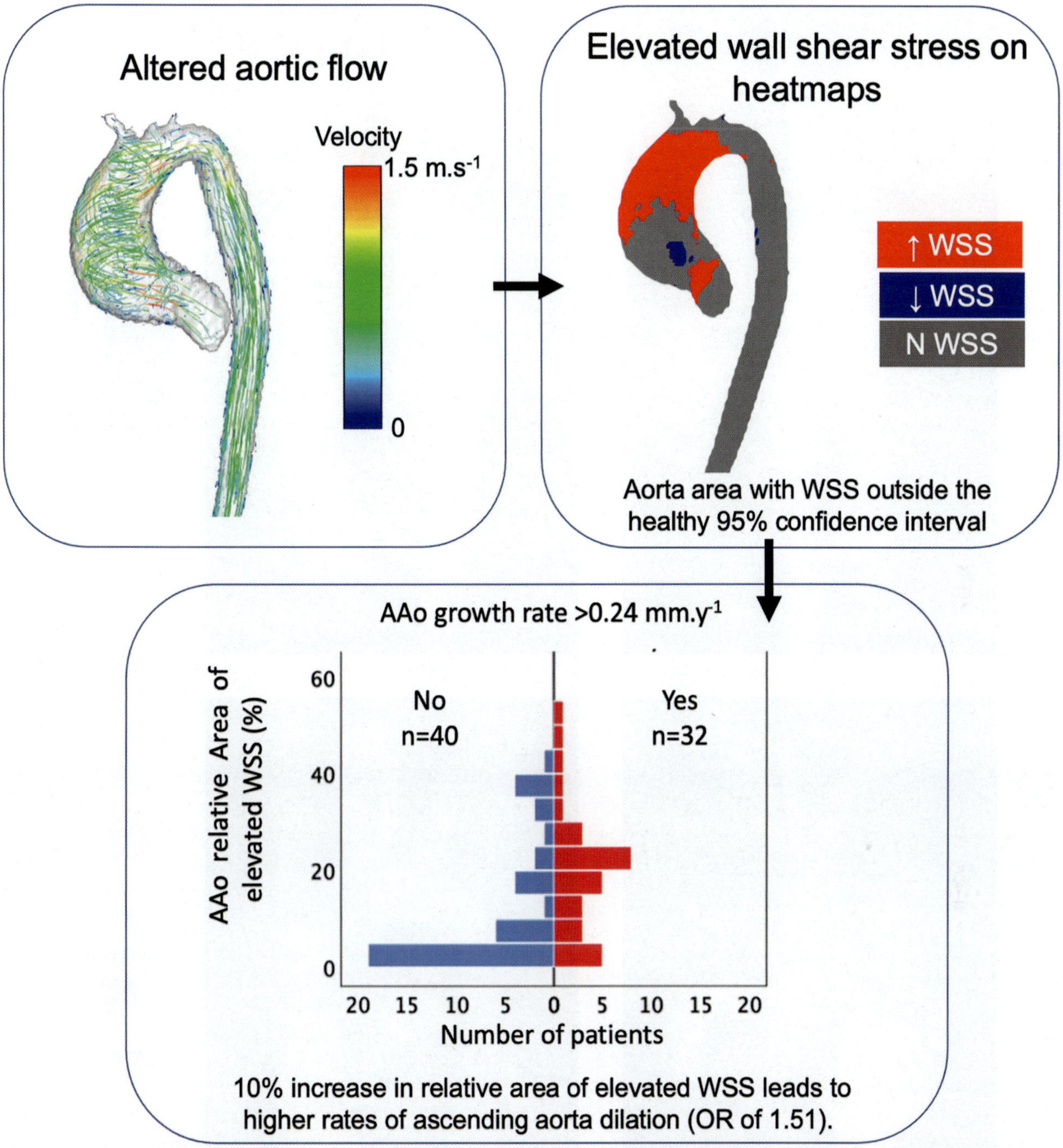

FIG. 5.10 Four-dimensional (4D) flow MRI visualization and wall shear stress (*WSS*) assessment in bicuspid aortic valve disease. *Top left*: example of flow visualization using systolic streamlines demonstrates abnormal flow patterns in the ascending aorta in a patient with bicuspid aortic valve disease. *Top right*: assessment in the same patient demonstrates regions of elevated WSS (*red*) compared to age- and sex-matched controls. *Bottom*: summary boxplot of WSS and aortic growth rate shows results from the entire study cohort, demonstrating that elevated WSS in the ascending aorta was associated with progressive aortic dilation. (Courtesy Gilles Soulat, MD, PhD. From Soulat G, Scott MB, Allen BD, et al. Association of regional wall shear stress and progressive ascending aorta dilation in bicuspid aortic valve. *JACC Cardiovasc Imaging*. 2022;15:33–42.)

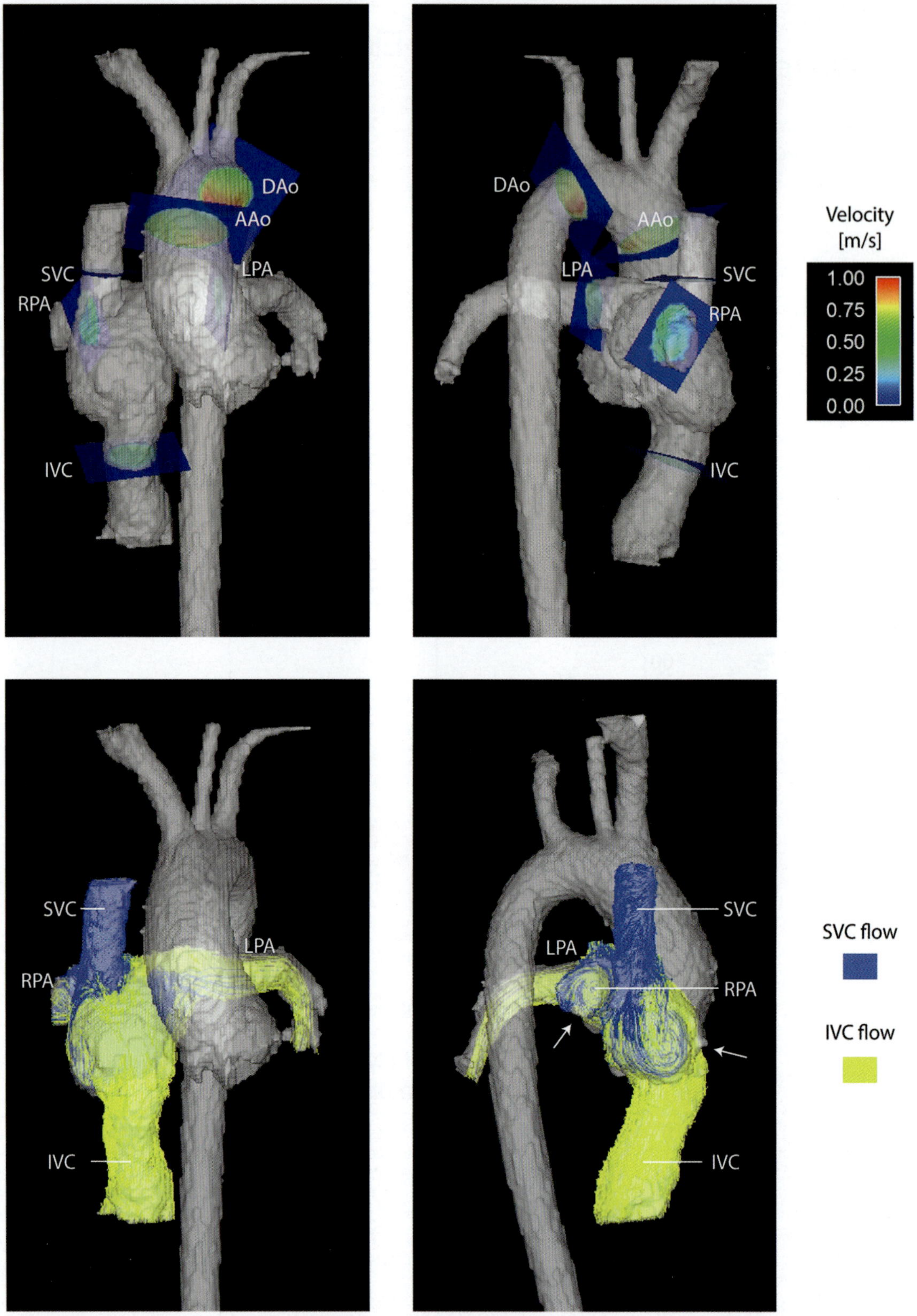

FIG. 5.11 Example of four-dimensional (*4D*) flow MRI in a patient with complex congenital heart disease. *Top*: analysis planes were placed in the AAo, DAo, superior vena cave (SVC), inferior vena cave (IVC), right (RPA), and left pulmonary artery LPA where net flow was 69 mL/cycle, 54 mL/cycle, 12 mL/cycle, 68 mL/cycle, 33 mL/cycle, and 32 mL/cycle, respectively. *Bottom*: path lines depict vortex flow (*arrows*) in the IVC and RPA. For both rows, two views of the imaging volume are shown (*left* and *right* columns). The mismatch of flow from the caval veins to the pulmonary arteries may be explained by the complex flow situation, including possible fenestration and venovenous collaterals. *AAo*, Ascending aorta; *DAo*, descending aorta.

REFERENCES

1. Carr HY, Purcell EM. Effects of diffusion on free precession in nuclear magnetic resonance experiments. *Phys Rev*. 1954;94:630–638.
2. Hahn E. Detection of sea water motion by nuclear precession. *J Geophys Res*. 1960;65.
3. Bryant DJ, Payne JA, Firmin DN, Longmore DB. Measurement of flow with NMR imaging using a gradient pulse and phase difference technique. *J Comput Assist Tomogr*. 1984;8:588–593.
4. Moran PR. A flow velocity zeugmatographic interlace for NMR imaging in humans. *Magn Reson Imaging*. 1982;1:197–203.
5. Nayler GL, Firmin DN, Longmore DB. Blood flow imaging by cine magnetic resonance. *J Comput Assist Tomogr*. 1986;10:715–722.
6. van Dijk P. Direct cardiac NMR imaging of heart wall and blood flow velocity. *J Comput Assist Tomogr*. 1984;8:429–436.
7. Chai P, Mohiaddin R. How we perform cardiovascular magnetic resonance flow assessment using phase-contrast velocity mapping. *J Cardiovasc Magn Reson*. 2005;7:705–716.
8. Pelc NJ, Herfkens RJ, Shimakawa A, Enzmann DR. Phase contrast cine magnetic resonance imaging. *Magn Reson Q*. 1991;7:229–254.
9. Feinberg DA, Crooks LE, Sheldon P, Hoenninger 3rd J, Watts J, Arakawa M. Magnetic resonance imaging the velocity vector components of fluid flow. *Magn Reson Med*. 1985;2:555–566.
10. Firmin DN, Nayler GL, Klipstein RH, Underwood SR, Rees RS, Longmore DB. In vivo validation of MR velocity imaging. *J Comput Assist Tomogr*. 1987;11:751–756.
11. Markl M, Kilner PJ, Ebbers T. Comprehensive 4D velocity mapping of the heart and great vessels by cardiovascular magnetic resonance. *J Cardiovasc Magn Reson Off J Soc Cardiovasc Magn Reson*. 2011;13:7.
12. Dyverfeldt P, Bissell M, Barker AJ, et al. 4D flow cardiovascular magnetic resonance consensus statement. *J Cardiovasc Magn Reson Off J Soc Cardiovasc Magn Reson*. 2015;17:72.
13. Azarine A, Garçon P, Stansal A, et al. Four-dimensional flow MRI: principles and cardiovascular applications. *Radiographics*. 2019;39:632–648.
14. Jacobs K, Hahn L, Horowitz M, Kligerman S, Vasanawala S, Hsiao A. Hemodynamic assessment of structural heart disease using 4D flow MRI: how we do it. *AJR Am J Roentgenol*. 2021;217:1322–1332.
15. Maroun A, Quinn S, Dushfunian D, et al. Clinical applications of four-dimensional flow MRI. *Magn Reson Imaging Clin*. 2023. https://doi.org/j.mric.2023.04.005.
16. Wieben O, Roberts GS, Corrado PA, Johnson KM, Roldán-Alzate A. Four-dimensional flow MR imaging: technique and advances. *Magn Reson Imaging Clin N Am*. 2023;31:433–449.
17. Bernstein MA, Shimakawa A, Pelc NJ. Minimizing TE in moment-nulled or flow-encoded two- and three-dimensional gradient-echo imaging. *J Magn Reson Imaging*. 1992;2:583–588.
18. Dall'Armellina E, Hamilton CA, Hundley WG. Assessment of blood flow and valvular heart disease using phase-contrast cardiovascular magnetic resonance. *Echocardiography*. 2007;24:207–216.
19. Kilner PJ, Gatehouse PD, Firmin DN. Flow measurement by magnetic resonance: a unique asset worth optimising. *J Cardiovasc Magn Reson Off J Soc Cardiovasc Magn Reson*. 2007;9:723–728.
20. Nayak KS, Nielsen JF, Bernstein MA, et al. Cardiovascular magnetic resonance phase contrast imaging. *J Cardiovasc Magn Reson*. 2015;17:71.
21. DeGroff CG, Shandas R, Kwon J, Valdes-Cruz L. Accuracy of the Bernoulli equation for estimation of pressure gradient across stenotic Blalock-Taussig shunts: an in vitro and numerical study. *Pediatr Cardiol*. 2000;21:439–447.
22. Firstenberg MS, Vandervoort PM, Greenberg NL, et al. Noninvasive estimation of transmitral pressure drop across the normal mitral valve in humans: importance of convective and inertial forces during left ventricular filling. *J Am Coll Cardiol*. 2000;36:1942–1949.
23. Oshinski JN, Parks WJ, Markou CP, et al. Improved measurement of pressure gradients in aortic coarctation by magnetic resonance imaging. *J Am Coll Cardiol*. 1996;28:1818–1826.
24. Andersen AH, Kirsch JE. Analysis of noise in phase contrast MR imaging. *Med Phys*. 1996;23:857–869.
25. Walker PG, Cranney GB, Scheidegger MB, Waseleski G, Pohost GM, Yoganathan AP. Semiautomated method for noise reduction and background phase error correction in MR phase velocity data. *J Magn Reson Imaging*. 1993;3:521–530.
26. Bernstein MA, Zhou XJ, Polzin JA, et al. Concomitant gradient terms in phase contrast MR: analysis and correction. *Magn Reson Med*. 1998;39:300–308.
27. Markl M, Bammer R, Alley MT, et al. Generalized reconstruction of phase contrast MRI: analysis and correction of the effect of gradient field distortions. *Magn Reson Med*. 2003;50:791–801.
28. Didier D. Assessment of valve disease: qualitative and quantitative. *Magn Reson Imaging Clin N Am*. 2003;11:115–134, vii.
29. Beerbaum P, Korperich H, Barth P, Esdorn H, Gieseke J, Meyer H. Noninvasive quantification of left-to-right shunt in pediatric patients: phase-contrast cine magnetic resonance imaging compared with invasive oximetry. *Circulation*. 2001;103:2476–2482.
30. Gatehouse PD, Keegan J, Crowe LA, et al. Applications of phase-contrast flow and velocity imaging in cardiovascular MRI. *Eur Radiol*. 2005;15:2172–2184.
31. Underwood SR, Firmin DN, Rees RS, Longmore DB. Magnetic resonance velocity mapping. *Clin Phys Physiol Meas*. 1990;11:37–43.
32. Kowallick JT, Joseph AA, Unterberg-Buchwald C, et al. Real-time phase-contrast flow MRI of the ascending aorta and superior vena cava as a function of intrathoracic pressure (Valsalva manoeuvre). *Br J Radiol*. 2014;87:20140401.
33. Thavendiranathan P, Verhaert D, Walls MC, et al. Simultaneous right and left heart real-time, free-breathing CMR flow quantification identifies constrictive physiology. *JACC Cardiovasc Imaging*. 2012;5:15–24.
34. Untenberger M, Tan Z, Voit D, et al. Advances in real-time phase-contrast flow MRI using asymmetric radial gradient echoes. *Magn Reson Med*. 2015. https://doi.org/10.1002/mrm.25696.
35. Kellman P, Epstein FH, McVeigh ER. Adaptive sensitivity encoding incorporating temporal filtering (TSENSE). *Magn Reson Med*. 2001;45:846–852.
36. Lin HY, Bender JA, Ding Y, et al. Shared velocity encoding: a method to improve the temporal resolution of phase-contrast velocity measurements. *Magn Reson Med*. 2012;68:703–710.
37. Hope MD, Sedlic T, Dyverfeldt P. Cardiothoracic magnetic resonance flow imaging. *J Thorac Imaging*. 2013;28:217–230.
38. Markl M, Frydrychowicz A, Kozerke S, Hope M, Wieben O. 4D flow MRI. *J Magn Reson Imaging*. 2012;36:1015–1036.
39. Bissell MM, Raimondi F, Ait Ali L, et al. 4D flow cardiovascular magnetic resonance consensus statement: 2023 update. *J Cardiovasc Magn Reson Off J Soc Cardiovasc Magn Reson*. 2023;25:40.
40. Markl M, Harloff A, Bley TA, et al. Time-resolved 3D MR velocity mapping at 3T: improved navigator-gated assessment of vascular anatomy and blood flow. *J Magn Reson Imaging*. 2007;25:824–831.
41. Griswold MA, Jakob PM, Heidemann RM, et al. Generalized autocalibrating partially parallel acquisitions (GRAPPA). *Magn Reson Med*. 2002;47:1202–1210.
42. Huang F, Akao J, Vijayakumar S, Duensing GR, Limkeman M. k-t GRAPPA: a k-space implementation for dynamic MRI with high reduction factor. *Magn Reson Med*. 2005;54:1172–1184.
43. Schnell S, Markl M, Entezari P, et al. k-t GRAPPA accelerated four-dimensional flow MRI in the aorta: effect on scan time, image quality, and quantification of flow and wall shear stress. *Magn Reson Med*. 2014;72:522–533.
44. Lustig M, Donoho D, Pauly JM. Sparse MRI: the application of compressed sensing for rapid MR imaging. *Magn Reson Med*. 2007;58:1182–1195.
45. Ma LE, Markl M, Chow K, et al. Aortic 4D flow MRI in 2 minutes using compressed sensing, respiratory controlled adaptive k-space reordering, and inline reconstruction. *Magn Reson Med*. 2019;81:3675–3690.
46. Kim D, Jen ML, Eisenmenger LB, Johnson KM. Accelerated 4D-flow MRI with 3-point encoding enabled by machine learning. *Magn Reson Med*. 2023;89:800–811.
47. Peper ES, van Ooij P, Jung B, Huber A, Gräni C, Bastiaansen JAM. Advances in machine learning applications for cardiovascular 4D flow MRI. *Front Cardiovasc Med*. 2022;9:1052068.
48. Bock J, Frydrychowicz A, Stalder AF, et al. 4D phase contrast MRI at 3 T: effect of standard and blood-pool contrast agents on SNR, PC-MRA, and blood flow visualization. *Magn Reson Med*. 2010;63:330–338.
49. Berhane H, Scott M, Elbaz M, et al. Fully automated 3D aortic segmentation of 4D flow MRI for hemodynamic analysis using deep learning. *Magn Reson Med*. 2020. https://doi.org/10.1002/mrm.28257.
50. Berhane H, Scott MB, Barker AJ, et al. Deep learning-based velocity antialiasing of 4D-flow MRI. *Magn Reson Med*. 2022;88:449–463.
51. Rose MJ, Jarvis K, Chowdhary V, et al. Efficient method for volumetric assessment of peak blood flow velocity using 4D flow MRI. *J Magn Reson Imaging*. 2016. https://doi.org/10.1002/jmri.25305.
52. Barker AJ, Markl M, Burk J, et al. Bicuspid aortic valve is associated with altered wall shear stress in the ascending aorta. *Circ Cardiovasc Imaging*. 2012;5:457–466.
53. Soulat G, Scott MB, Allen BD, et al. Association of regional wall shear stress and progressive ascending aorta dilation in bicuspid aortic valve. *JACC Cardiovasc Imaging*. 2022;15:33–42.
54. van Ooij P, Potters WV, Collins J, et al. Characterization of abnormal wall shear stress using 4D flow MRI in human bicuspid aortopathy. *Ann Biomed Eng*. 2015;43:1385–1397.
55. Qin JJ, Obeidy P, Gok M, Gholipour A, Grieve SM. 4D-flow MRI derived wall shear stress for the risk stratification of bicuspid aortic valve aortopathy: a systematic review. *Front Cardiovasc Med*. 2022;9:1075833.
56. Binter C, Gotschy A, Sundermann SH, et al. Turbulent kinetic energy assessed by multipoint 4-dimensional flow magnetic resonance imaging provides additional information relative to echocardiography for the determination of aortic stenosis severity. *Circ Cardiovasc Imaging*. 2017;10.
57. Dyverfeldt P, Hope MD, Tseng EE, Saloner D. Magnetic resonance measurement of turbulent kinetic energy for the estimation of irreversible pressure loss in aortic stenosis. *JACC Cardiovasc Imaging*. 2013;6:64–71.
58. Ha H, Kvitting JP, Dyverfeldt P, Ebbers T. Validation of pressure drop assessment using 4D flow MRI-based turbulence production in various shapes of aortic stenoses. *Magn Reson Med*. 2019;81:893–906.
59. Wentland AL, Grist TM, Wieben O. Review of MRI-based measurements of pulse wave velocity: a biomarker of arterial stiffness. *Cardiovasc Diagn Ther*. 2014;4:193–206.
60. Harloff A, Mirzaee H, Lodemann T, et al. Determination of aortic stiffness using 4D flow cardiovascular magnetic resonance—a population-based study. *J Cardiovasc Magn Reson Off J Soc Cardiovasc Magn Reson*. 2018;20:43.
61. Jarvis K, Scott MB, Soulat G, et al. Aortic pulse wave velocity evaluated by 4D flow MRI across the adult lifespan. *J Magn Reson Imaging*. 2022. https://doi.org/10.1002/jmri.28045.
62. Soulat G, Gencer U, Kachenoura N, et al. Changes in segmental pulse wave velocity of the thoracic aorta with age and left ventricular remodelling. An MRI 4D flow study. *J Hypertens*. 2020;38:118–126.

63. Hope MD, Hope TA, Meadows AK, et al. Bicuspid aortic valve: four-dimensional MR evaluation of ascending aortic systolic flow patterns. *Radiology*. 2010;255:53–61.
64. Allen BD, Aouad PJ, Burris NS, et al. Detection and hemodynamic evaluation of flap fenestrations in type B aortic dissection with 4D flow MRI: comparison with conventional MRI and CT angiography. *Radiol Cardiothorac Imaging*. 2019;1:e180009.
65. Burris NS, Nordsletten DA, Sotelo JA, et al. False lumen ejection fraction predicts growth in type B aortic dissection: preliminary results. *Eur J Cardio-Thorac Surg Off J Eur Assoc Cardio-Thorac Surg*. 2020;57:896–903.
66. Feneis JF, Kyubwa E, Atianzar K, et al. 4D flow MRI quantification of mitral and tricuspid regurgitation: reproducibility and consistency relative to conventional MRI. *J Magn Reson Imaging*. 2018;48:1147–1158.
67. Zhuang B, Sirajuddin A, Zhao S, Lu M. The role of 4D flow MRI for clinical applications in cardiovascular disease: current status and future perspectives. *Quant Imaging Med Surg*. 2021;11:4193–4210.
68. Roes SD, Hammer S, van der Geest RJ, et al. Flow assessment through four heart valves simultaneously using 3-dimensional 3-directional velocity-encoded magnetic resonance imaging with retrospective valve tracking in healthy volunteers and patients with valvular regurgitation. *Invest Radiol*. 2009;44:669–675.
69. Kamphuis VP, Roest AAW, Ajmone Marsan N, et al. Automated cardiac valve tracking for flow quantification with four-dimensional flow MRI. *Radiology*. 2019;290:70–78.
70. Bachler P, Valverde I, Pinochet N, et al. Caval blood flow distribution in patients with Fontan circulation: quantification by using particle traces from 4D flow MR imaging. *Radiology*. 2013;267:67–75.
71. Jarvis K, Schnell S, Barker AJ, et al. Evaluation of blood flow distribution asymmetry and vascular geometry in patients with Fontan circulation using 4-D flow MRI. *Pediatr Radiol*. 2016;46:1507–1519.
72. Kamphuis VP, Elbaz MSM, van den Boogaard PJ, et al. Disproportionate intraventricular viscous energy loss in Fontan patients: analysis by 4D flow MRI. *Eur Heart J Cardiovas Imaging*. 2019;20:323–333.
73. Sjoberg P, Heiberg E, Wingren P, et al. Decreased diastolic ventricular kinetic energy in young patients with Fontan circulation demonstrated by four-dimensional cardiac magnetic resonance imaging. *Pediatr Cardiol*. 2017;38:669–680.
74. Geiger J, Hirtler D, Burk J, et al. Postoperative pulmonary and aortic 3D haemodynamics in patients after repair of transposition of the great arteries. *Eur Radiol*. 2014;24:200–208.
75. Jarvis K, Vonder M, Barker AJ, et al. Hemodynamic evaluation in patients with transposition of the great arteries after the arterial switch operation: 4D flow and 2D phase contrast cardiovascular magnetic resonance compared with Doppler echocardiography. *J Cardiovasc Magn Reson Off J Soc Cardiovasc Magn Reson*. 2016;18:59.
76. Francois CJ, Srinivasan S, Schiebler ML, et al. 4D cardiovascular magnetic resonance velocity mapping of alterations of right heart flow patterns and main pulmonary artery hemodynamics in tetralogy of Fallot. *J Cardiovasc Magn Reson Off J Soc Cardiovasc Magn Reson*. 2012;14:16.
77. Fredriksson A, Trzebiatowska-Krzynska A, Dyverfeldt P, Engvall J, Ebbers T, Carlhäll CJ. Turbulent kinetic energy in the right ventricle: potential MR marker for risk stratification of adults with repaired Tetralogy of Fallot. *J Magn Reson Imaging*. 2018;47:1043–1053.
78. Sjoberg P, Bidhult S, Bock J, et al. Disturbed left and right ventricular kinetic energy in patients with repaired tetralogy of Fallot: pathophysiological insights using 4D-flow MRI. *Eur Radiol*. 2018;28:4066–4076.
79. Hofman MB, Visser FC, van Rossum AC, Vink QM, Sprenger M, Westerhof N. In vivo validation of magnetic resonance blood volume flow measurements with limited spatial resolution in small vessels. *Magn Reson Med*. 1995;33:778–784.
80. Fratz S, Chung T, Greil GF, et al. Guidelines and protocols for cardiovascular magnetic resonance in children and adults with congenital heart disease: SCMR expert consensus group on congenital heart disease. *J Cardiovasc Magn Reson Off J Soc Cardiovasc Magn Reson*. 2013;15:51.

6 Myocardial Imaging: Advanced Techniques

DAVID WENDELL, ENN-LING CHEN, AND RAYMOND J. KIM

INTRODUCTION

In this chapter we discuss advanced techniques that are works in progress, but which are readily available and appear to have immediate clinical utility. In the section "Dark-Blood Delayed-Enhancement Imaging," other emerging technologies are presented that, while promising, require additional development and/or validation prior to routine clinical use. As an example of the requirement for additional development, there are techniques that work well in volunteers who can perform long breath-holds and/or have a perfectly regular heart rate and rhythm, but perform poorly when these conditions are not met. In our experience, up to 50% of patients have trouble holding their breath and/or have an irregular rhythm or poor ECG gating. This means that an emerging technique—particularly one that requires several minutes for image acquisition—may be abandoned if deemed insufficiently reliable for clinical practice. The techniques presented in this chapter can accommodate most clinical patients, including those with arrhythmias and those with difficulty holding their breath. We focus on two specific areas of myocardial imaging: 1) the improved detection of myocardial infarction and/or scarring, and 2) the discrimination of intramyocardial fat.

DARK-BLOOD DELAYED-ENHANCEMENT IMAGING

Conventional bright-blood delayed-enhancement cardiac magnetic resonance (DE-CMR) has become the reference standard for the in vivo detection of myocardial infarction given its ability to generate high-resolution spatial maps of infarcted and viable myocardium.[1,2] Accordingly, its use is increasing in clinical practice and in randomized trials evaluating novel myocardial infarction (MI) treatments to provide a measure of therapeutic efficacy.[3] One important limitation of DE-CMR, however, is that infarcted myocardium and the left ventricle (LV) blood pool often hyperenhance to a similar degree following administration of contrast media.[4] Hence, infarcted myocardium may be hidden when immediately adjacent to the LV cavity because there is poor delineation between "bright" (i.e., hyperenhanced) tissue and bright blood pool (Fig. 6.1). This may explain the results of the first multicenter international trial evaluating the performance of DE-CMR for the detection of MI.[5] While, overall, the sensitivity of DE-CMR was quite high, reaching 99% and 94% in acute and chronic MI, respectively, results were worse in certain cohorts. For instance, among those with non-Q wave MI, up to 21% of chronic infarcts were missed (Fig. 6.2), most likely because these patients had small subendocardial infarcts. Here, it is important to note that the detection of any infarct, no matter how small, is associated with worse short- and long-term prognosis, and the diagnosis of MI is essential because there are proven therapies that can improve outcome.[6]

To address the issue of subendocardial MI with poor blood-pool contrast, a number of approaches have been proposed. We will provide a brief overview of these approaches and discuss the contrast mechanism and complexities of each method. The bulk of the discussion, however, will be on a novel Flow-Independent Dark-blood DeLayed Enhancement technique known as FIDDLE, which allows visualization of tissue contrast enhancement while simultaneously suppressing blood-pool signal (Fig. 6.3). The magnetization preparation scheme will be illustrated, the experimental and clinical validation data presented, and clinical scenarios in which FIDDLE may be helpful will be discussed.

Methods to Improve Myocardial Infarction-to-Blood Contrast

Conventional "black blood" magnetic resonance imaging (MRI) techniques, such as double or triple inversion recovery (IR) turbo spin echo,[7,8] provide improved delineation of anatomy by suppressing signal from the blood pool of vascular structures. However, these techniques depend on the long T1 (longitudinal relaxation time) of blood (c.a. 2 seconds at 3 T) and sufficient blood flow within this time period to generate black-blood images. Hence, these techniques were not designed to work after contrast media administration (which greatly shortens blood T1), and cannot be used to provide contrast-enhanced, black-blood images of tissues (Fig. 6.3).

More recently, blood flow–sensitive techniques have been introduced that can theoretically function after contrast media administration.[9] However, these techniques remain susceptible to "slow blood flow" artifacts. An important limitation is that stagnant blood may have similar "motion" to adjacent diseased myocardium, and it is patients with disease—those with ischemic or nonischemic cardiomyopathy—who are most likely to have areas with a stagnant cavity blood pool. Additional limitations include reduced signal-to-noise ratio (SNR) compared with conventional delayed-enhancement imaging, and for some sequences the difficulty of setting multiple precise inversion times.

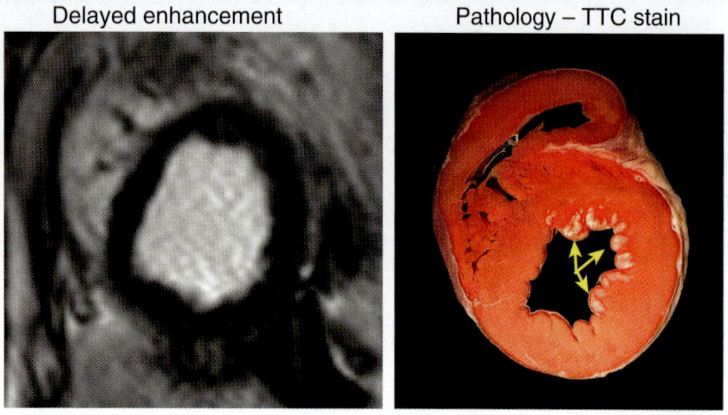

FIG. 6.1 In many patients, myocardial hyperenhancement on delayed-enhancement cardiac magnetic resonance (DE-CMR) may be hidden because there is poor delineation between hyperenhanced tissue and bright blood pool. Left panel shows example of DE-CMR image in which there is no obvious hyperenhancement, however, the triphenyl-tetrazolium chloride (*TTC*)-stained pathology slice (which delineates viable tissue in *red* and infarcted myocardium in *white*) clearly shows a subendocardial infarct in the anterior and anterolateral wall (*arrows*).

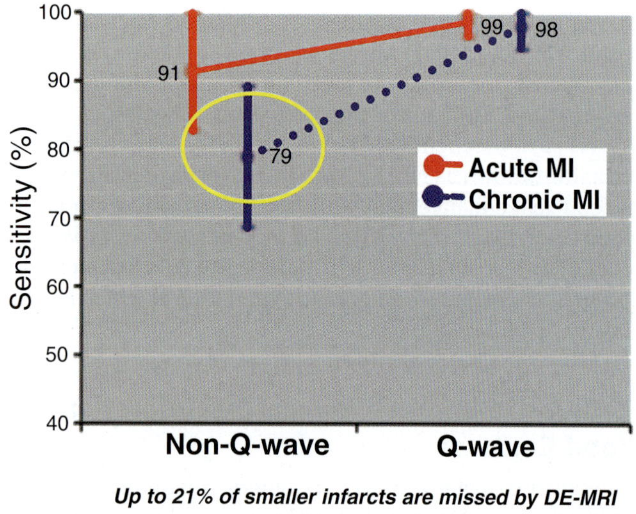

FIG. 6.2 A multicenter trial evaluating the performance of delayed-enhancement cardiac magnetic resonance demonstrated that up to 21% of infarcts may be missed in select patient cohorts such as those with non-Q-wave chronic myocardial infarction (*MI*). *DE-MRI*, Delayed-enhancement magnetic resonance imaging. (From Kim RJ, Albert TS, Wible JH, et al. Performance of delayed-enhancement magnetic resonance imaging with gadoversetamide contrast for the detection and assessment of myocardial infarction: an international, multicenter, double-blinded, randomized trial. *Circulation*. 2008;117:629–637.)

A simple but indirect method to address the issue of subendocardial MI with poor blood-pool contrast is to use steady-state free precession (SSFP) cine images acquired before contrast administration in conjunction with delayed-enhancement images. SSFP cine images offer excellent contrast between blood pool and myocardium and a region for which wall thickness on DE imaging appears to be "thinner" than that seen on cine imaging, which could represent a subendocardial infarct (Fig. 6.4). Although this comparison can be helpful, multiple factors limit the practicality of this approach. Cine and DE images are acquired on separate breath-holds and at different time points during the examination, and patient movement can be a problem. Additionally, there are significant differences in temporal resolution and comparing regional wall thickness on a single cine frame to the corresponding DE image could be problematic since the latter has far worse temporal resolution (readout time: cine frame, 35–40 ms; DE, 160–180 ms). One method that alleviates some of these issues was described by Kellman et al. in 2005.[10] Their multicontrast delayed enhancement (MCODE) approach combines a conventional phase-sensitive inversion recovery (PSIR) acquisition with an extra T2-weighted image that is acquired in the same breath-hold. The function of the T2 image is similar to that of a cine image, however, without the issue of patient motion and differences in spatial and temporal resolution. Nonetheless, even with this improvement, comparing two separate images to make a determination of subendocardial infarction can be difficult and time consuming, and small differences may be impossible to resolve. In a follow-up study in 2012, MCODE was found to have modestly improved diagnostic sensitivity compared with DE imaging alone, but specificity was not improved.[11] In a cohort of 73 patients, conventional delayed-enhancement imaging had two false-positive MIs, whereas MCODE had three false-positive MIs.

Instead of acquiring an extra T2-weighted image, T2 preparation can be incorporated into the delayed-enhancement sequence itself to produce a blood pool–suppressed image. Liu et al.[12] described a technique in which a T2 preparation module is placed immediately prior to each inversion pulse in an otherwise conventional segmented delayed-enhancement sequence. As we will see later in the section describing FIDDLE, the T2 preparation followed by an inversion pulse results in a less negative magnetization vector for infarcted myocardium compared to blood pool. After an inversion time is chosen to null normal myocardium, the blood-pool signal is then usually suppressed relative to infarcted myocardium. In nine patients with MI, Liu et al. demonstrated that this technique resulted in a modest 22% increase in infarct-blood contrast-to-noise ratio (CNR) compared to conventional imaging.

Another way to increase infarct-blood CNR is to null a range of T1 values and not just the T1 that relates to healthy myocardium. Peel et al.[13] implemented a dual IR sequence that was optimized to suppress a wide range of T1s so that only very short T1 species had high signal intensity. The hypothesis being that as long as the T1 of infarction is shorter than that of blood pool, the dual IR sequence will allow visualization of infarction as bright tissue while suppressing the background signal that also includes blood signal. In 12 patients with MI, the dual IR sequence resulted in improved infarct-blood CNR, but at the expense of lower infarct—normal myocardium and blood—normal myocardium CNR. A limitation of the study is that only patients in whom conventional DE imaging had already detected MI were enrolled. Hence, patients with subendocardial and/or patchy infarcts that were difficult to detect (or were missed) with conventional DE imaging (e.g., the group in whom blood-suppressed delayed-enhancement imaging would have its greatest use) were not included, and the reported tissue CNR measurements likely reflected some level of sampling bias.

Additional magnetization preparations, such as the use of multiple inversion pulses, will generally reduce tissue

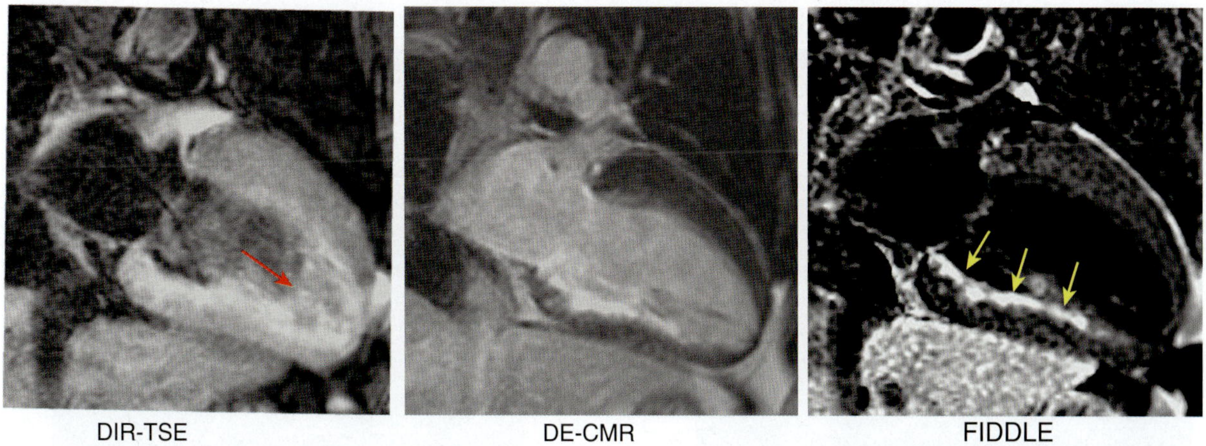

FIG. 6.3 Examples of slow-flow artifacts (*red arrows*) in double-inversion recovery turbo spin echo (*DIR-TSE*) sequences due to poor blood exchange within the imaging slice (*left*). Conventional delayed-enhancement cardiac magnetic resonance (*DE-CMR*) imaging (*center*) without slow-flow artifacts within the left ventricle; however, bright blood pool partially obscures the infarct/blood-pool border. Flow-independent dark-blood delayed enhancement (*FIDDLE*) (*right*) demonstrates uniform blood suppression natively without slow-flow artifacts and simultaneously demonstrates enhanced myocardium in the region of infarction (*arrows*).

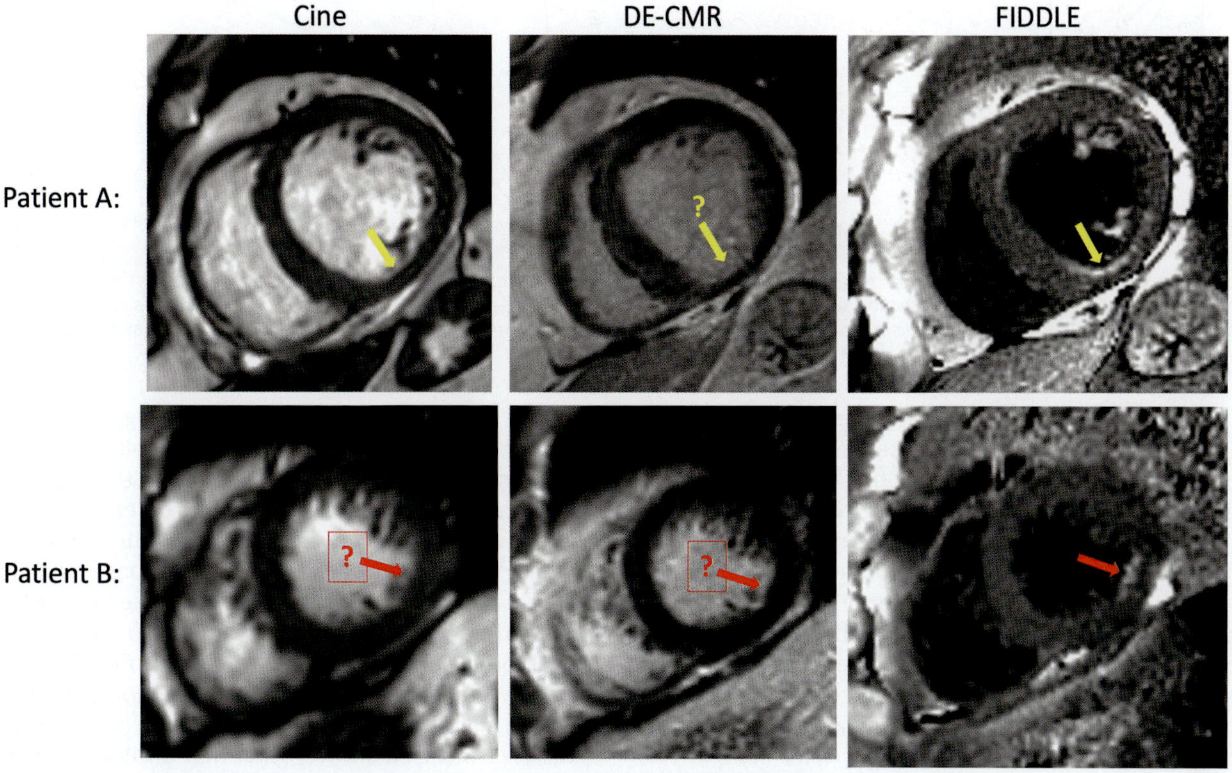

FIG. 6.4 An indirect method to overcome the issue of subendocardial myocardial infarction with poor blood-pool contrast is to compare the delayed-enhancement cardiac magnetic resonance (*DE-CMR*) image against a steady-state free precession cine image acquired before contrast at the same slice location. Patient A shows an example of a subendocardial infarct in the inferior wall, which is clearly seen on the flow-independent dark-blood delayed-enhancement (*FIDDLE*) image (*right*). The infarct is more indistinct on DE-CMR, but assuming that an infarct is not present would suggest that the inferior wall (black, viable layer) is very thin in this patient. Comparison with the cine image acquired at the same location (*left*) shows a thicker wall. This indicates that there is subendocardial hyperenhancement in the DE-CMR image that is obscured by the bright blood pool. This indirect method of comparing DE-CMR with cine images has limitations. In patient B there does not appear to be an infarct in the DE-CMR image (*center*), and the wall does not appear to be appreciably thinner in the cine image (*left*). However, FIDDLE shows a subendocardial infarct in the inferolateral wall (*right*).

SNR. In 2017, Holtackers et al. investigated the feasibility of leveraging a standard PSIR sequence without additional magnetization preparation to suppress blood-pool signal. The key is to use a short inversion time to null the blood pool rather than normal myocardium. This results in the blood pool appearing black in the magnitude image but gray in the phase-sensitive reconstructed image since normal myocardium has a longer T1 relaxation time and thus a lower (negative) magnetization vector (Fig. 6.5). Therefore, PSIR is required to interpret the delayed enhancement

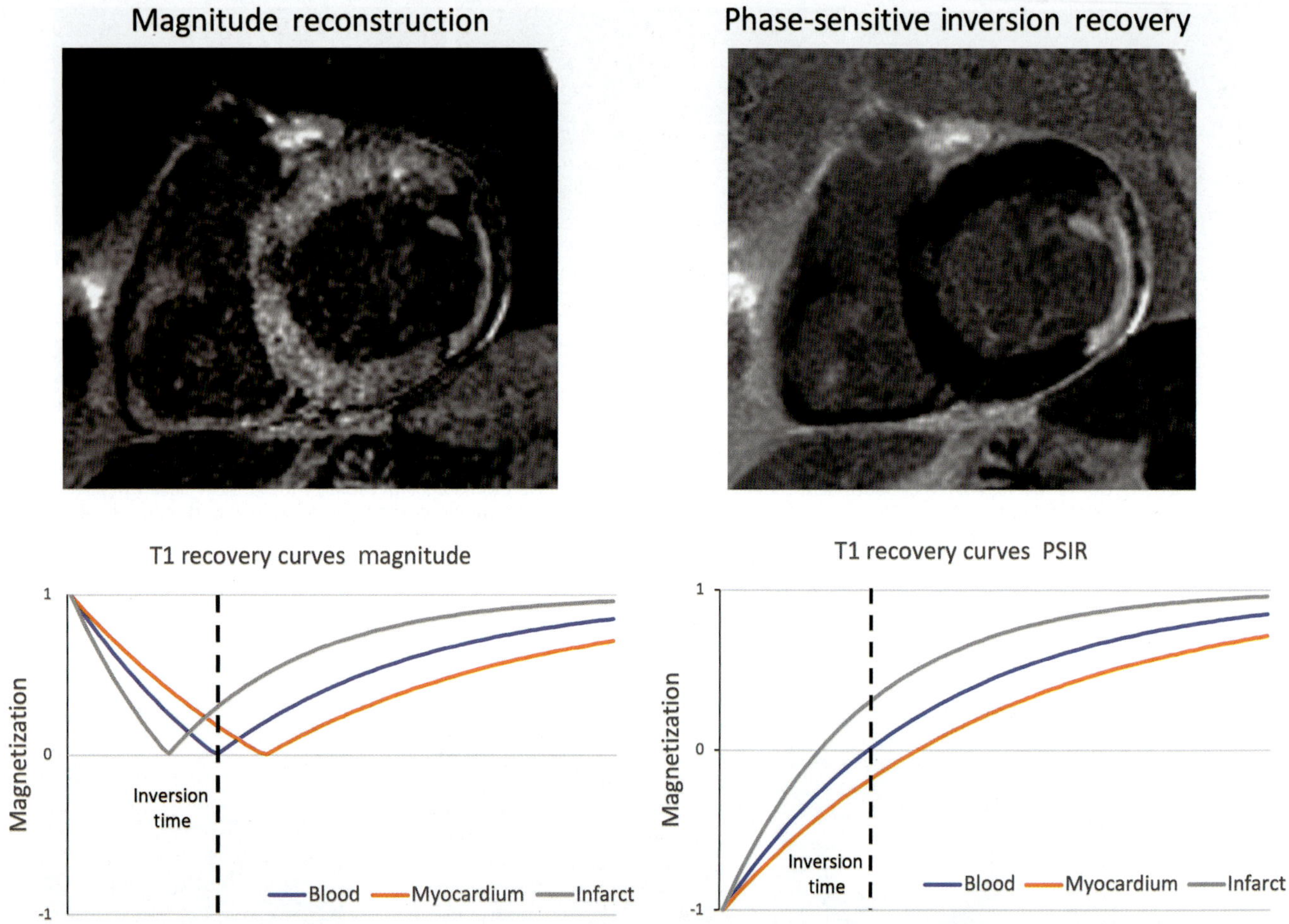

FIG. 6.5 Blood-nulled phase-sensitive inversion recovery (*PSIR*) magnitude (*left*) and PSIR (*right*) images. The magnitude image shows the inversion time (TI) is selected to null the blood pool: the blood curve (*blue line*) is at zero and the left ventricle cavity is dark. The lateral wall infarct has shorter T1 (*gray line*) and normal myocardium has longer T1 (*red line*) than blood. Therefore, after phase-sensitive reconstruction, the PSIR image shows that normal myocardium is now black, blood is gray, and the infarct is bright. See text for details.

data, and in this study the blood-nulled PSIR technique (BN-PSIR) resulted in a 99% increase in infarct-blood CNR compared to conventional imaging. In a follow-up study of an unselected cohort of 300 patients, BN-PSIR led to an 8% increase in the rate of scar detection and a 10% increase in total scar burden compared with conventional imaging.[14] However, it should be noted that there was no reference standard for the diagnosis of MI or ischemic scar, hence, diagnostic performance (sensitivity, specificity, and accuracy) could not be calculated. More recently, in 2021, BN-PSIR was evaluated against histology in a porcine model of MI. In 5 pigs, there were 24 matched slices for comparison with histology. Although Bland-Altman analyses demonstrated high levels of agreement with histology for both DE methods, conventional imaging showed a small bias to underestimate infarct size, whereas BN-PSIR did not. Unfortunately, very few infarcts were small (e.g., less than 10% of the pathology slice), perhaps due to the small sample size. Hence, although diagnostic performance was not reported, the Bland-Altman plots indicate that test sensitivity was 100% for both conventional and BN-PSIR techniques (i.e., no DE technique measured an infarct size of zero) and test specificity could not be calculated since there were no pathology slices with an infarct size of zero.[15]

Similar to the method of Peel et al., a key limitation of the BN-PSIR technique is the assumption that infarct (or scar) T1 is shorter than blood-pool T1 (Fig. 6.6A). By using an inversion time that nulls the blood pool, BN-PSIR accentuates infarcts with a T1 that is different than blood pool. However, this means that if there is no difference in T1 then there is nothing to accentuate, and infarction may be invisible (Fig. 6.6B). Moreover, if infarct T1 is longer than blood-pool T1, then it will resemble the interface between blood pool and normal myocardium, which also has a longer T1 than blood (due to the long T1 of normal myocardium and partial volume effect), and again infarction will be invisible. The major problem then, is that there is no reason why infarct T1 must be shorter than that of blood. Depending on the severity and duration of ischemia, anywhere from 1% to 100% of the myocytes in the infarct-related artery perfusion territory may be infarcted, and that region could have a postcontrast T1 that ranges from just shorter than normal myocardium (i.e., T1 that is far longer than blood) to shorter than that of blood.

A related issue is the importance of appropriately categorizing blood suppression techniques. The methods of Liu, Peel, and Holtackers result in images with gray blood pool but (similar to conventional DE imaging) normal myocardium that is black. Contrast this with FIDDLE (described in detail in the following section) in which the blood is black and normal myocardium is gray. This distinction is important because there is a fundamental difference between a

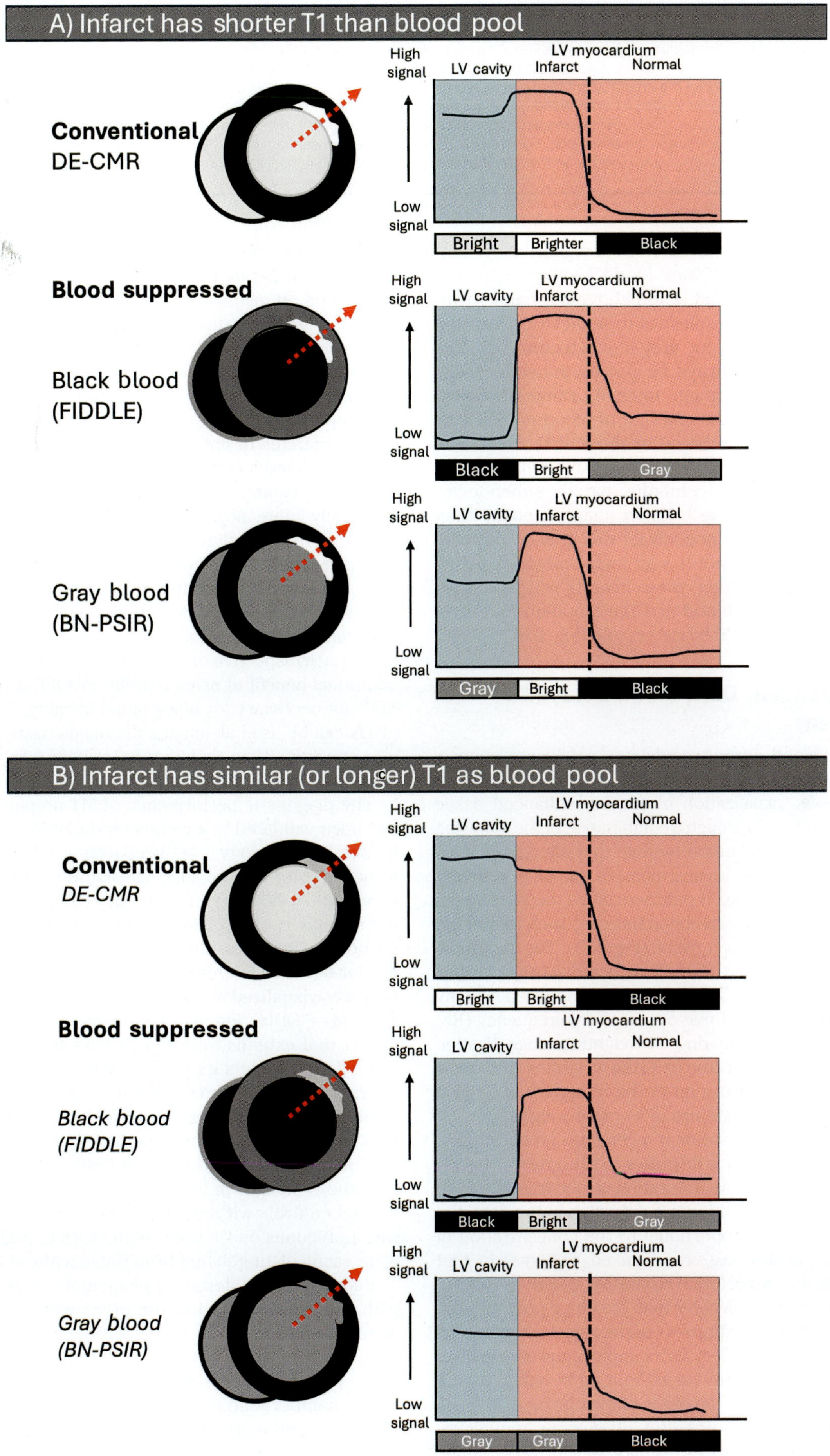

Caption on next page

FIG. 6.6 A schematic comparing conventional bright-blood delayed-enhancement cardiac magnetic resonance (*DE-CMR*) and two blood suppression techniques: flow-independent dark-blood delayed enhancement (*FIDDLE*), which is usually run with a black-blood implementation and blood-nulled PSIR (*BN-PSIR*), which is a gray-blood technique. Representative line intensity profiles are shown for the three techniques with the interrogation line drawn from the left ventricle (*LV*) cavity blood pool moving toward then through the subendocardial infarct to the epicardial layer. If the infarct has shorter T1 than blood (panel A), all techniques depict the infarct with blood suppression techniques accentuating the difference in signal between infarct and blood pool. However, if the infarct has similar (*or longer*) T1 than blood (panel B), the infarct is difficult to visualize with conventional DE-CMR, and conspicuity is not improved with BN-DE. In this situation only FIDDLE allows depiction of the infarct-blood border. The schematic also shows that there is a fundamental difference between a technique that reduces the blood-pool signal below that of normal myocardium ("black blood") versus one that results in blood signal that is still above normal myocardium ("gray blood"). See text for details. *DE-PSIR*, Delayed-enhancement phase-sensitive inversion recovery.

technique that reduces the blood-pool signal below that of normal myocardium ("black blood") versus one that results in a blood signal that is still above normal myocardium ("gray blood"). Regardless of the exact T1 relaxation times of various tissues, for gray-blood techniques, this means that there can always be patchy subendocardial infarcts for which their image intensity ranges between that of normal myocardium and that of blood pool. These infarcts will resemble the blood or the interface between blood and normal myocardium and will be invisible (Fig. 6.6B). For a black-blood technique, patchy subendocardial infarcts will again have brighter image intensity than normal myocardium. But in contrast to a gray-blood technique, since the blood pool has an image intensity below that of normal myocardium, these infarcts will be clearly distinguished from the blood and the blood-normal myocardium interface and will be detectable (Fig. 6.6).

Flow-Independent Dark-Blood Delayed Enhancement

A new class of blood-suppressed delayed-enhancement imaging known as FIDDLE was developed in 2011.[16] FIDDLE allows for simultaneous visualization of contrast-enhanced tissue and a black blood pool through a combination of the following components: 1) a preparation module that affects the magnetization of tissue (e.g., myocardium) in a manner different than blood, 2) an IR pulse, 3) phase-sensitive reconstruction, and 4) the selection of an inversion time (TI) such that blood magnetization is lower than tissue (Fig. 6.7).[17] For the preparation module, the goal is to reduce myocardial tissue magnetization more than blood. This may be accomplished in many ways, including the use of one or more radiofrequency (RF) pulses that impart T2 weighting, T1 weighting, magnetization transfer (MT) weighting, T2rho or T1rho weighting (i.e., transverse or longitudinal relaxation in the rotating frame), or a combination of these weightings or by other weightings.

The MT-preparation module is a common preparation. It uses a train of off-resonance RF pulses to saturate the macromolecular proton pool. This saturation is then transferred to the main water pool, resulting in a reduction in the detected magnetization that is proportional to the concentration of large macromolecules (e.g., cross-linked proteins) in that tissue.[18] Given that myocardial tissue has a higher concentration of large macromolecules than the blood pool, the MT-preparation module will suppress tissue signal while leaving blood relatively undisturbed. An example of the effects of an MT-preparation module (alone without an IR pulse) on the magnetization of cardiac tissues is shown in Fig. 6.8. Imaging was performed 15 minutes after intravenous administration of gadolinium contrast (0.15 mmol/kg gadoversetamide to mimic the conditions of clinical delayed-enhancement imaging). Increasing train length, increasing flip angle, and decreasing off-resonance frequency of the MT-preparation module steadily reduced signal intensity for all tissues. However, the effect was substantially larger for myocardial tissue compared to the blood pool, and differences between normal and infarcted myocardium were negligible. Since the MT-preparation module suppresses myocardial tissue signal (either infarcted or not) more than blood, following the MT-preparation module with an inversion pulse (i.e., as occurs in FIDDLE) results in the magnetization of blood (Mz), which is initially more negative than normal myocardium (i.e., blood Mz < myocardial Mz). Phase-sensitive reconstruction will then render the blood in the cardiac chambers darker than the myocardium after remapping the magnetization to positive-only values. Here, it is useful to understand that PSIR renders the most negative magnetization as the darkest signal irrespective of the absolute value of the signal. An additional benefit of using PSIR for FIDDLE is that a precise TI is not necessary for black-blood imaging, rather, a range of TIs can be used as long as the magnetization of blood is more negative than that of myocardium (aka "black-blood condition" in Fig. 6.8).

The diagnostic performance of MT-preparation FIDDLE has been validated in a canine model of MI with direct reference to pathology.[17] MT-preparation FIDDLE was found to be superior to conventional DE-CMR with a higher sensitivity (96% vs. 85%) and accuracy (95% vs. 87%) and similar specificity (both 92%). In infarcts that were identified by both techniques, the entire length of the endocardial border between infarcted myocardium and adjacent blood pool was visualized in only 33% for DE-CMR compared with 100% for FIDDLE. Fig. 6.9 demonstrates an example of an infarct that extends from the LV base to nearly the apical cap. FIDDLE depicts its endocardial border throughout its course, whereas with DE-CMR it is unclear if an infarct is even present at multiple short-axis levels. In patients, findings were similar. FIDDLE demonstrated a higher accuracy for the diagnosis of MI than DE-CMR (100% vs. 84%). Fig. 6.10 shows images in five patients (three with MI and two normal controls without MI) in whom the diagnosis of MI was ambiguous on DE-CMR. With FIDDLE, patients with MI were easily distinguished from those without MI.

Recently, two different implementations of FIDDLE, one with MT preparation and the other with T2 preparation, were compared at 3 and 1.5 T.[19] Although diagnostic-quality images were usually obtained with both techniques, bright blood-pool artifacts were frequently observed in the left atrial chamber (and occasionally extending into the chamber of the left ventricle) with T2-preparation FIDDLE, particularly at 3 T (Fig. 6.11A). These blood "in-flow" artifacts, reflecting incomplete blood-pool suppression, highlight a disadvantage of T2 preparation, which is more sensitive to field inhomogeneities and regions with rapid blood flow than MT preparation. Another inherent limitation of T2 preparation is nonuniform blood-pool suppression in right- versus left-sided cardiac chambers. Differences in O_2 saturation between venous and arterial blood result in different native T2 relaxation times between right- and left-sided chambers, which in turn leads to an elevated right ventricular blood-pool signal compared to the left ventricular signal on T2-preparation FIDDLE (Fig. 6.11B). Given these findings, the study concluded that MT preparation was superior to T2 preparation for flow-independent, black-blood, delayed-enhancement imaging of the heart.

The FIDDLE sequence can be adapted to a wide range of clinical settings (such as irregular cardiac rhythms, poor breath holding, etc.). Fig. 6.12 shows example images from various implementations, all using MT preparation.

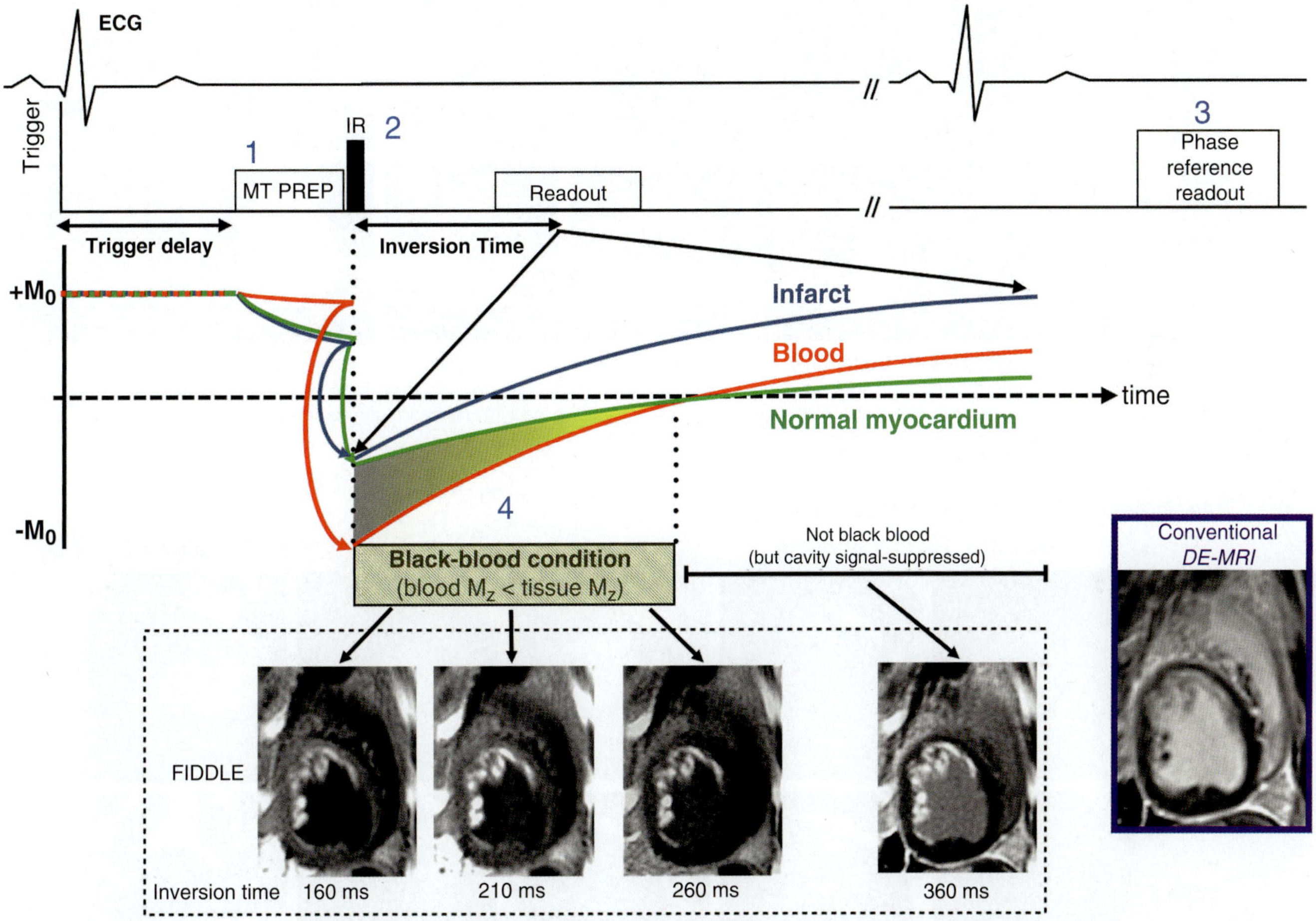

FIG. 6.7 Flow-independent dark-blood delayed enhancement (*FIDDLE*) timing diagram: Primary components are: (1) preparatory module, (2) inversion recovery pulse, (3) phase-sensitive reconstruction, and (4) inversion time such that blood magnetization is less than tissue magnetization (referred to as "black-blood condition"). Even with inversion times outside the black-blood condition, blood-pool signal is suppressed (i.e., gray-blood FIDDLE) compared with conventional, bright-blood delayed-enhancement cardiac magnetic resonance, which improves the conspicuity of infarcted myocardium (M_0 = baseline longitudinal magnetization; Mz = blood or tissue magnetization). *DE-MRI*, Delayed-enhancement magnetic resonance imaging; *MT-PREP*, magnetization transfer preparation. (From Kim HW, Rehwald WG, Jenista ER, et al. Dark-blood delayed enhancement cardiac magnetic resonance of myocardial infarction. *JACC Cardiovasc Imaging*. 2018;11:1758–1769.)

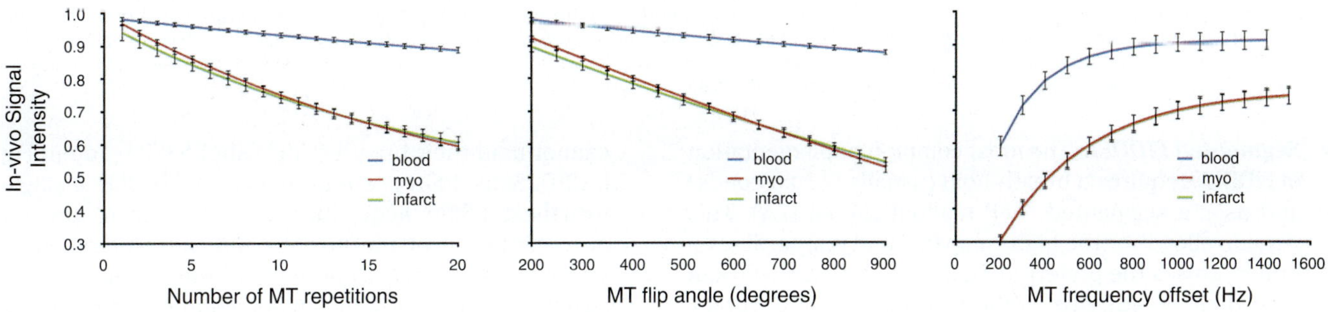

FIG. 6.8 In vivo characterization of a magnetization transfer (*MT*)-preparation module in a canine model of myocardial infarction. Increasing train length, holding flip angle, and frequency offset constant (600 degrees and 800 Hz) reduced signal, particularly for normal myocardium (myo) and infarcted myocardium (*left panel*). Increasing flip angle, holding train length, and frequency offset constant (14 and 800 Hz) reduced signal, again especially for myocardial tissue (*middle panel*). Increasing frequency offset, holding train length, and flip angle constant (14 and 600 degrees) led to increased signal for myocardium and blood (*right panel*). (From Kim HW, Rehwald WG, Jenista ER et al. Dark-blood delayed enhancement cardiac magnetic resonance of myocardial infarction. *JACC Cardiovasc Imaging*. 2018; 11:1758–1769.)

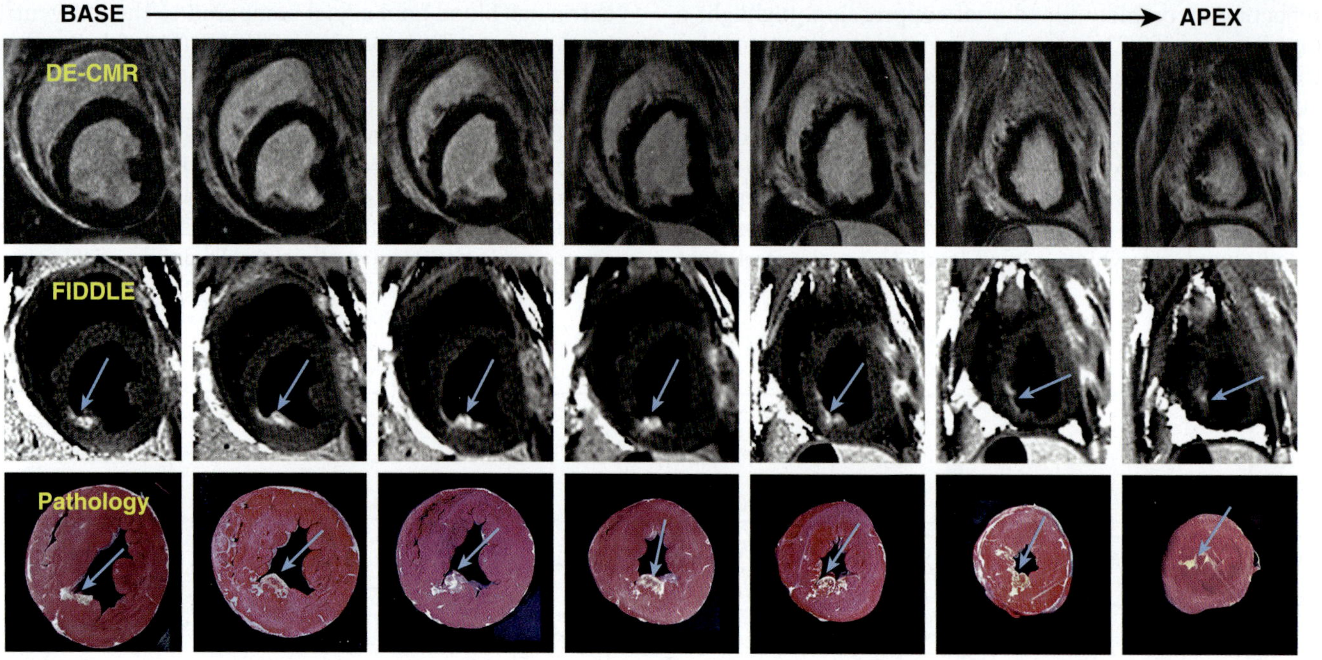

FIG. 6.9 Matched delayed-enhancement cardiac magnetic resonance (*DE-CMR*), flow-independent dark-blood delayed enhancement (*FIDDLE*), and pathology images in a subject with an inferoseptal wall subendocardial infarct (*blue arrows*) that extends from base to nearly the apical cap. See text for details. (From Kim HW, Rehwald WG, Jenista ER, et al. Dark-blood delayed enhancement cardiac magnetic resonance of myocardial infarction. *JACC Cardiovasc Imaging*. 2018;11:1758–1769.)

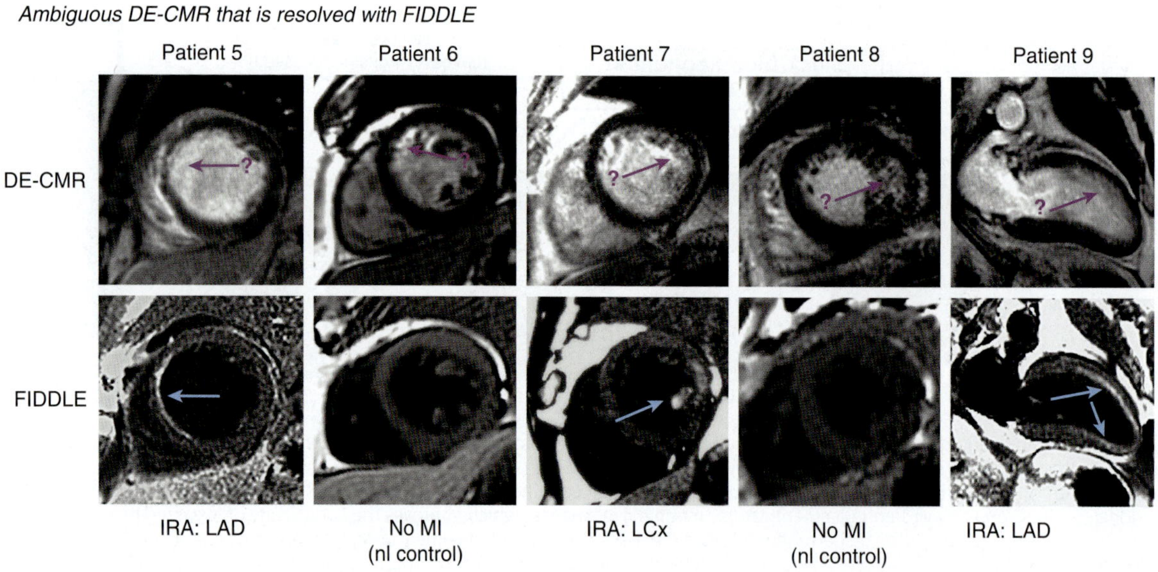

FIG. 6.10 Images in 5 patients (3 with myocardial infarction [MI] and 2 normal controls without MI) in whom the diagnosis of MI is ambiguous on delayed-enhancement cardiac magnetic resonance (*DE-CMR*). In patients #5 and #6, there is possibly anteroseptal wall hyperenhancement on DE-CMR (*purple arrows*). However, flow-independent dark-blood delayed enhancement (*FIDDLE*) shows no hyperenhancement and correctly identifies patient 6 as a normal control. In patients #7 and #8, FIDDLE identifies the fact that patient #8 is a normal control. In patient #9, FIDDLE clearly demonstrates not only a subendocardial infarct in the anterior wall but also extension into the inferoapical wall (*blue arrows*). *IRA,* Infarct-related artery; *LAD,* left anterior descending; *LCx,* left circumflex; *MI,* myocardial infarction; *RCA,* right coronary artery. (From Kim HW, Rehwald WG, Jenista ER, et al. Dark-blood delayed enhancement cardiac magnetic resonance of myocardial infarction. *JACC Cardiovasc Imaging*. 2018;11:1758–1769.)

- ***Segmented FIDDLE:*** The most common implementation of FIDDLE requires a breath-hold (usually 5–10 seconds) and uses a segmented SSFP readout (Fig. 6.12A). This version allows for the highest spatial and temporal resolution. This is the preferred method in patients who can hold their breath, due to the high diagnostic accuracy for assessment of myocardial injury.
- ***Single-heartbeat FIDDLE:*** This implementation provides subsecond, real-time imaging for a patient who cannot hold their breath (single-shot SSFP readout; Fig. 6.12B). Since PSIR is a requirement of FIDDLE, a single-heartbeat PSIR[20] acquisition can be used to prevent misregistration of the IR data and the proton-density reference data used to perform phase-sensitive reconstruction. A typical PSIR implementation acquires the phase reference data one heartbeat after the IR data, which may result in phase misregistration for free-breathing applications.

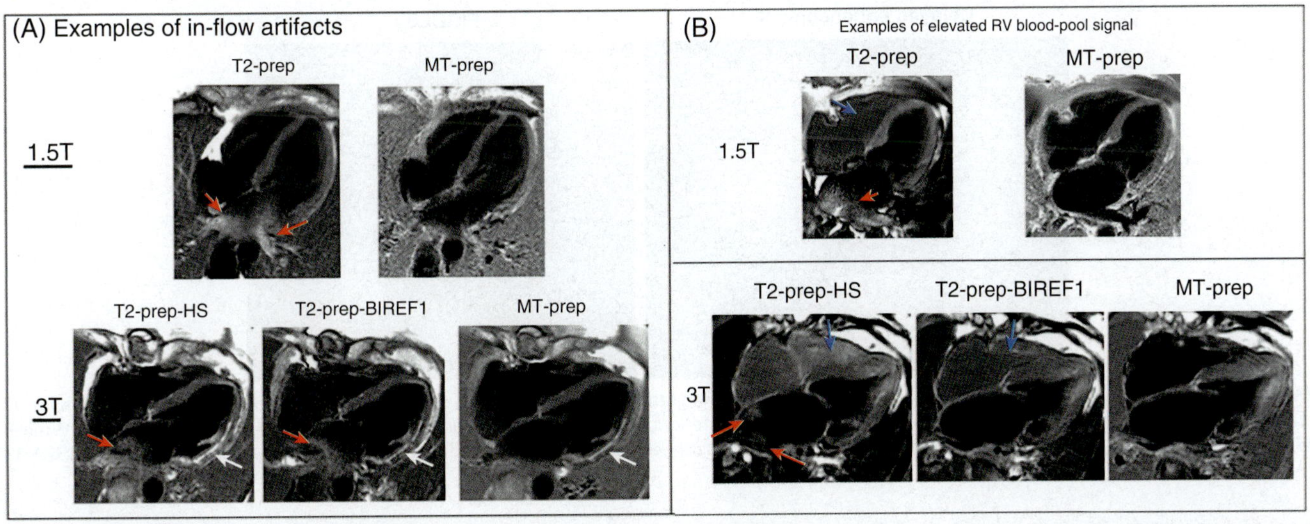

FIG. 6.11 (A) Typical examples of inflow artifacts. T2-preparation flow-independent dark-blood delayed enhancement (FIDDLE) images acquired at 1.5 T (*top row*) and 3 T (*bottom row*) show bright artifacts (*red arrows*), reflecting poor blood-pool suppression involving the origin of the pulmonary veins and extending to adjacent regions in the left atrium. In-flow artifacts are absent with magnetization transfer (*MT*)-preparation FIDDLE. At 3 T, artifacts appear slightly worse with hyperbolic secant (*HS*) compared with B_1-insensitive refocusing (*BIREF1*) adiabatic pulses used for T2 preparation. (B) Examples of different blood-pool suppression between right- and left-sided cardiac chambers. Elevated right ventricular (*RV*) blood-pool signal (*blue arrows*) is seen on the T2-preparation FIDDLE images, acquired either at 1.5 T (*top row*) or 3 T (*bottom row*). In general, elevation of RV blood signal was more prominent at 3 T than 1.5 T, and with T2-preparation-HS than T2-preparation-BIREF1. By contrast, MT-preparation FIDDLE demonstrates uniform blood-pool suppression throughout all cardiac chambers. See text for details. (From Jenista ER, Wendell DC, Kim HW, et al. Comparison of magnetization transfer-preparation and T2-preparation for dark-blood delayed-enhancement imaging. *NMR in Biomed*. 2020;33[11]:e4396.)

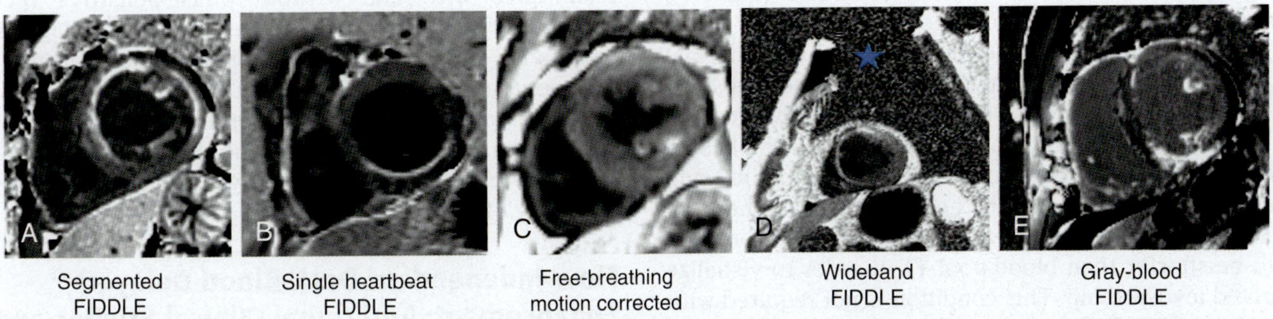

FIG. 6.12 (A) Segmented readout acquisition. (B) Single-shot single heartbeat acquisition (inversion recovery [IR] data and phase reference data occur in one heartbeat). (C) Free-breathing motion corrected with signal averaging. (D) A wideband IR pulse with high bandwidth gradient-echo readout for a patient with an implantable cardiac device (the *blue star* indicates the location of the device in the image). (E) MT-preparation flow-independent dark-blood delayed enhancement (*FIDDLE*) with inversion time set to be "long" (i.e., greater than the black-blood condition) to produce gray-blood images. See text for details.

- ***Motion-corrected, free-breathing, high spatial resolution FIDDLE*:** This implementation is useful for patients with ectopic beats and other irregular cardiac rhythms. It acquires multiple high spatial resolution, single-shot images during free-breathing and uses motion correction and signal averaging to boost the SNR.[19,21] The motion-correction algorithm corrects for in-plane motion between acquisitions and reduces artifacts from misregistration (Fig. 6.12C).
- ***Wideband FIDDLE for use with implanted cardiac devices*:** This implementation uses a wideband (stretched adiabatic) IR pulse, which provides a uniform inversion even in the presence of metal (prosthetic valves, implanted cardiac devices, etc.).[22] The MT module is intrinsically robust toward poor B_0 inhomogeneity since the MT pulses are applied off-resonance. In addition, the wideband protocol is run with a high bandwidth gradient-recalled echo (GRE) readout to further reduce sensitivity to field inhomogeneities (Fig. 6.12D).

Flow-Independent Dark-Blood Delayed Enhancement Variants and Alternatives

The modular design of FIDDLE is flexible and can accommodate different preparation modules, execution orders, readout times, and scan durations. A variety of different implementations were described in the prior section. Here, we discuss some specific variations in more detail and some alternatives to FIDDLE that have been reported in the literature.

The position of the preparation module relative to the IR pulse is flexible and can be placed before (prep-IR), or after the IR pulse (IR-prep). If there is no wait time between the two pulses, the order of execution should result in minimal differences in tissue magnetization by the end of the two pulses. However, the IR-preparation variant is more limited since the duration of the preparation module itself limits the shortest inversion time that can be set. Depending on contrast dose, type, and imaging time after contrast

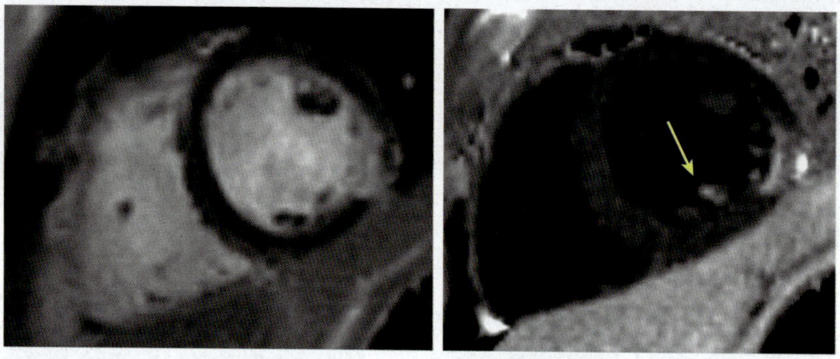

FIG. 6.13 Comparison of conventional delayed-enhancement cardiac magnetic resonance with flow-independent dark-blood delayed enhancement (*FIDDLE*) in a patient with an inferolateral wall myocardial infarction (MI). Posterior papillary muscle MI (*yellow arrow*) is identified only by FIDDLE. (From Wendell D, Jenista E, Kim HW, et al. Assessment of papillary muscle infarction with dark-blood delayed enhancement cardiac MRI in canines and humans. *Radiology*. 2022;305[2]:329–338.)

administration, the minimum achievable inversion time may be inadequate (i.e., too long) to generate black-blood images. Nevertheless, Kellman et al. have shown that IR-T2-preparation FIDDLE with motion-corrected averaging of free-breathing, single-shot images can increase the conspicuity of myocardial regions likely to represent subendocardial fibrosis[23,24] and detect more segments with hyperenhancement than conventional DE-CMR.[23]

If the inversion time for FIDDLE is longer than that necessary to fulfill the "black-blood condition" (Fig. 6.7), a gray-blood image will result (see also Fig. 6.12E). While the blood-pool signal will be higher than that of normal myocardium, gray-blood imaging can still be helpful since the blood-pool signal will be attenuated relative to conventional DE-CMR. Additionally, gray-blood FIDDLE has an important advantage compared to other gray-blood techniques. As discussed earlier, the gray-blood methods of Peel et al.[13] and Holtackers et al.[25] require infarct (or scar) T1 to be shorter than blood-pool T1 in order to visualize infarcted myocardium. This condition is not required with gray-blood FIDDLE. The preparation module of FIDDLE produces a directional difference in magnetization between infarcted myocardium and blood pool that results in a higher signal for infarcted myocardium, despite a T1 that may be similar or even slightly longer for infarcted myocardium compared to the blood pool.

As described above, FIDDLE uses PSIR reconstruction in order to reveal negative magnetization levels during signal readout. If reference phase data are not acquired, scan time is potentially reduced. However, without PSIR, negative magnetization levels are visualized as positive levels of the same magnitude, which often decreases tissue contrast. With this alternative form of dark-blood delayed-enhancement imaging (i.e., without PSIR), it is far more difficult to adjust the signal of normal myocardium separate from that of blood, and usually one can only get a black-blood image if normal myocardium is also black. In other words, the contrast-to-noise ratio between normal myocardium and blood pool is nearly zero. Basha et al.[26] used an IR-T2-preparation sequence without PSIR to obtain black-blood images in a heterogeneous group of patients with a variety of cardiac disorders. They reported that the contrast between myocardial scar and blood pool was high. However, the simultaneous nulling of normal myocardium as well as blood pool potentially enhances noise/artifact in patients without scarring, and assessment of scar transmurality becomes difficult. Hence, the same group later reported that a gray-blood implementation of their IR-T2-preparation sequence improved the ability to identify and localize myocardial scarring compared to their black-blood implementation (both without PSIR).[27] These studies highlight the difference between black-blood delayed-enhancement techniques with and without phase-sensitive reconstruction. Finally, it should be mentioned that diagnostic sensitivity and specificity have been reported only for MT-preparation FIDDLE (as of 2025). For the majority of other techniques, although differences in the detection rate of scar is often reported, neither a clinical- nor a histology-based truth standard was used to confirm the accuracy of the findings.

Flow-Independent Dark-Blood Delayed Enhancement: Additional Clinical Studies and Scenarios

With acute MI, necrosis may extend into one or both left ventricular papillary muscles. Recently, MT-preparation FIDDLE has been validated against pathology for the diagnosis of papillary muscle infarction.[28] Unlike conventional DE-CMR, FIDDLE was shown to be highly accurate in the detection of papillary muscle infarction with the test sensitivity reaching nearly double that of conventional imaging. Unlike the left ventricular wall, the papillary muscles are often completely encircled by bright blood pool on conventional DE-CMR, making visualization of hyperenhancement even more difficult (Fig. 6.13). In patients with MI, these findings may have clinical impact because papillary muscle MI may lead to potentially fatal complications such as papillary muscle rupture, severe mitral regurgitation, and malignant ventricular tachyarrhythmias.

Papillary muscle scarring (papSCAR) can also occur without epicardial coronary artery disease (CAD), likely from microvascular dysfunction.[29] Nonischemic dilated cardiomyopathy (DCM) has been associated with microvascular dysfunction, as studies have demonstrated impaired myocardial perfusion reserve in the absence of epicardial CAD.[30] The prevalence and prognostic significance of

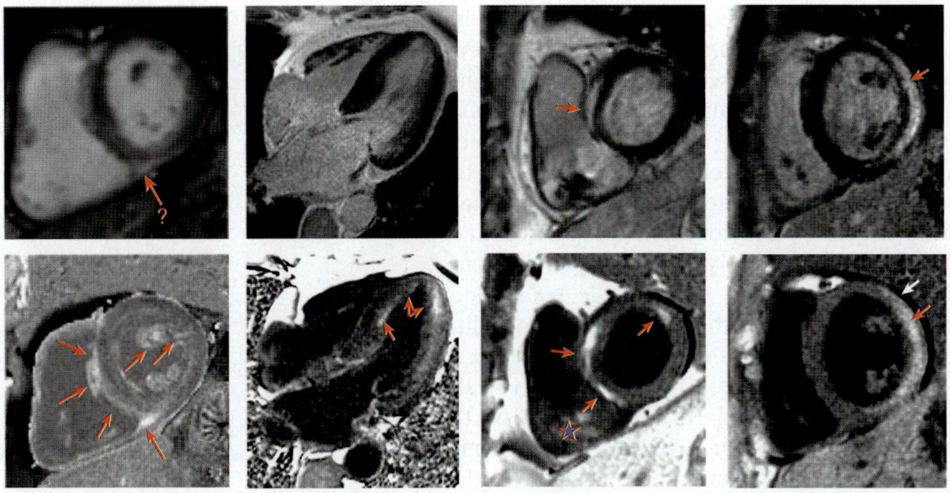

FIG. 6.14 Example images in different nonischemic cardiomyopathies. In many of these cases, blood-pool suppression improves the appreciation of the location and extent of hyperenhancement. *Red arrows* indicate regions of hyperenhancement. In (C) the *red star* indicates the right ventricular (RV) lead from an implanted pacemaker, which appears black on the conventional bright-blood delayed-enhancement cardiac magnetic resonance image, and bright on the flow-independent dark-blood delayed enhancement (*FIDDLE*) image. In (D) the *white arrow* highlights that the phase-sensitive inversion recovery reconstruction used with FIDDLE has the added benefit of rendering fluid (in this case pericardial effusion) black, enabling better visualization of the epicardial surface. See text for additional details. *DE-MRI*, Delayed-enhancement magnetic resonance imaging; *HCM*, hypertrophic cardiomyopathy; *NICM*, non-ischemic cardiomyopathy.

papSCAR in DCM patients are unclear. In this context, a recent study has reported that papSCAR, as detected by MT-preparation FIDDLE, is present in approximately one-third of patients with DCM and serves as an independent predictor of cardiac death.[31] Moreover, the presence of papSCAR in the cohort with hypokinetic nondilated cardiomyopathy—an early subtype of DCM characterized by left ventricular dysfunction despite the absence of left ventricular dilatation—was also associated with an elevated risk for cardiac mortality. Overall, the study findings show that papSCAR provides prognostic value across the spectrum of patients with DCM and suggest that papSCAR may be an early marker of risk.

Currently, there are limited data regarding the diagnostic performance of FIDDLE in other nonischemic disorders. That said, anecdotal case studies suggest that FIDDLE may provide incremental value to conventional DE-CMR for visualizing abnormalities. Fig. 6.14 shows a series of examples of FIDDLE versus DE-CMR in different nonischemic cardiomyopathies. In many cases, suppression of the blood pool allows for improved appreciation of the location and extent of hyperenhancement. For example, in cardiac amyloidosis FIDDLE shows multiple regions of hyperenhancement including the subendocardium and the right ventricular (RV) side of the septum (Fig. 6.14A). In hypertrophic cardiomyopathy FIDDLE is useful when the hyperenhancement pattern is diffuse and subendocardial (Fig. 6.14B). In cardiac sarcoidosis blood-pool suppression is particularly helpful when assessing hyperenhancement on the RV side of the septum near the base (Fig. 6.14C). Finally, in myocarditis (Fig. 6.14D) both DE-CMR and FIDDLE show epicardial hyperenhancement, but the fluid suppression due to the PSIR readout in FIDDLE helps differentiate epicardial hyperenhancement from the bright signal from the pericardial effusion.

MYOCARDIAL FAT

Fatty infiltration of the myocardium, also known as lipomatous metaplasia, may occur in over 80% of healed MIs, depending on the infarct age.[32] Moreover, it represents a typical finding in arrhythmogenic right ventricular cardiomyopathy, and it can occur in a variety of other nonischemic disorders, including primary dilated cardiomyopathy and chronic valvulopathy.[33] The deposition of intramyocardial fat has been postulated to be part of the healing cascade following myocardial injury. Its detection may be important because fatty infiltration can alter the electrophysiological properties of the myocardium and may serve as substrate for ventricular arrhythmias and sudden death.[34–36]

In addition to its pathophysiological significance, the discrimination of fat is essential because it may be a confounding factor in image interpretation. Specifically, fatty infiltration may cause image artifacts or signal changes that may be misinterpreted if the presence of fat is not recognized. This can occur for many of the sequences in a routine cardiac examination including SSFP, delayed-enhancement imaging, first-pass perfusion, and T1 and T2 mapping. Examples and mechanisms of these will be described below.

Physics of Fat-Water Imaging

In clinical MRI, the major contribution to the proton (^1H) signal is either from water or fat, the latter of which exists in tissues primarily as triglycerides, although other lipids such as free fatty acids, cholesterol, and phospholipids are usually also present at less abundant levels. For fat, the signal is a composite of a number of distinct chemical contributions including the protons in the methylene group ($[-CH_2-]_n$), the terminal methyl ($[-CH_3]$), and olefinic groups ([–HC=CH–]), which are components of long-chain fatty acids. At a given field strength (B_0), all hydrogen nuclei do not resonate at precisely their Larmor frequency (e.g., 63.87 MHz at 1.5 T). Instead, there are small differences in resonance frequency (called *chemical shifts*) due to alterations in the local magnetic field, which itself is dependent on the local chemical environment. For water molecules, the electronegative oxygen atom pulls the shielding electron clouds away from the ^{1}H nucleus, exposing them to the full force of B_0. For many of the hydrogen atoms of fat (but not all), there is greater electronic shielding and hence they usually resonate at a slightly lower frequency than that of water. Fig. 6.15 depicts a ^{1}H magnetic resonance (MR) spectrum of a fat-water mixture. By convention, different resonance frequencies are displayed relative to a highly shielded reference proton moiety (tetramethylsilane), which is arbitrarily assigned the frequency of 0 parts per million (ppm). Using this scale, which is independent of B_0, water [–OH] protons resonate at 4.7 ppm and methylene [–CH_2–] protons at 1.3 ppm at body temperature (Table 6.1). For in vivo imaging at clinical field strengths (e.g., 1.5 T or 3 T) there is insufficient spectral resolution to delineate each proton moiety, and some of the peaks merge together. Here, it is important to note that the "methylene" peak at 1.3 ppm contains nearly 10 times the signal of any other fat peak,[37] and it is usually reasonable for clinical purposes to consider fat as a single peak that resonates 3.4 ppm away from water (i.e., 4.7–1.3 = 3.4). This translates into a chemical shift of −217 Hz for fat at 1.5 T (i.e., 3.4 Hz per 1 × 63.87 MHz), where the negative sign signifies that fat precesses more slowly than water. The actual MRI signal is, of course, dependent not only on fat content (proton density of fat) but also on the T1 and T2 of fat (Table 6.2) and the imaging pulse sequence. Fat molecules are much

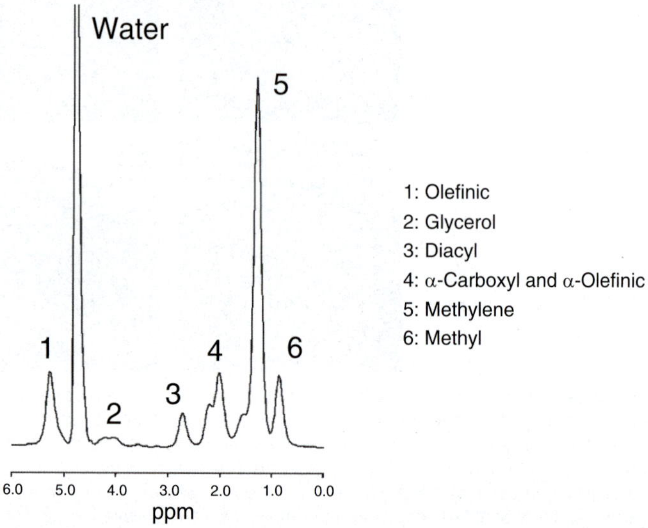

FIG. 6.15 ^{1}H magnetic resonance spectrum of a fat-water mixture showing the relative fat peaks typically seen in vivo. Of the six fat peaks resolvable by spectroscopy at 3 T, in vivo peaks one and two are buried within the water peak. *ppm*, Parts per million (Adapted from Hamilton G, Yokoo T, Bydder M, et al. In vivo characterization of the liver fat ^{1}H MR spectrum. *NMR Biomed*. 2011;24[7]:784–790.)

TABLE 6.1 Proton magnetic resonance spectrum of liver fat as measured by Hamilton et al.[38] and Reeder et al.[39].

PEAK	IN VIVO PPM	EX VIVO PPM	CHEMICAL ENVIRONMENT	TYPE	T1 (MS)	T2 (MS)	RELATIVE MAGNITUDE
1	5.3	5.29 5.19	–CH=CH– –CH-O-CO–	Olefinic Glycerol	421 n/a	44 n/a	4.7%
Water	4.7	4.7	H_2O	–			–
2	4.2	4.2	–CH_2–O–CO–	Glycerol	154	n/a	3.9%
3	2.75	2.75	–CH=CH–CH_2– CH=CH–	Diacyl	284	46	0.6%
4	2.1	2.24 2.02	–CH–CH_2–CH_2– –CH_2–CH=CH– CH_2–	α-Carboxyl α-Olefinic	202 249	52 52	12.0%
5	1.3	1.6 1.3	–CO–CH_2–CH_2 –$(CH_2)_n$–	β-Carboxyl Methylene	240 280	55 55	70.0%
6	0.9	0.9	–$(CH_2)_n$–CH_3	Methyl	543	80	8.80%

TABLE 6.2 Native T1 and T2 values for different tissue types at 1.5 and 3.0 T.

	T1-3T (MS)		T2-3T (MS)		T1-1.5T (MS)		T2-1.5T (MS)	
TISSUE	EX VIVO	IN VIVO	EX VIVO	IN VIVO	EX VIVO	IN VIVO	EX VIVO	IN VIVO
Skeletal muscle	1412 ± 13	1420	50 ± 4	32	1008 ± 20	880–1003	44 ± 6	30–39
Myocardium	1471 ± 31	1122–1309	47 ± 11	44–54	1030 ± 34	933–1020	44 ± 6	54–59
Blood	1932 ± 85	1664	275 ± 50	n/a	1441 ± 120	1480–1499	290 ± 30	n/a
Liver	812 ± 64	751–781	42 ± 3	34–48	576 ± 30	575–645	46 ± 6	36–54
Kidney	1194 ± 27	1057–1514	56 ± 4	78	690 ± 30	1049	55 ± 3	47
Spleen	n/a	1221–1328	n/a	61 ± 9	n/a	1178–1240	n/a	76–103

Note: for myocardium and blood, these values represent the water protons of myocardium and blood. Also, "blood" in this case refers to "arterial" blood.[41,61]

larger than water; their motions are slower with components that occur near the Larmor frequency. This results in more effective dipole-dipole interactions producing relaxation, and hence a shorter T1 than water protons in either myocardium or blood.[38,39] The T2 of fat (methylene moiety) is between the T2 of water protons in myocardium and that of blood.[40,41]

Conventional Methods for Fat-Water Imaging

There are a wide variety of approaches to detecting and/or suppressing tissue fat. These can be divided into three groups depending on whether they exploit differences in T1 relaxation times, resonance frequency (i.e., chemical shift), or both. The short tau inversion recovery (STIR) sequence uses a nonfrequency selective (but usually spatially selective) IR pulse that is coordinated to play at a specific time to null fat (short T1) at the beginning of a fast spin-echo readout. STIR suppresses fat relatively homogeneously because it is based on the longitudinal relaxation time of fat; it is insensitive to B_0 field inhomogeneity since it does not depend on chemical shift. On the other hand, due to the IR pulse and the requirement for a specific, short inversion time, it is restrictive in the choice of imaging parameters, has reduced SNR, has T1 weighting for the remaining water signal (which may not be desirable), and the signal suppression is not specific to fat since it suppresses all tissues with a similar T1 relaxation time as fat. Because of the latter, STIR has limited utility in conjunction with paramagnetic contrast agents.

Chemically selective excitation techniques take advantage of the resonance frequency difference between water and methylene protons. The saturation of fat is usually through a narrow bandwidth, fat frequency–selective saturation pulse (90-degree pulse then application of spoiling gradients) followed immediately by a standard imaging sequence. A major limitation of this technique is that it is highly sensitive to B_0 and B_1 field inhomogeneities. This can result in failed fat suppression and even inadvertent water suppression. In addition, due to the short T1 of fat and the long duration often needed for data acquisition, a significant portion of the fat magnetization may have already recovered from an adequate fat saturation pulse, again resulting in poor fat suppression. In general, uniform suppression of fat signal throughout the entire field of view is rare.

The spectral presaturation inversion recovery (SPIR) and spectral selection attenuated inversion recovery (SPAIR) sequences work similarly to STIR but the nonfrequency-selective IR pulse is replaced by a fat frequency–selective pulse. Compared to the STIR sequence, these sequences make the signal suppression more specific to fat, but an important limitation, similar to chemical fat saturation techniques, is that B_0 and B_1 field inhomogeneities make complete suppression of fat throughout the heart difficult. The SPAIR technique compared to SPIR is more resistant to B_1 inhomogeneity by utilizing an adiabatic inversion pulse, but sensitivity to B_0 inhomogeneity remains a significant problem.

Chemical shift–based "Dixon" methods separate the MR signal into water and fat components by acquiring GRE images at two or more echo times (TEs). Rather than suppressing fat signal or selectively exciting water, this class of techniques relies on phase shifts created by fat-water resonance frequency differences to separate fat from water. By strategically acquiring images at two or more specific TE values, the combined signal from a voxel containing fat and water signals can be decomposed into separate fat and water images. The original approach required only two TEs, one in which fat and water were "in-phase" and one "out-of-phase," thus it is also known as the "two-point" Dixon method. A limitation of the two-point Dixon method is that it is highly sensitive to B_0 inhomogeneities, which results in spatial variations in resonant frequencies and thus an error term in the phase accumulated during TE. This phase error term can result in a type of artifact known as "fat-water swapping," in which a voxel containing mostly fat can be misidentified as mostly water and vice versa. These errors can be fairly dramatic and water signals in a fairly large area such as an entire organ can be mislabeled as fat.[42]

More recently, multipoint Dixon methods leverage acquisitions at multiple TEs with full complex data sets (rather than just magnitude data) and utilize sophisticated estimation methods to more accurately separate the fat and water signals. These methods, such as IDEAL[39] and VARPRO,[43] impose a spatial smoothness constraint in estimating the B_0 field inhomogeneities, and the resulting "field map" allows unambiguous fat-water signal separation. An additional benefit is that methods can be used with arbitrary echo times, which allows for more flexible protocols. Conversely, the requirement of three or more echoes increases scan time, the specific absorption rate (the rate at which RF energy is absorbed), and reconstruction time.

A significant limitation with all of the imaging techniques described so far is that obtaining images using these methods takes time to set up and run these additional sequences—time which is often limited for clinical MRI protocols. Hence, even though these fat-specific sequences are available, it would be impractical to routinely use these techniques as a part of a regular cardiac core exam. Not surprisingly, clinical CMR protocols generally do not include sequences specifically dedicated to imaging fat; these sequences are only "optional" and run in the rare situation that there is a specific clinical inquiry related to the detection of fat, such as for the evaluation of cardiac masses.

Fortunately, SSFP sequences are often an indispensable part of standard clinical protocols since they provide a high SNR, reliable tissue contrast, and are rapid. For example, SSFP sequences are widely used for noncontrast MR angiography of the chest and abdomen, and SSFP cine sequences are part of the conventional cardiac core exam. SSFP cine sequences depict large regions of homogeneous fat, such as subcutaneous or epicardial fat, as bright tissue (Fig. 6.16A). Large areas of homogeneous fat within the myocardium may present as a central bright region encircled by a dark low-signal line: the familiar "India-ink" pattern (Fig. 6.16B) that has been reported in the literature as a way to diagnose lipomatous metaplasia.[44,45]

However, there are several issues with using conventional SSFP sequences to diagnose fatty infiltration of

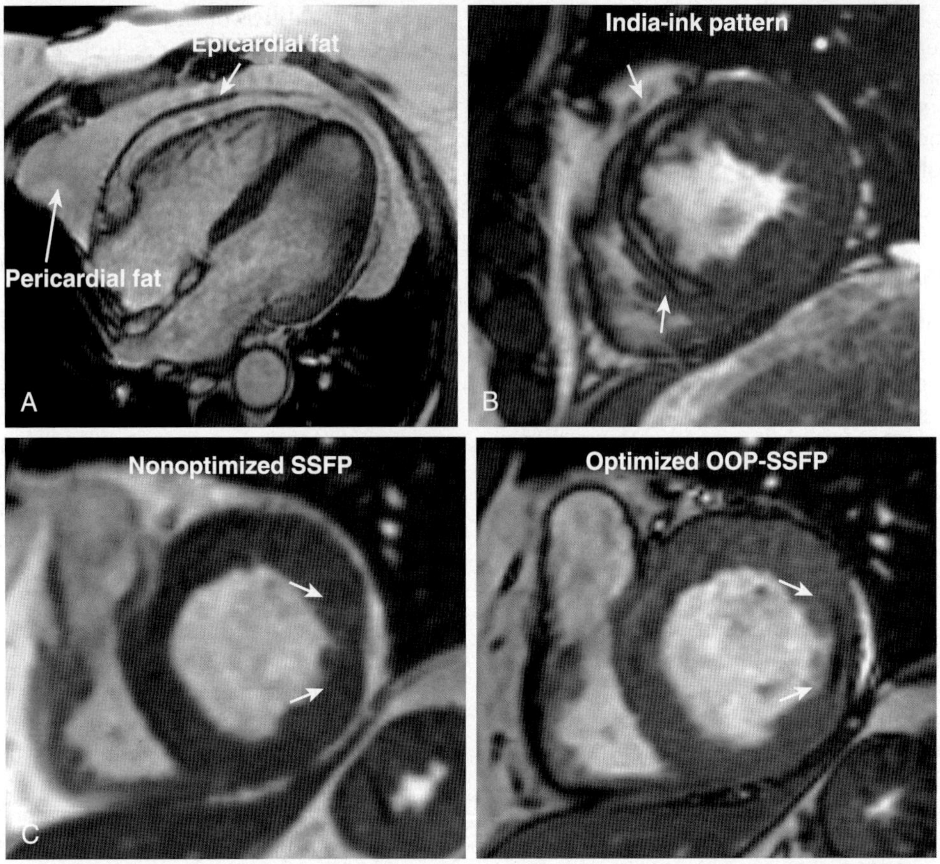

FIG. 6.16 Detection of fat in cardiac imaging. (A) Large regions of homogeneous fat, such as subcutaneous or epicardial fat (*arrows*), are easily detected on steady-state free precession (*SSFP*) cine images as bright tissue. (B) Large areas of homogenous fat within the myocardium may present as a central bright region encircled by a dark low-signal line, the so-called India-ink pattern (*arrows*). (C) Lipomatous metaplasia usually consists of an admixture of fat and fibrous tissue, which often results in voxels of tissue that are only partially fat throughout the infiltrated region. The region of partial fat may be undetectable using nonoptimized conventional SSFP cine imaging (*arrows, left panel*). However, partial fat may become readily identifiable as a paradoxically dark intramyocardial region if the SSFP cine sequence is optimized so that fat signal is consistently "out of phase" (*OOP*) with water throughout the heart (*arrows, right panel*).

tissues. First, it is important to recognize that the India-ink pattern is *not* a constant feature of SSFP imaging.[46] Specifically, the dark line at the border that represents the fat-water interface only occurs when fat and water resonances have opposite phase and there is destructive interference of fat and water signals through a partial volume effect. Unfortunately, prior studies employing SSFP imaging to diagnose lipomatous metaplasia assume that signal cancellation at fat-water interfaces is an inherent feature of SSFP sequences and does not require any special conditions or consideration of sequence parameters,[44,45] or there is an incorrect belief that simply setting TE = TR/2 (where TR is the repetition time) will result in an SSFP sequence for which fat and water are out of phase.[47]

A second issue for using conventional SSFP sequences to diagnose lipomatous metaplasia is that only the India-ink appearance has been described. However, pathology studies report that a large central zone of homogeneous fat is relatively rare and lipomatous metaplasia more commonly consists of an admixture of fat and fibrous tissue throughout.[48,49] Hence, lipomatous metaplasia may consist entirely of voxels of tissue, all of which contain a partial amount of fat. The area with partial fat may be difficult to detect with conventional SSFP cine imaging (Fig. 6.16C, left panel). However, if the sequence were optimized so that the fat signal is consistently "out of phase" with water throughout the heart, then the area of partial fat—the lipomatous metaplasia—could become visible as an intramyocardial region that is entirely dark throughout (Fig. 6.16C, right panel). The appearance of partial fat as dark is paradoxical to that of homogeneous fat, which is bright, however, note that this strategy allows the detection of all regions of intramyocardial fat, partial or complete, since the outer border of fatty metaplasia will always consist of a transition zone of voxels of tissue that contain partial fat. To ensure that the area with partial fat is consistently detected and thus recognized, an optimization process for SSFP imaging is necessary, as described in the following section.

Out-of-Phase Steady-State Free Precession Imaging

A unique feature of SSFP imaging is the repeating "passband" behavior of the magnetization. The period of these repeating bands is 1/TR, and the phase of the signals in adjacent pass bands alternates between 0 and 180 degrees.[50] When fat and water are in passbands of opposite phase, voxels containing a mixture of fat and water will have reduced or no signal. Hence, in order to be able to detect partial fat

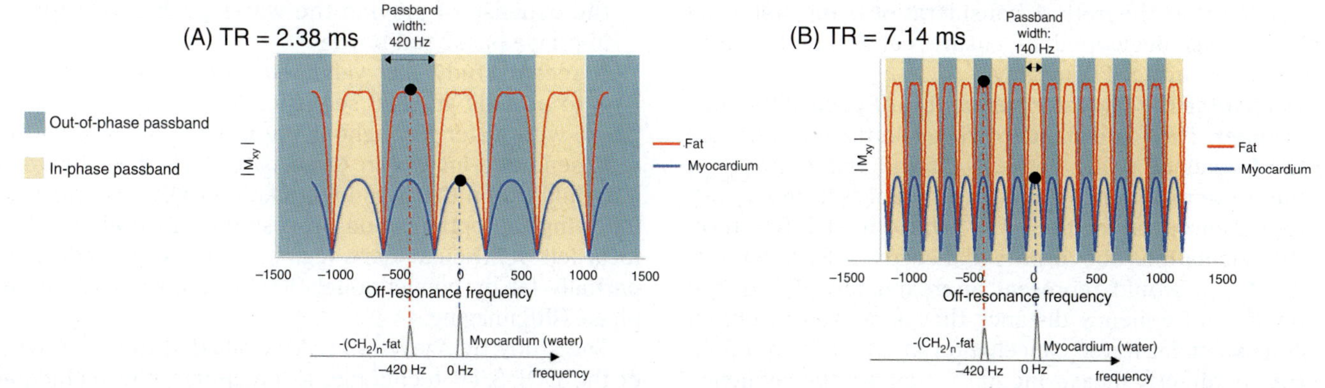

FIG. 6.17 Steady-state free precession off-resonance response of myocardium (*blue line*) and fat (*red line*) at 3T. Tan and blue colors represent in-phase (0-degree phase shift relative to water) and out-of-phase (180 degrees phase shift relative to water) passbands, respectively. (A) With a repetition time (*TR*) of 2.38 ms (assuming a fat-water frequency difference of 420 Hz), the main fat peak is centered in the first out-of-phase passband immediately adjacent to water. The passband width is 420 Hz, and the distance from the fat peak to the border of the passband is 210 Hz. (B) With a TR of 7.14 ms, the fat peak is centered in the second out-of-phase passband. The passband width is reduced to 140 Hz, and the distance to the passband border is reduced to 70 Hz. (Adapted from Azevedo CF, Jenista ER, Kaolawanich Y, et al. Assessment of myocardial lipomatous metaplasia using an optimized out-of-phase cine steady-state free-precession sequence: validation and clinical implementation. *NMR Biomed*. 2022;35[10]:e4777.)

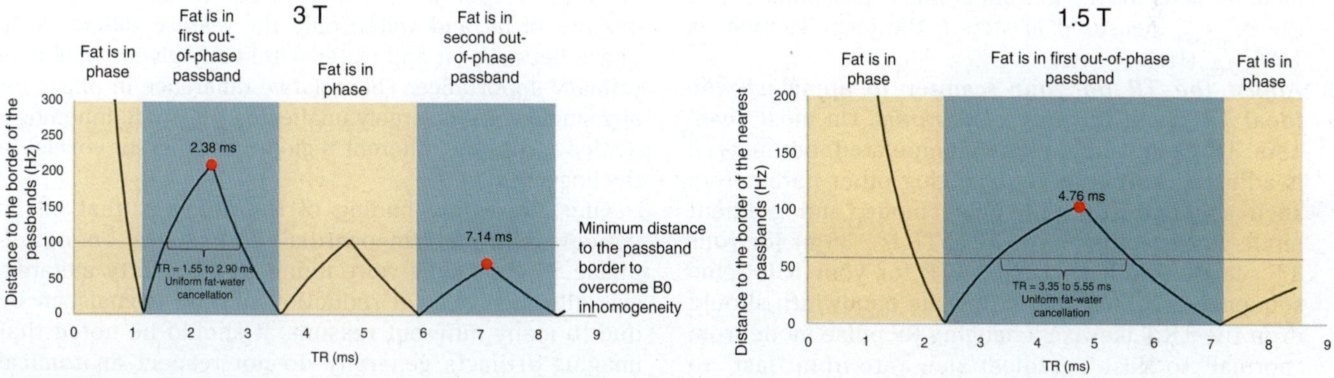

FIG. 6.18 Relationship between repetition time (*TR*) and the distance in frequency from the fat peak to the nearest passband border. The *red dots* show the TR that places the fat peak optimally in the center of each out-of-phase passband (assuming a fat-water frequency difference of 420 Hz at 3T, and 210 Hz at 1.5T). At 1.5T, only the first out-of-phase passband is shown, as the second requires prohibitively long TRs (>12 ms) that will result in image artifacts and signal loss. The *dashed line* displays the minimum distance condition that is necessary to obtain consistent fat-water cancellation throughout the heart. (Adapted from Azevedo CF, Jenista ER, Kaolawanich Y, et al. Assessment of myocardial lipomatous metaplasia using an optimized out-of-phase cine steady-state free-precession sequence: validation and clinical implementation. *NMR Biomed*. 2022;35[10]:e4777.)

within the myocardium as focal regions with reduced signal, the SSFP sequence has to be adjusted so that the fat peak (methylene protons) is in a passband that is out of phase (OOP) with water (i.e., myocardium without fat).

Fig. 6.17 shows the off-resonance response of fat and myocardium (without fat) at 3T. Given that the frequency difference between fat and water is fixed for a given field strength, different choices of TR will center the main fat peak in different OOP passbands. For example, assuming a fat-water frequency difference of 420 Hz at 3T, TRs of 2.38 and 7.14 ms will place the fat peak in the first and second OOP passbands, respectively. However, longer TRs result in narrower passbands and consequently imaging becomes more sensitive to B_0 inhomogeneity because the frequency spread of fat across the heart may be greater than the passband width.

Fig. 6.18 shows the relationship between TR and the distance in frequency from the fat peak (optimally centered in an OOP passband) to the nearest passband border. This distance dictates how much frequency spread due to B_0 inhomogeneity can occur before some of the fat within the heart crosses the passband border into an in-phase passband, failing to cancel the signals.

Prior studies suggest that B_0 inhomogeneity can result in a frequency variation across the heart of up to 200 Hz at 3T and 120 Hz at 1.5T.[51] Thus, to first order, the minimum distance that is needed to obtain consistent fat-water cancellation throughout the heart (dashed line, Fig. 6.18) would be half of the maximum frequency spread (~100 Hz at 3T, ~60 Hz at 1.5T). Calculation of the range of acceptable TRs (ms) to meet this condition is given by the expression:

$$\frac{1}{2(\Delta f_{\text{fat-water}} - \mathit{MinDistanceCondition})} \le \text{TR} \le \frac{3}{2(\Delta f_{\text{fat-water}} + \mathit{MinDistanceCondition})}$$

Assuming the accuracy of the above values of B_0 inhomogeneity across the heart imaging area, acceptable TRs can range from 1.55 to 2.90 ms at 3T, and from 3.35 to 5.55 ms at 1.5T. Note that none of the TRs that place the fat peak in the second OOP passband meet this condition because the passband width is now too narrow (see Fig. 6.18).

Given these theoretical considerations, the following protocol was developed to ensure consistent fat-water cancellation with SSFP imaging.

1 ***Determine the fat-water frequency difference for your scanner.*** There are standard values in the literature for the frequency offset between fat and water ($\Delta f_{\text{fat-water}}$), but in our experience there are differences from scanner to scanner even for the same vendor model. Based on the calculations above, note that even a 10 Hz difference in $\Delta f_{\text{fat-water}}$ would represent approximately 10% of the minimum frequency distance that is needed to obtain consistent fat-water cancellation at 3T (17% at 1.5 T). Hence, directly measuring $\Delta f_{\text{fat-water}}$ allows the sequence to be specifically tailored to the scanner and provide more robust fat-water signal cancellation. On Siemens scanners this is done by using the "Confirm Frequency" function and measuring the distance from the water peak to the fat peak.

2 ***Calculate the ideal TR.*** The ideal TR will maximize robustness to B_0 inhomogeneity by centering the main fat peak in the first out-of-phase passband. Using the $\Delta f_{\text{fat-water}}$ measured in step 1, the ideal TR (ms) is $1/\Delta f_{\text{fat-water}}$ (Hz).

3 ***Adjust the TR on your scanner to approach the ideal TR given imaging constraints.*** On most scanners, TR cannot be directly manipulated, but instead is adjusted indirectly by changing other parameters such as bandwidth, RF pulse mode, and gradient mode. For example, if the ideal TR is 2.38 ms for your 3 T scanner, and the current TR for your SSFP cine sequence is 3.2 ms, increasing the bandwidth should drop the TR. Likewise, changing RF pulse mode from "normal" to "fast," gradient slew rate from "fast" to "performance," or turning on asymmetric echo will also reduce the TR. Unfortunately, many of these changes will affect image quality, and there are also hardware constraints. Hence, the goal is to approach the ideal TR while maintaining image quality, and TRs in the range that result in the main fat peak being more than the minimum distance condition (Fig. 6.18) from the nearest passband border should provide uniform fat-water cancellation throughout the heart. The minimum distance condition should be at least 100 Hz at 3 T and 60 Hz at 1.5 T, as described above.

4 ***Center the water peak of the heart for individual patients.*** For individual patients, a second-order shim should be performed over a local volume (box) encompassing just the heart. Even after localized shimming, myocardial water can be off-resonance up to 75 Hz at 3 T and 50 Hz at 1.5 T.[52] Given that the frequency difference between fat and water is fixed for a given field strength, centering the water peak of the heart (by directly changing the scanner center frequency) is crucial in calculating accurate frequency distances from the fat peak to the out-of-phase passband border. On the other hand, if an appropriate TR cannot be reached in step 3 because of hardware or other constraints, then an additional option is to directly change the scanner center frequency for individual patients. This can move the fat peak to a more central location in the out-of-phase passband, but at the expense of moving the water peak closer to the in-phase passband border.

A recent study has validated this optimization process to provide an SSFP sequence for which fat is out of phase with water throughout the heart.[48] Fig. 6.19 shows representative images in three patients with myocardial fatty infiltration that was identified on OOP-SSFP imaging, following the optimization process described above. The focal left ventricular dark regions were confirmed to be partially fat by conventional DIXON in-phase and out-of-phase GRE imaging.

The study by Azevedo et al.[48] evaluated the sensitivity of the OOP-SSFP technique. In phantoms, the technique was able to discern fat fractions as low as 2%, which is in line with previously described techniques based on multiecho GRE fat-water–separated imaging.[53] Moreover, of the patients enrolled, there were none in whom additional regions of fatty metaplasia were detected by conventional Dixon imaging but missed by OOP-SSFP imaging. An additional benefit is that fat-water swapping is not an issue. Since the technique is based on detecting voxels with a mixture of fat and water, only the *relative* difference in phase between fat and water within any given voxel is of primary importance. This relative difference in phase for any single voxel is largely unaffected by any B_0 inhomogeneities across the different regions (or different voxels) in the imaging slice.

One interesting finding of the study is that all 50 patients with intramyocardial dark zones on out-of-phase SSFP imaging were found to have fatty metaplasia. Although a focal reduction in SSFP signal can be due to many different reasons, it should be noted that imaging artifacts generally do not respect anatomical boundaries (e.g., remain localized to just the intramyocardial space). Linear stripes of SSFP "dark-band" artifacts crossing the myocardium are easily identified and patients with these artifacts were excluded from the study. Likewise, dark regions could be due to intramyocardial iron or calcium deposition, however, the study by Azevedo et al. excluded patients with recent (<1 year) myocardial infarction as well as patients with mitral annular calcification or cardiac tumor. Hence, the study results suggest that when artifact is excluded and the patient does not have a recent MI, mitral annular calcification, or cardiac tumor, a focal intramyocardial dark region is highly likely to represent fatty metaplasia on out-of-phase SSFP imaging.

In summary, the study by Azevedo et al. demonstrates that through an appropriate optimization process, it is possible to incorporate robust myocardial fat assessment into routine SSFP cine imaging, without the need for additional time-consuming dedicated pulse sequences. Indeed, through routine myocardial fat assessment of consecutive patients referred for clinical CMR exams, it is notable that Azevedo et al. reported that only 34% of intramyocardial dark regions identified on OOP-SSFP imaging displayed an India-ink pattern, whereas 66% were entirely dark throughout. This suggests that prior studies utilizing SSFP cine imaging—which all relied on detecting just the India-ink pattern[44,45,47]—substantially underestimated the true prevalence of myocardial fatty metaplasia.

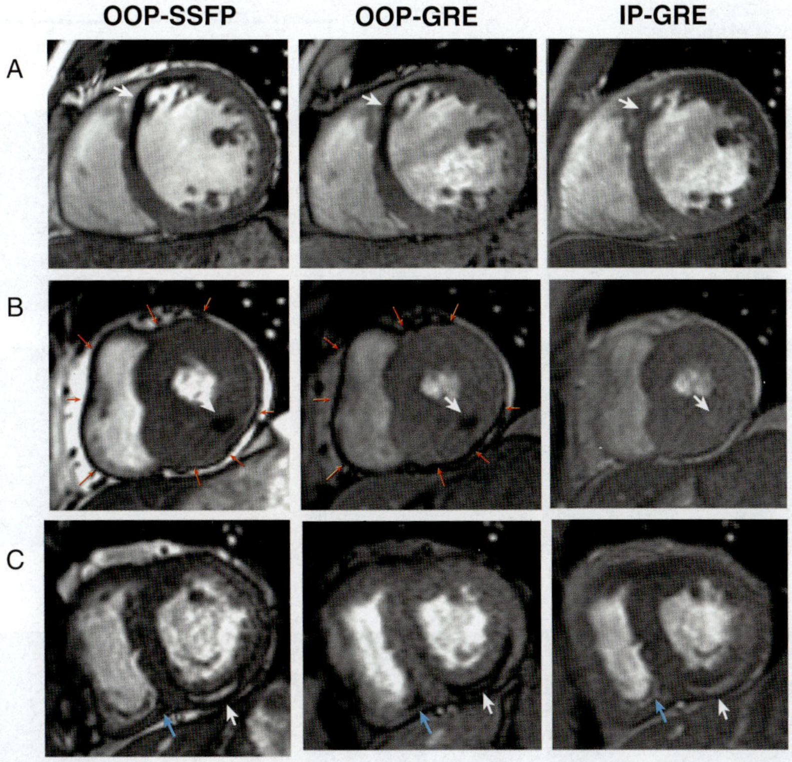

FIG. 6.19 Representative examples of patients with intramyocardial fatty infiltration identified on out-of-phase (*OOP*) steady-state free precession (*SSFP*) images. Dark myocardial regions on OOP-SSFP images were found to be present in the exact same location on OOP gradient-recalled echo (*GRE*) images and to be absent on in-phase GRE images (*white arrows*), confirming that they represent areas of intramyocardial fatty metaplasia. Dark regions on OOP-SSFP were dark throughout (A and B) or encircled a central bright region in the familiar "India-ink" pattern (C). Note that there is also a small region of fatty metaplasia in the right ventricular (RV) diaphragmatic wall in example C (*blue arrow*). Moreover, a dark line of signal cancellation was seen along the entire interface between myocardium and epicardial fat on both OOP-SSFP and OOP-GRE images (highlighted by *small red arrows* in row B) but was absent on in-phase GRE images. (A and C: 3T scanner; B: 1.5T scanner). (Adapted from Azevedo CF, Jenista ER, Kaolawanich Y, et al. Assessment of myocardial lipomatous metaplasia using an optimized out-of-phase cine steady-state free-precession sequence: validation and clinical implementation. *NMR Biomed.* 2022;35[10]:e4777.)

Fat as a Confounding Factor in Image Interpretation

In addition to its pathophysiological significance, the discrimination of fat is essential because it may be a confounding factor in image interpretation. One important situation in which fat can cause misinterpretation of CMR images occurs with native T1 mapping. In expert reviews and society consensus statements, native T1 mapping has been touted as a useful technique to diagnose chronic MI without the need for gadolinium contrast.[54–56] This is based on studies reporting that native T1 mapping is highly accurate in detecting the myocardial replacement fibrosis that occurs in patients with chronic MI.[57,58] However, an investigation by Kellman et al.[53] raised an important concern—which is that the measurement of myocardial T1 by widely used mapping protocols incorporating the SSFP readout is subject to artifactual bias when there is a mixture of water and fat in the myocardium. This is problematic since fatty metaplasia of replacement fibrosis is commonly seen in chronic MI.[32,59,60] In other words, T1 measurements can be erroneous in the presence of intramyocardial fat, and native T1 maps could be detecting an artifact due to partial fatty metaplasia of chronic MI, rather than fibrosis. Indeed, Kellman et al. have demonstrated that native T1 of chronic MI can be artifactually elevated—sometimes by as much as 1000 ms—when there is fatty metaplasia of replacement fibrosis.

A recent study by Kaolawanich et al.[49] examined the use of native T1 mapping for the diagnosis of chronic MI, with careful attention paid to the presence of myocardial fat. The study reported that chronic MI was not detectable by native T1 mapping unless fatty metaplasia was present. Furthermore, in subjects with fatty metaplasia, the MI size based on native T1 mapping was underestimated compared with delayed-enhancement images, reflecting the fact that native T1 mapping was actually measuring the extent of fat that is generally in the core of the MI. Fig. 6.20 shows typical images of chronic MI with and without fatty metaplasia. Note that native T1 maps show elevated T1 only in the infarcts with fatty metaplasia, with the location and extent of abnormal T1 regions matching the areas of fatty metaplasia. Hence, abnormal T1 regions are smaller than the corresponding infarcted regions.

Although native T1 mapping was shown to be insensitive at detecting replacement fibrosis, the study by Kaolawanich et al. suggests that it could still be useful in identifying chronic MI if there is associated fatty metaplasia. However, it is important to note that Kaolawanich et al. performed T1 mapping at 3T, where the polarity of fat signal with respect to myocardial water will generally be out of phase and a mixture of fat and water will lead to artifactually elevated T1. At 1.5T, where fat has a smaller chemical shift, fat may be in phase or out of phase or switch between the two across different

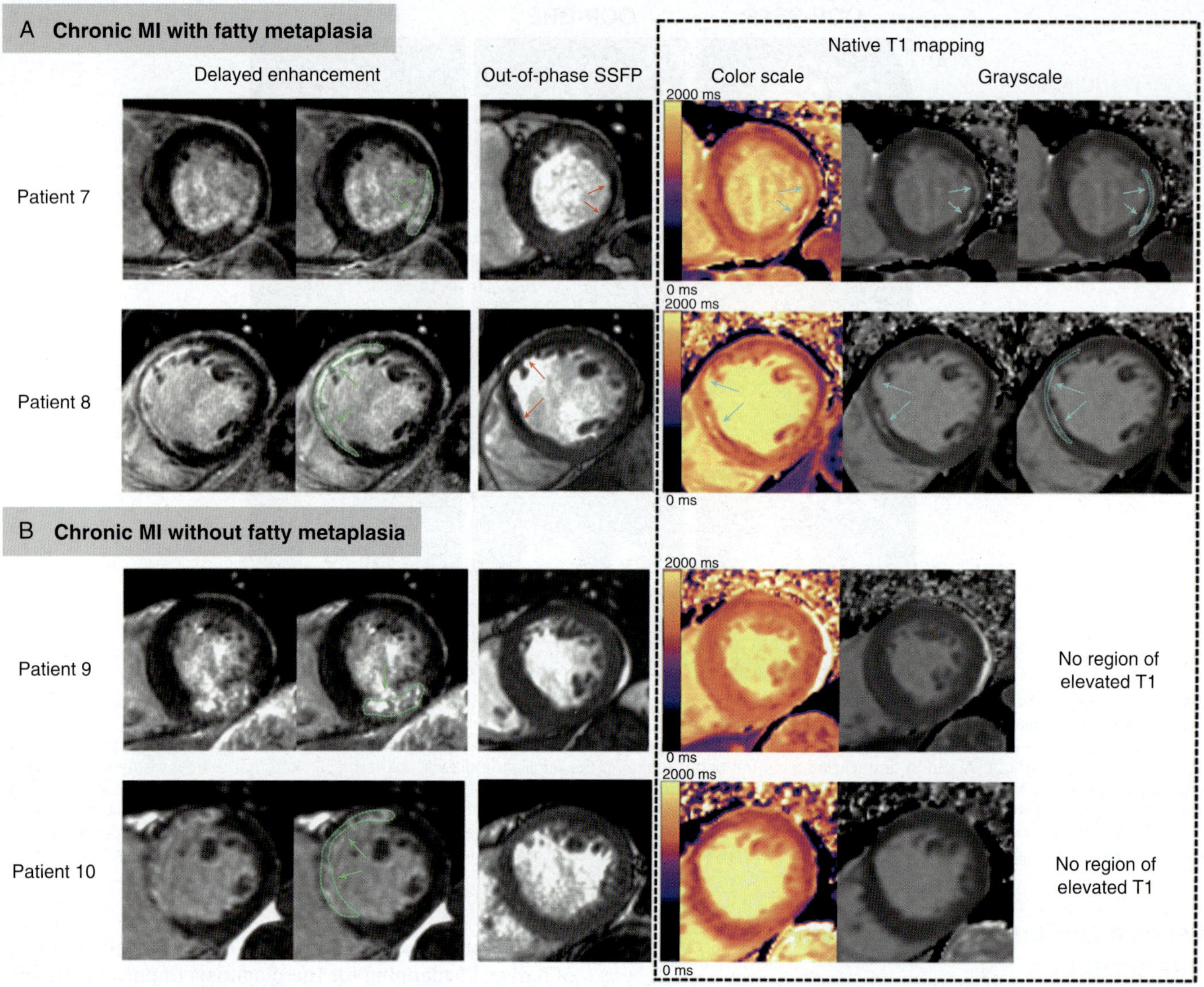

FIG. 6.20 (A) Regions of fatty metaplasia (*red arrows* on out-of-phase cine images) localize to infarcted regions (*green arrows* on DE-CMR) but the size is smaller. Native T1 maps show elevated T1 (*blue arrows*) in the infarcts with fatty metaplasia, with the location and extent of abnormal T1 regions (*dashed blue region* of interest) matching the areas of fatty metaplasia. (B) Native T1 maps do not show any myocardial regions with elevated T1 in patients without fatty metaplasia. *DE-CMR,* Delayed-enhancement cardiac magnetic resonance; *MI,* myocardial infarction; *SSFP,* steady-state free precession. (Adapted from Kaolawanich Y, Azevedo CF, Kim HW, et al. Native T1 Mapping for the diagnosis of myocardial fibrosis in patients with chronic myocardial infarction. *JACC Cardiovasc Imaging.* 2022;15[12]:2069–2079.)

regions of the heart depending on small off-resonance variations caused by an imperfect shim. Hence, at 1.5T the sensitivity of native T1 mapping for detecting fatty metaplasia will be significantly reduced, and accordingly, the sensitivity for detecting chronic MI even with associated fatty metaplasia may be poor.

The study by Kaolawanich et al. dispels the notion that native T1 mapping with currently used methods can detect the focal replacement fibrosis that occurs with chronic MI. There are other types of myocardial fibrosis—such as reactive interstitial fibrosis, which can occur in hypertensive heart disease and primary dilated cardiomyopathy—which were not evaluated. Nonetheless, it is difficult to conceive of a mechanism by which native T1 mapping can detect a fine microscopic distribution of diffuse interstitial fibrosis yet is insensitive to the dense macroscopic fibrosis of infarct scars. The findings, therefore, suggest that native T1 mapping for the diagnosis and/or characterization of any type of myocardial fibrosis would be unreliable.

Finally, the study highlights the potential for misinterpreting CMR images when the presence of fat is not recognized. Although the focus was on the misinterpretation of native T1 maps, any sequence utilizing SSFP or GRE readout could be problematic if there are tissue voxels with partial fat and the local B_0 along with the sequence settings (perhaps unbeknownst to the operator) render fat as out of phase to water. Without knowledge that there is partial fatty metaplasia, the paradoxically dark intramyocardial regions could be misinterpreted as image artifact, myocardial calcification, iron, or hemorrhage.

On conventional delayed-enhancement images, fat usually appears bright due to its short T1. Hence, in patients with chronic MI, myocardial hyperenhancement is not specific to replacement fibrosis but can reflect both replacement fibrosis and fatty metaplasia. That said, this finding

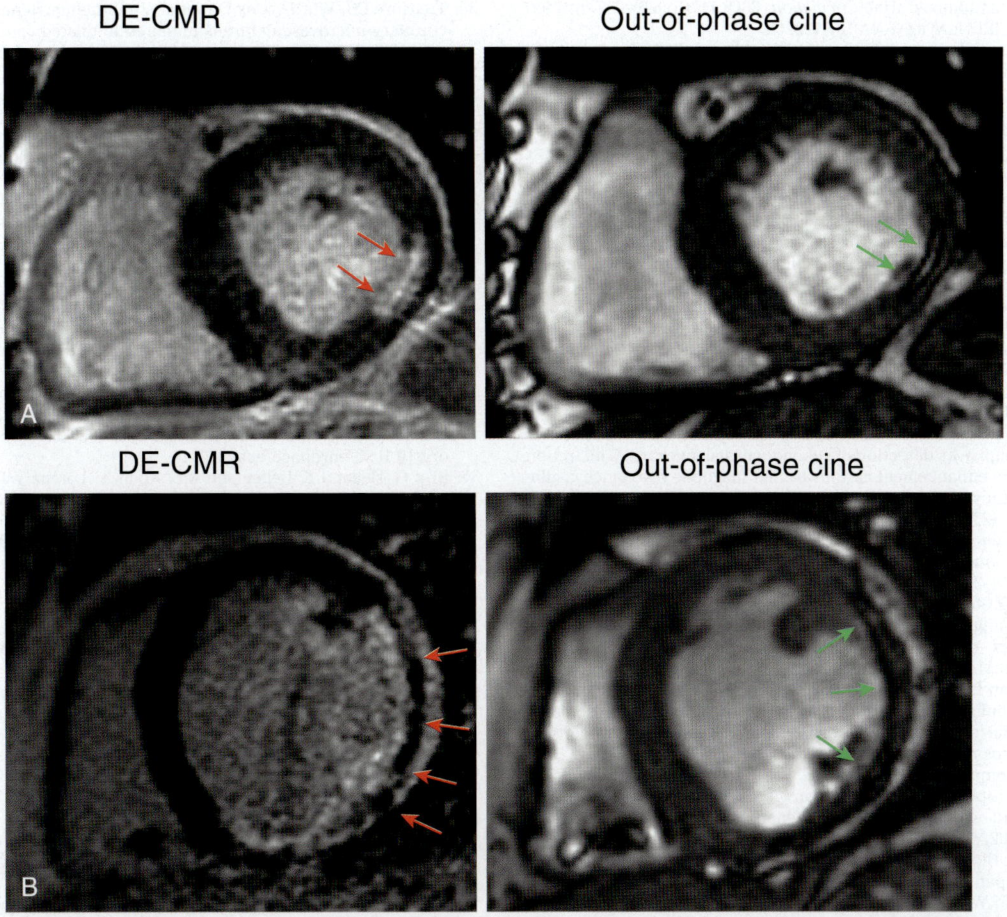

FIG. 6.21 Patient with frequent episodes of ventricular tachycardia requiring placement of an implantable cardioverter-defibrillator (ICD) who was scanned at 1.5 T. Delayed-enhancement imaging was performed at a relatively high bandwidth to reduce ICD artifact. The resultant echo time was 1.6 ms, for which fat is in the out-of-phase regime. (A) Short-axis delayed-enhancement image suggests that a significant portion of the lateral wall is dark (i.e., not hyperenhanced) and therefore "viable" (*red arrows*). (B) Out-of-phase cine image frame demonstrates fatty metaplasia throughout the lateral wall (*green arrows*) indicating little viability. See text for details. *DE-CMR*, Delayed-enhancement cardiac magnetic resonance.

is dependent on the sequence settings, and it is important to note that TE is often automatically set by many vendors to be at a "minimum" (to maximize SNR) depending on the choice of the other sequence parameters. If TE happened to be set so that fat is out of phase with water and the post-gadolinium T1 of scar is similar to that of fat, then again there may be a paradoxically dark myocardial region, even though the region consists entirely of scar and fat and is devoid of viable myocardium (Fig. 6.21). The examples in this section demonstrate the limitations of current clinical protocols for which fat-specific sequences are "optional" and run only when one already suspects that myocardial fat may be present.

CONCLUSION

Despite the large range of imaging techniques available for diagnosing cardiac disease, image-based diagnosis can still be difficult. Using new yet reliable imaging methods can improve study interpretation, risk stratification, decision making, and management. FIDDLE performs consistently in the presence of patient variability, and can increase the confidence of clinical decision making with dark-blood delayed-enhancement imaging in both ischemic and nonischemic cardiomyopathies. In addition to its pathophysiological significance, the discrimination of fat is essential because it may be a confounding factor in image interpretation. With an optimized out-of-phase SSFP cine sequence, it is possible to incorporate robust myocardial fat assessment into routine SSFP cine imaging, without the need for additional time-consuming fat-specific sequences.

REFERENCES

1. Fieno DSKR, Chen EL, Lomasney JW, Klocke FJ, Judd RM. Contrast-enhanced magnetic resonance imaging of myocardium at risk: distinction between reversible and irreversible injury throughout infarct healing. *J Am Coll Cardiol*. 2000;36(6):1985–1991.
2. Kim RJ, Fieno DS, Parrish TB, et al. Relationship of MRI delayed contrast enhancement to irreversible injury, infarct age, and Contractile function. *Circulation*. 1999;100(19):1992–2002. https://doi.org/10.1161/01.CIR.100.19.1992.
3. Kim HW, Farzaneh-Far A, Kim RJ. Cardiovascular magnetic resonance in patients with myocardial infarction: current and emerging applications. *J Am Coll Cardiol*. 2009;55(1):1–16. https://doi.org/10.1016/j.jacc.2009.06.059.
4. Sievers B, Elliott MD, Hurwitz LM, et al. Rapid detection of myocardial infarction by subsecond, free-breathing delayed contrast-enhancement cardiovascular magnetic resonance. *Circulation*. 2007;115(2):236–244. https://doi.org/10.1161/CIRCULATIONAHA.106.635409.
5. Kim RJ, Albert TS, Wible JH, et al. Performance of delayed-enhancement magnetic resonance imaging with gadoversetamide contrast for the detection and assessment of myocardial infarction: an international, multicenter,

double-blinded, randomized trial. *Circulation*. 2008;117(5):629–637. https://doi.org/10.1161/CIRCULATIONAHA.107.723262.
6. Alpert JS, Thygesen K, Antman E, Bassand JP. Myocardial infarction redefined-a consensus document of the Joint European Society of Cardiology/American College of Cardiology Committee for the redefinition of myocardial infarction. *J Am Coll Cardiol*. 2000;36(3):959–969. https://doi.org/10.1016/s0735-1097(00)00804-4.
7. Edelman RR, Chien D, Kim D. Fast selective black blood MR imaging. *Radiology*. 1991;181(3):655–660. https://doi.org/10.1148/radiology.181.3.1947077.
8. Simonetti OP, Finn JP, White RD, Laub G, Henry DA. "Black blood" T2-weighted inversion-recovery MR imaging of the heart. *Radiology*. 1996;199(1):49–57. https://doi.org/10.1148/radiology.199.1.8633172.
9. Farrelly C, Rehwald W, Salerno M, et al. Improved detection of subendocardial hyperenhancement in myocardial infarction using dark blood-pool delayed enhancement MRI. *AJR Am J Roentgenol*. 2011;196(2):339–348. https://doi.org/10.2214/AJR.10.4418.
10. Kellman P, Chung YC, Simonetti OP, McVeigh ER, Arai AE. Multi-contrast delayed enhancement provides improved contrast between myocardial infarction and blood pool. *J Magn Reson Imaging*. 2005;22(5):605–613. https://doi.org/10.1002/jmri.20426.
11. Bandettini WP, Kellman P, Mancini C, et al. MultiContrast Delayed Enhancement (MCODE) improves detection of subendocardial myocardial infarction by late gadolinium enhancement cardiovascular magnetic resonance: a clinical validation study. *J Cardiovasc Magn Reson*. 2012;14(1):83. https://doi.org/10.1186/1532-429X-14-83.
12. Liu CY, Bley TA, Wieben O, Brittain JH, Reeder SB. Flow-independent T(2)-prepared inversion recovery black-blood MR imaging. *J Magn Reson Imaging*. 2010;31(1):248–254. https://doi.org/10.1002/jmri.21986.
13. Peel SA, Morton G, Chiribiri A, Schuster A, Nagel E, Botnar RM. Dual inversion-recovery mr imaging sequence for reduced blood signal on late gadolinium-enhanced images of myocardial scar. *Radiology*. 2012;264(1):242–249. https://doi.org/10.1148/radiol.12112004.
14. Holtackers RJ, Van De Heyning CM, Nazir MS, et al. Clinical value of dark-blood late gadolinium enhancement cardiovascular magnetic resonance without additional magnetization preparation. *J Cardiovasc Magn Reson*. 2019;21(1):44. https://doi.org/10.1186/s12968-019-0556-1.
15. Holtackers RJ, Gommers S, Heckman LIB, Van De Heyning CM, Chiribiri A, Prinzen FW. Histopathological validation of dark-blood late gadolinium enhancement MRI without additional magnetization preparation. *J Magn Reson Imaging*. 2022;55(1):190–197. https://doi.org/10.1002/jmri.27805.
16. Kim RJ, inventor; Blood signal suppressed contrast enhanced magnetic resonance imaging. patent application US9131870B2. 2015.
17. Kim HW, Rehwald WG, Jenista ER, et al. Dark-blood delayed enhancement cardiac magnetic resonance of myocardial infarction. *JACC Cardiovasc Imaging*. 2018;11(12):1758–1769. https://doi.org/10.1016/j.jcmg.2017.09.021.
18. Henkelman RM, Stanisz GJ, Graham SJ. Magnetization transfer in MRI: a review. *NMR Biomed*. 2001;14(2):57–64. https://doi.org/10.1002/nbm.683.
19. Jenista ER, Wendell DC, Kim HW, et al. Comparison of magnetization transfer-preparation and T2-preparation for dark-blood delayed-enhancement imaging. *NMR in Biomedicine*. 2020;33(11):e4396. https://doi.org/10.1002/nbm.4396.
20. Rehwald W, Wendell, DC., Jenista ER., Chen EL., Kim RJ., inventor; Systems and methods for phase-sensitive inversion recovery MR imaging with reduced sensitivity to cardiac motion USA patent application US10591568B2. 2020.
21. Munoz C, Bustin A, Neji R, et al. Motion-corrected 3D whole-heart water-fat high-resolution late gadolinium enhancement cardiovascular magnetic resonance imaging. *J Cardiovasc Magn Reson*. 2020;22(1):53. https://doi.org/10.1186/s12968-020-00649-5.
22. Rehwald W, Wendell DC, Jenista ER, Kim RJ. A Novel Single-Cardiac Cycle Phase Sensitive Inversion Recovery (PSIR) Method improves Free Breathing Single Shot Flow Independent Dark Blood Delayed Enhancement (FIDDLE). *JCMR*. 2017:386.
23. Kellman P. Dark-blood late-enhancement imaging improves detection of myocardial infarction. *JACC Cardiovasc Imaging*. 2018;11(12):1770–1772. https://doi.org/10.1016/j.jcmg.2017.10.014.
24. Kellman P, Xue H, Olivieri LJ, et al. Dark blood late enhancement imaging. *J Cardiovasc Magn Reson*. 2016;18(1):77. https://doi.org/10.1186/s12968-016-0297-3.
25. Holtackers RJ, Chiribiri A, Schneider T, Higgins DM, Botnar RM. Dark-blood late gadolinium enhancement without additional magnetization preparation. *J Cardiovasc Magn Reson*. 2017;19(1):64. https://doi.org/10.1186/s12968-017-0372-4.
26. Basha TA, Tang MC, Tsao C, et al. Improved dark blood late gadolinium enhancement (DB-LGE) imaging using an optimized joint inversion preparation and T(2) magnetization preparation. *Magn Reson Med*. 2018;79(1):351–360. https://doi.org/10.1002/mrm.26692.
27. Fahmy AS, Neisius U, Tsao CW, et al. Gray blood late gadolinium enhancement cardiovascular magnetic resonance for improved detection of myocardial scar. *J Cardiovasc Magn Reson*. 2018;20(1):22. https://doi.org/10.1186/s12968-018-0442-2.
28. Wendell D, Jenista E, Kim HW, et al. Assessment of papillary muscle infarction with dark-blood delayed enhancement cardiac MRI in canines and Humans. *Radiology*. 2022;305(2):329–338. https://doi.org/10.1148/radiol.220251.
29. Roberts WC, Cohen LS. Left ventricular papillary muscles. *Circulation*. 1972;46(1):138–154. https://doi.org/10.1161/01.CIR.46.1.138.
30. Treasure CB, Vita JA, Cox DA, et al. Endothelium-dependent dilation of the coronary microvasculature is impaired in dilated cardiomyopathy. *Circulation*. 1990;81(3):772–779. https://doi.org/10.1161/01.cir.81.3.772.
31. Kaolawanich Y, Wendell DC, Kim HW, et al. Prognostic value of papillary muscle scarring in patients with dilated cardiomyopathy. *JAMA Cardiol*. 2025;10(12):1267–1275. https://doi.org/10.1001/jamacardio.2025.3822.
32. Ichikawa Y, Kitagawa K, Chino S, et al. Adipose tissue detected by multislice computed tomography in patients after myocardial infarction. *JACC Cardiovasc Imaging*. 2009;2(5):548–555. https://doi.org/10.1016/j.jcmg.2009.01.010.
33. Baroldi G, Silver MD, De Maria R, Parodi O, Pellegrini A. Lipomatous metaplasia in left ventricular scar. *Can J Cardiol*. 1997;13(1):65–71.
34. Sung E, Prakosa A, Zhou S, et al. Fat infiltration in the infarcted heart as a paradigm for ventricular arrhythmias. *Nat Cardiovasc Res*. 2022;1(10):933–945. https://doi.org/10.1038/s44161-022-00133-6.
35. Xu L, Khoshknab M, Berger RD, et al. Lipomatous metaplasia enables ventricular tachycardia by reducing current loss within the protected corridor. *JACC Clin Electrophysiol*. 2022;8(10):1274–1285. https://doi.org/10.1016/j.jacep.2022.07.005.
36. Xu L, Zahid S, Khoshknab M, et al. Lipomatous metaplasia prolongs repolarization and increases repolarization dispersion within post-infarct ventricular tachycardia circuit cites. *Europace*. 2023;25(2):496–505. https://doi.org/10.1093/europace/euac222.
37. Brix G, Heiland S, Bellemann ME, Koch T, Lorenz WJ. MR imaging of fat-containing tissues: valuation of two quantitative imaging techniques in comparison with localized proton spectroscopy. *Magn Reson Imaging*. 1993;11(7):977–991. https://doi.org/10.1016/0730-725x(93)90217-2.
38. Hamilton G, Yokoo T, Bydder M, et al. In vivo characterization of the liver fat (1)H MR spectrum. *NMR Biomed*. 2011;24(7):784–790. https://doi.org/10.1002/nbm.1622.
39. Reeder SB, McKenzie CA, Pineda AR, et al. Water-fat separation with IDEAL gradient-echo imaging. *J Magn Reson Imaging*. 2007;25(3):644–652. https://doi.org/10.1002/jmri.20831.
40. Peterson P, Trinh L, Mansson S. Quantitative (1) H MRI and MRS of fatty acid composition. *Magn Reson Med*. 2021;85(1):49–67. https://doi.org/10.1002/mrm.28471.
41. Stanisz GJ, Odrobina EE, Pun J, et al. T1, T2 relaxation and magnetization transfer in tissue at 3T. *Magn Reson Med*. 2005;54(3):507–512. https://doi.org/10.1002/mrm.20605.
42. Glocker BKE, Lavdas I, Iglesias E, Aboagye E, Rockall A, Rueckert D. Correction of fat-water swaps in Dixon MRI. *Lecture Notes in Computer Science*. 2016:9902.
43. Hernando D, Haldar JP, Sutton BP, Ma J, Kellman P, Liang ZP. Joint estimation of water/fat images and field inhomogeneity map. *Magn Reson Med*. 2008;59(3):571–580. https://doi.org/10.1002/mrm.21522.
44. Lucke C, Schindler K, Lehmkuhl L, et al. Prevalence and functional impact of lipomatous metaplasia in scar tissue following myocardial infarction evaluated by MRI. *Eur Radiol*. 2010;20(9):2074–2083. https://doi.org/10.1007/s00330-010-1791-x.
45. Shriki JE, Surti KS, Farvid AF, et al. Chemical shift artifact on steady-state free precession cardiac magnetic resonance sequences as a result of lipomatous metaplasia: a novel finding in chronic myocardial infarctions. *Can J Cardiol*. 2011;27(5):664 e17–23. https://doi.org/10.1016/j.cjca.2010.12.074.
46. Bley TA, Wieben O, Francois CJ, Brittain JH, Reeder SB. Fat and water magnetic resonance imaging. *J Magn Reson Imaging*. 2010;31(1):4–18. https://doi.org/10.1002/jmri.21895.
47. Aquaro GD, Todiere G, Strata E, Barison A, Di Bella G, Lombardi M. Usefulness of India ink artifact in steady-state free precession pulse sequences for detection and quantification of intramyocardial fat. *J Magn Reson Imaging*. 2014;40(1):126–132. https://doi.org/10.1002/jmri.24335.
48. Azevedo CF, Jenista ER, Kaolawanich Y, et al. Assessment of myocardial lipomatous metaplasia using an optimized out-of-phase cine steady-state free-precession sequence: validation and clinical implementation. *NMR Biomed*. 2022;35(10):e4777. https://doi.org/10.1002/nbm.4777.
49. Kaolawanich Y, Azevedo CF, Kim HW, et al. Native T1 mapping for the diagnosis of myocardial fibrosis in patients with chronic myocardial infarction. *JACC Cardiovasc Imaging*. 2022;15(12):2069–2079. https://doi.org/10.1016/j.jcmg.2022.09.011.
50. Hargreaves BA, Vasanawala SS, Pauly JM, Nishimura DG. Characterization and reduction of the transient response in steady-state MR imaging. *Magn Reson Med*. 2001;46(1):149–158. https://doi.org/10.1002/mrm.1170.
51. Kellman P, Hansen MS. T1-mapping in the heart: accuracy and precision. *J Cardiovasc Magn Reson*. 2014;16(1):2. https://doi.org/10.1186/1532-429X-16-2.
52. Kellman P, Herzka DA, Arai AE, Hansen MS. Influence of Off-resonance in myocardial T1-mapping using SSFP based MOLLI method. *J Cardiovasc Magn Reson*. 2013;15(1):63. https://doi.org/10.1186/1532-429X-15-63.
53. Kellman P, Bandettini WP, Mancini C, Hammer-Hansen S, Hansen MS, Arai AE. Characterization of myocardial T1-mapping bias caused by intramyocardial fat in inversion recovery and saturation recovery techniques. *J Cardiovasc Magn Reson*. 2015;17(1):33. https://doi.org/10.1186/s12968-015-0136-y.
54. Baxa J, Ferda J, Hromadka M. T1 mapping of the ischemic myocardium: review of potential clinical use. *Eur J Radiol*. 2016;85(10):1922–1928. https://doi.org/10.1016/j.ejrad.2016.04.010.
55. Haaf P, Garg P, Messroghli DR, Broadbent DA, Greenwood JP, Plein S. Cardiac T1 Mapping and Extracellular Volume (ECV) in clinical practice: a comprehensive review. *J Cardiovasc Magn Reson*. 2016;18(1):89. https://doi.org/10.1186/s12968-016-0308-4.

56. Karamitsos TD, Arvanitaki A, Karvounis H, Neubauer S, Ferreira VM. Myocardial tissue characterization and fibrosis by imaging. *JACC Cardiovasc Imaging.* 2020;13(5):1221–1234. https://doi.org/10.1016/j.jcmg.2019.06.030.
57. Kali A, Cokic I, Tang RL, et al. Determination of location, size, and transmurality of chronic myocardial infarction without exogenous contrast media by using cardiac magnetic resonance imaging at 3 T. *Circ Cardiovasc Imaging.* 2014;7(3):471–481. https://doi.org/10.1161/CIRCIMAGING.113.001541.
58. Wang G, Lee SE, Yang Q, et al. Multicenter study on the diagnostic performance of native-T1 cardiac magnetic resonance of chronic myocardial infarctions at 3T. *Circ Cardiovasc Imaging.* 2020;13(6):e009894. https://doi.org/10.1161/CIRCIMAGING.119.009894.
59. Fishbein MC, Maclean D, Maroko PR. The histopathologic evolution of myocardial infarction. *Chest.* 1978;73(6):843–849. https://doi.org/10.1378/chest.73.6.843.
60. Mordi I, Radjenovic A, Stanton T, et al. Prevalence and prognostic significance of lipomatous metaplasia in patients with prior myocardial infarction. *JACC Cardiovasc Imaging.* 2015;8(9):1111–1112. https://doi.org/10.1016/j.jcmg.2014.07.024.
61. Gold GE, Han E, Stainsby J, Wright G, Brittain J, Beaulieu C. Musculoskeletal MRI at 3.0 T: relaxation times and image contrast. *AJR Am J Roentgenol.* 2004;183(2):343–351. https://doi.org/10.2214/ajr.183.2.1830343.

7 Myocardial Perfusion Imaging—Techniques

SVEN PLEIN, MANISH MOTWANI, AND MICHAEL JEROSCH-HEROLD

INTRODUCTION

Physiological Basis for Measuring Myocardial Perfusion

The term myocardial perfusion describes the delivery of blood in myocardial tissue via the coronary vasculature to maintain an adequate supply of oxygen and metabolites under varying demand conditions. The coronary arterial system consists of the epicardial coronary arteries (diameter ca 0.5–5 mm), the prearterioles (diameter ca. 100 to 500 μm), the intramural arterioles (diameter <100 μm), and the capillary bed (Fig. 7.1). An intricate interplay between these three compartments of the coronary arterial system continuously autoregulates blood flow to meet myocardial demand over a wide range of physiological conditions. Mechanisms determining these autoregulatory processes include tissue pressure, coronary perfusion pressure, and metabolic, neural, and hormonal factors. Regulation of blood flow is mostly achieved by controlling the diameter of resistance vessels that are smaller than approximately 300 μm in diameter, generally termed the myocardial microvasculature. In response to increased demand or reduced flow, these resistance vessels dilate, which allows an increase in coronary blood flow over baseline of up to fivefold in health. In the presence of epicardial coronary artery disease with up to 80% narrowing, compensatory vasodilation of resistance vessels maintains adequate myocardial blood flow under resting conditions.[1,2] With more severe narrowing in an epicardial vessel, and in the absence of significant collateral flow, the distal perfusion bed is fully vasodilated, even at resting conditions. Under conditions of increased demand, such as physical exercise or pharmacologically induced vasodilatation, further augmentation of blood flow is limited in the presence of severe epicardial coronary stenosis, and to a lesser extent myocardial microvascular dysfunction, and myocardial ischemia can ensue. This means that assessment of myocardial ischemia generally requires stress perfusion testing to achieve maximal vasodilation.[1,2]

Blood flow across the myocardial wall is not uniform, reflecting the differences in workload and oxygen consumption in the different myocardial layers. The subendocardial layer has the highest demand and capillary density, allowing higher blood flow to this layer compared with the subepicardium.[3,4] Under normal conditions the ratio of subendocardial to subepicardial blood flow is on the order of 1.15:1 at rest.[5] At maximal vasodilation, blood flow equalizes between the myocardial layers and the subendocardial to subepicardial blood flow is closer to 1. In the presence of significant epicardial coronary artery stenosis, blood flow is first diverted away from the subendocardial layer and the subendocardial-to-epicardial blood flow ratio is often <1:1, in particular under stress.[5,6]

Methods for Measuring Myocardial Perfusion

Myocardial perfusion can be assessed with a wide range of invasive and noninvasive methods. In clinical practice, myocardial perfusion assessment is mostly used to detect the presence and determine the functional significance of epicardial coronary artery disease and, less commonly, to detect the presence of microvascular myocardial dysfunction. The cross-sectional narrowing from a lesion impinging on the vessel lumen has been widely used as an anatomical measure of stenosis severity from coronary angiography, but can be an unreliable measure of functional significance. Coronary stenosis also results in a pressure drop across the lesion; the pressure distal to the stenosis during maximal vasodilation, normalized by aortic pressure, is referred to as fractional flow reserve (FFR) and is an invasive measure of the functional significance of a stenosis. FFR is theoretically equal to 1 in epicardial vessels that normally have negligible conduit resistance. FFR is considered the invasive reference standard for clinical decision making, resulting in less stenting and better long-term clinical outcomes.[7] Furthermore, FFR accounts for myocardial perfusion from collateral vessels, which can lessen the functional significance of an epicardial lesion. The functional impact of epicardial stenosis can also be quantified by the coronary flow reserve (CFR), defined as the ratio of maximal hyperemic coronary blood flow to resting coronary blood flow. At the tissue level, myocardial perfusion can be measured with noninvasive imaging methods that assess the delivery and distribution of a method-specific tracer to the myocardium. Established methods for myocardial perfusion imaging include positron emission tomography (PET), single photon emission computed tomography, cardiovascular magnetic resonance (CMR), as well as echocardiography and computed tomography (CT). In principle, all these methods can depict myocardial perfusion for visual analysis, and some, most notably PET and CMR, also allow quantitative estimates of myocardial blood flow (MBF). The ratio of stress over rest MBF defines the myocardial perfusion reserve, a measure that is in principle equivalent to the CFR in the absence of collateral flow. The sensitivity of a myocardial perfusion imaging technique is directly related to its contrast-to-noise ratio,

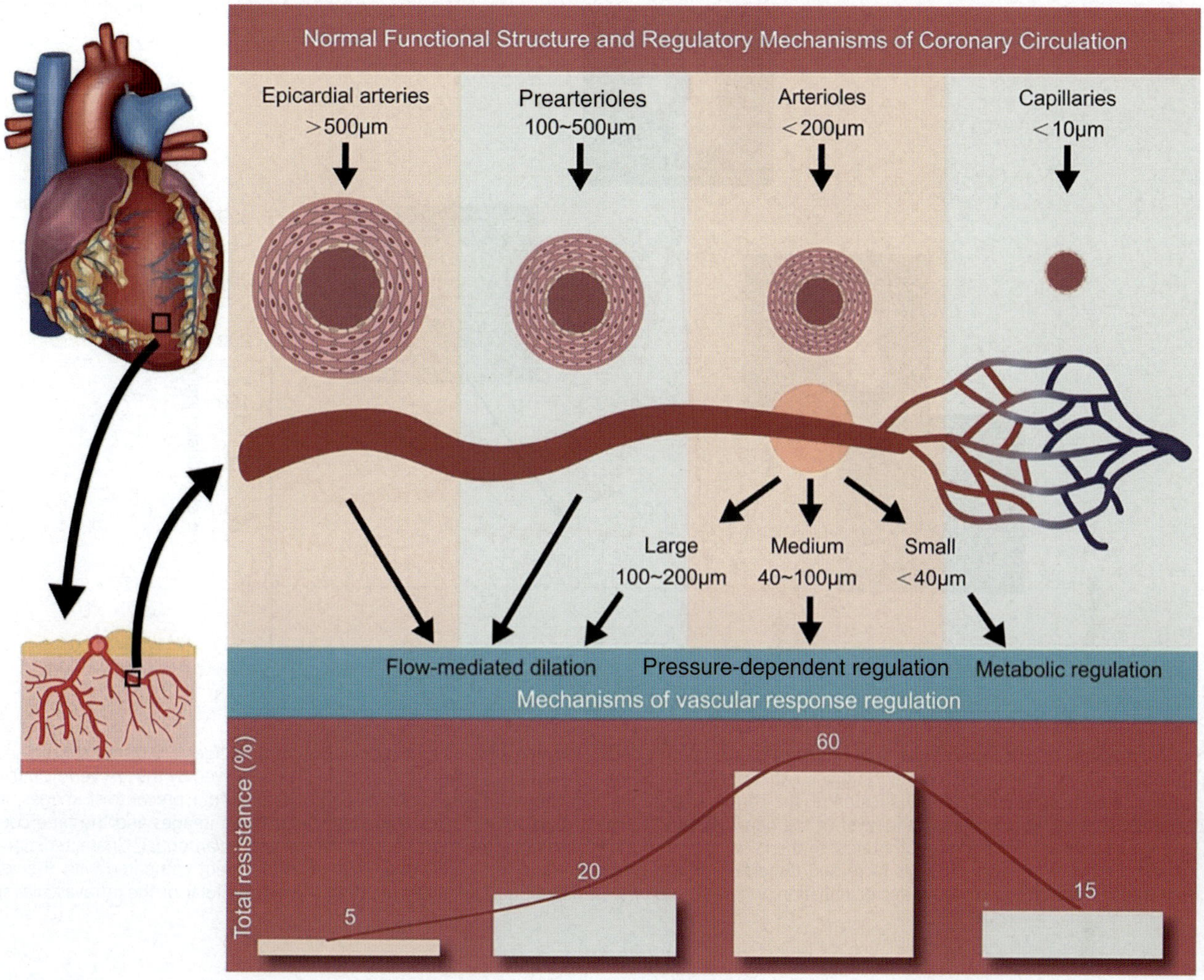

FIG. 7.1 Coronary microvascular structure and regulatory mechanisms. (Reproduced from Yang Z, Liu Y, Li Z, et al. Coronary microvascular dysfunction and cardiovascular disease: pathogenesis, associations and treatment strategies. *Biomed Pharmacother*. 2023;164:115011. Copyright © 2023 Elsevier Masson SAS. All rights reserved.)

spatial resolution, and the ability to discern transmural variations of flow.[8,9] With CMR it has become feasible to detect flow impairments limited or most accentuated in the subendocardial layer.[10] Furthermore, CMR offers the unique possibility of quantitatively assessing perfusion, viability, and function with high accuracy to distinguish stunned, hibernating, and infarcted myocardium.[11,12]

MYOCARDIAL PERFUSION MAGNETIC RESONANCE IMAGING TECHNIQUE

Principles of Myocardial Perfusion Cardiovascular Magnetic Resonance

The default method for myocardial perfusion assessment with CMR is dynamic first-pass perfusion imaging, in which an exogenous tracer is injected into the bloodstream and its first passage through the heart is tracked with an appropriately designed T1-weighted image acquisition method. The resulting dynamic image series can be interpreted visually or quantified to estimate myocardial blood flow. Perfusion methods using endogenous tracers, such as arterial spin labeling, can in principle also be used for myocardial perfusion imaging, but currently play no role in clinical practice (Fig. 7.2).

The basic characteristics of a dynamic first-pass perfusion CMR method include the choice of contrast agent, dose, and delivery; an imaging sequence sensitive to the contrast agent; the ability to track the contrast agent with high spatial and temporal resolution; and freedom from cardiac and respiratory motion compromise or availability of corrective methods (Table 7.1).

Contrast Agents and Administration

Most contrast agents used in clinical practice are gadolinium-based chelates, which are characterized by their strong T1-shortening properties. These contrast agents shorten the T1 relaxation rates (1/T1) of blood proportionally to their concentration, but the relationship between T1-weighted signal and contrast concentration is only approximately linear. Commercially available gadolinium-based contrast agents differ in their T1 relaxivity, meaning their T1-shortening effects are not all the same. Furthermore, the most commonly available contrast agents are extravascular and disperse into the interstitial space even during the first myocardial passage. These

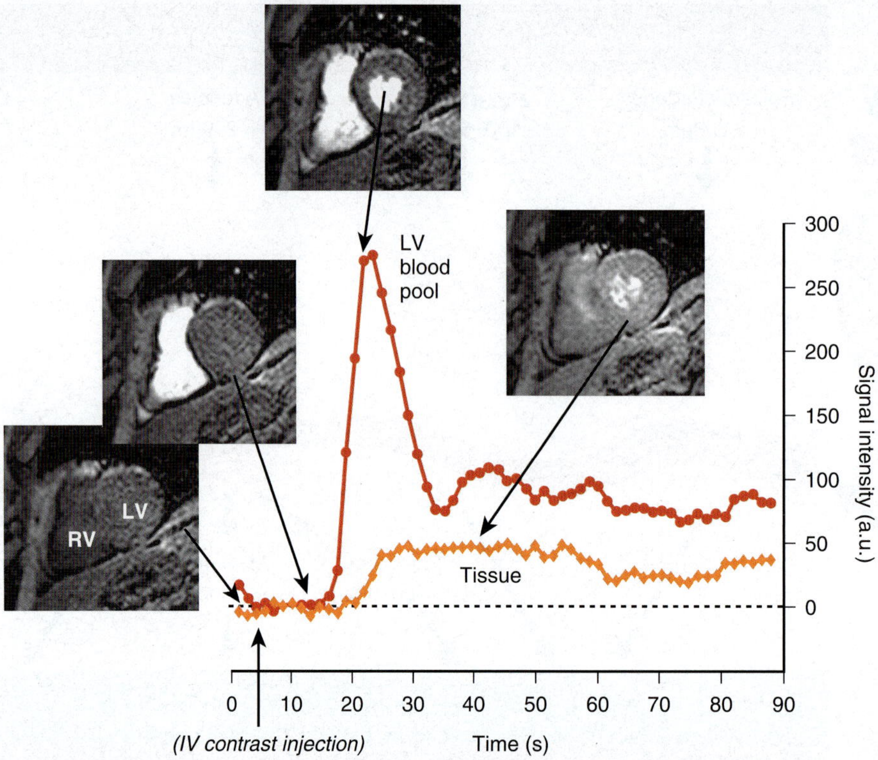

FIG. 7.2 The gradient echo cardiovascular magnetic resonance images depict the first pass of an extracellular contrast agent (0.03 mmol/kg of gadodiamide/Omniscan, GE Healthcare) in a healthy subject, with appearance of the contrast first in the right ventricle *(RV)*, followed by the left ventricle *(LV)*, and finally leading to myocardial contrast enhancement. The contrast agent was injected after acquisition of approximately four precontrast images. Images were acquired in the short-axis view at the level of the papillary muscle. The arrows show the correspondence between images and the time course of changes in signal intensity for a region of interest in the LV *(circles)* and a myocardial segment in the inferolateral wall *(diamonds)*. Characteristics of the signal curve for a tissue region such as its increased dispersion, lower amplitude, and reduced rate of signal enhancement compared with the ventricle result from transit through the coronary microcirculation, where the volume of distribution is limited to either the extracellular or the intravascular space.

TABLE 7.1 Basic characteristics of myocardial perfusion CMR methods.

Contrast agents, dose, and administration regime	Gadolinium-based contrast agent bolus 0.05–0.1 mmol/kg (@3–7 mL/s) followed by at least 30 mL saline flush (@3–7 mL/s)
Respiratory compensation	Breath-hold during first contrast passage through aorta and myocardium *or* Free breathing with respiratory motion correction performed with image reconstruction
Cardiac motion compensation	ECG or pulse oxymeter gating
Pulse sequence	Saturation recovery imaging with readout: • Spoiled GRE • GRE-echo planar hybrid • Steady-state free precession
Acceleration method	Parallel imaging, EPI, other
Temporal resolution	Every heartbeat
Readout temporal resolution (= acquisition shot duration)	~100–125 ms or shorter as available
No. of dynamics	Typically, 40–50 heartbeats; more in very poor LVEF
No. of slices	At least 3 short-axis slices
In-plane spatial resolution	<3 mm
Slice thickness	8–10 mm

CMR, Cardiovascular magnetic resonance; *EPI*, echoplanar imaging; *GRE*, gradient echo; *LV*, left ventricular; *LVEF*, left-ventricular ejection fraction.

properties need to be considered when interpreting first-pass myocardial perfusion CMR images.

International practice guidelines recommend that gadolinium contrast is administered at a dose of 0.05–0.1 mmol/kg and with an injection rate of 3–7 mL/s, followed by at least a 30 mL saline flush at the same injection rate.[13] Use of a power injector is recommended to deliver a compact and reproducible bolus. The contrast injection is usually administered to a vein in the antecubital fossa. Following bolus injection, the contrast agent will pass through the right heart chambers into the pulmonary circulation and then into the left heart chambers, followed by myocardial distribution. This transit time is determined by various factors including filling pressures and cardiac function.

For visual interpretation of myocardial perfusion CMR, injection of a single-contrast bolus is sufficient. However, for quantitative analysis, measurements need to be taken from the blood pool (which provides the arterial input function [AIF]) and the myocardium (the tissue response compartment); however, because the relationship between contrast agent dose and signal becomes increasingly nonlinear with higher contrast doses and contrast agent concentrations in the blood pool are higher than in the myocardium, a single bolus regime cannot deliver reliable data for both compartments. Accordingly, dual-bolus protocols, in which a lower-concentration prebolus (designed to allow measurement of the AIF) is followed by

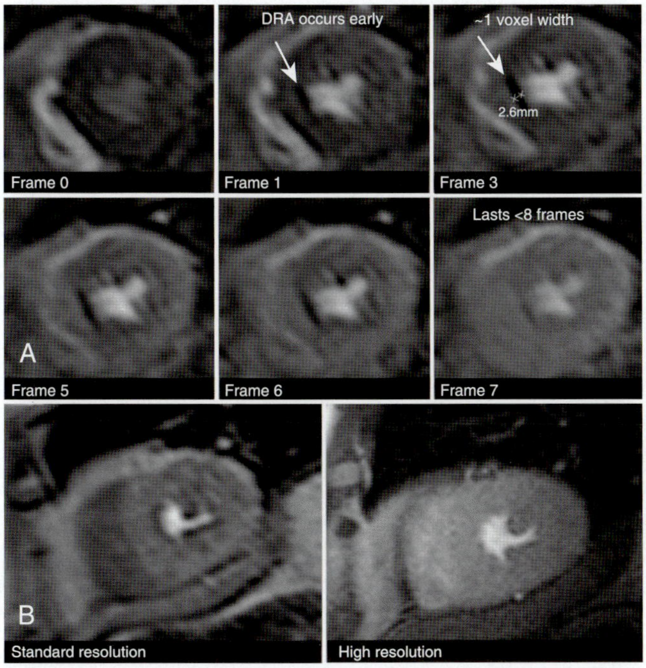

FIG. 7.4 Dark rim artifact. (A) Dark rim artifact (*DRA*) (*arrows*) is a frequent finding in standard-resolution perfusion cardiovascular magnetic resonance (CMR) and relates to several factors, including cardiac motion, Gibb's ringing, susceptibility, and partial volume cancellation between the myocardium and blood pool. Although DRAs may mimic perfusion defects, they can be distinguished by characteristic features: they occur at the arrival of contrast in the left ventricular cavity and before its arrival in the myocardium (Frame 1); they tend to disappear within 8 to 10 frames (Frame 7); their location is usually typical for a particular pulse sequence; and their width roughly equates to the in-plane spatial resolution, which was 2.5 mm in this example (Frame 3). (B) A 60-year-old male with suspected angina underwent stress perfusion CMR at 1.5 T with both standard-resolution (2.5 mm in-plane) and high-resolution (1.5 mm in-plane) acquisition (8 × *k-t* BLAST). There was no perfusion defect seen with either acquisition but there was significant DRA on the standard-resolution images (*arrows*). X-ray angiography confirmed normal coronary arteries.

T2* decay throughout the echo train can reduce the quality of images. Therefore, a hybrid EPI technique in which shorter echo trains are obtained by applying multiple RF pulses to acquire k-space segments is typically employed for perfusion imaging—this reduces the detrimental effect of T2* decay, enhancing image quality while keeping the speed advantage of the EPI technique.

BALANCED STEADY-STATE FREE PRECESSION

Instead of spoiling interference from transverse magnetization like with FGE, bSSFP pulse sequences apply additional balancing gradients to rephase the MR signal before each subsequent RF pulse. After multiple repetitions, a steady-state equilibrium arises in which the transverse magnetization from the successive repetitions accumulates to generate a much higher signal. The higher signal allows the use of higher receiver bandwidths, resulting in a shorter TE and TR compared to gradient echo pulse sequences and therefore improved imaging efficiency. However, if the magnetic field is not homogenous, the transverse magnetization cannot be rephased at the end of each TR, resulting in signal loss. For this reason, bSSFP is also more susceptible to signal loss at the endocardial border during peak enhancement in the blood pool, resulting in a dark rim artifact. DRAs can be minimized by using a TR that is as short as possible. If opting for bSSFP perfusion sequences for signal gain, it is important to ensure the magnetic field over the myocardial region of interest is as uniform as possible by performing B0 shimming.

1.5-T versus 3.0-T Field Strength

In the clinical setting, perfusion CMR is usually performed at 1.5-T or 3.0-T field strengths, with 1.5-T being more widely available. A major advantage of perfusion CMR at 3 T is the superior signal-to-noise ration (SNR) and contrast enhancement that can be obtained, with reported improved diagnostic accuracy for the detection of single vessel and multivessel CAD.[16-18] However, perfusion CMR at 3 T can be hampered by susceptibility artifacts related to the higher field strength such as magnetic field inhomogeneities as well as restrictions related to local energy deposition. Use of a GRE readout as opposed to a bSSFP readout is therefore often preferred at 3 T to minimize these artifacts.[19] Although these challenges at 3-T can be overcome, for example with more attention to RF-shimming in the region of interest and the introduction of multitransmit radiofrequency technology, the trade-offs are additional calibration sequences and increased operator dependence for image quality.[20]

HIGHLY ACCELERATED PERFUSION CARDIOVASCULAR MAGNETIC RESONANCE

Image acquisition during first-pass perfusion requires very fast pulse sequences to acquire high spatial and temporal resolution with optimal volume coverage and high SNR. Therefore, the need for higher spatial and temporal resolution in dynamic CMR has prompted the development of several dedicated imaging speed-up techniques. Effects on SNR and increasing artifacts limit the practically achievable acceleration to approximately two to threefold using standard acceleration techniques such as echo planar or parallel imaging. Data acquisition can be further accelerated with methods that exploit both temporal and spatial correlations, capitalizing on significant spatiotemporal redundancy within imaging data, which is particularly relevant to first-pass perfusion imaging.[21-24] Several of these advanced acceleration approaches have been used to improve the in-plane spatial resolution of myocardial perfusion CMR to <2 mm (high-resolution perfusion CMR) with reductions in DRA, better detection of subendocardial ischemia, better defect registration with cine and late gadolinium enhancement images (similar spatial resolution), and possible improvements in diagnostic accuracy versus standard resolution acquisition (Fig. 7.5).[22,25-29] Others have used speed-up to increase spatial coverage, with acquisition of more than three slices or even whole-heart three-dimensional (3D) acquisition (3D perfusion CMR), permitting more reliable calculation of the total myocardial ischemic burden, akin to nuclear myocardial perfusion imaging (Figs. 7.6 and 7.7).[21,30-35] Additionally, 3D perfusion CMR with whole-heart coverage includes the true apex of the heart, which is not conventionally imaged with 2D methods.

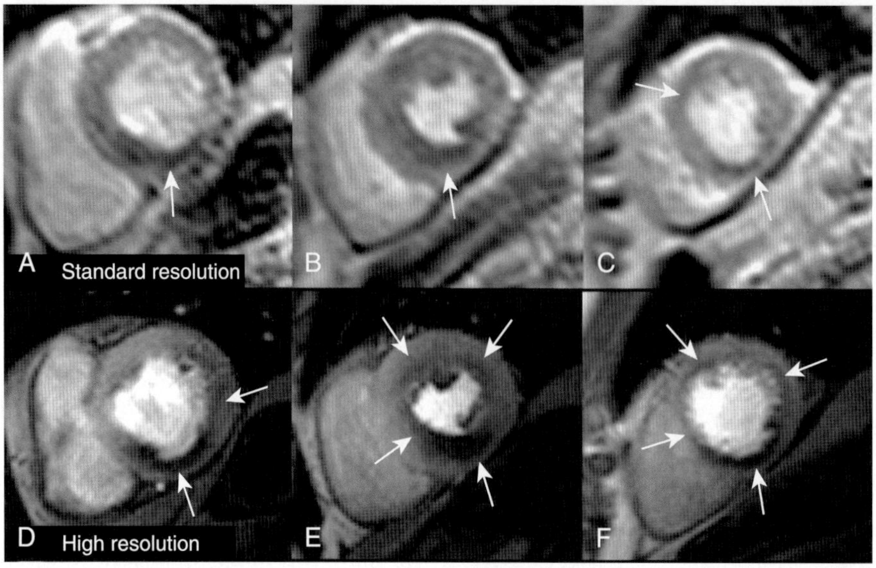

FIG. 7.5 High-resolution perfusion cardiovascular magnetic resonance (CMR). Standard (A–C) and high-resolution (D–F) stress perfusion CMR in a patient with three-vessel coronary artery disease. Standard resolution shows perfusion defects *(arrows)* in the basal-inferior (A), midinferior, midinferoseptal (B), apical-anterior, and apical-inferior segments (C). High resolution shows a similar distribution of perfusion defects but demonstrates additional ischemia in the basal-lateral (D), midanterior, and midanterolateral segments (E), with a circumferential defect in the apical slice (F). Perfusion defects are also better delineated at high resolution and the transmural extent of ischemia more clearly seen. (From Motwani M, Maredia N, Fairbairn TA, et al. Assessment of ischaemic burden in angiographic three-vessel coronary artery disease with high-resolution myocardial perfusion cardiovascular magnetic resonance imaging. Eur Heart J Cardiovasc Imaging. 2014;15(6):701–708.)

In practice, advanced acceleration techniques add complexity to the acquisition of perfusion CMR and often require research software. Reconstruction processes can be demanding on computing hardware and are therefore often lengthy and performed offline. Methods that include temporal undersampling are more sensitive to respiratory motion and cardiac arrhythmias. In many of the published studies, breathing-related artifacts were minimized by acquiring fewer than standard dynamics (in many studies only 30 dynamics), which requires very precise breath-holding and contrast injection timing to ensure that the main contrast bolus is imaged.[25] For these reasons, despite the theoretical advantages and diagnostic accuracy seen with these methods in several small studies, further technical advances are needed before they become practical for routine clinical practice, as well as studies to determine the clinically optimal balance between spatial resolution and spatial coverage afforded.

PRIOR KNOWLEDGE TECHNIQUES

Most studies reporting high-resolution or 3D perfusion CMR have used techniques based on "prior knowledge" to derive the required acceleration factors for data acquisition.[22,25,27,30,33,34] Prior-knowledge methods are based on the observation that image datasets exhibit considerable correlation in space and time.[23] Perfusion CMR datasets contain a high degree of temporal redundancy, because data are acquired at a single time point in the cardiac cycle using ECG gating and during breath-holding—this means that most of the image is static and the predominant change between neighboring time frames is related to the passage of contrast. This image redundancy can be taken advantage of by undersampling data in the time *(t)* domain as well as the more conventional undersampling in the spatial (*k*-space) domain. With some of the acceleration schemes discussed, data acquisition can be accelerated up to a factor of 10 times.

The *k-t* broad linear acquisition speed-up technique (*k-t* BLAST) is a prior-knowledge spatiotemporal *(k-t)* undersampling technique that has gained common use. In *k-t* BLAST, undersampling is applied along *k*-space and time, while a low spatial resolution image ("training data") is obtained in an interleaved fashion during the acquisition.[36] A nonaliased, full image series is then reconstructed using prior knowledge derived from the training data (Fig. 7.8). The signal aliasing is resolved by an adaptive filtering process in which the aliased signal is distributed according to a low-resolution estimate of the signal covariance, as derived from the training images. A particular advantage of this approach is that it allows some overlapping of the aliased object, thereby permitting higher acceleration factors. However, the inherent temporal filtering reduces temporal fidelity, which can lead to reconstruction errors or limit the reduction in data acquisition achieved.

A further limitation of *k-t* BLAST is that the reconstruction problem is intrinsically underdetermined (i.e., there are fewer equations than unknowns), which reflects its dependence on the estimated signal covariance from training data. One method of improving this is to incorporate sensitivity-encoding information into the reconstruction—this is the *k-t* SENSE method.[37,38] A further extension of *k-t* BLAST or *k-t* SENSE, known as *k-t* PCA, allows even higher acceleration factors by constraining reconstruction using a standard data compression technique, called principal component analysis (PCA)—this is a commonly used mathematical algorithm that reduces highly dimensional datasets to lower

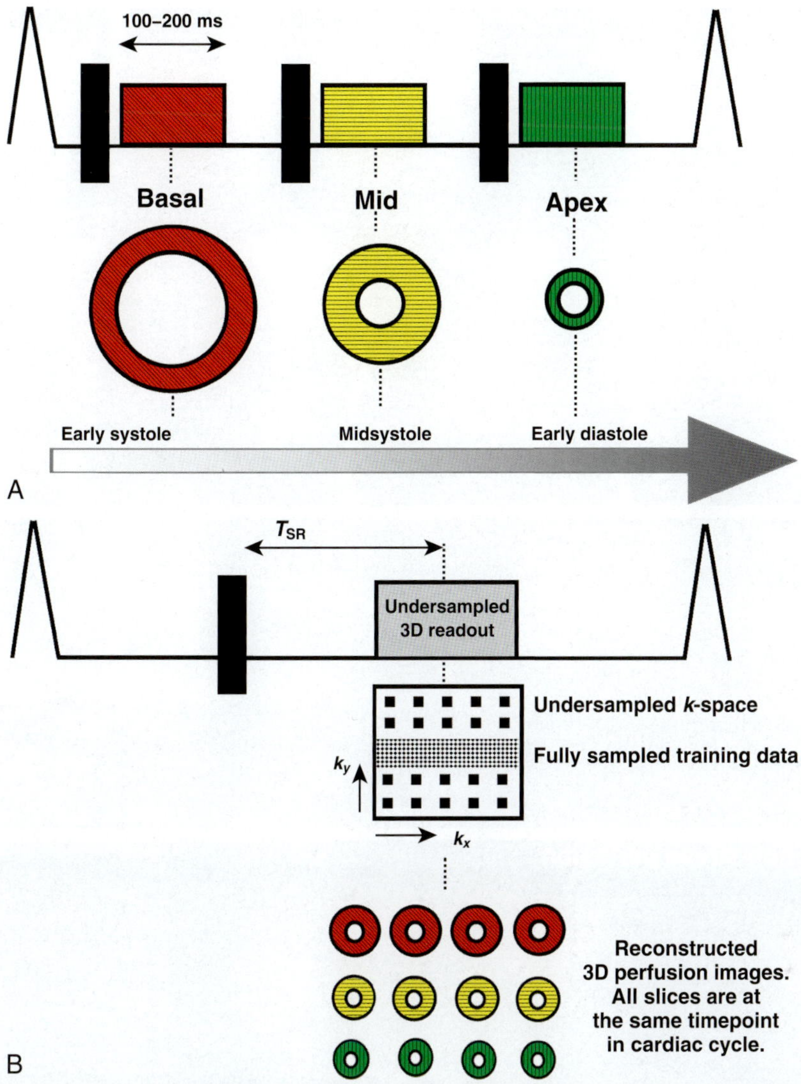

FIG. 7.6 Pulse sequence diagrams for two-dimensional (2D) and three-dimensional (3D) perfusion cardiovascular magnetic resonance (CMR). (A) In 2D perfusion CMR, three to four noncontiguous slices are acquired in different phases of the cardiac cycle to maximize spatial coverage. Each slice is acquired after a saturation prepulse *(black bar)*. (B) In 3D-perfusion CMR, a single saturation prepulse is followed by a saturation recovery time and undersampled 3D perfusion data readout. The use of advanced spatiotemporal undersampling allows sufficient data acquisition to reconstruct 16 contiguous slices (whole-heart coverage). The "training data" is acquired with the undersampled data in an interleaved fashion. Because all perfusion data in the 3D technique are acquired at the same point in the cardiac cycle, the reconstructed slices all appear in the same cardiac phase. (From Motwani M, Jogiya R, Kozerke S, et al. Advanced cardiovascular magnetic resonance myocardial perfusion imaging: high-spatial resolution versus 3-dimensional whole-heart coverage. *Clin Cardiovasc Imaging.* 2013; 6:339–348.)

dimensionality by extracting and exploiting relevant correlations within the data.[38]

Compressed Sensing

An alternative method for reconstruction of undersampled data permitting acceleration is compressed sensing (CS), which is based upon the principle that an image with a sparse representation in a known transform domain can be recovered from randomly undersampled *k*-space data using a nonlinear reconstruction (Fig. 7.9).[39,40] Sparsity in this context describes a matrix of pixels with predominantly zero values in a single image or series of images. CS is therefore readily applicable to perfusion CMR because the signal is sparse in the combined temporal frequency (f) and spatial domain with only portions of the field of view requiring full temporal bandwidth and the other regions having only static information or low temporal frequencies.

Unlike *k-t* BLAST and *k-t* SENSE, CS does not require training data, and, as a result, it may be less sensitive to inconsistencies between training and imaging data. Application of CS to dynamic CMR has been presented in methods such as *k-t* SPARSE and *k-t* FOCUSS using the temporal fast Fourier transform as the sparsifying transform and k_y-*t* random undersampling.[39,41-43] The maximum acceleration rate in CS is determined by image sparsity, and in practice the number of required samples is approximately three to five times the number of nonzero coefficients in the image.[39,42] CS can also be combined with parallel imaging or non-Cartesian techniques to obtain higher accelerations.

Non-Cartesian Techniques

Another approach to advanced acceleration involves data acquisition along non-Cartesian patterns such as radial trajectories through the center of *k*-space (Fig. 7.10). Spatial and

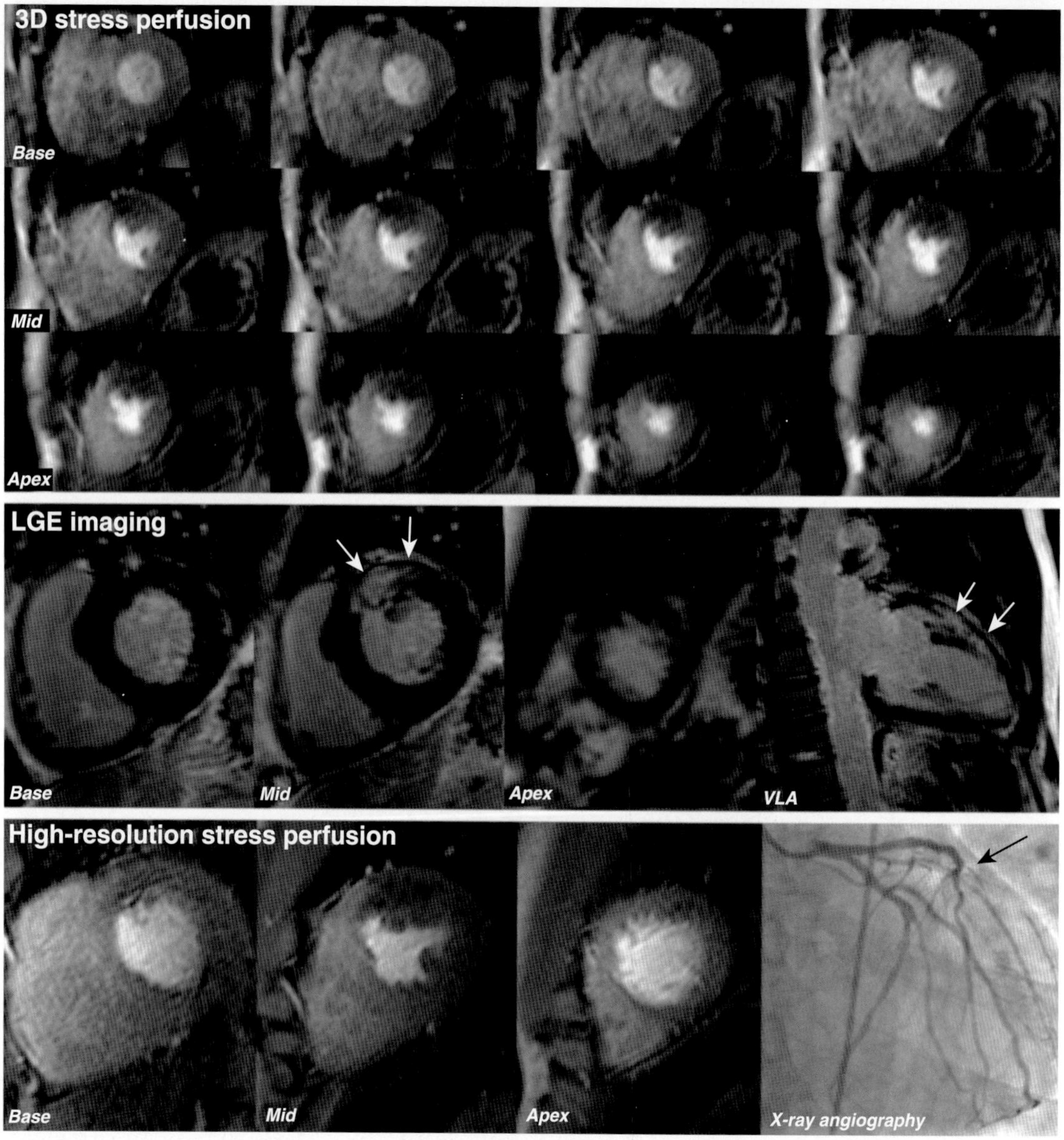

FIG. 7.7 Case example 2. A 45-year-old male with prior percutaneous coronary intervention of the left anterior descending presented with significant angina. The top panel shows 3D perfusion cardiovascular magnetic resonance (CMR) (12 slices) at stress; the middle panel shows late-gadolinium enhancement *(LGE)* imaging, and the bottom panel shows high-resolution (1.1 mm in-plane) stress perfusion CMR, all performed at 3.0 T. Three-dimensional *(3D)* perfusion CMR shows stress-induced hypoperfusion throughout the anterior wall from base to apex—that is, well beyond the area of scar seen in the midanterior wall on LGE imaging *(arrows)*. This example shows the benefit of whole-heart coverage with the 3D acquisition, as the 3-slice high-resolution techniques did not demonstrate any significant ischemia beyond the established scar in the midventricle. Invasive coronary angiography confirmed a subtotal occlusion of a large diagonal branch, accounting for the anterior ischemia *(black arrow)*. *VLA,* Vertical long axis. (From Motwani M, Jogiya R, Kozerke S, et al. Advanced cardiovascular magnetic resonance myocardial perfusion imaging: high-spatial resolution versus 3-dimensional whole-heart coverage. *Clin Cardiovasc Imaging*. 2013;6:339–348.)

temporal redundancy are exploited serially and the altered geometry of *k*-space coverage facilitates greater efficiency compared with conventional Cartesian techniques by collecting more data with each RF excitation.[23,37,44] Non-Cartesian sampling techniques such as radial or spiral imaging have shown particular benefits in minimizing dark-rim artifact reduction because of their robustness to motion and Gibbs ringing effects.[15,45] Non-Cartesian techniques may also be combined with parallel imaging and compressed sensing techniques, and therefore hold potential for very large gains in spatial-temporal resolution.[21] Radial perfusion CMR is also well suited for continuous acquisition and self-gating, effectively eliminating the need for ECG gating, and therefore has the potential to achieve high diagnostic accuracy in arrhythmic patients. However, these techniques are largely experimental and have not been fully validated clinically.

MYOCARDIAL PERFUSION ANALYSIS

Visual Analysis of Perfusion Cardiovascular Magnetic Resonance

Dynamic myocardial perfusion CMR images can be displayed and viewed as cine loops. Visual analysis of these images compares myocardial signal intensity changes over time between different myocardial regions. Visual analysis considers the arrival time of the contrast bolus

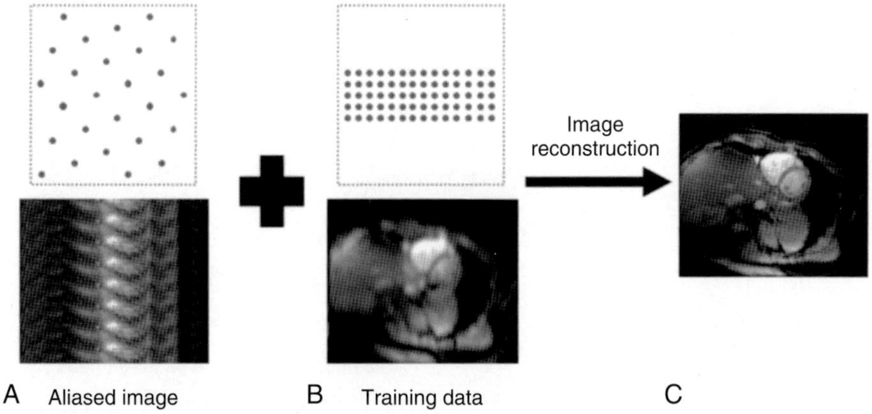

FIG. 7.8 *k-t* undersampling acceleration techniques. (A) In the *k-t* broad linear speed-up technique (BLAST) and *k-t* sensitivity encoding (SENSE), data acquisition is accelerated by undersampling along the spatial encoding *(k)* and time *(t)* axes, which leads to an aliased image. (B) Low-resolution "training data" is also obtained to determine data correlations, that is, "prior-knowledge." (C) Finally, a nonaliased full image series is reconstructed using a statistical model derived from the training data. (From Motwani M, Jogiya R, Kozerke S, et al. Advanced cardiovascular magnetic resonance myocardial perfusion imaging: high-spatial resolution versus 3-dimensional whole-heart coverage. *Clin Cardiovasc Imaging*. 2013; 6:339–348.)

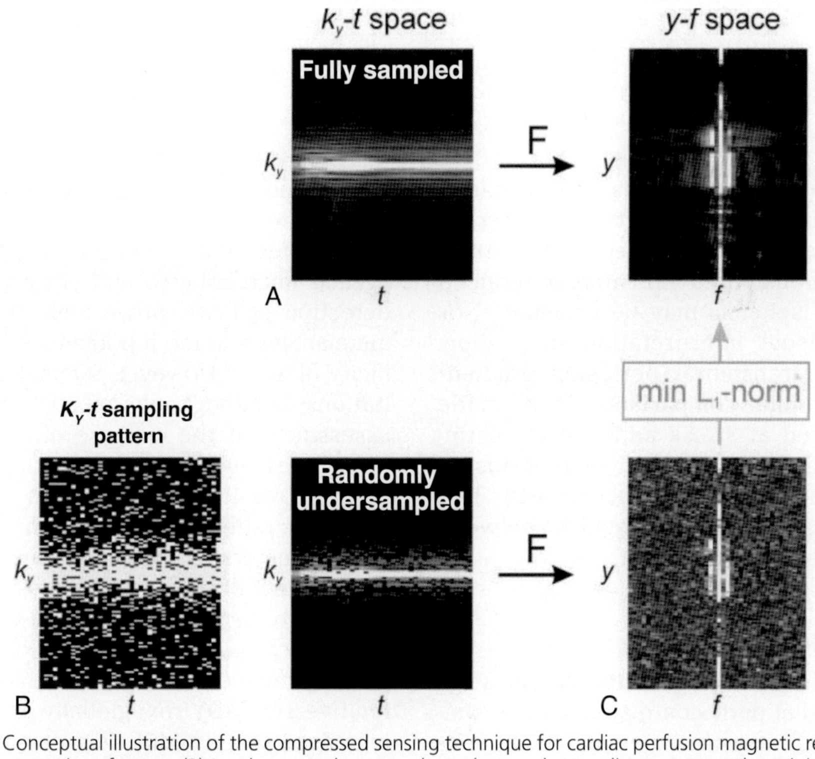

FIG. 7.9 Compressed sensing. Conceptual illustration of the compressed sensing technique for cardiac perfusion magnetic resonance imaging. (A) Sparsity: The fully sampled *ky-t* data is sparse in *y-f* space. (B) Incoherence: *ky-t* pseudorandom undersampling preserves the original sparse representation in *y-f* space and presents artifacts that look like additive noise (pseudonoise). (C) Nonlinear reconstruction: The sparse coefficients in *y-f* space can be recovered with a nonlinear reconstruction that minimizes the number of nonzero coefficients (minimum L1-norm). *F*, Fourier transform. (From Otazo R, Kim D, Axel L, et al. Combina-tion of compressed sensing and parallel imaging for highly accelerated first-pass cardiac perfusion MRI. *Magn Reson Med*. 2010; 64:767–776.)

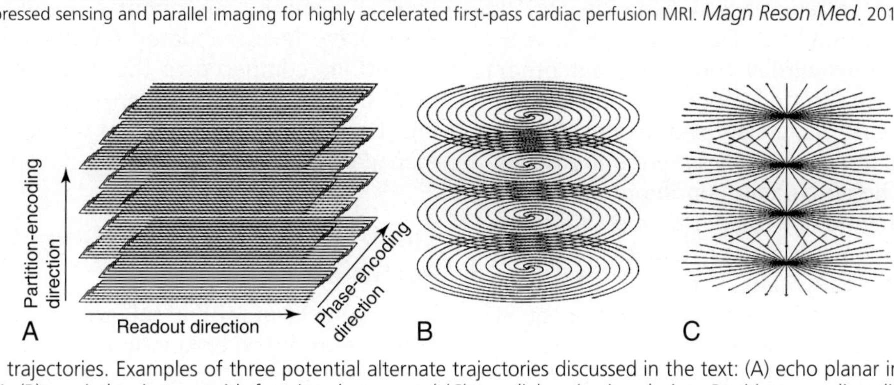

FIG. 7.10 Non-Cartesian trajectories. Examples of three potential alternate trajectories discussed in the text: (A) echo planar imaging demonstrated with an echo train length of 4, (B) a spiral trajectory with four interleaves, and (C) a radial projection design. Partition encoding direction in (B) and (C) is the same as for (A). (From Fair MJ, Gatehouse PD, DiBella EV, et al. A review of 3D first-pass, whole-heart, myocardial perfusion cardio-vascular magnetic resonance. *J Cardiovasc Magn Reson*. 2015;17:68.)

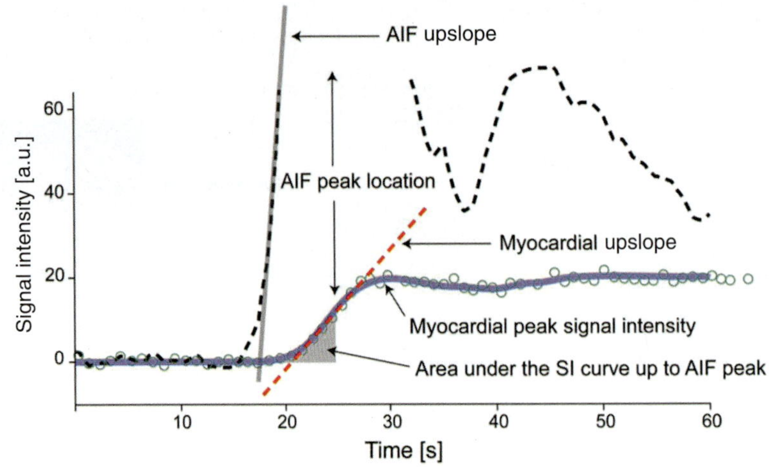

FIG. 7.11 The characteristics of myocardial contrast enhancement. The characteristics of myocardial contrast enhancement have been assessed in the literature using several parameters, as illustrated in this example, showing the signal intensity (SI) changes in the left ventricular (LV) blood pool (arterial input function ℵ [*AIF*]), and in an anterior segment of the left ventricle (*green circles*). The *blue line* shows the fit to the measured data with a two-space distributed model. The *dashed red line* is commonly referred to as the upslope parameter and gives the initial rate of contrast enhancement. It is often normalized by the upslope of the AIF as an empirical correction factor to account for hemodynamic changes between rest and stress. The area under the tissue curve (*gray shaded area*), up to the location in time where the peak of the AIF is observed, has been proposed as an alternative parameter to assess perfusion and the perfusion reserve. The myocardial peak signal intensity during the first pass of the contrast bolus in the LV is arguably the least flow-sensitive parameter, and therefore is only used to assess contrast to noise, but not changes or differences in myocardial perfusion. (From Jerosch-Herold M. Quantification of myocardial perfusion by cardiovascular magnetic resonance. *J Cardiovasc Magn Reson*. 2010;12(1):57. doi: 10.1186/1532-429X-12-57. PMID: 20932314; PMCID: PMC2964700.)

in each region, the rate of signal increase, the maximal signal, and the washout of the contrast bolus after its first myocardial passage. Delayed and reduced contrast uptake in any region is considered indicative of reduced perfusion or ischemia. Ischemia may be transmural or subendocardial and visual interpretation may allow the identification of a transmural perfusion gradient as another sign of ischemia. Comparison can be made between images acquired at stress and rest to distinguish perfusion defects from artifact, and perfusion imaging is usually analyzed in conjunction with late gadolinium-enhanced images to distinguish between scar and ischemia in viable myocardium.

Semiquantitative Analysis

Before recent computational developments that facilitate fully automated myocardial perfusion quantification, simpler semiquantitative (SQ) measures of myocardial perfusion were often utilized. SQ methods describe features of myocardial time-signal intensity (SI) curves during first-pass perfusion without attempting to estimate MBF in ml/g/min (i.e., 'full quantitation'). The most common SQ parameter is maximal myocardial "upslope", but others including "upslope integral ratio," "contrast enhancement ratio," and "time to peak" have also been evaluated (Fig. 7.11).[46-48] SQ myocardial perfusion parameters are dependent upon underlying hemodynamic conditions, and therefore require normalizing before comparing rest and stress values, or values between individuals. Hemodynamic conditions are reflected by the shape of the AIF, which can measured from the LV blood pool; normalization of SQ myocardial parameters is therefore achieved by dividing by the equivalent AIF parameter such as the "upslope of the AIF". The ratio of normalized stress and rest SQ perfusion parameters is known as the myocardial perfusion reserve index (MPRI), a noninvasive surrogate for CFR and an indicator of ischemia severity.[2,47,48]

SQ myocardial perfusion analysis has been validated against microspheres and coronary angiography for the detection of CAD with a high diagnostic accuracy[49-51]; a meta-analysis found a pooled sensitivity of 77% and specificity of 84%.[52] However, SQ analysis also has several limitations including: only minimal gains compared to visual assessment at the expense of a significant time penalty for processing[53]; underestimation of perfusion at flow rates above 1.5 mL/g/min when validated against microspheres[46]; differing MPRI ischemic thresholds for different SQ parameters as well as for invasively measured CFR[47]; requirement of both stress and rest acquisitions for MPRI, counter to the trend of reducing scan duration by omitting routine rest perfusion; and MPRI is unable to distinguish globally reduced stress MBF with normal resting MBF (e.g., multivessel CAD) from globally preserved stress MBF with increased resting MBF (e.g., hypertension with left ventricular hypertrophy (LVH))—only a full quantification of stress and rest MBF would resolve these very different clinical scenarios. In summary, while SQ perfusion measures have been validated for detecting CAD, they have limitations compared to the quantification of myocardial perfusion in absolute units (e.g., ml/min/g)—understanding these trade-offs is crucial for accurate diagnosis and management.

Full Quantitative Evaluation of Myocardial Perfusion

Measurement of MBF in mL/g/min is possible through the application of tracer-kinetic models to the perfusion data (Fig. 7.12). Several different methodologies for perfusion quantification have been developed based on the technical principles summarized below. Contemporary, fully

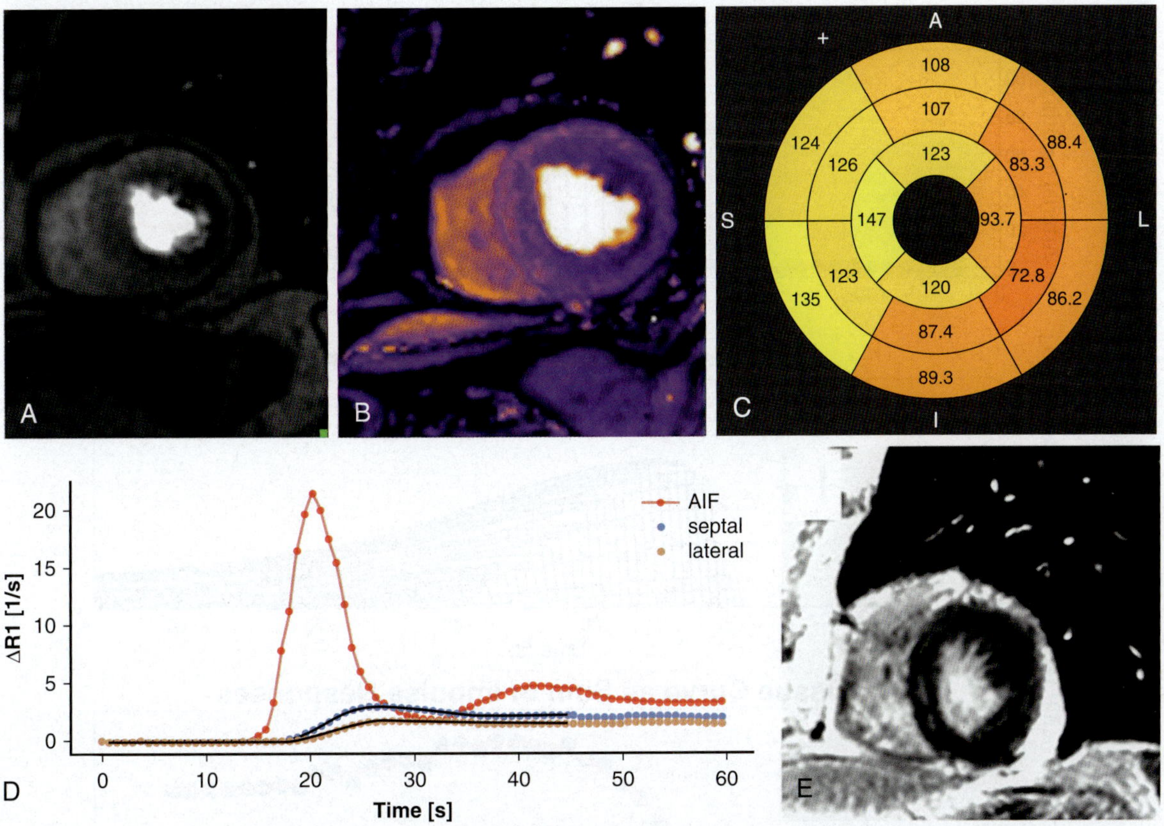

FIG. 7.12 Quantitative pixelwise myocardial perfusion with segmental bullseye representation of myocardial blood flow values. This case illustrates stress-induced perfusion defects in the lateral wall. *AIF*, arterial input function.(A) shows one image of the dynamic stress perfusion series acquired at the mid ventricular short axis location with a perfusion defect in the lateral wall. (B) shows the corresponding colour coded stress myocardial blood flow map. (C) is a bulls eye plot of myocardial blood flow values in all three slices of the stress perfusion acquisition in ml/mg/min. (D) represents the time intensity profiles for the arterial input function (AIF) taken from a region of interest in the left ventricular blood pool and regions of interest in the septal and lateral myocardium. (E) is a corresponding late gadolinium enhanced image at mid ventricular level showing absence of infarction in the lateral wall with mid-wall enhancement in the septum.

automated perfusion quantification pipelines can provide an accessible, observer-independent analysis with superior diagnostic and prognostic performance, particularly in patients with complex multivessel CAD and microvascular disease (MVD).

The myocardial contrast enhancement during the first pass of an intravenously injected contrast agent bolus through the heart can be used to determine myocardial blood. Though the myocardial contrast enhancement may be blood flow–sensitive it still reflects the time course of the arterial input to a region of interest in the myocardium. Injecting the contrast agent rapidly as a bolus is a condition for contrast enhancement to be sufficiently sensitive to coronary flow and not to the rate at which contrast is injected. This requirement for rapid contrast injection is of particular importance at higher myocardial blood flows achieved during hyperemia, as the rate of injection can then be a more limiting factor for myocardial contrast enhancement than at rest.

The concentrations of the blood-borne contrast agent at the arterial input and in a myocardial region of interest are related in a way that is mathematically expressed as a convolution integral of the arterial input with what is called the tissue impulse response. The tissue impulse response is a characteristic that is independent of the arterial input shape or duration and provides a measure of myocardial blood flow. It is useful to think here of the arterial input as composed of a series of very narrow pulses whose peaks trace out the shape of the arterial input (Fig. 7.13). Convolution means that for each of these essentially instantaneous arterial pulses there is a response of the tissue (impulse response) that extends forward in time. In evaluating the convolution integral, these overlapping responses are added at each time point. The result is a function (of time) that represents the tissue response to the arterial input.

The tissue impulse response has some useful properties for the quantification of myocardial blood flow: its initial amplitude is a measure of blood flow. This property of the impulse response is independent of the vascular and compartmental structure inside the tissue region of interest or the properties of barriers such as their permeability. For example, leakage of a contrast agent from the capillaries into the interstitial space produces a redistribution of the contrast agent *within* the region of interest but does not contribute to flow in and out of the region of interest, if transport by diffusion and convection is much slower than by blood flow. For an MR contrast agent such as gadolinium diethylenetriamine-pentaacetic acid (Gd-DTPA) these assumptions hold up well, but for freely diffusible tracers they may not always hold.

This model of the relationship between arterial input and tissue response is the basis of what has become known as Zierler's Central Volume theorem, and which is expressed mathematically by said convolution integral (Eq. E1):

$$C_{\text{tissue}}(t) = \int_0^t \text{AIF}(\tau).R_F(t-\tau).d\tau = \text{AIF}(t) * R_F(t) \quad (1)$$

The flow-weighted tissue impulse response is denoted by $R_F\ (t)$, AIF(t) is the arterial input, and the ⋆

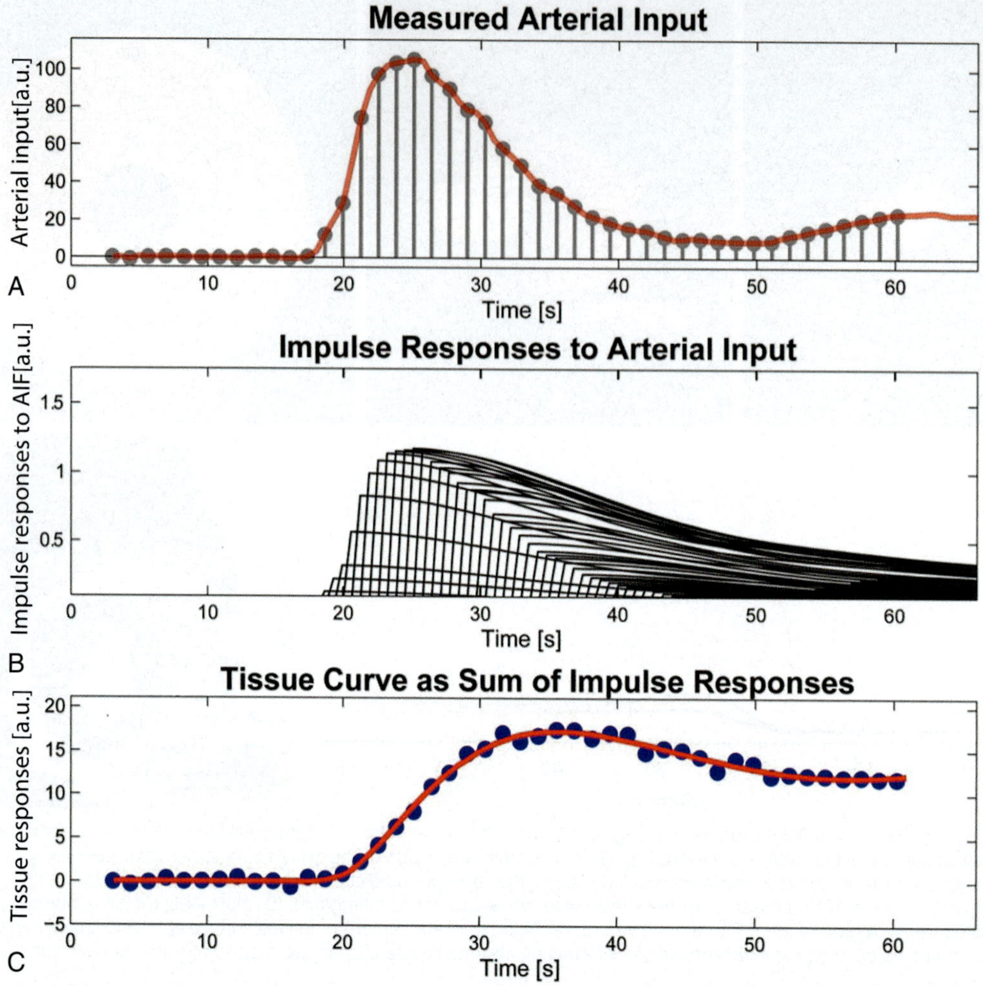

FIG. 7.13 (A) The arterial input of contrast (*red continuous line*) can be decomposed into an equivalent series of very narrow pulses (*stems with circles at end*) with amplitudes that trace out the shape of the *measured* arterial input. (There should be no gaps between the individual pulses, which was omitted here to simplify the graphical representation.) (B) For each of these essentially instantaneous arterial pulses there is a response of the tissue (impulse response) that extends forward in time. For this example, the impulse response was modeled as a Fermi function. (C) Summing at each time point the contributions from the overlapping impulse responses gives the tissue response. This mathematical operation of summing time-shifted impulse responses scaled by the arterial input amplitude is referred to as convolution of the arterial input with the impulse response. The calculated tissue response can be compared to the *measured* tissue curves to determine optimal values for the Fermi function by least squares optimization. *AIF*, arterial input function.

is a shorthand for the convolution operation. $R_F(t-\tau)$ is the impulse response shifted by τ, and by summing or integrating over this time-shift impulse response one adds up tissue responses for each "pulse" of the arterial input.

To obtain the impulse response, $R_F(t)$, whose amplitude equals myocardial blood flow, one has to perform a *deconvolution* of the measured tissue residue curve with the arterial input curve, that is, perform the inverse of the convolution operation shown in Eq. (E2). The deconvolution analysis is quite sensitive to noise in the data, and one therefore needs to constrain the deconvolution operation to get results not dominated by random noise. A Fermi function has been used as an empirical model for the impulse response to fit the first pass portion of the signal curves (Fig. 7.14).[54,55] The Fermi model of the impulse response has the following equation:

$$R_F(t) = \frac{A}{1+\exp[(t-\mu)/\tau]} \qquad (2)$$

where A, μ and τ are model parameters. The parameter μ can be interpreted as the average time before any contrast exits the tissue region of interest, and τ is related to the dispersion of contrast residence times within the region. From an empirical standpoint, the shape of the Fermi function provides a reasonable approximation to the shape of the impulse response of an *intravascular* tracer. The portion of the signal-intensity curves up to the peak has higher sensitivity to flow changes than later phases of contrast enhancement. The early enhancement is relatively insensitive to capillary leakage of contrast agent and therefore not that different between extracellular and intravascular tracers. This early part of the signal intensity curve can be approximated well by the Fermi function model to assess blood flow. The Fermi model for the quantification of myocardial perfusion and the perfusion reserve was validated by comparison to blood flow measurements with labeled microspheres[46,56] and also by comparison to invasive CFR measurements.[55]

A more general approach for deconvolution of the measured tissue contrast enhancement imposes conditions on

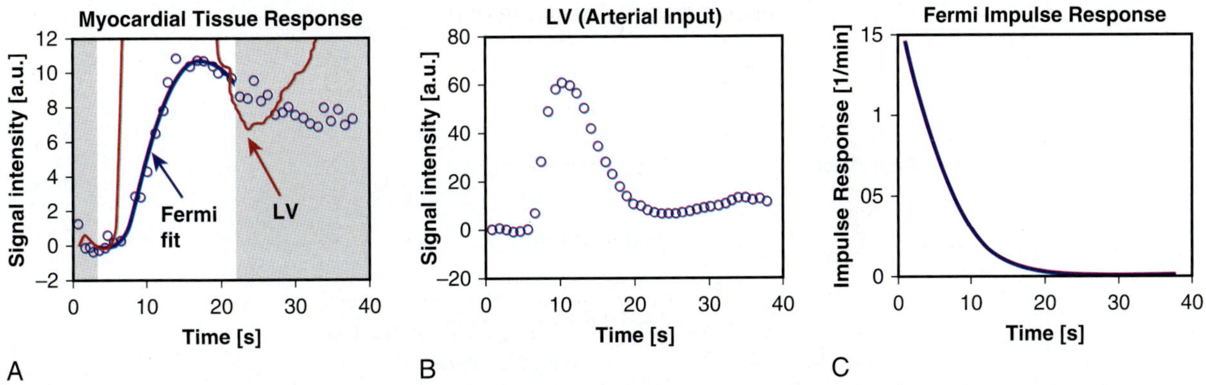

FIG. 7.14 Deconvolution of the measured signal intensity curve (*blue circles* in A) with the arterial input (B) in the left ventricle (LV) was performed with a Fermi function model of the impulse response (C). Deconvolution of the measured myocardial signal intensity curve (*blue circles*) with the arterial input shown in (B) was performed with a Fermi function model of the impulse response as in (C). The time window for the fit excluded the portion of the signal intensity curve after the first pass in the blood pool (*grayed out*). Also, the initial transition of the myocardial signal to a steady-state level, before injection of contrast, was excluded (*grayed out*). The best fit to the measured data, shown as a *solid blue line* in (A), was obtained by nonlinear least-squares fitting using a Marquardt-Levenberg algorithm in the Matlab environment (Mathworks, Natick, MA, USA). The fitting function is calculated by convolution of the Fermi function with the measured arterial input. The impulse response shape corresponding to this best fit is shown in panel (C). The myocardial blood flow is estimated from the initial amplitude of the Fermi impulse response. (From Jerosch-Herold M. Quantification of myocardial perfusion by cardiovascular magnetic resonance. *J Cardiovasc Magn Reson*. 2010;12(1):57. doi: 10.1186/1532-429X-12-57. PMID: 20932314; PMCID: PMC2964700.)

the impulse response that are consistent with the physiological basis of the contrast enhancement, rather than specifying a specific functional form:

a) The impulse response must be a monotonically decaying function of time because no additional tracer enters the tissue region after the initial contrast input, and after this initial impulse input of contrast, the concentration in tissue can only remain constant as long as all contrast remains within the region being analyzed, or decline.
b) A second condition is that the impulse response shape changes smoothly. Smoothness of the impulse response follows to the degree that the magnitudes of flow, diffusion, and permeation in the heart impose time scales that exclude abrupt signal intensity changes in myocardial tissue after contrast agent injection. Such smoothness constraints can be imposed by representing the impulse response as a sum of smooth cubic spline basis functions.

The deconvolution algorithms that use these physiological constraints without assuming a specific shape of the impulse response have been termed "model-independent" deconvolution[57] to distinguish them from the approach in which a parameterized representation of the impulse response (e.g., Fermi model) is used. The advantage of this more general approach is that extended clearance of contrast (e.g., from interstitial clearance of extracellular contrast agent) does not compromise data fitting for the quantification of MBF.

TRACER KINETIC MODELS FOR MYOCARDIAL CONTRAST ENHANCEMENT

As an alternative to the deconvolution analysis, one can build a mathematical model of tracer transport through tissue. For an extracellular contrast agent, this involves the exchange of tracer between vascular and interstitial spaces. For a lumped parameter model, which reduces the subspaces to nodes within which tracer mixes instantaneously, one neglects the spatial variation of tracer concentration (e.g., along a vascular unit from the arterial to the venous side). The advantage of such models is that they have fewer parameters than distributed models, though blood flow estimates can be biased because of this simplification. The rapid injection of a tracer will create a tracer concentration gradient from the arterial to the venous side. Spatially distributed models are described by *partial* differential equations that account for the variation of tracer concentrations within each tissue region as a function of time *and* at least one spatial variable.[58,59] The number of parameters in these models tends to be larger than with lumped models. Sensitivity analysis is needed to determine which (hopefully few) model parameters need to be adjusted for a best fit of the measured residue curves. The number of degrees of freedom can be reduced using an intravascular contrast agent.[59,60] An example of the use of a tracer kinetic model for analysis of a CMR perfusion study is shown in Fig. 7.15, including an illustration of the Central Volume Principle based on model simulations derived from a spatially distributed model of blood tissue exchange.

Up to this point, the general terms arterial input and tissue response have been used without specifying what they exactly embody. The images acquired during a CMR perfusion scan form the basis for any quantitative analysis. From the images one can generate data for regions of interest or pixel locations that depict change of signal intensity as a function of time. With a fast T1-weighted gradient echo sequence and low-contrast agent dosages (e.g., 0.03 mmol/kg of Gd-DTPA for an intravenous bolus injection into an antecubital vein), the T1-weighted signal intensity is approximately proportional to the R_1 relaxation rate. R_1 and contrast concentration (c_Gd) are exchangeable quantities for the quantitative analysis as contrast agent concentration multiplied by contrast agent relaxivity equals the R_1 relaxation rate. The units do not matter here, but the variable representing contrast enhancement should follow the same linear relationship in the tissue and blood pool with contrast

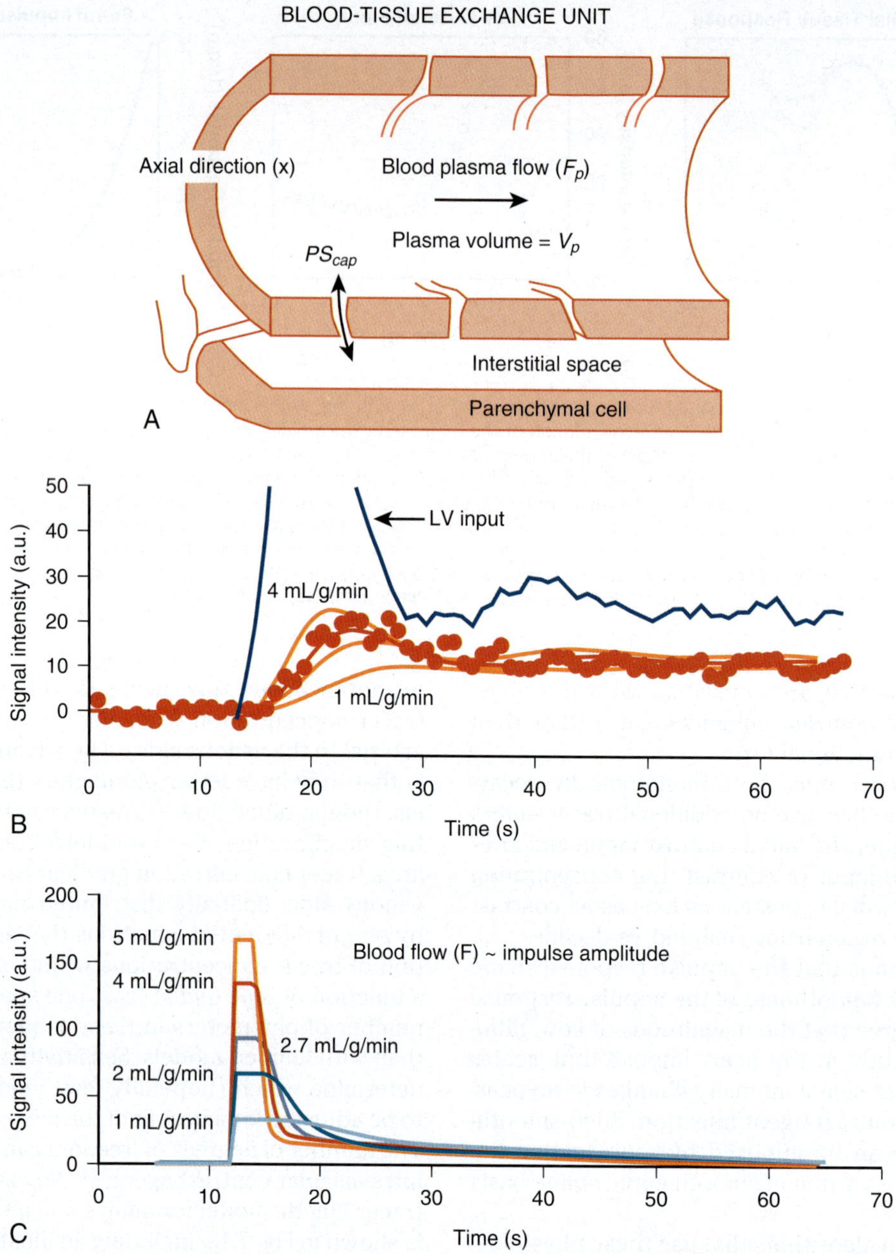

FIG. 7.15 (A) Conceptual diagram of the spatially distributed, two-region model that was implemented in the JSim simulation environment (http://www.physiome.org/jsim/) for analysis of tracer residue curves and quantification of myocardial blood flow. The following model parameters are optimized for fitting to experimental data: plasma flow (*Fp*), plasma volume (*Vp*), and capillary permeability surface area product (*PScap*). (B) A tissue contrast residue curve measured in a 56-year-old healthy female during vasodilation with adenosine *(circles)* was analyzed with the model described in A, and the best fit corresponding to a tissue blood flow of 2.8 mL/g/min is shown as a *solid line*. Additional model curves for flows of 1, 2, and 4 mL/g/min and otherwise unchanged model parameters are shown as *dashed lines* to illustrate the sensitivity of the initial contrast enhancement to blood flow. The rate of the initial contrast enhancement ("upslope") changes as the flow is varied, whereas the curves cluster together after the first pass, when sensitivity to flow changes is low. Also note that for equal increments of blood flow, the peak contrast enhancement changes less as the absolute magnitude of flow increases. (C) The measured arterial input was replaced by an impulse input, with approximately the same area under the curve. Now the amplitude of the simulated tissue response to the impulse input increases in proportion to the blood flow (F ~ impulse amplitude), as predicted by Zierler's central volume principle. *LV,* Left ventricular.

concentration—enhancement in the tissue is interpreted relative to the enhancement in the blood pool, and the units for contrast uptake effectively cancel out when tissue blood flow is estimated.

Arterial Input Function

Quantification of myocardial blood flow generally requires the measurement of an arterial input function, which serves as a reference for analysis of the myocardial contrast enhancement. Under ideal conditions the input function would be measured in a "feeding artery" adjacent to the region in the myocardium that is being analyzed to determine the tissue blood flow, but with CMR it is not feasible to reliably measure the arterial input even in the epicardial vessels. One therefore must settle for a measurement at a more upstream location, either near the aortic root or in the left ventricle.

One consequence of measuring the arterial input at a relatively large distance from the tissue region of interest is that the true arterial input is delayed compared to the true arterial input. This issue can be dealt with relatively easily by including a time-shift operator, applied to the measured arterial input, in the analysis. This arterial input delay parameter was found to be particularly noticeable in myocardial regions that depend on collateral blood supply. In fact, an abnormally delayed start of contrast enhancement in a myocardial segment, as shown in the example from a patient with a right coronary artery occlusion in Fig. 7.16, has been used to identify myocardial regions that depend significantly on blood supply through collateral vessels. In collateral-dependent segments the myocardial blood flow under resting conditions is often still within the normal range, and the delayed arrival of contrast may provide the only indication of collaterization.[61] The presence and extent of collateral circulation in the heart is associated with lower mortality in patients with chronic coronary artery disease.[62]

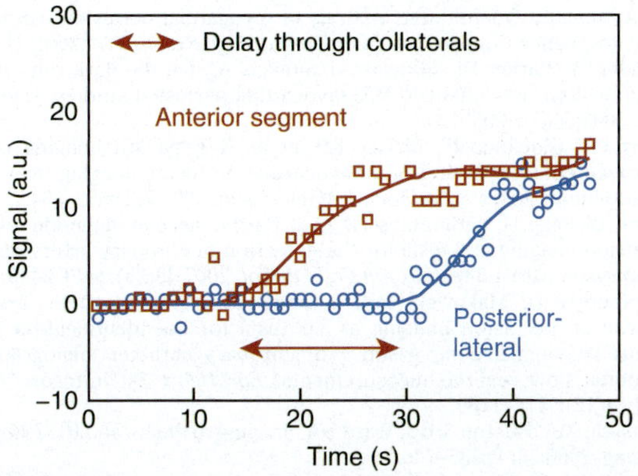

FIG. 7.16 A male patient with an occluded right coronary artery on catheter-based angiography and a right-dominant coronary distribution. A cardiovascular magnetic resonance first-pass perfusion study during resting conditions showed a significantly delayed contrast enhancement in the inferolateral and inferior segments *(blue circles)*, compared with contrast enhancement in the anterior segment *(red squares)* supplied by the left coronary artery. A quantitative analysis showed that resting blood flow was similar in these segments, suggesting that during resting conditions the delay in the arrival of the arterial input of contrast was an important marker for identifying collateral-dependent segments.

A more significant challenge for obtaining an accurate measure of the arterial input is the fact that during the transit of the arterial input from the measurement location (e.g., the center of the LV blood pool at the basal level) through the epicardial vessels one can expect that dispersion of the contrast bolus will broaden the arterial input before it enters a tissue region of interest. This is schematically illustrated in Fig. 7.17. The degree of bolus dispersion during the transit through the epicardial vessels can only be guessed or estimated from computational models. Neglecting bolus dispersion will result in an underestimation of the myocardial blood flow, because the measured arterial input is narrower and has a higher peak value than the true input. The *true* input therefore produces less contrast enhancement in a myocardial segment than would be expected for a certain tissue blood flow level based on the *measured* arterial input. Based on comparisons of estimates of myocardial blood flow obtained with the CMR first-pass technique and estimates of blood flow from injected microspheres, one can arguably conclude that the neglect of the bolus dispersion does not appear to create a major bias to underestimate myocardial blood flow under normal conditions, unless both methods would suffer from systematic bias in the same direction. In patients with bypass grafts any dispersion of the arterial input in the bypass graft appears to be small enough that at least under resting conditions it does not lead to significant bias of the

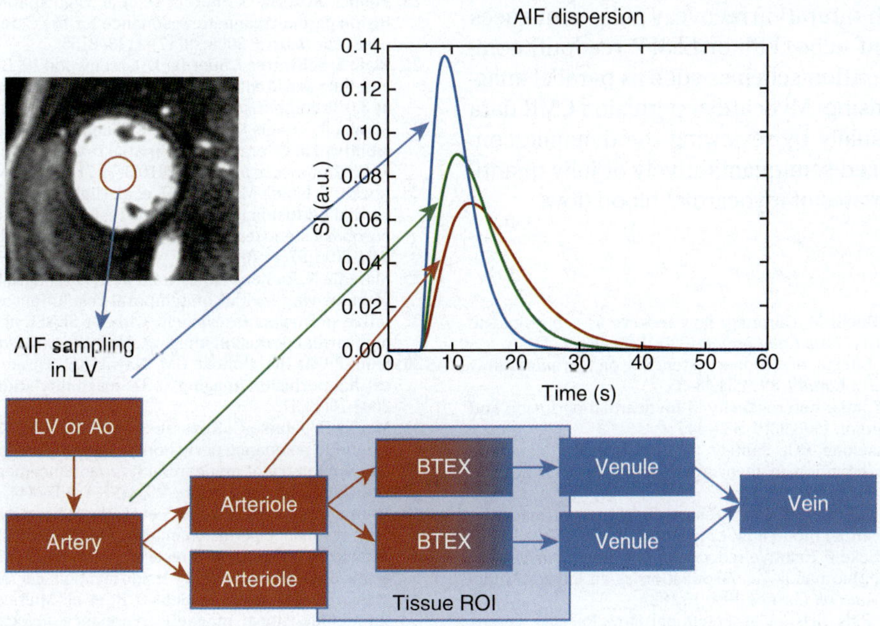

FIG. 7.17 Conceptual illustration of the change in the shape of the arterial input between the location where it is routinely measured in cardiac magnetic resonance perfusion studies (e.g., at basal level in the center of the left ventricular [*LV*] blood pool) and the tissue region of interest (*ROI*) where perfusion is quantified with the measured arterial input. Ideally, one would use the true immediate arterial input to the ROI, which, because of dispersion, is broader and has a lower peak value than the arterial input measured in the LV blood pool. Neglect of the described dispersion of the arterial input can lead to a systematic underestimate of myocardial blood flow. *Ao*, Aorta; *AIF*, arterial input function; *BTEX*, blood tissue exchange.

blood flow estimate.[63] But with a significant epicardial stenosis it is unlikely that the passage of the bolus through the vessel narrowing could not lead to some significant bolus dispersion. The uncertainties surrounding the true shape of the arterial input to a tissue region of interest therefore continue to represent a significant limitation of "first-pass" perfusion imaging. The increasing capabilities for imaging of the epicardial vessels create an opportunity to combine this information about vessel geometry with computational modeling to estimate changes in the arterial input between the LV or aorta and myocardial tissue regions of interest. Arterial spin labeling, which represents a method in which the arterial input of blood can be "shaped" by the pulse sequence, probably represents the most conceptually elegant approach to avoid uncertainties in the estimate of tissue blood flow that would result from a poorly characterized arterial input.

It may be possible in the future to control the arterial input of an injected contrast agent in a manner similar to the approach used by arterial spin labeling, or in myocardial contrast echocardiography with echogenic bubbles that can be destroyed by ultrasound pulses. For MRI, hyperpolarized contrast media [64] could be one possible approach, as it is relatively easy to selectively quench the hyperpolarized signal.

CONCLUSIONS

Myocardial perfusion assessment with CMR uses dynamic first-pass contrast-enhanced methods with injection of an exogenous gadolinium-based contrast agent. Pulse sequences for myocardial perfusion CMR must meet several competing requirements, including high contrast-to-noise ratio, high spatial and temporal resolution, and resilience to variable heart rate and hemodynamic conditions. This is typically achieved with saturation recovery pulse sequences with a spoiled gradient echo, EPI, or bSSFP readout, combined with data acceleration schemes such as parallel imaging or compressed sensing. Myocardial perfusion CMR data can be interpreted visually by reviewing the dynamic contrast passage or analyzed semiquantitatively or fully quantitatively to derive estimates of myocardial blood flow.

REFERENCES

1. Gould KL, Kirkeeide RL, Buchi M. Coronary flow reserve as a physiologic measure of stenosis severity. *J Am Coll Cardiol*. 1990;15(2):459–474.
2. Gould KL, Lipscomb K. Effects of coronary stenosis on coronary flow reserve and resistance. *Am J Cardiol*. 1974;34:48–55.
3. Decking UK, Schrader J. Spatial heterogeneity of myocardial perfusion and metabolism. *Basic Res Cardiol*. 1998;93(6):439–445.
4. Arai AE, Grauer SE, Anselone CG, Pantely GA, Bristow JD. Metabolic adaptation to a gradual reduction in myocardial blood flow. *Circulation*. 1995;92(2):244–252.
5. Bache RJ, Schwartz JS. Effect of perfusion pressure distal to a coronary stenosis on transmural myocardial blood flow. *Circulation*. 1982;65(5):928–935.
6. Canty JJ, Piotrowski B, Klocke F. Relative reductions in subendocardial and full-thickness flow during pharmacologic vasodilation as an index of functional stenosis seventy. *J Am Coll Cardiol*. 1990;15:182A.
7. Tonino PAL, Bruyne BD, Pijls NHJ, et al. Fractional Flow Reserve versus Angiography for Guiding Percutaneous Coronary Intervention. *N Engl J Med*. 2009;360(3):213–224.
8. Schwitter J, Nanz D, Kneifel S, et al. Assessment of myocardial perfusion in coronary artery disease by magnetic resonance: a comparison with positron emission tomography and coronary angiography. *Circulation*. 2001;103(18):2230–2235.
9. Wagner A, Mahrholdt H, Holly TA, et al. Contrast-enhanced MRI and routine single photon emission computed tomography (SPECT) perfusion imaging for detection of subendocardial myocardial infarcts: an imaging study. *Lancet*. 2003;361(9355):374–379.
10. Muehling OM, Panse P, Jerosch-Herold M, et al. Cardiac magnetic resonance perfusion imaging identifies transplant arteriopathy by a reduced endomyocardial resting perfusion. *J Heart Lung Transplant*. 2005;24(8):1122–1123.
11. Bolli R, Zhu W-X, Thornby JI, O'Neill PG, Roberts R. Time course and determinants of recovery of function after reversible ischemia in conscious dogs. *Am J Physiol*. 1988;254:H102–H114.
12. Tarantini G, Cacciavillani L, Corbetti F, et al. Duration of ischemia is a major determinant of transmurality and severe microvascular obstruction after primary angioplasty: a study performed with contrast-enhanced magnetic resonance. *J Am Coll Cardiol*. 2005;46(7):1229–1235.
13. Kramer CM, Barkhausen J, Bucciarelli-Ducci C, Flamm SD, Kim RJ, Nagel E. Standardized cardiovascular magnetic resonance imaging (CMR) protocols: 2020 update. *J Cardiovasc Magn Reson*. 2020;22(1):17.
14. Chong EYS, Wang H, Leung KHG, et al. Comparison of dual-bolus versus dual-sequence techniques for determining myocardial blood flow and myocardial perfusion reserve by cardiac magnetic resonance stress perfusion: From the Automated Quantitative analysis of myocardial perfusion cardiac Magnetic Resonance Consortium. *J Cardiovasc Magn Reson*. 2024;26(2):101085.
15. Di Bella EV, Parker DL, Sinusas AJ, Sinusas AJ. On the dark rim artifact in dynamic contrast-enhanced MRI myocardial perfusion studies. *Magn Reson Med*. 2005;54(5):1295–1299.
16. Araoz PA, Glockner JF, McGee KP, et al. 3 Tesla MR imaging provides improved contrast in first-pass myocardial perfusion imaging over a range of gadolinium doses. *J Cardiovasc Magn Reson*. 2005;7(3):559–564.
17. Cheng AS, Pegg Tj, Karamitsos TD, et al. Cardiovascular magnetic resonance perfusion imaging at 3-tesla for the detection of coronary artery disease: a comparison with 1.5-tesla. *J Am Coll Cardiol*. 2007;49(25):2440–2449.
18. Ebersberger U, Makowski MR, Schoepf UJ, et al. Magnetic resonance myocardial perfusion imaging at 3.0 Tesla for the identification of myocardial ischaemia: comparison with coronary catheter angiography and fractional flow reserve measurements. *Eur Heart J Cardiovasc Imaging*. 2013;14(12):1174–1180.
19. Bernstein MA, Huston 3rd J, Ward HA. Imaging artifacts at 3.0T. *J Mag Reson Imaging*. 2006;24(4):735–746.
20. Willinek WA, Gieseke J, Kukuk GM, et al. Dual-source parallel radiofrequency excitation body MR imaging compared with standard MR imaging at 3.0 T: initial clinical experience. *Radiology*. 2010;256(3):966–975.
21. Fair MJ, Gatehouse PD, DiBella EV, Firmin DN. A review of 3D first-pass, whole-heart, myocardial perfusion cardiovascular magnetic resonance. *J Cardiovasc Magn Reson*. 2015;17(1):68.
22. Motwani M, Maredia N, Fairbairn TA, et al. High-resolution versus standard-resolution cardiovascular MR myocardial perfusion imaging for the detection of coronary artery disease. *Circ Cardiovasc Imaging*. 2012;5(3):306–313.
23. Kozerke S, Plein S. Accelerated CMR using zonal, parallel and prior knowledge driven imaging methods. *J Cardiovasc Magn Reson*. 2008;10(1):29.
24. Tsao J, Kozerke S. MRI temporal acceleration techniques. *J Magn Reson Imaging*. 2012;36(3):543–560.
25. Plein S, Kozerke S, Suerder D, et al. High spatial resolution myocardial perfusion cardiac magnetic resonance for the detection of coronary artery disease. *Eur Heart J*. 2008;29(17):2148–2155.
26. Plein S, Schwitter J, Suerder D, Greenwood JP, Boesiger P, Kozerke S. k-space and time sensitivity encoding-accelerated myocardial perfusion MR imaging at 3.0 T: comparison with 1.5 T. *Radiology*. 2008;249(2):493–500.
27. Manka R, Vitanis V, Boesiger P, Flammer AJ, Plein S, Kozerke S. Clinical feasibility of accelerated, high spatial resolution myocardial perfusion imaging. *JACC Cardiovasc Imaging*. 2010;3(7):710–717.
28. Lockie T, Ishida M, Perera D, et al. High-resolution magnetic resonance myocardial perfusion imaging at 3.0-Tesla to detect hemodynamically significant coronary stenoses as determined by fractional flow reserve. *J Am Coll Cardiol*. 2011;57(1):70–75.
29. Maredia N, Radjenovic A, Kozerke S, Larghat A, Greenwood JP, Plein S. Effect of improving spatial or temporal resolution on image quality and quantitative perfusion assessment with k-t SENSE acceleration in first-pass CMR myocardial perfusion imaging. *Magn Reson Med*. 2010;64(6):1616–1624.
30. Shin T, Hu HH, Pohost GM, Nayak KS. Three dimensional first-pass myocardial perfusion imaging at 3T: feasibility study. *J Cardiovasc Magn Reson*. 2008;10(1):57.
31. Manka R, Jahnke C, Kozerke S, et al. Dynamic 3-dimensional stress cardiac magnetic resonance perfusion imaging: detection of coronary artery disease and volumetry of myocardial hypoenhancement before and after coronary stenting. *J Am Coll Cardiol*. 2011;57(4):437–444.
32. Manka R, Paetsch I, Kozerke S, et al. Whole-heart dynamic three-dimensional magnetic resonance perfusion imaging for the detection of coronary artery disease defined by fractional flow reserve: determination of volumetric myocardial ischaemic burden and coronary lesion location. *Eur Heart J*. 2012;33(16):2016–2024.
33. Manka R, Wissmann L, Gebker R, et al. Multicenter evaluation of dynamic three-dimensional magnetic resonance myocardial perfusion imaging for the detection of coronary artery disease defined by fractional flow reserve. *Circ Cardiovasc Imaging*. 2015;8(5):e003061.
34. Jogiya R, Kozerke S, Morton G, et al. Validation of dynamic 3-dimensional whole heart magnetic resonance myocardial perfusion imaging against fractional flow reserve for the detection of significant coronary artery disease. *J Am Coll Cardiol*. 2012;60(8):756–765.

35. Jogiya R, Morton G, De Silva K, et al. Ischemic burden by 3-dimensional myocardial perfusion cardiovascular magnetic resonance: comparison with myocardial perfusion scintigraphy. *Circ Cardiovasc Imaging.* 2014;7(4):647–654.
36. Plein S, Ryf S, Schwitter J, Radjenovic A, Boesiger P, Kozerke S. Dynamic contrast-enhanced myocardial perfusion MRI accelerated with k-t sense. *Magn Reson Med.* 2007;58(4):777–785.
37. Tsao J, Boesiger P, Pruessmann KP. k-t BLAST and k-t SENSE: dynamic MRI with high frame rate exploiting spatiotemporal correlations. *Magn Reson Med.* 2003;50(5):1031–1042.
38. Pedersen H, Kozerke S, Ringgaard S, Nehrke K, Kim WY. k-t PCA: temporally constrained k-t BLAST reconstruction using principal component analysis. *Magn Reson Med.* 2009;62(3):706–716.
39. Otazo R, Kim D, Axel L, Sodickson DK. Combination of compressed sensing and parallel imaging for highly accelerated first-pass cardiac perfusion MRI. *Magn Reson Med.* 2010;64(3):767–776.
40. Lustig M, Donoho D, Pauly JM. Sparse MRI: The application of compressed sensing for rapid MR imaging. *Magn Reson Med.* 2007;58(6):1182–1195.
41. Feng L, Srichai MB, Lim RP, et al. Highly accelerated real-time cardiac cine MRI using k-t SPARSE-SENSE. *Magn Reson Med.* 2013;70(1):64–74.
42. Gamper U, Boesiger P, Kozerke S. Compressed sensing in dynamic MRI. *Magn Reson Med.* 2008;59(2):365–373.
43. Jung H, Sung K, Nayak KS, Kim EY, Ye JC. k-t FOCUSS: a general compressed sensing framework for high resolution dynamic MRI. *Magn Reson Med.* 2009;61(1):103–116.
44. Ge L, Kino A, Griswold M, Mistretta C, Carr JC, Li D. Myocardial perfusion MRI with sliding-window conjugate-gradient HYPR. *Magn Reson Med.* 2009;62(4):835–839.
45. Sharif B, Dharmakumar R, LaBounty T, et al. Towards elimination of the dark-rim artifact in first-pass myocardial perfusion MRI: removing Gibbs ringing effects using optimized radial imaging. *Magn Reson Med.* 2014;72(1):124–136.
46. Christian TF, Rettmann DW, Aletras AH, et al. Absolute myocardial perfusion in canines measured by using dual-bolus first-pass MR imaging. *Radiology.* 2004;232(3):677–684.
47. Jerosch-Herold M. Quantification of myocardial perfusion by cardiovascular magnetic resonance. *J Cardiovasc Magn Reson.* 2010;12(1):57.
48. Cullen JH, Horsfield MA, Reek CR, Cherryman GR, Barnett DB, Samani NJ. A myocardial perfusion reserve index in humans using first-pass contrast-enhanced magnetic resonance imaging. *J Am Coll Cardiol.* 1999;33(5):1386–1394.
49. Klocke FJ, Simonetti OP, Judd RM, et al. Limits of detection of regional differences in vasodilated flow in viable myocardium by first-pass magnetic resonance perfusion imaging. *Circulation.* 2001;104(20):2412–2416.
50. Nagel E, Klein C, Paetsch I, et al. Magnetic resonance perfusion measurements for the noninvasive detection of coronary artery disease. *Circulation.* 2003;108(4):432–437.
51. Al-Saadi N, Nagel E, Gross M, et al. Noninvasive detection of myocardial ischemia from perfusion reserve based on cardiovascular magnetic resonance. *Circulation.* 2000;101(12):1379–1383.
52. van Dijk R, van Assen M, Vliegenthart R, de Bock GH, van der Harst P, Oudkerk M. Diagnostic performance of semi-quantitative and quantitative stress CMR perfusion analysis: a meta-analysis. *J Cardiovasc Magn Reson.* 2017;19(1):92.
53. Knott KD, Fernandes JL, Moon JC. Automated quantitative stress perfusion in a clinical routine. *Magn Reson Imaging Clin N Am.* 2019;27(3):507–520.
54. Axel L. Tissue mean transit time from dynamic computed tomography by a simple deconvolution technique. *Invest Radiol.* 1983;18(1):94–99.
55. Jerosch-Herold M, Wilke N, Stillman AE, Wilson RF. MR quantification of the myocardial perfusion reserve with a Fermi function model for constrained deconvolution. *Med Phys.* 1998;25(1):73–84.
56. Mühling OM, Wang Y, Panse P, et al. Transmyocardial laser revascularization preserves regional myocardial perfusion: an MRI first pass perfusion study. *Cardiovasc Res.* 2003;57(1):63–70.
57. Jerosch-Herold M, Swingen C, Seethamraju RT. Myocardial blood flow quantification with MRI by model-independent deconvolution. *Med Phys.* 2002;29(5):886–897.
58. Bassingthwaigthe JB, Raymond GR, Chan JIS. Principles of tracer kinetics. In: Zaret BL, Beller GA, eds. *Nuclear Cardiology: State of the Art and Future Directions.* Mosby-Year Book; 1993:3–23.
59. Kroll K, Wilke N, Jerosch-Herold M, et al. Accuracy of modeling of regional myocardial flows from residue functions of an intravascular indicator. *Am J Physiol.* 1996;40:H1643–H1655.
60. Jerosch-Herold M, Wilke N, Wang Y, et al. Direct comparison of an intravascular and an extracellular contrast agent for quantification of myocardial perfusion. *Int J Card Imaging.* 1999;15(6):453–464.
61. Muehling OM, Huber A, Cyran C, et al. The delay of contrast arrival in magnetic resonance first-pass perfusion imaging: a novel non-invasive parameter detecting collateral-dependent myocardium. *Heart.* 2007;93(7):842–847.
62. Seiler C, Engler R, Berner L, et al. Prognostic relevance of coronary collateral function: confounded or causal relationship? *Heart.* 2013;99(19):1408–1414.
63. Arnold JR, Francis JM, Karamitsos TD, et al. Myocardial perfusion imaging after coronary artery bypass surgery using cardiovascular magnetic resonance: a validation study. *Circ Cardiovasc Imaging.* 2011;4(3):312–318.
64. Johansson E, Mansson S, Wirestam R, et al. Cerebral perfusion assessment by bolus tracking using hyperpolarized 13C. *Magn Reson Med.* 2004;51(3):464–472.

8 Cardiac Magnetic Resonance Image Artifacts

MICHAEL SALERNO

INTRODUCTION

Cardiac magnetic resonance (CMR) imaging is an important diagnostic tool for evaluating the anatomy and function of the heart and cardiovascular system. Over the past 3 decades, there have been significant improvements in magnetic resonance imaging (MRI) hardware and pulse sequences that have considerably improved image quality. Despite advances in MRI technology, CMR, like all imaging techniques, can still suffer from image artifacts that can compromise image quality and reduce diagnostic accuracy. It is vital for cardiovascular imagers to be able to differentiate image artifacts from cardiovascular pathology. Understanding the etiology of specific CMR artifacts is important for determining how the artifacts can be mitigated. This chapter aims to highlight common cardiac MRI artifacts, explore their causes, and offer strategies to address them.

CMR artifacts can be characterized into different categories, as described in Table 8.1. Hardware artifacts include radiofrequency (RF) interference from equipment within the scanner room or from improper shielding of signals outside of the scanner room, or RF coil voltage spikes from improper connection of coils. Physiological artifacts can result from poor breath-holding; poor ECG gating; cardiac arrhythmias such as atrial fibrillation, atrial premature beats, or ventricular premature beats; and blood flow–related artifacts. Operator-related imaging artifacts include wrap artifacts due to improper field of view (FOV) or phase-encoding (PE) direction selection, signal dropout from improper coil selection, India-ink artifacts from improper inversion time selection for late gadolinium enhancement (LGE), and velocity aliasing artifacts due to improper velocity encoding selection. Patient-related artifacts can result from implanted metallic hardware, B_0 or B_1 inhomogeneity, or parallel imaging artifacts due to patient geometric factors. Specific pulse sequences can also have characteristic artifacts such as banding artifacts on SSFP (steady state free precession) images or dark-rim artifacts on myocardial perfusion images. Other artifacts may result from improper image registration such as in the fitting of parametric T1 or T2 maps.

Hardware-Related Artifacts

Hardware artifacts can occur when there are malfunctions of the CMR imaging hardware, or if the coils are picking up spurious signals in the radiofrequency range.

RADIOFREQUENCY INTERFERENCE ARTIFACTS

RF interference artifacts occur when the RF coils receive radiofrequency signals originating from either within or outside of the MRI shielding. The MRI scanner room is enclosed by a metallic mesh cage, which isolates the MRI scanner from outside electrical interference. Occasionally, monitoring equipment or other electronic equipment in the magnetic resonance (MR) scanner room can give off RF signals that can be detected by the scanner. The other common etiology for this artifact is not having the MRI scanner room door closed. In rare cases these types of artifacts can be indicative of a problem with the room's RF shielding. This can occur, for example, when the metal on the edges of the MRI scanner door is not making a proper connection. This artifact typically appears as one or more lines perpendicular to the frequency-encoding direction in the image (Fig. 8.1). This is because this type of interference often has a constant frequency such as 60 Hz noise originating from the AC power grid.

RADIOFREQUENCY SPIKES

When there is an RF spike that occurs during acquisition of the MRI data, there is a characteristic artifact called the corduroy artifact (Fig. 8.2). This artifact is a superposition of the actual image and the wave pattern resulting from a voltage spike at a particular location in *k*-space. Each location in *k*-space corresponds to a wave pattern in image space. The location of the *k*-space voltage spike will determine the frequency and orientation of this wave pattern. We can think of this artifact of the superposition of the actual image with the Fourier transform of the signal resulting from the voltage spike. This type of artifact sometimes occurs when an RF coil's plug is not properly inserted. Sometimes unplugging and reinserting the coil plug will resolve this artifact. In other instances, this artifact can occur with a damaged RF receive coil.

PHYSIOLOGICAL MONITORING ERRORS

Sometimes there may be issues with the physiological monitoring equipment that can cause issues with cardiac gating. Most typically these occur when one of the electrodes is not appropriately placed on the chest, or if there is poor contact with the skin such as in people who have hairy chests. Ensuring that the leads are appropriately attached to the patient will typically mitigate this issue. Sometimes moving the leads to different locations may help. Another issue with gating is the magnetohydrodynamic effect.[1] When a charged particle is moving through a magnetic field it will experience a force perpendicular to the magnetic field, and these will

TABLE 8.1 Cardiac Magnetic Resonance Artifacts and How to Fix Them.

ARTIFACTS	REMEDY
Hardware Artifacts	
RF interference artifacts	Check equipment in room; check if door is closed
RF coil voltage spikes—corduroy artifact	Make sure coils are plugged in correctly
Physiological Artifacts	
Respiratory motion artifacts	Ensure proper breath-holding, real-time imaging
Cardiac gating/triggering artifacts	Ensure proper gating, prospective, real time
Flow/ghosting artifacts	SSFP—check shim, change PE direction
Imaging Artifacts	
Operator-Related Artifacts	
Improper coil selection	Turn appropriate receive coils on
Wrap artifacts	Increase the FOV
Late gadolinium enhancement TI too short	Utilize PSIR, increase TI
Velocity-encoding aliasing artifacts	Increase velocity-encoding max velocity
Sequence-Related Artifacts	
SSFP banding artifacts	Check shim, local shim, frequency scout
Dark-rim artifacts	Check temporal and spatial resolution
Dark-blood spin echo imaging artifacts	Optimize dark-blood preparation, timing in RR interval
Patient-Related Artifacts	
Metallic implant artifacts	Utilize GRE sequences, wide-band pulses
B_0 and B_1 inhomogeneity artifacts	Gradient shimming, RF shimming
Parallel imaging artifacts	Reduce acceleration, optimize coil selection
Postprocessing Artifacts	
Motion correction artifacts	Visualize noncorrected series, repeat imaging
Poor-fitting artifacts	Visualize images and repeat imaging if needed

B_0, main magnetic Field; B_1, RF transmit field; *FOV*, field of view; *GRE*, gradient echo; *PE*, phase encoding; *RF*, radiofrequency; *RR*, R to R interval; *SSFP*, steady state free precession; *TI*, inversion time

have opposite directions depending on whether the charge is positive or negative. This effect is most prominent due to the motion of blood in the aorta. This phenomenon results in a voltage signal that will be superimposed on the ECG tracing, causing distortion of the ECG signal. This effect is directly proportional to the field strength and is typically more of a problem at 3T. Sometimes repositioning of the leads or choosing a different lead to trigger from can reduce the effect of this artifact.

Physiological Artifacts

Standard CMR images are typically acquired during breath-holding to eliminate respiratory-induced motion and using ECG gating to properly time the imaging to the cardiac cycle. Standard CMR images typically use segmented acquisitions in which part of the data is acquired in a particular phase of the cardiac cycle over multiple heartbeats during a breath-hold to create each image. Physiological artifacts manifest as ghosting and/or blurring artifacts resulting from respiratory motion due to improper breath-holding, cardiac motion due to improper ECG gating, or cardiac arrythmias during segmented acquisitions (Fig. 8.3).

RESPIRATORY MOTION ARTIFACTS

To understand respiratory motion artifacts, we need to recall image acquisition modes for cardiac MRI. Images are typically acquired in either a single shot (all *k*-space lines are acquired at one time, typically during a single heartbeat) or in a segmented mode (a subset of *k*-space lines are acquired in each heartbeat over a breath-hold). For single-shot images such as myocardial perfusion images, single-shot LGE images, or real-time cine, all of the *k*-space lines needed to make each image are typically acquired in a 50–200 ms time frame. As these times are short compared to respiratory motion, these types of images typically do not suffer from respiratory motion, which is the reason that they are used in patients with difficulty holding their breath. For segmented images, such as those used for cine, LGE, and dark-blood turbo-spin echo, a certain number of raw data lines are acquired over each heartbeat during a breath-hold. When a patient is not holding their breath, the chest will not be in the same position for each heartbeat, which will result in ghosting of the chest wall in the image. Respiratory artifacts typically lead to ghosting, which will include the heart, diaphragm, and chest wall (Fig. 8.3), whereas cardiac-related motion artifacts are typically isolated to cardiac structures. When respiratory motion artifacts are present, there are a few things to check: (1) make sure the patient has not fallen asleep, (2) make sure that the patient is able to hear the breathing instructions, (3) make sure that the patient is not moving their chest during the breath-hold, and (4) make sure the breath-hold duration is not too long for the patient. In some cases, switching between expiratory and inspiratory breath-holding may be helpful, particularly in patients that are short of breath and having difficulty holding their breath for the duration of the sequence. Reviewing the breathing instructions with the patient and reinforcing the importance of not moving their chest can also help. Other approaches may include shortening the breath-hold duration, though this will typically be at the expense of worsening temporal and/or spatial resolution. In patients with very shallow breathing, sometimes multiple acquisitions (NEX), typically 3, within free breathing will adequately average over respiratory positions, resulting in images with acceptable diagnostic image quality. In patients who are not able to hold their breath at all, free-breathing acquisition techniques can be used. Typically, these images will also have limited spatial and/or temporal resolution. More recently, techniques using respiratory navigation or self-navigation, which either gate based on or compensate for respiratory motion, can be used to acquire high-quality images during free breathing.

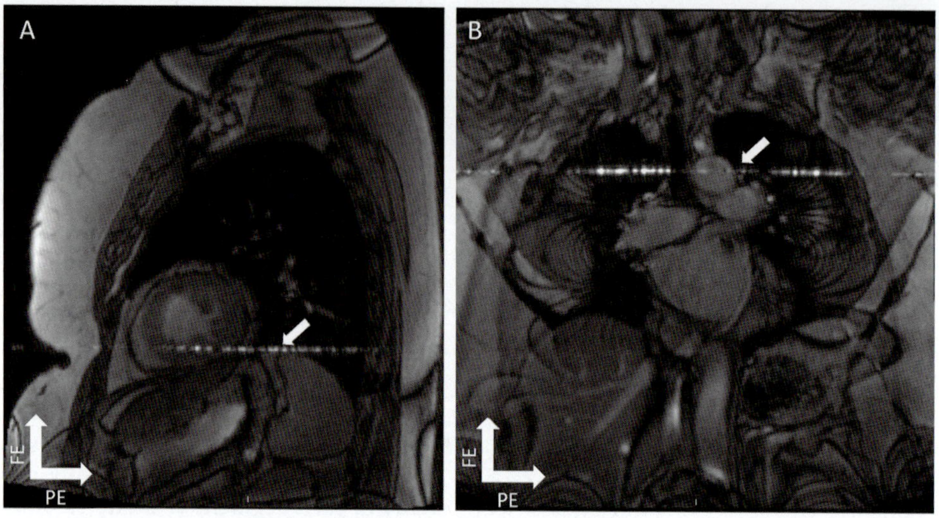

FIG. 8.1 Constant-frequency noise artifacts. (A) Sagittal image with phase encoding (*PE*) in the A–P (Anterior-Posterior) direction. Note the line in the image along the PE direction in the image perpendicular to the frequency-encoding (*FE*) direction (*arrow*) corresponding to a constant-frequency noise at a single frequency. (B) Coronal image with PE in the L-R (Left-Right) direction with a constant-frequency noise artifact (*arrow*).

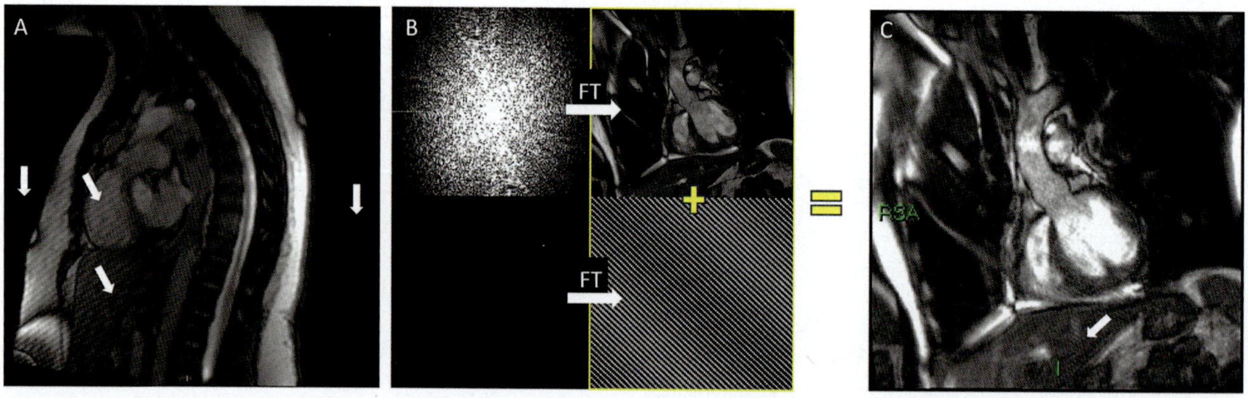

FIG. 8.2 Corduroy artifacts from radiofrequency spikes. (A) Corduroy artifacts in multiple directions resulting from multiple voltage spikes during acquisition. (B) The origin of this artifact can be understood as the superposition of the raw *k*-space data (*top*) and a bright signal occurring due to an RF voltage spike when acquiring a specific *k*-space point (*bottom*) corresponding to a particular spatial frequency. The Fourier transform (*FT*) of the raw data produces the image, while the FT of the voltage spike causes a corduroy pattern. (C) Superposition of these two images yields the image with the corduroy artifact. In this case the artifact was resolved by unplugging and replugging the RF coil connector.

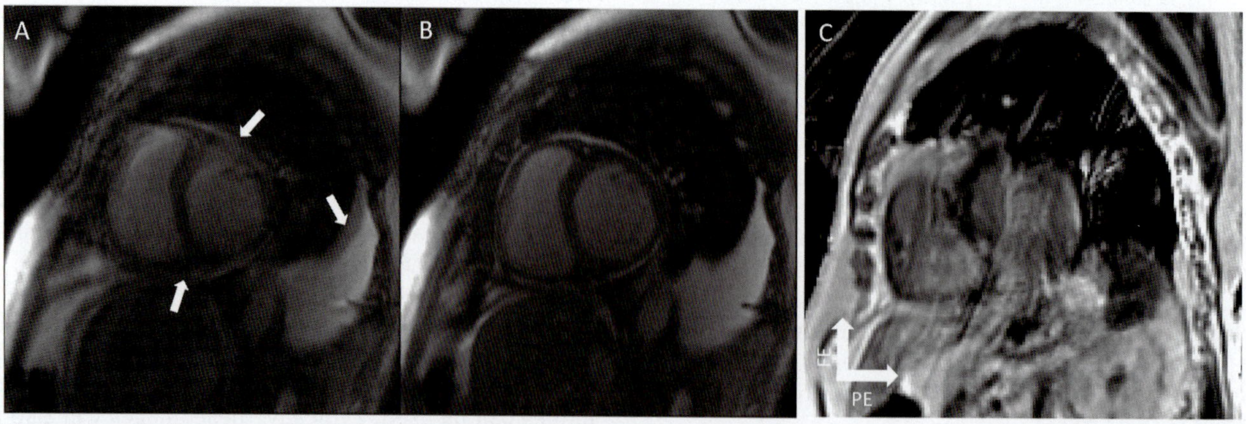

FIG. 8.3 Respiratory motion artifacts. (A) Blurring and ghosting from respiratory motion can be seen across the cine images including ghosting of the pleural effusion. (B) Acquisition was repeated with a better breath-hold resulting in resolution of these artifacts. (C) Respiratory motion artifacts in a late gadolinium enhancement image due to improper breath-holding resulting in ghosting of the chest wall across the image in the phase-encoding direction.

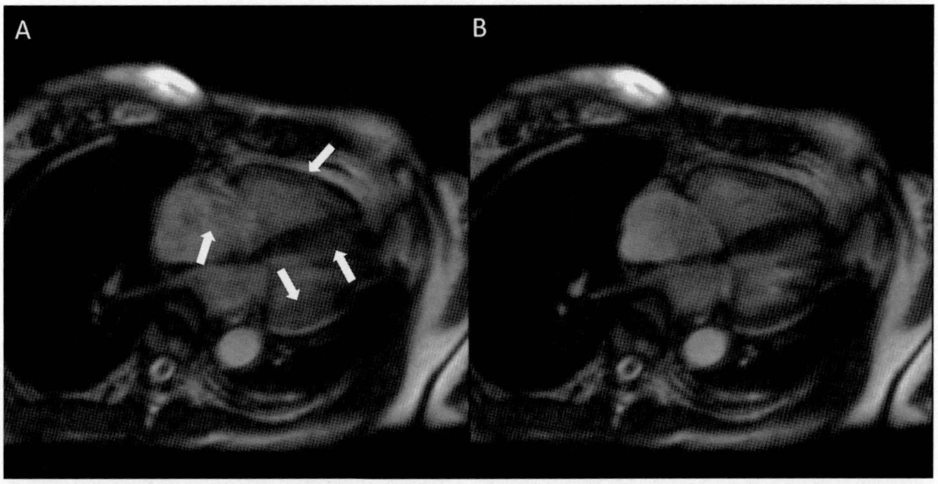

FIG. 8.4 Cardiac motion artifacts resulting from a premature ventricular contraction. (A) Blurring can be seen most obviously in the LV (left ventricle) walls, RV (right ventricle) free wall, and atrial blood pool. (B) Acquisition was repeated, showing less blurring of the ventricular walls at the same phase of the cardiac cycle.

Another sequence that is sensitive to respiratory motion is contrast-enhanced magnetic resonance angiography (MRA). For these types of acquisition, the technologist can ask the patient to take a few breaths in and out before the image acquisition, and images can be acquired on inspiration. Trying to minimize the FOV in the slice and phase direction, and choosing appropriate combinations of slice thickness, spatial resolution, and parallel imaging factor can be used to shorten the breath-hold duration.

CARDIAC MOTION ARTIFACTS

For segmented image acquisition, irregular cardiac motion can also result in ghosting artifacts (Fig. 8.4). We will briefly review retrospective versus prospective acquisition modes to explain how these types of artifacts occur. For a segmented cine image, data is acquired during multiple heartbeats during a breath-hold to create a single cine movie. In retrospective imaging, each heartbeat is divided into a fixed number of equally spaced bins, and the data from different phases of the cardiac cycle from each heartbeat will be distributed to each of the bins. During image reconstruction data from each bin will be reconstructed to provide a single frame of the cine image. This type of acquisition assumes that the heart has the same motion on each heartbeat during the acquisition. Thus, any disturbance in the cardiac rhythm could potentially result in artifacts from mismatch of the cardiac data in each bin. Typical arrythmias that can be problematic include atrial premature contractions, premature ventricular contractions, and atrial fibrillation, particularly with irregular RR intervals. Gating errors such as missed triggers will also result in ghosting artifacts for retrospective segmented cine imaging. Arrhythmia rejection techniques, which throw out data from irregular heartbeats, can be used, but typically these techniques prolong the breath-hold by the number of irregular beats. In some cases, such as atrial fibrillation with a slow ventricular response, switching to prospective imaging can be helpful to mitigate ghosting artifacts. For prospective imaging, the temporal resolution for each phase and the number of phases are fixed and chosen to be shorter than the RR duration. With irregular heart rates the systolic portion of the cycle is preserved with variation in the duration of diastole. While you cannot acquire the whole cardiac cycle with prospective imaging, these images will typically enable assessment of systolic function. Again, if adequate image quality cannot be obtained due to heart rhythm irregularities, free-breathing cine images can be acquired, typically at the expense of reductions in temporal and/or spatial resolution. Most recently, compressed sensing techniques[2] and deep-learning techniques[3] have been used to acquire high temporal and spatial resolution images within a single heartbeat or a small number of heartbeats. Free-breathing[4] and self-gated techniques[5] may also be used to mitigate cardiac motion–related artifacts.

BLOOD FLOW–RELATED ARTIFACTS

Certain types of sequences can be sensitive to effects from blood flow. SSFP cine sequences can have flow-related artifacts, particularly in the setting of off-resonance.[6] Flow voids seen in turbulent flows resulting from valvular stenosis or regurgitation result from dephasing of the transverse magnetization, resulting in signal loss. For the off-resonance SSFP flow artifacts, using a localized shim can sometimes mitigate the artifacts. For gradient echo images, minimizing the echo time (TE) will typically reduce the appearance of dephasing artifacts. Ghosting artifacts can also be seen when acquiring GRE (gradient echo) images with very long echo times such as for T2* mapping.

Imaging Artifacts

OPERATOR-RELATED ARTIFACTS

Some artifacts can result from improper parameter choices made in the user interface. Many of these artifacts can be resolved by adjusting parameters in the user interface and repeating the imaging.

IMPROPER COIL SELECTION

In some cases, the user may inadvertently shut off or misselect coil elements of a phased array coil. As phased-array

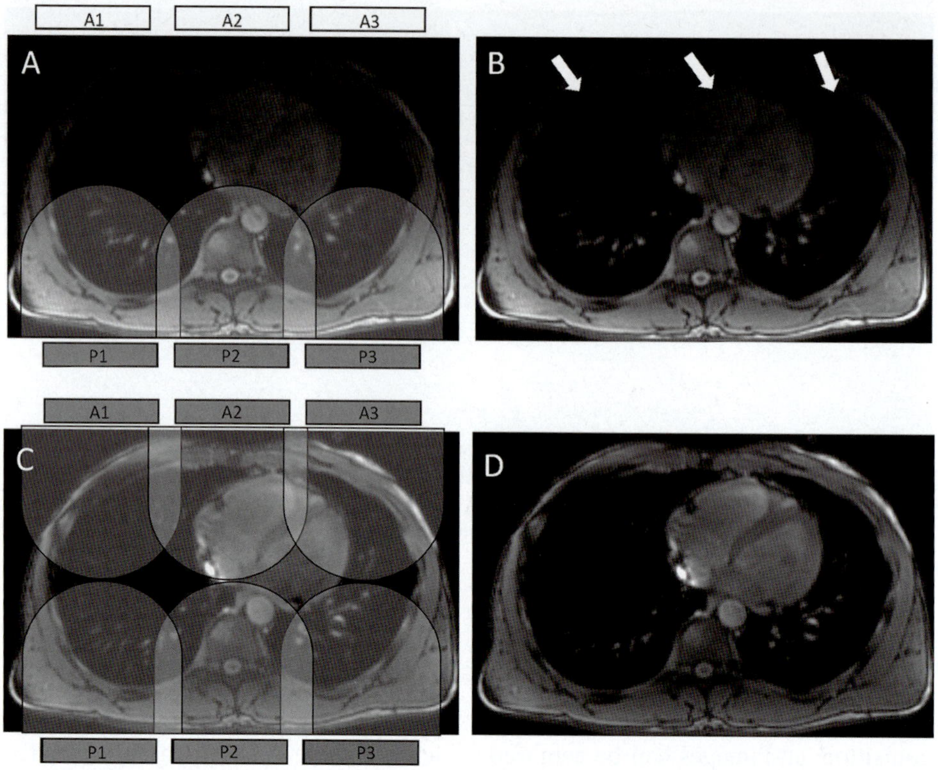

FIG. 8.5 Improper coil selection. (A) The image was acquired with the anterior coil elements (A1–A3) off, but with the posterior coil elements (P1–P3) turned on. (B) This results in lower signal intensity in the anterior region of the body. (C) By turning on the anterior and posterior coil elements, (D) the signal is more uniform throughout the imaged region.

coils have multiple coil elements, each with differing localized sensitivity regions, the signal will be darker in regions that are remote from the coil elements (Fig. 8.5). This can also occasionally occur when the plug from the phased array coil is not plugged in properly. This problem can usually be resolved by choosing the correct coils in the user interface.

WRAP ARTIFACTS

Wrap artifacts occur when the chosen FOV in the PE direction is too small, resulting in aliasing of the image (Fig. 8.6A,B). Typically, this will appear as the back of the body wrapping around into the front of the image or vice versa. Due to the discrete Fourier transform that is used for image reconstruction, the image is periodic in the image domain with a spacing equal to the FOV. This means that if the body is larger than the FOV in the PE direction, the signal will alias into the FOV in this direction. This artifact can be alleviated by increasing the FOV in the PE direction, or by utilizing phase oversampling. It is important to note that increasing the FOV in the PE direction increases the amount of data that needs to be acquired to create the image, which is proportional to the chosen FOV in the PE direction. Phase oversampling eliminates aliasing by increasing the effective FOV in the PE direction, thus this additional time also needs to be considered. Of note, wrap artifacts in practice occur only in the PE direction. In the readout direction, the FOV can be extended by increasing the sampling frequency of the ADC (analog to digital converter) without any time penalty. Typically, twofold oversampling is utilized in the readout direction, which results in 2× the FOV in the frequency-encoding direction. During image reconstruction the FOV in the frequency-encoding direction is reduced to the desired FOV. A similar related artifact is the "Phantom arm" artifact, which can result when the arm is outside of the FOV and aliases into the FOV, as can particularly be seen on oblique short-axis images (Fig. 8.6C,D). Sometimes this artifact can be mitigated by rotating the FOV slightly counterclockwise, which can move the arm out of the slice plane. Another FOV artifact that can occur is aliasing of misencoded signal from the edges of the FOV where the gradients are nonlinear. These will result in aliasing of distorted signals from the edge of the FOV. This can typically be mitigated by increasing the FOV.

LATE GADOLINIUM ENHANCEMENT INVERSION TIME-RELATED ARTIFACTS

LGE images are acquired using an inversion recovery (IR) pulse sequence, which imparts T1-weighted contrast in the image.[7] Following the inversion, the magnetization is initially negative, then passes through its null point where its magnitude is zero, and then becomes positive as it recovers to equilibrium. Typically, the inversion time is set to null the normal myocardium, as this is the point in the curve that maximizes the contrast between the myocardium and scar. The inversion time that will null the myocardial signal can be approximated using a technique called a TI (inversion time) scout or Cine-IR. A TI scout obtains images at multiple points along the T1-recovery curve and a time after the myocardium is black is chosen for the subsequent delayed-enhancement images. Artifacts

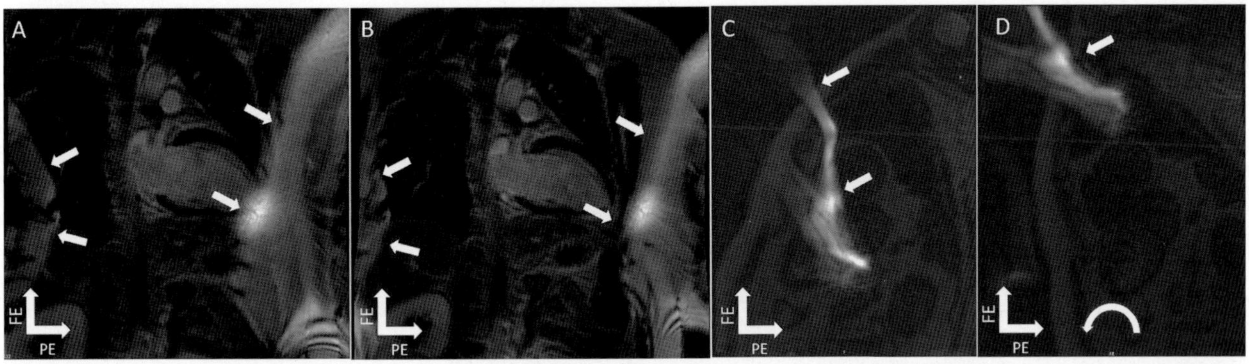

FIG. 8.6 Wrap artifacts. (A) Two-chamber late gadolinium enhancement image with wrap covering the apex of the left ventricle. (B) The field of view (FOV) was increased, eliminating the wrap over the LV apex. (C) Phantom arm wrap artifact on a short-axis perfusion image. (D) In this case, the location of the wrap from the arm was displaced to a different location by rotating the FOV counterclockwise. *FE*, frequency encoding; *PE*, phase encoding.

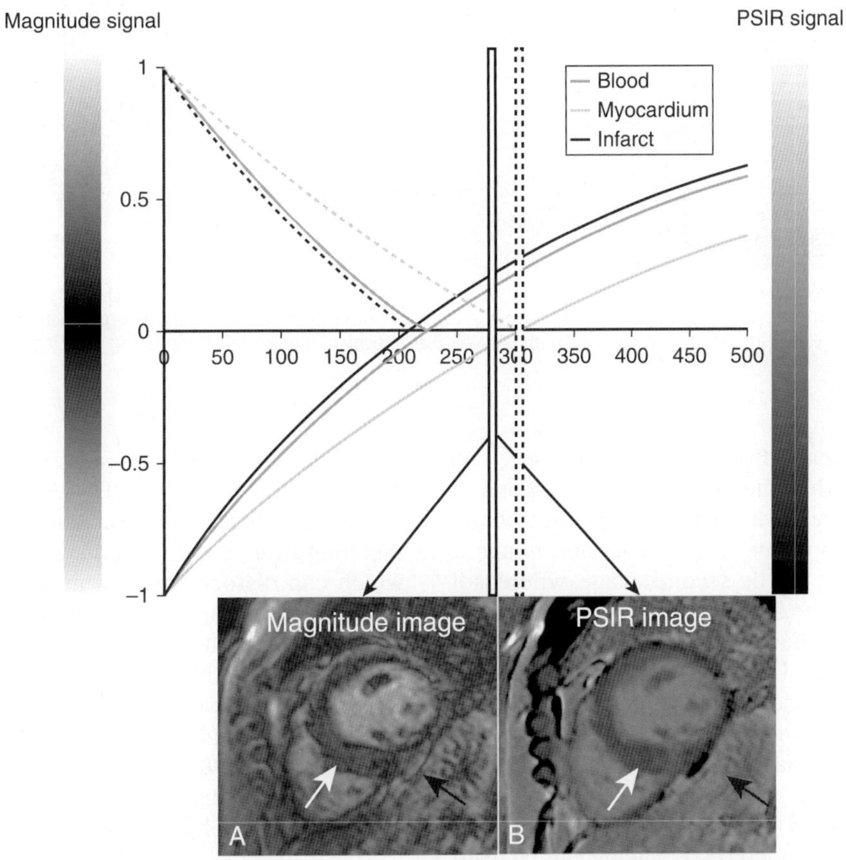

FIG. 8.7 Inversion recovery curves for blood, myocardium, and infarct show recovery of longitudinal magnetization following an inversion pulse. Note the signal in the magnitude image (*dotted line*) is the absolute value of the magnetization so both +1 and −1 will be white (*scale on left*). (A) If the inversion time is set shorter than the null of the myocardium it will appear bright on the magnitude image (*white arrow*) and can be mistaken for fibrosis. (B) Phase-sensitive inversion recovery (*PSIR*) restores the polarity of the magnetization such that +1 will be bright whereas −1 will be black (*scale on right*). The artifactual signal seen in A is corrected in the PSIR image. Note this could also be corrected by increasing the inversion time to properly null the myocardium (*dotted box*).

can occur in magnitude LGE images when the inversion time is set shorter than the null time of the myocardium and the myocardial magnetization is negative (Fig. 8.7) In the magnitude image, both negative and positive magnetization will appear bright in the image, and the bright signal can be mistaken for scar in the myocardium. This problem can be resolved by increasing the inversion time such that the myocardium has passed its null point, or by utilizing phase-sensitive inversion recovery techniques that restore the polarity of the signal, eliminating this artifact.[8] For PSIR (phase sensitive inversion recovery), an inversion pulse is played followed by a TI and an image is acquired in the diastolic phase of the same cardiac cycle. In the following heartbeat, an image is acquired in the same diastolic

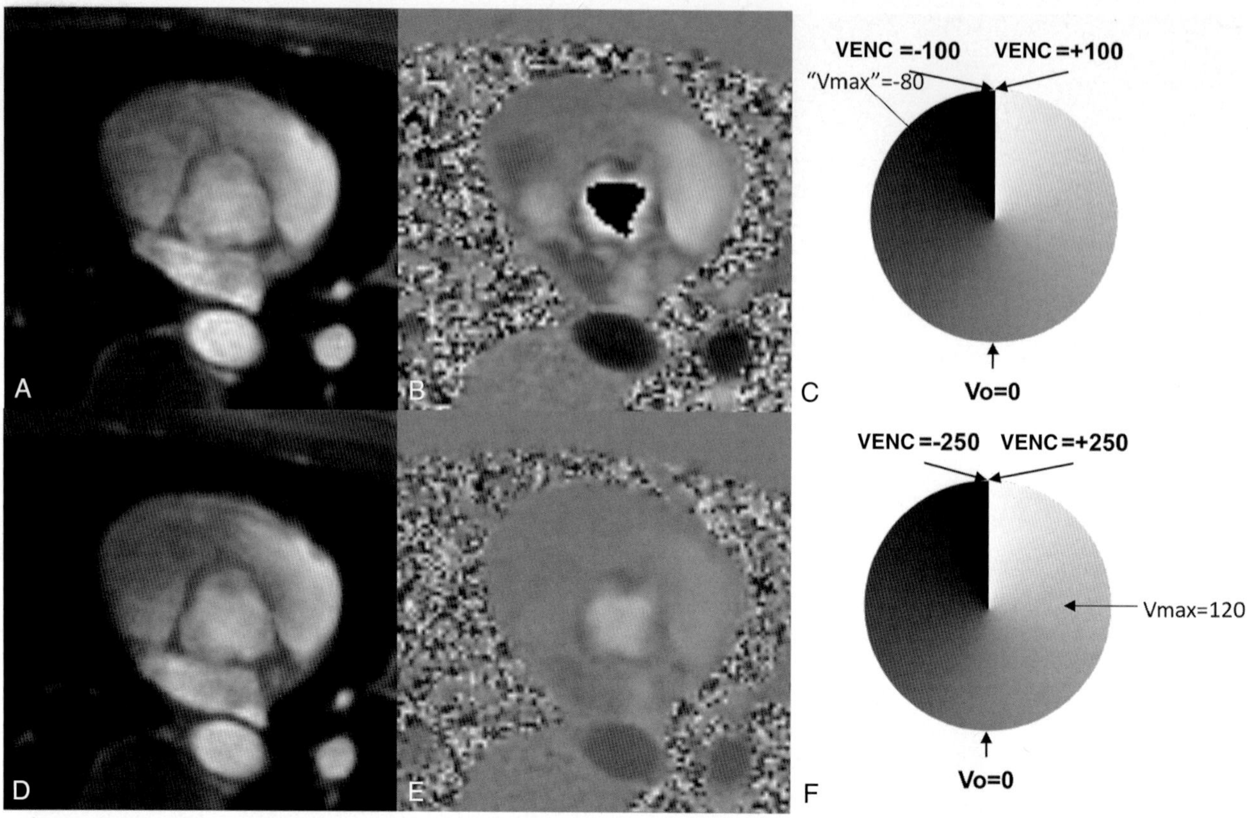

FIG. 8.8 Maximum encoding velocity (*VENC*) set too low. (A) Magnitude and (B) phase velocity image with VENC = 100 cm/s. (C) As the velocity is over 100 cm/s across the aortic valve there is aliasing, with an apparent peak velocity of −80 cm/s showing as a black region within the aortic valve during systole. (D) Magnitude and (E) phase velocity image with VENC = 250 cm/c. (F) As the velocity is lower than the aliasing velocity, the aortic valve has continuous positive velocities during systole.

phase without the application of the inversion pulse. The assumption for PSIR is that the signal from all regions of the image will be positive during the second image acquisition. If its signal was positive on the inversion image it will have the same phase on the second image, whereas if the signal is negative on the first image and positive on the second image, the signal phase between the images will be approximately 180 degrees. In this way the signal polarity can be corrected in the phase-sensitive image. Of note, the TI that nulls myocardium will still be optimal in terms of contrast to noise for both magnitude IR and PSIR.

VELOCITY-ENCODING ARTIFACTS

Phase contrast velocity-encoded (PC) imaging can be used to assess blood flow and velocities within the myocardium and cavities.[9] PC encodes the velocity in a chosen direction in the phase of the MRI signal. For typical CMR images, the magnitude of the signal is what is visualized. However, for PC images, the phase images are visualized to look at the direction and magnitude of velocity. When using PC velocity-encoding imaging, aliasing artifacts in the phase images can occur from improper selection of the maximum encoding velocity (Fig. 8.8). The maximum encoding velocity (VENC) determines the maximum velocity that can be faithfully visualized on the phase contrast images without aliasing. The aliasing in the velocities is periodic in +/- VENC. This artifact can be seen as a strong negative flow in the middle of a positive flow, such as can be seen in the ascending aorta in the presence of aortic stenosis where flow velocities are increased. This artifact can be eliminated by increasing the VENC. Other artifacts that can be problematic for velocity imaging are off-resonance artifacts resulting from metallic implants such as prosthetic valves, which can distort the local magnetic field and cause artifacts in the measured velocity. In patients with prosthetic valves, the flow may need to be measured away from the valve such as in the ascending aorta for patients with prosthetic aortic valves. Other artifacts include effects from eddy currents and concomitant magnetic fields, which are often corrected during postprocessing by fitting a bias field to the static background tissue. Errors in these corrections can also result in bias of the measured velocity values.

Other Pulse Sequence–Related Artifacts

STEADY-STATE FREE PRECESSION-RELATED ARTIFACTS

SSFP pulse sequences are frequently used for CMR due to their high signal-to-noise ratio and high contrast between the myocardium and blood pool.[10] However, SSFP pulse sequences are particularly sensitive to off-resonance effects (Fig. 8.9). For SSFP there is a periodic modulation of the signal intensity as a function of resonance frequency with periodic nulls in the signal response, which can appear as dark bands in SSFP images (Fig. 8.9A,B).[10] The frequency separation between bands is inversely proportional to the repetition time (TR) between the acquisition RF pulses (Fig. 8.9A). This means that the appearance of

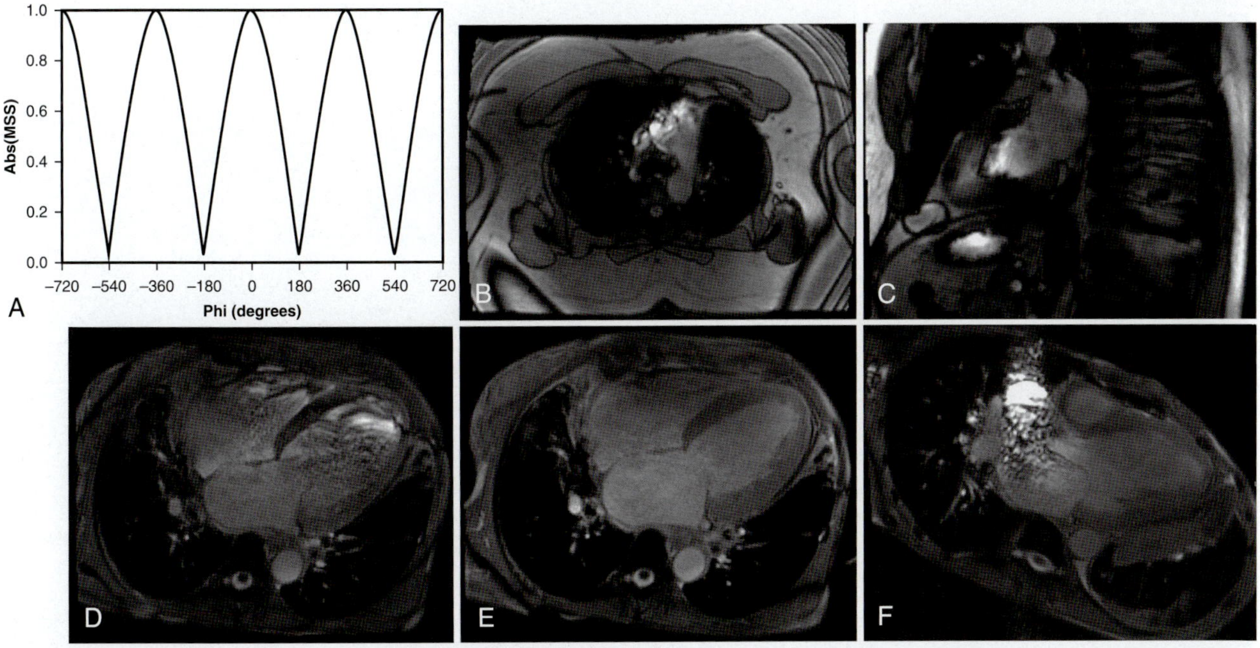

FIG. 8.9 SSFP (steady state free precession) artifacts: (A) SSFP demonstrates a periodic signal response as a function of the off-resonance frequency. (B) In regions of steep magnetic field gradients, the bands appear close together, similar to a topographic map. Sometimes banding artifacts (C) or other SSFP artifacts (D) will obscure anatomy of interest. This can be mitigated by either localized shimming to make the magnetic field more homogeneous or shifting the center frequency (E) so that the SSFP artifacts are outside of the anatomy of interest. (F) Flow can cause coherent ghosting artifacts in regions of field inhomogeneity.

banding artifacts will be worse for sequences with longer TRs or at higher field strengths. Banding artifacts are more severe and more closely spaced when there are strong gradients in the background magnetic field, such as near the edges of the subject (Fig. 8.9B), near air-filled structures, and near metallic implants. Banding artifacts can sometimes be reduced or eliminated across the region of interest by utilizing localized shimming. This reduces banding artifacts by making the field more homogeneous so there is less off-resonance frequency variation across the desired part of the image. A second approach is to use a frequency scout, which obtains images at multiple off-resonance frequencies, typically ranging from -500 to 500 Hz off-resonance. The images can be viewed and the frequency offset with the least banding over the anatomy of interest, which can be selected and set for the pulse sequence (Fig. 8.9D,E). This approach does not lessen the background off-resonance frequencies, but instead shifts the frequency offset of the null so it is not over the anatomy of interest. As mentioned in the prior section, significant magnetic field variations can also cause flow-related artifacts (Fig. 8.9F). SSFP images are also sensitive to off-resonance and out-of-plane flow as described for physiological artifacts above. Again, this can usually be lessened by localized shimming.

PERFUSION DARK-RIM ARTIFACTS

Dark-rim artifacts (DRA) can appear as a subendocardial dark region that can be mistaken for a myocardial perfusion abnormality. Although the reasons for this artifact are multifactorial and can include effects related to off-resonance and Gibbs ringing due to limited spatial resolution, the major contributor to this artifact is the interaction between linear data collection and cardiac motion.[11] It has been shown that an edge moving at a constant velocity can result in a bandlike dark artifact, and this has subsequently also been demonstrated for cardiac imaging.[12] The main ways to mitigate the dark rim artifacts (DRA) are to acquire images with a high spatial resolution (typically <2.5 mm) and to utilize a short temporal footprint (typically <120 ms) to acquire each image. Of note, the DRA may appear slightly different at stress compared to rest as there is increased contractility and hence increased cardiac motion (Fig. 8.10). The DRA can also vary at different parts of the cardiac cycle and is typically worse during systole compared to diastole. Shorter temporal footprints can be achieved by increasing the bandwidth, utilizing asymmetric echo (both reduce TR), or reducing the number of phase-encoding lines using parallel imaging or a rectangular FOV. Non-Cartesian pulse sequences such as radial and spiral techniques can also reduce this artifact as they acquire the image data using different trajectories that are less sensitive to cardiac motion.[13] However, these techniques are not widely available clinically and have sensitivities to other factors such as off-resonance.

DARK-BLOOD TURBO SPIN ECHO IMAGING ARTIFACTS

Dark-blood turbo spin echo pulse sequences are typically used for anatomic imaging and can suffer from multiple types of artifacts.[14] These pulse sequences are sensitive to cardiac motion and thus are typically acquired in quiescent parts of the cardiac cycle. These artifacts typically manifest as signal dropout or signal variations and may complicate assessment of T2 weighting. A second artifact results in incomplete suppression of signal in the cavity due to the dark-blood preparation. The dark-blood preparation consists of a nonselective inversion pulse to impart T1 weighting of the blood, followed by a slice-selective

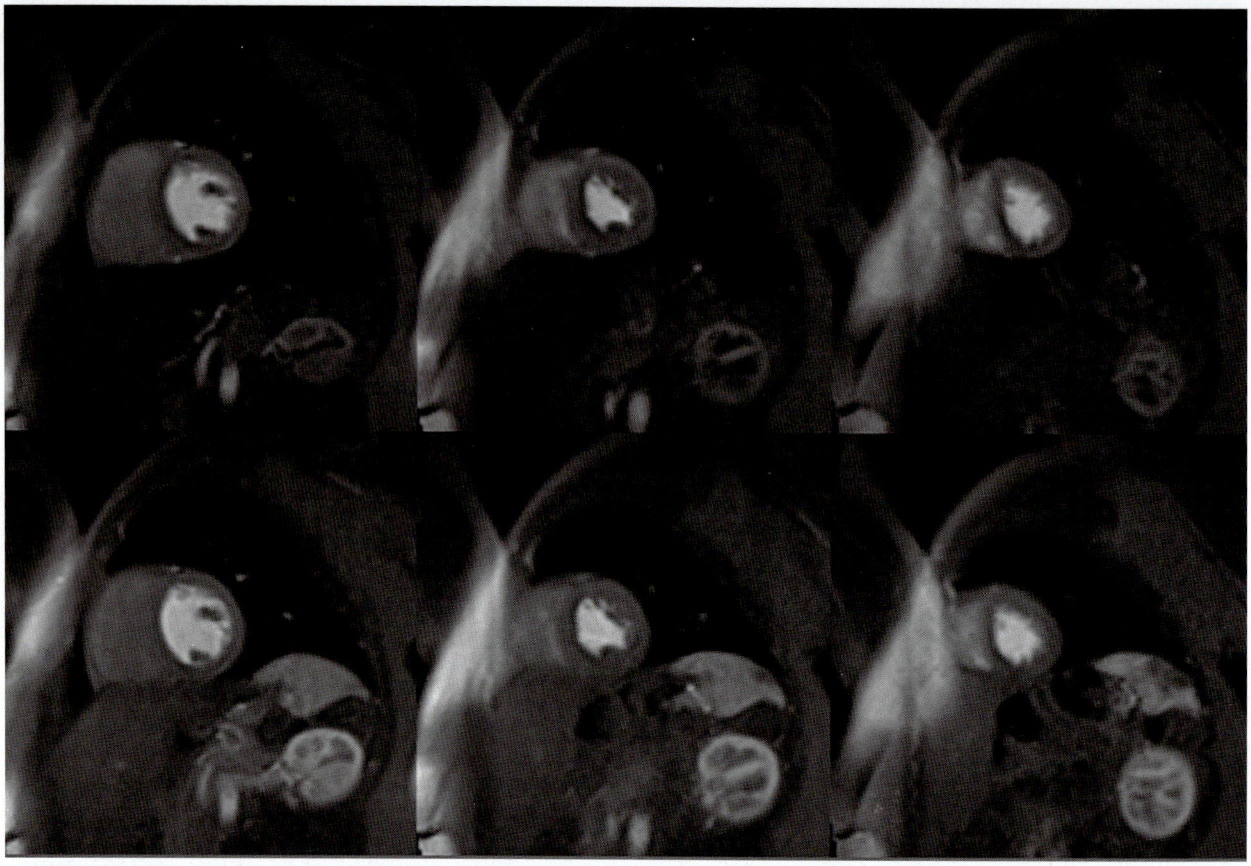

FIG. 8.10 Dark-rim artifacts. Stress images (*top row*) show an endocardial dark signal that is circumferential and more prominent along the phase-encoding direction. On the most basal slice the adjacent blood pool also appears black. At rest (*bottom row*) similar defects are seen, but of note appear somewhat less pronounced. These images are from a normal volunteer and are consistent with dark-rim artifacts rather than true perfusion defects.

inversion pulse on the slice of interest (Fig. 8.11A). Following this preparation, the longitudinal magnetization within the slice of interest (including the blood pool and myocardium) effectively has been restored to its initial magnetization. A period corresponding to the null time of the blood outside of the slice of interest then elapses during which the blood inside the slice of interest flows out of the slice, while inverted blood from outside of the slice flows into the slice of interest. Imaging commences at this time and the signal from the blood pool will be nulled and appear black. In regions of slow flow, such as in regions of cardiac dysfunction or hypertrabeculation, the signal may appear bright in the blood pool due to failure of reinverted blood failing to leave the slice of interest (Fig. 8.8B). This effect is also worse for long-axis images compared to short-axis images because the flow is not perpendicular to the slice of interest, and is worse in regions of cardiac dysfunction, as in this patient with takotsubo cardiomyopathy (Fig. 8.11B–D).

METALLIC IMPLANT ARTIFACTS

Implanted hardware such as cardiac pacemakers, ICDs (implantable cardiac defibrillator), and devices such as mitral clips can significantly impact magnetic field inhomogeneity, resulting in significant signal drop-out artifacts, particularly for SSFP-based pulse sequences (Fig. 8.12A,B). Utilization of turbo spin echo anatomic imaging and gradient-echo cine imaging can significantly reduce these artifacts. For patients with pacemakers or ICDs, having the patient put their arm above their head can move the device away from the heart, significantly reducing signal drop-out artifacts.

A second issue that arises when imaging patients with pacemakers and ICDs is improper inversion for LGE images, resulting in significant artifacts that can be mistaken for myocardial fibrosis or can obscure segments of myocardium. This effect is due to the large range of off-resonance frequencies due to the metallic implant. This type of artifact can be mitigated using so-called wide-band LGE pulse sequences.[15] These techniques use an inversion pulse, which is robust over a wide band of off-resonance frequencies. These types of sequences are available from all vendors and have become standard of care for imaging patients with pacemakers and ICDs. Similarly, wide-band inversion pulses can also be used for myocardial T1 mapping.[16]

B1 INHOMOGENEITY ARTIFACTS

At higher field strengths the RF field and resulting B_1 field can also have inhomogeneities. Most 3T systems have multiple RF transmitters, which allows for B_1 shimming. In certain patients, such as those with large pleural or pericardial effusions or in some larger patients, there may be signal variations due to differences in B_1, resulting in

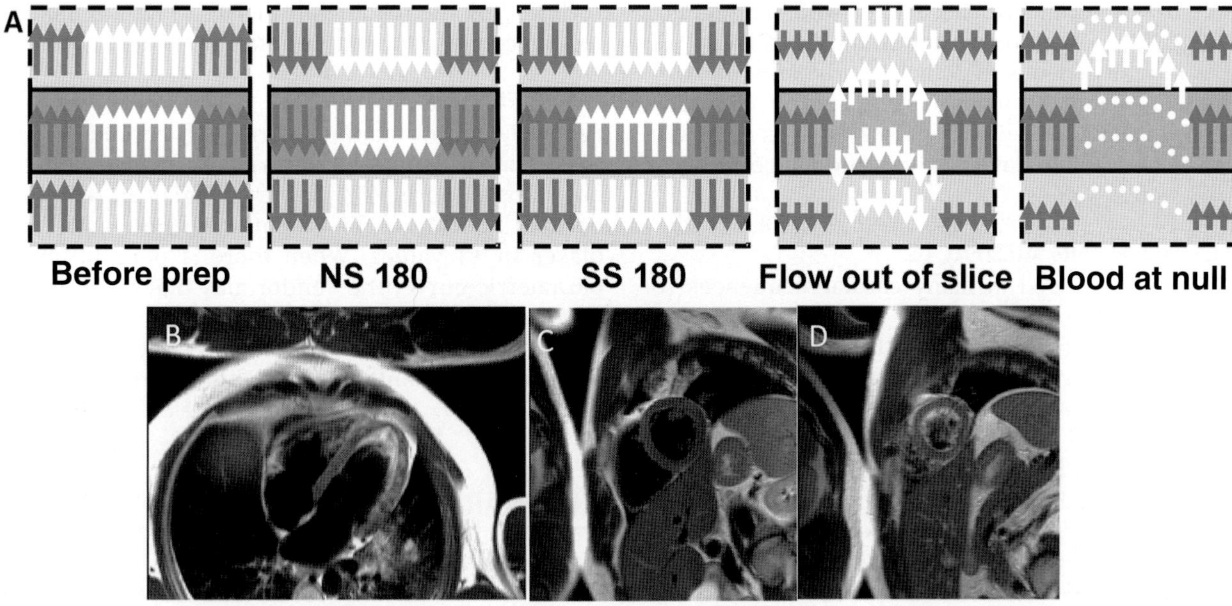

FIG. 8.11 (A) Dark-blood preparation. Before the preparation both myocardial (*gray*) and blood-pool magnetization are fully recovered to equilibrium. Slice of interest is shown in *light gray*. Following the nonselective inversion pulse, all magnetization is inverted. The slice-selective inversion restores the magnetization in the slice of interest. During an inversion recovery time, blood from outside of the slice of interest moves into the slice of interest and blood in the slice of interest flows out of the slice. At the inversion time for the blood, all of the blood from outside of the slice that has flowed into the slice of interest will be at null and will appear black in the image. (B) In a case where there is reduced flow, such as this patient with takotsubo cardiomyopathy, there can be a bright signal artifact resulting from slow flow of reinverted blood out of the slice of interest, particularly for in-plane magnetization. This tends to be worse for long-axis images compared to short-axis images (C–D). *NS*, non-selective; *SS*, slice selective.

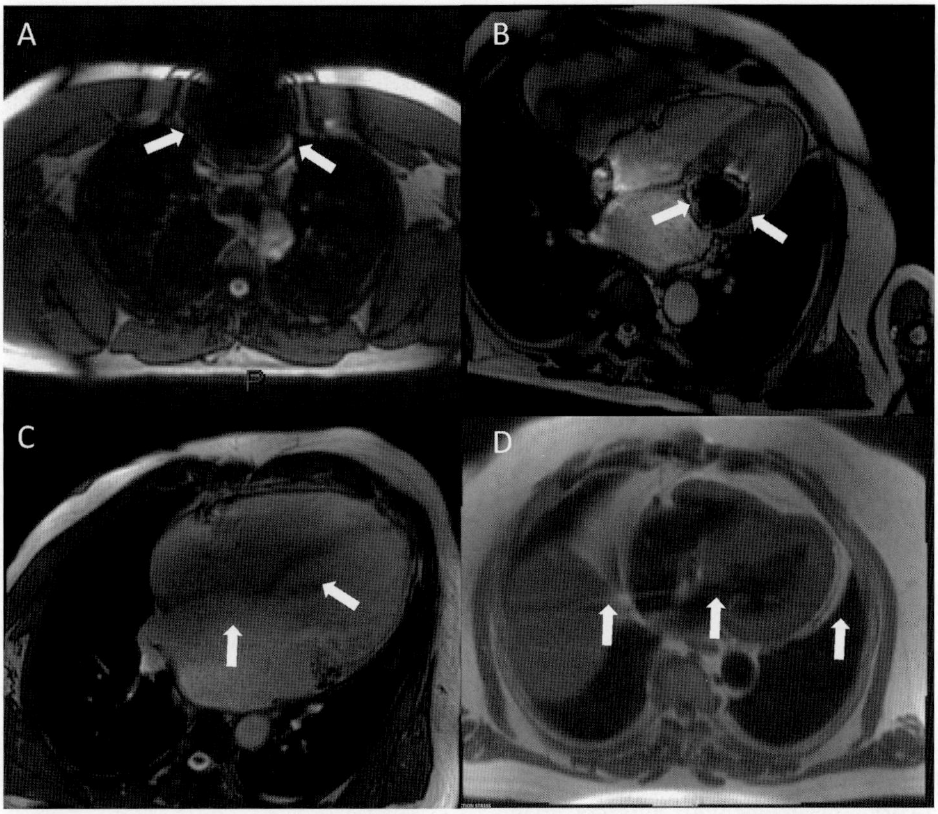

FIG. 8.12 Miscellaneous artifacts. (A) Signal void from sternal wires. (B) Signal void from mitral clip. (C) Shading artifact from B_1 inhomogeneity in a large patient at 3 T. (D) Parallel imaging artifact shows high-frequency aliasing of the chest wall.

different parts of the image being excited with different flip angles (Fig. 8.12C). The other manifestation of this type of artifact is inhomogeneous IR, which can be seen as hazy signal in delayed-enhancement images. This effect can be mitigated by using B_1-insensitive pulses, such as adiabatic inversion pulses, which have better performance across a range of B_1 and B_0 values.

PARALLEL IMAGING ARTIFACTS

Parallel imaging is used in many cardiac sequences to reduce the number of lines needed to acquire an image. The acceleration factor describes the reduction in the number of lines that needs to be acquired. For example, if the matrix was 256, with parallel imaging at R = 2, only 128 lines would need to be acquired (assuming that data for calibration is acquired separately). In the simplest form, this is achieved by sampling every other raw data line in *k*-space. As the spacing between the lines in *k*-space determines the FOV, this would result in a reduction of the FOV in the PE direction by a factor of 2. If the images were visualized without using parallel imaging there would be aliasing in the image. Parallel imaging uses the fact that each coil in a phased-array coil has a slightly different sensitivity over the imaged volume. This information can be used to unalias the images, resulting in images that have an original unaliased FOV. This is how SENSE (sensitivity encoding)-based parallel imaging works. Sometimes, high-frequency/high-amplitude signal from the chest wall will not be adequately dealiased (Fig. 8.12C,D). This artifact is more likely to be seen when the PE direction is anterior-posterior, particularly in larger patients because there is less coil overlap and variation along this direction. This can typically be mitigated by decreasing the parallel imaging acceleration factor. For *k*-space–based parallel imaging such as GeneRalized Autocalibrating Partial Parallel Acquisition (GRAPPA) or related techniques, the main effect of parallel imaging will be noise enhancement in the image, which varies spatially due to the coil configuration. This enhancement in noise is characterized by the G-factor of the phased-array coil. The severity of this noise enhancement will increase with the acceleration factor. If this noise is particularly problematic over a region of interest, it can be reduced by decreasing the parallel imaging factor and can sometimes be moved in the image by changing the FOV or rotating the PE direction.

Postprocessing Artifacts

MOTION CORRECTION ARTIFACTS T1, T2, AND T2* MAPPING

Pixelwise mapping of myocardial T1, T2, and T2* have become important components of a comprehensive CMR exam. To perform pixelwise maps, the anatomy must be stationary across a series of images with different image weighting. If the patient has inadequate breath-holding, or if the images are acquired during free breathing, then motion correction is mandatory. Motion artifacts are best determined by looking at the raw weighted images that were used to create the parametric maps. Images without and with motion correction should ideally be provided and reviewed by the reading physician. Failure of motion correction can result in biases in the T1 values.

POOR-FITTING ARTIFACTS

Secondly, for T1 mapping care must be taken to ensure that there is accurate triggering so that heartbeats are not skipped during the IR curve. This can result in suboptimal spacing of T1-weighted images, again causing biases in T1 values. When there is poor fitting of the parametric curve, the vendor may black out pixels that have poor fitting. This can manifest as an image with a bunch of small holes or black pixels. Images with poor fitting or significant uncorrectable motion artifacts must be reacquired.

SUMMARY

In this chapter we have summarized the major cardiac MRI artifacts that may result from a variety of factors. Specifically, we discussed hardware artifacts, physiologic artifacts, user-related artifacts, specific sequence-related artifacts, and postprocessing artifacts. Recognition of artifacts is paramount to both differentiate artifacts from cardiac pathology and to optimize acquisition to minimize or eliminate imaging artifacts.

REFERENCES

1. Dimick RN, Hedlund LW, Herfkens RJ, Fram EK, Utz J. Optimizing electrocardiograph electrode placement for cardiac-gated magnetic resonance imaging. *Investig Radiol*. 1987;22:17–22.
2. Lin ACW, Strugnell W, Riley R, et al. Higher resolution cine imaging with compressed sensing for accelerated clinical left ventricular evaluation. *J Magn Reson Imaging*. 2017;45:1693–1699.
3. Monteuuis D, Bouzerar R, Dantoing C, Poujol J, Bohbot Y, Renard C. Prospective comparison of free-breathing accelerated cine deep learning reconstruction versus standard breath-hold cardiac mri sequences in patients with ischemic heart disease. *AJR Am J Roentgenol*. 2024;222:e2330272.
4. Xue H, Kellman P, Larocca G, Arai AE, Hansen MS. High spatial and temporal resolution retrospective cine cardiovascular magnetic resonance from shortened free breathing real-time acquisitions. *J Cardiovasc Magn Reson*. 2013;15:102.
5. Larson AC, White RD, Laub G, McVeigh ER, Li D, Simonetti OP. Self-gated cardiac cine MRI. *Magn Reson Med*. 2004;51:93–102.
6. Li W, Storey P, Chen Q, Li BS, Prasad PV, Edelman RR. Dark flow artifacts with steady-state free precession cine MR technique: causes and implications for cardiac MR imaging. *Radiology*. 2004;230:569–575.
7. Simonetti OP, Kim RJ, Fieno DS, et al. An improved MR imaging technique for the visualization of myocardial infarction. *Radiology*. 2001;218:215–223.
8. Kellman P, Arai AE, McVeigh ER, Aletras AH. Phase-sensitive inversion recovery for detecting myocardial infarction using gadolinium-delayed hyperenhancement. *Magn Reson Med*. 2002;47:372–383.
9. Bryant DJ, Payne JA, Firmin DN, Longmore DB. Measurement of flow with NMR imaging using a gradient pulse and phase difference technique. *J Comput Assist Tomogr*. 1984;8:588–593.
10. Scheffler K, Lehnhardt S. Principles and applications of balanced SSFP techniques. *Eur Radiol*. 2003;13:2409–2418.
11. Meloni A, Al-Saadi N, Torheim G, et al. Myocardial first-pass perfusion: influence of spatial resolution and heart rate on the dark rim artifact. *Magn Reson Med*. 2011;66:1731–1738.
12. Storey P, Chen Q, Li W, Edelman RR, Prasad PV. Band artifacts due to bulk motion. *Magn Reson Med*. 2002;48:1028–1036.
13. Salerno M, Sica C, Kramer CM, Meyer CH. Improved first-pass spiral myocardial perfusion imaging with variable density trajectories. *Magn Reson Med*. 2013;70:1369–1379.
14. Simonetti OP, Finn JP, White RD, Laub G, Henry DA. "Black blood" T2-weighted inversion-recovery MR imaging of the heart. *Radiology*. 1996;199:49–57.
15. Rashid S, Rapacchi S, Shivkumar K, Plotnik A, Finn JP, Hu P. Modified wideband three-dimensional late gadolinium enhancement MRI for patients with implantable cardiac devices. *Magn Reson Med*. 2016;75:572–584.
16. Shao J, Rashid S, Renella P, Nguyen KL, Hu P. Myocardial T1 mapping for patients with implanted cardiac devices using wideband inversion recovery spoiled gradient echo readout. *Magn Reson Med*. 2017;77:1495–1504.

SECTION II EMERGING TECHNOLOGY WITH REQUIREMENTS FOR CLINICAL USE

9 Artificial Intelligence: Promises, Pitfalls, and Ethical Considerations

NAY AUNG, CAROLINE RONEY, DAVID LESLIE, GREGORY SLABAUGH, AND STEFFEN E. PETERSEN

INTRODUCTION

In the last few years, the field of artificial intelligence (AI) has made remarkable strides in revolutionizing cardiovascular magnetic resonance (CMR) imaging. Recent review articles[1-3] have highlighted the potential of AI in advancing various aspects of CMR, ranging from image acquisition and reconstruction to segmentation, classification, and prognosis. These advancements have the potential to transform the clinical pathway of CMR, offering new opportunities for improved patient care and outcomes.

In this chapter, we endeavor to present a detailed summary of progress made to date, with particular focus on the challenges associated with the integration of AI in CMR along the clinical pathway. We will discuss issues related to biases in AI algorithms, distribution shifts, and the need for AI auditing and continual learning to ensure the reliability and generalizability of AI models. Ethical considerations surrounding the use of AI in CMR will be explored, along with system-wide issues including the reliance on AI tools, energy costs, climate impact, and importance of maintaining the human perspective and touch in patient care.

Overall, this chapter aims to provide a comprehensive understanding of the current state, potential, and challenges of AI in CMR. By emphasizing the pitfalls, we hope to foster a balanced perspective compared to the hype in the AI literature related to CMR and guide future research and implementation of AI technologies in cardiovascular imaging.

ARTIFICIAL INTELLIGENCE IN THE CLINICAL CARE PATHWAY AND CARDIOVASCULAR MAGNETIC RESONANCE

Administrative and Noninterpretative Tasks

A patient care pathway in cardiac imaging begins at the time of referral initiated by a clinician. Inputs from administrative and clinical staff are required to ensure that scheduling of an imaging test is done at the right time for the right patient with the right indication at the right cost. Electronic and verbal information exchange occurs across multiple channels encompassing several key stakeholders including the ordering physician, imaging physician, administrator, nurse, radiographer, and patient/family. Given the complexity and multiplicity of technical and human factors involved in this process, built-in sources of inefficiencies are prevalent, which are ripe for targeted improvements by AI tools—in particular, advanced natural language processing (NLP) techniques offered by foundation models[4]—under the broad aim of workflow optimization. Several pitfalls should, however, be acknowledged. Firstly, the information provided by the referrer is often limited (sometimes to a few words!), which prevents meaningful application of powerful AI tools. Electronic health records (EHRs) hold a richer set of unstructured text which in theory could be mined with the assistance of NLP. Efficiency improvement was highlighted in several reports[5-8] outlining the potentials of AI in radiology protocolling. Despite these promises, many healthcare institutions deploy under-resourced and poorly integrated informatic systems (e.g., EHRs, radiological information systems, outpatient notes, scanned records). This restricts the widespread application of NLP beyond larger, well-resourced institutes and can lead to the exacerbation of existing digital inequalities and healthcare inequity.

Even in the optimal scenario where a seamless, fully centralized, and fully digitized electronic data repository is in operation, nuances in the referral's intention, subspecialty requirements (e.g., cardiomyopathy vs. electrophysiology), and patient preference will not be accounted for in the AI's decision-making. Arguably, key safety information is already protocolized in the current workflow (e.g., checking creatinine, metallic implant), and the use of 'intelligent' rules is not scalable to capture a wider range of clinical variables that inform the scheduling process.[9] While AI-assisted clinical decision support systems[10,11] built on the appropriate use criteria[12] and the Choosing Wisely initiative[13] have been proposed to aid scan triaging, their real-world application is substantially hindered by the incomplete coverage of the appropriate use criteria on the entire spectrum of clinical indications.

Image Acquisition

AI tools have made major inroads into planning, optimizing image quality, reducing artifacts, and shortening scan time.[14-16] A 'single-click' CMR acquisition AI software has recently been approved by the Food and Drug Administration.[17] SonicDL from GE Healthcare uses deep learning algorithms integrated within their scanners to decrease scan times by up to 83%, reducing motion artifacts by collecting one cardiac cycle per slice in a single heartbeat.[18] Other applications include the use of deep learning to learn late gadolinium enhancement intensities from magnetic resonance imaging (MRI) without the use of contrast agents.[19] Undoubtedly, these solutions will be adopted widely in the near future given the strong case for scan-time efficiency and consistency as well as enhanced quality and patient experience. It should be noted that key processes in scanning such as patient positioning in the magnet, electrode and surface coil placement, and two-way communications during the scan still require interface with human technicians. Over recent years, despite advancement in software solutions, innovations in robotics have lagged in healthcare, limiting the complete automation of image acquisition.

Image Reconstruction: Risks of Hallucination

Deep learning approaches can be used to reconstruct images, reducing the amount of data required and reducing the scan time by enabling higher undersampling factors in k-space. These approaches can generate imaging slices at higher resolution or in different orientations, leveraging prior information extracted from training data. However, there is a risk of hallucination,[20] which means that false image features are introduced because an imperfect or inaccurate prior model is used. This can occur when the training and testing datasets have different distributions. For example, Antun et al. demonstrated that adding small perturbations in the acquired k-space could introduce large artifacts in the final image reconstruction, and that small features like tumors may not be captured in the reconstruction.[21] These issues are likely to pose a further challenge for congenital cases. There is ongoing research into identifying and minimizing hallucinations, for example by using interpretability approaches, by encoding disease-related information,[22] and by using maps to identify where hallucinations may be induced from sparse k-space sampling.[23] This research is crucial to ensure we can trust image reconstruction in the absence of ground truth data. Nonetheless, further study is needed to understand the extent to which distributional discrepancies between training and testing datasets lead to differential performance for population subgroups who are underrepresented in the training data. As with other instances of sampling and representation bias in datasets,[24-26] such discrepancies could disproportionately harm historically marginalized, minoritized, or underserved communities, augmenting existing patterns of inequity and discrimination.[27-29]

Artificial Intelligence for Segmentation: the Potential of Full Automation

Deep learning approaches achieve state-of-the-art accuracy for segmenting cardiac structures including the ventricular myocardium, atrial and ventricular blood pools, and aorta. El-Taraboulsi et al. provide a comprehensive review of deep learning in cardiac image segmentation in which they discuss Swin transformers, image-to-image translation, and weakly supervised learning as exciting areas of future research.[30]

Despite the clear advantages of automated segmentation in terms of reducing human error and saving large amounts of time, there is a current debate on whether cardiac segmentation should be fully automated or allow for corrections in contouring. Human oversight and intervention are still likely required to ensure accuracy and reliability. This may be particularly true for segmentation of unusual cases or congenital cases in which there is more variability and less training data available to ensure accuracy of the AI algorithms. Tandon et al. retrained a convolutional neural network contouring algorithm developed for structurally normal hearts on repaired tetralogy of Fallot training cases, which improved the ability of the algorithm to segment repaired tetralogy of Fallot cases.[31] Similar approaches could be used to improve automated segmentation approaches for other forms of congenital heart disease.

For some applications, AI may provide a more consistent and standardized assessment as it is not prone to variability like human measurement. For example, Augusto et al. developed an algorithm for left ventricular maximum wall thickness and compared its reproducibility with that of 11 international experts.[32] Their algorithm demonstrated superior reproducibility, with the implication that a clinical trial to detect a 2 mm change in maximum wall thickness would need 2.3 times fewer patients when using this algorithm compared to human assessment.

Classification and Reporting

Recent developments in the field of large vision-language models show promising abilities for producing imaging reports directly from images. An example is GPT-4V(ision), which has been tested by Yang et al. on many examples, including radiology examples.[33] Although the methodology correctly reported some examples, including an abdominal x-ray and a knee MRI, it missed a distal radial fracture on a hand and wrist x-ray. For a chest computed tomography (CT) example, GPT-4V reported a nodule on the left side rather than the right side, and it hallucinated measurements. As such, these approaches have the potential to save time by generating a template report; however, these generated reports will need to be checked and corrected by radiologists or cardiologists. This emphasizes the need for human-AI collaboration in using such tools in the clinical workflow.

Van Veen et al. adapted large language models to summarize clinical text.[34] They applied their domain adaptation methods to four tasks: radiology reports, patient questions, progress notes, and doctor-patient dialogue, and demonstrated more complete and correct summaries from their model than from human experts. Again, these methodologies require all reports to be readily available, and will miss any verbal information given to a clinician that is not documented.

AI-supported templates are likely to improve structure of reports and ensure consistency; however, clinicians may prefer to write the final summary sentence themselves. There is a lot of variation between clinicians in their style and they may prefer to retain this autonomy and the personal aspect of the message. Reports are likely to be framed depending on who the report is for; for example, there may be differences when reporting for an electrophysiologist compared to a heart failure or cardiomyopathy expert. These human nuances and uniqueness may not be captured by AI.

Prognosis

AI has already demonstrated prognostic value in CMR for numerous conditions including myocardial infarction,[1] heart failure,[35] and pulmonary hypertension.[36] Often, such machine learning approaches will be based on biomarkers extracted from the images and used to make predictive models. For many conditions, improved prognostication may be achieved by including additional modalities beyond CMR. For example, Chen et al. predicted 1-year cardiovascular events in patients with severe dilated cardiomyopathy using features derived from CMR, electrocardiography, echocardiography, and other clinical data.[37] The study demonstrated that multimodal data is more effective in estimating prognostic risk than CMR-derived features alone. More broadly, realizing the benefits of AI for accurate prognostication may require the availability of additional modalities such as longitudinal data, multiomics, or features derived from digital twin models that replicate a patient's cardiology in silico. However, harmonizing data across modalities, handling missing values, and fusing the data effectively remain open challenges and active areas of research.[38,39]

Relatedly, patients with multimorbidities present challenges in prognostication. Multimorbidity often leads to complex clinical presentations in which symptoms and signs may overlap or influence each other. Interpreting CMR in this context requires a nuanced understanding of how multiple conditions might affect cardiac structure and function—sometimes in opposing directions. These factors can confound the interpretation of CMR images, making it difficult for an AI system trained to detect specific features attributable to a single or few cardiac pathologies. Coordinating CMR findings with other diagnostic tools to form a comprehensive view of the patient's cardiac health may be beyond the scope of an AI system trained solely to assess CMR.

BIAS OF ARTIFICIAL INTELLIGENCE IN CARDIOVASCULAR MAGNETIC RESONANCE

A key challenge for the future of AI in CMR is addressing issues introduced by various biases to ensure that AI tools do not provide worse performance for different subpopulations, depending on characteristics such as age, race or ethnicity, sex, or socioeconomic status. Recent healthcare examples have highlighted this ethical problem. For example, an AI algorithm for diagnosing diabetic retinopathy demonstrated a large difference in diagnostic accuracy depending on skin color (light skin 73% vs. darker skin 60.5%) because the dataset used for training was imbalanced.[40] A further example demonstrated that an AI model for pathology classification from chest radiography data exhibited worse performance on underserved subpopulations, including Black patients.[28] A consequence of this type of bias could be that such patients are more likely to be discharged without receiving the care that they need. Similarly, Puyol-Antón et al. showed that cardiac MRI segmentation algorithms exhibit worse performance on Black patients when using a training database that is sex-balanced but not race-balanced (e.g., UK Biobank).[41]

Bias can occur throughout various stages of the imaging process due to imbalances in data and AI models and human predilections. For example, biases can occur at the data collection stage because of the patient population included in the datasets used to train AI models.[42] Specifically, if the training dataset primarily represents certain demographics (e.g., age, race, sex), it might not adequately reflect variations in disease presentation across diverse populations, leading to incorrect diagnoses.[28] Larrazabal et al. demonstrated that x-ray image datasets used to diagnose thoracic diseases decrease in performance when they do not fulfill sex balance conditions.[43] This can be further impacted by inequalities in access to healthcare, including reduced access to medical imaging equipment, lack of advanced imaging or computational technologies, disparities in the quality of care received by different demographics, and lack of research funding in some countries. Furthermore, socioeconomic status may impact the likelihood of seeking medical care and the quality of care received. This can introduce biases in imaging results, as patients from different socioeconomic backgrounds might have different disease presentations or access to follow-up care. Many studies do not disclose data on race, socioeconomic status, or other protected attributes. Certain countries such as France and Germany do not currently gather ethnicity statistics in routinely collected healthcare data, which further limits efforts to actively augment the training datasets with underrepresented ethnicities. This also makes it challenging to conduct thorough checks to demonstrate AI systems are not biased, particularly for minority groups for whom there may be less available data.

Bias also exists in AI models. For example, AI models may apply a type of shortcut learning in which extra features on images (e.g., chest tubes) are used for prediction instead of identifying the true pathology, which may introduce bias into the model.[44] Cognitive bias occurs at the image interpretation stage since radiologists' interpretations can be influenced by implicit biases, leading to disparities in diagnosis or treatment recommendations. This might manifest as overdiagnosis or underdiagnosis of conditions based on preconceived stereotypes associated with certain patient groups. These cognitive biases are challenging to identify and overcome. These cognitive biases could be built into the training data, which could further exacerbate and propagate the problem.

To mitigate these biases, there are multiple possible approaches. First, datasets used for training AI models or establishing diagnostic criteria should be sufficiently diverse and representative of the population these models are designed to serve. Second, efforts to improve access to healthcare resources are paramount, including to imaging technology across different demographics, geographic locations, and socioeconomic groups. Third, procedural guidelines and protocols to standardize interpretations and reduce subjective biases should be implemented. These ethical guidelines should ensure adherence to fairness principles and patient privacy and include regulatory requirements to prevent discrimination and biases in healthcare practices. This can be reinforced by training radiologists and cardiologists to recognize and mitigate biases through education, awareness, and ongoing evaluation of decision-making processes. Ultimately, this is crucial to ensure accurate diagnoses, equitable care, and improved patient outcomes.

There are also approaches focused on the algorithm side, including the development of interpretable models that provide explanations for their decision-making processes, which helps imaging physicians understand how the AI arrives at its conclusions, facilitating trust and identification of biases. Tools can be implemented to detect and mitigate biases in imaging physicians' interpretations. AI algorithms should be regularly audited for bias and their performance evaluated across diverse populations to ensure fairness. Novel algorithms could be developed that are robust to imbalances in the dataset.[43] Before training, a dataset could be rebalanced by oversampling data from underrepresented patient groups, but this is challenging in medical imaging due to consent, cost, and potentially low prevalence of a disease. Alternative approaches during algorithm training are data augmentation[45] and adversarial training.[46] Recently, generative methods have been used for data augmentation, and adversarial schemes provide a way to calibrate a prediction across subgroups.[47] Finally, it is important to establish feedback mechanisms to continuously assess and improve algorithms and practices based on real-world outcomes and feedback from diverse patient populations. These approaches to improve algorithmic fairness are challenging to apply in such a way as to not decrease model performance and often require careful compromises and ethical considerations.

Several national and international agencies have published standards on training data composition and evaluation strategies to ensure generalizability as well as explainability and traceability. For example, the recommended practice for the quality management of medical AI datasets, produced by the Institute of Electrical and Electronics Engineers, outlined best practices for dataset lifecycle, quality control, privacy, and security.[48] The US National Institute of Standards and Technology AI Risk Management Framework[49] and the upcoming European Union AI Act[50] are designed to promote responsible and safe use of AI applications by providing a set of key regulatory principles to mitigate risks.

DISTRIBUTION SHIFTS, ARTIFICIAL INTELLIGENCE AUDITING, AND CONTINUAL LEARNING

Despite the remarkable performance AI systems have demonstrated in laboratory environments, they may underperform on live data captured in the clinical environment, particularly when the data seen in the clinic has differences compared to the data used to train the AI system. This phenomenon is well known in the AI community as a generalization problem: the AI model may underperform as the data distribution has shifted, that is, changed between training and deployment. Distribution shifts can result from multiple sources, including differences in scanners used to acquire the data or clinical acquisition protocols. For example, Li et al. demonstrated substantial degradation of performance when training CMR image segmentation approaches on data from one clinical site and evaluating data from another clinical site, characterizing generalization performance as "very limited".[51]

This generalization problem is more nuanced, as distribution shifts can occur over time as well. An AI system may have excellent performance when initially deployed, but if there are real-time changes in the clinical environment that affect the data, the AI performance may suffer. Pianykh et al.[52] demonstrated significant inaccuracies of a machine learning model trained on "ageing" radiological data, with models becoming unreliable 8 months postdeployment as the distribution of live data shifted from the data used to train the AI. de Vries et al.[53] observed large degradation in AI performance in a deployed breast mammography system due to a software upgrade on the mammography equipment, highlighting that AI is a part of an interconnected system and that changes to the clinical environment may affect the AI performance.

Therefore, there is a clear need for iterative auditing of an AI system to check that, once deployed, it continues to perform as expected. The World Health Organization (WHO) recently published regulatory considerations on AI for health tools[54] that consider risks across the entire AI lifecycle from idea to postdeployment. The latter considers new risks that may appear once AI tools are implemented in specific real-world environments with users with varying levels of experience. This can be achieved with periodic safety checks to report any potential harm and timely reporting of adverse events associated with the use of software medical devices to relevant regulators.

AI technology is implemented as software, and therefore can be upgraded with an updated version that has enhanced capabilities or performance. Continual learning takes this further, where the AI updates automatically, adapting continuously to changes in the local data environment. This way, the AI system can more flexibly respond to distribution shifts.[52] Implementing continual learning requires updating an already deployed AI system on real-time data streams from the clinical environment, rather than "static" datasets captured at a particular point in time. This may require feedback loops wherein clinicians score AI findings (e.g., accept or reject) and the feedback is used to update the AI system. A well-known challenge in continual learning is "catastrophic forgetting," when a continual-learning AI method focuses on the latest data input to the model, forgetting what it has learned before. However, there are numerous techniques to address catastrophic forgetting including regularization, rehearsal, and parameter isolation.[55] Continual learning poses additional complexity from a regulatory point of view. This can be managed through change control mechanisms.[54,56] Nonetheless, regulatory and governance challenges remain a concern insofar as dynamic, continual learning models break the mold of conventional precautionary processes of validation and clinical trialing. Unlike in the case of continuous learning models, the latter establish an objective, predeployment basis for assurance of the safety and reliability of static systems that do not change or evolve when operating 'in the wild'.

SYSTEM-WIDE ISSUES POSED BY ARTIFICIAL INTELLIGENCE

Reliance on Artificial Intelligence Tools—Automation Bias and Loss of Human Expertise

Automated AI tools in CMR have the potential to save radiologists and cardiologists time, meaning they have more time available for interacting with patients and for complex cases. However, this use must be balanced with the risk of overreliance on AI resulting in the potential loss of human expertise, automation bias, and lack of innovation. Li and Little proposed a framework for radiology trainees to use AI tools appropriately, requiring trainees to develop skills to use AI safely.[57] Dratsch et al. investigated the impact of an AI system used in mammography on radiologists' performance to check for the presence of automation bias in which radiologists favor suggestions from AI systems.[58] They found that radiologists across all experience levels were prone to automation bias, and the percentage of mammograms that were correctly labelled by the radiologist was significantly impacted by the correctness of the AI prediction. Mehrizi et al. investigated whether providing explainability or priming interventions could negate these automation bias effects but found these had a limited effect on overcoming the influence of AI suggestions.[59] This suggests that innovative approaches are required to overcome these automation biases in human-machine interactions.

Agarwal et al. investigated how to optimize the use of human expertise with AI, reaching the disappointing conclusion that performances were typically improved by either using expert diagnosis or AI diagnosis but rarely by humans assisted by AI.[60] Interestingly, they found that providing AI predictions does not uniformly increase diagnostic quality and similarly providing contextual information does not improve quality. Their explanation was that radiologists may not put enough weight on the information provided by the AI, and they also do not account for the correlation between their own information and the AI prediction. This suggests that improving outcomes for humans assisted by AI requires imaging physicians to carefully consider the importance of different sets of information.

A final risk is the overreliance on AI resulting in the potential loss of human expertise. This is particularly important when considering innovation in research, which requires humans with a high level of training and expertise. The development of innovative treatments requires research by scientists at the frontiers of the field; these developments will not be made by AI alone.

Energy Costs and Climate Impact

A potentially limiting factor for AI applications is energy costs and the associated environmental impact. While companies such as Siemens aim to reduce energy consumption of MRI scanners, there must be a similar drive to reduce energy consumption of AI algorithms. Importantly, deep learning algorithms are costly to train due to the cost of hardware and electricity or cloud compute time and environmentally costly due to the carbon footprint, but once trained and deployed in hospitals, the inference stage is less computationally demanding. Strubell et al. highlighted the importance of considering the utility of these technologies while keeping their environmental costs in mind by showing that training a neural network for NLP produced an amount of carbon dioxide equivalent to nearly the lifetime emission of five average American cars.[61] Bloomfield et al. provide recommendations for policymakers, climate researchers, and AI developers to consider as part of achieving a net zero National Health Service (NHS) by 2040 in the UK, including implementing standardized measures for quantifying the impact on the climate of AI tools in healthcare.[62]

The Human Perspective and Touch

At present, AI deployments consist of specific and narrow tasks, such as performing a segmentation of specific cardiac anatomies. However, clinical decision-making is often nuanced, particularly when dealing with ambiguous cases. For example, clinical experts may look at additional imaging sequences, patient history, and a possible clinical diagnosis to finalize a segmentation, which is challenging for an AI algorithm as there is considerable hidden information that AI may not know how to interpret given its specific training regime. Cardiologists often encounter novel patient cases that require creative problem-solving skills. For an AI algorithm, such out-of-distribution cases may produce unreliable results.

AI systems also lack the ability to empathize with patients on a human level. Emotional support and reassurance provided by a healthcare professional is a vital aspect of patient care. Relatedly, AI currently lacks the ability to navigate complex ethical dilemmas and make value-based decisions that align with those of a patient. Physicians, unlike AI, often serve as advocates for their patients, ensuring they receive the best care and have their concerns addressed.

ETHICAL VALUES AND PRINCIPLES RELEVANT TO CARDIOVASCULAR MAGNETIC RESONANCE

This chapter has, so far, touched on various ethical challenges that arise both across the AI innovation lifecycle in CMR and within the broader clinical and sociotechnical contexts in which AI applications in CMR are embedded, including issues surrounding explainability, algorithmic bias, digital inequality, healthcare inequity, physician autonomy, patient privacy, environmental harm, and

TABLE 9.1 Key Ethical Considerations for Cardiovascular Artificial Intelligence.

	WHO AI ETHICS PRINCIPLE	DESCRIPTION
1	*Protecting human autonomy*	Humans should remain in control of healthcare systems and medical decisions.
2	*Promoting human well-being and safety and public interest*	The designers of artificial intelligence (AI) technologies should satisfy regulatory requirements for safety, accuracy, and efficacy for well-defined use cases or indications.
3	*Ensuring transparency, explainability, and intelligibility*	Transparency necessitates the publication or documentation of sufficient information prior to the design or implementation of an AI technology.
4	*Fostering responsibility and accountability*	It is the responsibility of stakeholders to ensure that AI technologies are used under appropriate conditions and by appropriately trained people.
5	*Ensuring inclusiveness and equity*	Inclusiveness requires that AI for health must be designed to encourage the widest possible equitable use and access, irrespective of age, sex, gender, income, race, ethnicity, sexual orientation, ability, or other characteristics protected under human rights codes.
6	*Promoting AI that is responsive and sustainable*	Developers should continuously and transparently assess AI applications during actual use to determine whether AI responds adequately and appropriately to expectations and requirements.

the importance of empathy and solidarity in the doctor-patient relationship. Much significant work has been done over the past several years to map out and articulate the values and principles that are needed to ensure that the full range of potential adverse impacts and ethical risks posed by health-related AI technologies are anticipated and addressed.[63-65] Such a body of research and guidance has included the European and North American Multistate Statement on the Ethics of AI in Radiology (2019),[66] which consolidates the ethical values and practical principles contained in recommendations from professional, regulatory, and academic bodies across several different sectors. The statement distills these values and principles down to three imperatives:

1. Promote well-being, minimize harm, and ensure that the benefits and harms are distributed among the possible stakeholders in a just manner.
2. Respect human rights and freedoms, including dignity and privacy.
3. Be transparent and dependable, curtailing bias and decision, while ensuring that the locus of responsibility and accountability remains with their human designers or operators.

More recently, in a review of prospects for the use of AI in cardiovascular medicine, Kodera et al. drew directly from the WHO's six AI ethics principles to provide a useful précis of the range of ethical considerations that are salient for cardiovascular AI[67] (Table 9.1).

Putting Ethical Considerations Into Practice

The high-level descriptions of principles and values contained in the European and North American Multistate Statement on the Ethics of AI in Radiology[66] and the WHO AI ethics and governance guidance[63] provide a good aerial view of the spectrum of ethical considerations that are important for CMR. However, these descriptions provide only a preliminary picture of the conceptual machinery that is needed for ethical, equitable, and responsible AI innovation to be realized *in practice*. That is, they do not yet provide substantial direction on how to move from the "what" of abstract ethical values and principles to the "how" of real-world AI governance mechanisms that can be put into use in the design, development, and deployment contexts of AI for CMR.[68] Rectifying this practical deficit has been the object of much research over last few years in applied AI ethics, where growing attention has been paid to how to move from "principles to practice."[69,70] A more practice-centered and process-driven approach to AI ethics focuses on setting in place clear and actionable governance mechanisms that can facilitate the operationalization of values and principles from the initial steps of AI project horizon scanning and planning to the later stages of AI system deployment, monitoring, and retirement.

The move from principles to practice in applied AI ethics for CMR, however, requires more than just the development and implementation of a portfolio of governance tools. First and foremost, it demands that each of the communities of practices that are involved in the AI research, innovation, and application lifecycle are culturally oriented (or reoriented) to the priority of habits of responsible research and innovation (RRI) across AI project workflows.[71] Namely, it requires that the data scientists, AI researchers, and technologists who are conceptualizing and building the systems, as well as the clinicians and medical practitioners who are using them incorporate end-to-end practices of RRI into all their activities. An RRI perspective provides researchers and practitioners with an awareness that all processes of scientific discovery, problem solving, and application possess ethical consequences and sociotechnical aspects (i.e., interactions between social factors and scientific practices that influence technical choices, decisions, and outcomes). Rather than conceiving AI research, development, and application as independent from human norms, interests, institutions, and values, an RRI point of view regards these activities as sociotechnical practices that are often shaped by social biases, potentially fallible human judgments, and potentially unjust societal structures. These practices therefore bear a responsibility for *anticipatory and critical self-reflection* about the role that norms, interests, institutions, and values play in AI research, development, and application processes and in considerations of the societal impacts that these processes yield.[72]

Over the last decade, research in science and technology studies and applied technology ethics has transformed this RRI view of 'science with and for society' into actionable guidance that provides a helpful reference point for moving from AI ethics principles to responsible AI-enabled CMR practice. Starting with the UK Engineering and Physical Science Research Council's (EPSRC's) 2013 AREA (anticipate, reflect, engage, act) framework and the 2014 Rome Declaration, this RRI guidance has focused, in particular, on the role that anticipatory reflection, public engagement, and transparent and justifiable action should play across the research, innovation, and application lifecycles. More recently, EPSRC's AREA principles have been extended into the fields of data science and AI in the biomedical context by the CARE & Act Framework, which consists of five guiding maxims: consider context; anticipate impacts; reflect on purposes, positionality, and power; engage inclusively; and act responsibly and transparently.

The application of the CARE & Act principles to the use of AI in CMR provides a handy device to enable researchers and practitioners to continuously sense check the social and ethical implications of their research, innovation, and application practices and to establish and sustain habits of responsible scientific investigation, technology design and development, model reporting, and deployment in clinical and other operational contexts. Putting the CARE & Act Framework into practice involves taking its several guiding maxims as a launching pad both for continuously deliberate choice making across the research, innovation, and application workflow and for the reflective adoption of governance mechanisms that can support the assurance

TABLE 9.2 Overview of the CARE & Act maxims.

CARE & ACT MAXIM	DESCRIPTION	GOVERNANCE CONSIDERATIONS AND ACTIONS FOR AI IN CMR CONTEXT
Consider context	Think about the conditions and circumstances surrounding your research and innovation project and its application. Take into account the specific domain and environment in which its applications are situated and reflect on the expectations of affected stakeholders that derive therefrom. Center analysis of the social determinants of health as relevant contextual factors in project design and data analysis.	• Bring together an **interdisciplinary team** of data scientists, AI researchers, social scientists, ethicists, clinicians, patients, and other domain experts from the start to identify the **salient contextual factors across complex healthcare processes and environments** that may determine the appropriateness of developing and using AI solutions for the specific use case under consideration. • Draw on this interdisciplinary team to identify contextual factors in healthcare processes that may function as **confounding variables** for the models being developed. • Put in place **iterative auditing and revisitation processes** that consider changes in the environments in which the AI system operates, so that **shifts in underlying data distributions** can be detected and models can be updated or retired in a timely fashion.
Anticipate impacts	Describe and analyze the impacts, intended or not, that might arise from your project. This does not seek to predict but rather to support an exploration of possible risks and implications that may otherwise remain uncovered and little discussed.	• Carry out an **ethical and human rights impact assessment** at the earliest stage of the AI project and revisit it iteratively across the project lifecycle, drawing on existing AI impact assessment methodologies from UNESCO,[73] the NHS,[74] the council of Europe,[75] and the Alan Turing Institute.[76] • Ensure appropriate **patient and public involvement and engagement (PPIE),** from start to finish, in impact-assessment processes. • Ensure that impact assessment processes are **contextually responsive to and include scrutiny of CMR-specific concerns** such as the loss of physician and patient autonomy, the harm of patient-healthcare provider solidarity and empathy, and the exacerbation of existing digital, health and healthcare inequalities. This should also include, in every case, considerations of environmental impacts and biospheric sustainability.
Reflect on purposes, positionality, and power	Reflect on the goals of and motivations for the project; scrutinize the way that potential perspectival limitations could exercise influence on the equity, integrity, and inclusiveness of the project; reflect on the power imbalances that could exist between the project team and the communities impacted by your project: How, if at all, could these power imbalances result in the injustice or harm?	• Carry out **structured positionality reflection**[77] to identify potential cultural and socioeconomic biases on the project team and to identify impacted stakeholders, whose perspectives should be included in the design, development, and deployment of the AI system. • Draw on the global partnership on AI's data justice in practice guidance for developers[78] to **analyze and address power imbalances that may affect the equity, integrity, and inclusiveness** of the project's research, innovation, and application processes and its products.
Engage inclusively	Open up AI project design and impact assessment processes to broader deliberation, dialogue, engagement, and debate in an inclusive way. Embrace peer review at all levels and welcome different views.	• Set up thorough **PPIE and stakeholder engagement processes**[77,79-81] to ensure an appropriate and proportionate degree of public consent, social license, and democratic governance of the AI project. • Follow **PPIE best practices** to ensure meaningful participation that does not harm or adversely affect members of historically marginalized, discriminated against, or vulnerable communities.

Continued

TABLE 9.2 Overview of the CARE & Act maxims.—cont'd

CARE & ACT MAXIM	DESCRIPTION	GOVERNANCE CONSIDERATIONS AND ACTIONS FOR AI IN CMR CONTEXT
Act responsibly & transparently	Use these processes to influence the direction and trajectory of the research and innovation process itself. Produce research that is both scientifically and ethically justifiable and provide transparent documentation, following best governance, self-assessment, and reporting practices.	• Set up governance processes that ensure end-to-end diligence in addressing **SSAFE-D concerns**[65,82-88]: **Sustainability** (project is continuously responsive to real-world impacts); **safety** (project is technically accurate, performant, reliable, secure, and robust); **accountability** (project has comprehensive answerability, auditability, and transparent reporting mechanisms); **fairness** (project is not discriminatory, advances equity, diversity, and inclusiveness, and mitigates unfair biases); **explainability** (project outputs are sufficiently interpretable and research, innovation, and application processes are sufficiently transparent to warrant justified public trust); **data stewardship** (project has assured sufficient data quality, data integrity, data privacy, and data protection). • Corresponding governance processes should include: **impact assessment; safety and performance self-assessment and risk management** (including testing of differential performance for different demographic groups); **governance logging protocols** to ensure process transparency and diligent documentation; **transparent model reporting** (for instance, following AI reporting protocols like TRIPOD-AI[89], PROBAST-AI[89], STARD-AI[90], CLAIM[91], CONSORT-AI[92], and SPIRIT-AI[93]); **bias self-assessment and risk management**; and **data documentation protocols** to transparently report the provenance of data and the data lifecycle such as data factsheets or datasheets for datasets.[94,95]

AI, Artificial Intelligence; *CLAIM,* Checklist for Artificial Intelligence in Medical Imaging; *CMR,* Cardiovascular Magnetic Resonance; *CONSORT-AI,* Consolidated Standards of Reporting Trials–Artificial Intelligence; *NHS,* National Health Service; *PPIE,* Patient and Public Involvement and Engagement; *PROBAST-AI,* Prediction model Risk Of Bias ASsessment Tool–Artificial Intelligence; *SPIRIT-AI,* Standard Protocol Items: Recommendations for Interventional Trials–Artificial Intelligence; *SSAFE-D,* Sustainability, Safety, Accountability, Fairness, Explainability, Data stewardship; *STARD-AI,* Standards for Reporting Diagnostic Accuracy–Artificial Intelligence; *TRIPOD-AI,* Transparent Reporting of a multivariable prediction model for Individual Prognosis Or Diagnosis–Artificial Intelligence; *UNESCO,* United Nations Educational, Scientific and Cultural Organization

of responsible and trustworthy technology development and use. Table 9.2 provides an overview of the CARE & Act maxims alongside corresponding governance considerations, actions, and mechanisms in the AI in CMR context.

CONCLUSION

AI approaches have made great strides across the entire CMR imaging workflow, from image acquisition to interpretation, prognosis, and treatment. Given the rapid development in the field, it is expected that AI methods will continue to increase performance and utility in clinical workflows. However, there are many reasons including technical, human, societal, and ethical factors that should caution against the overoptimistic view portrayed at times that AI will be taking over medical healthcare related to CMR.

Taken altogether, AI is best used as a tool to enhance healthcare rather than a replacement for the human expertise, empathy, and ethical judgement that are crucial components of cardiology and patient care.

REFERENCES

1. Chong JH, Abdulkareem M, Petersen SE, Khanji MY. Artificial intelligence and cardiovascular magnetic resonance imaging in myocardial infarction patients. *Curr Probl Cardiol.* 2022;47:101330.
2. Leiner T, et al. Machine learning in cardiovascular magnetic resonance: basic concepts and applications. *J Cardiovasc Magn Reson Off J Soc Cardiovasc Magn Reson.* 2019;21:61.
3. Taylor AM. The role of artificial intelligence in paediatric cardiovascular magnetic resonance imaging. *Pediatr Radiol.* 2022;52:2131–2138.
4. Moor M, et al. Foundation models for generalist medical artificial intelligence. *Nature.* 2023;616:259–265.
5. Brown AD, Marotta TR. Using machine learning for sequence-level automated MRI protocol selection in neuroradiology. *J Am Med Inform Assoc JAMIA.* 2017;25:568–571.
6. Brown AD, Marotta TR. A natural language processing-based model to automate MRI brain protocol selection and prioritization. *Acad Radiol.* 2017;24:160–166.
7. Kalra A, Chakraborty A, Fine B, Reicher J. Machine learning for automation of radiology protocols for quality and efficiency improvement. *J Am Coll Radiol JACR.* 2020;17:1149–1158.
8. Lee YH. Efficiency improvement in a busy radiology practice: determination of musculoskeletal magnetic resonance imaging protocol using deep-learning convolutional neural networks. *J Digit Imaging.* 2018;31:604–610.
9. Agniel D, Kohane IS, Weber GM. Biases in electronic health record data due to processes within the healthcare system: retrospective observational study. *BMJ.* 2018;361:k1479.
10. Bizzo BC, Almeida RR, Michalski MH, Alkasab TK. Artificial intelligence and clinical decision support for radiologists and referring providers. *J Am Coll Radiol.* 2019;16:1351–1356.
11. Chaudhari GR, et al. Clinical language search algorithm from free-text: facilitating appropriate imaging. *BMC Med Imaging.* 2022;22:18.
12. Hundley WG, et al. Society for cardiovascular magnetic resonance (SCMR) guidelines for reporting cardiovascular magnetic resonance examinations. *J Cardiovasc Magn Reson.* 2022;24:29.
13. Cassel CK, Guest JA. Choosing wisely: helping physicians and patients make smart decisions about their care. *JAMA.* 2012;307:1801–1802.
14. Nitta S, et al. Automatic slice alignment method for cardiac magnetic resonance imaging. *Magn Reson Mater Phys Biol Med.* 2013;26:451–461.
15. Lu X, et al. Automatic view planning for cardiac MRI acquisition. In: *Med Image Comput Comput Assist Interv–MICCAI 2011* Fichtinger G, Martel A, Peters T, eds. Springer; 2011:479–486. https://doi.org/10.1007/978-3-642-23626-6_59.
16. Argentiero A, et al. The applications of artificial intelligence in cardiovascular magnetic resonance—a comprehensive review. *J Clin Med.* 2022;11:2866.
17. HeartVista Receives FDA 510(k) Clearance for One Click™ Cardiac MRI Package, the First AI-assisted Cardiac MRI Scan Solution. (2019). https://www.businesswire.com/news/home/20191029005333/en/HeartVista-Receives-FDA-510-k-Clearance-for-One-Click%E2%84%A2-Cardiac-MRI-Package-the-First-AI-assisted-Cardiac-MRI-Scan-Solution.
18. Life-speed imaging with Sonic DL™ deep learning MRI acceleration. https://www.gehealthcare.co.uk/products/magnetic-resonance-imaging/sonic-dl-deep-learning-mri-acceleration.
19. Zhang Q, et al. Artificial intelligence for contrast-free MRI: scar assessment in myocardial infarction using deep learning–based virtual native enhancement. *Circulation.* 2022;146:1492–1503.
20. Muckley MJ, et al. Results of the 2020 fastMRI challenge for machine learning MR image reconstruction. *IEEE Trans Med Imaging.* 2021;40:2306–2317.

21. Antun V, Renna F, Poon C, Adcock B, Hansen AC. On instabilities of deep learning in image reconstruction and the potential costs of AI. *Proc Natl Acad Sci U S A*. 2020;117:30088–30095.
22. Zhou X. et al. Adversarial learning for MRI reconstruction and classification of cognitively Impaired individuals. 2023.11.13.23298477 Preprint at https://doi.org/10.1101/2023.11.13.23298477 (2023).
23. Bhadra S, Kelkar VA, Brooks FJ, Anastasio MA. On hallucinations in tomographic image reconstruction. *IEEE Trans Med Imaging*. 2021;40:3249–3260.
24. Feng Q, Du M, Zou N, Hu X. Fair machine learning in healthcare: a review. Preprint at 10.48550/arXiv.2206.14397 (2022).
25. Mehrabi N, Morstatter F, Saxena N, Lerman K, Galstyan A. A survey on bias and fairness in machine learning. *ACM Comput Surv*. 2021;54:35.
26. Suresh, H. & Guttag, J. A Framework for Understanding Unintended Consequences of Machine Learning. ArXiv (2019).
27. Goyal M, Knackstedt T, Yan S, Hassanpour S. Artificial intelligence-based image classification methods for diagnosis of skin cancer: challenges and opportunities. *Comput Biol Med*. 2020;127:104065.
28. Seyyed-Kalantari L, Zhang H, McDermott MBA, Chen IY, Ghassemi M. Underdiagnosis bias of artificial intelligence algorithms applied to chest radiographs in under-served patient populations. *Nat Med*. 2021;27:2176–2182.
29. Gijsberts CM, et al. Race/ethnic differences in the associations of the framingham risk factors with carotid IMT and cardiovascular events. *PLOS ONE*. 2015;10:e0132321.
30. El-Taraboulsi J, Cabrera CP, Roney C, Aung N. Deep neural network architectures for cardiac image segmentation. *Artif Intell Life Sci*. 2023;4:100083.
31. Tandon A, et al. Retraining convolutional neural networks for specialized cardiovascular imaging tasks: lessons from tetralogy of fallot. *Pediatr Cardiol*. 2021;42:578–589.
32. Augusto JB, et al. Diagnosis and risk stratification in hypertrophic cardiomyopathy using machine learning wall thickness measurement: a comparison with human test-retest performance. *Lancet Digit Health*. 2021;3:e20–e28.
33. Yang Z. et al. The Dawn of LMMs: preliminary explorations with GPT-4V(ision). Preprint at 10.48550/arXiv.2309.17421 (2023).
34. Van Veen D, et al. Clinical text summarization: adapting large language models can outperform human experts. *Res Sq*. 2023;rs.3:rs-3483777. https://doi.org/10.21203/rs.3.rs-3483777/v1.
35. Pezel T, et al. AI-based fully automated left atrioventricular coupling index as a prognostic marker in patients undergoing stress CMR. *JACC Cardiovasc Imaging*. 2023;16:1288–1302.
36. Dawes TJW, et al. Machine learning of three-dimensional right ventricular motion enables outcome prediction in pulmonary hypertension: a cardiac MR imaging study. *Radiology*. 2017;283:381–390.
37. Chen R, et al. Using machine learning to predict one-year cardiovascular events in patients with severe dilated cardiomyopathy. *Eur J Radiol*. 2019;117:178–183.
38. Alwazzan O, Khan A, Patras I, Slabaugh G. MOAB: multi-modal outer arithmetic block for fusion of histopathological images and genetic data for brain tumor grading. in 2023 IEEE 20th International Symposium on Biomedical Imaging (ISBI) 1–5 (2023) https://doi.org/10.1109/ISBI53787.2023.10230698.
39. Antikainen E, et al. Transformers for cardiac patient mortality risk prediction from heterogeneous electronic health records. *Sci Rep*. 2023;13:3517.
40. Burlina P, Joshi N, Paul W, Pacheco KD, Bressler NM. Addressing Artificial Intelligence Bias in Retinal Diagnostics. *Transl Vis Sci Technol*. 2021;10:13.
41. Puyol-Antón E, et al. Fairness in cardiac magnetic resonance imaging: assessing sex and racial bias in deep learning-based segmentation. *Front Cardiovasc Med*. 2022;9:859310.
42. Burlina P, Joshi N, Paul W, Pacheco KD, Bressler NM. Addressing artificial intelligence bias in retinal diagnostics. *Transl Vis Sci Technol*. 2021;10:13.
43. Larrazabal AJ, Nieto N, Peterson V, Milone DH, Ferrante E. Gender imbalance in medical imaging datasets produces biased classifiers for computer-aided diagnosis. *Proc Natl Acad Sci*. 2020;117:12592–12594.
44. Banerjee I, et al. "Shortcuts" causing bias in radiology artificial intelligence: causes, evaluation, and mitigation. *J Am Coll Radiol*. 2023;20:842–851.
45. Joshi N. & Burlina, P. AI fairness via domain adaptation. Preprint at https://doi.org/10.48550/arXiv.2104.01109 (2021).
46. Correa R. et al. Two-step adversarial debiasing with partial learning–medical image case-studies. Preprint at https://doi.org/10.48550/arXiv.2111.08711 (2021).
47. Ricci Lara MA, Echeveste R, Ferrante E. Addressing fairness in artificial intelligence for medical imaging. *Nat Commun*. 2022;13:4581.
48. IEEE Standards Association. IEEE Standards Association. https://standards.ieee.org.
49. Team, N. A. NIST AIRC - AIRMF. https://airc.nist.gov/AI_RMF_Knowledge_Base/AI_RMF.
50. Artificial intelligence act: Council and Parliament strike a deal on the first rules for AI in the world. https://www.consilium.europa.eu/en/press/press-releases/2023/12/09/artificial-intelligence-act-council-and-parliament-strike-a-deal-on-the-first-worldwide-rules-for-ai/.
51. Li L, Zimmer VA, Schnabel JA, Zhuang X. AtrialGeneral: domain generalization for left atrial segmentation of multi-center LGE MRIs. In: de Bruijne M, et al., ed. *Medical Image Computing and Computer Assisted Intervention–MICCAI 2021*. Springer International Publishing; 2021:557–566. https://doi.org/10.1007/978-3-030-87231-1_54.
52. Pianykh OS, et al. Continuous learning AI in radiology: implementation principles and early applications. *Radiology*. 2020;297:6–14.
53. de Vries CF, et al. Impact of different mammography systems on artificial intelligence performance in breast cancer screening. *Radiol Artif Intell*. 2023;5:e220146.
54. WHO outlines considerations for regulation of artificial intelligence for health. https://www.who.int/news/item/19-10-2023-who-outlines-considerations-for-regulation-of-artificial-intelligence-for-health.
55. De Lange M, et al. A continual learning survey: defying forgetting in classification tasks. *IEEE Trans Pattern Anal Mach Intell*. 2022;44:3366–3385.
56. Pianykh OS, et al. Continuous learning ai in radiology: implementation principles and early applications. *Radiology*. 2020;297:6–14.
57. Li MD, Little BP. Appropriate reliance on artificial intelligence in radiology education. *J Am Coll Radiol JACR*. 2023;20:1126–1130.
58. Dratsch T, et al. Automation bias in mammography: the impact of artificial intelligence BI-RADS suggestions on reader performance. *Radiology*. 2023;307:e222176.
59. Rezazade Mehrizi MH, et al. The impact of AI suggestions on radiologists' decisions: a pilot study of explainability and attitudinal priming interventions in mammography examination. *Sci Rep*. 2023;13:9230.
60. Combining Human Expertise with Artificial Intelligence: Experimental Evidence from Radiology. Blueprint Labs. https://blueprintlabs.mit.edu/research/combining-human-expertise-with-artificial-intelligence-experimental-evidence-from-radiology/.
61. Strubell E, Ganesh A, McCallum A. Energy and Policy Considerations for Deep Learning in NLP. Preprint at 10.48550/arXiv.1906.02243 (2019).
62. Bloomfield P, Clutton-Brock P, Pencheon E, Magnusson J, Karpathakis K. Artificial intelligence in the NHS: climate and emissions. *J Clim Change Health*. 2021;4:100056.
63. Ethics and governance of artificial intelligence for health. https://www.who.int/publications-detail-redirect/9789240029200.
64. Morley J, et al. The ethics of AI in health care: a mapping review. *Soc Sci Med*. 2020;260:113172.
65. Leslie D. Tackling COVID-19 through responsible AI innovation: five steps in the right direction. *Harv Data Sci Rev*. 2020. https://doi.org/10.1162/99608f92.4bb9d7a7.
66. Geis JR, et al. Ethics of artificial intelligence in radiology: summary of the joint european and north american multisociety statement. *J Am Coll Radiol*. 2019;16:1516–1521.
67. Kodera S, Akazawa H, Morita H, Komuro I. Prospects for cardiovascular medicine using artificial intelligence. *J Cardiol*. 2022;79:319–325.
68. Morley J, Floridi L, Kinsey L, Elhalal A. From what to how: an initial review of publicly available AI ethics tools, methods and research to translate principles into practices. *Sci Eng Ethics*. 2020;26:2141–2168.
69. Mittelstadt B. Principles alone cannot guarantee ethical AI. *Nat Mach Intell*. 2019;1:501–507.
70. Burr C, Leslie D. Ethical assurance: a practical approach to the responsible design, development, and deployment of data-driven technologies. *AI Ethics*. 2023;3:73–98.
71. AI Ethics and Governance in Practice. *The Alan Turing Institute*. https://www.turing.ac.uk/research/research-projects/ai-ethics-and-governance-practice.
72. Leslie, D. Don't 'research fast and break things': on the ethics of computational social Science. https://doi.org/10.5281/zenodo.6635569 (2022).
73. Ethical Impact Assessment: A Tool of the Recommendation on the Ethics of Artificial Intelligence | UNESCO. https://www.unesco.org/en/articles/ethical-impact-assessment-tool-recommendation-ethics-artificial-intelligence.
74. Artificial Intelligence: How to get it right. NHS Transformation Directorate https://transform.england.nhs.uk/ai-lab/explore-all-resources/understand-ai/artificial-intelligence-how-get-it-right/(2019).
75. Leslie D. et al. Human rights, democracy, and the rule of law assurance framework for AI systems: a proposal. http://arxiv.org/abs/2202.02776 https://doi.org/10.5281/zenodo.5981676 (2022).
76. AI Ethics and Governance in Practice: AI Sustainability in Practice Part Two: Sustainability Throughout the AI Workflow. *The Alan Turing Institute*. https://www.turing.ac.uk/news/publications/ai-ethics-and-governance-practice-ai-sustainability-practice-part-two.
77. AI Ethics and Governance in Practice: AI Sustainability in Practice Part One: Foundations for Sustainable AI Projects. *The Alan Turing Institute*. https://www.turing.ac.uk/news/publications/ai-ethics-and-governance-practice-ai-sustainability-practice-part-one-foundations.
78. Data Justice in Practice: A Guide for Developers. *The Alan Turing Institute*. https://www.turing.ac.uk/news/publications/data-justice-practice-guide-developers.
79. Nine principles of effective deliberative public engagement | Involve. https://www.involve.org.uk/resources/knowledge-base/what-are-qualities-good-participatory-process/nine-principles-effective.
80. de Freitas C, Martin G. Inclusive public participation in health: Policy, practice and theoretical contributions to promote the involvement of marginalised groups in healthcare. *Soc Sci Med*. 2015;135:31–39.
81. Community Planning Toolkit - Community Engagement. https://www.communitycommons.org/entities/c99aece3-4159-4fd1-a504-2155d69f3605.
82. Fenech ME, Buston O. AI in cardiac imaging: A UK-Based perspective on addressing the ethical, social, and political challenges. *Front Cardiovasc Med*. 2020;7:54.
83. Fisher E, Rip A. Responsible innovation: multi-level dynamics and soft intervention practices. *Responsible Innovation: Managing the Responsible Emergence of Science and Innovation in Society* Wiley; 2013:165–183. https://doi.org/10.1002/9781118551424.ch9.
84. Owen R. The UK engineering and physical sciences research council's commitment to a framework for responsible innovation. *J Responsible Innov*. 2014;1:113–117.

85. Owen R, Macnaghten P, Stilgoe J. Responsible research and innovation: From science in society to science for society, with society. *Sci Public Policy*. 2012;39:751–760.
86. Owen R, et al. A framework for responsible innovation. In: *Responsible Innovation 27–50*. John Wiley & Sons, Ltd; 2013. https://doi.org/10.1002/9781118551424.ch2.
87. Stilgoe J, Watson M, Kuo K. Public engagement with biotechnologies offers lessons for the governance of geoengineering research and beyond. *PLOS Biol*. 2013;11:e1001707.
88. AI Ethics and Governance in Practice: An Introduction. *The Alan Turing Institute*. https://www.turing.ac.uk/news/publications/ai-ethics-and-governance-practice-introduction.
89. Collins GS, et al. Protocol for development of a reporting guideline (TRIPOD-AI) and risk of bias tool (PROBAST-AI) for diagnostic and prognostic prediction model studies based on artificial intelligence. *BMJ Open*. 2021;11:e048008.
90. Sounderajah V, et al. Developing a reporting guideline for artificial intelligence-centred diagnostic test accuracy studies: the STARD-AI protocol. *BMJ Open*. 2021;11:e047709.
91. Mongan J, Moy L, Kahn CE. Checklist for artificial intelligence in medical imaging (CLAIM): a guide for authors and reviewers. *Radiol Artif Intell*. 2020;2:e200029.
92. Liu X, Rivera SC, Moher D, Calvert MJ, Denniston AK. Reporting guidelines for clinical trial reports for interventions involving artificial intelligence: the CONSORT-AI extension. *BMJ*. 2020;370:m3164.
93. Rivera SC, et al. Guidelines for clinical trial protocols for interventions involving artificial intelligence: the SPIRIT-AI extension. *Lancet Digit Health*. 2020;2:e549–e560.
94. Understanding artificial intelligence ethics and safety. *The Alan Turing Institute*. https://www.turing.ac.uk/news/publications/understanding-artificial-intelligence-ethics-and-safety.
95. Gebru T. et al. Datasheets for Datasets. Preprint at https://doi.org/10.48550/arXiv.1803.09010 (2021).

10 Mid-Field Cardiovascular Magnetic Resonance Imaging

ORLANDO P. SIMONETTI AND JULIET VARGHESE

INTRODUCTION

Cardiac magnetic resonance imaging (MRI) is predominantly performed on systems with B_0 field strengths of 1.5 T or 3 T. With signal-to-noise ratio (SNR) being approximately linearly proportional to B_0, 1.5 T and 3 T systems have been found to offer sufficient SNR to support all cardiovascular imaging applications. While not routinely used for clinical imaging, field strengths above and below this range have been explored to expand the scope of cardiac imaging. Ultra-high field (>3 T) MRI, by virtue of greater magnetic resonance (MR) signal, provides superior SNR, which can be effectively traded for higher spatial and temporal resolution and acquisition speed. However, higher-field systems also come with substantial challenges. These include high installation and operational costs, field inhomogeneity, tissue heating due to high specific absorption ratio (SAR), acoustic noise, distortion of the electrocardiogram, and strong susceptibility artifacts around metallic implants. While mid-field MRI (ranging from 0.3T to 1.0 T) inherently offers less SNR, many of the challenges of a higher field are reduced.

This chapter explores the opportunities, challenges, and clinical applications of mid-field MRI for cardiovascular imaging, highlighting its growing relevance in both routine and specialized cardiology practice.

OPPORTUNITIES MOTIVATING THE DEVELOPMENT OF MID-FIELD CARDIAC MAGNETIC RESONANCE IMAGING

MR systems operating at 1.5 T and 3 T have become the de facto standard for cardiac imaging over prior generation lower field units due to a superior SNR that supports higher spatial and temporal resolution and image quality. However, the high costs of installation, operation, and maintenance of contemporary 1.5 T and 3 T systems remain significant barriers to widespread adoption and utilization of cardiovascular magnetic resonance (CMR), particularly in resource-limited settings.[1] Recent advancements in hardware and pulse sequence design and image reconstruction and denoising methods, combined with some inherent physics advantages, may substantially offset the SNR limitations of mid fields (Fig. 10.1).[2] Together, these factors have generated renewed interest in mid-field CMR as a sustainable lower cost solution for expanding access to advanced imaging including routine CMR in underserved regions. Mid-field MRI presents a range of opportunities that potentially make it an attractive alternative or complement to high-field imaging systems, particularly in specific clinical and operational contexts.

Magnetic Resonance System Siting and Infrastructure

Mid-field MRI systems require less superconducting material, and therefore less cryogen to cool the magnet. These factors alone make them substantially more affordable than higher field units. Mid-field MRI scanners are smaller and lighter due to these reduced hardware and material demands.[3] In addition, recent technological advancements like the "dry cool" technology significantly reduces the volume of liquid helium required for cooling and seals the cryogen within the system, thereby eliminating the need for a quench pipe and reducing the complexity in site construction and infrastructure demands. Siting and installation of a mid-field MR system is thus easier, and these factors reduce overall costs that extend beyond the purchase price, making them more affordable.[4,5]

The smaller footprint and reduced infrastructure requirements can potentially enable the integration of mid-field MRI into nontraditional environments for immediate advanced imaging access. Emergent imaging in emergency departments or intensive care units could be performed, reducing the logistical challenges associated with transporting unstable patients to dedicated imaging facilities. The increased flexibility in siting could facilitate MRI in outpatient and satellite health care clinics where installation of higher field systems may not be feasible.

Patient Comfort and Accessibility

Increased patient comfort and accessibility are also major drivers for mid-field cardiac MRI (Table 10.1). High-field MRI scanners are typically designed to have longer and narrower bores to address the challenge of maintaining homogeneity within the imaging volume at higher fields. Imaging larger patients poses safety concerns as the proximity of the body to the radiofrequency (RF) transmitter coil can increase the risk of heating and burns. The gradient systems also generate loud acoustic noise at a level that scales with B_0 field strength. These factors can induce anxiety, claustrophobia, and discomfort, particularly in larger patients, and can prevent successful completion of the CMR exam. Homogeneity is easier to achieve at lower fields, providing greater flexibility in magnet design and

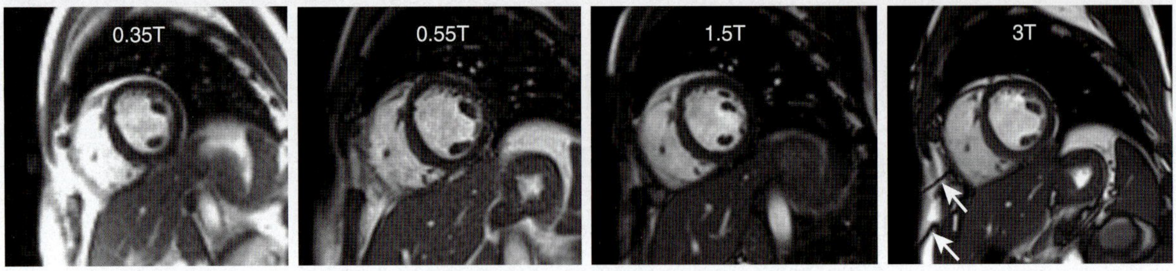

FIG. 10.1 End-diastolic frame from balanced steady-state free precession (bSSFP) cine images acquired in a volunteer at field strengths of 0.35 T, 0.55 T, 1.5 T, and 3 T on contemporary magnetic resonance systems. While there is increasing signal-to-noise ratio with increasing B_0, the images acquired at every field strength are adequate for qualitative and quantitative assessment of cardiac structure and function. bSSFP banding artifacts at 3 T (*white arrows*) are not evident in the examples acquired at lower field.

TABLE 10.1 Magnetic field and hardware benefits and challenges of high- and mid-field systems.

	HIGH FIELD (>1 T)	MID FIELD (<1 T)
System and siting requirements	Expenses limit affordability and access	Cost effectiveness facilitates broader use in various healthcare settings
B_0 homogeneity	Challenging to maintain over large imaging volume	Easier to maintain
B_1 homogeneity	Radiofrequency (RF) wavelength approaches body dimensions, leading to signal heterogeneity	RF wavelength is ~130 cm at 0.55 T, homogeneous contrast and signal-to-noise ratio over imaging volume
Bore size	Restricted to maintain B_0 and B_1 field homogeneity	Wider bore possible increasing imaging access and patient comfort
Acoustic noise	Increased force on gradient coil windings leads to increased noise	Reduced, improving patient comfort
Physiologic effects	Increased possibility of tissue heating, vertigo	Reduced concerns for physiologic effects
Electrocardiogram (ECG)	Increased magnetohydrodynamic (MHD) effects pose challenges for ECG monitoring and cardiac gating	Reduced MHD effects leads to improved ECG quality for monitoring and gating

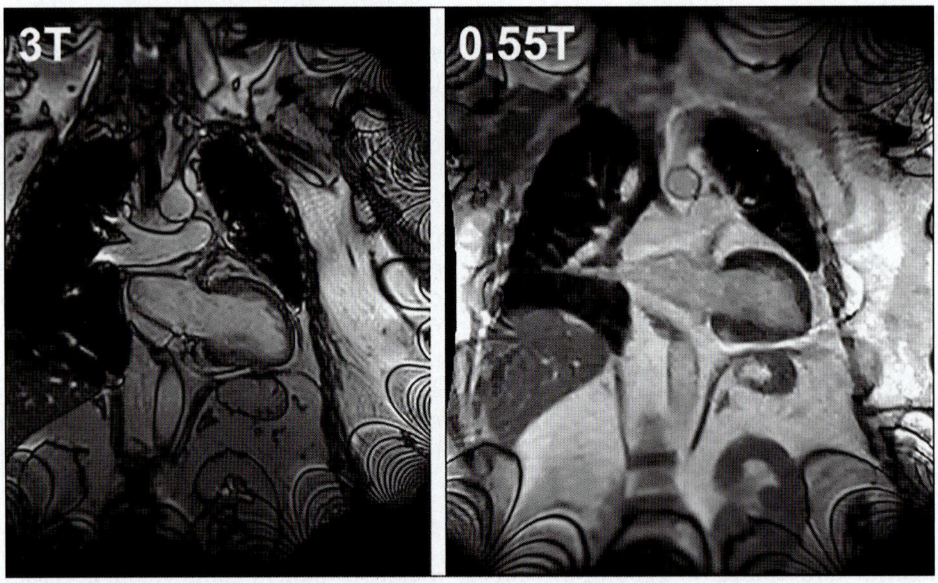

FIG. 10.2 End-diastolic frame from balanced steady-state free precession cine images acquired in a patient with height 175 cm, weight 155 kg, and a body mass index of 50.6 kg/m^2. The cardiovascular magnetic resonance (CMR) examination had to be discontinued in the 70 cm bore 3 T system due to patient discomfort and claustrophobia, while the patient was able to comfortably complete the examination on the 80 cm bore 0.55 T system. While there is some loss of resolution and signal-to-noise at 0.55 T compared to 3 T, cardiac structures can still be visualized. Most importantly, the wider bore allowed the CMR examination to be completed in this patient who could not proceed with the study in a 70 cm bore.

making wider bore systems possible while maintaining cost effectiveness. Mid-field systems with wider conventional closed-bore (up to 80 cm) or open magnet designs can more comfortably and safely accommodate severely obese patients and those with claustrophobia, enhancing patient comfort (Fig. 10.2). A mid field system can also offer quieter operation, further reducing anxiety.[4] These factors can contribute to a more tolerable and less intimidating patient experience.

Patient Safety

Safety, both to the patient and personnel, is another critical consideration motivating the development of mid-field

TABLE 10.2 Safety benefits and challenges of high- and low-field systems.

	HIGH FIELD (>1 T)	MID FIELD (<1 T)
Specific absorption rate (SAR)	Scales with B_0^2, increased risk of device and tissue heating, limits image acquisition parameters	Lower SAR makes it possible to achieve higher flip angles and more slices; diminishes device, implant, and tissue heating concerns
Projectiles	Scales with $B_0 dB_0/dr$, increasing projectile risks	Reduced projectile risk, improving personnel safety

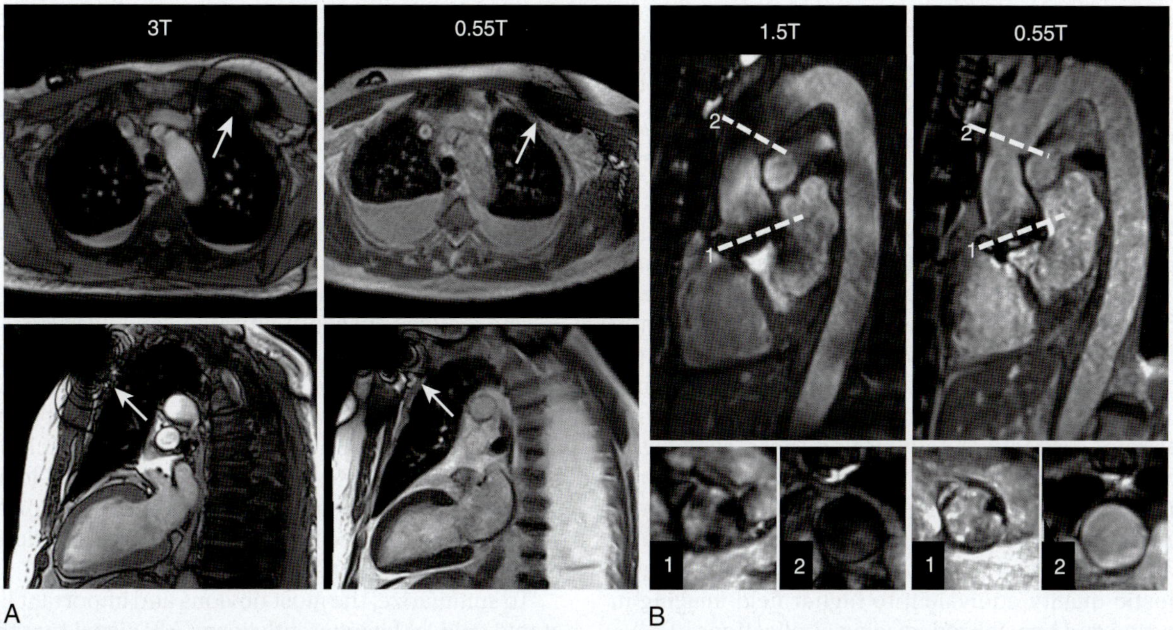

FIG. 10.3 (A) The extent of susceptibility artifacts in balanced steady-state free precession images caused by orthopedic plate and screws in the left clavicle of a patient is shown. The artifacts are significantly reduced at 0.55 T compared to 3 T. The increased bilateral pleural effusion observed in the 0.55 T images is due to a change in clinical status between scans. (B) Multiplanar reformatted angiographic images of the thoracic aorta acquired in a different patient with a bioprosthetic aortic valve and sternal wires. Dephasing artifacts impacting the blood pool signal are distinctly reduced in the images acquired at 0.55 T compared to 1.5 T. Higher blood signal is shown in the cross-sectional images of the aorta, leading to increased confidence in aortic diameter measurement.

cardiac MRI (Table 10.2). With advances in healthcare contributing to longer lifespan, the presence of both noncardiac implanted devices such as orthopedic implants and cardiac implanted electronic devices (CIEDs) such as pacemakers and defibrillators have become increasingly prevalent. At higher fields, the risks of device heating, magnetic interference, and susceptibility artifacts caused by metallic components can limit accessibility and the diagnostic value of CMR. While most safety risks associated with implanted devices can be effectively managed, and it has been shown that patients with CIEDs can be safely scanned at higher fields, the potential for RF-induced device heating remains.[6,7] RF power scales with the square of field strength and is therefore substantially reduced on lower field systems, reducing the risks of device heating.

Given that a growing percentage of patients with cardiovascular disease are treated with CIEDs, the presence of metallic sternal wires from the implant procedure and the proximity of these implanted devices and lead wires to the heart and great vessels can cause significant local image artifacts. This is especially problematic for cardiac MRI, as artifacts in and around the heart can limit the diagnostic value of the images. At lower B_0 fields, susceptibility artifacts near metal can be reduced, potentially providing more accurate imaging for patients with implanted devices (Fig. 10.3). Thus, mid-field systems can theoretically mitigate both device imaging risks and artifacts, providing safer and more effective CMR for the growing population of patients with CIEDs. However, at the time of writing, this has yet to be proven in any published studies, as will be needed before mid-field CMR of patients with CIEDs can be widely adopted.

The safety advantages of mid-field MRI also extend to the growing field of MRI-guided cardiovascular interventions using catheters and guidewires, which are prone to heating at higher fields. The benefits of nonradiation based, image-guided interventions can thus begin to be utilized on a broader clinical scale beyond their current use within a limited number of academic centers.

These imaging applications highlight the unique strengths of mid-field systems in scenarios where high-field imaging would be impractical or unsafe.

Motivation

The potential advantages of reduced cost, increased accessibility, and increased patient safety and comfort have provided sufficient motivation for both researchers and manufacturers to explore low-field CMR, aligning with global efforts to make advanced diagnostic imaging more equitable and accessible. It is to be noted that mid-field cardiac MRI should not currently be viewed as a substitute

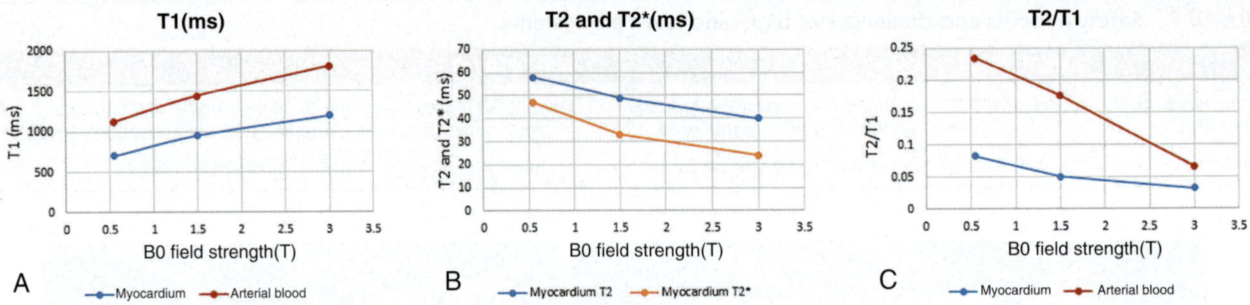

FIG. 10.4 Relaxation time characteristics at three different field strengths (0.55 T, 1.5 T, and 3 T) are shown for (A) myocardium and arterial blood T1, (B) myocardial T2 and T2*, and (C) T2/T1 ratio for myocardium and arterial blood[10,11]. (Data from Campbell-Washburn AE, Ramasawmy R, Restivo MC, et al. Opportunities in interventional and diagnostic imaging by using high-performance low-field-strength MRI. *Radiology*. 2019:190452. doi:10.1148/radiol.2019190452 and Varghese J, Craft J, Crabtree CD, et al. Assessment of cardiac function, blood flow and myocardial tissue relaxation parameters at 0.35 T. *NMR Biomed*. 2020:e4317. doi:10.1002/nbm.4317.)

for higher field systems, but as a complementary modality that can address specific clinical and logistical constraints. If lower field scanners are to provide a viable alternative to higher field systems, the primary challenge of inherently reduced SNR must be overcome. Contemporary technological advancements in iterative and artificial intelligence (AI)-based image reconstruction and denoising are playing a pivotal role in effectively addressing these challenges. These innovations are showing the potential to elevate the performance of mid-field systems to no longer be viewed as a compromise, but instead as a purposeful choice in cardiovascular imaging and in helping to achieve a level of diagnostic quality equivalent to higher field imaging in many routine and specialized imaging applications.[8,9]

MID-FIELD PHYSICS: BENEFITS AND CHALLENGES FOR CARDIAC MAGNETIC RESONANCE

In addition to being a key factor in driving the MR system design, static magnetic field strength also determines the image characteristics. While reduced B_0 results in lower achievable SNR, proton relaxation time properties and reduced susceptibility effects can be leveraged to achieve diagnostic quality cardiac imaging.[2,10] In particular, T1 relaxation time is shorter while T2 and T2* relaxation times are longer with lower field strengths (Fig. 10.4A, B). These factors are favorable for balanced steady-state free precession (bSSFP) cardiac imaging, in which the increased T2/T1 weighting at lower fields can improve blood-myocardium contrast (Fig. 10.4C). Additionally, higher flip angles can be utilized to further boost SNR at lower fields, whereas flip angle can be limited at higher field strengths due to the increased SAR. The longer T2 and T2* relaxation times at lower fields also imply that longer echo (TE) and repetition times (TR) can be used for imaging without significant loss of MR signal, allowing the efficient use of non-Cartesian k-space trajectories such as spiral and radial readouts.[12–14]

The shorter T1 times reduce tissue contrast in T1-weighted imaging and can affect gradient-recalled echo (GRE) applications including exogenous contrast-enhanced techniques like GRE-based perfusion and late gadolinium enhancement (LGE) imaging. However, at lower fields, SSFP-based imaging can serve as an alternative to many magnetization-prepared GRE-based applications. The longer T2 and T2* can enhance the dynamic range of tissue characterization techniques based on these transverse relaxation time constants, although sensitivity to mild changes may also be reduced.

The reduced susceptibility at lower fields also favors the possibility of lung parenchymal imaging,[9,15,16] whereas the reduced spectral separation between fat and water may pose challenges to the implementation of fat-suppressed and fat-water–separated cardiac imaging techniques. A brief overview of the mid-field, physics-based image quality and image application considerations are provided in Table 10.3, and specific applications are additionally discussed in the sections below.

To summarize, the most obvious and important limitation at mid field is the inherently lower MR signal that translates into reduced SNR compared to higher field systems. This can directly impact image quality, as efforts to boost SNR can lead to extended scan times and indirectly limit the spatial and temporal resolution of the images. Limited SNR can also make advanced cardiac imaging applications challenging at mid field, as techniques such as first-pass perfusion, 4D flow, spectroscopy, and diffusion tensor imaging rely on the higher SNR and imaging speed provided by high-field systems. Despite these obstacles, recent advances in acquisition, reconstruction, and denoising strategies can overcome the limited SNR, thereby improving the diagnostic quality of mid-field images and making advanced applications feasible. These include optimized acquisition techniques such as spiral readouts, compressed-sensing reconstruction methods, and AI-based denoising algorithms.

Apart from technical limitations, perhaps the most significant barrier to its widespread clinical application is the perception of mid-field MRI as an inferior imaging modality (Fig. 10.5). This is partly historic, as initial MR systems were of lower field strength, and since 1.5 T and 3 T became the clinical standard, lower field strength units have been associated with reduced image quality and performance. Despite the technological advancements that have occurred over the past four decades since the advent of MRI, this bias still exists among many physicians. This perception will likely slow the adoption of contemporary mid-field systems, even where they may be the most appropriate choice for specific clinical scenarios. Addressing this bias requires robust validation studies that clearly demonstrate the diagnostic equivalence of mid-field MRI for routine cardiovascular imaging. Limited studies comparing the performance of mid-field and high-field systems for basic techniques including cine, flow, and LGE imaging

TABLE 10.3 Image quality and image application considerations at high and low field strengths.

	HIGH FIELD (>1 T)	MID FIELD (<1 T)
Image quality		
Signal-to-noise ratio (SNR)	Greater polarization leads to higher signal; can be traded to increase image resolution and acquisition speed	Lower; ongoing studies demonstrate adequacy for clinical imaging
Contrast-to-noise ratio (CNR)	Improved for angiography, functional MRI (fMRI) and susceptibility-weighted imaging (SWI) applications	Angiography is possible, may reduce sensitivity for fMRI and SWI
Susceptibility and artifacts	Scales with B_0; susceptibility gradients caused by air-tissue interfaces regions can be challenging; artifacts can be severe surrounding metallic implants and devices	Reduced, creating opportunities for MR-guided interventions and improved exam quality for patients with implants and devices
Imaging Applications		
T1 relaxation time	Longer T1 improves image contrast for T1-weighted applications	Shorter T1 leads to reduced T1 contrast, but can increase signal
T2 and T2* relaxation time	Shorter T2 and T2* can be advantageous for QSM and BOLD imaging	Longer T2 and T2* can be advantageous for lung imaging
Spectral separation	Greater spectral separation may be offset by increased B_0 inhomogeneity	Less spectral separation can make fat suppression challenging
Metabolic imaging	High SNR facilitates ^{23}Na MRI, ^{31}P MRS, CEST, DTI	^{1}H imaging primarily possible

B0, Main magnetic field; *CEST,* chemical exchange saturation transfer; *CNR,* Contrast-to-noise ratio; *DTI,* diffusion tensor imaging; *fMRI,* functional magnetic resonance imaging; *^{1}H,* hydrogen; *MR,* magnetic resonance; *MRS,* magnetic resonance spectroscopy; *^{23}Na,* sodium; *^{31}P,* phosphorus; *QSM,* quantitative susceptibility mapping; *SNR,* signal-to-noise ratio; *SWI,* susceptibility weighted imaging.

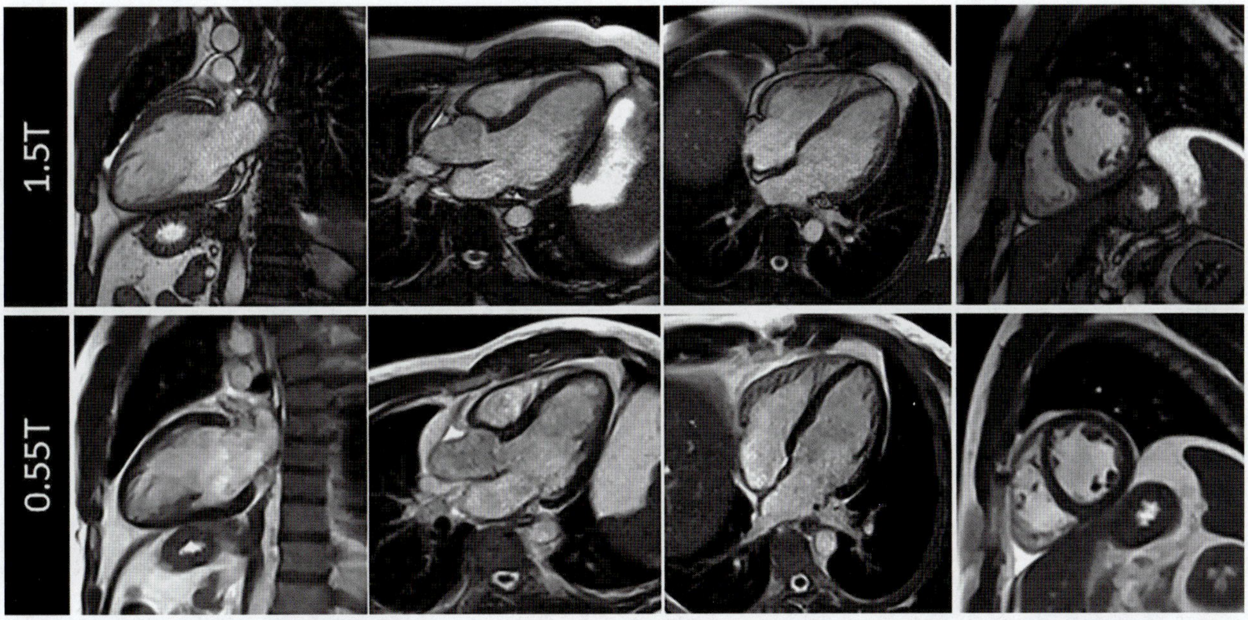

FIG. 10.5 End-diastole frame from balanced steady-state free precession cine images acquired in the same individual at 1.5 T (*top row*) and 0.55 T (*bottom row*) in multiple cardiac imaging planes (from left to right: two, three and four chamber views, mid short-axis view). Although magnetic resonance signal scales with B_0, contemporary advances in radiofrequency coils and receiver electronics, in addition to the utilization of compressed sensing-based image reconstruction techniques, demonstrates that excellent image quality can be achieved on a current generation 0.55 T system when compared to images from the older generation 1.5 T system. Additionally, a flip angle of 108° was achievable at 0.55 T in contrast to a maximum of 65° at 1.5 T, further boosting the low-field signal.

have already shown promising results,[17,18] providing the evidence needed to support larger scale studies and ultimately broader clinical acceptance.

APPLICATIONS OF MID-FIELD CARDIAC MAGNETIC RESONANCE IMAGING

Routine Cardiovascular Magnetic Resonance

The clinical applications of mid-field cardiac MRI are extensive and growing, driven by advancements in hardware and software that make these systems increasingly capable. For mid-field systems to provide a lower cost alternative in resource-limited regions, routine cardiac MRI sequences must generate adequate diagnostic quality (Fig. 10.6). Cine, flow, MR angiography, and LGE imaging are the most frequently used sequences that form the core of the cardiac MRI exam. In addition to published studies that have demonstrated the diagnostic quality of routine cine, flow, and LGE imaging in limited numbers of patients,[19,20] larger studies are needed to validate the performance of standard techniques at

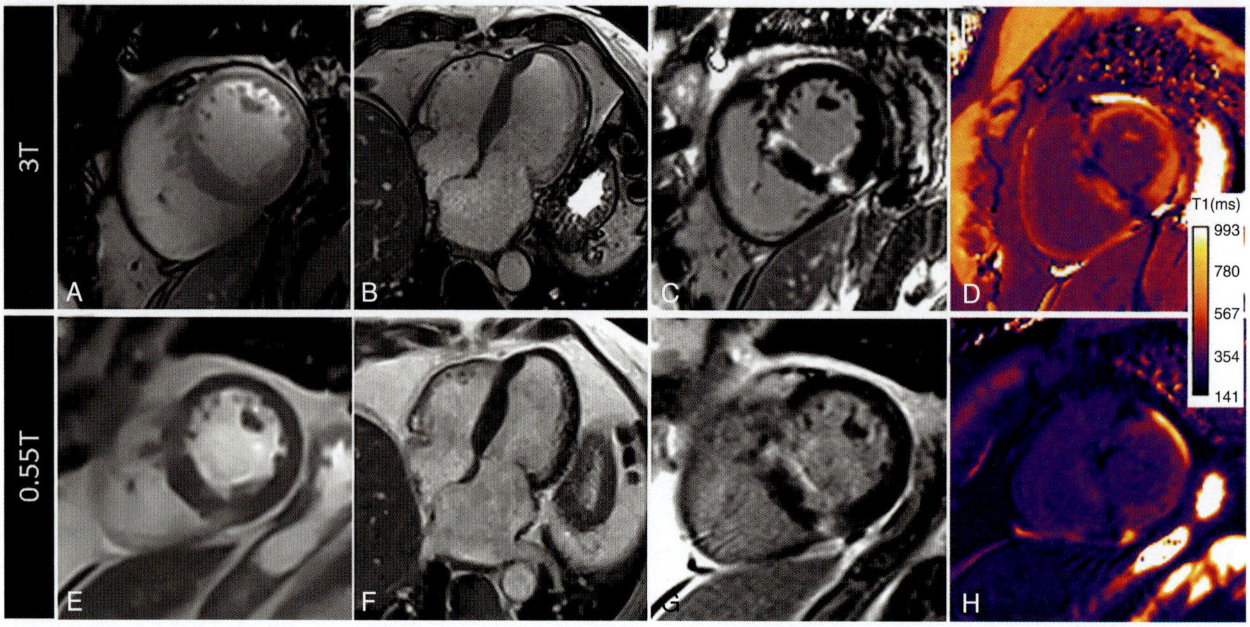

FIG. 10.6 Cardiovascular magnetic resonance images acquired at 3 T (*top row*) and 0.55 T (*bottom row*) in a patient with hypertrophic cardiomyopathy. Asymmetric basal septal left ventricular hypertrophy is observed on the short-axis (A, E) and four-chamber cine (B, F) frames. Prominent midwall scar along the septal and inferior walls is observed on the late gadolinium enhanced (C, G) and postcontrast T1 maps (D, H) at both field strengths.

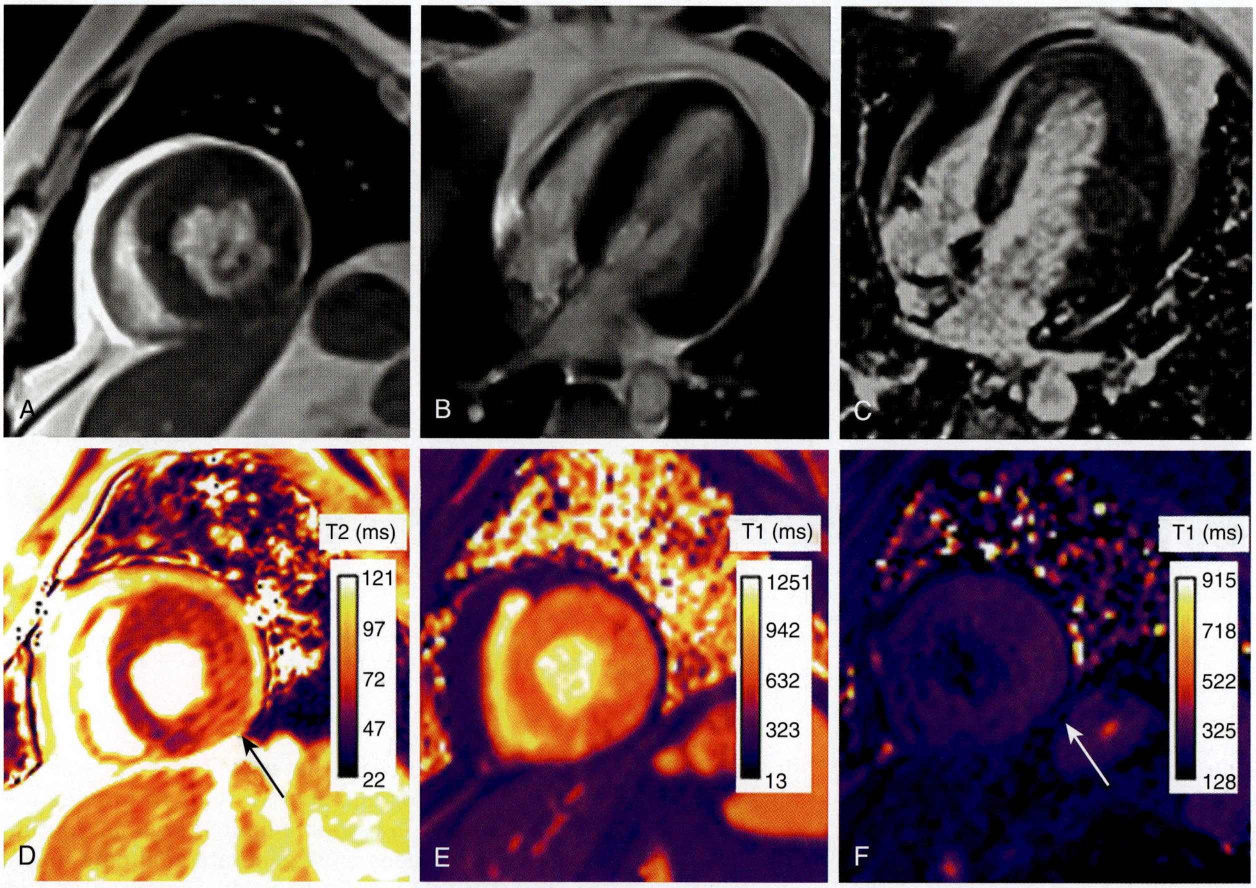

FIG. 10.7 Cardiovascular magnetic resonance examination acquired at 0.55 T in a patient with anxiety and claustrophobia showed severely hypertrophied left ventricle and severe systolic dysfunction on balanced steady-state free precession cine (A, B), prominent midwall nonischemic fibrosis in the septum on late gadolinium enhanced imaging (C), lateral wall T2 elevation indicating edema/inflammation (D), along with native (E) and postcontrast T1 (F) maps.

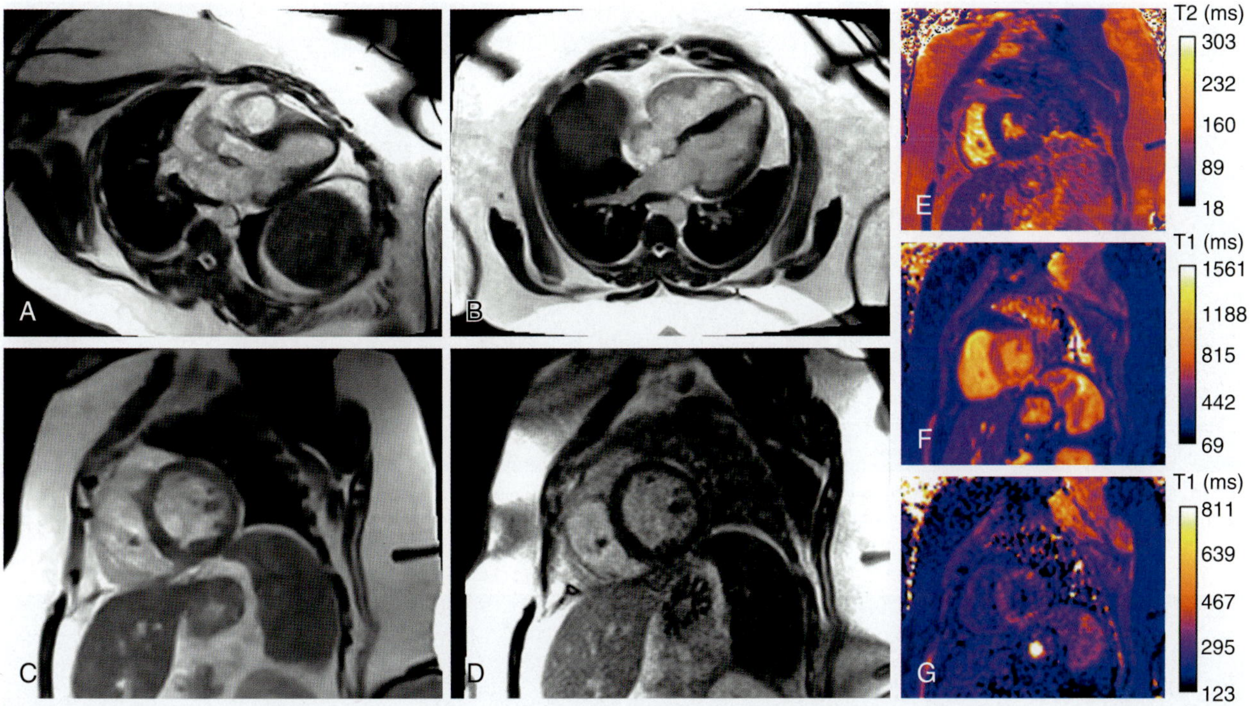

FIG. 10.8 Cardiovascular magnetic resonance examination at 0.55 T in a patient with a body mass index of 75 kg/m^2 (weight 188 kg, height 158 cm) with hypertension, obstructive sleep apnea, hypoxemia, and palpitations. (A) Three-chamber balanced steady-state free precession cine indicates a sclerotic aortic valve. Cine imaging (B, C) determined normal biventricular systolic function, while no significant fibrosis was seen on late gadolinium enhanced images (D). Additionally, parametric maps (E–T2, F–native T1, and G–postcontrast T1) did not demonstrate edema or fibrosis. The examination ruled out infiltrative/inflammatory cardiomyopathy and arrhythmogenic right ventricular cardiomyopathy.

mid field. More advanced techniques such as T1 and T2 myocardial parameter mapping have also been successfully demonstrated, although further optimization may be needed, especially in patients unable to breath-hold (Fig. 10.7).

Imaging Different Patient Populations

The larger, more open patient bore available on mid-field scanners affords the potential to scan certain patient populations—those who are severely obese, pregnant, or have health conditions restricting body flexibility and mobility—that cannot fit safely and comfortably into a higher field system with a standard bore diameter of 60 to 70 cm (Fig. 10.8). While larger body habitus can further contribute to the SNR challenge of mid fields, and additional sequence optimization may be needed to improve image quality, the ability to offer even the most basic routine CMR techniques to severely obese patients could offer a major advantage over other cardiac imaging modalities.[18,21] Echocardiography and nuclear single photon emission computed tomography (SPECT) image quality can be substantially degraded, and cardiac computed tomography (CT) can require a significantly higher radiation dose to achieve adequate image quality in severely obese patients. Mid-field MRI with a larger bore could therefore offer an important cardiac imaging alternative for these patients.

The better accommodation of the larger body habitus with a wider bore system improves patient comfort and facilitates advanced imaging applications for maternal-fetal CMR imaging. As susceptibility is reduced at lower fields, B_0 homogeneity becomes easier to maintain across the maternal abdomen, which has bowel air in proximity to the fetal tissue. B_1 homogeneity, which is a challenge at higher fields due to the large conductive volumes of amniotic fluid, is also easier to achieve at lower fields, translating to reduced image artifacts and better image quality.[22–24]

Pulmonary Imaging

Similarly, susceptibility gradients can be problematic at the air-tissue interfaces of the heart and lung, leading to localized signal loss and image artifacts. The superior B_0 field homogeneity and the longer T2 and T2* relaxation times reduce these effects at mid fields. These physics advantages extend to the possibility of morphological and functional imaging of the lung tissue itself (Fig. 10.9), whereas imaging the lung at higher fields is impacted by severe susceptibility gradients and signal loss. Mid fields thus offer the potential to not only image lung parenchyma, but also potential techniques that offer functional assessment of lung ventilation and perfusion as well as lung water mapping, which are being evaluated.[15,16,25,26] These techniques could be particularly important for patients with conditions including heart failure or pulmonary hypertension and dyspnea, for whom simultaneous evaluation of cardiac and respiratory function can provide a more comprehensive understanding of disease mechanisms and treatment efficacy.

Magnetic Resonance–Guided Cardiovascular Interventions

One of the more important future applications for mid field is in MRI-guided interventions (Fig. 10.10). Interventional cardiovascular magnetic resonance (iCMR) avoids radiation exposure to both the patient and the interventionalist

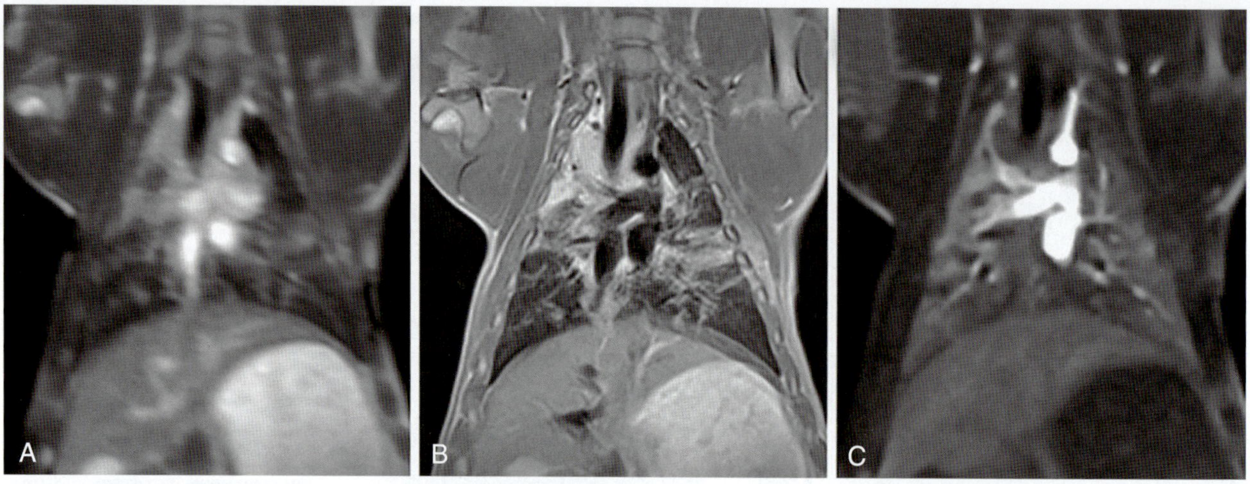

FIG. 10.9 (A) Single-shot balanced steady-state free precession and (B) proton density–weighted turbo spin echo coronal images acquired in a pig at 0.55 T with coincident respiratory illness at the time of imaging demonstrate regional signal heterogeneity in the lung. Contrast-enhanced first pass perfusion image (C) shows normal perfusion.

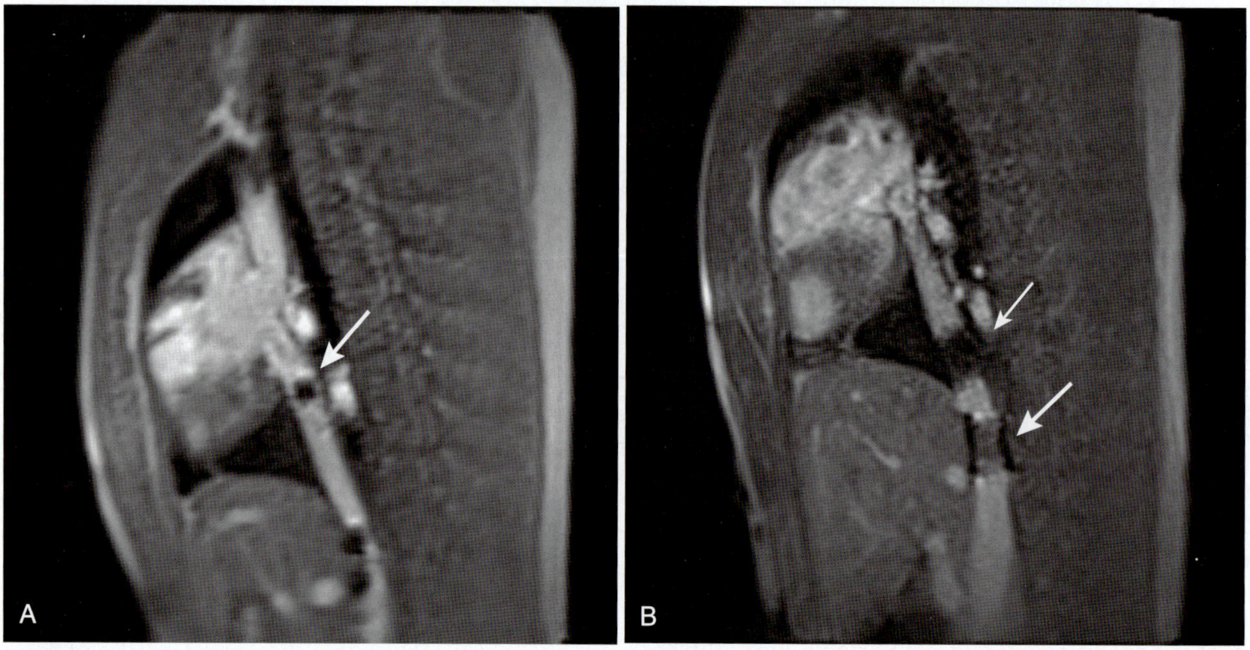

FIG. 10.10 Inferior vena cava (IVC) stenting procedure. (A) Air-filled balloon of a 7 French wedge catheter in IVC (*white arrow*) used for right heart catheterization. (B) After stent deployment and balloon removal, an implanted platinum-iridium–covered Cheatham Platinum (CP) stent with significant image artifact (*thin white arrow*) and an implanted 316L stainless steel 36mm long Mega Large Diameter (LD) stent with good wall apposition demonstrated (*thick white arrow*). (Figure adapted from Armstrong AK, Liu Y, Kelly JM, et al. Feasibility of MRI-guided cardiac catheterization, angioplasty, and stenting in a commercial wide-bore 0.55 T scanner. *J Cardiovasc Magn Reson*. 2025:101858. 10.1016/j.jocmr.2025.101858.)

and provides superior soft tissue contrast and the ability to immediately assess the effects of interventions.[27] The concept of iCMR is not new, and a few centers are already performing routine procedures such as right heart catheterization under MRI guidance in children at 1.5 T.[28,29] However, catheters and guidewires can heat up at 1.5 T and above unless specifically designed for MRI use, and the lack of such equipment has been a major factor limiting the development of MRI-guided interventions.

The reduced RF power and longer RF wavelength at lower fields minimizes device and tissue heating during the prolonged scans needed for interventional guidance, making mid-field systems safer and more practical for MRI-guided cardiovascular interventions, including catheterization and ablation procedures.[10,30] The reduced risk of device heating potentially allows for the safe use of off-the-shelf commercial devices designed for use with X-ray fluoroscopy.[10,31] The fast imaging techniques needed for real-time guidance of interventional procedures can be challenging to implement, given the reduced SNR of mid fields. Advances in image acquisition and reconstruction and image denoising techniques (Fig. 10.11) are therefore essential to generate images at the quality and speed required for iCMR applications.

TECHNOLOGICAL INNOVATIONS AND FUTURE DIRECTIONS

The resurgence of mid-field MRI has been fueled by technological innovations that focus on addressing its core

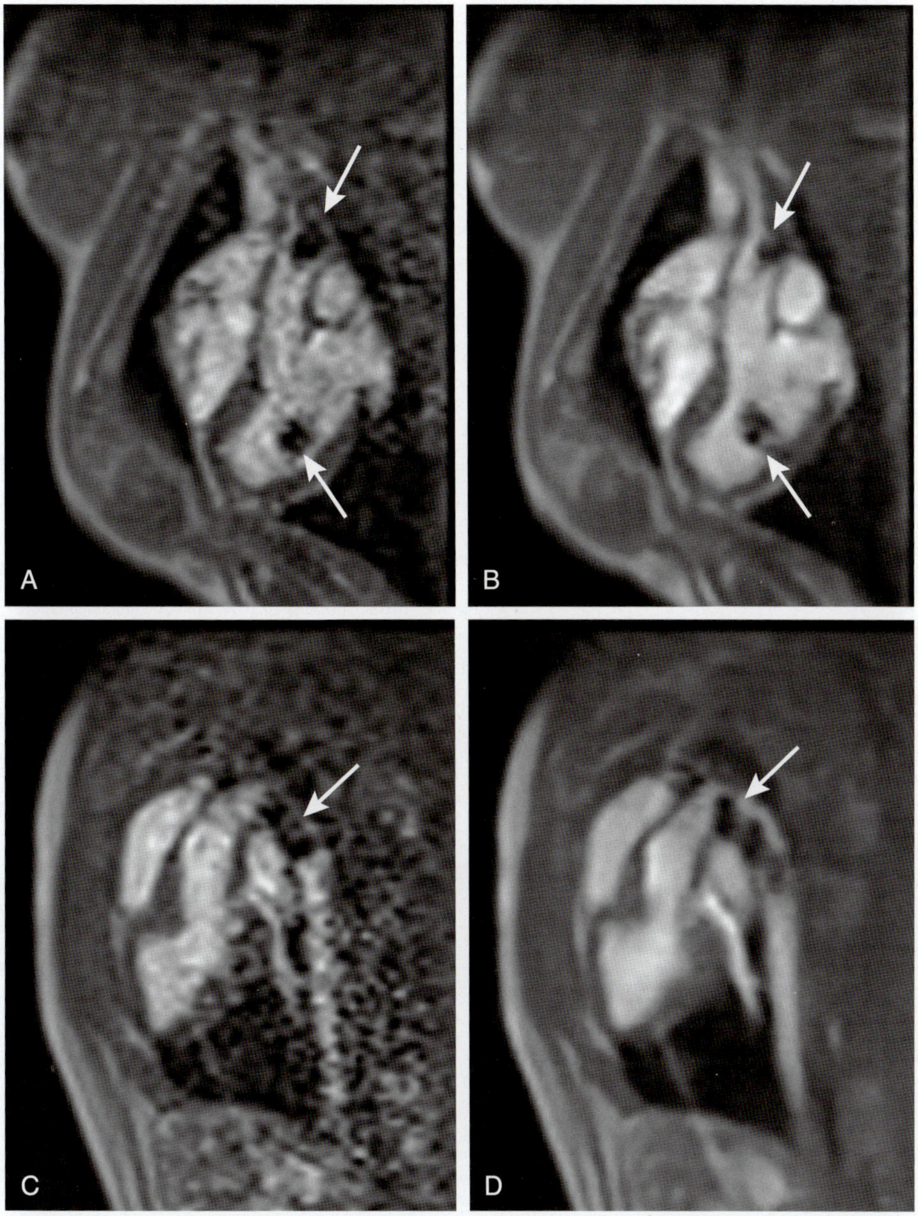

FIG. 10.11 The images on the left (A, C) show real-time spoiled gradient echo images from a magnetic resonance (MR)-guided left heart catheterization procedure performed in a pig at 0.55 T.[30] The tip of a guidewire with three MR-visible markers is seen (*white arrows*) in the left ventricle (A, B) and aortic arch (C, D). The images were acquired with an acceleration rate of four to achieve a temporal resolution of 100 ms, resulting in low signal-to-ratio (SNR). The images on the right (B, D) show recovery of SNR through machine learning–based denoising, providing good visualization of the guidewire markers (*white arrows*) in the left ventricle in the top row (A, B) and in the aortic arch in the bottom row (C, D).

limitation of reduced SNR. The favorable physics properties of mid fields include shorter native T1 and longer T2 and T2* relaxation times, along with higher field homogeneity and reduced susceptibility induced signal loss and artifact. Acquisition techniques such as bSSFP and spiral readouts benefit from these relationships, making them ideally suited for mid field and partially offsetting the SNR disadvantage. The potential for AI to enhance mid-field image quality is beginning to show promise, particularly in the realm of image reconstruction and denoising. AI-based algorithms can effectively reconstruct and denoise images using undersampled data, further compensating for the inherently lower SNR at mid field. These acquisition and reconstruction strategies are enabling mid-field systems to achieve diagnostic image quality without extending scan times, improving efficiency, cost effectiveness, and patient comfort.

CONCLUSION

While clinical validation studies are still needed to verify its transformative potential, there is growing evidence that mid-field cardiovascular MRI will soon begin to play an important role in expanding cardiac MRI access to underserved regions, patient populations, and healthcare settings. By leveraging technological advancements and innovative applications, mid-field systems have the potential to address long-standing challenges in cost, accessibility, and patient safety.

REFERENCES

1. Qin C, Murali S, Lee E, et al. Sustainable low-field cardiovascular magnetic resonance in changing healthcare systems. *Eur Heart J Cardiovasc Imaging.* 2022;23(6):e246–e260. https://doi.org/10.1093/ehjci/jeab286.
2. Simonetti OP, Ahmad R. Low-field cardiac magnetic resonance imaging: a compelling case for cardiac magnetic resonance's future. *Circ Cardiovasc Imaging.* 2017;10(6):e005446. https://doi.org/10.1161/CIRCIMAGING.117.005446.

3. Marques JP, Simonis FFJ, Webb AG. Low-field MRI: an MR physics perspective. *J Magn Reson Imaging*. 2019;49(6):1528–1542. https://doi.org/10.1002/jmri.26637.
4. Rusche T, Vosshenrich J, Winkel DJ, et al. More space, less noise-new-generation low-field magnetic resonance imaging systems can improve patient comfort: a prospective 0.55 T-1.5 T-scanner comparison. *J Clin Med*. 2022;11(22). https://doi.org/10.3390/jcm11226705.
5. Vosshenrich J, Breit HC, Bach M, Merkle EM. Economic aspects of low-field magnetic resonance imaging: acquisition, installation, and maintenance costs of 0.55 T systems. *Radiologe*. 2022;62(5):400–404. https://doi.org/10.1007/s00117-022-00986-9.
6. Schwitter J, Gold MR, Al Fagih A, et al. Image quality of cardiac magnetic resonance imaging in patients with an implantable cardioverter defibrillator system designed for the magnetic resonance imaging environment. *Circ Cardiovasc Imaging*. 2016;9(5):e004025. https://doi.org/10.1161/CIRCIMAGING.115.004025.
7. Simonetti OP, Gross DC. Cardiovascular magnetic resonance in patients with magnetic resonance-conditional cardiac implantable electronic devices: what can we see? *Circ Cardiovasc Imaging*. 2016;9(5):e004970. https://doi.org/10.1161/CIRCIMAGING.116.004970.
8. Strach K, Naehle CP, Muhlsteffen A, et al. Low-field magnetic resonance imaging: increased safety for pacemaker patients? *Europace*. 2010;12(7):952–960. https://doi.org/10.1093/europace/euq081.
9. Tian Y, Nayak KS. New clinical opportunities of low-field MRI: heart, lung, body, and musculoskeletal. *MAGMA*. 2024;37(1):1–14. https://doi.org/10.1007/s10334-023-01123-w.
10. Campbell-Washburn AE, Ramasawmy R, Restivo MC, et al. Opportunities in interventional and diagnostic imaging by using high-performance low-field-strength MRI. *Radiology*. 2019;293:190452. https://doi.org/10.1148/radiol.2019190452.
11. Varghese J, Craft J, Crabtree CD, et al. Assessment of cardiac function, blood flow and myocardial tissue relaxation parameters at 0.35 T. *NMR Biomed*. 2020;33:e4317. https://doi.org/10.1002/nbm.4317.
12. Ramasawmy R, Herzka DA, Lederman RJ, Campbell-Washburn AE. Spiral bSSFP Phase-contrast Flow at 0.55 T. Presented at: Proceedings of the ISMRM Annual Meeting 2020; 1332.
13. Hamilton JI, Seiberlich N. Real-Time Spiral bSSFP Functional Cardiac MRI on a 0.55 T Scanner Using a Deep Image Prior Reconstruction with GROG. Presented at: Proceedings of the ISMRM Annual Meeting; 2022; 1761.
14. Tian Y, Lim Y, Nayak KS. Real-Time Water Fat Imaging at 0.55 T with Spiral Out-In-Out-In Sampling. Presented at: Proceedings of the ISMRM Annual Meeting; 2022; 0516.
15. Campbell-Washburn AE, Malayeri AA, Jones EC, et al. T2-weighted lung imaging using a 0.55-T MRI system. *Radiol Cardiothorac Imaging*. 2021;3(3):e200611. https://doi.org/10.1148/ryct.2021200611.
16. Bhattacharya I, Ramasawmy R, Javed A, et al. Assessment of lung structure and regional function using 0.55 T MRI in patients with lymphangioleiomyomatosis. *Investig Radiol*. 2022;57(3):178–186. https://doi.org/10.1097/RLI.0000000000000832.
17. Campbell-Washburn AE, Varghese J, Nayak KS, Ramasawmy R, Simonetti OP. Cardiac MRI at low field strengths. *J Magn Reson Imaging*. 2024;59(2):412–430. https://doi.org/10.1002/jmri.28890.
18. Varghese J, Jin N, Giese D, et al. Building a comprehensive cardiovascular magnetic resonance exam on a commercial 0.55 T system: a pictorial essay on potential applications. *Front Cardiovasc Med*. 2023;10:1120982. https://doi.org/10.3389/fcvm.2023.1120982.
19. Bandettini WP, Shanbhag SM, Mancini C, et al. Evaluation of myocardial infarction by cardiovascular magnetic resonance at 0.55-T compared to 1.5-T. *JACC Cardiovasc Imaging*. 2021;14(9):1866–1868. https://doi.org/10.1016/j.jcmg.2021.02.024.
20. Bandettini WP, Shanbhag SM, Mancini C, et al. A comparison of cine CMR imaging at 0.55 T and 1.5 T. *J Cardiovasc Magn Reson*. 2020;22(1):37. https://doi.org/10.1186/s12968-020-00618-y.
21. Goyal A, Crabtree CD, Lee BC, et al. The impact of severe obesity on image quality and ventricular function assessment in echocardiography and cardiac MRI. *Int J Cardiovasc Imaging*. 2024;40(5):1081–1094. https://doi.org/10.1007/s10554-024-03078-y.
22. Tian Y, Detterich J, Pruetz JD, Yagiz E, Wood JC, Nayak KS. Feasibility of fetal cardiac function and anatomy assessment by real-time spiral balanced steady-state free precession magnetic resonance imaging at 0.55 T. *J Cardiovasc Magn Reson*. 2024;27(1):101130. https://doi.org/10.1016/j.jocmr.2024.101130.
23. Aviles Verdera J, Story L, Hall M, et al. Reliability and feasibility of low-field-strength fetal MRI at 0.55 T during pregnancy. *Radiology*. 2023;309(1):e223050. https://doi.org/10.1148/radiol.223050.
24. Zhang CY, Cleri M, Woodgate T, et al. Structural and functional fetal cardiac imaging using low field (0.55 T) MRI. *Front Pediatr*. 2024;12:1418645. https://doi.org/10.3389/fped.2024.1418645.
25. Wieslander B, Seemann F, Javed A, et al. Impact of vasodilation on oxygen-enhanced functional lung MRI at 0.55 T. *Investig Radiol*. 2023;58(9):663–672. https://doi.org/10.1097/RLI.0000000000000958.
26. Tian Y, Lee NG, Zhao Z, Wilcox AG, Nieva JJ, Nayak KS. Single breath-hold volumetric lung imaging at 0.55 T using stack-of-spiral (SoS) out-in balanced SSFP. *Magn Reson Med*. 2024;93:1999–2007. https://doi.org/10.1002/mrm.30386.
27. Rogers T, Campbell-Washburn AE, Ramasawmy R, et al. Interventional cardiovascular magnetic resonance: state-of-the-art. *J Cardiovasc Magn Reson*. 2023;25(1):48. https://doi.org/10.1186/s12968-023-00956-7.
28. Ratnayaka K, Kanter JP, Faranesh AZ, et al. Radiation-free CMR diagnostic heart catheterization in children. *J Cardiovasc Magn Reson*. 2017;19(1):65. https://doi.org/10.1186/s12968-017-0374-2.
29. Rogers T, Ratnayaka K, Khan JM, et al. CMR fluoroscopy right heart catheterization for cardiac output and pulmonary vascular resistance: results in 102 patients. *J Cardiovasc Magn Reson*. 2017;19(1):54. https://doi.org/10.1186/s12968-017-0366-2.
30. Armstrong AK, Liu Y, Kelly JM, et al. Feasibility of MRI-Guided cardiac catheterization, angioplasty, and stenting in a commercial wide-bore 0.55 T scanner. *J Cardiovasc Magn Reson*. 2025;27:101858. https://doi.org/10.1016/j.jocmr.2025.101858.
31. Basar B, Sonmez M, Yildirim DK, et al. Susceptibility artifacts from metallic markers and cardiac catheterization devices on a high-performance 0.55 T MRI system. *Magn Reson Imaging*. 2021;77:14–20. https://doi.org/10.1016/j.mri.2020.12.002.

11 Cardiac Magnetic Resonance Spectroscopy

LADISLAV VALKOVIČ, STEFAN NEUBAUER, AND OLIVER J. RIDER

PREAMBLE

Cardiac magnetic resonance imaging (MRI) uses the ^{1}H nucleus in water (H_2O) and fat (CH_2 and CH_3 groups) molecules as its only signal source, and therefore offers little insight into the biochemical state of cardiac tissue. In contrast, cardiac magnetic resonance spectroscopy (MRS) allows the study of many other nuclei. It is the only available method for the noninvasive assessment of cardiac metabolism without the need for external radioactive tracers. Information on the major nuclei of interest for the metabolic study of cardiac tissue by MRS is given in Table 11.1, including ^{1}H, ^{13}C, and ^{31}P. While, theoretically, many clinical questions can be answered with cardiac MRS, the main reason why MRS has not yet fulfilled its potential in clinical cardiology is related to the fundamental physical limitations of the method. MRS is often used to study non-^{1}H nuclei, which have a much lower intrinsic magnetic resonance (MR) sensitivity than ^{1}H. Furthermore, metabolite concentrations in vivo are typically in the mM range, which is several orders of magnitude lower than that for water (approx. 80 M) or fat (often >1 M). Therefore, the temporal and spatial resolution of MRS has so far remained far behind that of MRI. However, the new technique of hyperpolarized MRS is now starting to overcome this major limitation—this method has been called "the light at the end of the tunnel" for clinical cardiac spectroscopy. In addition, MRS is likely to become a clinical tool in situations where its unique metabolic insights are more important than obtaining high spatial or temporal resolution.

This chapter focuses on the clinical development and application of MRS, but the method has also been widely used in experimental cardiology, ever since the first ^{31}P-MR spectrum from an isolated heart was obtained by Radda's group in the 1970s.[1] Since then, experimental MRS studies have offered numerous fundamental insights into cardiac metabolism. For those interested in experimental MRS and a more detailed methodological background, comprehensive reviews of the subject are available elsewhere.[2–4] Complementary clinical reviews include Holloway et al.[5] or Hudsmith et al.[6]

PHYSICAL PRINCIPLES

The basic principles of MRS (see Refs. [7–9] for textbooks on the general physical principles of MRI and MRS) are, from the perspective of the organ of interest here (i.e., the human heart), best explained in terms of the most extensively studied nucleus (^{31}P), but these principles apply to MRS of all nuclei. An MR system used for in vivo MRS consists of a high-field superconducting magnet (currently up to 14 T, but usually 1.5 or 3 T, where tesla (T) is the unit of magnetic field strength) with a bore size ranging between ~60 and 80 cm. The nucleus-specific radiofrequency (RF) coils, which are used for MR excitation and signal reception, are seated within the magnet bore. The magnet is interfaced with a computer, a magnetic field gradient system, and an RF transmitter and receiver. MRS requires much higher magnetic field homogeneity than common MRI. Therefore, before any MRS experiment, the magnetic field must first be homogenized with shim gradients. Spin excitation is achieved by transmitting a radiofrequency pulse through the RF coils into the subject. The resulting MR signal, known as the free induction decay (FID), is then received from the subject by the RF coils and recorded by the scanner. The signal (or FID) oscillates with time, but within an overall exponentially decaying "envelope". It typically reaches negligible levels after tens of milliseconds. An MR spectrum is then computed from the acquired FID (by applying the discrete Fourier transform formula[10]), which is the main difference from MRI, for which only the first point of the FID is used. The MR spectrum describes the signal intensity as a function of resonance frequency. Because of the low sensitivity of MRS, in practice, many FIDs are averaged to obtain MR spectra with an adequate "signal-to-noise ratio" (SNR; i.e., the magnitude of the first point in time for the metabolite-specific response of a selected peak in the spectrum, divided by the standard deviation of noise[11]). The required number of averages depends on the concentration of the metabolite under investigation, its MR relaxation times (T_1, T_2, T^*_2), the "filling factor" (the mass of the heart in the interrogated voxel relative to the coil size), the natural abundance of the nuclear isotope studied, its relative MR sensitivity (Table 11.1), the excitation pulse angle, and the pulse repetition time (TR). For a human heart study at ≥3 T, over 400 localized FIDs are typically acquired. To quantify metabolite concentrations from MR spectra, it is vital to correct for partial saturation, which depends on the selected pulse angles and TR. This is because the maximum MR signal is only obtained when nuclei are excited from a fully relaxed spin state, that is, when a time of at least $5 \times T_1$ has passed since a previous excitation (e.g., T_1 of phosphocreatine [PCr] at 7 T is ~3 s, requiring a TR of ≥15 s; at 1.5 T the PCr T_1 is ~ 4.4 s, requiring a TR of ≥22 s). Acquisition of fully relaxed MR spectra thus leads to prohibitively long acquisition times. In practice, we take advantage of the fact that the initial part of the FID contains most of the signal. Use of shorter TRs with optimized pulse angles therefore yields spectra with higher signal to noise for a given acquisition time, but some of the signal is lost due to saturation (i.e., spectra are "partially saturated"). The extent of saturation also varies for different ^{31}P resonances, because the T_1 s of ^{31}P metabolites such as PCr and adenosine triphosphate (ATP) are significantly different (T_1 of PCr is 2–3 × longer than T_1 of ATP). Therefore, for metabolite quantification from partially saturated spectra, the spectral peak areas are determined (e.g., fitted using AMARES[12,13] or LCModel[14]), and then correction factors are applied to obtain the metabolite concentrations. By comparing fully relaxed and saturated spectra, these factors can be determined for each metabolite. In practice, TRs and pulse angles for MRS are chosen to yield acceptable measurement times at an ~20–50% degree of saturation. Larger degrees of saturation, resulting from the use of extremely short TRs, make quantification of spectra challenging due to uncertainties in the metabolite T_1 values and confounders from the dynamic chemical reactions involving these metabolites.

Sample ^{31}P-MR spectra from the septum of the human heart, obtained at 1.5 T, 3 T, and 7 T with a TR of 1 s and a pulse angle of ~40°, are depicted in Fig. 11.1. A typical cardiac in vivo ^{31}P spectrum shows eight resonances, corresponding to the three (γ, α, and β) ^{31}P atoms of ATP (the resonance at the right shoulder of the α-ATP peak represents the P atom of nicotinamide adenine dinucleotide in its oxidized and reduced form [NAD^+ and NADH, respectively]), PCr, phosphodiesters (mostly representing glycerol phosphocholine and glycerol phosphoethanolamine), and 2,3-diphosphoglycerate (2,3-DPG; originating from the red blood cells in the blood pool).[9] The reason why only a small number of ^{31}P resonances are detectable, in spite of many more ^{31}P-containing metabolites are present in the heart, is that, for ^{31}P nuclei to be visible, they must be present above a certain concentration threshold of ~600 μM, they must be free to tumble in solution, and they cannot be obscured by larger signals (e.g., as is the case for inorganic phosphate [Pi] covered by 2,3-DPG). Largely immobilized metabolites such as plasma membrane phospholipids do not yield a quantifiable MR signal due to their very short T_2 values; instead, these metabolites contribute to the broad "baseline hump" of ^{31}P spectra, which is particularly pronounced in the brain and at lower field strengths. Due to the phenomenon termed "chemical shift", different metabolites resonate at distinct frequencies, allowing their discrimination from each other. Chemical shift is given in units of parts per million (ppm) relative to the resonance frequency of a reference compound (e.g., phosphoric acid [H_3PO_4] or PCr in vivo experiments). ^{31}P-metabolite resonances extend over a range of ~30 ppm.[9] The physical basis of chemical shift is that nuclei at different positions in the molecule have different spatial distributions of electrons around them, which interact differently with the scanner's magnetic field.[15] Fitting of spectral peak areas (e.g., with AMARES) and saturation correction yields metabolite concentrations in arbitrary units. Often, metabolite ratios such as the PCr/ATP ratio are then calculated—implicitly assuming that the concentration of the metabolite in the denominator (ATP here) is tightly regulated to act as an endogenous reference. Alternatively, using an exogenous

TABLE 11.1 Nuclei most frequently studied by magnetic resonance spectroscopy.

NUCLEUS	NATURAL ABUNDANCE (%)	RELATIVE MR SENSITIVITY (%)	MYOCARDIAL TISSUE CONCENTRATIONS
^{1}H	99.98	100	H_2O 110 M; up to ~ 90 mM (CH_3-^{1}H of creatine)
^{13}C	1.1	1.6	Labelled compounds, several mM
^{31}P	100	6.6	Up to ~ 18 mM (PCr)

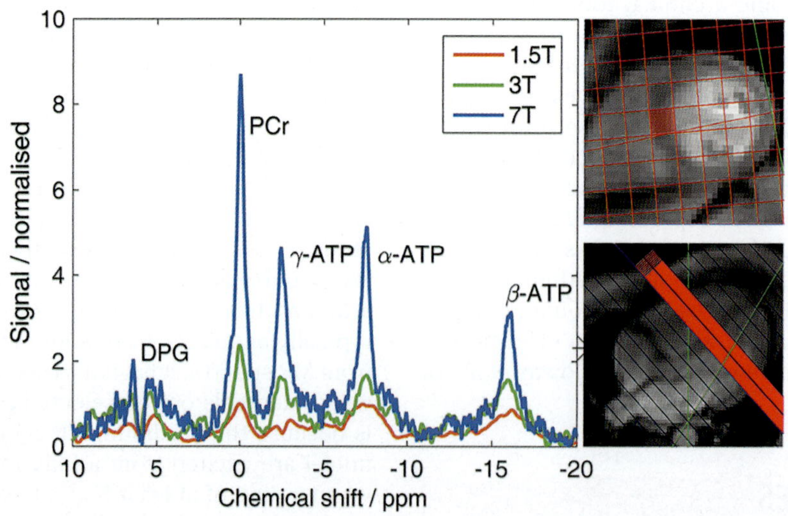

FIG. 11.1 Left: ^{31}P magnetic resonance spectra from the interventricular septum of the same volunteer recorded at 1.5 T, 3 T, and 7 T using a 3D magnetic resonance spectroscopy imaging (MRSI) sequence. Field-of-view 240 × 240 × 200 mm^3 with a 12 × 8 × 8 matrix with 32 averages at 1.5 T in 22 min and a 16 × 16 × 8 matrix with 10 averages at 3 T and 7 T in 28 min. To facilitate comparison, the spectra are normalized to the baseline noise level, apodized, and the 1.5 T spectrum is scaled to account for its larger voxel size and shorter acquisition. Right: corresponding short-axis and four-chamber localizer images recorded by ^{1}H magnetic resonance imaging at 3 T. The 3D-MRSI voxel grid is overlaid. The voxel corresponding to the ^{31}P spectra is highlighted. *DPG*, 2,3-diphosphoglycerate (*from blood*); *PCr*, phosphocreatine; *γ-, α-, β-ATP*, the three phosphorus atoms of adenosine triphosphate.

reference phantom, absolute metabolite concentrations can be computed.[16,17] Frequently, phenylphosphonic acid is used for this purpose, as this generates an additional peak in the spectrum that does not overlap with the cardiac ^{31}P resonances.[18] The most significant advantage of MRS over destructive methods, such as traditional biochemical assays in which the tissue has to be frozen and extracted, is that the MRS measurement is noninvasive. Therefore, spectra can be acquired sequentially, and the response of energy metabolites to, for example, ischemia, hypoxia, or inotropic stimulation can be followed longitudinally in the same tissue.

NUCLEI FOR CARDIAC MAGNETIC RESONANCE SPECTROSCOPY

^{31}P Magnetic Resonance Spectroscopy

With ^{31}P-MRS, cardiac high-energy phosphate metabolism (i.e., the energetic state of the heart) can be monitored noninvasively. ATP is the direct energy source for all energy-consuming reactions in the heart. PCr acts as a temporal energy buffer and as an energy transport molecule in the "creatine kinase (CK)/PCr energy shuttle"[19] (Fig. 11.2). For this, the high-energy phosphate group is transferred from ATP to creatine in the mitochondria (where ATP is produced by ATP synthase), yielding PCr and adenosine diphosphate (ADP) in a reaction catalyzed by the mitochondrial CK isoenzyme (CK_{mito}). PCr diffuses through the cytoplasm to the site of ATP utilization (the myofibrils), where the back reaction (catalyzed by the myofibrillar-bound CK-MM isoenzymes) occurs and ATP is reformed and used for contraction. Free creatine then diffuses back to the mitochondria. The reaction rates at the CK isoenzymes complement each other to maintain this steady state.[20] The second important function of PCr and CK is to control the thermodynamic state of the cell, that is, to maintain free cytosolic ADP at a low concentration during times of increased energy demand, and instead raise ADP and consume Cr in the mitochondrial space, thereby upregulating oxidative phosphorylation.[21] This is a requirement for normal cardiac function, because ADP determines the free energy change of ATP hydrolysis (ΔG; kJ/mol), which is a measure of the maximum amount of energy released from hydrolyzing ATP (see[22] for details on the calculation of free ADP and ΔG from CK shuttle metabolites). In the normal heart, ΔG is ~ −58 kJ/mol. Many intracellular enzymes such as SR-Ca^{++}-ATPase and others will not function properly above a threshold value for ΔG of about −52 kJ/mol. CK has also been implicated in minimizing cellular ADP loss, maintaining intracellular pH, and activating glycogenolysis and glycolysis.[21]

Inorganic phosphate (Pi) is formed when ATP is hydrolyzed: ATP ADP + Pi. Pi increases when ATP utilization exceeds ATP production (e.g., during ischemia). Intracellular pH (pH_i) can also be measured with ^{31}P-MRS, from the chemical shift difference between PCr and Pi, which is pH sensitive due to shifts in the equilibrium $H_2PO_4^- \rightleftharpoons HPO_4^{2-} + H^+$ near pH 7. Furthermore, the chemical shift difference between PCr and β-ATP or between α-ATP and β-ATP can be used to measure the intracellular magnesium ion concentration.[23,24]

Cardiac energy metabolism has been investigated by ^{31}P-MRS under various study conditions. For example, the effect of changes in cardiac workload on energetics have been examined. PCr levels do not change with moderate changes in workload,[25] but decline with substantial increases in cardiac work.[26] ATP content remains nearly constant with varying workload and during the cardiac cycle, because the CK equilibrium favors ATP synthesis over PCr synthesis by a factor of ~100.[27–29] Thus, for any acute myocardial stress situation, including ischemia, ATP only decreases when PCr levels are substantially depleted.[30] This is the fundamental reason why the PCr/ATP ratio is a highly sensitive indicator of the energetic state of the heart.

With the magnetization (saturation) transfer method,[31–33] the exchange rate of the CK reaction, a measure of ATP transfer from mitochondria to myofibrils, can be measured in vivo. This technique uses selective irradiation of a metabolite involved in the reaction (i.e., ATP) and measures the effect on its exchange partner (i.e., PCr). In other words, due to the forward flux in the CK reaction, saturation of the γ-ATP resonance frequency causes a reduction in measurable PCr signal, which is proportional to the rate of CK flux. Besides knowing the difference in PCr signal amplitude from saturated and control spectra, the knowledge of apparent relaxation time (i.e., the T_1 of PCr measured during the saturation of γ-ATP) is needed for CK rate calculation[34].

^{1}H Magnetic Resonance Spectroscopy

Other than ^{31}P, the nuclei with the greatest potential for clinical cardiac MRS are ^{1}H and hyperpolarized ^{13}C (see more below). Protons have the highest MR sensitivity of all

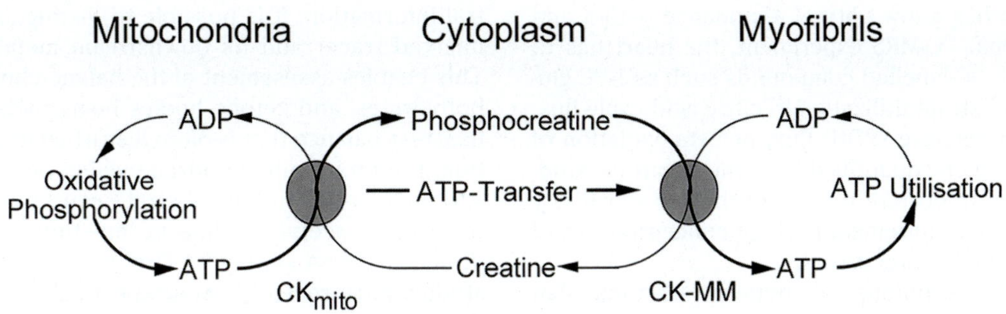

FIG. 11.2 Creatine kinase-phosphocreatine energy shuttle. For details, see text. *ADP*, *Adenosine diphosphate; ATP, adenosine triphosphate;* CK_{mito}, *mitochondrial creatine kinase; CK-MM, myofibrilar bound CK*

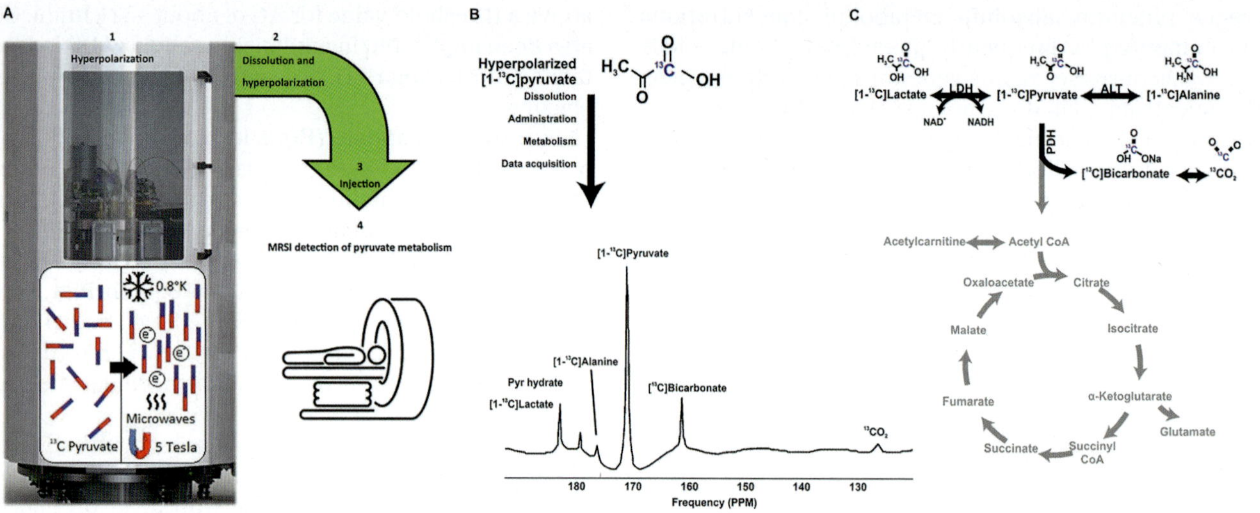

FIG. 11.3 (A) Illustration of the dissolution dynamic nuclear polarization process in the clinical hyperpolarizer "SPINlab". First (1), up to four samples of [1-13C] pyruvate are placed in the SPINlab and the combination of a free radical, low temperature (0.8°K), microwave irradiation, and a magnetic field of 5 T results in hyperpolarization of the ^{13}C nuclei. Second (2), the [1-13C] pyruvate is dissolved and a quality control module ensures that temperature, pH, concentration, and polarization level are acceptable for (3) injection. Fourth (4), immediately after injection into the patient, spectra and/or images of the pyruvate metabolism can be acquired. (B) Hyperpolarized [1-13C] pyruvate molecule and the resulting spectrum following label incorporation in the heart using hyperpolarized [1-13C] pyruvate. (C) Biochemical basis for label exchange and resulting spectrum in the heart. *ALT*, Alanine aminotransferase; *LDH*, lactate dehydrogenase; *NAD*+, Oxidised form of nicotinamide adenine dinucleotide; *NADH*, reduced form of nicotinamide adenine dinucleotide; *MRSI*, magnetic resonance spectroscopic imaging; *PDH*, pyruvate dehydrogenase. (Adapted from Jørgensen SH, Bogh N, Hansen E, et al. Hyperpolarized MRI—an update and future perspectives. *Semin Nucl Med*. 2022;52(3):374–381; and Lewis AJ, Tyler DJ, Rider OJ. Clinical cardiovascular applications of hyperpolarized magnetic resonance. *Cardiovasc Drugs Ther*. 2020;34(2):231–240; both under the Creative Commons Attribution Licence.)

MR-detectable nuclei as well as a high natural abundance (Table 11.1). ^{1}H is contained in a large number of metabolites, for example creatine, lactate, carnitine, taurine, and $-CH_3$ and $-CH_2$ resonances of lipids.[35,36] Since water content can be considered stable under most conditions, water is often used as an internal concentration reference for metabolite concentration and lipid content quantification. Measurement of total creatine by single voxel spectroscopy[37–40] or navigator-gated echo-planar spectroscopic imaging[41] or potentially by creatine chemical exchange saturation transfer imaging[42] should, in conjunction with ^{31}P-MRS, allow the noninvasive determination of free ADP and ΔG of ATP hydrolysis, as demonstrated by Bottomley et al.[43,44] Technical challenges for ^{1}H-MRS include the need for suppression of the strong ^{1}H signal from water and the complexity of ^{1}H spectra with overlapping resonances, many of which remain to be characterized, and which also means that excellent shimming, frequency alignment, and motion compensation are needed.[45,46]

^{13}C Magnetic Resonance Spectroscopy

The ^{13}C nucleus has a low natural abundance (~1%), and for a conventional ^{13}C-MRS experiment, the heart has to be supplied with ^{13}C-labelled compounds such as 1-^{13}C glucose. Cardiac substrate utilization,[173] citric acid cycle flux, pyruvate dehydrogenase (PDH) flux, or beta-oxidation of fatty acids can then be quantified.[47,48] Clinical cardiac studies have yet to be reported because of the low sensitivity of ^{13}C-MRS and the requirement for high concentrations of exogenous ^{13}C-labelled precursors.

However, the technique of hyperpolarization can increase the SNR of ^{13}C experiments by a factor of up to 10,000× for a few minutes, until the magnetization decays by T_1 relaxation back to thermal equilibrium.[49,50] The detailed physics of dissolution by dynamic nuclear polarization (DNP), which is the most widely used method for hyperpolarization, is beyond the scope of this chapter. Briefly, the DNP method transfers the high polarization levels from electron spins of a free radical to ^{13}C-labelled agents in an extremely cold environment (0.8 °K) in a strong magnetic field (~5 T) using microwave irradiation (Fig. 11.3). The polarization level of >20%, equivalent to a 10^5-fold enhancement, requires a polarization time that is dependent on the magnetic field and the sample, which is typically ~2 hours.[51,52]

DNP is currently a very active area of research, as new pulse sequences, analysis methods, and injectable hyperpolarized agents are developed to capitalize on this extraordinary but brief burst of enhanced signal to noise. [1-^{13}C]Pyruvate[53,54] is a particularly attractive molecule to hyperpolarize, because it plays a pivotal role in substrate uptake preceding oxidative phosphorylation, enabling fluxes into acetyl- CoA, lactate, and bicarbonate to be quantified (Fig. 11.4). By encoding spatial and spectral information, it is possible to distinguish between the injected tracer and its downstream metabolic products. This enables assessment of the balance between fats, carbohydrates, and ketone bodies being metabolized by the heart—a balance that is often disturbed in disease. In addition, the rapid mitochondrial cycling between acetyl-CoA and an acetylcarnitine substrate can be used to uncover the role of acetylcarnitine in 'fine-tuning' the mitochondrial acetyl-CoA supply.[55,56] First human hyperpolarization studies have recently been reported,[57] which focused on PDH flux changes in diabetes and infarction.[58,59]

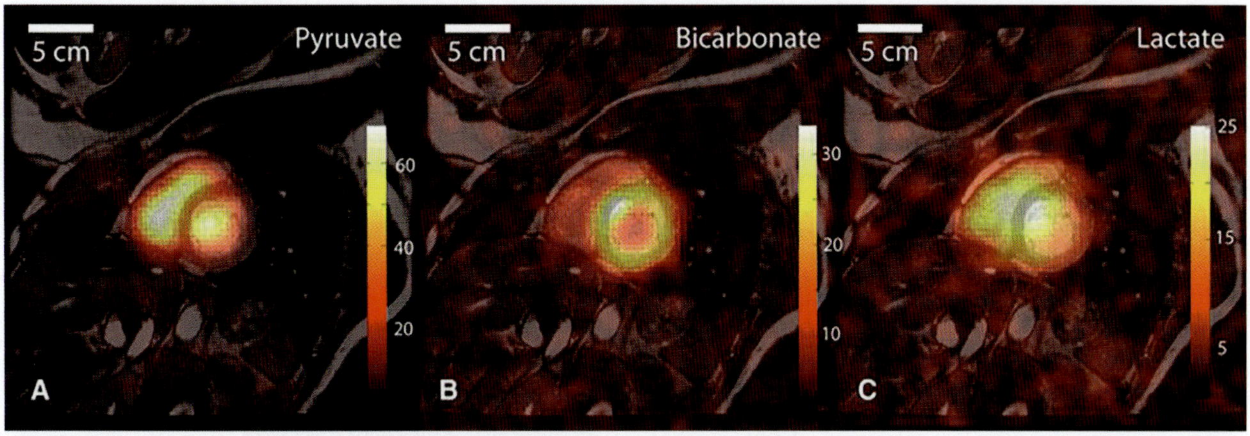

FIG. 11.4 Initial human experience using hyperpolarized [1-^{13}C] pyruvate to image the heart. Pyruvate and its downstream metabolites can be detected with relatively high spatial resolution. Representative 13C images displayed as color overlays on top of grayscale anatomic images in a short-axis midventricular (LV) slice. The [1-^{13}C] pyruvate substrate is seen mainly in the blood pool within the cardiac chambers. (A). Flux of pyruvate through the pyruvate dehydrogenase complex is reflected in the ^{13}C-bicarbonate image (B) with signal predominantly in the LV wall. The [1-^{13}C] lactate signal (C) appears covering both heart muscle and chambers. (Adapted from Cunningham CH, Lau JY, Chen AP, et al. Hyperpolarized ^{13}C metabolic MRI of the human heart: initial experience. Circ Res. 2016;119:1177-1182. doi: 10.1161/CIRCRESAHA.116.309769 under the Creative Commons Attribution Licence)

HOW TO GET STARTED WITH MAGNETIC RESONANCE SPECTROSCOPY

Hardware Requirements

While ^{1}H-MRS does not require additional hardware and can be used on any clinical MR system, ^{31}P and ^{13}C have several specific hardware requirements. In particular, a dedicated broadband RF power amplifier is needed to provide excitation pulses at the ^{31}P or ^{13}C frequency. To deliver these pulses (and receive the resulting FID), dedicated RF coils tuned to the frequency of ^{31}P and ^{13}C are also needed, since the MR systems have an integrated transmit coil for ^{1}H only. When selecting the RF coil, several aspects need to be considered, in particular, the shape and size of the coil, which depends on which position the MRS scans will be acquired in. Historically, ^{31}P- and ^{13}C-MRS studies have been performed in the prone position rather than supine, as this reduces breathing motion artifacts and may slightly reduce the distance of the heart from the surface coil, thereby improving sensitivity. However, for 3 T and 7 T systems with modern sensitive RF coils, the supine position is recommended, as it is much more comfortable for the patient, and thus minimizes involuntary motion. Another aspect to consider is the number of receive elements, since modern coil designs often allow two or more receive elements to be used, thus providing increased SNR. Hyperpolarized ^{13}C-MRS additionally requires a clinical hyperpolarizer (Fig. 11.3), which provides a sterile hyperpolarized substrate (e.g., [1-^{13}C]pyruvate). This needs to pass a quick quality assessment (polarization level, pH, pyruvate concentration, and temperature) before being cleared for injection into a patient. The so-called SPINlab (GE Healthcare) has automated all these processes and is currently the only commercially available hyperpolarizer to be used in a clinical setting.[51]

Magnetic Resonance Spectroscopy Data Acquisition

The heart is a rapidly moving organ, thus signal localization to the relatively small voxels used for ^{1}H-MRS currently requires gating to the ECG and, when resolution is further improved, ultimately to respiration as well.[60] Most clinical ^{31}P-MRS studies were performed at 1.5 T until the early 2000s and, since then, mostly at 3 T, with a few most recently at 7 T.[61,62] The cardiac muscle lies behind the chest wall skeletal muscle, which creates a strong ^{31}P signal that must be suppressed by spectral localization techniques, outer volume suppression,[63] or surface-spoiling gradient coils.[64] Besides skeletal muscle, liver tissue also has to be avoided and/or suppressed as it does not express CK. Typical localization methods include DRESS (**d**epth-**re**solved **s**urface coil **s**pectroscopy), 1D-MRSI (MRS imaging), ISIS (**i**mage-**s**elected **i**n vivo **s**pectroscopy), and 2D/3D-MRSI (Fig. 11.5). These methods are reviewed in detail elsewhere.[65] Bottomley et al.[66–68] pioneered most of the early methodological development of human cardiac MRS. A variety of recently proposed non-Cartesian acquisition methods, such as compressed sensing (CS) spectroscopy,[69] spiral ^{31}P-MRS,[70] and concentric ring ^{31}P-MRS,[71] enable a smooth trade-off between acquisition time, spatial resolution, and spectral resolution. Most spectroscopic techniques require a stack of ^{1}H scout images to be obtained first, which are used to select the spectroscopic volume(s). The low sensitivity of ^{31}P-MRS requires relatively large voxel sizes, typically nominally ~20–70 mL (and often rather larger if one considers the "true" integrated point-spread-function volume), either encompassing all of the heart or localized to the septum.[61] Due to this, ECG gating is less effective and rarely used in ^{31}P-MRS.[72] A set of ^{31}P-MRS spectra acquired from a healthy volunteer with 3D-MRSI at 1.5 T, 3 T, and 7 T is shown in Fig. 11.1. Even though the spectral bandwidth also increases with field strength, the 2,3-DPG peaks overlap with the Pi resonance in human ^{31}P-MR spectra at all field strengths. Thus, intracellular pH is typically difficult to determine; however, recent results show that Pi and pH become detectable in human myocardium at 7 T when flip angle and TR are increased or STEAM (STimulated Echo Acquisition Mode) single voxel localization is used.[73,74]

STEAM and PRESS (point-resolved spectroscopy) techniques are typically used for cardiac ^{1}H-MRS, with the voxel again placed in the septum. In addition to ECG

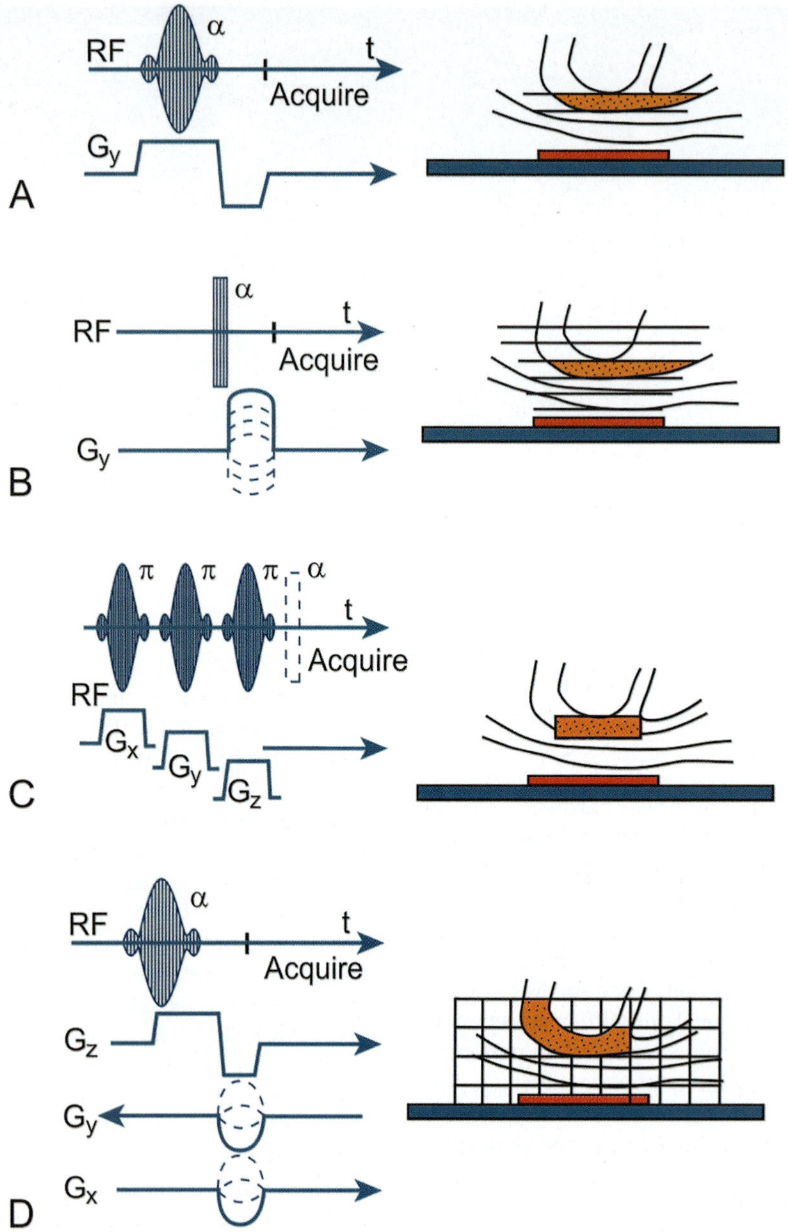

FIG. 11.5 Basic pulse sequences for localized cardiac spectroscopy with surface coils. (A) "Depth-resolved surface coil spectroscopy". A single section parallel to the plane of the surface coil is selected by applying a magnetic resonance (MR) imaging gradient (*G*) in the presence of a modulated radiofrequency (*RF*) excitation pulse of flip angle α. (B) The "one-dimensional chemical shift imaging" method similarly encodes multiple sections but uses an MR imaging gradient whose amplitude is stepped. (C) The "image-selected in vivo spectroscopy" method localizes to a single volume with selective inversion pulses applied with G_x, G_y, and G_z MR imaging gradients. All eight combinations of the three pulses must be applied and the resultant signals added and subtracted. (D) A section-selective "three-dimensional chemical shift imaging" sequence employs MR imaging section selection in one dimension and phase encoding in two dimensions. (From: Bottomley PA. MR spectroscopy of the human heart: the status and the challenges. Radiology. 1994;191:593-612. doi: 10.1148/radiology.191.3.8184033. Adapted with permission from the Radiological Society of North America.)

gating, acquisition is typically performed at breath-hold[75] or using navigator gating[60] to avoid breathing motion artifacts. In case of hyperpolarized ^{13}C, acquisition speed is essential as the hyperpolarization decreases rapidly. The high amounts of signal, on the other hand, allow fast spectrally selective imaging,[76] thus, providing maps of metabolic activity instead of individual spectra. Using multiband selective pulses with a variable flip angle setting for individual resonances[77] allows simultaneous acquisition of multiple metabolite maps. The required high temporal resolution is secured by using echo-planar imaging[77] or spiral trajectory readouts.[76] These can either be single-shot readouts,[57] which provide the highest temporal resolution, or multishot readouts,[76] which eventually provide higher spatial resolution. Variable density spirals can also be used to shorten the readout and minimize motion artifacts,[78] but potentially lead to noise amplification.

Vendor-Specific Acquisition Aspects

It is important to note that it is not possible to simply transfer MRS methods from one MR system to another if they are not from the same manufacturer—just like it would not be possible to do that for imaging sequences. Still, the three main MR system manufacturers (i.e., Siemens Healthineers, Philips Healthcare, and GE HealthCare) provide similar basic product sequences (i.e., PRESS and STEAM) and 2D/3D MRSI. However, the product sequences and protocols are primarily designed for brain ^{1}H-MRS, so they often need some modifications to be practical for cardiac applications. These modifications include enabling ECG gating, which is essential for cardiac ^{1}H-MRS, or potentially including MRI packages that allow diaphragm position monitoring using navigators. This typically requires getting a work in progress package from the vendor, getting the optimized sequence from another site, or doing some sequence programming. Luckily, these three manufacturers support sequence transfer between sites with appropriate research agreements, so getting a sequence from another center using similar MR systems is usually straightforward.

One noteworthy difference between the vendor single-voxel sequences is the ability of the Philips systems to visualize the spatial displacement between two metabolites of interest (e.g., between water and CH_2 lipids) caused by imperfect pulses. This ability allows for suppression of the signals from non-overlapping volumes, ensuring that all metabolic information originates from the same position (e.g., the septum). The other vendors provide an alternative approach for this by enabling a shift in the excitation pulse frequency to the metabolites of interest between acquisitions (e.g., to -3.5 ppm for CH_2 lipids and to 0 ppm for water).

Given the typical voxel size used in ^{31}P-MRS, the application of product MRSI techniques with a FID readout is much more straightforward. However, these are far from optimized for cardiac ^{31}P-MRS. For example, by minimizing the time between excitation and acquisition, significant signal increase can be gained and first-order phase impact can be reduced. To reduce MRSI scan times, acquisition weighting is often used. This is provided as standard on Siemens and Philips systems, and can also be available on GE systems as a part of the flexible research pack called the "FIDall" extension.

As mentioned above, the only clinically approved commercial hyperpolarizer is made by GE. It is, therefore, not surprising that the majority of hyperpolarized ^{13}C research is done on GE systems. Furthermore, while the basic product sequences do not offer the temporal resolution needed, FIDall facilitates more complex and rapid MRS acquisitions, and the community sharing provides a good range of ready-to-use sequences.

To summarize, while there are some differences between the acquisition techniques provided by the vendors, with sequence sharing between sites and in-house support for pulse programming, it is possible to close these gaps. Hence, while planning multicenter studies with sites using similar MR systems from the same vendor is simpler, cross-vendor studies are technically possible and needed for future development of the field. However, these will first require standardization efforts to ensure that quantitative spectroscopy results obtained on different MR systems are indeed equivalent.

Magnetic Resonance Spectroscopy Data Analysis

As discussed under "Physical principles", acquired spectra need to be fitted (e.g., using the AMARES fitting algorithm) and resulting signals corrected for partial saturation. This number then needs to be normalized to ensure it is comparable for different patients and research sites. Since ATP is considered stable until the late stages of heart failure (HF), ^{31}P-MRS can use ATP as an internal reference. By calculating the PCr/ATP peak area ratios, relative quantification of human ^{31}P spectra is straightforward. PCr/ATP is a powerful index of the energetic state of the heart (see section on specific MRS nuclei). ^{31}P resonances must be corrected for partial saturation using measured or literature T_1 values,[2,61] as described above. Intrinsic ^{31}P-T_1 values most likely remain constant in the presence of cardiac disease,[79] although observed T_1 values can change due to the effects of chemical exchange via the CK system.[80] Furthermore, ^{31}P-spectra require correction for blood contamination: blood contributes signal to the ATP, 2,3-diphosphoglycerate, and phosphodiester resonances. As human blood spectra have an ATP/2,3-diphosphoglycerate area ratio of ~0.15 and a phosphodiester/2,3-diphosphoglycerate area ratio of ~0.19, for blood correction, the ATP resonance area of cardiac spectra is reduced by 15% of the 2,3-diphosphoglycerate resonance area, and the phosphodiester resonance area is reduced by 19% of the 2,3-diphosphoglycerate resonance area.[81]

Absolute quantification of PCr and ATP is technically challenging, but is desirable, as the PCr/ATP ratio does not detect simultaneous decreases of both PCr and ATP, which occur in the failing[82] or infarcted nonviable myocardium.[83] Absolute ^{31}P metabolite levels can be obtained by acquiring signal from a ^{31}P standard as well as estimates of myocardial mass from MRI.[67,84] A different approach calibrates the ^{31}P signal to the tissue water proton content, measured by ^{1}H-MRS.[68] Modern "non-Fourier" methods for the determination of metabolite concentrations solve the powerful "inverse problem" mathematical formulation. For example, SLOOP (Spatial LOcalization with Optimal Pointspread function)[85] postprocessing can deliver concentrations in noncuboidal compartments (e.g., myocardium). SLAM (Spectroscopy with Linear Algebraic Modeling)[86–88] accelerates the acquisition steps to focus the scan time most effectively and assess concentrations in a predetermined compartment (e.g., segmented from a ^{1}H image).

A long-term goal for human cardiac MRS is to combine ^{31}P and ^{1}H spectroscopy to measure free ADP and ΔG of ATP hydrolysis, as described in canine myocardium by Bottomley et al.[37] Another relevant energetic parameter is the rate and extent of ATP transfer ("CK-flux"; see experimental section). Bottomley et al.[89] developed the "four-angle saturation transfer" (FAST) method, which allows measurement of CK flux in ~30 min at 1.5 T. More recently, Bottomley et al. introduced the Triple Repetition Time Saturation Transfer (TRiST)[32] (illustrated in Fig. 11.6) and later the Two Repetition Time Saturation Transfer (TwiST)[79] methods to measure CK flux at 3 T based on dual-TR T_1 measurements[90] during saturation, and we have introduced Bloch-Siegert four Angle Saturation Transfer (BOAST) to measure 3D-resolved CK flux at 7 T.[33]

The methods of ^{31}P-MRS are still being improved. Nevertheless, a major effort to standardize protocols and make advanced RF coils and pulse sequences at ultra-high field strengths routinely available will be required to bring cardiac MRS into clinical practice.

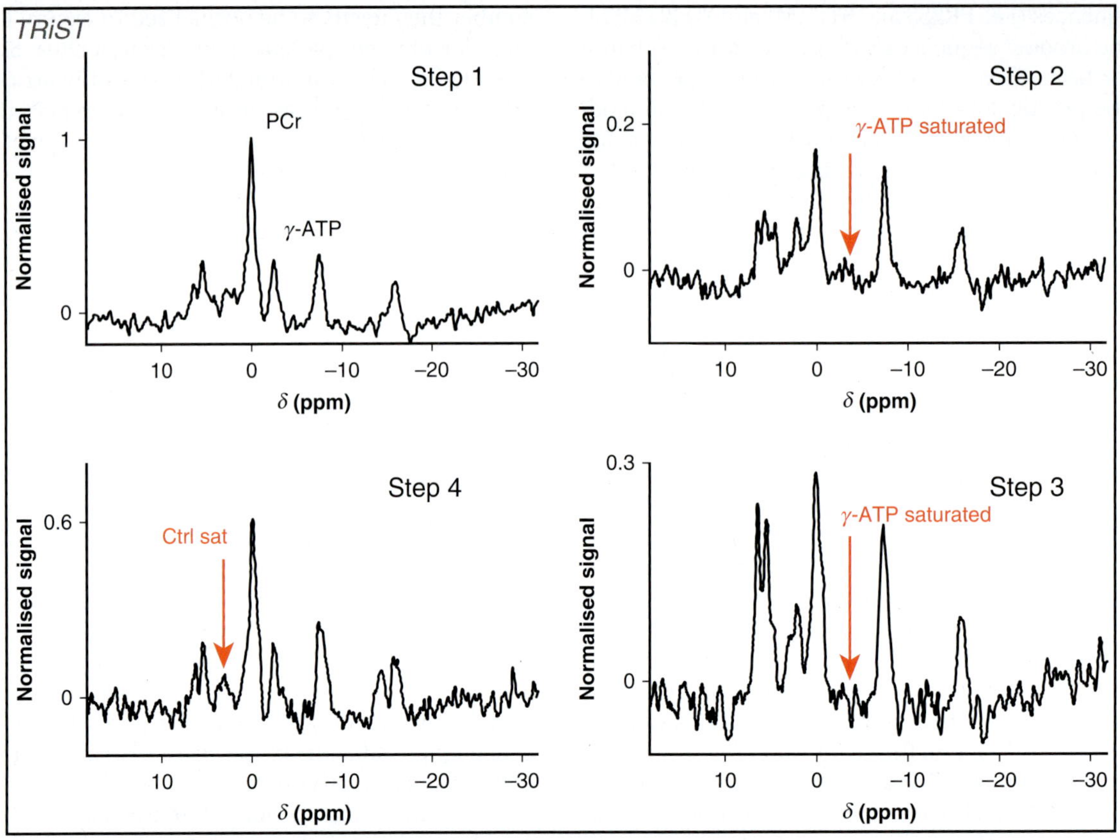

FIG. 11.6 Illustration of data used to measure the creatine-kinase rate constant k_f at 3 T with the Triple Repetition Time Saturation Transfer (TRiST) protocol. (Step 1) 9-min acquisition without any saturation used to determine M_0 from the peak height of the phosphocreatine (*PCr*) peak. This spectrum is also used to determine the saturation frequency of the γ-adenosine triphosphate (*ATP*) peak in the heart. (Step 2) 11-min acquisition with γ-ATP saturation at the frequency indicated by the *red arrow* and short repetition time (TR) used to determine the $M'(TR_{short})$. (Step 3) 21-min acquisition with γ-ATP saturation (*red arrow*) and long TR used to determine the $M'(TR_{long})$. (Step 4) This 9-min acquisition acquired fully relaxed with control saturation (*red arrow*) used to determine the $M_0^{control}$. (Adapted from Clarke WT, Peterzan MA, Rayner JJ, et al. Localized rest and stress human cardiac creatine kinase reaction kinetics at 3 T. *NMR Biomed.* 2019;32(6):e4085; under its Creative Commons Attribution Licence.)

CARDIAC MAGNETIC RESONANCE SPECTROSCOPY AT 3 T AND 7 T

Apart from hyperpolarization, the most promising route for the improvement of spatial and temporal resolution of MRS is the use of higher magnetic field strengths, because MRS methods are fundamentally still signal-to-noise limited.

Early attempts to increase the field strength[91,92] were limited by the technical prototype nature of the magnets available at that time. From 2009, significant (~2×) gains were demonstrated for ^{31}P MRS at 3 T compared to 1.5 T in volunteers[63,93,94] and in patients with hypertrophic cardiomyopathy (HCM).[115] Proton ^{1}H-MRS also improves significantly at 3 T.[75,95] Over the past decade, methods for absolute metabolite quantitation[90] and for measuring the CK forward rate constant k_f and ATP flux[32,79] have also been developed. To date, 3 T ^{31}P-MRS has been used in dozens of patient studies.

Since 2011, we have pioneered the use of ultra-high field 7 T scanners for cardiac ^{31}P-MRS. We observed further 2.8x gains in SNR (compared to 3 T) in volunteers,[61] and a similar 2.6x gain in patients with dilated cardiomyopathy (DCM).[62] This SNR boost translates to significantly improved repeatability of results,[96] even with superfast 2.5-minute long protocols,[71] and can be pushed even further by using a SLAM reconstruction algorithm[88]. We have also showcased adiabatic excitation,[97] made the first 3D-resolved cardiac CK k_f measurements,[33] and demonstrated robust cardiac Pi measurements[73,74] using the 7 T system. Realizing the full potential of 7 T scanners will require significant continuing technical and methodological development[64] to utilize the increased SNR, while avoiding excessive RF heating, line broadening, and spatial inhomogeneity. One step towards this realization was recently completed with the design of birdcage transmit RF coils that promise assessment of cardiac energetics from the whole heart.[98,99] X-nuclear MR spectroscopy and imaging is expected to be one of the principal beneficiaries of ultra-high field MR systems, as exemplified in Fig. 11.1.[100,101]

CLINICAL MAGNETIC RESONANCE SPECTROSCOPY STUDIES

Regardless of the etiology, many cardiac diseases eventually manifest in one final common phenotype of left ventricular (LV) systolic dysfunction. As delivery of ATP to the myocardium is essential for normal contractile function, it follows that a reduction in ATP delivery could serve as the final common pathway that allows many different etiologies to manifest as the same end phenotype (i.e., systolic failure). ^{31}P-MRS is the only noninvasive way to quantify high-energy phosphate metabolites in the human heart and is becoming more commonly used in clinical studies to interrogate energy metabolism in heart disease.

Left Ventricular Hypertrophy

MRS has made considerable progress in phenotyping the hypertrophied heart. This chapter will cover two aspects of hypertrophy for which MRS has been most insightful, firstly using spectroscopy to discriminate pressure-load hypertrophy (hypertension and aortic stenosis) from hypertrophic cardiomyopathy or athletic remodeling, and secondly the use of spectroscopy to understand the mechanisms of transition to LV failure.

Discriminating Different Forms of Left Ventricular Hypertrophy

All forms of hypertrophic remodeling have morphological, electrical, and metabolic dimensions that depend on the underlying cause. While the etiology of the extreme cases of hypertrophy are seldom a clinical conundrum, the increased use of CMR has now allowed detection of milder phenotypes of hypertrophic, dilated, and arrhythmogenic cardiomyopathy, such that extents of wall thickness increase or chamber dilation may now overlap with those seen in athletic hypertrophy. Furthermore, given the development of new causal therapeutic approaches, identification of early phenotypes (e.g., in HCM) is becoming increasingly important. MRS offers the opportunity to noninvasively investigate the metabolic phenotype and improve the discrimination in these milder or early cases. In contrast to all other forms of hypertrophy, despite demonstrable changes in ventricular mass and volume, physiological hypertrophy does not impair myocardial metabolism. Whereas the PCr/ATP ratio in all other causes of hypertrophy has been shown to be reduced, with further reductions seen during increased workload, in physiological hypertrophy PCr/ATP is normal at rest and remains unchanged during catecholamine stress.[102,103] In addition, while cardiac lipid content is elevated in pressure overload hypertrophy[104] and related to concentric remodeling in hypertrophic cardiomyopathy,[105] it is lower in the athletic heart than in the normal heart.[106] As such, low myocardial lipid and normal PCr/ATP, which remains stable during increased workload, may aid the discrimination of physiological hypertrophy from pathological hypertrophy.

Transition From Left Ventricular Hypertrophy to Heart Failure

Cardiac metabolism culminates in the delivery of ATP to sites of utilization, where the free energy change of ATP hydrolysis drives contraction and relaxation. This free energy varies with local reactant and product concentrations, which are, in turn, regulated by the creatine kinase (CK) system. As pressure overload left ventricular hypertrophy increases the energetic cost of contraction, a mismatch in myocardial energy supply and demand occurs, which contributes to the development of heart failure in left ventricular hypertrophy. Currently, identifying all those who will go on to develop systolic decline in the face of pressure overload is not possible. Using ^{31}P-MRS, it has been shown that not only is the PCr/ATP ratio reduced in aortic stenosis[107] and hypertension,[108] but also the delivery of ATP through CK is reduced in the hypertrophied[107] and failing pressure-overloaded heart.[109] As such, ^{31}P-MRS has the potential to probe changes in the CK system to identify those at risk of transition to systolic failure.

Hypertrophic Cardiomyopathy

Energetic derangement due to the inefficiency of the actin myosin interaction has been suggested as the common pathophysiologic mechanism underlying all forms of HCM.[110] Human studies in HCM[111–115] have uniformly shown reduced PCr/ATP ratios across the clinical spectrum of HCM, including early in the disease process in young, asymptomatic patients.[116] In addition, patients with a familial history of HCM appear to have a more pronounced derangement of energetics than those patients without a definable family history.[117] In patients with HCM caused by a point mutation of Arg403Gln, reduced myocardial phosphocreatine, CK kf, and forward CK flux have been seen.[118] The lack of a relationship between energetic and contractile abnormalities in this study suggest that the impaired energetics result from sarcomeric mutation and are not a late consequence of mechanical dysfunction. During exercise, this preexisting energetic deficit in HCM is further exacerbated, which is associated with worsening diastolic function, and is seen to be independent of hypertrophy, perfusion reserve, or degree of fibrosis.[119] Myocardial intracellular pH, assessed by ^{31}P-MRS, is unchanged in HCM at rest.[73] In addition to the reduced PCr/ATP, an increased Pi/PCr ratio has been observed in HCM patients compared to healthy subjects.[73,113,116] Using ^{1}H-MRS, reduced total creatine content in patients with HCM has been reported.[120] Energetics appear to be a promising therapeutic target, with perhexiline treatment resulting in increased PCr/ATP ratios in patients with HCM.[121] In the future, MRS may contribute to identifying early phenotypes of HCM, assessing which patients are most suitable for novel treatments such as myosin inhibitors or gene therapy, using a personalized medicine approach, and evaluating the efficacy of novel drugs/therapies in clinical HCM trials.

Valvular Heart Disease

Clinical MRS studies of valve disease have focused on the associations between metabolism and disease severity, symptoms, susceptibility to transition to systolic failure, and resolution of changes with valve intervention.

PCr/ATP has previously been shown to be reduced in mitral valve regurgitation.[122] Even when left ventricular ejection fraction (LVEF)[172] is normal, severe mitral regurgitation is associated with reduced PCr/ATP, CK k_f, and CK flux. Overall, these findings suggest that energetic depletion exists before LVEF declines in severe mitral regurgitation. As such, targeting CK capacity and/or flux may be a therapeutic strategy to prevent/treat systolic failure in mitral regurgitation and/or delay the need for valve replacement.

Energetic depletion is also observed in both aortic valve stenosis[123,124] and regurgitation.[125] In the setting of aortic valve disease, when matched for the degree of heart failure, energy metabolism appears more susceptible to decline with pressure overload from aortic stenosis than with volume overload from aortic regurgitation, with altered energetics correlating with LV end diastolic pressures,[126] LV perfusion, oxygenation, and systolic strain.[127] In line with this, it has been shown that significant energetic impairment is already established in moderate aortic stenosis, with both PCr/ATP and CK k_f being reduced. As such, a reduction in ATP delivery via CK flux does not appear to be a necessary step to cause the transition to systolic failure, but more likely, as ATP demands increase with valve stenotic severity, this increases susceptibility to systolic failure.[107] In patients with aortic stenosis, there is a relationship between reduced energetics and symptoms, with PCr/ATP only being reduced in those with New York Heart Association (NYHA) class III-IV but not in those with NYHA class I-II symptoms.[125,126] In the absence of significant comorbidities, cardiac energetic changes are reversible following aortic valve replacement.[124,127] However, preexisting type 2 diabetes mellitus is associated with persistent abnormalities in myocardial PCr/ATP following Aortic Valve Replacement (AVR).[128] Proton spectroscopy has also provided further insights into the pathophysiology of valve disease. Myocardial steatosis is present early in aortic stenosis,[129] is universally reported in severe aortic stenosis (AS) regardless of symptoms, and is independently associated with the degree of LV strain impairment.[130] In the setting of moderate or severe AS, cardiac lipid content remains modifiable, and reduction with fenofibrate was seen to be accompanied by improvement in cardiac energetics[131].

MRS provides clinicians with a more detailed understanding of myocardial metabolism in valve disease. Monitoring myocardial ATP metabolism may help early detection of subclinical myocardial dysfunction, before the onset of overt heart failure symptoms. As such, myocardial energetics may act as an early biomarker of impending systolic failure in asymptomatic severe AS or mitral regurgitation and inform the timing of valve repair or replacement. In addition, MRS data provides a rationale for drugs that modulate cardiac metabolism, aiming to improve energy efficiency, or those that alleviate the metabolic consequences of hypertrophy, which can potentially be used to treat, delay, or prevent heart failure in patients with AS or mitral regurgitation.

Obesity and Diabetes

As continual ATP delivery to the myocardium is required for both contraction and relaxation, the increased ATP demand in the context of metabolic inefficiency in obesity is a potential explanation for the increased risk of heart failure with reduced LVEF (HFrEF) and heart failure with preserved ejection fraction (HFpEF) in those with obesity and/or diabetes. In line with this, using ^{31}P-MRS, the PCr/ATP ratio was shown to be lower in obesity, and it is also correlated with diastolic dysfunction.[132] A similar energetic depletion is seen in type 2 diabetes,[133] in the presence or absence of obesity.[134,135] However, in obesity, forward flux through the CK reaction has been shown to be increased, thus compensating for the reduced PCr/ATP ratio and maintaining ATP delivery at rest. This compensation at rest, however, results in reduced energetic[132] and systolic reserve during higher workloads (Fig. 11.7).[136] Given this, altered myocardial energetics in obesity may be a pathophysiological mechanism responsible for the increased incidence of heart failure in this population. Successful and intentional weight loss is associated with reduced CK flux,[136] increased PCr/ATP,[137] and normalization of CK flux in patients with obesity and HFrEF.[138] In type 2 diabetes, treatment with an Sodium-Glucose Co-transporter 2 (SGLT2) inhibitor improved cardiac energetics and was associated with improved LV function.[139]

Whether significant lipotoxicity occurs in human obesity remains unclear, but increased levels of intramyocardial lipid have been demonstrated in humans with obesity, diabetes, and HF,[140] and also in obesity without diabetes, hypertension, or HF, where the degree of steatosis was related to concentric LV remodeling and diastolic impairment.[141] This would suggest that ectopic myocardial triglyceride is playing a role in cardiac dysfunction and remodeling in the diabetic myocardium. This concept is supported by results from dietary intervention studies that have shown that myocardial triglyceride is modifiable and related to cardiac function in obesity[142] and diabetes.[143–145]

More recent clinical studies using hyperpolarized ^{13}C MRS have confirmed that the energetic impairment and lipid accumulation seen on ^{31}P and ^{1}H-MRS in the diabetic myocardium is accompanied by reduced pyruvate dehydrogenase flux and increased lactate production via lactate dehydrogenase. This study showed that the ability to switch fuel use from fatty acids to glucose during the fasted fed transition is impaired in diabetes.[58]

Altered myocardial metabolism plays a central role in the cardiac complication of diabetes, obesity, and metabolic syndrome. Novel therapeutics that improve outcomes in diabetes and obesity (SGLT2 inhibitors, Glucagon-like Peptide-1 [GLP1] agonists) also improve cardiac metabolism. As such, MRS provides a basis for further drug development and monitoring treatment response. Given the intertwined relationship between diabetes/obesity and heart failure, the ability to measure cardiac metabolism will become increasingly important in tailoring interventions to individual patients (personalized medicine) and ensuring optimal patient outcomes.

Heart Failure Including Dilated Cardiomyopathy

^{31}P-MRS studies have substantially contributed to our understanding of the role of energetics in heart failure.[31,146] Independent of the etiology of heart failure, the failing myocardium shows reduced PCr, unchanged or moderately (by less than 30%) reduced ATP, unchanged or increased Pi, and substantially reduced CK reaction velocity and flux. These changes are likely to contribute to the impairment of contractile reserve in failing myocardium due to the inability to maintain appropriate ΔG values during inotropic stimulation.[147]

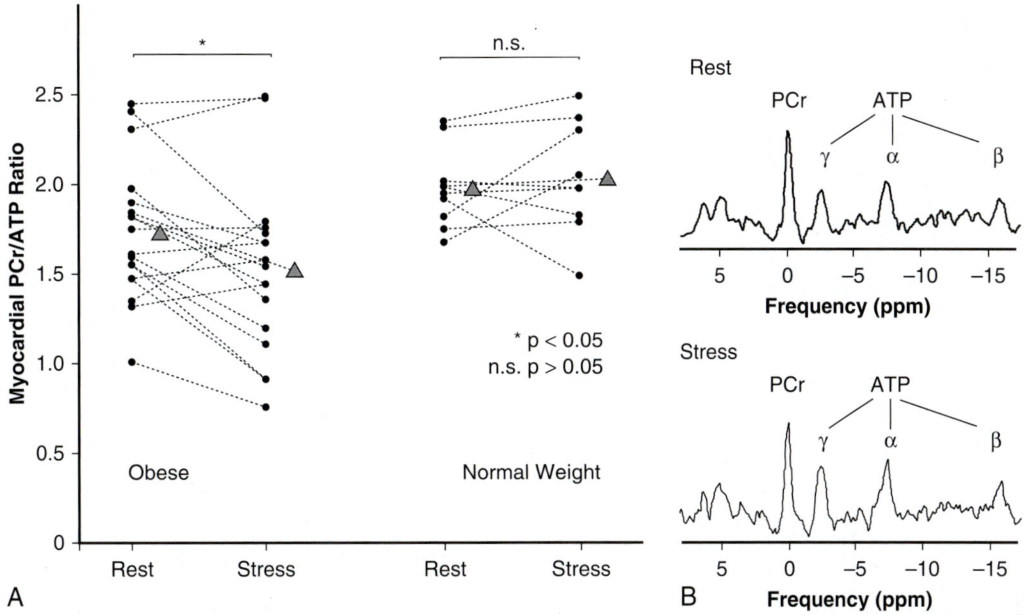

FIG. 11.7 (A) The effect of catecholamine stress on myocardial energetics in normal-weight and obese subjects (*large gray triangles*, mean ± SD values). (B) Example ^{31}P magnetic resonance spectra in an obese subject at rest and in the same subject during stress, showing a significant decrease in the phosphocreatine (*PCr*)/adenosine triphosphate (*ATP*) ratio. (Reproduced from Rider OJ, Francis JM, Ali MK, et al. Effects of catecholamine stress on diastolic function and myocardial energetics in obesity. Circulation. 2012;125:1511-1519. doi: 10.1161/CIRCULATIONAHA.111.069518 under its Creative Commons Attribution Licence.)

There is now a wealth of studies that have established altered energy metabolism as a hallmark of heart failure. The creatine kinase (CK) reaction is the prime energy reserve of the heart, providing a rapid source of ATP and enhancing its delivery from mitochondrial sites of production to sites of use, including the myofibrils.[148] As such, it is not surprising that ^{31}P-MRS measures have been shown to be clinically relevant in heart failure. Not only is a significant reduction in the myocardial PCr/ATP ratio seen in patients with HFrEF[123,149–151], but the PCr/ATP ratio is also correlated with NYHA class and LV ejection fraction[149] and is worsened by the presence of iron deficiency.[152] Furthermore, the PCr/ATP ratio has been shown to hold prognostic information on the survival of heart failure patients.[150] In HFpEF, PCr/ATP is also reduced (Fig. 11.8) and is related to diastolic function and transient pulmonary edema during exercise.[153,154]

However, the cardiac PCr/ATP ratio itself cannot detect ATP depletion or reductions in the rate of ATP delivery, which are more sensitive and important indices of cardiac energy metabolism. More recent advances in ^{31}P-MRS using saturation transfer (ST) methods have also permitted quantification of the pseudo first-order forward reaction rate constant (k_f) for the CK reaction in the human heart,[155] allowing interrogation of myocardial ATP delivery rate. Patient studies combining both ST and concentration measurements have demonstrated not only that [PCr] is reduced, but also that the reduction in the rate of ATP synthesis through CK (CK flux), given by the product k_f [PCr], is disproportionately greater (up to 70%) than the reduction in the PCr/ATP ratio (up to 20%) in patients with nonischemic DCM.[43] In addition, in the setting of reduced PCr/ATP, the coexistence of a reduced CK k_f phase has been associated with transition to HFrEF in hypertensive heart disease.[109] Reduced CK-mediated ATP delivery rate impairs contractile function,[156] and ^{31}P-MRS–recorded CK flux has emerged as an independent predictor of mortality in HFrEF.[146] While in patients with DCM and normal body weight this pattern suggests reduced resting myocardial ATP delivery as the cause of dysfunction, in obesity cardiomyopathy, ATP forward flux through CK is greater than normal, suggesting that reduced efficiency or increased energy utilization drives contractile dysfunction.[138] This compensatory mechanism[138] also suggests that a reduction in CK activity is not the cause for transition to systolic failure in obesity, identifying the pathological separation of this reversible form of heart failure from dilated cardiomyopathy.[142,154] Importantly, energetics are modifiable in HFrEF, with intravenous administration of the xanthine oxidase inhibitor allopurinol[44] and increased cardiac fatty acid utilisation[158] both improving ATP flux through CK in the failing human heart as direct evidence that myofibrillar CK energy delivery can be pharmacologically augmented in the failing human heart, with the latter resulting in significant increases in LVEF. Furthermore, both perhexiline[157] and trimetazidine[159] improved PCr/ATP in dilated cardiomyopathy.

In addition to ^{31}P-MRS, ^{1}H-MRS is capable of measuring cardiac total creatine (creatine + phosphocreatine) and lipid content. Myocardial lipid accumulation may induce cardiomyopathy. Exposure of the heart to high levels of fatty acids can cause accumulation of lipids and cardiac lipotoxicity. The general hypothesis of cardiac lipotoxicity is that excessive accumulation of lipids within cardiomyocytes increases the intracellular pool of long-chain fatty acyl-CoA, which provides a fatty acid substrate for nonoxidative processes, including triacylglycerol, diacylglycerol, and ceramide synthesis, which can lead to cell dysfunction, insulin resistance, and potentially apoptotic cell death. Lipid accumulation within the myocardium, or "cardiac steatosis", is attributable to an imbalance between fatty acid uptake and oxidation. Many risk factors

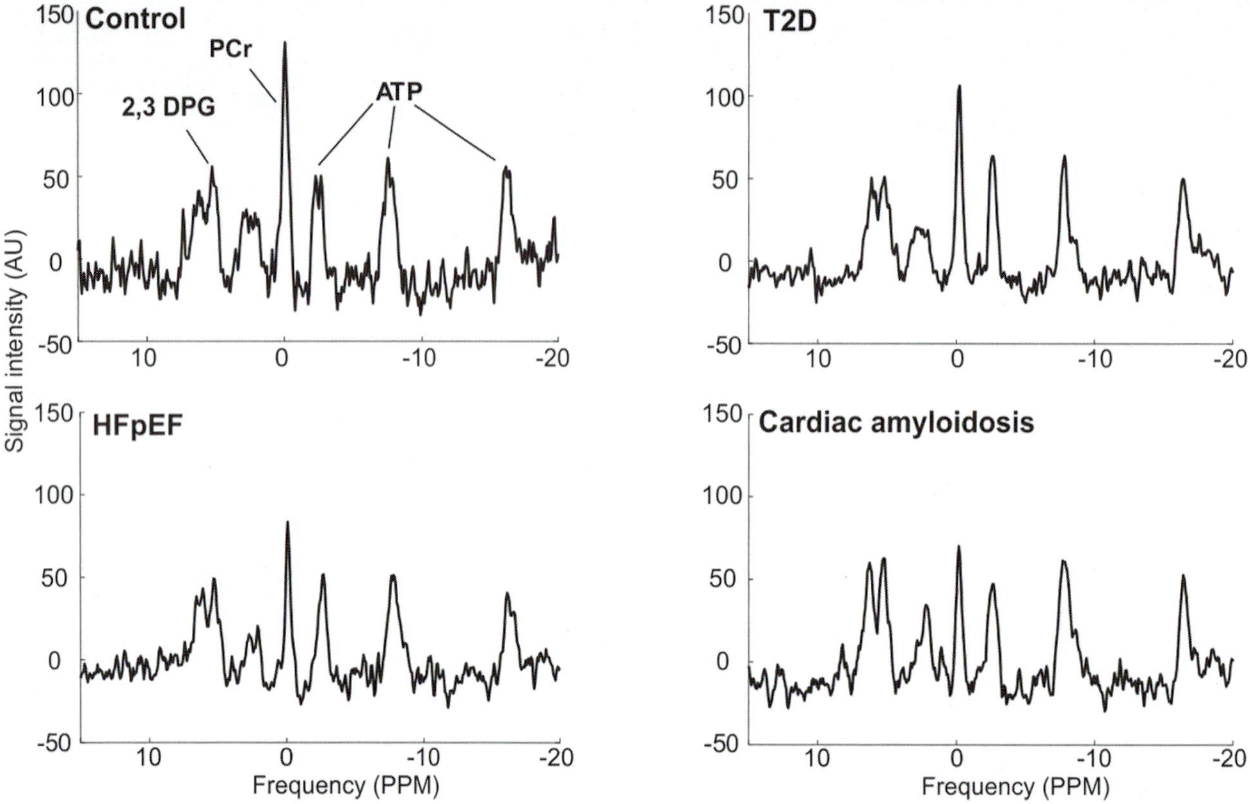

FIG. 11.8 Representative cardiac ^{31}P spectra across the range of diastolic dysfunction showing progressive decrease of phosphocreatine (*PCr*)/adenosine triphosphate (*ATP*) from healthy heart through type 2 diabetes to heart failure with preserved ejection fraction (*HFpEF*) and cardiac amyloidosis. *2,3-DPG*, 2,3-diphosphoglycerol; *T2D*, Type 2 diabetes. (Reproduced from Burrage MK, Hundertmark M, Valkovič L, et al. Energetic basis for exercise-induced pulmonary congestion in heart failure with preserved ejection fraction. Circulation. 2021;144:1664–1678. doi: 10.1161/CIRCULATIONAHA.121.054858 under its Creative Commons Attribution Licence.)

such as obesity[142] and diabetes[134] show elevated plasma triglycerides (TG) levels, and in line with this, myocardial TG is elevated immediately following hospital admission with acute heart failure and is related to the severity of the underlying HF.[160] ^{1}H-MRS–measured myocardial TG content was also shown to be significantly associated with readmission in hospitalized patients with acute heart failure.[161]

Even in mild HFpEF, myocardial steatosis is seen and is independently associated with impaired diastolic function.[154] In dilated cardiomyopathy, cardiac total creatine is depleted and is significantly correlated with LVEF,[120,162] with evidence that creatine has a closer correlative relationship to heart failure severity than TG.[163]

Therefore, ^{31}P and ^{1}H-MRS provide valuable insights into cardiac metabolism in heart failure and its clinical endpoints. These noninvasive imaging methods allow for the measurement of several metabolites that define alteration in energy production and utilization, which are central not only to heart failure risk, but also its progression and severity. Integration of ^{31}P-MRS and ^{1}H-MRS into the clinical phenotyping of heart failure may allow better disease classification, improved etiology assessment, more reliable prognostication, and a more detailed assessment of treatment response. As the next generation of drug development moves away from addressing the generalized neurohormonal dysregulation in heart failure and pivots towards targeting the underlying myocardial pathobiology, tools that can go beyond simply assessing function and scar burden to assessing fundamental aspects of metabolism will become increasingly important.

ENDPOINTS IN CLINICAL TRIALS

Numerous studies emphasizing the significance of assessing metabolism in cardiovascular disease, combined with consistent advancements in the precision and reliability of MRS techniques, have shown promise for use as primary endpoints in clinical trials for investigational medicinal products.

The advantage that MRS brings to drug development is that it can determine drug target organ engagement, confirm mechanisms of action, and provide surrogate biomarkers of improvement in small, cost-effective early phase II trials of metabolically active drugs, thereby accelerating, and vice versa derisking, drug development. ^{31}P-MRS readouts are increasingly used as endpoints in phase II clinical trials, with sodium glucose transporter 2 inhibitors,[139,164] trimetazidine,[159,165] perhexiline,[121,157] and GLP-1 agonists[166] trials already completed, and future trials planned or ongoing (e.g., with trientine[167] and novel mitotropic agents).[168] The application of ^{1}H-MRS in clinical trials is currently less well developed and remains in the preclinical and early clinical research phase.

FUTURE DIRECTIONS: ^{13}C HYPERPOLARIZED MAGNETIC RESONANCE SPECTROSCOPY

Although current cardiovascular MRS techniques offer a detailed evaluation of cardiac metabolism, the effectiveness of ^{31}P and ^{1}H-MRS in examining the metabolic processes that drive changes in cardiac function during health and disease is inherently constrained due to their MR insensitivity (i.e., low SNR for detecting the relevant metabolites). Hyperpolarized MR with DNP is a new technology that overcomes this limitation, generating molecular contrast agents with up to 10,000-fold signal enhancement. One key tracer, hyperpolarized [1-^{13}C] pyruvate, shows particular promise for the assessment of cardiac energy metabolism and other fundamental biological processes in cardiovascular disease. This molecule has numerous potential applications of clinical relevance in cardiology and has now been translated to human use in early clinical studies.

The fate of pyruvate metabolism after glycolysis depends on the prevailing metabolic conditions and thus has the potential to be used diagnostically, with equilibrium between PDH and lactate dehydrogenase (LDH) activity indicating a balance between aerobic and anaerobic metabolism. This allows the characteristic metabolic signatures of ischemia (lactate production) and viability (bicarbonate production) to be directly imaged. As such, DNP imaging of the downstream metabolism of [1-^{13}C]pyruvate might surpass the diagnostic capabilities of contemporary ischemia and viability testing.

After preliminary animal work demonstrated that PDH and LDH flux could be studied noninvasively using [1-^{13}C] pyruvate,[169] anatomical localization of ischemia and metabolic signatures of viability have been demonstrated in large animal infarct models,[170,171] and anatomical localization of these metabolites with metabolic maps is now in early clinical translation to humans, as reported in a small case series of patients with ischemic heart disease.[59]

The advent of hyperpolarized ^{13}C MRS and the ability to truly detect ischemia (with lactate production) and viability (retained myocellular bicarbonate production) brings the possibility to refine the current diagnostic and treatment strategies used in cardiology trials.

For metabolic heart disease, clinical studies of hyperpolarized [1-^{13}C] pyruvate have been conducted in diabetes[58] and also in the clinical trial of a new metabolic modulator[168]. Considering the significance of altered fuel selection in the development of heart failure and cardiac hypertrophy, the utilization of hyperpolarized ^{13}C imaging is expected to grow. Ongoing early clinical studies demonstrate the potential of hyperpolarized MRI to offer fresh perspectives compared to current MRS techniques across various cardiovascular conditions, such as ischemic heart disease, cardiac hypertrophy, and heart failure. Furthermore, multiple additional hyperpolarized compounds have been developed such as fumarate, which, when converted to malate in cells, can inform on necrosis. Many of these new compounds may well be suitable for clinical translation in the foreseeable future.

PERSPECTIVE AND GENERAL CONCLUSIONS

MRS allows for the noninvasive assessment of many aspects of cardiac metabolism in the normal and diseased heart, providing a wealth of information that may, in the future, be clinically relevant for patient management. Significant technical advances have recently been made, including ultra-high field and hyperpolarization methods, in overcoming the main obstacle for the widespread implementation of cardiac MRS (its limited spatial and temporal resolution), and these efforts are likely to progress further in the coming years. The main potential clinical applications of cardiac MRS are also becoming clearer, such as the distinction of different forms of cardiomyopathy, including better prognostication; the assessment of metabolic effects of novel heart failure treatments, potentially enabling early acceleration and derisking of drug development; and ischemia and viability testing based on cellular metabolic processes. After the early enthusiasm in the 1980s gave way to a long period of slow progress, the future of MRS now seems brighter than it has for a long time.

ACKNOWLEDGEMENTS

SN acknowledges support from the Oxford NIHR Biomedical Research Centre and from the Oxford British Heart Foundation Centre of Research Excellence. OJR also acknowledges support from the BHF Senior Clinical Research Fellowship (FS/SCRF/22/32014). LV acknowledges support from the Sir Henry Dale Fellowship awarded jointly by the Wellcome Trust and the Royal Society (221805/Z/20/Z).

REFERENCES

1. Garlick PB, Radda GK, Seeley PJ. Phosphorus NMR studies on perfused heart. *Biochem Biophys Res Commun*. 1977;74:1256–1262.
2. Bottomley PA. NMR Spectroscopy of the human heart. In: Harris RK, Wasylishen RE, eds. *Encyclopedia of Magnetic Resonance*. John Wiley; 2009.
3. Bizino MB, Hammer S, Lamb HJ. Metabolic imaging of the human heart: clinical application of magnetic resonance spectroscopy. *Heart*. 2014;100:881–890. https://doi.org/10.1136/heartjnl-2012-302546.
4. van Ewijk PA, Schrauwen-Hinderling VB, Bekkers SC, Glatz JF, Wildberger JE, Kooi ME. MRS: a noninvasive window into cardiac metabolism. *NMR Biomed*. 2015;28:747–766. https://doi.org/10.1002/nbm.3320.
5. Holloway CJ, Suttie J, Dass S, Neubauer S. Clinical cardiac magnetic resonance spectroscopy. *Prog Cardiovasc Dis*. 2011;54:320–327. https://doi.org/10.1016/j.pcad.2011.08.002.
6. Hudsmith LE, Neubauer S. Magnetic resonance spectroscopy in myocardial disease. *JACC Cardiovasc Imaging*. 2009;2:87–96. https://doi.org/10.1016/j.jcmg.2008.08.005.
7. Westbrook C. *MRI at a glance*. Blackwell Science; 2002.
8. Gadian DG. *NMR and its applications to living systems*. 2nd ed. Oxford University Press; 1995.
9. De Graaf RA. *In vivo NMR spectroscopy: principles and techniques*. 2nd ed. John Wiley & Sons; 2007.
10. Bracewell RN. *The Fourier transform and its applications*. 3rd ed. WCB/McGraw Hill; 2000.
11. Kreis R, Boer V, Choi IY, et al. Terminology and concepts for the characterization of in vivo MR spectroscopy methods and MR spectra: background and experts' consensus recommendations. *NMR Biomed*. 2020;34:e4347. https://doi.org/10.1002/nbm.4347.
12. Vanhamme L, van den Boogaart A, Van Huffel S. Improved method for accurate and efficient quantification of MRS data with use of prior knowledge. *J Magn Reson*. 1997;129:35–43.
13. Purvis LAB, Clarke WT, Biasiolli L, Valkovič L, Robson MD, Rodgers CT. OXSA: An open-source magnetic resonance spectroscopy analysis toolbox in MATLAB. *PLoS One*. 2017;12:e0185356. https://doi.org/10.1371/journal.pone.0185356.
14. Provencher SW. Estimation of metabolite concentrations from localized in-Vivo Proton NMR-Spectra. *Magn Reson Med*. 1993;30:672–679. https://doi.org/10.1002/mrm.1910300604.
15. Levitt MH. *Spin Dynamics: Basics Of Nuclear Magnetic Resonance*. 2nd ed. John Wiley & Sons; 2008.
16. El-Sharkawy AMM, Gabr RE, Schär M, Weiss RG, Bottomley PA. Quantification of human high-energy phosphate metabolite concentrations at 3 T with partial volume and sensitivity corrections. *NMR Biomed*. 2013;26:1363–1371. https://doi.org/10.1002/nbm.2961.
17. Purvis LAB, Valkovič L, Robson MD, Rodgers CT. Feasibility of absolute quantification for (31) P MRS at 7 T. *Magn Reson Med*. 2019;82:49–61. https://doi.org/10.1002/mrm.27729.
18. Ingwall JS. Phosphorus nuclear magnetic resonance spectroscopy of cardiac and skeletal muscles. *Am J Physiol*. 1982;242:H729–H744.
19. Bessman SP, Geiger PJ. Transport of energy in muscle: the phosphorylcreatine shuttle. *Science*. 1981;211:448–452.
20. vanDorsten FA, Reese T, Gellerich JF, et al. Fluxes through cytosolic and mitochondrial creatine kinase, measured by P-31 NMR. *Mol Cell Biochem*. 1997;174:33–42. https://doi.org/10.1023/A:1006847605088.
21. Greenhaff PL. The creatine-phosphocreatine system: there's more than one song in its repertoire. *J Physiol*. 2001;537:657.
22. Neubauer S. Cardiac magnetic resonance spectroscopy. In: Fayad Z, Chronos N, Fuster V, eds. *In Cardiovascular Magnetic Resonance Established And Emerging Applications A Lardo*. Martin Dunitz; 2003:39–60.
23. Iotti S, Frassineti C, Alderighi L, Sabatini A, Vacca A, Barbiroli B. In vivo assessment of free magnesium concentration in human brain by P-31 MRS. A new calibration curve based on a mathematical algorithm. *NMR Biomed*. 1996;9:24–32. https://doi.org/10.1002/(Sici)1099-1492(199602)9:1<24::Aid-Nbm392>3.0.Co;2-B.

24. Iotti S, Frassineti C, Alderighi L, Sabatini A, Vacca A, Barbiroli B. In vivo P-31-MRS assessment of cytosolic [Mg2+] in the human skeletal muscle in different metabolic conditions. *Magn Reson Imaging*. 2000;18:607–614. https://doi.org/10.1016/S0730-725x(00)00132-6.
25. Balaban RS, Kantor HL, Katz LA, Briggs RW. Relation between work and phosphate metabolite in the in vivo paced mammalian heart. *Science*. 1986;232:1121–1123.
26. Zhang J, Duncker DJ, Xu Y, et al. Transmural bioenergetic responses of normal myocardium to high workstates. *Am J Physiol*. 1995;268:H1891–H1905.
27. Wu F, Beard DA. Roles of the creatine kinase system and myoglobin in maintaining energetic state in the working heart. *BMC Syst Biol*. 2009;3:22. https://doi.org/10.1186/1752-0509-3-22.
28. Saks V, Schlattner U, Tokarska-Schlattner M, et al. Systems level regulation of cardiac energy fluxes via metabolic cycles: role of creatine, phosphotransfer pathways, and AMPK signaling. *Springer Ser Biophys*. 2014;16:261–320. https://doi.org/10.1007/978-3-642-38505-6_11.
29. Weiss K, Bottomley PA, Weiss RG. On the theoretical limits of detecting cyclic changes in cardiac high-energy phosphates and creatine kinase reaction kinetics using in vivo P-31 MRS. *NMR Biomed*. 2015;28:694–705. https://doi.org/10.1002/nbm.3302.
30. Clarke K, O'Connor AJ, Willis RJ. Temporal relation between energy-metabolism and myocardial-function during ischemia and reperfusion. *Am J Physiol*. 1987;253:H412–H421.
31. Neubauer S, Horn M, Naumann A, et al. Impairment of energy metabolism in intact residual myocardium of rat hearts with chronic myocardial infarction. *J Clin Investig*. 1995;95:1092–1100. https://doi.org/10.1172/JCI117756.
32. Schar M, El-Sharkawy AMM, Weiss RG, Bottomley PA. Triple repetition time saturation transfer (TRiST) P-31 spectroscopy for measuring human creatine kinase reaction kinetics. *Magn Reson Med*. 2010;63:1493–1501. https://doi.org/10.1002/Mrm.22347.
33. Clarke WT, Robson MD, Rodgers CT. 3D resolved human cardiac creatine kinase rate from 31P-MRS at 7 T. In: ISMRM2016. 2016.
34. Valkovič L, Chmelík M, Krššák M. In-vivo(31)P-MRS of skeletal muscle and liver: a way for non-invasive assessment of their metabolism. *Anal Biochem*. 2017;529:193–215. https://doi.org/10.1016/j.ab.2017.01.018.
35. Ugurbil K, Petein M, Madian R, Michurski S, Cohn JN, From AH. High resolution proton NMR studies of perfused rat hearts. *FEBS Lett*. 1984;167:73–78.
36. Balschi JA, Hai JO, Wolkowicz PE, et al. 1H NMR measurement of triacylglycerol accumulation in the post-ischemic canine heart after transient increase of plasma lipids. *J Mol Cell Cardiol*. 1997;29:471–480.
37. Bottomley PA, Weiss RG. Noninvasive localized MR quantification of creatine kinase metabolites in normal and infarcted canine myocardium. *Radiology*. 2001;219:411–418.
38. Schneider J, Fekete E, Weisser A, Neubauer S, von Kienlin M. Reduced (1)H-NMR visibility of creatine in isolated rat hearts. *Magn Reson Med*. 2000;43:497–502.
39. Bottomley PA, Weiss RG. Non-invasive magnetic-resonance detection of creatine depletion in non-viable infarcted myocardium. *Lancet*. 1998;351:714–718.
40. Ding B, Peterzan M, Mozes FE, Rider OJ, Valkovič L, Rodgers CT. Water-suppression cycling 3-T cardiac (1) H-MRS detects altered creatine and choline in patients with aortic or mitral stenosis. *NMR Biomed*. 2021;34:e4513. https://doi.org/10.1002/nbm.4513.
41. Weiss K, Martini N, Boesiger P, Kozerke S. Metabolic MR imaging of regional triglyceride and creatine content in the human heart. *Magn Reson Med*. 2012;68:1696–1704. https://doi.org/10.1002/mrm.24178.
42. Haris M, Singh A, Cai KJ, et al. A technique for in vivo mapping of myocardial creatine kinase metabolism. *Nat Med*. 2014;20:209–214. https://doi.org/10.1038/nm.3436.
43. Weiss RG, Gerstenblith G, Bottomley PA. ATP flux through creatine kinase in the normal, stressed, and failing human heart. *Proc Natl Acad Sci USA*. 2005;102:808–813. https://doi.org/10.1073/pnas.0408962102.
44. Hirsch GA, Bottomley PA, Gerstenblith G, Weiss RG. Allopurinol acutely increases adenosine triphospate energy delivery in failing human hearts. *J Am Coll Cardiol*. 2012;59:802–808. https://doi.org/10.1016/j.jacc.2011.10.895.
45. de Heer P, Bizino MB, Lamb HJ, Webb AG. Parameter optimization for reproducible cardiac 1H-MR spectroscopy at 3 Tesla. *J Magn Reson Imaging*. 2016;44:1151–1158. https://doi.org/10.1002/jmri.25254.
46. Fuetterer M, Stoeck CT, Kozerke S. Second-order motion compensated PRESS for cardiac spectroscopy. *Magn Reson Med*. 2016;77:57–64. https://doi.org/10.1002/mrm.26099.
47. Lewandowski ED. Cardiac carbon 13 magnetic resonance spectroscopy: on the horizon or over the rainbow? *J Nucl Cardiol*. 2002;9:419–428.
48. Weiss RG. 13C-NMR for the study of intermediary metabolism. *MAGMA*. 1998;6:132.
49. Schroeder MA, Clarke K, Neubauer S, Tyler DJ. Hyperpolarized magnetic resonance a novel technique for the in vivo assessment of cardiovascular disease. *Circulation*. 2011;124:1580–1594. https://doi.org/10.1161/Circulationaha.111.024919.
50. Rider OJ, Tyler DJ. Clinical implications of cardiac hyperpolarized magnetic resonance imaging. *J Cardiov Magn Reson*. 2013;15:93. https://doi.org/10.1186/1532-429x-15-93.
51. Ardenkjaer-Larsen JH. On the present and future of dissolution-DNP. *J Magn Reson*. 2016;264:3–12. https://doi.org/10.1016/j.jmr.2016.01.015.
52. Jorgensen SH, Bogh N, Hansen E, Vaeggemose M, Wiggers H, Laustsen C. Hyperpolarized MRI - an update and future perspectives. *Semin Nucl Med*. 2022;52:374–381. https://doi.org/10.1053/j.semnuclmed.2021.09.001.
53. Atherton H, Schroeder M, Dodd M, et al. Real-Time assessment of krebs cycle metabolism with hyperpolarised [2-13c]pyruvate. *Heart*. 2010;96. https://doi.org/10.1136/hrt.2009.191049c.
54. Dodd M, Atherton H, Schroeder M, et al. Investigating metabolic flux in the hyperthyroid heart using hyperpolarised magnetic resonance. *Heart*. 2010;96. https://doi.org/10.1136/hrt.2009.191064c.
55. Schroeder MA, Atherton HJ, Dodd MS, et al. The cycling of acetyl-coenzyme A through acetylcarnitine buffers cardiac substrate supply: a hyperpolarized 13C magnetic resonance study. *Circ Cardiovasc Imaging*. 2012;5:201–209. https://doi.org/10.1161/CIRCIMAGING.111.969451.
56. Schroeder MA, Clarke K, Neubauer S, Tyler DJ. Hyperpolarized magnetic resonance: a novel technique for the in vivo assessment of cardiovascular disease. *Circulation*. 2011;124:1580–1594. https://doi.org/10.1161/CIRCULATIONAHA.111.024919.
57. Cunningham CH, Lau JY, Chen AP, et al. Hyperpolarized 13C metabolic MRI of the human heart: initial experience. *Circ Res*. 2016;119:1177–1182. https://doi.org/10.1161/CIRCRESAHA.116.309769.
58. Rider OJ, Apps A, Miller J, et al. Noninvasive in vivo assessment of cardiac metabolism in the healthy and diabetic human heart using hyperpolarized (13)C MRI. *Circ Res*. 2020;126:725–736. https://doi.org/10.1161/CIRCRESAHA.119.316260.
59. Apps A, Lau JYC, Miller J, et al. Proof-of-Principle demonstration of direct metabolic imaging following myocardial infarction using hyperpolarized 13C CMR. *JACC Cardiovasc Imaging*. 2021;14:1285–1288. https://doi.org/10.1016/j.jcmg.2020.12.023.
60. Schar M, Kozerke S, Boesiger P. Navigator gating and volume tracking for double-triggered cardiac proton spectroscopy at 3 Tesla. *Magn Reson Med*. 2004;51:1091–1095. https://doi.org/10.1002/mrm.20123.
61. Rodgers CT, Clarke WT, Snyder C, Vaughan JT, Neubauer S, Robson MD. Human cardiac ^{31}P magnetic resonance spectroscopy at 7 tesla. *Magn Reson Med*. 2014;72:304–315. https://doi.org/10.1002/mrm.24922.
62. Stoll VM, Clarke WT, Levelt E, et al. Phosphorus (31P) magnetic resonance spectroscopy at 7 tesla in patients with dilated cardiomyopathy. *Radiology*. 2016.
63. Tyler DJ, Emmanuel Y, Cochlin LE, et al. Reproducibility of ^{31}P cardiac magnetic resonance spectroscopy at 3 T. *NMR Biomed*. 2009;22:405–413. https://doi.org/10.1002/Nbm.1350.
64. Schaller B, Clarke WT, Neubauer S, Robson MD, Rodgers CT. Suppression of skeletal muscle signal using a crusher coil: a human cardiac 31p-MR spectroscopy study at 7 tesla. *Magn Reson Med*. 2016;75:962–972. https://doi.org/10.1002/mrm.25755.
65. Bottomley PA. MR spectroscopy of the human heart: the status and the challenges. *Radiology*. 1994;191:593–612. https://doi.org/10.1148/radiology.191.3.8184033.
66. Bottomley PA. Noninvasive study of high-energy phosphate metabolism in human heart by depth-resolved 31P NMR spectroscopy. *Science*. 1985;229:769–772.
67. Bottomley PA, Hardy CJ, Roemer PB. Phosphate metabolite imaging and concentration measurements in human heart by nuclear magnetic resonance. *Magn Reson Med*. 1990;14:425–434.
68. Bottomley PA, Atalar E, Weiss RG. Human cardiac high-energy phosphate metabolite concentrations by 1D-resolved NMR spectroscopy. *Magn Reson Med*. 1996;35:664–670.
69. Maguire ML, Geethanath S, Lygate CA, Kodibagkar VD, Schneider JE. Compressed sensing to accelerate magnetic resonance spectroscopic imaging: evaluation and application to Na-23-imaging of mouse hearts. *J Cardiov Magn Reson*. 2015;17:45. https://doi.org/10.1186/s12968-015-0149-6.
70. Valkovič L, Chmelík M, Meyerspeer M, et al. Dynamic (31) P-MRSI using spiral spectroscopic imaging can map mitochondrial capacity in muscles of the human calf during plantar flexion exercise at 7 T. *NMR Biomed*. 2016;29:1825–1834. https://doi.org/10.1002/nbm.3662.
71. Clarke WT, Hingerl L, Strasser B, Bogner W, Valkovič L, Rodgers CT. Three-dimensional, 2.5-minute, 7 T phosphorus magnetic resonance spectroscopic imaging of the human heart using concentric rings. *NMR Biomed*. 2023;36:e4813. https://doi.org/10.1002/nbm.4813.
72. Wampl S, Korner T, Valkovič L, et al. Investigating the effect of trigger delay on cardiac 31P-MRS signals. *Sci Rep*. 2021;11:9268. https://doi.org/10.1038/s41598-021-87063-8.
73. Valkovič L., Clarke WT, Schmid AI, et al. Measuring inorganic phosphate and intracellular pH in the healthy and hypertrophic cardiomyopathy hearts by in vivo 7 T (31)P-cardiovascular magnetic resonance spectroscopy. *J Cardiovasc Magn Reson*. 2019;21:19. https://doi.org/10.1186/s12968-019-0529-4.
74. Apps A, Valkovič L, Peterzan M, et al. Quantifying the effect of dobutamine stress on myocardial Pi and pH in healthy volunteers: a (31) P MRS study at 7 T. *Magn Reson Med*. 2021;85:1147–1159. https://doi.org/10.1002/mrm.28494.
75. Rial B, Robson MD, Neubauer S, Schneider JE. Rapid quantification of myocardial lipid content in humans using single breath-hold 1H MRS at 3 Tesla. *Magn Reson Med*. 2011;66:619–624. https://doi.org/10.1002/mrm.23011.
76. Tyler A, Lau JYC, Ball V, et al. A 3D hybrid-shot spiral sequence for hyperpolarized 13C imaging. *Magn Reson Med*. 2021;85:790–801. https://doi.org/10.1002/mrm.28462.
77. Miller JJ, Lau AZ, Teh I, et al. Robust and high resolution hyperpolarized metabolic imaging of the rat heart at 7 T with 3D spectral-spatial EPI. *Magn Reson Med*. 2016;75:1515–1524. https://doi.org/10.1002/mrm.25730.
78. Liao JR, Pauly JM, Brosnan TJ, Pelc NJ. Reduction of motion artifacts in cine MRI using variable-density spiral trajectories. *Magn Reson Med*. 1997;37:569–575. https://doi.org/10.1002/mrm.1910370416.
79. Schar M, Gabr RE, El-Sharkawy AM, Steinberg A, Bottomley PA, Weiss RG. Two repetition time saturation transfer (TwiST) with spill-over correction to measure creatine kinase reaction rates in human hearts. *J Cardiov Magn Reson*. 2015;17:70. https://doi.org/10.1186/s12968-015-0175-4.
80. Ouwerkerk R, Bottomley PA. On neglecting chemical exchange effects when correcting in vivo P-31 MRS data for partial saturation. *J Magn Reson*. 2001;148:425–435. https://doi.org/10.1006/jmre.2000.2166.
81. Neubauer S, Krahe T, Schindler R, et al. 31P magnetic resonance spectroscopy in dilated cardiomyopathy and coronary artery disease. Altered cardiac high-energy phosphate metabolism in heart failure. *Circulation*. 1992;86:1810–1818.
82. Beer M, Sandstede J, Landschütz W, et al. Absolute concentrations of myocardial high-energy phosphate metabolites in normal, hypertrophied and failing human myocardium, measured non-invasively with 31P-SLOOP-magnetic resonance spectroscopy. *J Am Coll Cardiol*. 2002;40:1267–1274.
83. Yabe T, Mitsunami K, Inubushi T, Kinoshita M. Quantitative measurements of cardiac phosphorus metabolites in coronary artery disease by 31P magnetic resonance spectroscopy [see comments]. *Circulation*. 1995;92:15–23.
84. Bottomley PA, Hardy CJ. Rapid, reliable in vivo assays of human phosphate metabolitesby nuclear magnetic resonance. *Clin Chem*. 1989;35/3.
85. von Kienlin M, Beer M, Greiser A, et al. Advances in human cardiac P-31-MR spectroscopy: SLOOP and clinical applications. *J Magn Reson Imaging*. 2001;13:521–527.
86. Zhang Y, Gabr RE, Schar M, Weiss RG, Bottomley PA. Magnetic resonance spectroscopy with linear algebraic modeling (SLAM) for higher speed and sensitivity. *J Magn Reson*. 2012;218:66–76. https://doi.org/10.1016/j.jmr.2012.03.008.
87. Zhang Y, Gabr RE, Zhou J, Weiss RG, Bottomley PA. Highly-accelerated quantitative 2D and 3D localized spectroscopy with linear algebraic modeling (SLAM) and sensitivity encoding. *J Magn Reson*. 2013;237:125–138. https://doi.org/10.1016/j.jmr.2013.09.018.
88. Tyler A, Ellis J, Lau JYC, et al. Compartment-based reconstruction of 3D acquisition-weighted (31) P cardiac magnetic resonance spectroscopic imaging at 7 T: A reproducibility study. *NMR Biomed*. 2023;36:e4950. https://doi.org/10.1002/nbm.4950.
89. Bottomley PA, Ouwerkerk R, Lee RF, Weiss RG. Four-angle saturation transfer (FAST) method for measuring creatine kinase reaction rates in vivo. *Magn Reson Med*. 2002;47:850–863.
90. El-Sharkawy AM, Schar M, Ouwerkerk R, Weiss RG, Bottomley PA. Quantitative Cardiac P-31 spectroscopy at 3 tesla using adiabatic pulses. *Magn Reson Med*. 2009;61:785–795. https://doi.org/10.1002/Mrm.21867.
91. Menon RS, Hendrich K. 31P NMR spectroscopy of human heart at 4 T: detection of substantially uncontaminated cardiac spectra and differentiation of subepicardium and subendocardium. *Magn Reson Med*. 1992;26:368–376.
92. Hetherington HP, Luney DJ, Vaughan JT, et al. 3D 31P spectroscopic imaging of the human heart at 4.1 T. *Magn Reson Med*. 1995;33:427–431.
93. Tyler DJ, Hudsmith LE, Clarke K, Neubauer S, Robson MD. A comparison of cardiac ^{31}P MRS at 1.5 and 3 T. *NMR Biomed*. 2008;21:793–798. https://doi.org/10.1002/Nbm.1255.
94. Rodgers CT, Cochlin LE, Tyler DJ, Neubauer S, Robson MD. In: *Performance of a Phased Array for 31P Cardiac MR Spectroscopy*. ISMRM; 2010.
95. Schar M, Kozerke S, Boesiger P. Navigator gating and volume tracking for double-triggered cardiac proton spectroscopy at 3 tesla. *Magn Reson Med*. 2004;51:1091–1095. https://doi.org/10.1002/Mrm.20123.
96. Ellis J, Valkovič L, Purvis LAB, Clarke WT, Rodgers CT. Reproducibility of human cardiac phosphorus MRS ((31) P-MRS) at 7 T. *NMR Biomed*. 2019;32:e4095. https://doi.org/10.1002/nbm.4095.
97. Valkovič L, Clarke WT, Purvis LAB, et al. Adiabatic excitation for ^{31}P MR spectroscopy in the human heart at 7 T: A feasibility study. *Magn Reson Med*. 2017;78(5):1667–1673. https://doi.org/10.1002/mrm.26576.
98. Loring J, van der Kemp WJ, Almujayyaz S, van Oorschot JW, Luijten PR, Klomp DW. Whole-body radiofrequency coil for (31) P MRSI at 7 T. *NMR Biomed*. 2016;29:709–720. https://doi.org/10.1002/nbm.3517.
99. Valkovič L, Dragonu I, Almujayyaz S, et al. Using a whole-body 31P birdcage transmit coil and 16-element receive array for human cardiac metabolic imaging at 7 T. *PLoS One*. 2017;12:e0187153. https://doi.org/10.1371/journal.pone.0187153.

100. Niendorf T, Paul K, Oezerdem C, et al. W(h)ither human cardiac and body magnetic resonance at ultrahigh fields? Technical advances, practical considerations, applications, and clinical opportunities. *NMR Biomed*. 2015;29:1173–1197. https://doi.org/10.1002/nbm.3268.
101. Trattnig S, Bogner W, Gruber S, et al. Clinical applications at ultrahigh field (7 T). Where does it make the difference? *NMR Biomed*. 2015;29:1316–1334. https://doi.org/10.1002/nbm.3272.
102. Perseghin G, De Cobelli F, Esposito A, et al. Effect of the sporting discipline on the right and left ventricular morphology and function of elite male track runners: a magnetic resonance imaging and phosphorus 31 spectroscopy study. *Am Heart J*. 2007;154:937–942. https://doi.org/10.1016/j.ahj.2007.06.039.
103. Pluim BM, Chin JC, De Roos A, et al. Cardiac anatomy, function and metabolism in elite cyclists assessed by magnetic resonance imaging and spectroscopy. *Eur Heart J*. 1996;17:1271–1278. https://doi.org/10.1093/oxfordjournals.eurheartj.a015046.
104. Monga S, Valkovič L, Tyler D, et al. Insights into the metabolic aspects of aortic stenosis with the use of magnetic resonance imaging. *JACC Cardiovasc Imaging*. 2022;15:2112–2126. https://doi.org/10.1016/j.jcmg.2022.04.025.
105. Sai E, Shimada K, Yokoyama T, et al. Myocardial triglyceride content in patients with left ventricular hypertrophy: comparison between hypertensive heart disease and hypertrophic cardiomyopathy. *Heart Vessel*. 2017;32:166–174. https://doi.org/10.1007/s00380-016-0844-8.
106. Sai E, Shimada K, Yokoyama T, et al. Association between myocardial triglyceride content and cardiac function in healthy subjects and endurance athletes. *PLoS One*. 2013;8:e61604. https://doi.org/10.1371/journal.pone.0061604.
107. Peterzan MA, Clarke WT, Lygate CA, et al. Cardiac energetics in patients with aortic stenosis and preserved versus reduced ejection fraction. *Circulation*. 2020;141:1971–1985. https://doi.org/10.1161/CIRCULATIONAHA.119.043450.
108. Lamb HJ, Beyerbacht HP, van der Laarse A, et al. Diastolic dysfunction in hypertensive heart disease is associated with altered myocardial metabolism. *Circulation*. 1999;99:2261–2267. https://doi.org/10.1161/01.cir.99.17.2261.
109. Smith CS, Bottomley PA, Schulman SP, Gerstenblith G, Weiss RG. Altered creatine kinase adenosine triphosphate kinetics in failing hypertrophied human myocardium. *Circulation*. 2006;114:1151–1158. https://doi.org/10.1161/CIRCULATIONAHA.106.613646.
110. Ashrafian H, Redwood C, Blair E, Watkins H. Hypertrophic cardiomyopathy:a paradigm for myocardial energy depletion. *Trends Genet*. 2003;19:263–268. https://doi.org/10.1016/s0168-9525(03)00081-7.
111. de Roos A, Doornbos J, Luyten PR, Oosterwaal LJ, van der Wall EE, den Hollander JA. Cardiac metabolism in patients with dilated and hypertrophic cardiomyopathy: assessment with proton-decoupled P-31 MR spectroscopy. *J Magn Reson Imaging*. 1992;2:711–719.
112. Sakuma H, Takeda K, Tagami T, et al. 31P MR spectroscopy in hypertrophic cardiomyopathy: comparison with Tl-201 myocardial perfusion imaging. *Am Heart J*. 1993;125:1323–1328.
113. Sieverding L, Jung WI, Breuer J, et al. Proton-decoupled myocardial 31P NMR spectroscopy reveals decreased PCr/Pi in patients with severe hypertrophic cardiomyopathy. *Am J Cardiol*. 1997;80(3A):34A–40A.
114. Crilley JG, Boehm EA, Blair E, et al. Hypertrophic cardiomyopathy due to sarcomeric gene mutations is characterized by impaired energy metabolism irrespective of the degree of hypertrophy. *J Am Coll Cardiol*. 2003;41:1776–1782.
115. Shivu GN, Abozguia K, Phan TT, Ahmed I, Henning A, Frenneaux M. P-31 magnetic resonance spectroscopy to measure in vivo cardiac energetics in normal myocardium and hypertrophic cardiomyopathy: experiences at 3 T. *Eur J Radiol*. 2010;73:255–259. https://doi.org/10.1016/j.ejrad.2008.10.018.
116. Jung WI, Sieverding L, Breuer J, et al. 31P NMR spectroscopy detects metabolic abnormalities in asymptomatic patients with hypertrophic cardiomyopathy. *Circulation*. 1998;97:2536–2542.
117. Jung WI, Hoess T, Bunse M, et al. Differences in cardiac energetics between patients with familial and nonfamilial hypertrophic cardiomyopathy. *Circulation*. 2000;101:E121.
118. Abraham MR, Bottomley PA, Dimaano VL, et al. Creatine kinase adenosine triphosphate and phosphocreatine energy supply in a single kindred of patients with hypertrophic cardiomyopathy. *Am J Cardiol*. 2013;112:861–866. https://doi.org/10.1016/j.amjcard.2013.05.017.
119. Dass S, Cochlin LE, Suttie JJ, et al. Exacerbation of cardiac energetic impairment during exercise in hypertrophic cardiomyopathy: a potential mechanism for diastolic dysfunction. *Eur Heart J*. 2015;36:1547–1554. https://doi.org/10.1093/eurheartj/ehv120.
120. Nakae I, Mitsunami K, Omura T, et al. Proton magnetic resonance spectroscopy can detect creatine depletion associated with the progression of heart failure in cardiomyopathy. *J Am Coll Cardiol*. 2003;42:1587–1593. https://doi.org/10.1016/j.jacc.2003.05.005.
121. Abozguia K, Elliott P, McKenna W, et al. Metabolic modulator perhexiline corrects energy deficiency and improves exercise capacity in symptomatic hypertrophic cardiomyopathy. *Circulation*. 2010;122:1562–1569. https://doi.org/10.1161/CIRCULATIONAHA.109.934059.
122. Conway MA, Bottomley PA, Ouwerkerk R, Radda GK, Rajagopalan B. Mitral regurgitation: impaired systolic function, eccentric hypertrophy, and increased severity are linked to lower phosphocreatine/ATP ratios in humans. *Circulation*. 1998;97:1716–1723. https://doi.org/10.1161/01.cir.97.17.1716.
123. Beer M, Seyfarth T, Sandstede J, et al. Absolute concentrations of high-energy phosphate metabolites in normal, hypertrophied, and failing human myocardium measured noninvasively with (31)P-SLOOP magnetic resonance spectroscopy. *J Am Coll Cardiol*. 2002;40:1267–1274. https://doi.org/10.1016/s0735-1097(02)02160-5.
124. Beyerbacht HP, Lamb HJ, van Der Laarse A, et al. Aortic valve replacement in patients with aortic valve stenosis improves myocardial metabolism and diastolic function. *Radiology*. 2001;219:637–643.
125. Conway MA, Allis J, Ouwerkerk R, Niioka T, Rajagopalan B, Radda GK. Detection of low phosphocreatine to ATP ratio in failing hypertrophied human myocardium by 31P magnetic resonance spectroscopy. *Lancet*. 1991;338:973–976.
126. Neubauer S, Horn M, Pabst T, et al. Cardiac high-energy phosphate metabolism in patients with aortic valve disease assessed by 31P-magnetic resonance spectroscopy. *J Investig Med*. 1997;45:453–462.
127. Mahmod M, Francis JM, Pal N, et al. Myocardial perfusion and oxygenation are impaired during stress in severe aortic stenosis and correlate with impaired energetics and subclinical left ventricular dysfunction. *J Cardiov Magn Reson*. 2014;16:29. https://doi.org/10.1186/1532-429x-16-29.
128. Jex N, Greenwood JP, Cubbon RM, et al. Association between type 2 diabetes and changes in myocardial structure, contractile function, energetics, and blood flow before and after aortic valve replacement in patients with severe aortic stenosis. *Circulation*. 2023;148:1138–1153. https://doi.org/10.1161/CIRCULATIONAHA.122.063444.
129. Monga S, Valkovič L, Myerson SG, Neubauer S, Mahmod M, Rider OJ. Role of cardiac energetics in aortic stenosis disease progression: identifying the high-risk metabolic phenotype. *Circ Cardiovasc Imaging*. 2023;16:e014863. https://doi.org/10.1161/CIRCIMAGING.122.014863.
130. Mahmod M, Bull S, Suttie JJ, et al. Myocardial steatosis and left ventricular contractile dysfunction in patients with severe aortic stenosis. *Circ Cardiovasc Imaging*. 2013;6:808–816. https://doi.org/10.1161/CIRCIMAGING.113.000559.
131. Monga S, Valkovič L, Myerson SG, Neubauer S, Mahmod M, Rider OJ. A randomised double-blind placebo-controlled study of fenofibrate as a metabolic modulator to augment cardiac physiology in moderate-severe aortic stenosis. *Heart*. 2023;109:A23–A24. https://doi.org/10.1136/heartjnl-2022-BSCMR.29.
132. Rider OJ, Francis JM, Ali MK, et al. Effects of catecholamine stress on diastolic function and myocardial energetics in obesity. *Circulation*. 2012;125:1511–1519. https://doi.org/10.1161/CIRCULATIONAHA.111.069518.
133. Chowdhary A, Javed W, Thirunavukarasu S, et al. Cardiac adaptations to acute hemodynamic stress in function, perfusion, and energetics in Type 2 diabetes with overweight and obesity. *Diabetes Care*. 2022;45:e176–e178. https://doi.org/10.2337/dc22-0887.
134. Levelt E, Mahmod M, Piechnik SK, et al. Relationship between left ventricular structural and metabolic remodeling in type 2 diabetes. *Diabetes*. 2016;65:44–52. https://doi.org/10.2337/db15-0627.
135. Levelt E, Neubauer S. Reply: ectopic fat deposition and diabetes mellitus. *J Am Coll Cardiol*. 2016;68:2595. https://doi.org/10.1016/j.jacc.2016.09.939.
136. Rayner JJ, Peterzan MA, Watson WD, et al. Myocardial energetics in obesity: enhanced ATP delivery through creatine kinase with blunted stress response. *Circulation*. 2020;141:1152–1163. https://doi.org/10.1161/CIRCULATIONAHA.119.042770.
137. Rider OJ, Francis JM, Tyler D, Byrne J, Clarke K, Neubauer S. Effects of weight loss on myocardial energetics and diastolic function in obesity. *Int J Cardiovasc Imaging*. 2013;29:1043–1050. https://doi.org/10.1007/s10554-012-0174-6.
138. Rayner JJ, Peterzan MA, Clarke WT, Rodgers CT, Neubauer S, Rider OJ. Obesity modifies the energetic phenotype of dilated cardiomyopathy. *Eur Heart J*. 2021;43:868–877. https://doi.org/10.1093/eurheartj/ehab663.
139. Thirunavukarasu S, Jex N, Chowdhary A, et al. Empagliflozin treatment is associated with improvements in cardiac energetics and function and reductions in myocardial cellular volume in patients with type 2 diabetes. *Diabetes*. 2021;70:2810–2822. https://doi.org/10.2337/db21-0270.
140. Sharma S, Adrogue JV, Golfman L, et al. Intramyocardial lipid accumulation in the failing human heart resembles the lipotoxic rat heart. *FASEB J*. 2004;18:1692–1700. https://doi.org/10.1096/fj.04-2263com.
141. Banerjee R, Rial B, Holloway CJ, et al. Evidence of a direct effect of myocardial steatosis on LV hypertrophy and diastolic dysfunction in adult and adolescent obesity. *JACC cardiovasc Imaging*. 2015;8:1468–1470. https://doi.org/10.1016/j.jcmg.2014.12.019.
142. Rayner JJ, Abdesselam I, Peterzan MA, et al. Very low calorie diets are associated with transient ventricular impairment before reversal of diastolic dysfunction in obesity. *Int J Obes*. 2019;43:2536–2544. https://doi.org/10.1038/s41366-018-0263-2.
143. Hexeberg S, Hessevik I, Hexeberg E. Intravenous lipid infusion results in myocardial lipid droplet accumulation combined with reduced myocardial performance in heparinized rabbits. *Acta Physiol Scand*. 1995;153:159–168. https://doi.org/10.1111/j.1748-1716.1995.tb09847.x.
144. Ge F, Hu C, Hyodo E, et al. Cardiomyocyte triglyceride accumulation and reduced ventricular function in mice with obesity reflect increased long chain fatty acid uptake and de novo fatty acid synthesis. *J Obes*. 2012;2012:205648. https://doi.org/10.1155/2012/205648.
145. Jonker JT, Djaberi R, et al. Very-low-calorie diet increases myocardial triglyceride content and decreases diastolic left ventricular function in type 2 diabetes with cardiac complications. *Diabetes Care*. 2014;37:e1–e2. https://doi.org/10.2337/dc13-1423.
146. Bottomley PA, Panjrath GS, et al. Metabolic rates of ATP transfer through creatine kinase (CK Flux) predict clinical heart failure events and death. *Sci Transl Med*. 2013;5:215re213. https://doi.org/10.1126/scitranslmed.3007328.
147. Ingwall JS. Is cardiac failure a consequence of decreased energy reserve? *Circulation*. 1993;87(Suppl.VII):58–62.
148. Ingwall JS, Kramer MF, Fifer MA, et al. The creatine kinase system in normal and diseased human myocardium. *N Engl J Med*. 1985;313:1050–1054. https://doi.org/10.1056/NEJM198510243131704.
149. Neubauer S, Horn M, Pabst T, et al. Contributions of 31P-magnetic resonance spectroscopy to the understanding of dilated heart muscle disease. *Eur Heart J*. 1995;16(Suppl O):115–118. https://doi.org/10.1093/eurheartj/16.suppl_o.115.
150. Neubauer S, Horn M, Cramer M, et al. Myocardial phosphocreatine-to-ATP ratio is a predictor of mortality in patients with dilated cardiomyopathy. *Circulation*. 1997;96:2190–2196. https://doi.org/10.1161/01.cir.96.7.2190.
151. Hansch A, Rzanny R, Heyne JP, Leder U, Reichenbach JR, Kaiser WA. Noninvasive measurements of cardiac high-energy phosphate metabolites in dilated cardiomyopathy by using 31P spectroscopic chemical shift imaging. *Eur Radiol*. 2005;15:319–323. https://doi.org/10.1007/s00330-004-2504-0.
152. Papalia F, Jouhra F, Amin-Youssef G, Shah AM, Charles-Edwards G, Okonko DO. Cardiac energetics in patients with chronic heart failure and iron deficiency: an in-vivo (31) P magnetic resonance spectroscopy study. *Eur J Heart Fail*. 2022;24:716–723. https://doi.org/10.1002/ejhf.2454.
153. Burrage MK, Hundertmark M, Valkovič L, et al. Energetic basis for exercise-induced pulmonary congestion in heart failure with preserved ejection fraction. *Circulation*. 2021;144:1664–1678. https://doi.org/10.1161/CIRCULATIONAHA.121.054858.
154. Mahmod M, Pal N, Rayner J, et al. The interplay between metabolic alterations, diastolic strain rate and exercise capacity in mild heart failure with preserved ejection fraction: a cardiovascular magnetic resonance study. *J Cardiovasc Magn Reson*. 2018;20:88. https://doi.org/10.1186/s12968-018-0511-6.
155. Schar M, El-Sharkawy AMM, Weiss RG, Bottomley PA. Triple repetition time saturation transfer (TRiST) (31)P spectroscopy for measuring human creatine kinase reaction kinetics. *Magn Reson Med*. 2010;63:1493–1501. https://doi.org/10.1002/Mrm.22347.
156. Gupta A, Akki A, Wang Y, et al. Creatine kinase-mediated improvement of function in failing mouse hearts provides causal evidence the failing heart is energy starved. *J Clin Investig*. 2012;122:291–302. https://doi.org/10.1172/JCI57426.
157. Beadle RM, Williams LK, Kuehl M, et al. Improvement in cardiac energetics by perhexiline in heart failure due to dilated cardiomyopathy. *JACC Heart Fail*. 2015;3:202–211. https://doi.org/10.1016/j.jchf.2014.09.009.
158. Watson WD, Green PG, Lewis AJM, et al. Retained metabolic flexibility of the failing human heart. *Circulation*. 2023;148:109–123. https://doi.org/10.1161/CIRCULATIONAHA.122.062166.
159. Fragasso G, Perseghin G, De Cobelli F, et al. Effects of metabolic modulation by trimetazidine on left ventricular function and phosphocreatine/adenosine triphosphate ratio in patients with heart failure. *Eur Heart J*. 2006;27:942–948. https://doi.org/10.1093/eurheartj/ehi816.
160. Liao PA, Lin G, Tsai SY, et al. Myocardial triglyceride content at 3 T cardiovascular magnetic resonance and left ventricular systolic function: a cross-sectional study in patients hospitalized with acute heart failure. *J Cardiovasc Magn Reson*. 2016;18:9. https://doi.org/10.1186/s12968-016-0228-3.
161. Chang KF, Lin G, Huang PC, et al. Left ventricular function and myocardial triglyceride content on 3 T Cardiac MR predict major cardiovascular adverse events and readmission in patients hospitalized with acute heart failure. *J Clin Med*. 2020;9:169. https://doi.org/10.3390/jcm9010169.
162. Walecki J, Michalak MJ, Michalak E, Bilinska ZT, Ruzyllo W. Usefulness of 1H MR spectroscopy in the evaluation of myocardial metabolism in patients with dilated idiopathic cardiomyopathy: pilot study. *Acad Radiol*. 2003;10:1187–1192. https://doi.org/10.1016/s1076-6332(03)00104-1.
163. Nakae I, Mitsunami K, Yoshino T, et al. Clinical features of myocardial triglyceride in different types of cardiomyopathy assessed by proton magnetic resonance spectroscopy: comparison with myocardial creatine. *J Card Fail*. 2010;16:812–822. https://doi.org/10.1016/j.cardfail.2010.05.006.
164. Hundertmark MJ, Adler A, Antoniades C, et al. Assessment of cardiac energy metabolism, function, and physiology in patients with heart failure taking empagliflozin: the randomized,

controlled EMPA-VISION trial. *Circulation*. 2023;147:1654–1669. https://doi.org/10.1161/CIRCULATIONAHA.122.062021.

165. van de Bovenkamp AA, Bakermans AJ, Allaart CP, et al. TrimetaziDine as a Performance-enhancING drug in heart failure with preserved ejection fraction (DoPING-HFpEF): rationale and design of a placebo-controlled cross-over intervention study. *Neth Heart J*. 2020;28:312–319. https://doi.org/10.1007/s12471-020-01407-z.
166. Lepore JJ, Olson E, Demopoulos L, et al. Effects of the novel long-acting GLP-1 Agonist, albiglutide, on cardiac function, cardiac metabolism, and exercise capacity in patients with chronic heart failure and reduced ejection fraction. *JACC Heart Fail*. 2016;4:559–566. https://doi.org/10.1016/j.jchf.2016.01.008.
167. Farrant J, Dodd S, Vaughan C, et al. Rationale and design of a randomised trial of trientine in patients with hypertrophic cardiomyopathy. *Heart*. 2023;109:1175–1182. https://doi.org/10.1136/heartjnl-2022-322271.
168. Hundertmark MJ, Birkhoelzer SM, Portwood C, et al. IMPROVE-DiCE, a 2-Part, Open-Label, Phase 2a Trial Evaluating the Safety and Effectiveness of Ninerafaxstat in Patients With Cardiometabolic Syndromes. *Circulation*. 2025. https://doi.org/10.1161/CIRCULATIONAHA.125.074041. In press.
169. Schroeder MA, Cochlin LE, Heather LC, Clarke K, Radda GK, Tyler DJ. DIABETES PDH FED In vivo assessment of pyruvate dehydrogenase flux in the heart using hyperpolarized carbon-13 magnetic resonance. *Proc Natl Acad Sci U S A*. 2008;105:12051–12056. https://doi.org/10.1073/pnas.0805953105.
170. Ball DR, Cruickshank R, Carr CA, et al. Metabolic imaging of acute and chronic infarction in the perfused rat heart using hyperpolarised [1–13C] pyruvate. *NMR Biomed*. 2013;26:1441–1450.
171. O h-Ici D, Wespi P, Busch J, et al. Hyperpolarized metabolic MR imaging of acute myocardial changes and recovery after ischemia-reperfusion in a small-animal model. *Radiology*. 2015;278:742–751.
172. Peterzan M, Clarke W, Lake H, et al. Cardiac energetics in severe mitral regurgitation: relationship with eccentric hypertrophy, stroke volume, and effects of valve repair. *Eur Heart J Imaging Methods Pract*. 2025;3(4). https://doi.org/10.1093/ehjimp/qyaf146. In this issue.
173. Malloy CR, Jones JG, Jeffrey FM, Jessen ME, Sherry AD. Contribution of various substrates to total citric acid cycle flux and anaplerosis as determined by 13C isotopomer analysis and O2 consumption in the heart. *MAGMA*. 1996;4(1):35–46. https://doi.org/10.1007/BF01759778.

12 Special Considerations for Cardiovascular Magnetic Resonance: Safety, Electrocardiographic Setup, Monitoring, and Contraindications

EIKE NAGEL

SAFETY OF CARDIOVASCULAR MAGNETIC RESONANCE

General Issues

A cardiovascular magnetic resonance (CMR) study usually takes between 15 and 60 minutes, depending on the number of modules used, the need for stress imaging, the availability of rapid imaging methods such as real-time or compressed sensing, the amount of automation, and operator skills. Placement of the patient in a partially enclosed environment with strong magnetic fields, separated from the operator, may pose potential safety concerns that can be summarized as follows:

1. Biologic effects
2. Ferromagnetism
3. Potential effects on the relatively slow time-varying magnetic field gradients
4. Effects of rapidly switched magnetic fields
5. Radiofrequency time-varying fields
6. Noise
7. Claustrophobia
8. Contrast agents
9. Stress conditions
10. Implants, especially cardiac implantable electronic devices (CIEDs)

Biologic Effects

Overall, the biologic effects of the static magnetic field on human cells and tissue are negligible. Even though two preliminary studies reported that lymphocytes from blood samples obtained in humans exposed to a 1.5 T field demonstrated DNA double-strand breaks and changes consistent with mild inflammation,[1,2] these studies had significant limitations, and several more recent reports have found no such DNA damage[3–6] or only minimal alterations after several magnetic resonance (MR) scans on a level below harmful effects for humans.[7]

There is general acceptance that, whenever possible, clinicians should choose an imaging modality during pregnancy that has little or no ionizing radiation, such as ultrasonography or magnetic resonance imaging (MRI). MRI during pregnancy is generally thought to be safe for the fetus, especially in the second or third trimester.[8] Earlier concerns about the safety of MRI exposure in the first trimester due to the heating of sensitive tissues by radiofrequency fields and exposure to the loud acoustic environment[9] have been alleviated by more recent data.[10,11] However, of note, the safety of MRI at field strengths higher than 1.5 T (i.e., 3 T, 7 T) during pregnancy has not been thoroughly assessed and is still not fully understood, even though no reproducible harmful effects of exposure of the mother or developing fetus to the 3 T or weaker magnetic fields used in routine clinical MRI have been shown.[12–17]

According to the latest American College of Radiology (ACR) safety statement,[18] 3 T MR examinations performed within the normal operating mode for durations of less than 30 minutes should be considered safe in pregnant patients.

Ferromagnetism

Ferromagnetic objects are attracted by static magnetic fields, resulting in a potential health hazard. Most modern MR scanners are actively shielded, leading to a sudden and potentially unexpected attraction of ferromagnetic objects in the vicinity of a scanner.

The primary concern is the force exerted on a ferromagnetic object, which can lead to rotational (torque) or translational (attraction) motion of the object. Within the human body, a ferromagnetic metallic structure may be sufficiently attracted, or have enough torque exerted, to create a hazardous situation, particularly if the device is in a potentially dangerous area of the body, where movement or dislodgment of the device could injure the patient. Prime examples are splinters in or within the vicinity of the eyes or certain aneurysm clips in the brain. Outside the human body, ferromagnetic objects can be attracted with sufficient force to accelerate significantly and accumulate kinetic energy, which on impact with the patient or their environment may cause irreversible damage or death. The

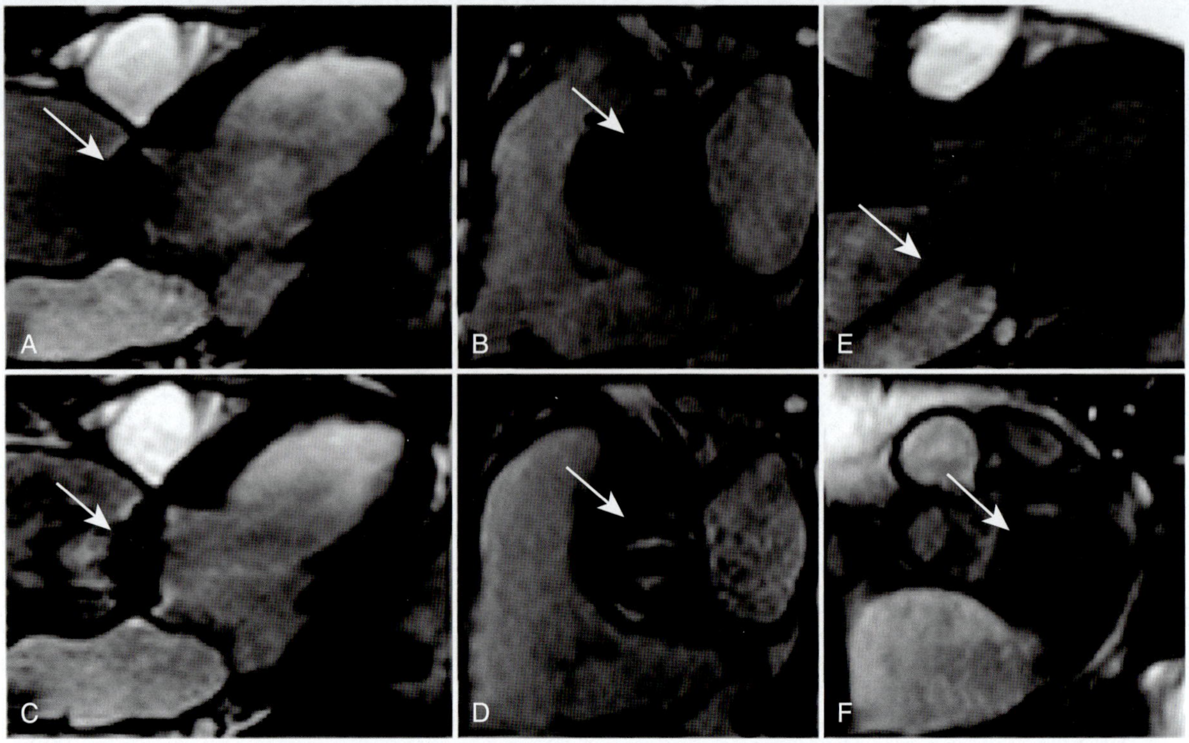

FIG. 12.1 Bileaflet, tilting disc, mechanical aortic valve prosthesis (*arrow*) during diastole on steady-state free precession (SSFP) imaging (A). Short-axis view of the same prosthesis (*arrow*) as in a during diastole, clearly demonstrating an artifact (B). Systolic image of the prosthesis (*arrow*) in (C). Systolic, short-axis view of the same prosthesis *(arrow)* in B, with both leaflets visible in the open position (D). Bileaflet, tilting disc, mechanical mitral valve prosthesis during systole on an SSFP image, demonstrating a regurgitant jet (*arrow*) (E). Short-axis view of the same prosthesis (*arrow*) in E (F). (From Von Knobelsdorff-Brenkenhoff F, Trauzeddel RF, Schulz-Menger J. Cardiovascular magnetic resonance in adults with previous cardiovascular surgery. *Eur Heart J Cardiovasc Imaging*. 2014;15(3):235–248).

data has been compiled extensively[19] and the core reference manual for the effects of various field strengths on specific metallic implants is found at www.mrisafety.com. Stainless steel is not ferromagnetic, and as such patients with stainless steel implants can be imaged safely with very few exceptions. Stainless steel implants will cause distortion of the magnetic field visible as signal loss (e.g., around metallic prosthetic valves and sternal wires after bypass surgery) (Figs. 12.1 and 12.2).[20]

The second concern is adverse effects of the magnetic field on sensitive equipment, such as pacemakers and implantable cardioverter defibrillators (ICDs). While significant effort has been made over the last decade to make these devices MR conditional, there are still many implants that are not MR safe. In any case, the examination of patients with pacemakers or other devices needs special consideration, as, for example, the sensing function can be overrun by placing a magnet on the thorax[21] and the same effect is created in the CMR environment. The safety of pacemakers and ICDs is discussed later in this chapter.

Effect of Rapidly Switched Magnetic Fields

The rapid changes in magnetic gradients during imaging can generate currents within any conductive material, such as the human body (according to Faraday's law). The magnitude of these currents is influenced by the rate of magnetic field change (dB/dt), the cross-sectional area of the conductive tissue loop, and the tissue's conductivity.

These currents—also called eddy currents—can lead to heating of loop structures at the point of the highest resistance, for example, the patient legs touching each other at the feet or the contact between the patient's hand and body core. To avoid such body loops, patients should not be allowed to cross their legs or let their hands touch their body and operators should place pillows or cloth to prevent such body loops. Other potential loops are the cables from the ECG leads. To avoid burns between the ECG electrode and the skin, carbon fiber electrodes should be used. In addition, it is important to use fresh electrodes with sufficient lubrication and to not reuse electrodes at a different position, as less lubrication will increase the resistance, which in turn may cause heating.

Rapidly switching magnetic fields can also induce nonthermal effects such as the excitation of nerve or muscle cells,[22] known as peripheral neural stimulation (PNS). The current levels required to stimulate nerves or induce ventricular fibrillation are considerably higher than the currents typically induced under standard clinical CMR conditions. However, with the introduction of faster gradient systems to the market, this concern becomes more pertinent, and the MRI system may issue a warning to the user about the potential for PNS. The user than can choose to stay in 'normal mode' and reduce the speed of the gradient system or to allow 'first-level controlled operating mode,' which has a higher likelihood to induce PNS, but which is still rare for cardiac examinations and slightly more common for peripheral MR angiographies.

Radiofrequency Time-Varying Field

Transmitted radiofrequencies (RFs) create nonthermal effects that are negligible—at least for a patient with

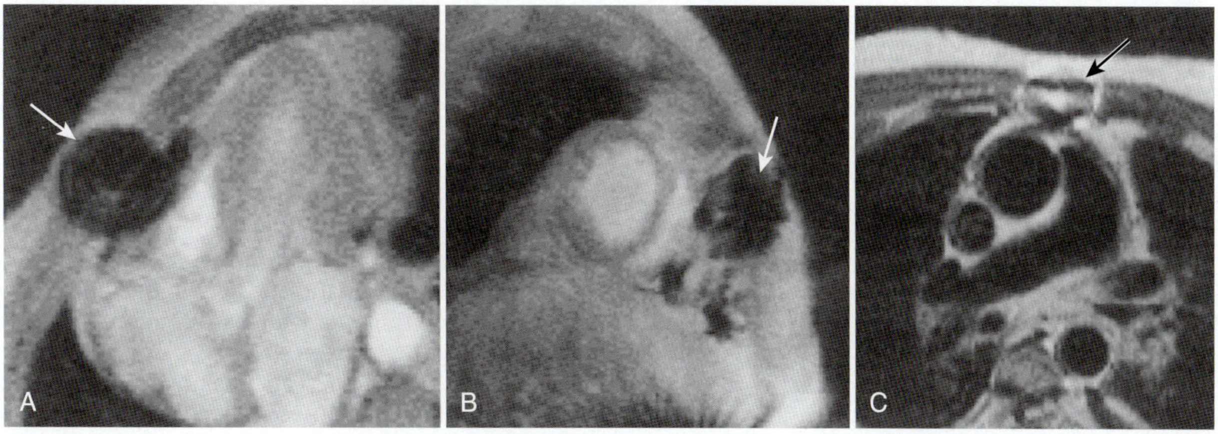

FIG. 12.2 Cardiovascular magnetic resonance image of a patient with sternal wires after bypass grafting. The artifact is clearly seen (*arrows*) on the horizontal long-axis (A) and short-axis (B) gradient echo cine images, and to a much lesser extent, on the transaxial spin echo image (C). (Courtesy Dr. Dudley Pennell, Royal Brompton Hospital, London).

short-term exposure—as well as thermal effects, which work like a microwave (but with much lower frequencies), leading to some warming within the patient's tissue. The heating effect of the RF is modeled as the specific absorption rate (SAR) or specific energy dose for the specific imaging sequence used and a limit for maximal safe SAR is set (e.g., by the US Food and Drug Administration). As these models generally do not take cardiac triggering (with potential wait times between RF transmission) or breath-holding (with no RF transmission during the breathing period) into account, they restrict SAR very conservatively for current cardiac examinations. To restrict SAR, the energy of the imaging sequence may be reduced automatically by the scanner software or manually after user interaction (e.g., by reducing the flip angle or spatial resolution).

A specific mechanism of heating is the antenna effect, which occurs at the ends of implants, such as pacemaker or ICD wires, and can lead to considerable heating, as discussed later in this chapter.

Noise Considerations

During CMR, the gradient coils produce a loud noise that must be considered when imaging a patient. The amplitude of this noise depends on factors such as the physical configuration of the magnet, the pulse sequence type, timing specifications of the pulse sequence, and the amount of current passing through these coils[23] and can reach 100 dB, which is about the same level as a disco. Irreversible damage may occur from longer exposure to 85 dB or above. Short-term exposure to 100 dB can cause temporary hearing impairment and should be avoided by using magnet-safe headphones, which can also be used to communicate with the patient, or wax earplugs.[24]

Claustrophobia

Claustrophobia may be encountered in some patients undergoing CMR, with incidences ranging between <1% and 10% depending on location and age group. In general, explanation and reassurance minimize this issue. We have had good experience with a member of the staff holding the patient by the shoulder during the beginning of scanning and talking to them from the head opening of the scanner. The use of light sedation with, for example, 2–5 mg intravenous (IV) diazepam or use of a mirror system have been reported as beneficial for the few patients who cannot tolerate the restrictive space of the magnet bore.[25–27]

Safety Considerations Associated With Cardiovascular Magnetic Resonance Contrast Agents

The safety profile of contrast agents containing gadolinium currently on the market is extremely good,[28,29] considerably better than that for x-ray contrast agents, with a large margin between diagnostic dose (around 0.1 mmol/kg body weight) and lethal dose for gadopentetate dimeglumine (Gd-DTPA) of 10 mmol/kg. In general, the prevalence of side effects is low (0.1%–2%) and includes headache, nausea, vomiting, local burning or cool sensation, and hives.[30] Rare incidents of anaphylactoid reactions associated with IV injection happen in approximately 1 per 100,000 doses.[31] The main concerns with gadolinium-based agents are nephrogenic systemic fibrosis and accumulation in the brain. The former has occurred in high doses in combination with severely impaired kidney function and has practically been eliminated by adapting the dose or type of agent to the patient's renal function (i.e., using more stable agents in those with reduced kidney function).[32] It is important to know that the more stable gadolinium chelates can be safely given in patients with severely reduced kidney function. Since gadolinium contrast agents are not nephrotoxic, they are preferrable to x-ray contrast agents in these patients. Gadolinium accumulation in the brain has not been related to any negative outcome and is correlated with the total amount of gadolinium contrast given[33]; and the European Medical Agency has withdrawn market authorization for the more susceptible lower stability linear contrast agents as a precautionary measure.

In pregnancy, gadolinium-containing contrast agents should be avoided as the risk for adverse events is small but not negligible.[11]

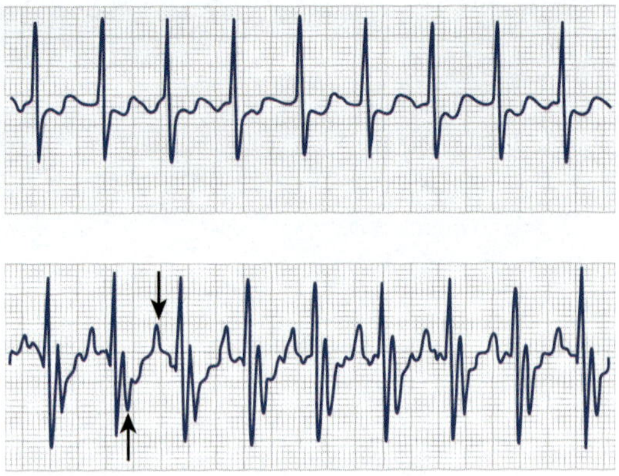

FIG. 12.3 The magnetohydrodynamic effect. The top trace was recorded in a patient with atrial fibrillation outside of the magnet, and the bottom trace, inside. Note the distortion of the ST segment (*arrows*) caused by added potentials arising from systolic flow in the aorta. (Courtesy Dr. Dudley Pennell, Royal Brompton Hospital, London).

Patient Safety During Stress Conditions

An early concern with stress CMR was the more difficult monitoring of patients in the MR environment, especially as ECG tracings are not diagnostic for ST-segment evaluation within the scanner (Fig. 12.3).[34] This is especially important for high-dose dobutamine stress CMR in patients with reduced left ventricular ejection fraction, as high-dose dobutamine can provoke true myocardial ischemia in patients with coronary artery disease. In these patients, observation of wall motion during scanning is essential, as a new wall motion abnormality or a biphasic response is the first sign of myocardial ischemia.[35] High-dose dobutamine, however, has been replaced by vasodilator stress in the vast majority of patients, and vasodilator stress does not cause myocardial ischemia, but rather an increase of blood flow to areas subtended by nonstenotic coronary arteries. Only in cases with severe collateralization, a steal phenomenon may reduce blood flow to areas subtended by stenotic coronary arteries, but—in contrast to dobutamine—the lack of chronotropic (increasing heart rate) and inotropic (increasing contractility) stimulation leads to a much less pronounced ischemic response.

Vasodilators share similar side effects, such as flush, heaviness of the head and legs, hypotension, tachycardia, and, in rare cases, arrhythmias or bradycardia. As such, the patient needs to be prepared to expect these symptoms and blood pressure and heart rate should be monitored. During pharmacologic stress CMR procedures, an experienced physician must be present and appropriate treatments for potential complications must be readily accessible.

Adenosine has a half-life of 10 seconds and acts on A_{2A} receptors, which mediate coronary and peripheral vasodilation, as well as on A_1, A_{2B}, and A_3 receptors, which cause bronchoconstriction and atrioventricular (AV) block.[36]

Dipyridamole, a phosphodiesterase enzyme inhibitor, boosts myocardial perfusion indirectly by preserving cyclic adenosine monophosphate and impeding cellular adenosine reuptake. This leads to a significant rise in circulating adenosine levels with the same mechanism as adenosine. Peak vasodilation typically occurs about 6.5 minutes after dipyridamole infusion, with the effect lasting over 50 minutes, given its half-life of 30 to 45 minutes. Dipyridamole is metabolized in the liver and the strength and duration of its effect depend on liver function.

Due to the bronchoconstrictive side effects of adenosine and dipyridamole, they should not be given in patients with severe asthma (e.g., requiring oral medication or hospitalization for status asthmaticus within the previous 6 months). They are also contraindicated in patients with second- or third-degree AV block or sick sinus syndrome. However, AV block during vasodilation is rare. It is typically asymptomatic and self-limited and—in case of adenosine—rhythm can usually be restored quickly after discontinuing the infusion.

Regadenoson is an A2A adenosine receptor agonist with a half-life of about 3 minutes. Due to the longer half-life than adenosine it can be administered as a bolus, and therefore does not require a CMR-compatible infusion pump[36] or second IV line. Due to its more selective action on A2A receptors it is considered safe for patients with asthma and chronic obstructive pulmonary disease. Regadenoson, however, is not available in all countries and the higher costs of the drug need to be assessed versus the reduced costs of equipment, scanner time, and personnel.

Aminophylline is a suitable antagonist to dipyridamole, adenosine, and regadenoson and can be administered slowly at an initial dose of 50 mg IV up to a maximum dose of 250 mg if necessary, following local protocols. In cases of persistent advanced heart block, IV atropine can be given at a dose of 0.5 mg initially, up to a total dose of 3 mg.

Dobutamine (half-life 2 minutes) is a beta-agonist, leading to an increase in cardiac inotropy (contractility) and chronotropy (heart rate). Common side effects are palpitations and, less commonly, arrhythmias such as supraventricular tachycardia and (nonsustained) ventricular tachycardia. Dobutamine is safe for patients with asthma[37] and can be counteracted by IV administration of a short-acting, beta-blocking agent like esmolol.

In cases of cardiac arrest or ventricular fibrillation, guidelines such as those provided by the European Resuscitation Council[18,38,39] should be followed. Each CMR facility should have an alarm system and a written emergency flow chart readily available. It is crucial to evacuate patients from the examination room promptly (ideally within 20 seconds) to an area where emergency treatment can be safely administered away from magnetic field hazards. Having a nonferromagnetic stretcher or a detachable scanner table stored in the scanner room is recommended. If there is a cardiac arrest, chest compression should be started in the examination room in cases where quick transfer is not possible. If more extensive treatment is required in the scanner room, a decision to resuscitate in the MR environment can be made. In these cases, a quench to shut down the magnetic field is required as most emergency equipment, such as automated external defibrillators, are not allowed inside the examination room while the magnetic field is on. Additionally, a cardiac arrest trolley should be kept nearby, and staff should undergo regular training in cardiopulmonary resuscitation techniques. Moreover, routine checks of resuscitation equipment and alarm systems are necessary.

We have had very good experience with prepacked asthma and anaphylaxis boxes in addition to the standard resuscitation equipment. These boxes contain the latest flow chart for treating asthma or anaphylaxis as well as adequate medication (according to local rules and regulations) for treating these conditions. Since the two conditions mentioned above constitute almost all emergencies in a CMR service, specific boxes significantly increase the likelihood of adequate and timely response as well as contribute to reducing the stress level of staff.

PATIENT MONITORING AND ELECTROCARDIOGRAPHIC SETUP

Patient monitoring in the MR environment used to be a cumbersome issue, with early sites developing their own monitoring equipment and adapting it to the specific needs of the magnetic field and frequency shielding. Modern equipment has overcome these issues, and multiple MR-compatible setups are available from various vendors, including ECG triggering and monitoring, noise-canceling headphones, monitors for blood pressure, breathing excursion and oxygen saturation, infusion pumps for adenosine or dobutamine, and injection pumps for contrast agent. Some of these modules provide several functions in one piece of equipment, potentially reducing overall costs.

Modern MR ECG equipment is based on fiberoptic and wireless transmission and carbon-fiber electrodes. To avoid large effects from the gradients and keep the wires reasonably short, the electrodes are usually attached relatively close together on the left side of the chest. It is important to obtain a high-quality ECG outside the scanner and check again once the patient is inside the magnet bore. It is better to invest time before scanning to optimize this, rather than needing to remove the patient in the middle of the scan to redo the electrodes. Most vendors now offer vectorcardiography, which calculates a vector from the ECG tracings that points to a different direction than the vector induced by gradient switching to separate the two electronic signals.[40]

SAFETY CONSIDERATIONS OF IMPLANTS FOR CARDIOVASCULAR MAGNETIC RESONANCE

Even though the frequency of MR-incompatible implants has been reduced over the last decade with the development of MR-conditional devices, it remains mandatory to assess potential contraindications in every single patient before every single examination. Patient reports ("I had an MR scan last month and everything was fine") are as insufficient as a telephone call from the surgeon ("All implants are MR safe"), since the final responsibility for the safety of the patient lies with the physician (or in some instances the radiographer) performing the examination, and frequently the referring physician is not trained to evaluate MR safety. Every implant needs to be checked. MR-safe implants pose no hazard, MR-unsafe implants cannot be examined, and for MR-conditional devices the exact specification needs to be obtained and followed (e.g., by looking up the device at http://www.mrisafety.com/). All information on the specifics of a patient's implant needs to be documented in writing by an MR safety pass, in the hospital record or a written statement. Conditions for MR safety may include the field strength (e.g., up to 1.5T), the gradient speed, or the body area that can be safely examined. Every part of an implant needs to be assessed separately (e.g., pacemaker and pacemaker electrode). Focus must be placed on redundant implants, such as remaining pacemaker electrodes.

Cerebral aneurysm clips manufactured after 1995 are not ferromagnetic and are safe, but earlier versions may not be. As such, the exact type of clip used must be fully ascertained from the implanting center before an MR scan can be performed.

Metallic splinters in the eye must be removed before an MR scan; clarity can be obtained with an orbital x-ray.

Orthopedic implants are usually made from titanium and are MR safe, but—as with every implant—must be checked individually before placing the patient in the magnet.

Some clothing materials, especially those containing metallic elements like antimicrobial silver or copper, have been linked to thermal injuries during MRI scans. To prevent thermal issues, it is advised to gown patients in MR-safe, pocketless garments provided by the imaging facility, especially for areas exposed to RF fields during scans.

Although thermal risks associated with individual small dermal implants (i.e., skin staples, superficial metallic sutures, piercings that cannot be removed) are quite small, dermal implants in close proximity to each other may increase the risk of thermal injury. If the items are inside the MR bore, a transmit-receive coil should be used to avoid RF irradiation of the dermal implants. In addition, the patient should be instructed to report warmth or burning sensations during the study immediately. They should be specifically instructed not to wait with this until the end of the imaging sequence.

Tattoos used to be an issue when they were based on metal-containing dyes. Modern tattoos are pigment based and pose no problem. However, large, dark tattoos may increase the potential for RF heating and again, the patient should be instructed to use the emergency signal if they feel warmth or burning sensations.

If possible, drug delivery patches should be removed. Exceptions may be made if constant drug delivery is required, transmit-receive coils are used, and the patch is in a different location than the scan.

Electronic implants pose the other major safety problem. They are at risk of malfunctioning or being damaged by CMR. This applies to cochlear implants, neurostimulation systems, non-MR–conditional pacemakers/ICDs, and several other modern implants. In general, the main rule to observe is to determine the risk-benefit ratio for the proposed procedure. If the information is only obtainable by CMR, and if it is of great importance, the risk-benefit ratio may be positive for some patients (as is increasingly shown in patients with pacemakers). Reference texts on the safety of specific devices are available (e.g., http://www.mrisafety.com/).

SPECIFIC SAFETY CONSIDERATIONS AFTER DEVICE IMPLANTATION

The specific patient group frequently examined with CMR tends to have a higher likelihood for implanted devices than the general population. Swan-Ganz catheters and temporary pacing wires preclude CMR examinations, except under very specific circumstances to be defined on a case-by-case basis. Sternal wires and vascular clips on grafts do not present safety problems but do produce localized artifacts on the images.

Typically, patients with nonferromagnetic "passive" implants made from materials like titanium or nitinol, without MR-related heating concerns, can undergo MRI immediately after implantation. The timing for MRI after weakly ferromagnetic device implantation remains uncertain and contentious. While there is a theoretical risk of device displacement during MRI due to weak ferromagnetism, some firmly implanted devices, like intravascular coils and stents, should be securely anchored by tissue and resist hemodynamic forces that are often greater than those from MRI. Sometimes it is suggested to wait around 6 weeks postimplantation to allow for tissue healing and increased device stability before MRI, but there is no strong evidence for this.

Coronary Artery and Peripheral Vascular Stents

Most stents are made from stainless steel or nitinol with variable amounts of platinum, cobalt alloy, gold, tantalum, MP35N, or other materials that are nonferromagnetic or weakly ferromagnetic. Their metallic structure raises concerns about stent dislodgment as well as possible heating effects during CMR, which has led to the recommendation to wait 6 to 8 weeks before CMR imaging to allow for tissue ingrowth.[41] Except for a strongly debated case report,[42] all published data on coronary artery stents has demonstrated minimal deflection or heating up to 7 T[43] field strength with no MR-induced complications.[44–46] Consequently, while the waiting time may theoretically increase safety, a risk-benefit analysis would usually tend toward CMR scanning—even immediately after stent implantation if there is an adequate clinical indication. Since there are occasional stents or grafts that may require a more careful approach (e.g., the Zenith AAA endovascular graft), local rules and individual safety assessment remain a central requirement.

VALVULAR PROSTHESES AND STRUCTURAL HEART DISEASE INTERVENTION DEVICES

Based on the most recent recommendations, all heart valve prostheses are considered safe for CMR. Studies using up to 3 T static magnetic fields have shown that, for a number of prosthetic valves, there is no hazardous deflection during exposure to the magnetic field.[47–49] In general, a waiting period of 6 weeks is advocated for valvular prostheses and structural heart disease devices (allowing tissue to heal) before CMR evaluation.[41] Heating of small metallic implants was tested, exposing them to changing magnetic fields 6.4 times stronger than those commonly used in the CMR scanner, with no significant increase in temperature.[50] As a result, there is no contraindication to CMR in patients with currently used prosthetic valves.[51–53] Image artifacts around the valves are localized and usually still allow measurement of flow or detection of paravalvular leaks.[52]

Transcatheter aortic valve replacement (TAVR) and percutaneous mitral valve repair are increasingly used in clinical practice. Similar to surgically replaced valves, TAVR devices[54–56] and MitraClips are considered MR safe or MR conditional.[57–59] While artifacts due to TAVRs are rather small (Fig. 12.4A,B and D), allowing flow measurements within the value,[60,61] the MitraClip device creates a significant artifact in the mitral valve area, disallowing accurate evaluation of the mitral valve leaflet morphology and residual postimplant regurgitation.[62]

Even though left atrial occluder devices contain metal, such as nitinol mesh, they have been scanned safely at 1.5 T and 3 T (Fig. 12.4C).[41,63,64] Septal occlusion devices containing nitinol and cobalt have shown no torque, a maximum deflection of 4°, and a temperature increase of 0.4°C in vitro at 3 T.[59] These devices may therefore be considered safe for CMR.[59]

CARDIAC IMPLANTABLE ELECTRONIC DEVICES

The number and variety of CIEDs continue to increase and include cardiac pacemakers, implantable cardiovascular monitors, implantable loop recorders, ICDs, and cardiac resynchronization therapy.

The issues surrounding CMR of pacemakers and ICDs are complex and require a specific setup in every center. While some imaging departments scan patients with nonconditional devices after risk assessment and written informed consent, others avoid these patients. There are three reasons for this wide range of attitudes.

First, there are multiple possible interactions of the magnetic field or gradients that can cause potential problems:

- The static magnetic fields exert mechanical forces on the ferromagnetic components of the devices, such as the pacemaker and the leads.
- The static magnetic fields may induce asynchronous pacing.
- The RF field may induce oversensing.
- The RF field may induce currents in the leads, resulting in thermal damage at the tissue-electrode interface.
- The gradient magnetic fields may induce voltages on leads, resulting in over and undersensing.
- The device may be damaged by the MR environment.
- Pacemaker leads may serve as antennas, resulting in pacing from the imaging pulses. This could potentially lead to hypotension and dysrhythmias.
- The battery may be depleted faster.[65,66]

Some of these issues can be overcome by setting the pacing mode to asynchronous pacing in pacemaker-dependent patients,[67] or sense-only mode in patients with high intrinsic heart rates.[66,68] The specific set-up and conditions need to be checked and implemented for each device and may change over time. More detailed information can be found in the expert consensus statement from the Heart Rhythm Society.[69]

In clinical practice, these issues are rarely observed. In 438 patients with implanted cardiac devices, 555 scans were performed at 1.5 T using asynchronous mode in pacemaker-dependent patients.[67] In two patients (one ICD, one pacemaker), the settings reverted to the default mode.[67] At 3 T, 16% of devices reset to default mode with no negative consequences.[66] In another study of 201 ICD devices at 1.5 T, one reset occurred.[67] The beeper volume seems to be frequently affected by CMR scanning.[70] In the more recent Patient Registry of Magnetic Resonance

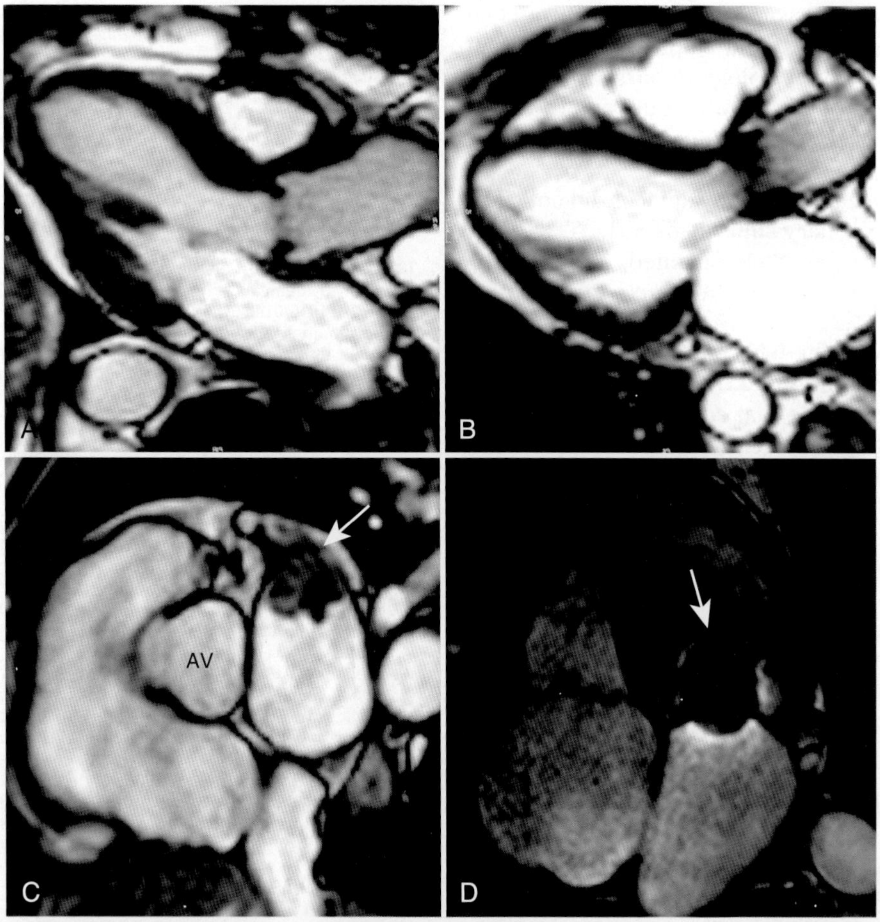

FIG. 12.4 Images of valvular prostheses and structural heart disease intervention devices. An aortic bioprosthesis is demonstrated in (A), with a transcatheter aortic valve replacement device in (B). A left atrial occlusion device (Watchman) is shown in situ in the left atrial appendage (*arrow*) (C). The *arrow* in (D) identifies a MitraClip device causing an artifact in the mitral valve area on a steady-state free precession image in a four-chamber view. *AV,* Atrioventricular. (A and B, From Crouch G, Tully PJ, Bennetts J, et al. Quantitative assessment of paravalvular regurgitation following transcatheter aortic valve replacement. *J Cardiovasc Magn Reson*. 2015;17:32. C, From Hong SN, Rahimi A, Kissinger KV, et al. Cardiac magnetic resonance imaging and the WATCHMAN device. *J Am Coll Cardiol*. 2010;55(24):2785. D, From Lurz P, Serpytis R, Blazek S, et al. Assessment of acute changes in ventricular volumes, function, and strain after interventional edge-to-edge repair of mitral regurgitation using cardiac magnetic resonance imaging. *Eur Heart J Cardiovasc Imaging*. 2015;16(12):1399–1404).

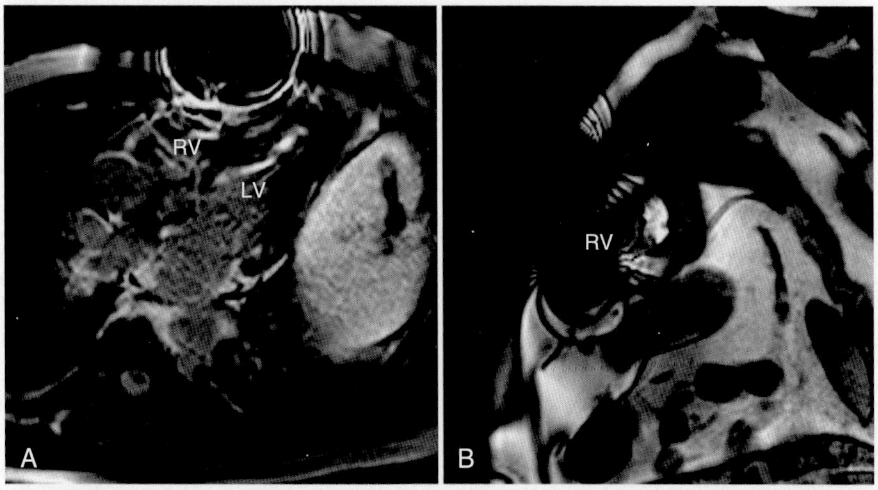

FIG. 12.5 A significant imaging artifact created by a cardiac implantable electronic device in a four-chamber view (A) and a short-axis view (B). *LV,* Left ventricle; *RV,* right ventricle. (From Nordbeck P, Ertl G, Ritter O. Magnetic resonance imaging safety in pacemaker and implantable cardioverter defibrillator patients: how far have we come? *Eur Heart J*. 2015;36(24):1505–1511).

Imaging in Mon-Approved Devices (PROMeNADEe), 532 patients with non-MRI–conditional CIEDs underwent 608 MRI scans at 1.5 T, of which 61 were cardiac MRIs.[71] No patient- or device-related complications were reported.

Second, image quality can be significantly disturbed in the proximity of the implant (Fig. 12.5A and B).[72] This can be overcome by using wide-band sequences and gradient echo instead of steady-state free precession (discussed elsewhere).

Third, patients with ICDs or pacemakers need a clear definition of responsibilities and supervision on their path between the electrophysiology department (e.g., to change the settings of a device to MR mode) and the imaging department and back for checking and resetting the device.

Cardiac resynchronization therapy devices did not show dislodgement of the coronary sinus leads at 1.5 T.[65,67,73]

Loop recorders may be safely scanned, although the device should be read before the MR scan to avoid potential data loss.[74,75]

Given the complexity, the high rate of potential issues, and the required adaptation to these specific circumstances, it is understandable that some centers with specific interests will set up a system to accommodate these patients, while others, having less patients, may not want to go through the effort. However, in summary, there is increasing confidence that even nonconditional CIEDs can be imaged safely at 1.5 T if adequate precautions are taken.[76] The European Society of Cardiology guideline on cardiac pacing and cardiac resynchronization therapy provides a class IIb recommendation for nonconditional CIED systems, and a class IIa recommendation for conditional devices.[68]

CONCLUSION

In general, CMR is safe, and no long-term adverse effects have been reported. The use of adequate precautions, local protocols, sufficient monitoring, and well-trained personnel make CMR safe even during stress conditions and in most cases with implants. Still, it does remain mandatory to assess the risk of every patient for every scan individually and to obtain written information on any metallic object that cannot be removed. In some circumstances, conditions such as restriction of the field strength to 1.5 T apply.

REFERENCES

1. Fiechter M, Stehli J, Fuchs TA, Dougoud S, Gaemperli O, Kaufmann PA. Impact of cardiac magnetic resonance imaging on human lymphocyte DNA integrity. *Eur Heart J*. 2013;34(30):2340–2345. https://doi.org/10.1093/eurheartj/eht184.
2. Brand M, Ellmann S, Sommer M, et al. Influence of cardiac MR imaging on DNA double-strand breaks in human blood lymphocytes. *Radiology*. 2015;277(2):406–412. https://doi.org/10.1148/radiol.2015150555.
3. Reddig A, Fatahi M, Friebe B, et al. Analysis of DNA double-strand breaks and cytotoxicity after 7 tesla magnetic resonance imaging of isolated human lymphocytes. *PLoS One*. 2015;10(7):e0132702. https://doi.org/10.1371/journal.pone.0132702.
4. Fatahi M, Reddig A, null Vijayalaxmi, et al. DNA double-strand breaks and micronuclei in human blood lymphocytes after repeated whole body exposures to 7T magnetic resonance imaging. *Neuroimage*. 2016;133:288–293. https://doi.org/10.1016/j.neuroimage.2016.03.023.
5. Reddig A, Fatahi M, Roggenbuck D, et al. Impact of in vivo high-field-strength and ultra-high-field-strength MR imaging on dna double-strand-break formation in human lymphocytes. *Radiology*. 2017;282(3):782–789. https://doi.org/10.1148/radiol.2016160794.
6. Ciet P, Litmanovich DE. MR safety issues particular to women. *Magn Reson Imaging Clin N Am*. 2015;23(1):59–67. https://doi.org/10.1016/j.mric.2014.09.002.
7. Herate C, Brochard P, De Vathaire F, et al. The effects of repeated brain MRI on chromosomal damage. *Eur Radiol Exp*. 2022;6(1):12. https://doi.org/10.1186/s41747-022-00264-2.
8. Jaffe TA, Miller CM, Merkle EM. Practice patterns in imaging of the pregnant patient with abdominal pain: a survey of academic centers. *AJR Am J Roentgenol*. 2007;189(5):1128–1134. https://doi.org/10.2214/AJR.07.2277.
9. Kanal E, Barkovich AJ, Bell C, et al. ACR guidance document for safe MR practices: 2007. *AJR Am J Roentgenol*. 2007;188(6):1447–1474. https://doi.org/10.2214/AJR.06.1616.
10. American College of Radiology. *ACR Manual on MR Safety*. American College of Radiology; 2020. https://www.acr.org/-/media/ACR/Files/Radiology-Safety/MR-Safety/Manual-on-MR-Safety.pdf. Accessed February 6, 2024. Accessed.
11. Ray JG, Vermeulen MJ, Bharatha A, Montanera WJ, Park AL. Association between MRI exposure during pregnancy and fetal and childhood outcomes. *JAMA*. 2016;316(9):952–961. https://doi.org/10.1001/jama.2016.12126.
12. UK Childhood Cancer Study Investigators. Exposure to power-frequency magnetic fields and the risk of childhood cancer. *Lancet*. 1999;354(9194):1925–1931.
13. Easterbrook PJ, Berlin JA, Gopalan R, Matthews DR. Publication bias in clinical research. *Lancet*. 1991;337(8746):867–872. https://doi.org/10.1016/0140-6736(91)90201-y.
14. Newnham JP, Evans SF, Michael CA, Stanley FJ, Landau LI. Effects of frequent ultrasound during pregnancy: a randomised controlled trial. *Lancet*. 1993;342(8876):887–891. https://doi.org/10.1016/0140-6736(93)91944-h.
15. Irnich W, Schmitt F. Magnetostimulation in MRI. *Magn Reson Med*. 1995;33(5):619–623. https://doi.org/10.1002/mrm.1910330506.
16. Hartnell GG, Spence L, Hughes LA, Cohen MC, Saouaf R, Buff B. Safety of MR imaging in patients who have retained metallic materials after cardiac surgery. *AJR Am J Roentgenol*. 1997;168(5):1157–1159. https://doi.org/10.2214/ajr.168.5.9129404.
17. Murphy KJ, Cohan RH, Ellis JH. MR imaging in patients with epicardial pacemaker wires. *AJR Am J Roentgenol*. 1999;172(3):727–728. https://doi.org/10.2214/ajr.172.3.10063869.
18. American College of Radiology. Draft ACR Manual on MR Safety. https://www.acr.org/-/media/ACR/NOINDEX/Radiology-Safety/MR-Safety/Draft-ACR-Manual-on-MR-Safety.pdf; 2023. Accessed February 6, 2024.
19. Shellock FG, Crues JV, Karacozoff AM, eds. *MRI Bioeffects, Safety, and Patient Management*. second edition. Biomedical Research Publ. Group; 2022.
20. Pavlicek W, Geisinger M, Castle L, et al. The effects of nuclear magnetic resonance on patients with cardiac pacemakers. *Radiology*. 1983;147(1):149–153. https://doi.org/10.1148/radiology.147.1.6828720.
21. Bottomley PA, Edelstein WA. Power deposition in whole-body NMR imaging. *Med Phys*. 1981;8(4):510–512. https://doi.org/10.1118/1.595000.
22. Ham CL, Engels JM, van de Wiel GT, Machielsen A. Peripheral nerve stimulation during MRI: effects of high gradient amplitudes and switching rates. *J Magn Reson Imaging*. 1997;7(5):933–937. https://doi.org/10.1002/jmri.1880070524.
23. Brummett RE, Talbot JM, Charuhas P. Potential hearing loss resulting from MR imaging. *Radiology*. 1988;169(2):539–540. https://doi.org/10.1148/radiology.169.2.3175004.
24. McJury M, Stewart RW, Crawford D, Toma E. The use of active noise control (ANC) to reduce acoustic noise generated during MRI scanning: some initial results. *Magn Reson Imaging*. 1997;15(3):319–322. https://doi.org/10.1016/s0730-725x(96)00337-2.
25. Francis JM, Pennell DJ. Treatment of claustrophobia for cardiovascular magnetic resonance: use and effectiveness of mild sedation. *J Cardiovasc Magn Reson*. 2000;2(2):139–141. https://doi.org/10.3109/10976640009148683.
26. Enders J, Zimmermann E, Rief M, et al. Reduction of claustrophobia during magnetic resonance imaging: methods and design of the "CLAUSTRO" randomized controlled trial. *BMC Med Imaging*. 2011;11:4. https://doi.org/10.1186/1471-2342-11-4.
27. Weinreb JC, Maravilla KR, Peshock R, Payne J. Magnetic resonance imaging: improving patient tolerance and safety. *AJR Am J Roentgenol*. 1984;143(6):1285–1287. https://doi.org/10.2214/ajr.143.6.1285.
28. Goldstein HA, Kashanian FK, Blumetti RF, Holyoak WL, Hugo FP, Blumenfield DM. Safety assessment of gadopentetate dimeglumine in U.S. clinical trials. *Radiology*. 1990;174(1):17–23. https://doi.org/10.1148/radiology.174.1.2403679.
29. Sullivan ME, Goldstein HA, Sansone KJ, Stoner SA, Holyoak WL, Wiggins JR. Hemodynamic effects of Gd-DTPA administered via rapid bolus or slow infusion: a study in dogs. *AJNR Am J Neuroradiol*. 1990;11(3):537–540.
30. Bruder O, Schneider S, Pilz G, et al. 2015 Update on Acute Adverse Reactions to Gadolinium based Contrast Agents in Cardiovascular MR. Large Multi-National and Multi-Ethnical Population Experience With 37788 Patients From the EuroCMR Registry. *J Cardiovasc Magn Reson*. 2015;17(1):58. https://doi.org/10.1186/s12968-015-0168-3.
31. Weiss KL. Severe anaphylactoid reaction after i.v. Gd-DTPA. *Magn Reson Imaging*. 1990;8(6):817–818. https://doi.org/10.1016/0730-725x(90)90019-x.
32. Reiter T, Ritter O, Prince MR, et al. Minimizing risk of nephrogenic systemic fibrosis in cardiovascular magnetic resonance. *J Cardiovasc Magn Reson*. 2012;14(1):31. https://doi.org/10.1186/1532-429X-14-31.
33. Malayeri AA, Brooks KM, Bryant LH, et al. National institutes of health perspective on reports of gadolinium deposition in the brain. *J Am Coll Radiol*. 2016;13(3):237–241. https://doi.org/10.1016/j.jacr.2015.11.009.
34. Nagel E, Lehmkuhl HB, Bocksch W, et al. Noninvasive diagnosis of ischemia-induced wall motion abnormalities with the use of high-dose dobutamine stress MRI: comparison with dobutamine stress echocardiography. *Circulation*. 1999;99(6):763–770. https://doi.org/10.1161/01.cir.99.6.763.
35. Wahl A, Paetsch I, Gollesch A, et al. Safety and feasibility of high-dose dobutamine-atropine stress cardiovascular magnetic resonance for diagnosis of myocardial ischaemia: experience in 1000 consecutive cases. *Eur Heart J*. 2004;25(14):1230–1236. https://doi.org/10.1016/j.ehj.2003.11.018.

36. Nguyen KL, Bandettini WP, Shanbhag S, Leung SW, Wilson JR, Arai AE. Safety and tolerability of regadenoson CMR. *Eur Heart J Cardiovasc Imaging.* 2014;15(7):753–760. https://doi.org/10.1093/ehjci/jet278.
37. Pennell DJ, Underwood SR, Ell PJ. Safety of dobutamine stress for thallium-201 myocardial perfusion tomography in patients with asthma. *Am J Cardiol.* 1993;71(15):1346–1350. https://doi.org/10.1016/0002-9149(93)90553-o.
38. Olasveengen TM, Semeraro F, Ristagno G, et al. European resuscitation council guidelines 2021: basic life support. *Resuscitation.* 2021;161:98–114. https://doi.org/10.1016/j.resuscitation.2021.02.009.
39. Soar J, Böttiger BW, Carli P, et al. European resuscitation council guidelines 2021: adult advanced life support. *Resuscitation.* 2021;161:115–151. https://doi.org/10.1016/j.resuscitation.2021.02.010.
40. Fischer SE, Wickline SA, Lorenz CH. Novel real-time R-wave detection algorithm based on the vectorcardiogram for accurate gated magnetic resonance acquisitions. *Magn Reson Med.* 1999;42(2):361–370. https://doi.org/10.1002/(sici)1522-2594(199908)42:2<361::aid-mrm18>3.0.co;2-9.
41. Levine GN, Gomes AS, Arai AE, et al. Safety of magnetic resonance imaging in patients with cardiovascular devices: an American Heart Association scientific statement from the Committee on Diagnostic and Interventional Cardiac Catheterization, Council on Clinical Cardiology, and the Council on Cardiovascular Radiology and Intervention: endorsed by the American College of Cardiology Foundation, the North American Society for Cardiac Imaging, and the Society for Cardiovascular Magnetic Resonance. *Circulation.* 2007;116(24):2878–2891. https://doi.org/10.1161/CIRCULATIONAHA.107.187256.
42. Parthasarathy H, Saeed O, Marcuzzi D, Cheema AN. MRI-induced stent dislodgment soon after left main coronary artery stenting. *Circ Cardiovasc Interv.* 2013;6(5):e58–e59. https://doi.org/10.1161/CIRCINTERVENTIONS.112.000790.
43. Santoro D, Winter L, Müller A, et al. Detailing radio frequency heating induced by coronary stents: a 7.0 Tesla magnetic resonance study. *PLoS One.* 2012;7(11):e49963. https://doi.org/10.1371/journal.pone.0049963.
44. Gerber TC, Fasseas P, Lennon RJ, et al. Clinical safety of magnetic resonance imaging early after coronary artery stent placement. *J Am Coll Cardiol.* 2003;42(7):1295–1298. https://doi.org/10.1016/s0735-1097(03)00993-8.
45. Nagel E, Hug J, Bünger S, et al. Coronary flow measurements for evaluation of patients after stent implantation. *MAGMA.* 1998;6(2-3):184–185. https://doi.org/10.1007/BF02660955.
46. Al-Saadi N, Nagel E, Gross M, et al. Improvement of myocardial perfusion reserve early after coronary intervention: assessment with cardiac magnetic resonance imaging. *J Am Coll Cardiol.* 2000;36(5):1557–1564. https://doi.org/10.1016/s0735-1097(00)00914-1.
47. Shellock FG. Biomedical implants and devices: assessment of magnetic field interactions with a 3.0-Tesla MR system. *J Magn Reson Imaging.* 2002;16(6):721–732. https://doi.org/10.1002/jmri.10207.
48. Hassler M, Le Bas JF, Wolf JE, Contamin C, Waksmann B, Coulomb M. [Effects of the magnetic field in magnetic resonance imaging on 15 tested cardiac valve prostheses]. *J Radiol.* 1986;67(10):661–666.
49. Soulen RL, Budinger TF, Higgins CB. Magnetic resonance imaging of prosthetic heart valves. *Radiology.* 1985;154(3):705–707. https://doi.org/10.1148/radiology.154.3.3969474.
50. Davis PL, Crooks L, Arakawa M, McRee R, Kaufman L, Margulis AR. Potential hazards in NMR imaging: heating effects of changing magnetic fields and RF fields on small metallic implants. *AJR Am J Roentgenol.* 1981;137(4):857–860. https://doi.org/10.2214/ajr.137.4.857.
51. Globits S, Higgins CB. Assessment of valvular heart disease by magnetic resonance imaging. *Am Heart J.* 1995;129(2):369–381. https://doi.org/10.1016/0002-8703(95)90020-9.
52. Bachmann R, Deutsch HJ, Jüngehülsing M, Sechtem U, Hilger HH, Schicha H. [Magnetic resonance tomography in patients with a heart valve prosthesis]. *Rofo.* 1991;155(6):499–505. https://doi.org/10.1055/s-2008-1033306.
53. Di Cesare E, Enrici RM, Paparoni S, et al. Low-field magnetic resonance imaging in the evaluation of mechanical and biological heart valve function. *Eur J Radiol.* 1995;20(3):224–228. https://doi.org/10.1016/0720-048x(95)00656-b.
54. Abdel-Wahab M, Mehilli J, Frerker C, et al. Comparison of balloon-expandable vs self-expandable valves in patients undergoing transcatheter aortic valve replacement: the CHOICE randomized clinical trial. *JAMA.* 2014;311(15):1503–1514. https://doi.org/10.1001/jama.2014.3316.
55. Merten C, Beurich HW, Zachow D, et al. Aortic regurgitation and left ventricular remodeling after transcatheter aortic valve implantation: a serial cardiac magnetic resonance imaging study. *Circ Cardiovasc Interv.* 2013;6(4):476–483. https://doi.org/10.1161/CIRCINTERVENTIONS.112.000115.
56. Hartlage GR, Babaliaros VC, Thourani VH, et al. The role of cardiovascular magnetic resonance in stratifying paravalvular leak severity after transcatheter aortic valve replacement: an observational outcome study. *J Cardiovasc Magn Reson.* 2014;16(1):93. https://doi.org/10.1186/s12968-014-0093-x.
57. Saeedi M, Thomas A, Shellock FG. Evaluation of MRI issues at 3-Tesla for a transcatheter aortic valve replacement (TAVR) bioprosthesis. *Magn Reson Imaging.* 2015;33(4):497–501. https://doi.org/10.1016/j.mri.2015.01.012.
58. Krumm P, Zuern CS, Wurster TH, et al. Cardiac magnetic resonance imaging in patients undergoing percutaneous mitral valve repair with the MitraClip system. *Clin Res Cardiol.* 2014;103(5):397–404. https://doi.org/10.1007/s00392-014-0670-x.
59. Radunski UK, Franzen O, Barmeyer A, et al. Cardiac remodeling following percutaneous mitral valve repair—initial results assessed by cardiovascular magnetic resonance imaging. *Rofo.* 2014;186(10):951–958. https://doi.org/10.1055/s-0034-1366216.
60. Crouch G, Tully PJ, Bennetts J, et al. Quantitative assessment of paravalvular regurgitation following transcatheter aortic valve replacement. *J Cardiovasc Magn Reson.* 2015;17(1):32. https://doi.org/10.1186/s12968-015-0134-0.
61. Hong SN, Rahimi A, Kissinger KV, Pedrosa I, Manning WJ, O'Halloran TD. Cardiac magnetic resonance imaging and the WATCHMAN device. *J Am Coll Cardiol.* 2010;55(24):2785. https://doi.org/10.1016/j.jacc.2010.03.027.
62. Lurz P, Serpytis R, Blazek S, et al. Assessment of acute changes in ventricular volumes, function, and strain after interventional edge-to-edge repair of mitral regurgitation using cardiac magnetic resonance imaging. *Eur Heart J Cardiovasc Imaging.* 2015;16(12):1399–1404. https://doi.org/10.1093/ehjci/jev115.
63. Mohrs OK, Wunderlich N, Petersen SE, Pottmeyer A, Kauczor HU. Contrast-enhanced CMR in patients after percutaneous closure of the left atrial appendage: a pilot study. *J Cardiovasc Magn Reson.* 2011;13(1):33. https://doi.org/10.1186/1532-429X-13-33.
64. Romero J, Perez IE, Krumerman A, Garcia MJ, Lucariello RJ. Left atrial appendage closure devices. *Clin Med Insights Cardiol.* 2014;8:45–52. https://doi.org/10.4137/CMC.S14043.
65. Cohen JD, Costa HS, Russo RJ. Determining the risks of magnetic resonance imaging at 1.5 tesla for patients with pacemakers and implantable cardioverter defibrillators. *Am J Cardiol.* 2012;110(11):1631–1636. https://doi.org/10.1016/j.amjcard.2012.07.030.
66. Naehle CP, Meyer C, Thomas D, et al. Safety of brain 3-T MR imaging with transmit-receive head coil in patients with cardiac pacemakers: pilot prospective study with 51 examinations. *Radiology.* 2008;249(3):991–1001. https://doi.org/10.1148/radiol.2493072195.
67. Nazarian S, Hansford R, Roguin A, et al. A prospective evaluation of a protocol for magnetic resonance imaging of patients with implanted cardiac devices. *Ann Intern Med.* 2011;155(7):415–424. https://doi.org/10.7326/0003-4819-155-7-201110040-00004.
68. Brignole M, Auricchio A, Baron-Esquivias G, et al. 2013 ESC guidelines on cardiac pacing and cardiac resynchronization therapy: the Task Force on cardiac pacing and resynchronization therapy of the European society of cardiology (ESC). Developed in collaboration with the European heart rhythm association (EHRA). *Eur Heart J.* 2013;34(29):2281–2329. https://doi.org/10.1093/eurheartj/eht150.
69. Indik JH, Gimbel JR, Abe H, et al. 2017 HRS expert consensus statement on magnetic resonance imaging and radiation exposure in patients with cardiovascular implantable electronic devices. *Heart Rhythm.* 2017;14(7):e97–e153. https://doi.org/10.1016/j.hrthm.2017.04.025.
70. Holtstiege V, Meier C, Bietenbeck M, et al. Clinical experience regarding safety and diagnostic value of cardiovascular magnetic resonance in patients with a subcutaneous implanted cardioverter/defibrillator (S-ICD) at 1.5 T. *J Cardiovasc Magn Reson.* 2020;22(1):35. https://doi.org/10.1186/s12968-020-00626-y.
71. Gupta SK, Ya'qoub L, Wimmer AP, Fisher S, Saeed IM. Safety and clinical impact of MRI in patients with non-MRI-conditional cardiac devices. *Radiol Cardiothorac Imaging.* 2020;2(5):e200086. https://doi.org/10.1148/ryct.2020200086.
72. Nordbeck P, Ertl G, Ritter O. Magnetic resonance imaging safety in pacemaker and implantable cardioverter defibrillator patients: how far have we come? *Eur Heart J.* 2015;36(24):1505–1511. https://doi.org/10.1093/eurheartj/ehv086.
73. Sheldon SH, Bunch TJ, Cogert GA, et al. Multicenter study of the safety and effects of magnetic resonance imaging in patients with coronary sinus left ventricular pacing leads. *Heart Rhythm.* 2015;12(2):345–349. https://doi.org/10.1016/j.hrthm.2014.11.037.
74. Gimbel JR, Zarghami J, Machado C, Wilkoff BL. Safe scanning, but frequent artifacts mimicking bradycardia and tachycardia during magnetic resonance imaging (MRI) in patients with an implantable loop recorder (ILR). *Ann Noninvasive Electrocardiol.* 2005;10(4):404–408. https://doi.org/10.1111/j.1542-474X.2005.00056.x.
75. Wong JA, Yee R, Gula LJ, et al. Feasibility of magnetic resonance imaging in patients with an implantable loop recorder. *Pacing Clin Electrophysiol.* 2008;31(3):333–337. https://doi.org/10.1111/j.1540-8159.2008.00994.x.
76. Yang E, Suzuki M, Nazarian S, Halperin HR. Magnetic resonance imaging safety in patients with cardiac implantable electronic devices. *Trends in Cardiovascular Medicine.* 2022;32(7):440–447. https://doi.org/10.1016/j.tcm.2021.08.001.

13 The Core Clinical Cardiovascular Magnetic Resonance Examination

HAN W. KIM, RAYMOND J. KIM, AND CLERIO F. AZEVEDO

INTRODUCTION

For clinical practitioners of cardiovascular magnetic resonance (CMR), a wide array of techniques are potentially available to assess patients with suspected cardiac and/or vascular disease. The breadth of pulse sequences, however, has the potential to create confusion when trying to prioritize which techniques are essential components of the core clinical examination versus those that are optional. The Society of Cardiovascular Magnetic Resonance (SCMR) regularly updates guidelines that address standardized imaging protocols[1] as well as postprocessing and image interpretation.[2]

The core clinical examination used at our center is shown in Fig. 13.1. Scouting, cine imaging, and late gadolinium enhancement (LGE) are the core components of the clinical examination, and are performed in the vast majority of patients. Scouting identifies the short- and long-axis views of the heart, which lie at arbitrary angles with respect to the axial, sagittal, and coronal planes. Cine imaging captures a movie of the beating heart to visualize its contractile function and measure volumes. Other anatomic features can also be viewed with high spatial and temporal resolution. LGE imaging is performed to visualize contrast enhancement of the myocardium, which can be used to identify myocardial infarction (MI) and nonischemic cardiomyopathies.

Depending on the clinical question, other sequences (Fig. 13.1, "Optional") may also be added to the examination to evaluate other characteristics such as velocity, native T1 and/or T2, and T2*, or to evaluate other anatomic abnormalities. If an assessment for ischemia is needed, the core examination may be modified to include first pass perfusion imaging during vasodilator stress and under resting conditions. Vasodilator first-pass perfusion imaging is performed after cine and other optional imaging sequences have been completed; rest perfusion imaging is usually performed following a short delay (~15 minutes).

In this chapter, we will build upon the information provided in the SCMR guidelines and describe the core clinical CMR examination currently in use at our center. Additionally, we will provide granular recommendations that can be incorporated into most CMR practices.

SCOUTING AND IMAGING PLANES

For CMR, the goal of scouting is to establish the short- and long-axis views of the heart. Importantly, both the short- and long-axis cardiac views lie at arbitrary angles with respect to scanner coordinates and are therefore referred to as double oblique planes. Due to variations in anatomy, these planes are identified on a per-patient basis following the acquisition of the initial thoracic localizing images in the standard scanner planes.

The process of selecting the short- and long-axis view is straightforward (Fig. 13.2). Using the best transverse (axial) localizer image that depicts a pseudo (off-axis) 4-chamber view, a 2-chamber scout is prescribed by selecting an imaging plane that bisects the center of the left ventricle (LV) and traverses through the LV apex (Fig. 13.2, step 1; yellow line). Using the just-acquired, 2-chamber scout image, an imaging plane is prescribed perpendicular through the center of the LV apex that bisects the LV and left atrium (LA) at the level of the mitral valve resulting in a double oblique 4-chamber (horizontal long-axis view) scout of the heart.

In our laboratory, we obtain the 2- and 4-chamber scout images using a single-shot steady-state free precession (SSFP) pulse sequence with the patient holding their breath at a relaxed point in end expiration. We perform breath-holding during acquisition of the scout images to ensure consistent positioning of the heart within the chest for the remainder of the examination and because we find that forced end-expiratory imaging can reduce patient tolerance to breath-holding.

Next, using both the 2-chamber and 4-chamber scouts, the short-axis imaging plane is prescribed, which is perpendicular to both the inferior wall on the 2-chamber scout and the interventricular septum on the 4-chamber scout (step 2; blue line), approximately 1–2 cm below the level of the atrioventricular valves (AV) valves. Like the long-axis scouts, the short-axis scout is obtained during a *relaxed* point in end expiration.

Once this basal short-axis scout plane has been identified, it is our practice to proceed to cine imaging and further refine the imaging planes. Other imaging planes (e.g., dedicated right ventricular views or valve planes) are generally localized from the subsequent cine image planes.

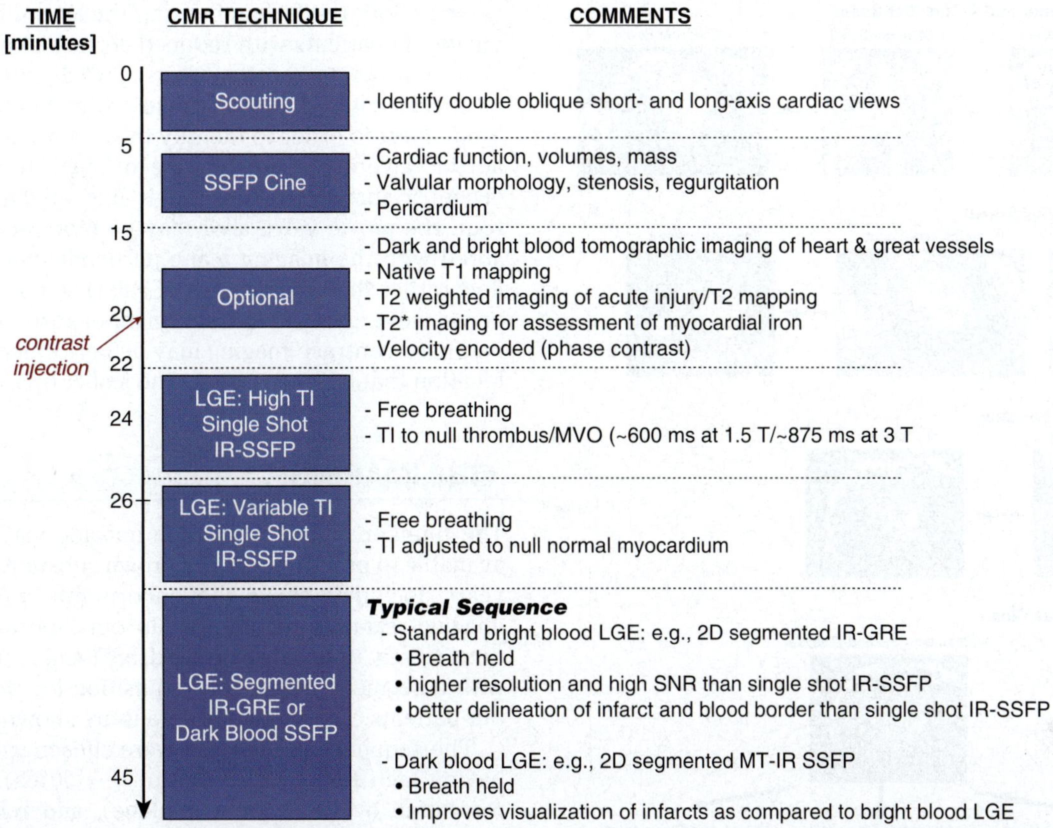

FIG. 13.1 Components and timeline of the core cardiovascular magnetic resonance examination. *SSFP*, steady-state free precession; *TI*, inversion time; *T*, Tesla; *LGE*, late gadolinium enhancement; *IR*, inversion recovery; *GRE*, gradient echo; *MT*, magnetization transfer; *2D*, two dimensional; *3D*, three dimensional.

From the short-axis scout, a long-axis 4-chamber cine CMR image is obtained by prescribing a perpendicular plane through the inferolateral wall of the right ventricle (RV) that intersects the septal wall below the left ventricular outflow tract (LVOT) and aortic valve and extends through the anterolateral wall of the LV (step 3; pink line). Similar to the scouts, we obtain all the cine images with the patient holding their breath at a relaxed point in end expiration.

Next, the short-axis cine images are prescribed from the 4-chamber cine (step 4; green lines). The orientation of the short-axis imaging plane is perpendicular to the interventricular septum at the insertion points of the mitral valve during diastole. We also rotate the field of view (FOV) so that the frequency-encoding direction is set to be parallel to the chest wall and use the smallest FOV that does not result in phase wrap artifacts within the region of interest.

In our laboratory, we perform separate, breath-held, short-axis cine images every 10 mm (8 mm slice thickness with 2 mm gap) from the mitral valve plane at the base to the tip of the apex. The total number of slices obtained varies depending on heart size. In patients with dilation of the right ventricle, additional slices may be needed (above the mitral annulus and past the LV apex) to capture the entire length of the RV. The number of slices acquired may be increased to also include full coverage of the atria if atrial pathology is suspected (e.g., atrial septal defects, masses).

The imaging planes for the 3- and 2-chamber cines are subsequently prescribed using the basal and apical short-axis cine images. For the 3-chamber cine, the imaging plane is perpendicular through the short-axis cine images at an angle going through the middle of the left ventricular outflow tract, through the inferolateral wall, and through the apex (step 5; purple line). For the 2-chamber cine, the imaging plane is perpendicular through the short-axis cine images at an angle going through the LV anterior and inferior walls at the base, and also passing through the apex (step 6; red line). If the LV apex is foreshortened (rounded in appearance) due to a curved shape of the LV in the 3- or 2-chamber cine, the angle of the imaging plane can be refined by tilting it back through the apex on the 4-chamber cine.

It is our practice to include dedicated long-axis views of the RV and right ventricular outflow tract (RVOT) in all patients (Fig. 13.3). These views aid in the assessment of RV function as well as visualization of tricuspid/pulmonic valve abnormalities. Moreover, when calculating RV volumes and RV ejection fraction from the short-axis cine images, these views allow readers to track the effect of through-plane motion on RV volume throughout the cardiac cycle and help in the discrimination of whether blood volume is part of the RV versus the right atrium, or part of the RV versus the pulmonary artery at end diastole and end systole.

For the RVOT cine, both the basal short-axis and 4-chamber cine images are used. The imaging plane is prescribed perpendicular through the basal short axis cine image at an angle that bisects the center of both the pulmonic and tricuspid valves. At the same time, the imaging plane is tilted toward the middle of the RV apex on the 4-chamber cine (step 7; yellow line). For the RV 2-chamber cine, a perpendicular plane is prescribed at an angle going through the middle of both the RV free wall and RV diaphragmatic wall using the basal and distal short-axis cine images (step 8; orange line). For patients with ventricular arrhythmias or suspected arrhythmogenic

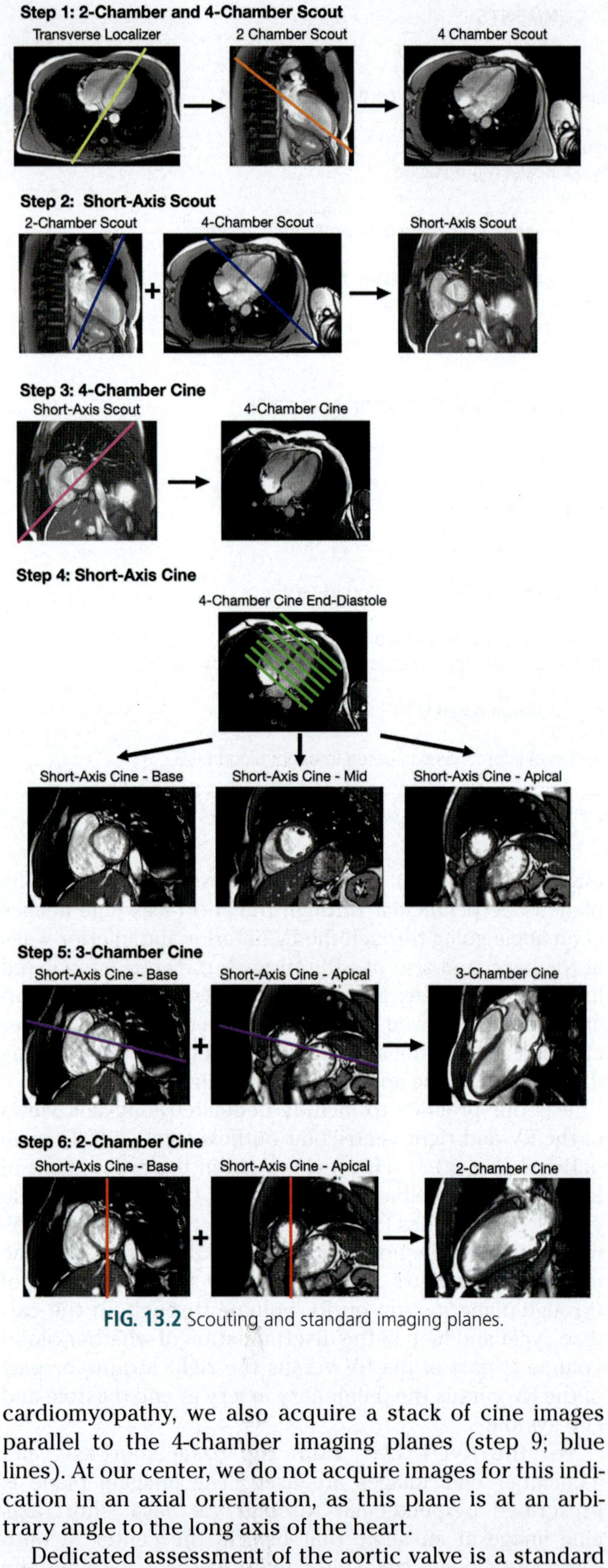

FIG. 13.2 Scouting and standard imaging planes.

cardiomyopathy, we also acquire a stack of cine images parallel to the 4-chamber imaging planes (step 9; blue lines). At our center, we do not acquire images for this indication in an axial orientation, as this plane is at an arbitrary angle to the long axis of the heart.

Dedicated assessment of the aortic valve is a standard part of our imaging protocol. Using the 3-chamber cine images as reference, an orthogonal image of the LV outflow tract is first acquired (Fig. 13.4). This plane is prescribed by bisecting the aortic valve in the 3-chamber view (step 10; pink line). Next, the plane of the aortic valve short axis is prescribed perpendicular to the long axis of the aortic valve in both the 3-chamber and the LV outflow tract cine images. In patients with reduced aortic valve leaflet excursion or suspected aortic stenosis, we acquire three parallel slices centered around the leaflet tips in peak systole ~ 3 mm apart in order to identify the minimum peak systolic aortic valve area (step 11; green lines). In patients with eccentric aortic valve flow that is angulated from the aortic root, the aortic valve area may be more accurately measured with the imaging plane perpendicular to the aortic flow rather than the sinuses of Valsalva. Planimetry of the aortic valve area and measurement of aortic valve velocity on phase-contrast imaging may be performed at the image location that best represents the leaflet tips.

CINE IMAGING

The number of cine sequence imaging variants that are available to practitioners has grown substantially in recent years, including those that incorporate advanced rapid imaging/real-time techniques. In our laboratory, we continue to rely upon a breath-held, SSFP cine pulse sequence with a segmented K-space acquisition for the majority of our patients. The sequence details are shown in Table 13.1.

The sequence parameters were chosen with the goal of having high temporal resolution (~< 50 ms), high spatial resolution (~<1.5 × 1.9 mm in-plane), and relatively short breath-hold times (~ < 6–8 heartbeats depending on the size of the FOV phase). We generally try to limit zero filling or interpolation in both the spatial and temporal domains. Additionally, the parameters have been purposefully selected to ensure that fat and water spins are centered in opposing passbands for SSFP imaging. This results in consistent “out-of-phase” behavior for fat and water across the entire imaging volume (see Chapter 7 for a full explanation). We find that most patients (even those who are admitted with dyspnea or heart failure) are able to adhere to breath-holding instructions with these parameters.

Our standard protocol is to acquire cine images using retrospective ECG gating. The average R to R interval is used to set the duration of retrospective acquisition (e.g., heart rate 80 bpm = R to R interval of 750 msec). This approach works well in patients with regular heart rhythm or in those with infrequent ectopy and has the advantage of capturing the entire cardiac cycle. We do not use prospective ECG gating in most patients because this approach ends the image acquisition prior to the end of diastole and truncates the visualization of the entire cardiac cycle (i.e., the last few frames of diastole). However, in patients with frequent ectopy or irregular heart rhythms, truncation of the acquisition can be advantageous, and this property can be used to capture the portions of the cardiac cycle that are relatively consistent (e.g., systole and the early part of diastole). For example, in patients with atrial fibrillation, the systolic portion of the cardiac cycle is relatively consistent from one heartbeat to another. With prospective gating, the acquisition time within the cardiac cycle can be set to less than the shortest R–R interval experienced by the patient, thus capturing only the consistent portion of the cardiac cycle and nearly none of the inconsistent portion that creates the majority of the artifacts (Fig. 13.5). This

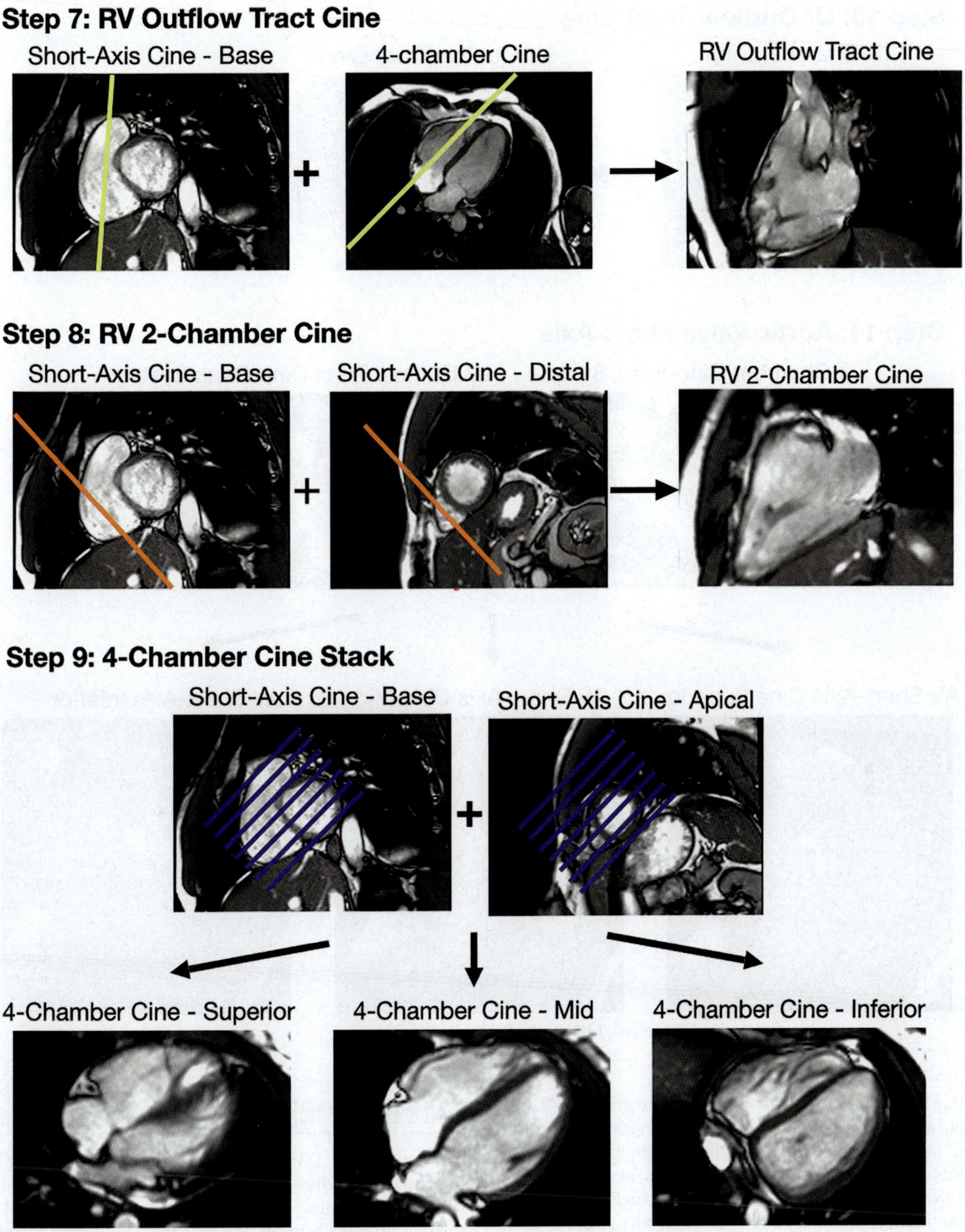

FIG. 13.3 Long-axis imaging planes for the right ventricle.

approach allows operators to acquire cine images using a breath-held segmented sequence, which provides better anatomic detail than real-time approaches. The disadvantage of this strategy is that events occurring in mid-to-late diastole may be missed. When adequate image quality cannot be obtained with this prospective segmented imaging strategy, real-time cine imaging can provide an alternative method (Table 13.2), but typically has worse spatial and temporal resolution than segmented approaches.

In patients with high heart rates (~>100 bpm), improving the temporal resolution of the sequence improves cine image quality. This is accomplished by reducing the

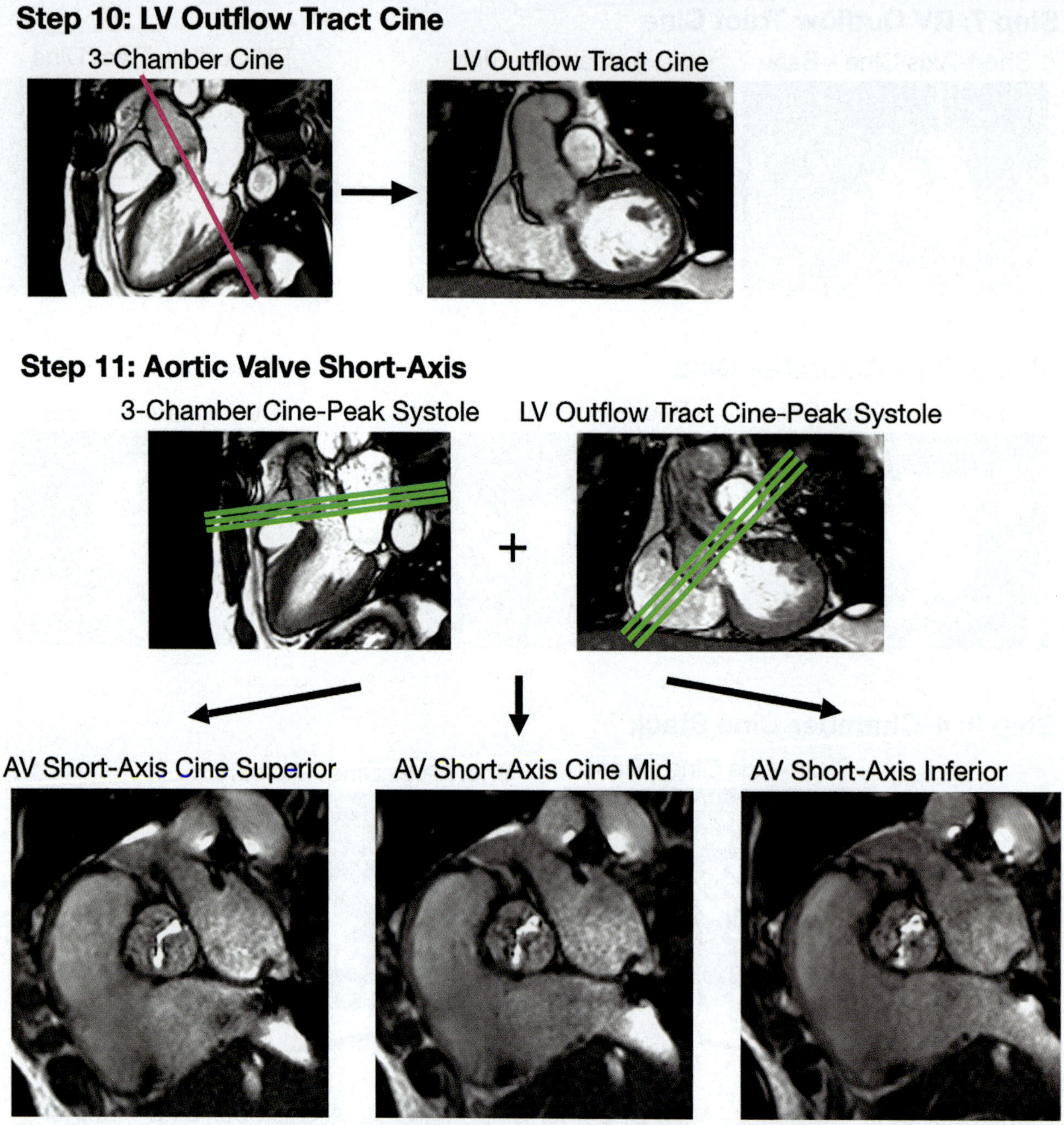

FIG. 13.4 Imaging planes for the aortic valve.

number of segments (K-space lines per segment). At our center, we acquire cine images with a temporal resolution of 48.2 msec, which corresponds to 11 segments for typical patients at 1.5 T (requiring six heart beats; see Table 13.1), but for patients with tachycardia, we instruct operators to reduce the number of segments to improve temporal resolution. For example, at a 100 bpm heart rate (R to R interval: 600 msec), acquiring cine images with seven segments (~4.4 msec per segment) would improve the temporal resolution to 30.7 msec (600 msec R–R interval/30.7 msec = ~20 frames over one cardiac cycle). A total of 10 heartbeats are needed to complete the acquisition, but the increased breath-hold time (relative to an acquisition of six segments at a heart rate of 80 bpm) is partially offset by the higher heart rate.

LATE GADOLINIUM ENHANCEMENT

At our center, LGE imaging is performed in the vast majority of studies. The inclusion of LGE imaging allows the simultaneous visualization of both infarcted and normal myocardium in patients with ischemic heart disease. In patients with nonischemic cardiac disease, the presence, location, and pattern of LGE provide clues to the extent of involvement and etiology of the pathologic process.

Contrast Dose and Type

We typically administer 0.15 mmol/kg of gadolinium contrast media for viability imaging alone or 0.2 mmol/kg in

TABLE 13.1 Typical parameters for 2D-segmented cine.

PARAMETER	1.5T	3.0T
FOV	300–380 mm	300–380 mm
In-plane voxel size	1.2–1.5 × 1.5–1.9 mm	1.2–1.5 × 1.4–1.7 mm
Matrix size	256 × 150	256 × 174
Slice thickness	8 mm	8 mm
Flip angle	55 degrees	42 degrees
Segments	11	14
Temporal resolution	48.2 msec	38.9 msec
Bandwidth	501 Hz/pixel	1302 Hz/pixel
TE (echo time)	2.21 msec	1.22 msec
TR (repetition time)	4.42 msec	2.78 msec
K-space ordering	Linear	Linear
Asymmetric echo	No	Yes
Acceleration	GRAPPA 2	GRAPPA 2
Breath-hold duration	6 heartbeats	6 heartbeats
Readout	SSFP	SSFP

2D, Two dimensional; *FOV,* field of view; *GRAPPA,* generalized autocalibrating partially parallel acquisitions; *Hz,* Hertz; *mm,* millimetre; *msec,* millisecond; *SSFP,* steady-state free precession; *T,* Tesla.

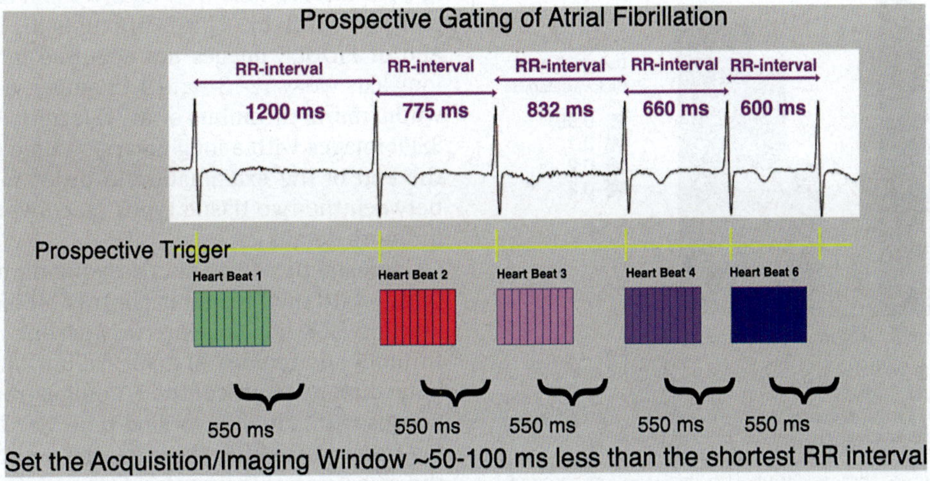

FIG. 13.5 Cine imaging with prospective ECG gating in patients with atrial fibrillation.

two divided doses during vasodilator stress and rest perfusion imaging. Lower doses of contrast media can be considered for viability imaging, however, this may reduce the diagnostic performance of the LGE imaging.[3] The relationship between LGE diagnostic accuracy and contrast dose was demonstrated in an international multicenter study that evaluated the performance of LGE for the detection of MI (Fig. 13.6). This study found a significant dose-response relationship (both $P < .0001$) of gadoversetamide with the sensitivity and accuracy for infarction location increasing with rising contrast dose.[3]

There are several factors that merit consideration when selecting a gadolinium-based contrast agent (GBCA) for LGE imaging. We use group II GBCAs due to their favorable safety profiles and few (if any) associated cases of nephrogenic systemic fibrosis.[4] We also find that the rate of contrast agent clearance from the blood pool is an important consideration when choosing a contrast agent for LGE. For example, albumin-binding GBCAs provide relatively persistent and high blood pool enhancement, often for more than 10-20 minutes following contrast administration. Although helpful for contrast-enhanced magnetic resonance (MR) angiography, the long duration of blood pool enhancement with albumin-binding GBCAs can be problematic for LGE imaging since the blood pool signal and adjacent subendocardial LGE (if present) will have similar (bright) image intensities, potentially leading to difficulty in consistently identifying subendocardial MI. At the other end of the spectrum, we have found that some GBCAs exhibit very rapid clearance from the body. The latter can be problematic (especially for less experienced operators) because there is a relatively short time window during which LGE images with optimal image contrast can be acquired. In instances for which image quality is insufficient, a small additional dose of contrast can be considered.

TABLE 13.2 Typical parameters for real-time cine.

PARAMETER	1.5T	3.0T
FOV	300–380 mm	300–380 mm
In-plane voxel size	2.3 × 3.0–3.0 × 3.8 mm	1.6 × 2.3 - 2.0 × 3.0 mm
Matrix size	128 × 60	192 × 88
Slice thickness	9 mm	8 mm
Flip angle	55 degrees	35 degrees
Segments	20	22
Temporal resolution[a]	44.8 msec	50.6 msec
Bandwidth	1184 Hz/pixel	1240 Hz/pixel
TE (echo time)	0.96 msec	1.11 msec
TR (repetition time)	2.24 msec	2.53 msec
K-space ordering	Linear	Linear
Asymmetric echo	Yes	Yes
Acceleration	GRAPPA 3	GRAPPA 4
Readout	SSFP	SSFP

[a]For real-time sequences, we try to fix the phase field of view (FOV) to 75% to ensure a constant temporal resolution. Increasing the FOV phase will worsen the temporal resolution. Conversely, reducing the FOV phase will improve the temporal resolution.

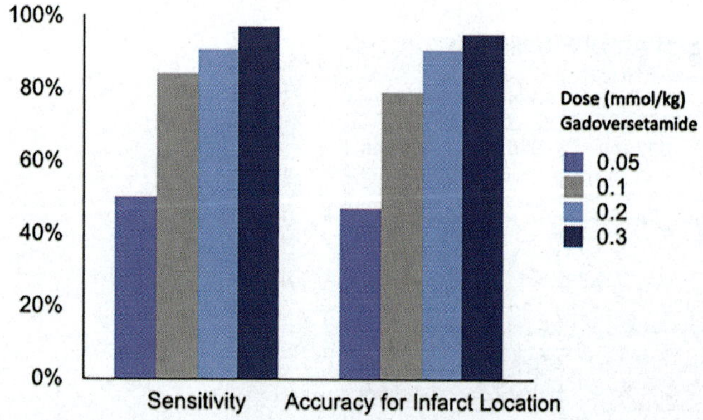

FIG. 13.6 The relationship between the diagnostic performance of late gadolinium enhancement and contrast (gadoversetamide) dose. (Adapted from Kim RJ, Albert TS, Wible JH, et al. Performance of delayed-enhancement magnetic resonance imaging with gadoversetamide contrast for the detection and assessment of myocardial infarction: an international, multicenter, double-blinded, randomized trial. *Circulation* 2008;117(5):629–637. DOI: 10.1161/CIRCULATIONAHA.107.723262.)

Late Gadolinium Enhancement Sequence Variants

Our imaging protocol for LGE utilizes the following pulse sequence variants for most patients:

(1) Bright-blood, 2D, free-breathing, single-shot inversion recovery steady-state free precession (SSIR-SSFP).

(2) Bright-blood, segmented, 2D, breath-held, inversion recovery fast gradient echo (IR-GRE) or segmented, 2D, breath-held, flow-independent dark blood-delayed enhancement (FIDDLE).

Our imaging protocol begins with the acquisition of SSIR-SSFP within 2-3 minutes of contrast administration (Fig. 13.1). Image stacks are prescribed in the short axis and in the LV 2-chamber orientation for full coverage of the heart, including both atria and ventricles. These images are acquired free breathing with a high or long inversion time (~600 ms at 1.5 T and ~875 ms at 3 T) in order to null thrombus or regions of myocardium with microvascular obstruction (MVO). Next, the imaging stacks are repeated in both orientations with an inversion time set to null normal myocardium. Third, breath-held, segmented IR-GRE and/or FIDDLE images are acquired in the LV short- and long-axis views (2-, 3-, and 4- chamber views). In patients in whom mural thrombus or MVO is initially suspected, SSIR-SSFP images with a long inversion time can be repeated at the end of the examination in order to help differentiate between the two tissue types (see Inversion Time section for more details).

Importantly, we do not use a standard or fixed wait time (e.g., ~8–10 minutes after contrast administration) before starting LGE imaging for two reasons. First, intracardiac thrombi and regions of myocardium with MVO are visible immediately after contrast administration on SSIR-SSFP images with a high inversion time. Second, when attempting to visualize LGE, there can be substantial variation in the clearance of the contrast agent from one individual to another, and using a fixed wait time before acquiring LGE images can result in missing the optimal imaging window in individuals with rapid contrast clearance. Accordingly, we instruct operators to begin high TI LGE imaging shortly after contrast administration.

We find that different pulse sequence variants for LGE imaging are complementary when performed in the same patient. With SSIR-SSFP, image acquisition is fast and does not require breath-holding, permitting a rapid survey of the heart. With the segmented implementation of LGE, spatial and temporal resolutions are higher than for SSIR-SSFP. However, breath-holding is required to eliminate image ghosts due to respiratory motion. The higher resolution leads to improved sensitivity for the detection of scar and better visualization of infarct transmurality compared to the single-shot variant.[5]

Over the last ~15 years, we have added dark blood delayed enhancement into our imaging protocol. This is because dark blood LGE techniques further improve the identification of myocardium with contrast enhancement.[6] In particular, with standard bright blood LGE techniques

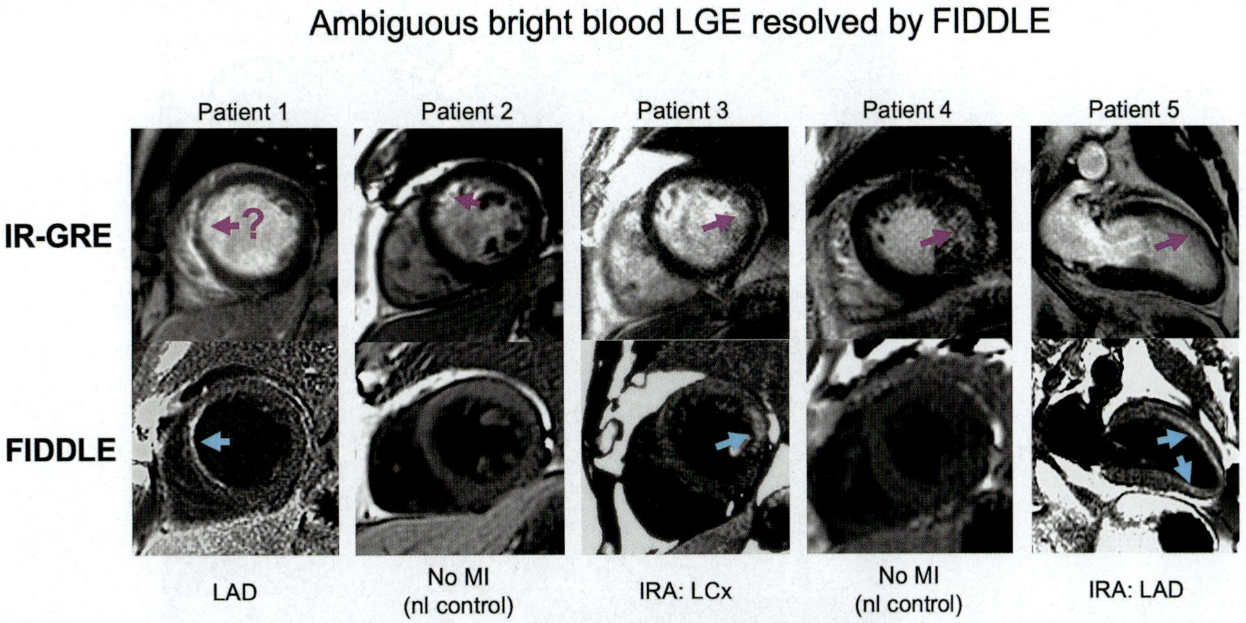

FIG. 13.7 Images in five patients ($n=3$ with myocardial infarction [*MI*], $n=2$ control patients without MI) in whom the diagnosis of MI was ambiguous on conventional bright blood LGE (IR-GRE). In patients 1 and 2, there is possibly anteroseptal wall LGE on IR-GRE. Flow-independent dark blood- delayed enhancement (*FIDDLE*) shows unequivocal LGE in patient 1, but also demonstrates no LGE in patient 2, who is a normal control. Similarly, in patients 3 and 4, there are ambiguous regions of LGE on the IR-GRE images involving the lateral wall. FIDDLE identifies that patient 3 has lateral wall infarct, while patient 4 is a normal control. In patient 5, FIDDLE demonstrates not only a subendocardial infarct in the anterior wall but also extension into the inferoapical wall. *IRA*, Infarct-related artery; *IR-GRE*, Inversion recovery gradient echo; *LAD*, Left anterior descending; *LCx*, Left circumflex; *MI*, myocardial infarction; *RCA*, Right coronary artery. (Adapted from Kim HW, Rehwald WG, Jenista ER, et al. Dark-blood delayed enhancement cardiac magnetic resonance of myocardial infarction. *JACC Cardiovasc Imaging* 2018;11(12):1758–1769. DOI: 10.1016/j.jcmg.2017.09.021.)

(SSIR-SSFP or IR-GRE), the hyperintense signal intensity of the LV cavity caused by the presence of intravascular contrast material reduces the contrast-to-noise ratio between blood and infarcted myocardium and hampers clear infarct delineation. In patients with subendocardial myocardial infarction or scarring, this is often problematic since the infarct can be indistinguishable from the adjacent blood pool, potentially leading to a missed or erroneous diagnosis (Fig. 13.7). In patients, FIDDLE has been shown to have improved diagnostic performance for the diagnosis of MI compared to conventional bright-blood IR-GRE (sensitivity: 96% vs 85%, respectively, $P=.002$; accuracy: 95% vs. 87%, $P=.01$).[6] In patients with nonischemic cardiomyopathies, we have also found that FIDDLE can be helpful in highlighting subtle regions of LGE (Fig. 13.8).

An alternative to segmented, breath-held, bright-blood IR-GRE is the acquisition of multiple SSIR-SSFP images that are subsequently motion corrected (MOCO), coregistered, and averaged.[7] This technique produces images that have hybrid characteristics of the SSIR-SSFP and segmented IR-GRE techniques. Similar to an individual SSIR-SSFP image acquisition, ghosting artifacts due to respiratory motion are not present, while the spatial and temporal resolutions are comparable to that of segmented IR-GRE through the application of parallel imaging. The signal-to-noise ratio (SNR) loss associated with higher resolution and the use of parallel imaging is offset through averaging of the images (typically 8 averages, acquired over 16 heart beats). In the LV short-axis orientation, MOCO is usually able to account for variations in the in-plane position of the heart, and the sequence provides overall image quality that is similar to that of segmented IR-GRE, but without the requirement for breath-holding. We have observed, however, that errors in the coregistration process can occur in patients with irregular or deep breathing patterns or in patients with significant pericardial/pleural effusions. Additionally, in the LV long-axis views, accurate image coregistration may not always be possible due to the through-plane motion of the heart during free breathing. Coregistration errors can lead to artifacts, which can be subtle in the composite image and not always apparent unless the source images are also reviewed. For these reasons we do not use these sequences in patients who are capable of breath-holding. Additionally, there may be little savings in scan time in these patients because the typical acquisition duration is ~20–30 seconds per slice (as compared to ~10–12 seconds for a single segmented IR-GRE acquisition). Nonetheless, the technique is very helpful in patients who are unable to comply with breath-holding instructions.

PULSE SEQUENCE PARAMETERS

In this section, we will discuss the parameters of the bright-blood and dark-blood pulse sequences used at our center and describe how we train operators to make patient-specific adjustments.

Bright-Blood Single-Shot Inversion Recovery Steady-State Free Precession and Segmented Inversion Recovery Fast Gradient Echo

Typical pulse sequence parameters at 1.5 T and 3 T for the segmented IR-GRE and SSIR-SSFP implementations used

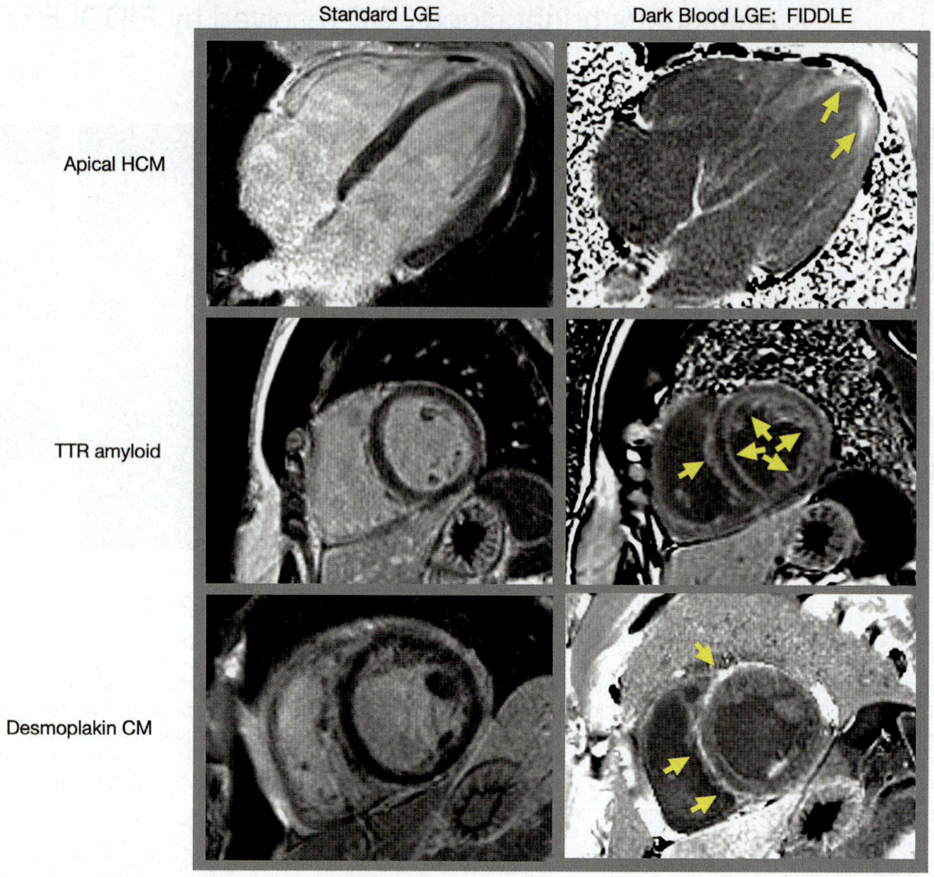

FIG. 13.8 Patient examples of dark-blood late gadolinium enhancement (*LGE*) (flow-independent dark blood-delayed enhancement [*FIDDLE*]) in three different types of nonischemic cardiomyopathy. The FIDDLE images (*left*) demonstrate regions of LGE (*yellow arrows*) that are difficult to appreciate on standard (*bright blood*) LGE imaging (*right*). *CM*, Cardiomyopathy; *HCM*, hypertrophic cardiomyopathy; *TTR*, transthyretin.

at our center are shown in Tables 13.3 and 13.4, respectively. In all patients, we attempt to obtain segmented IR-GRE images in the short-axis views (~8mm slice thickness, 2mm gap) and LV long axis in the same spatial locations as the cine images. For this sequence, we use an in-phase TE to reduce the effect of intravoxel dephasing that occurs within voxels containing an admixture of fat and water species. Intravoxel dephasing may cause an MI containing fatty metaplasia to appear 'nulled' or black. This artifact can lead to the affected voxels being mistakenly interpreted as viable tissue. One reason why we prefer the segmented IR-GRE implementation over SSFP variants (segmented or SSIR-SSFP with MOCO) is that setting the in-phase TE for GRE is straightforward. The operator simply selects the shortest possible in-phase echo time (TE). For SSFP, the process for reducing intravoxel dephasing is more complex (see Chapter 7) and more strongly influenced by factors such as field strength, magnetic field homogeneity, and patient anatomy. In some patients, selecting a repetition time (TR) in which fat and water spins are both consistently within an in-phase passband may not be possible. As the other technical details of the pulse sequences have been described elsewhere,[8–11] we will focus the remainder of this discussion upon the key parameters that our scan operators commonly adjust in order to improve image quality.

Data Acquisition Window

The time during which the image K-space data are acquired by the MRI scanner is the data acquisition window (Fig. 13.9). For both SSIR-SSFP and segmented IR-GRE implementations, the scan operator may adjust the location and/or duration of the acquisition window with the goal of limiting the impact of cardiac motion on image quality.

The location of the acquisition window is adjusted to occur in middiastole of the cardiac cycle when the heart is relatively motionless. Typically, the acquisition window is ~200ms in duration in patients with heart rates between ~45 and 100 bpm (Fig. 13.10). The end of the acquisition window corresponds to the end of the diastolic standstill period and usually occurs prior to the P wave of the ECG tracing. If there is ambiguity when LGE imaging should be performed (e.g., due to dyssynchronous contraction associated with left bundle branch block), operators can use cine imaging to identify the standstill location and duration more precisely.

The duration of the acquisition window is the temporal resolution for LGE imaging and is determined by the number of K-space lines (segments or view per segment) per heartbeat. There are several factors to consider when adjusting the duration of the acquisition window depending upon the sequence used.

TABLE 13.3 Typical parameters for 2D inversion recovery fast gradient echo.

PARAMETER	1.5T	3.0T
FOV	300–380 mm	300–380 mm
In-plane voxel size	1.2–1.5 × 1.5–2.0 mm	1.0–1.3 × 1.3–1.7 mm
Matrix size	256 × 146	256 × 230
Slice thickness	8 mm	8 mm
Flip angle	25 degrees	19 degrees
Segments	21	35
Inversion time (TI)	Variable	Variable
Bandwidth	130 Hz/pixel	347 Hz/pixel
TE (echo time)	4.76 msec	2.46 msec
TR (repetition time)	10.09 msec	5.25 msec
Gating factor	2	2
K-space ordering	Linear	Linear
Fat sat	No	No
Asymmetric echo	Yes	Yes
Grad moment refocusing	No	No
Parallel imaging factor	None	2
Temporal resolution	212 msec	183 msec

TABLE 13.4 Typical parameters for single-shot 2D IR-SSFP.[a]

PARAMETER	1.5T	3.0T
FOV	300–380 mm	300–380 mm
In-plane voxel size	1.4–1.8 × 2.0–2.5 mm	1.2–1.5 × 1.5–1.9 mm
Matrix size	208 × 150	256 × 200
Slice thickness	8 mm	8 mm
Flip angle	60 degrees	45 degrees
Segments	68	77
Inversion time (TI)	Variable	Variable
Bandwidth	601 Hz/pixel	977 Hz/pixel
TE (echo time)	1.24 msec	1.11 msec
TR (repetition time)	3.06 msec	2.64 msec
Gating factor	2	2
K-space ordering	Linear	Linear
Fat sat	No	No
Asymmetric echo	Yes	Yes
Parallel imaging	2	2

[a]For single shot sequences, we try to fix the phase field of view (FOV) to 75% to ensure a constant temporal resolution. Increasing the FOV phase will worsen the temporal resolution. Conversely, reducing the FOV phase will improve the temporal resolution.
2D, Two dimensional; *cm*, centimetre; *FOV*, field of view; *Hz*, Hertz; *IR*, inversion recovery; *mm*, millimetre; *msec*, millisecond; *SSFP*, steady-state free precession.

For segmented implementations, the acquisition of K-space occurs incrementally over several heartbeats. The number of phase-encoding lines acquired in each heartbeat determines temporal resolution (number of phase-encoding lines multiplied by repetition time; e.g., 21 lines × 10.09 ms = 212.1 ms). When fewer lines are acquired per heartbeat, the temporal resolution is shorter but the total number of heartbeats (and breath-hold time) to acquire the data needed for reconstruction is higher (matrix size divided by segments).

For single-shot implementations, all the K-space lines for an image are acquired in a single heartbeat. The temporal resolution is determined by the total number of K-space lines acquired in the phase-encoding direction and the parallel imaging acceleration factor. For any given matrix size and acceleration factor, the number of K-space lines acquired alters the temporal resolution (e.g., more lines/larger field of phase increases the readout duration). As such, single-shot implementations are typically limited by worse spatial resolution for the same temporal resolution compared to segmented implementations.

Altering the duration of the acquisition window or temporal resolution may be advantageous in specific instances for segmented K-space implementations (Fig. 13.10). For example, in patients with significant tachycardia (~>100 bpm), reducing the number of segments may

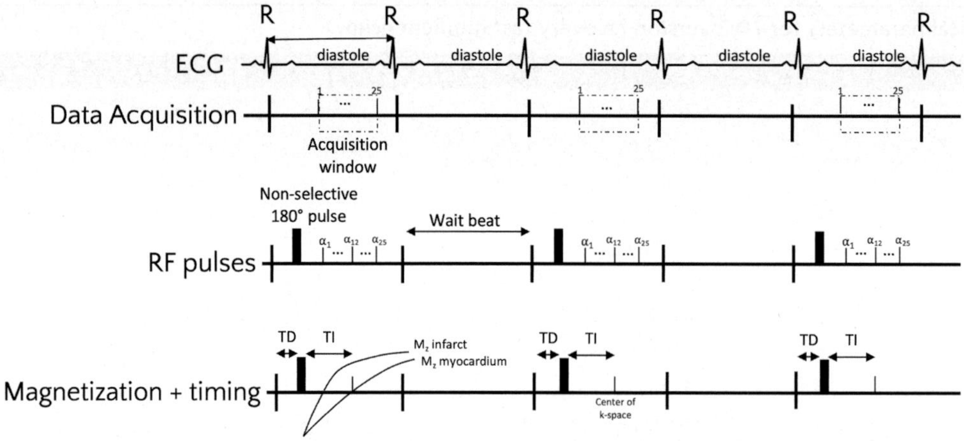

FIG. 13.9 Timing diagram of two-dimensional segmented inversion recovery fast gradient echo pulse sequence. ECG: The ECG tracing is used to trigger the image acquisition in mid-late diastole. Data acquisition: the *dashed box* indicates the time during which the data is acquired ("acquisition window"), which is controlled by the repetition time and the number of lines of k-space being acquired. RF pulses: The sequence begins with a nonselective 180° inversion pulse, followed by the readout pulses. The subsequent heartbeat is a "wait beat" to allow for magnetization recovery between inversion pulses. Magnetization: after detection of the R wave, there is a time delay before the inversion pulse is played. The inversion pulse inverts the magnetization, which recovers based on the tissue T1. The recovery curves for infarct and myocardium are shown to highlight the differences in magnetization recovery due to the differences in postcontrast T1. At the time when the center of k-space is acquired, the magnetization of the myocardium is at the zero crossing, while the infarct magnetization is above the zero crossing. The resulting image contrast is that the myocardium has very little signal (magnetization is near zero) while the infarct is bright (significantly above zero). *ECG*, electrocardiogram. *RF*, radiofrequency; *TD*, trigger delay; *TI*, inversion time delay; α, shallow flip angle excitation.

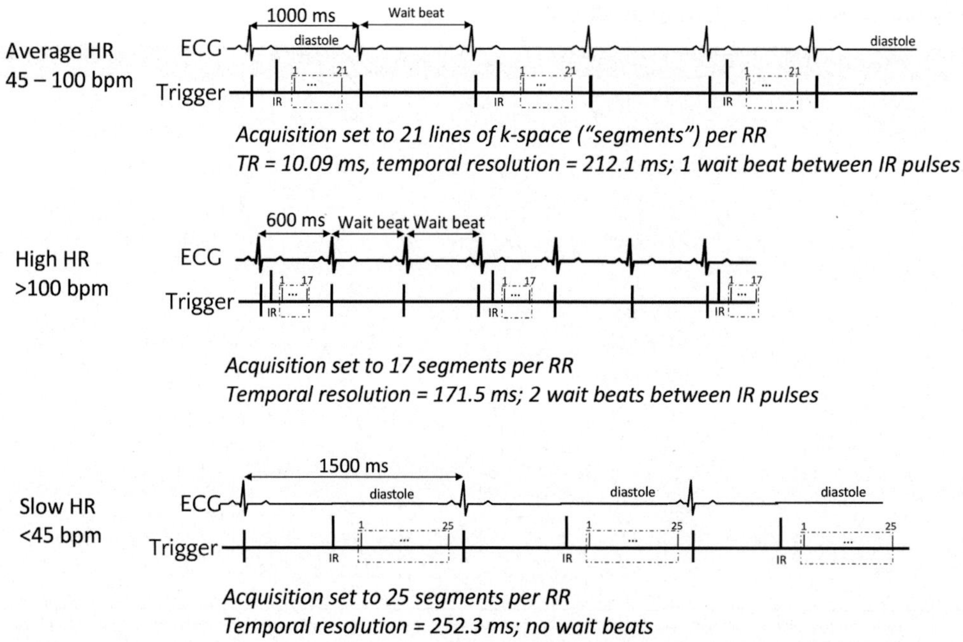

FIG. 13.10 Data acquisition duration and gating factor depending on heart rate (*HR*). TOP: ECG and readout timings for patients with typical heart rates seen in clinical practice (~45–100 bpm). Inversion pulses are played every other heartbeat to allow for longitudinal magnetization recovery between inversion pulses. MIDDLE: In patients with tachycardia (>100 bpm), two parameter adjustments may be considered. First, the duration of the readout may be reduced by lowering the number of segments (lines per segment), improving the temporal resolution. Second, two wait beats (gating factor of 3) may be used, which allows greater recovery of longitudinal magnetization between inversion pulses. BOTTOM: In patients with bradycardia (<45 bpm), a gating factor of 1 (no wait beats) can be considered. The time between inversion pulses is greater with very slow heart rates. Accordingly, there is sufficient recovery of longitudinal magnetization with no wait beats between inversion pulses. The duration of the acquisition window may be modestly increased to account for the longer period of the diastolic standstill period.

improve image sharpness since temporal resolution is improved (shorter; e.g., 17 segments × 10.09 ms = 171.5 ms). Conversely, increasing the number of segments (e.g., 25 segments × 10.09 ms = 252.3 ms) may provide acceptable temporal resolution with minimal change in image sharpness when the heart rate is slow (~<45 bpm) since the diastolic standstill period is longer. The latter change carries the additional benefit of reducing the overall breath-hold time.

Adjustments to the location of the acquisition window are typically required in patients with irregular arrhythmias, such as atrial fibrillation (AF). In patients with AF,

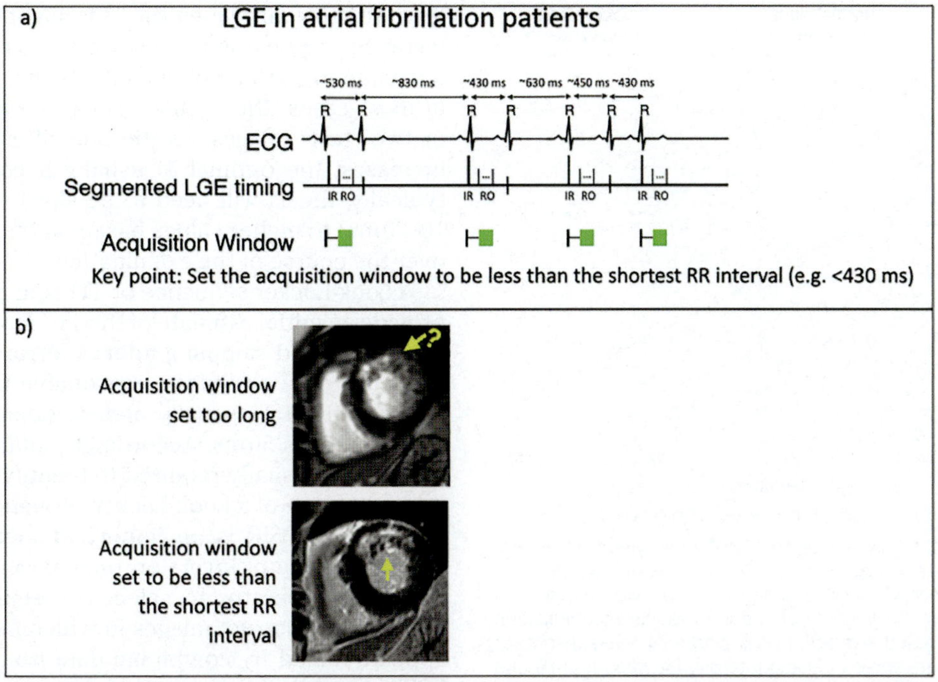

FIG. 13.11 Adjustment to the data acquisition window for patients with atrial fibrillation. (A) In patients with atrial fibrillation (or other irregular rhythms), we adjust the data acquisition window such that the imaging readout is completed prior to the end of the shortest R–R interval between heartbeats. (B) Examples of late gadolinium enhancement (*LGE*) images in a patient with atrial fibrillation. The top row shows a data acquisition window that was set too long (> than the shortest R–R interval). There is substantial blurring of the subendocardium, and it is not clear if an infarct is present. The bottom row is from the same patient in whom data acquisition was set to be less than the shortest R–R interval. Image sharpness is improved and the infarct is easily delineated from the blood pool and adjacent normal myocardium.

the length of the cardiac cycle is variable, and when one compares one R–R interval to another, the main difference between heartbeats is the duration of diastole (Fig. 13.11A). In other words, the duration of systole between heart rates in patients with AF is relatively similar, while the duration of diastole may be variable. Accordingly, at our center, we adjust the location of the data acquisition so that imaging occurs at the end of systole/early diastole. For most patients with AF, we adjust the timing such that the end of the image readout occurs prior to the end of the shortest R–R interval between heartbeats (Fig. 13.11B). This strategy can be adapted for other irregular heart rhythms and is compatible with both single-shot and segmented acquisitions.

Gating Factor

Since successive inversion recovery (IR) preparation pulses are used to impart T1 weighting, wait beats are used to allow the recovery of longitudinal magnetization between pulses (Fig. 13.9). The gating factor controls the number of heartbeats (or wait beats) between IR pulses. For patients with typical heart rates (~>45–<100 bpm), a gating factor of two (one wait beat between IR pulses) is sufficient to allow for the majority of the longitudinal magnetization to recover (Fig. 13.12). However, in patients with tachycardia, a gating factor of 3 (2 wait beats) is preferable since the time between IR pulses is shorter and image intensity differences between enhanced and normal myocardium are better maintained. Conversely, in patients with significant bradycardia, a gating factor of 1 (0 wait beats) can be sufficient to achieve recovery of longitudinal magnetization.

Inversion Time

The inversion time (TI) is defined as the time between the end of the nonselective inversion preparation to the center of k-space data acquisition (for a linear reordering, Fig. 13.9). Historically, the selection of TI for bright-blood LGE has been one of the more difficult parameters for operators to learn to adjust accurately. Fortunately, the development of phase-sensitive reconstruction (PSIR)[12] has greatly simplified the process. Using PSIR, operators are able to obtain high-quality LGE images without the need for precise optimization of the TI. Nonetheless, we find that an understanding of how the TI is manually selected has clinical utility, and this knowledge can be used to identify specific pathologies such as intracardiac thrombi or cardiac amyloidosis.

For manual selection of the TI, the goal is to select the TI so that the longitudinal magnetization of normal myocardium reaches just past the zero crossing (Fig. 13.13A), thereby 'nulling' normal myocardium. This TI also maximizes the difference in magnetization (and consequently, image intensity; Fig. 13.13B) between infarcted and normal myocardium.

Inaccurate selection of the TI may lead to missed detection of infarcts and incorrect infarct sizing, particularly if the TI selected is too short. In general, selection of TIs that are longer than the normal myocardium zero crossing maintains the difference in image intensities between

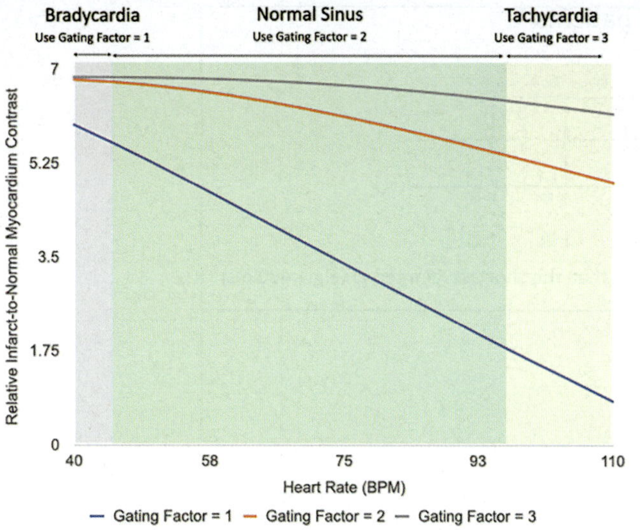

FIG. 13.12 Simulation of relative image contrast for infarcted myocardium as a function of heart rate and gating factor. For patients with typical heart rates (45–100 bpm, *green shading*), a gating factor of two (*orange line*) is sufficient to allow for the majority of the longitudinal magnetization to recover between repeated inversion pulses with minimal saturation of magnetization. Thus, differences in image intensity between normal and infarcted myocardium are high and relatively flat across these heart rates with a gating factor of 2. For patients with tachycardia (>100 bpm, *yellow shading*), a gating factor of 3 (*gray line*) is preferred since it maintains the time between repeated inversion pulses and allows longitudinal recovery to occur more fully. Compared to a gating factor of 2, the differences in image intensity between normal and infarcted myocardium are better maintained. The increase in total number of heartbeats required to complete the image is partially offset by the increase in heart rate. For patients with significant bradycardia (<45 bpm, *gray shading*), a gating factor of 1 (*blue line*) can be considered since the time between inversion pulses is longer and allows sufficient recovery between inversion pulses to occur. The decrease in number of heartbeats required to complete the image reduces the breath-hold time (assumes PSIR is not employed). Simulations using the Bloch equations assumed a gradient echo (GRE) readout with 23 lines of k-space per heartbeat, 19-degree readout flip angle, inversion time (TI) set to null normal myocardium, and an infarct T1 of 300 ms. *PSIR*, Phase-sensitive inversion recovery.

normal and infarcted myocardium over a reasonable range. However, selection of TIs that are shorter than the normal myocardium zero crossing may create ambiguity in the relative image intensities of normal and infarcted myocardium (Fig. 13.13, **red box**). Specifically, when inversion times that are somewhat shorter than the null time for normal myocardium are selected, differences in image intensity between normal and infarcted myocardium are variable or may even disappear. As a result, we train operators to select a slightly longer TI than the normal myocardium zero crossing in order to avoid acquiring images for which the TI may be too short (Fig. 13.13, **green box**).

At our center, our operators are trained to manually adjust the TI by imaging iteratively with different TIs. In general, a TI of 300 ms at 1.5 T or 400 ms at 3 T when using a linear K-space trajectory (50–100 ms shorter if centric) is a reasonable first estimate of the TI assuming a contrast dose 0.15 mmol/kg. One could consider reducing the initial TI estimate if a higher dose of contrast is given, imaging is performed earlier after contrast administration, or the rate of contrast clearance is anticipated to be reduced.

The process for iteratively selecting the TI is shown in Fig. 13.14. In particular, we recommend that operators learn to recognize when the TI is slightly too short. In this instance, myocardium will exhibit an 'etched' appearance due to partial volume effects (see Fig. 13.13 legend). In most cases, the optimal TI can be identified after one or two "test" images. As the time after contrast injection increases, the optimal TI usually becomes longer. Thus, typically, the TI will need to be slowly incremented (e.g., 10–20 ms) to higher values based on the image appearance over the course of the examination.

A Look-Locker sequence or TI scout can also be used to provide an initial estimate of the TI.[13] However, due to readout effects and sampling interval errors, the Look-Locker sequence only provides a reasonable first approximation of the optimal TI, usually underestimating the optimal TI by as much as 50 ms. Accordingly, additional manual iteration is still usually required to identify the optimal TI following the use of a Look-Locker sequence.

LGE with PSIR is an important method that reduces the complexity of inversion time selection.[12] The method allows the operator to select a "default" inversion time value to reconstruct images in which normal myocardium appears nulled by combining data from the conventional LGE acquisition with a second data acquisition (known as the 'reference'). The "reference" data is acquired during the wait beat and is used for the PSIR. The reference data are used to resolve the sign of longitudinal magnetization of a tissue species following the inversion preparation (e.g., used to determine if a tissue is at, above, or below the zero/null point). Accordingly, following PSIR, the image intensities on the PSIR image will be rendered based on the relative T1. Tissue species with the longest T1 (e.g., pericardial or pleural fluid) are displayed with the darkest image intensity. Viable myocardium has an intermediate relative T1 and is also dark but less dark than long T1 species. Tissue species with short T1s (e.g., myocardium with LGE or fat) will be displayed with the highest relative image intensity. Importantly, the differences in relative image intensity between normal myocardium and infarcted myocardium are maintained over a fairly wide range of inversion time times and obviates the problem of setting the inversion time too short.

As LGE imaging is typically acquired with a gating factor of two, the inclusion of PSIR comes at no cost in terms of breath-hold duration or SNR, and thus, our standard protocol includes PSIR. One caveat, however, is that a moderate degree of coregistration between the magnitude and reference data is required to avoid errors in the determination of phase for the PSIR image. Coregistration errors can occasionally occur in the PSIR image if large beat-to-beat changes in heart position occur due to respiratory motion or ectopy. In our experience, this is rarely an issue for breath-held implementations as the amount of misregistration is negligible. However, when using free-breathing, single-shot implementations, misregistration can be more common. The result can be inaccurate rendering of image intensity in the cardiac structures. Fortunately, in these instances, the magnitude reconstruction is still interpretable, provided that the TI was selected appropriately. For this reason, we teach operators to manually adjust the TI to null normal myocardium even when using PSIR, ensuring that both the magnitude and PSIR images are interpretable.

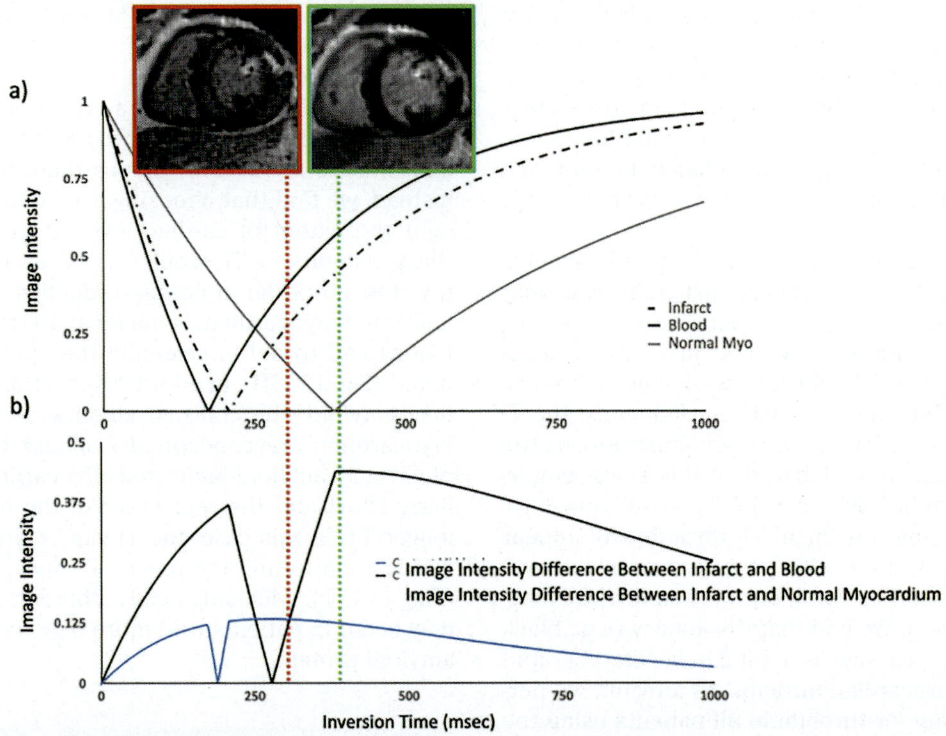

FIG. 13.13 (A) Image intensity of normal and infarcted myocardium as a function of inversion time (TI) for magnitude reconstruction late gadolinium enhancement (LGE). Simulations assumed a T1 of normal myocardium is 550 ms, infarcted myocardium is 350 ms, and blood is 300 ms. (B) Difference in image intensities between infarcted and normal myocardium as a function of TI for magnitude reconstruction LGE. The time at which the magnetization of normal myocardium crosses zero is defined as the TI to null normal myocardium. This TI is considered 'optimal' because the image intensity difference between infarcted and normal myocardium is maximized (*green box and line*). Selection of a TI that is shorter than the optimal time (*left of the green line*) is problematic because the image intensity difference between infarct and normal myocardium can be significantly reduced (or possibly eliminated), and the relationship with the selected TI time is not linear. An indication that the TI is set ~20–50 ms too short is the presence of 'etching' (*red box*), which occurs at the interface between the blood pool and subendocardium due to the partial volume effect. The voxels situated at this interface include both myocardium (which is below the zero crossing) and blood pool (which is above the zero crossing), leading to a net magnetization of zero; these voxels appear black. The adjacent midmyocardial voxels (below the zero crossing) and blood pool–only voxels (above the zero crossing) are bright. Because of this artifact, we recommend that operators systematically select a TI that is slightly longer than optimal (~30 ms). The image intensity difference between infarct and normal myocardium with these slightly longer TIs (*right of the green line*) is predictable and stable.

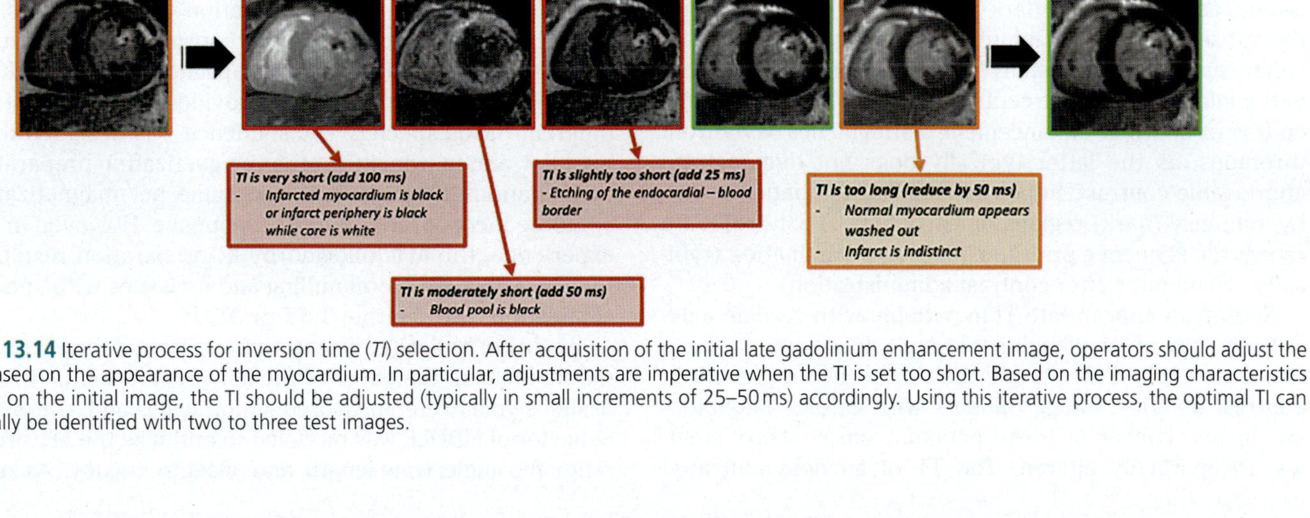

FIG. 13.14 Iterative process for inversion time (*TI*) selection. After acquisition of the initial late gadolinium enhancement image, operators should adjust the TI based on the appearance of the myocardium. In particular, adjustments are imperative when the TI is set too short. Based on the imaging characteristics seen on the initial image, the TI should be adjusted (typically in small increments of 25–50 ms) accordingly. Using this iterative process, the optimal TI can usually be identified with two to three test images.

As noted earlier, one advantage of having a high level of proficiency in adjusting the TI enables operators to easily adapt bright-blood LGE imaging to identify other pathologies, including intracardiac thrombi, microvascular obstruction associated with acute myocardial infarction, and cardiac amyloidosis. Typically, a change in approach to setting the TI can be used to highlight these pathologic findings.

Identification of intracardiac thrombi by LGE imaging exploits the principle that thrombi are generally avascular and do not display contrast enhancement.[14] In other words, while tissue species with perfusion take up contrast (leading to reduction in their T1), there is no significant change in the T1 of thrombus postcontrast. Consequently, the TI that nulls thrombus prior to contrast administration is the same TI postcontrast. In our laboratory, this TI was empirically determined to be ~600 ms at 1.5 T and ~875 ms at 3T (Fig. 13.15, top). Using this 'high' TI, thrombi will appear black, while other tissues with perfusion or blood will appear gray or bright (Fig. 13.15, bottom) on the LGE magnitude reconstruction. We find that this binary (e.g., black vs. bright) image appearance is helpful in facilitating rapid identification of intracardiac thrombi. As a result, we perform high TI imaging for thrombi in all patients using the SSIR-SSFP sequence variant in the short axis and 2-chamber image stacks shortly after contrast administration. Imaging in the 2-chamber orientation allows visualization of the left atrial appendage in a longitudinal axis. While thrombi can also be identified by standard LGE imaging using PSIR (e.g., without selecting a high TI), the image appearance will not be binary. Instead, since tissue species are rendered according to their relative T1, fluid, thrombus, and viable myocardium will all appear dark. Specifically, fluid will have the most negative relative image intensity value (e.g., most dark), followed by thrombus and then by viable myocardium (e.g., least dark). Adjusting the image window and level is often necessary to bring out differences in image intensities in these structures.

An added benefit of performing high TI SSIR-SSFP imaging is that it enables the identification of microvascular obstruction ("no-reflow"). The same high-TI LGE technique used for thrombus imaging can also serve to identify acute infarcts with damaged microvasculature. In infarcts with microvascular obstruction, there is minimal to no contrast enhancement early after contrast (e.g., the T1 in this region is long) and they appear dark (hypointense). However, over the subsequent ~10–60 minutes, there is gradual contrast enhancement (via diffusion) beginning from the outer rim of the infarct toward the central core (Fig. 13.16). The time course of contrast enhancement distinguishes MVO from thrombus, as the latter typically does not demonstrate appreciable contrast enhancement. Thus, in patients with hypointense (dark) regions on early high-TI SSIR-SSFP, we repeat the sequence prior to ending the examination (typically ~20 minutes after contrast administration).

Setting an appropriate TI in patients with cardiac amyloidosis may be challenging.[15] In our experience, we have found that this difficulty can be due to heterogeneity in contrast kinetics among patients with cardiac amyloidosis. In one subset of these patients, the contrast kinetics are markedly altered. The T1 of amyloid-infiltrated myocardium is significantly shorter than blood T1, even early after contrast administration (Fig. 13.17A). In this circumstance, operators will find that they are unable to 'null' the myocardium using a typical inversion time, perhaps because the majority of the myocardium is abnormal and there is no 'normal' myocardium that can be nulled. Instead, we find that choosing a TI to null blood will highlight the extent of cardiac involvement (Fig. 13.17B). In these patients, a TI scout can be used to quickly identify this alteration in contrast kinetics (e.g., the amyloid-infiltrated myocardium is nulled at a TI that is shorter than blood) and to aid in selecting the appropriate TI to null blood (Fig. 13.17B). In another subset of patients with cardiac amyloid, the contrast kinetics of amyloid-infiltrated myocardium are conceptually similar to scar: the T1 of blood and amyloid-infiltrated myocardium are both similarly short and the remainder of the myocardium has a longer T1. In this case, the TI can be adjusted in the normal fashion to null the longer T1 species of myocardium (Fig. 13.17C). Mechanistically, this latter pattern of LGE may occur in patients with more regional deposition of the amyloid protein.

DARK-BLOOD LATE GADOLINIUM ENHANCEMENT

Several dark-blood LGE sequences have been described in the literature.[16] In general, many of the pulse sequence parameters can be adjusted using the same guidelines as described above for bright-blood LGE (SSIR-SSFP and IR-GRE). However, since the mechanisms to generate image contrast between blood and infarcted myocardium are different, the process for selecting the optimal TI or other preparation time lengths to achieve dark-blood conditions are sequence specific. A recent review described the technical details of these sequences.[16] As discussed earlier, we use FIDDLE for dark-blood LGE, and now use it in place of segmented IR-GRE in many patients.

The typical pulse sequence parameters at 1.5 T and 3 T for segmented FIDDLE implementations used at our center are shown in Table 13.5. FIDDLE incorporates two preparation pulses with an SSFP readout with PSIR (Fig. 13.18).[6] First, a magnetization transfer (MT) preparation is used to reduce the magnetization of blood more than that of myocardium. Next, an IR preparation then separates the blood, infarcted myocardium, and normal myocardium on the basis of T1. Finally, with appropriate selection of the TI and PSIR, the resultant image provides separation of the different tissue species. The sequence was designed to be modular, and in principle, other magnetization preparation combinations that result in the same net magnetization could be incorporated into the sequence. However, in our experience, the MT followed by IR preparation results in the most uniform blood nulling and no issues with specific absorption rate at either 1.5 T or 3T.[6,17]

We do not typically adjust the parameters of the MT preparation. Instead, the effect of the MT preparation on in vivo tissue signal were measured empirically, and the signal behavior of FIDDLE was modeled to optimize the MT preparation flip angle, train length, and offset frequency.[6] As such,

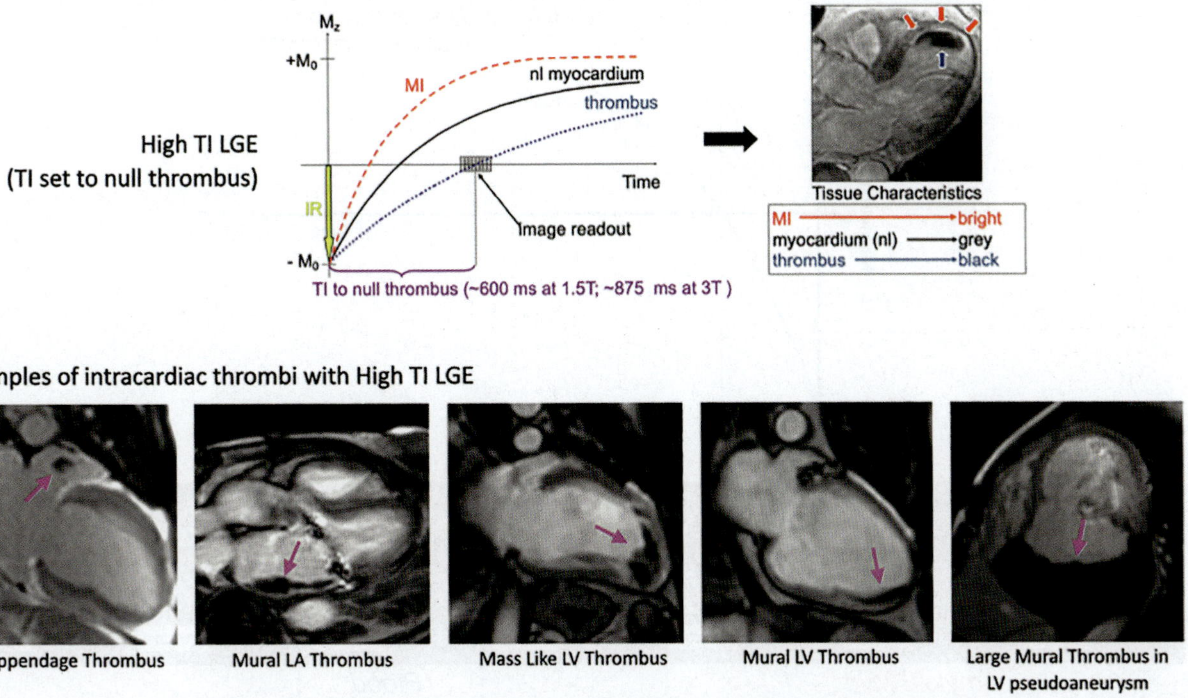

FIG. 13.15 High inversion time (*TI*) late gadolinium enhancement (*LGE*) imaging for intracardiac thrombi. TOP: Inversion recovery curves for myocardial infarction (*MI*), normal myocardium, and thrombus are shown. When a TI of 600 ms at 1.5 T or 875 ms at 3 T is used, intracardiac thrombi appear black, while other cardiac structures are gray or bright. BOTTOM: Examples of various intracardiac thrombi identified by high TI LGE are shown. *LA*, Left atrium; *LV*, left ventricle.

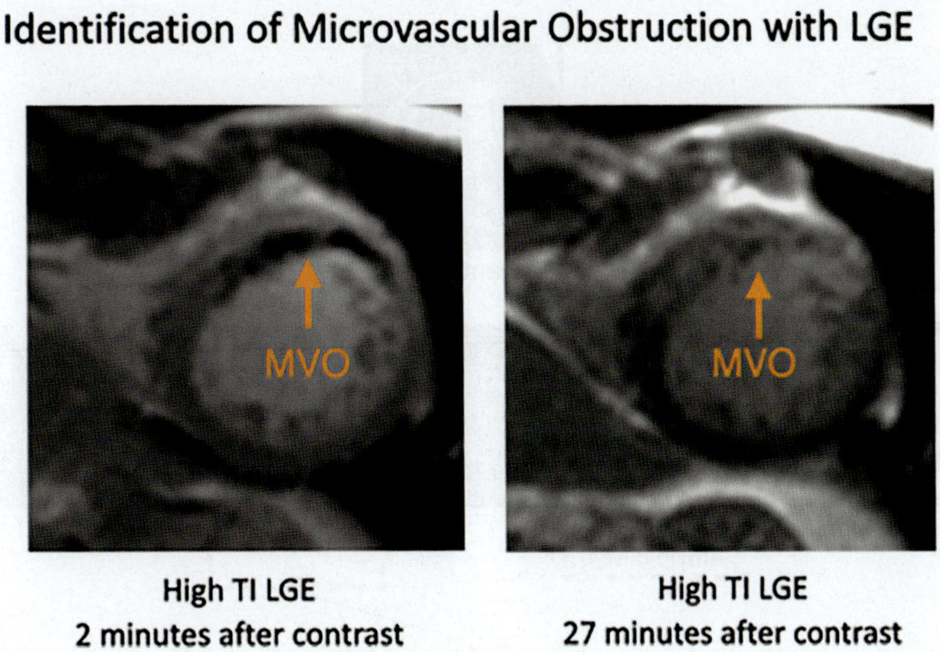

FIG. 13.16 High inversion time (*TI*) late gadolinium enhancement (*LGE*) imaging of microvascular obstruction (*MVO*). Early after contrast administration, the central core of an infarct with MVO (left) appears black on high TI LGE. MVO (right) can be differentiated from thrombus by repeat imaging using the same sequence toward the end of examination. Unlike thrombus, infarcts with MVO will eventually exhibit contrast enhancement.

the MT parameters values are not typically changed (Table 13.5). Analogous to conventional bright-blood LGE, however, we do manually adjust the FIDDLE TI (Fig. 13.18). We train the operators to pick a nominal TI (typically ~200 ms), and then based upon the image intensity of the blood pool, make an adjustment: if the blood pool is not black, the TI needs to be reduced, whereas, if the blood pool is black, then the TI should be increased to the maximum value that still results in black blood. Usually, one or two test images are sufficient to find the optimal TI. Importantly, operators should avoid setting a TI that is far too short, as this may result in reducing the difference in image intensity between

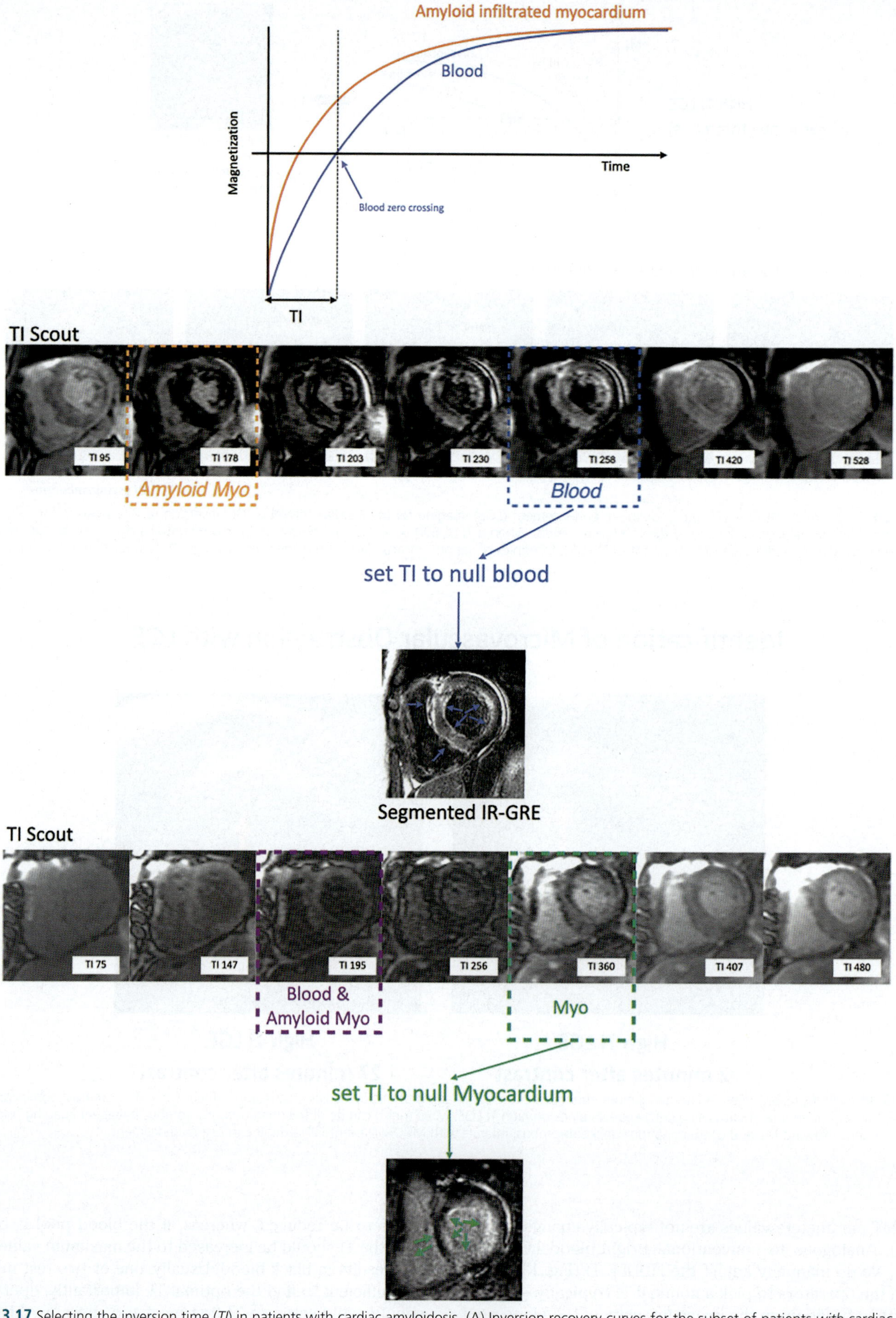

FIG. 13.17 Selecting the inversion time (*TI*) in patients with cardiac amyloidosis. (A) Inversion recovery curves for the subset of patients *with* cardiac amyloidosis *with* altered gadolinium kinetics. (B) A TI scout can be used to identify the subset of patients *with* altered gadolinium kinetics and to aid in the selection of the initial TI selection to null blood for subsequent late gadolinium imaging. (C) A TI scout can also be used to identify the subset of patients *without* altered gadolinium kinetics. In this group, the TI is selected in the normal fashion.

TABLE 13.5 Typical parameters for flow-independent dark blood-delayed enhancement.

PARAMETER	1.5T	3.0T
FOV	300–380	300–380
In-plane voxel size	1.1–1.7 × 1.1–1.7 mm	1.1–1.7 × 1.1–1.7 mm
Matrix size	256 × 205	256 × 205
Slice thickness	7 mm	7 mm
Flip angle	55 degrees	44 degrees
Segments	41	62
Inversion time (TI)	Variable	Variable
Bandwidth	514 Hz/px	930 Hz/px
TE (echo time)	1.92 ms	1.47 ms
TR (repetition time)	3.84 ms	2.94 ms
Gating factor	2	2
K-space ordering	Linear	Linear
Fat sat	None	None
Asymmetric echo	Yes	Yes
Parallel imaging	2	2
MT pulses	19	19
MT flip angle	500 degrees	400 degrees
MT offset frequency	600 Hz	800 Hz

FOV, Field of view; *Hz,* Hertz; *Mm,* millimetre; *ms,* millisecond; *px,* pixel.

myocardium with LGE compared to without (Fig. 13.19). For advanced users who become highly proficient in setting the dark-blood TI, operators may also opt to obtain images with longer TIs than necessary to create the dark-blood condition. The latter will generate blood-suppressed images (rather than dark blood) that are more highly T1 weighted, generating greater image contrast between normal and enhanced myocardium (Fig. 13.18). In our experience, some types of nonischemic LGE can be more conspicuous with these longer inversion times.

CARDIOVASCULAR MAGNETIC RESONANCE IN PATIENTS WITH CARDIAC DEVICES

In recent years, it has become consensus that performing CMR in patients with cardiac devices is safe and can provide high diagnostic image quality. At our center, patients with implanted cardiac devices constitute >20% of the 1.5 T scanner volume, which continues to grow. We routinely perform CMR in patients with MRI-conditional devices as well as perform off-label scans in patients that have devices that are not considered to be MRI conditional.

In our experience, patients undergoing off-label scans usually fall into three broad categories (listed in order of relatively higher to lower risk).

(1) Patients with abandoned generators, nonfunctioning/capped leads, recalled leads, or fractured leads.
(2) Patients with systems that are functioning normally but are not labeled for MRI.
(3) Patients with generators that are considered MRI conditional, but the leads are unlabeled or were manufactured by a different vendor.

We have found that CMR can be performed safely in all the patients described above. It is our practice to have more extensive discussions regarding benefit versus risk, develop patient-specific device programming plans, and use higher levels of monitoring during the scan in higher risk patients.

When performing CMR, cardiac devices cause signal voids and off-resonance artifacts by disrupting the homogeneity of the magnetic field. The artifacts are particularly problematic when the device is large or in very close proximity to the heart. For example, with levocardia, left-sided devices are more problematic than right-sided devices. Similarly, artifacts are typically worse with left-sided devices in patients with short stature (as compared to tall stature) as the device is typically closer to the heart. The presence of these artifacts necessitates some alterations to the standard core examination in patients with cardiac devices.

We have found that these artifacts can be mitigated by a combination of changing the positioning of the arms and changing the breath-holding instructions. Prior to the scan, we position the patient's left arm (with levocardia and a left-sided device) above the head and subsequently perform the scan with the arm in this location. This maneuver moves the device a short distance toward the head. To improve tolerance to this positioning, the patient's raised arm is supported with pillows for comfort. Some patients may also need periodic breaks from this position during the scan due to shoulder fatigue or discomfort. During the scan, we acquire the images during inspiration (rather than relaxed expiration). With this maneuver, the heart descends a short distance toward the feet. The combination can significantly reduce artifacts for both SSFP (Fig. 13.19A) and GRE (Fig. 13.19B) if enough separation between the device and the heart can be created.

Additional changes to the standard core examination may be needed if artifacts persist despite the simple maneuvers described above. In our experience, SSFP cine images are usually not completely free of signal voids or off-resonance artifacts in patients with devices. However, in a subset, the artifacts may only affect regions of the image outside the heart and do not significantly impede the assessment of cardiac morphology and function, and we obtain most or all of the cine images using an SSFP readout. In patients with more substantial artifacts, we obtain cine images using a GRE readout. GRE cine imaging is more resistant to off-resonance artifacts, but it may be necessary to reduce the echo spacing (TE) by increasing the receiver bandwidth if signal voids remain large or overlay the heart (Fig. 13.20). It should be remembered, however, that this change comes at the cost of a reduced SNR. To compensate, SNR can be improved by increasing the slice thickness, the number of phase-encoding lines acquired (i.e., the FOV phase), or the number of averages.

For LGE, we typically use gradient echo readouts in most patients. Like with GRE cine imaging, signal voids may affect the visualization of the myocardium when the device is situated close to the heart. Since standard IR-GRE sequences used for LGE typically employ a low receiver bandwidth (Table 13.3. 130 Hz/pixel at 1.5 T), signal voids tend to be large. Thus, when scanning a patient

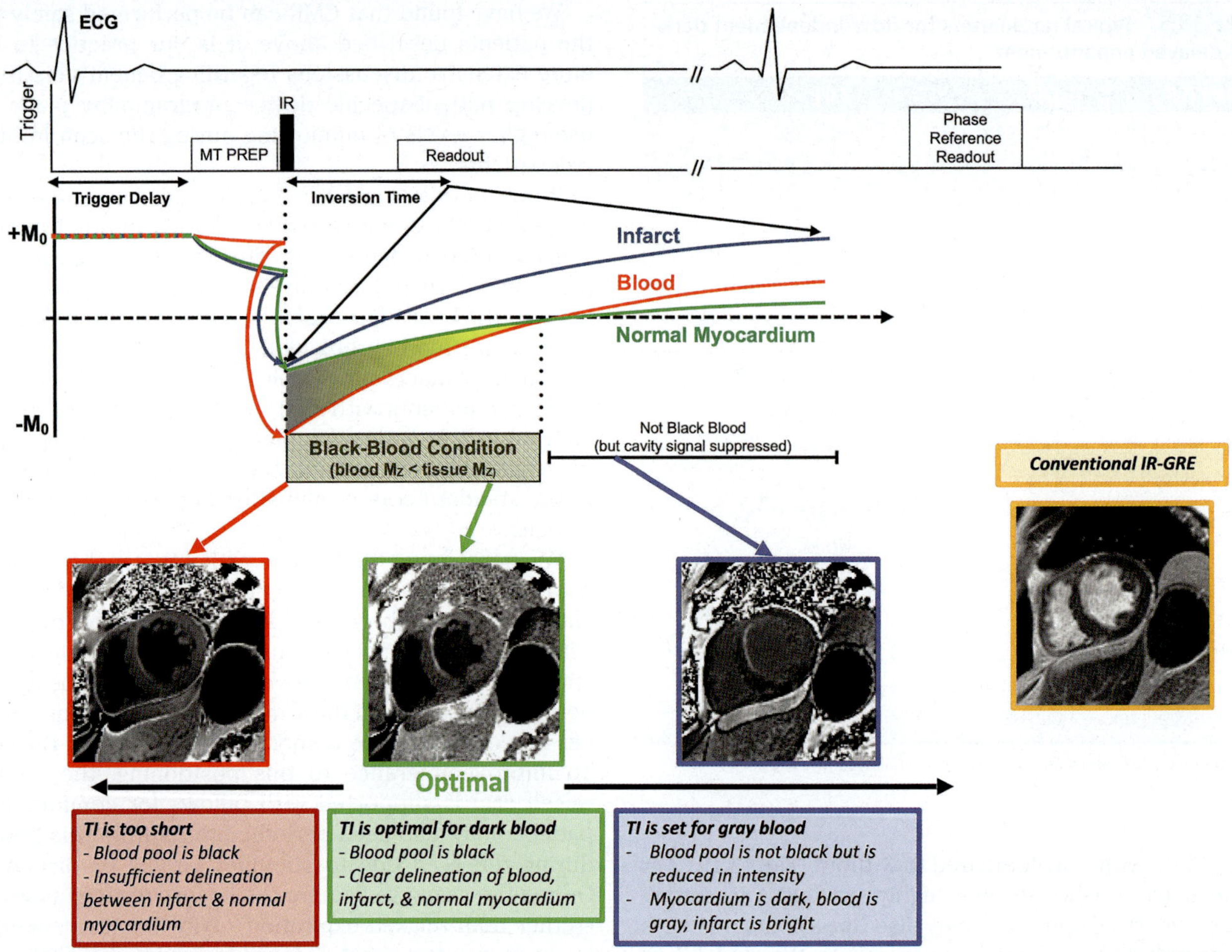

FIG. 13.18 TOP: Flow-independent dark blood-delayed enhancement pulse sequence timing diagram. The primary components are the: (1) preparatory module (magnetization transfer [*MT*] prep), (2) inversion recovery pulse, (3) phase-sensitive reconstruction, and (4) inversion time (*TI*), such that blood magnetization is less than tissue magnetization (black-blood condition). See text for details. BOTTOM: The adjustment of TI is based upon image appearance after the acquisition of the first test image using a nominal TI (e.g., ~200 ms). Operators can identify the optimal dark blood TI by identifying the maximum TI that results in a dark-blood image. *IR-GRE*, inversion recovery fast gradient echo.

with a device, we have changed our standard protocol by increasing the receiver bandwidth (300 Hz/pixel to start and adjusted higher if needed) and using the minimum possible TE to reduce the size of the signal void. Again, the SNR will be lower and changes are required to compensate (see above).

The second main source of artifacts for LGE comes from off-resonance effects. Although the GRE readout is relatively resistant, the standard IR preparation used for T1 weighting is susceptible to off-resonance effects from an implanted device. This is because a device near the heart leads to a wider distribution of resonance frequencies within the heart (~2000–6000 Hz when a device is present vs. 120 Hz when absent), which may exceed the spectral bandwidth of a standard inversion pulse (~1000 Hz).[18–20] Myocardium with resonance frequencies outside of the excitation bandwidth of the IR pulse are not inverted, thus creating an artifact that appears bright, irrespective of the presence of scar tissue (Fig. 13.21 left).

Fortunately, in recent years, wideband (broadband) inversion pulses have become increasingly available to address this problem. A wideband inversion preparation has a larger spectral bandwidth (~> 3000–4000 Hz) and is better able to tip down the full range of resonance frequencies within the heart when a device is present. Thus, normal myocardium can be uniformly nulled without the occurrence of bright artifacts due to this off-resonance effect (Fig. 13.21 right). As such, we employ wideband inversion pulses in patients with cardiac devices. It should be noted, however, that we do not use wideband inversions in all patients because they require more power (B1) than conventional inversion pulses and have a lower inversion efficiency.

SUMMARY

The core clinical examination is the basic building block for evaluation of cardiovascular disease by CMR. We describe the process for identifying the standard imaging planes and the standard protocols for cine and LGE imaging used at our center. We discuss sequence adjustments that can be applied to improve the imaging of challenging patients and how the protocols can be altered when imaging patients with cardiac devices.

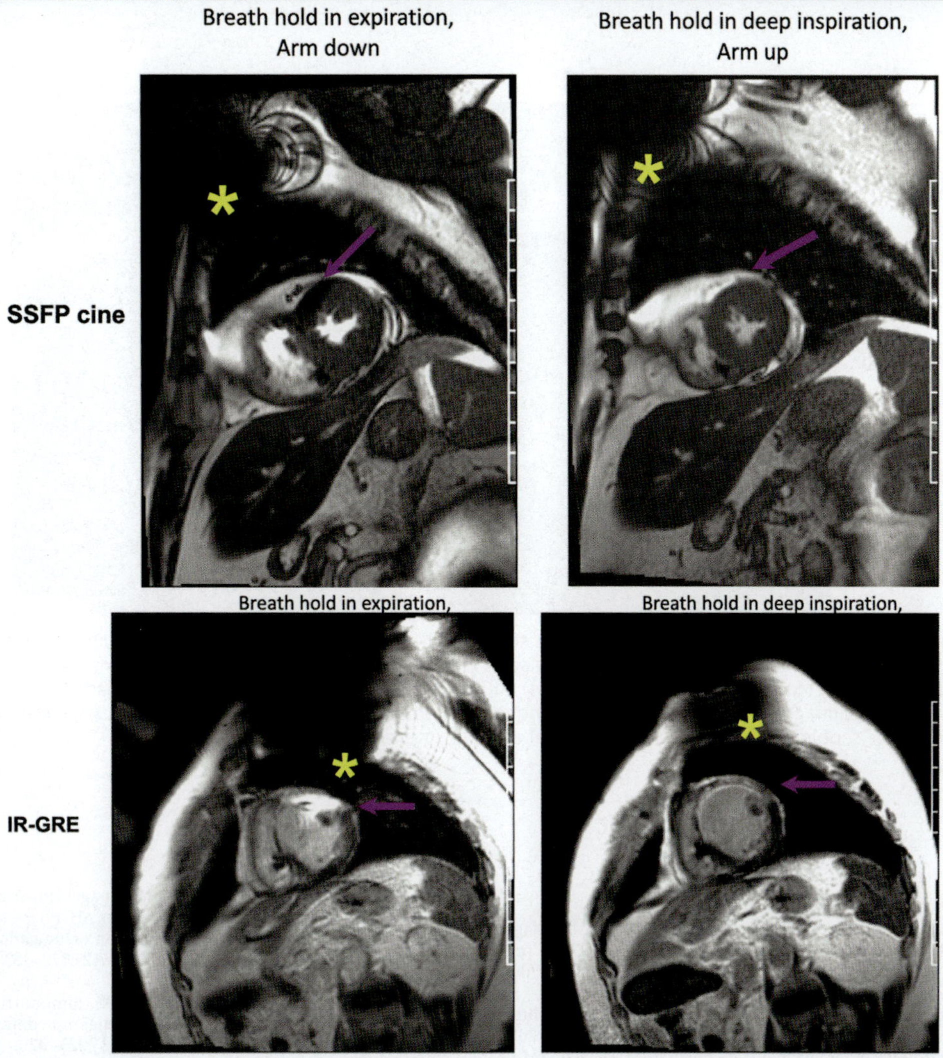

FIG. 13.19 Reducing device artifacts with changes to breath-holding phase and arm position. (A) LEFT: Steady-state free precession (SSFP) cine acquired during a breath-hold in expiration and arm down by the patient's side. An off-resonance artifact is seen overlying the anterior wall (*purple arrow*). RIGHT: SSFP cine acquired during a breath-hold in deep expiration and arm raised above the patient's head. The artifact is no longer present (*purple arrow*). (B) LEFT: Inversion recovery fast gradient echo (IR-GRE) acquired during a breath-hold in expiration and arm down by the patient's side. An off-resonance artifact is seen overlying the anterior wall (*purple arrow*). RIGHT: IR-GRE acquired during a breath-hold in deep expiration and arm raised above the patient's head. The artifact is no longer present (*purple arrow*). The yellow asterisks correspond to the signal void caused by the device located in the upper left chest.

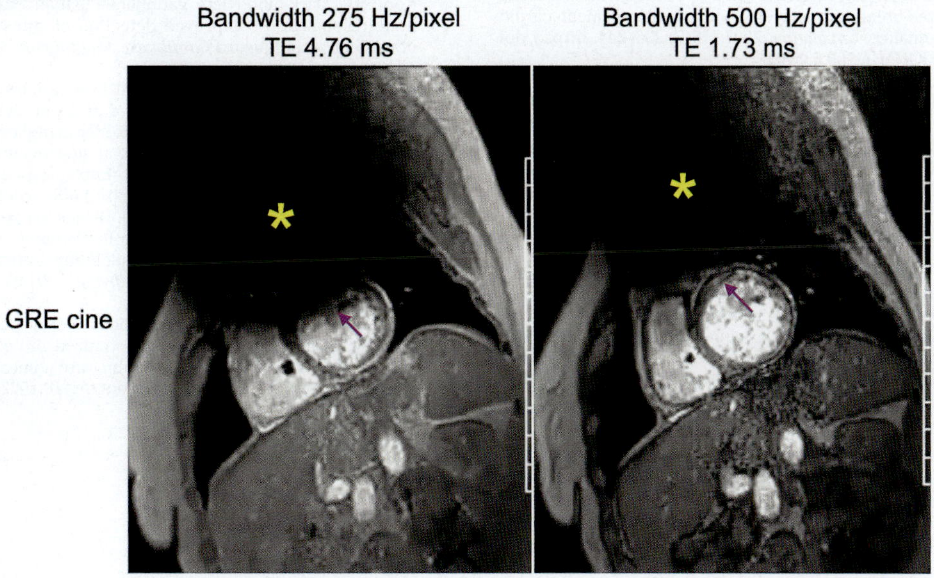

FIG. 13.20 The size of a signal void from a cardiac device can be reduced by increasing the receiver bandwidth (thereby reducing the echo spacing). With a bandwidth of 275 Hz/pixel and echo spacing (TE) of 4.75 msec (*LEFT*), the signal void (*yellow asterisk*) is large and obscures the anterior wall of the left ventricle. With a bandwidth of 500 Hz/pixel and echo spacing of 1.73 msec (*RIGHT*), the size of the signal void (*yellow asterisk*) is smaller and no longer affects the anterior wall of the left ventricle.

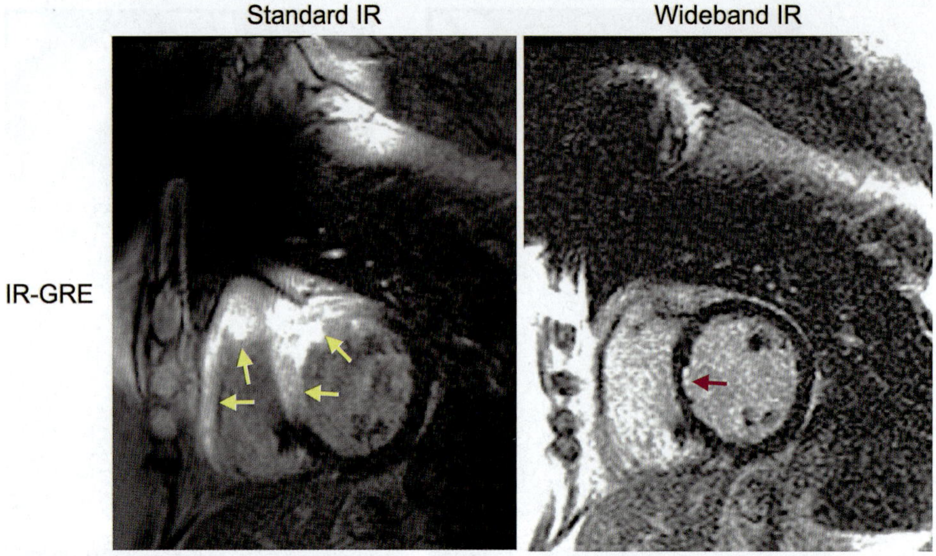

FIG. 13.21 LEFT: Late gadolinium enhancement (LGE) imaging with a standard inversion recovery (IR) preparation. Due to off-resonance effects from an implanted device, the standard IR preparation is not able to invert the spins in the septum, anterior wall of the left ventricle, right ventricle, and adjacent blood pool, leading to a bright artifact in these regions (*yellow arrows*). RIGHT: LGE imaging with a wideband IR preparation. The wideband preparation is able to tip down all the myocardium precessional frequencies, leading to a uniform inversion across the entire heart. As a result, a small subendocardial infarct could be visualized in the septum (*purple arrow*). *GRE*, Gradient echo; *IR*, inversion recovery.

REFERENCES

1. Kramer CM, Barkhausen J, Bucciarelli-Ducci C, Flamm SD, Kim RJ, Nagel E. Standardized cardiovascular magnetic resonance imaging (CMR) protocols: 2020 update. *J Cardiovasc Magn Reson*. 2020;22(1):17. https://doi.org/10.1186/s12968-020-00607-1.
2. Schulz-Menger J, Bluemke DA, Bremerich J, et al. Standardized image interpretation and post-processing in cardiovascular magnetic resonance - 2020 update: society for cardiovascular magnetic resonance (SCMR): board of trustees task force on standardized post-processing. *J Cardiovasc Magn Reson*. 2020;22(1):19. https://doi.org/10.1186/s12968-020-00610-6.
3. Kim RJ, Albert TS, Wible JH, et al. Performance of delayed-enhancement magnetic resonance imaging with gadoversetamide contrast for the detection and assessment of myocardial infarction: an international, multicenter, double-blinded, randomized trial. *Circulation*. 2008;117(5):629–637. https://doi.org/10.1161/CIRCULATIONAHA.107.723262.
4. The American College of Radiology. ACR Manual on Contrast Media Version 10.3 2018. Accessed May 24, 2019.
5. Sievers B, Elliott MD, Hurwitz LM, et al. Rapid detection of myocardial infarction by subsecond, free-breathing delayed contrast-enhancement cardiovascular magnetic resonance. *Circulation*. 2007;115(2):236–244. https://doi.org/10.1161/CIRCULATIONAHA.106.635409.
6. Kim HW, Rehwald WG, Jenista ER, et al. Dark-blood delayed enhancement cardiac magnetic resonance of myocardial infarction. *JACC Cardiovasc Imaging*. 2018;11(12):1758–1769. https://doi.org/10.1016/j.jcmg.2017.09.021.
7. Kellman P, Larson AC, Hsu LY, et al. Motion-corrected free-breathing delayed enhancement imaging of myocardial infarction. *Magn Reson Med*. 2005;53(1):194–200. https://doi.org/10.1002/mrm.20333.
8. Kim RJ, Shah DJ, Judd RM. How we perform delayed enhancement imaging. *J Cardiovasc Magn Reson*. 2003;5(3):505–514. https://doi.org/10.1081/jcmr-120022267.
9. Simonetti OP, Kim RJ, Fieno DS, et al. An improved MR imaging technique for the visualization of myocardial infarction. *Radiology*. 2001;218(1):215–223. https://doi.org/10.1148/radiology.218.1.r01ja50215.
10. Li W, Li BS, Polzin JA, Mai VM, Prasad PV, Edelman RR. Myocardial delayed enhancement imaging using inversion recovery single-shot steady-state free precession: initial experience. *J Magn Reson Imaging*. 2004;20(2):327–330. https://doi.org/10.1002/jmri.20095.
11. https://scmr.org/general/custom.asp?page=HowIDo).
12. Kellman P, Arai AE, McVeigh ER, Aletras AH. Phase-sensitive inversion recovery for detecting myocardial infarction using gadolinium-delayed hyperenhancement. *Magn Reson Med*. 2002;47(2):372–383. https://doi.org/10.1002/mrm.10051.
13. Gupta A, Lee VS, Chung YC, Babb JS, Simonetti OP. Myocardial infarction: optimization of inversion times at delayed contrast-enhanced MR imaging. *Radiology*. 2004;233(3):921–926. https://doi.org/10.1148/radiol.2333032004.
14. Weinsaft JW, Kim HW, Shah DJ, et al. Detection of left ventricular thrombus by delayed-enhancement cardiovascular magnetic resonance prevalence and markers in patients with systolic dysfunction. *J Am Coll Cardiol*. 2008;52(2):148–157. https://doi.org/10.1016/j.jacc.2008.03.041.
15. White JA, Kim HW, Shah D, et al. CMR imaging with rapid visual T1 assessment predicts mortality in patients suspected of cardiac amyloidosis. *JACC Cardiovasc Imaging*. 2014;7(2):143–156. https://doi.org/10.1016/j.jcmg.2013.09.019.
16. Holtackers RJ, Van De Heyning CM, Chiribiri A, Wildberger JE, Botnar RM, Kooi ME. Dark-blood late gadolinium enhancement cardiovascular magnetic resonance for improved detection of subendocardial scar: a review of current techniques. *J Cardiovasc Magn Reson*. 2021;23(1):96. https://doi.org/10.1186/s12968-021-00777-6.
17. Jenista ER, Wendell DC, Kim HW, et al. Comparison of magnetization transfer-preparation and T2-preparation for dark-blood delayed-enhancement imaging. *NMR Biomed*. 2020;33(11):e4396. https://doi.org/10.1002/nbm.4396.
18. Rashid S, Rapacchi S, Vaseghi M, et al. Improved late gadolinium enhancement MR imaging for patients with implanted cardiac devices. *Radiology*. 2014;270(1):269–274. https://doi.org/10.1148/radiol.13130942.
19. Stevens SM, Tung R, Rashid S, et al. Device artifact reduction for magnetic resonance imaging of patients with implantable cardioverter-defibrillators and ventricular tachycardia: late gadolinium enhancement correlation with electroanatomic mapping. *Heart Rhythm*. 2014;11(2):289–298. https://doi.org/10.1016/j.hrthm.2013.10.032.
20. Azevedo CF, Jenista ER, Kaolawanich Y, et al. Assessment of myocardial lipomatous metaplasia using an optimized out-of-phase cine steady-state free-precession sequence: Validation and clinical implementation. *NMR Biomed*. 2022;35(10):e4777. https://doi.org/10.1002/nbm.4777.

14 Scan Reporting and Registries

ROBERT M. JUDD AND ORLANDO P. SIMONETTI

INTRODUCTION

The physician-signed final cardiovascular magnetic resonance (CMR) report is the primary mechanism for communicating the results of an examination to the referring physician and their patient. As such, the CMR report is one of the most important aspects of the entire imaging procedure. Over the past two decades, the distribution of CMR reports has evolved from paper-based facsimile (fax) machines to hospital-wide electronic health record (EHR) systems. More recently, direct patient access to CMR reports via web browser portals has become increasingly common. In this chapter, we discuss the current state of the art of CMR reporting systems (Part I) and the large-scale aggregation of deidentified CMR reporting system data across healthcare providers for secondary purposes including quality control, education, and research (Part II).

PART I—REPORTING

The Society for Cardiovascular Magnetic Resonance (SCMR)[1] is the principal international, independent organization committed to the further development of CMR through education, quality assurance, research, and training, and plays an important role in defining the organization and content to be used for CMR reporting. For example, a recent SCMR guidance document[2] recommends that the CMR report contains specific data elements including site and equipment (e.g., hospital-based 1.5 T scanner), patient demographics (e.g., sex, age), indications for the study (e.g., chest pain, shortness of breath), and study performance (cines, stress perfusion, late gadolinium enhancement [LGE]). These CMR report sections typically appear near the beginning of the report, followed by the results of image postprocessing and the interpretation of the images and quantification results by the reading physician. An example of a typical user interface for CMR reporting is shown in Fig. 14.1.

The SCMR has published comprehensive guidance documents for both CMR image acquisition and subsequent postprocessing.[3,4] Protocols for image acquisition vary depending on the clinical question, and therefore the contents of the report will also vary. For example, evaluation of a patient with congenital heart disease may include sequences for heart and vascular structure, cardiac function, and flow quantification, while a protocol for evaluation of myocarditis could also add tissue characterization techniques including LGE, T1-mapping, and T2-mapping. A protocol designed for evaluation of ischemic heart disease would also likely include stress first-pass perfusion imaging; therefore, the particular indication will drive the contents of the CMR report. Nevertheless, virtually all reports should arguably include results of quantitative analysis of left ventricular (LV) and right ventricular (RV) structure and function based on cine CMR. An example format for reporting ventricular volumetric analyses is shown in Fig. 14.2. End-diastolic and end-systolic chamber volumes (EDV and ESV, respectively) are typically derived from a stack of six to eight short-axis cine images spaced 10 mm apart, where the endocardial borders have been defined either by manual or semiautomatic tracing of regions of interest (ROIs). The EDV and ESV ROIs are used to calculate stroke volume (SV), ejection fraction (EF), and cardiac output (CO). LV myocardial mass is also often reported, and requires additional ROIs for the epicardial borders. Most of these data elements can be reported as raw values or normalized to the patient's body surface area (BSA) in m^2. For many of these values, normal ranges have been published in the literature[5,6] and can be highlighted in red for those that lie outside the normal range (values within parentheses in Fig. 14.2). All of these quantitative values can easily be stored as structured data in a structured query language (SQL) database for later aggregation across patients (further detail below).

An important tool for CMR reporting is the 17-segment model or "bullseye plot," which is also widely used by other cardiac imaging modalities including echocardiography, nuclear cardiology, and cardiac computed tomography (CCT) to easily indicate the location of any abnormalities. CMR reporting systems typically include 17-segment model scores for wall motion, LGE, and stress perfusion, allowing for straightforward evaluation of the relationships between these metrics. For wall motion, a scale of 0–4 is typically used in a manner identical to echocardiography (0 is normal, 4 is dyskinetic). For LGE, a 0–4 scoring system is used, for which the value reflects the spatial extent of hyperenhancement (0 is none, 4 is 75%–100% of the surface area of that segment). The intramural distribution (e.g., subendocardial vs. midmyocardial) and pattern of LGE (e.g., focal vs. diffuse) can also be specified, and the specific pattern is indicative of an ischemic or nonischemic disease process. Similarly, the segmental scores for stress perfusion defects increase with increasing severity of the defect (0 is none, 4 is fully transmural defect). As for the volumetric data in Fig. 14.2, all of the 17-segment scores can easily be stored as structured data in an SQL database for later aggregation across patients.

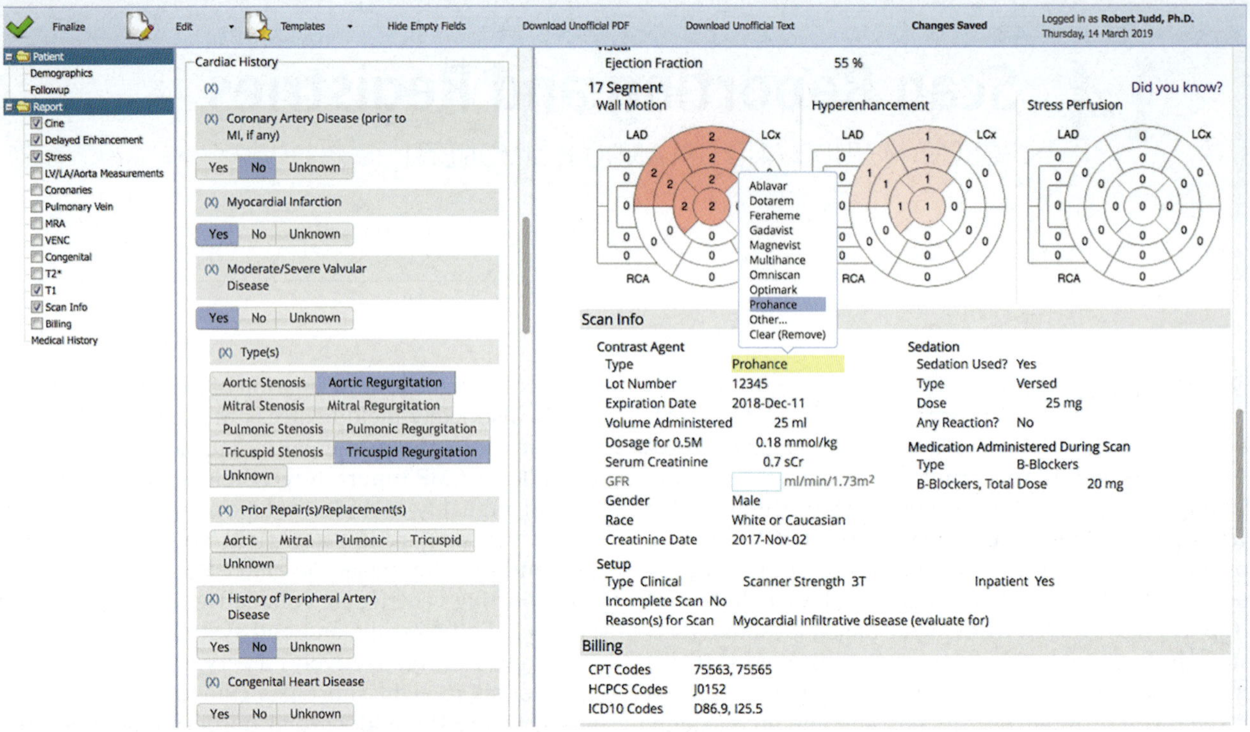

FIG. 14.1 Example of a user interface for a cardiovascular magnetic resonance reporting system.

		LV	(Reference)	RV	(Reference)
EDV	[ml]	245	(117-200)	284	(116-216)
	[ml/m²]	95	(64-99)	109	(62-108)
ESV	[ml]	122	(31-76)	159	(29-89)
	[ml/m²]	47	(17-38)	61	(16-45)
CO	[L/min]	7.99	(--)	8.17	(--)
	[L/min/m²]	3.08	(--)	3.14	(--)
MASS	[g]	80	(108-185)		(--)
	[g/m²]	31	(58-91)		(--)
SV	[ml]	123	(77-133)	126	(73-141)
	[ml/m²]	47	(42-66)	48	(39-71)
EF	[%]	50	(58-75)	44	(52-77)
Cardiac Output HR		65 BPM			

FIG. 14.2 Example of a table of cardiovascular magnetic resonance volumetric data. *CO*, Cardiac output; *EDV*, end diastolic volume; *EF*, ejection fraction; *ESV*, end systolic volume; *LV*, left ventricle; *RV*, right ventricle; *SV*, stroke volume.

Perhaps the most important aspect of the CMR report is the concluding statements that synthesize the results into a comprehensive diagnosis in a section typically labeled "Summary," "Conclusions," or "Final Impression." These concluding statements are typically typed or dictated into the user interface by the signing physician, and are intended to provide guidance for referring physicians planning patient treatments and interventions. Because these are entered manually as free text, these sections are somewhat less useful for aggregation across patients because they are not fully structured data. They can be searched for keywords, however, and are increasingly being used as training and testing data for exploratory artificial intelligence (AI) research projects. Preferably, CMR reports should also contain a discussion of prior studies, if applicable, in which the current results are compared to previous CMR examinations of the same patient.

The use of **structured data** is of fundamental importance to computerized storage of CMR reports. As opposed to unstructured data, structured CMR report data can be easily aggregated across all patients within a single health system and, with careful attention paid to patient privacy issues, across health systems on a national and international scale. Aggregation of CMR report data across patients and health systems greatly facilitates advancement of the field of CMR by providing insight into the practice of CMR across the world.

Dictation of CMR reports is an example of unstructured data. The resulting free text typically has no fixed format across patients for a single reading physician, no fixed format across physicians within a single health care organization, and no fixed format across healthcare organizations. The resulting volume of unstructured free text data is difficult to aggregate across providers. For example, performing a keyword search across thousands of dictated CMR reports in order to identify patients with myocarditis would include voluminous free text phrases with disparate meanings such as "patient has myocarditis," "patient has no evidence of myocarditis," "patient does not appear to have myocarditis," "myocarditis is present," "suspected myocarditis," or "rule out myocarditis." Accordingly, the use of unstructured data for CMR reporting systems effectively precludes automated aggregation of CMR data for quality control, education, and research purposes.

Conversely, entering and storing CMR report data in a structured format greatly facilitates aggregation across patients. For example, presenting physicians with a radio button list of contrast agent types for which only one

```
MariaDB> SELECT COUNT(*)
FROM cmr_reports
WHERE wall_motion > 2
AND lge > 0
AND contrast_agent='gadoteridol';

+----------+
| count(*) |
+----------+
|    69227 |
+----------+
1 row in set (0.63 sec)
```

FIG. 14.3 Example of a structured query language database query.

can be selected would represent collection of structured data. A *name-value* data structure might be defined as "name = contrast_agent" and "values = {Gadavist;Omniscan;Prohance}." Using this *name-value* structured data approach, the contrast agent cannot be inadvertently identified by its chemical name rather than its trade name, the name cannot be misspelled, and the values can easily be found programmatically by searching the underlying database for "name = contrast_agent." Fig. 14.1 shows an example of a CMR reporting system that uses structured data collection for contrast agent, ejection fraction, 17-segment scores, current procedural terminology (CPT) codes, and many other parameters. Structured data can be easily and conveniently stored as *name-value* pairs in an underlying database using SQL, such as MySQL or PostgreSQL. Fig. 14.3 shows how an SQL database can be easily searched for matching CMR reports.

Guidance documents such as those of the SCMR[2–4] are of great value in standardizing the content of CMR reports across healthcare providers. A major limitation of the current state of the art, however, is the lack of standards for specific data names and values that are to be used to define the row/column table schema of the underlying SQL database. For example, while the SCMR recommends identification of the contrast agent used during the CMR examination, there is no guidance regarding whether the associated data element name should be "contrast_agent," "contrast_type," "contrast_agent_type," or "agent_type." There is also no guidance on the specific values to offer the physician in the reporting system user interface (e.g., Gadavist;Omniscan;Prohance). A direct consequence of this lack of database-level specificity in the guidance documents means that commercial vendors of CMR reporting systems, of which there are dozens, use their own proprietary names and values within their underlying database schema. This variability of database schemas across reporting system vendors is a major impediment to data aggregation. While theoretically it is possible to create lookup tables that cross-reference vendor A's "contrast_agent" with vendor B's "contrast_type," the number of data name/value pairs within a typical CMR reporting system, the number of CMR reporting system vendors, and the ongoing introduction of new name/value data elements make lookup table creation and maintenance practically impossible.

> Chapter author opinion: The Society for Cardiovascular Magnetic Resonance (SCMR) should publish an additional guidance document that defines the underlying structured query language database schema in order to standardize cross-vendor storage of the existing SCMR-recommended data elements.

Once the authoring physician is satisfied with the contents of the CMR report, an electronic signature is typically used as the trigger for the CMR reporting system to transmit the final report to the hospital EHR for access by referring physicians and patients. This data transmission is typically achieved via Health Level Seven (HL7) computerized messaging. While the format and specifications of HL7 messages are beyond the scope of this chapter, it is useful for physicians to be aware that HL7 and its associated CMR report display systems often have significant practical limitations. For example, at some hospitals CMR reports can be sent to EHR systems as a PDF file, but it is not uncommon that PDF-formatted CMR reports cannot be accepted by the EHR. There are various reasons why PDF files cannot be accepted, including lack of EHR infrastructure to store PDF data and the use of intermediate "broker" systems that cannot pass PDF data from CMR reporting systems to EHRs. As a consequence, a significant percentage of hospital EHRs currently require that CMR reports be sent as a "block of text." The underlying concept is that the CMR report data must be formatted as if it were typed on a 20th century style typewriter, meaning no mechanism to display colors, graphs, images, italics, and other formatting elements that greatly improve the communicative value of CMR reports. Fig. 14.4 shows an example of three common display formats used by hospital EHRs. Panel A (PDF) is arguably ideal, but requires that the EHR accept PDF format. Panel B (fixed font) might be acceptable, but is more difficult for referring physicians to quickly recognize. Panel C (proportional font) is difficult to read and visually unattractive. The current state of the art is that roughly half of EHR systems in the United States cannot display the format of panel A (PDF) and use the format of Panel B instead (fixed font). This means no CMR images can be embedded into EHR reports; tables must be used for wall motion, LGE, and perfusion scores; and no italics or bold face type can be used. As a consequence, the state of the art for communication of CMR results is suboptimal at a significant number of healthcare providers, and undoubtedly has a small but finite negative effect on patient care.

> Chapter author opinion: All electronic health record systems should display cardiovascular magnetic resonance reports in PDF format.

Following transmission of the report to the EHR, most CMR reporting systems allow physicians to amend and/or addend the reports with an additional electronic signature. While the options and goals of modifying finalized CMR reports varies somewhat amongst healthcare providers, the main goal is to ensure that referring physicians see the most current results. Amended reports typically replace the original report in the EHR, and are displayed by default as soon as they are received. In some EHRs, the original report can be accessed with additional mouse clicks, but more commonly only the latest report version is available. Addended reports typically preserve the entire contents of the original report, but additionally display a block of text near the top of the report allowing the signing physician to draw the referring physician's attention to a corrected finding.

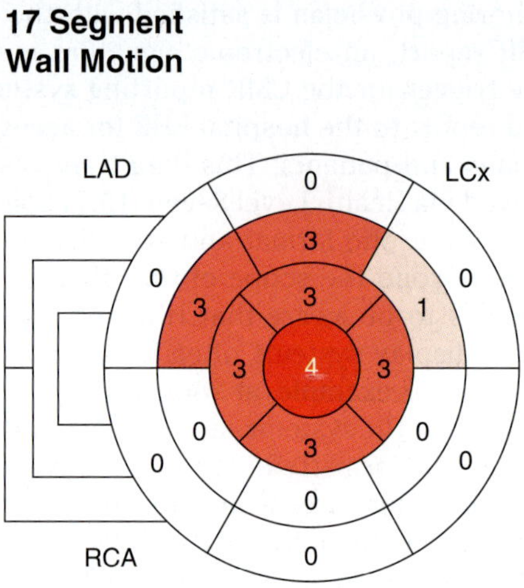

A

17 SEGMENT

Segments	Wall Motion
Base Anterior	Normal/Hyper
Base Anteroseptal	Normal/Hyper
Base Inferoseptal	Normal/Hyper
Base Inferior	Normal/Hyper
Base Inferolateral	Normal/Hyper
Base Anterolateral	Normal/Hyper
Mid Anterior	Akinetic
Mid Anteroseptal	Akinetic
Mid Inferoseptal	Normal/Hyper
Mid Inferior	Normal/Hyper
Mid Inferolateral	Normal/Hyper
Mid Anterolateral	Mild/Mod Hypo
Apical Anterior	Akinetic
Apical Septal	Akinetic
Apical Inferior	Akinetic
Apical Lateral	Akinetic
Apex	Dyskinetic

B

17 SEGMENT

Segments	Wall Motion
Base Anterior	Normal/Hyper
Base Anteroseptal	Normal/Hyper
Base Inferoseptal	Normal/Hyper
Base Inferior	Normal/Hyper
Base Inferolateral	Normal/Hyper
Base Anterolateral	Normal/Hyper
Mid Anterior	Akinetic
Mid Anteroseptal	Akinetic
Mid Inferoseptal	Normal/Hyper
Mid Inferior	Normal/Hyper
Mid Inferolateral	Normal/Hyper
Mid Anterolateral	Mild/Mod Hypo
Apical Anterior	Akinetic
Apical Septal	Akinetic
Apical Inferior	Akinetic
Apical Lateral	Akinetic
Apex	Dyskinetic

C

FIG. 14.4 Common electronic health record formats for display of identical 17-segment scores. (A) Graphical. (B) Fixed-font table. (C) Proportional-font table.

In addition to the use of structured data within the CMR report, another important concept of CMR reporting systems is the use of **unique identifiers**. In the United States, the use of social security numbers as unique identifiers for patients effectively disappeared in the early 21st century due to patient privacy concerns. Today, virtually every US hospital uses the patient medical record number (MRN) to uniquely identify patients, and each hospital maintains its own MRN pool. This means that combining CMR report data from the same patient across two different hospitals is intentionally impossible without some additional form of cross-referencing information. In addition, it is not uncommon for one healthcare provider to merge with or acquire another healthcare provider, in which case the differing MRN pools causes major problems when combining EHR systems if/when the MRN pools collide (two patients have the same MRN). Fortunately, with the exception of patient identifiers, the state of the art is such that widely accepted unique identifiers already exist for most if not all other data elements relevant to CMR reporting, including image pixel datasets (DICOM Study Instance ID), healthcare provider (National Provider Identifier), CMR reports (order ID or accession number), and billing codes (Common Procedure Code and International Classification of Diseases).

A final concept of comparable importance to structured data and unique identifiers is that of a **single source of truth** (SST), referring to the problem of the same piece of information being stored in two different computing systems for which the values may differ. For example, an imaging technician or nurse may populate patient history in the CMR reporting system (smoking, diabetes, high blood pressure, medications, etc.), but these same data elements are often already populated in the EHR, and there is no mechanism to ensure the values are synchronized across the two systems (CMR reporting database vs. EHR database). A better system design would be to designate the EHR as the SST and programmatically send updates to the CMR reporting system, or vice versa. Fortunately, the current state of the art now provides a mechanism for data transfers necessary for SST, namely the Fast Healthcare Interoperability Resources (FHIR) standard defined as an extension to the HL7 standard.[7] Currently, however, few if any CMR reporting systems incorporate FHIR to the extent needed for a single source of truth to exist even within a single healthcare provider.

> Chapter author opinion: All cardiovascular magnetic resonance reporting systems should use Fast Healthcare Interoperability Resources to synchronize database values with the hospital electronic health records whenever identical data elements exist on both systems.

While largely beyond the scope of this chapter, physicians should also be aware that software change control policies represent a necessary but burdensome aspect of improved CMR reporting systems. Most CMR reporting systems incorporate quantitative image postprocessing tools, and are therefore considered class II medical devices under federal laws. As a consequence, their underlying software is subject to initial regulatory 510(k) clearance followed by annual auditing by the US Food and Drug Administration (FDA) and/or comparable regulatory bodies in other countries. An important strength of these regulations is that medical errors secondary to software defects are minimized, but the burden and expense of compliance significantly slows the introduction of new and improved CMR reporting systems. Interestingly, unlike CMR reporting systems, most EHR systems are not considered to be a "medical device" under federal laws, apparently because they only exchange medical records and do not provide quantitative measurements on medical images. As a consequence, the current state of the art is such that CMR reporting systems are subject to software regulatory requirements that far exceed those of the hospital EHR systems that they subserve.

PART II - REGISTRIES

As discussed in Part I of this chapter, the use of structured data for CMR reporting systems greatly facilitates aggregation of data across patients and healthcare providers on a national and international scale. These aggregated data have many uses, including quality control, education, training, and research. Data aggregation is often organized into registries, where multiple healthcare providers contribute data to a single aggregated database for subsequent analyses.

A key requirement for a multicenter data registry is **deidentification** of patient data. Many registries satisfy this requirement by allowing participating sites to enter data into a secure website, in which case the patient identifier within that website is something unrelated to the patient's actual identity, such as "Patient 1," "Patient 2," etc. This approach works well at the moment of data entry, but if the site wants to update the registry data months or years later to add follow-up data or CMR report data for a subsequent imaging examination, it becomes necessary to know the true identity of "Patient 1," for example "William Jones." Storing this information within the registry itself defeats the goal of storing only deidentified data, but the participating site could maintain a local lookup table, unavailable to the registry, that lists "Patient 1" as being "William Jones." This approach is currently the most common method of patient deidentification in multicenter registries.

Deidentification becomes more complicated if DICOM image datasets are to be included in the registry. DICOM files contain metadata, stored as DICOM tags, that include detailed information related to patient identity including patient name, date of birth, medical record number, address, mother's maiden name, institution name, referring physician's name, and many others. In addition, Health Insurance Portability and Accountability Act (HIPAA) regulations specifically state that the date of the CMR examination must be removed, which is difficult because the DICOM tags are filled with dozens of dates including study date, series date, acquisition date, overlay date, etc. Moreover, postprocessed images known as DICOM "secondary captures" often contain patient identifiers burned directly into the image pixel data, independent of the DICOM tags, which is even more difficult to programmatically remove. Despite these complexities, automated deidentification of DICOM files is possible provided that software developers sufficiently address these issues.

The American College of Cardiology has organized the National Cardiovascular Data Registry (NCDR),[8] which is a suite of cardiovascular data registries helping hospitals and private practices measure and improve the quality of care they provide. The NCDR does not include a registry for CMR data, however. In the remainder of this chapter, we will focus on registries specifically designed to capture CMR data.

In the first decade of the 21st century the European Cardiovascular Magnetic Resonance (EuroCMR) organization created a multicenter registry to evaluate indications, image quality, safety, and impact on patient management with routine CMR. The EuroCMR Registry used a single website for data collection, allowing each participating healthcare provider to log into the website and enter data by hand. The website was intentionally designed to collect structured data for the reasons described in this chapter. In 2013, the results of data collection from 57 centers in 15 countries were published, representing more than 27,000 consecutive patients.[9] The EuroCMR Registry succeeded in demonstrating the power of aggregated CMR report data for research purposes, with a number of publications based on its multicenter data.[10,11] Of note, the EuroCMR Registry did not require submission of the raw image pixel data (DICOM) but rather primarily collected descriptive and interpretative data similar to that of routine clinical reports.

In the second decade of the 21st century, the SCMR created the Global Cardiovascular Magnetic Resonance (GCMR) Registry.[12] The technical and organizational structure of the GCMR was similar to that of the EuroCMR Registry, meaning data were entered by hand into a single secure website by each participating site, although aggregated data from some sites could be imported programmatically in batches, depending on the underlying CMR reporting system being used at each site; no image data were included. The GCMR Registry resulted in a number of high-quality publications in the literature, and the data were used in part to support FDA clearance of the first cardiac indication for a gadolinium-based contrast agent.

In 2019, the SCMR revised the technical and organizational infrastructure for the SCMR Registry, and that infrastructure remains in use currently. The remainder of this chapter discusses the organization of the current SCMR Registry.[13]

The currently stated overall goals of the SCMR Registry are:

- To promote evidence-based utilization of CMR through a collaborative global effort.
- To provide a web mechanism for CMR centers to upload deidentified patient data, CMR indications, and images that incorporates state-of-the-art data security and privacy standards.
- To provide a mechanism to automatically track patient outcomes (e.g., death, events).
- To support global access to registry data to the wider CMR research community.

The overall organization of the SCMR Registry is depicted in Fig. 14.5. An automated approach is used for data collection. Each participating site has software physically located on computer servers inside the internet firewall of their hospital (local system). These local systems are used clinically to author CMR reports, and the associated structured data are stored in a local SQL database. Each night at 01:00 am local time, software within the local system deidentifies the SQL data and transmits the CMR data to the SCMR Registry (cloud system). Importantly, the raw DICOM files are also deidentified locally and transmitted to the SCMR Registry. No patient identifiers leave the local system, ensuring that the cloud data cannot be used to learn a patient's true identity. Security policies are regularly audited by a registrar—BSI—to certify compliance to the ISO 27001:2013 standard, and are also SOC 2 type II certified. SOC 2 is an industry standard that provides detailed information and assurance about the controls at a service organization relevant to security, availability, and processing integrity of the systems used to process users' data, and the confidentiality and privacy of the information processed by these systems.

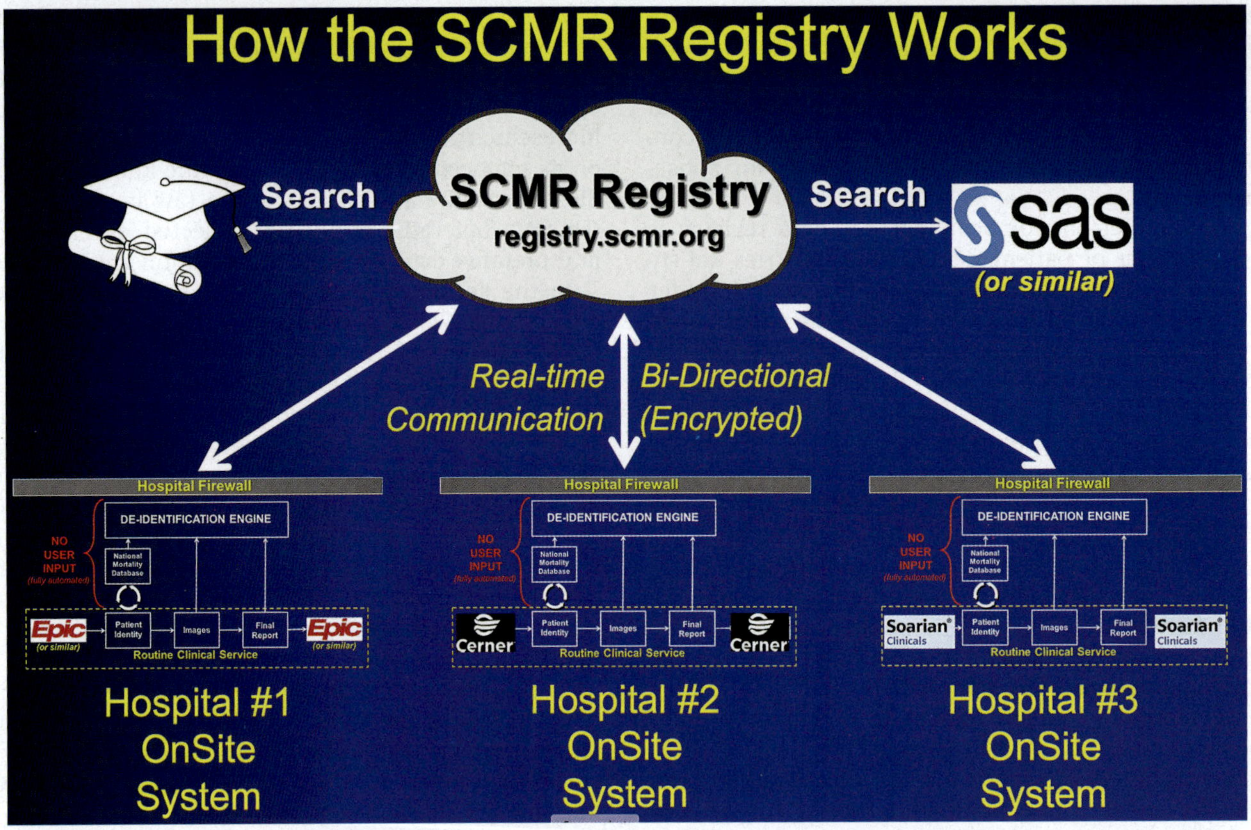

FIG. 14.5 Overview of Society for Cardiovascular Magnetic Resonance Registry.

In order to join the SCMR as a site, the SCMR Registry Participation Agreement document governing the submission and utilization of data is signed as a legal agreement by both the SCMR and the participating site. The Registry is designed in such a manner that submission of deidentified data is not considered "human subjects research" in the United States according to Health and Human Services guidelines,[14] although the local Insitutional Review Board (IRB) typically makes this determination. Contribution of data outside of the United States must be compliant with local institutional and national privacy laws. A data security review is generally required, which is performed by the local IT department. Once these tasks are completed, specialized software is installed on the site's local system in order to autonomously extract, deidentify, and upload both images and report data to the Registry from the existing picture archiving and communication system (PACS) and CMR reporting systems.

Local systems (hospital #2, etc., in Fig. 14.5) solve the problem of DICOM dates by shifting all dates by a random number of days. Importantly, local systems shift all dates within the same patient by the same (random) number of days. This means that the number of days between the patient's date of birth and the date of a CMR scan remains accurate because both underwent the same shift, yet neither date can be used to determine the patient's identity because the date shift is random.

Local systems solve the problem of associating multiple scans in the same patient by assigning a local identifier that is unique to each patient. For example, a patient with a hospital MRN of AB1234 would be internally assigned a deidentified MRN of 7023-9002-5515-4899. When the first CMR scan is transmitted to the SCMR Registry, the patient MRN in the deidentified dataset is set to 7023-9002-5515-4899. If the patient with MRN AB1234 returns for a second magnetic resonance imaging scan, the local software will assign the same deidentified MRN, namely 7023-9002-5515-4899, before transmission to the SCMR Registry. Upon receiving two scans with the same MRN (7023-9002-5515-4899), the SCMR Registry will correctly assign the two scans to the same cloud patient. Note that because local systems shift all dates within the same patient by the same (random) number of days, the relative time between the two scans will remain exactly correct within the SCMR Registry, even though neither date represents the actual date the patient was scanned.

One of the most innovative features of the SCMR Registry concerns ownership of Registry data. Rather than transferring ownership of the data from the site to the SCMR upon data submission, each participating site remains the legal owner of all data originating from that site even after the data physically leave their institution. This means that each slice of data within the overall pool of SCMR Registry data, stored in an Amazon Web Services data center, is owned by the participating sites rather than by the SCMR. Moreover, if/when the SCMR or another investigator wants to use Registry data for educational, research, or quality control projects, each site is asked for permission for use of their data on a project-by-project basis and can agree or decline to contribute their data. Using this approach, the sites remain in control of their own data even after data transmission outside their institution. This structure has supported the

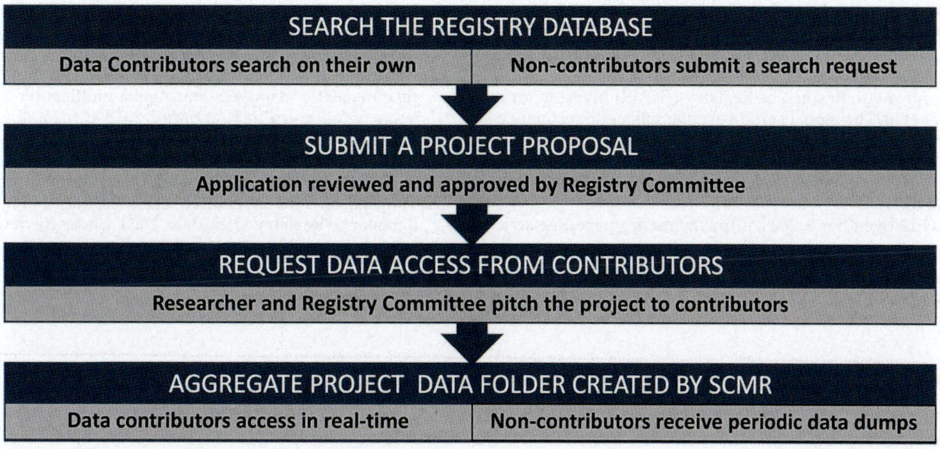

FIG. 14.6 Society for Cardiovascular Magnetic Resonance Registry Steering Committee project proposal review process.

publication of a growing number of investigations utilizing large-scale, real-world data aggregated across multiple centers to demonstrate the value of CMR.[15,16]

All-cause patient mortality is programmatically recorded based on information imported from local hospital EHR systems. Approximately once each year, individual sites provide a list of local patient MRNs corresponding to all patients that have undergone a CMR examination to their local hospital EHR data administrator, who subsequently returns a list of death dates to the local investigator. These death dates are programmatically imported into the local system, which then shifts the death date by the random date shift described above, and transmits this information to the SCMR Registry. Using this approach, large numbers of mortality events can be maintained within the Registry with minimal human effort. Additional patient follow-up data can also be added to the Registry, such as new myocardial infarction and interventions, but this information must be entered manually by local investigators.

The SCMR Registry is governed by a steering committee comprised of a chairperson and representatives of participating sites. The steering committee receives and reviews proposals for the use of SCMR Registry data for individual projects for a variety of purposes, including quality control, education, research, and training. The overall process of steering committee review of project proposals is depicted in Fig. 14.6.

As of November 2, 2023, there were 26 participating sites in the SCMR Registry that had collectively submitted 167,678 deidentified CMR final reports (SQL format), 322,052,200 deidentified CMR DICOM images (ca. 120 terabytes), and 457,276 patient-years of follow-up (all-cause mortality). Fig. 14.7 shows the growth of the SCMR Registry dataset over time.

A detailed description of the data available within the SCMR Registry appears in a recent publication by Tong et al.,[17] which provides a summary of the data held within the Registry when the number of datasets reached 150,000 (October 2022). The interested reader is encouraged to visit the SCMR website[12] and/or contact the SCMR Registry Steering Committee (contact information listed on the website) for additional information.

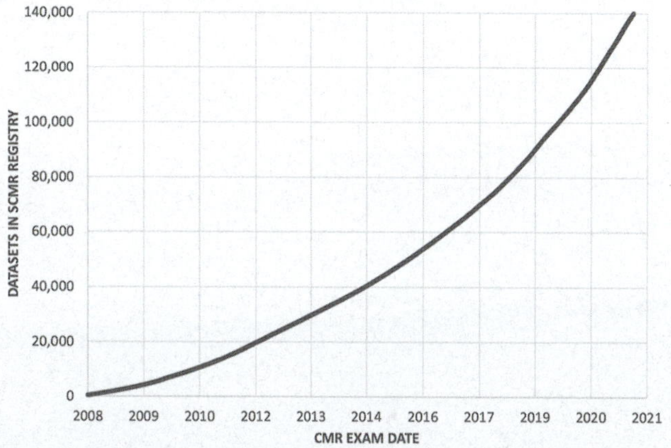

FIG. 14.7 Deidentified datasets in the Society for Cardiovascular Magnetic Resonance (*SCMR*) Registry. *CMR*, cardiovascular magnetic resonance.

REFERENCES

1. Society for Cardiovascular Magnetic Resonance. Accessed November 6, 2023. https://scmr.org/.
2. Hundley WG, Bluemke DA, Bogaert J, et al. Society for cardiovascular magnetic resonance (SCMR) guidelines for reporting cardiovascular magnetic resonance examinations. *J Cardiovasc Magn Reson*. 2022;24(1):29. Published 2022 Apr 28. https://doi.org/10.1186/s12968-021-00827-z.
3. Kramer CM, Barkhausen J, Bucciarelli-Ducci C, Flamm SD, Kim RJ, Nagel E. Standardized cardiovascular magnetic resonance imaging (CMR) protocols: 2020 update. *J Cardiovasc Magn Reson*. 2020;22(1):17. Published 2020 Feb 24. https://doi.org/10.1186/s12968-020-00607-1.
4. Schulz-Menger J, Bluemke DA, Bremerich J, et al. Standardized image interpretation and post-processing in cardiovascular magnetic resonance - 2020 update: society for cardiovascular magnetic resonance (SCMR): board of trustees task force on standardized post-processing. *J Cardiovasc Magn Reson*. 2020;22(1):19. Published 2020 Mar 12. https://doi.org/10.1186/s12968-020-00610-6.
5. Maceira AM, Prasad SK, Khan M, Pennell DJ. Reference right ventricular systolic and diastolic function normalized to age, gender and body surface area from steady-state free precession cardiovascular magnetic resonance. *Eur Heart J*. 2006;27(23):2879–2888. https://doi.org/10.1093/eurheartj/ehl336.
6. Kawel-Boehm N, Hetzel SJ, Ambale-Venkatesh B, et al. Reference ranges ("normal values") for cardiovascular magnetic resonance (CMR) in adults and children: 2020 update [published correction appears in J Cardiovasc Magn Reson. 2021 Oct 18;23(1):114]. *J Cardiovasc Magn Reson*. 2020;22(1):87. Published 2020 Dec 14. https://doi.org/10.1186/s12968-020-00683-3.
7. Fast Health Interoperability Resources, Accessed December 11, 2023. https://fhir.org/.
8. American College of Cardiology (ACC) National cardiovascular data registry (NCDR). Accessed November 8, 2023. https://cvquality.acc.org/NCDR-Home.
9. Bruder O, Wagner A, Lombardi M, et al. European cardiovascular magnetic resonance (EuroCMR) registry—multi national results from 57 centers in 15 countries. *J Cardiovasc Magn Reson*. 2013;15(1):9. Published 2013 Jan 18. https://doi.org/10.1186/1532-429X-15-9.
10. Klinke V, Muzzarelli S, Lauriers N, et al. Quality assessment of cardiovascular magnetic resonance in the setting of the European CMR registry: description and validation of standardized criteria. *J Cardiovasc Magn Reson*. 2013;15(1):55. Published 2013 Jun 20. https://doi.org/10.1186/1532-429X-15-55.

11. Moschetti K, Kwong RY, Petersen SE, et al. Cost-minimization analysis for cardiac revascularization in 12 health care systems based on the EuroCMR/SPINS registries. *JACC Cardiovasc Imaging*. 2022;15(4):607–625. https://doi.org/10.1016/j.jcmg.2021.11.008.
12. Global Cardiovascular Magnetic Resonance Registry (GCMR) Investigators, Kwong RY, Petersen SE, et al. The global cardiovascular magnetic resonance registry (GCMR) of the society for cardiovascular magnetic resonance (SCMR): its goals, rationale, data infrastructure, and current developments. *J Cardiovasc Magn Reson*. 2017;19(1):23. Published 2017 Jan 20. https://doi.org/10.1186/s12968-016-0321-7.
13. SCMR Registry. Accessed November 8, 2023. https://scmr.org/page/Registry.
14. U.S. Department of Health and Human Services, SCMR Registry. Accessed November 10, 2023. https://www.hhs.gov/ohrp/regulations-and-policy/decision-charts/index.html.
15. Heitner JF, Kim RJ, Kim HW, et al. Prognostic value of vasodilator stress cardiac magnetic resonance imaging: a multicenter study with 48,000 patient-years of follow-up. *JAMA Cardiol*. 2019;4(3):256–264.
16. Malahfji M, Crudo V, Kaolawanich Y, et al. Influence of cardiac remodeling on clinical outcomes in patients with aortic regurgitation. *J Am Coll Cardiol*. 2023;81(19):1885–1898. https://doi.org/10.1016/j.jacc.2023.03.001.
17. Tong MS, Slivnick JA, Sharif B, et al. The Society for Cardiovascular Magnetic Resonance Registry at 150,000. 2023. Under Review.

15 Cost-Effectiveness Analysis for Cardiovascular Magnetic Resonance Imaging

YIN GE, ANKUR PANDYA, JUERG SCHWITTER, VICTOR A. FERRARI, AND RAYMOND Y. KWONG

Explosive growth in medical imaging technology during the past few decades has provided physicians with an unparalleled ability to diagnose abnormalities of the cardiovascular system. The growth in available imaging technologies, in particular, has contributed to the continuous increase in healthcare spending since the 1970s. Despite a 50% reduction in deaths from coronary artery disease (CAD) over the past 40 years in the United States, cardiovascular disease remains, more than any other diagnosis, the leading source of healthcare expenditure, with a total estimated cost of $407 billion dollars in 2018–19.[1] An analysis of Medicare claims between 1999 and 2008 revealed that 78% of the growth in cardiovascular services was attributed to noninvasive testing—primarily nuclear stress imaging and echocardiography.[2] A comparison between imaging utilization in the United States and United Kingdom shows that the main driver of the nearly threefold increase in use of imaging in the United States was related to differences in reimbursement strategies (specifically the US fee-for-service system) rather than clinical practice guideline recommendations.[3] Legislation was enacted to reduce utilization of cardiac imaging, which resulted in decreased performance of nuclear imaging, echocardiography, cardiac computed tomography, and invasive coronary angiography; however, cardiovascular magnetic resonance studies increased, largely related to the technique's high diagnostic value and novel applications.[4]

Given these rising costs, there is increasing pressure worldwide from government agencies, insurance companies, and other stakeholders to demonstrate proof of value for all medical expenditures. Cost-effectiveness analysis (CEA) compares the costs and health outcomes of a new intervention with an existing alternative treatment, strategy, or intervention. The questions such analyses aim to answer are: would adopting a new intervention increase costs compared to current practice; is it more effective; and if so, what is the tradeoff between improved clinical outcomes and increased economic cost? By asking these types of questions, CEA provides the same information commonly used for making purchasing decisions in everyday life (Fig. 15.1). If a new strategy or intervention is more effective and less costly than the currently available option, it is almost certainly worth implementing, and in general such a strategy is called "dominant." Likewise, if the new strategy is less effective and more costly, no one is likely to use it. However, the typical scenario examined by a CEA relates to a new, more effective, yet more costly technology. A judgment must then be made as to whether the benefit obtained is worth the cost, and the certainty of that assessment. CEA provides a framework for making such decisions.

In this chapter, we will provide a brief overview of the techniques of CEA as applied to cardiovascular magnetic resonance (CMR) and review the current literature as it pertains to CMR in both US and European contexts.

BASIC TERMINOLOGY

A detailed review of the technical methods of CEA is beyond the scope of this chapter, and readers are referred elsewhere.[5–8] However, cardiovascular imaging physicians need to have a basic understanding of the terminology used in this field. CEA tries to provide a framework to compare different management strategies or treatments within the constraint of limited resources.[6] It aims to maximize health for a given budget. Although often used interchangeably, the terms "cost-minimization," "cost-benefit," "cost-effectiveness," and "cost-utility" have distinct definitions (Fig. 15.2).

Cost-Minimization Analysis

When clinical equivalence is demonstrated through rigorous trial data, then a cost-minimization analysis can be a useful economic tool. The rationale being that if two therapies (or management strategies) are equally effective, the cheaper one is favorable from an economic perspective. Often, it is difficult to determine clinical equivalence with high confidence, so caution must be used when interpreting results from such analyses.

Cost-Benefit Analysis

In a cost-benefit analysis, both the cost and the benefit, which in this case is improved health, are measured in monetary terms. This requires placing a dollar value on grades of health and duration of life. Although this methodology is appropriate in the analysis of many economic

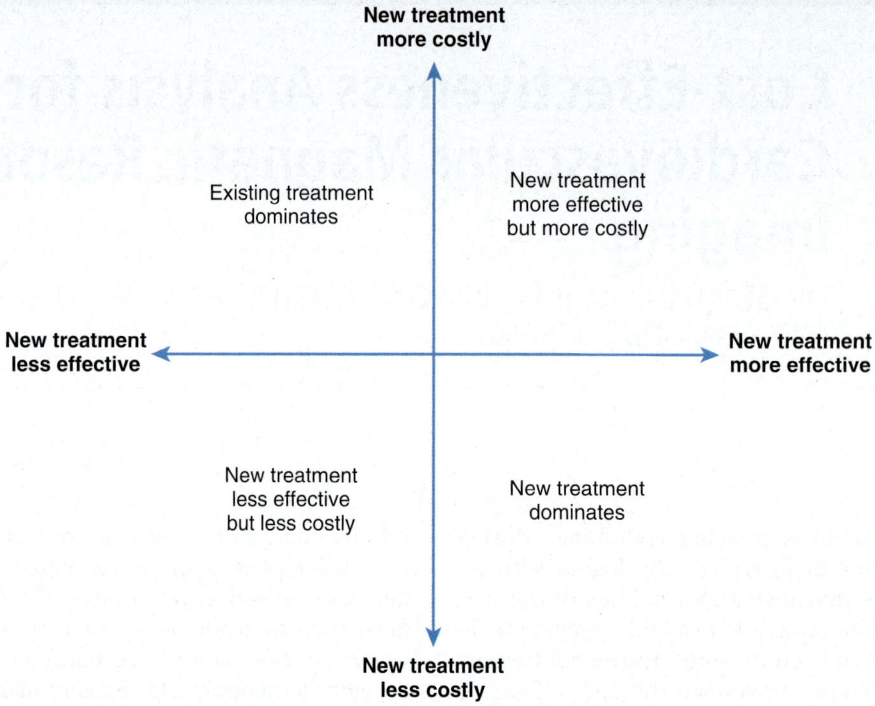

FIG. 15.1 Types of economic evaluations used in healthcare.

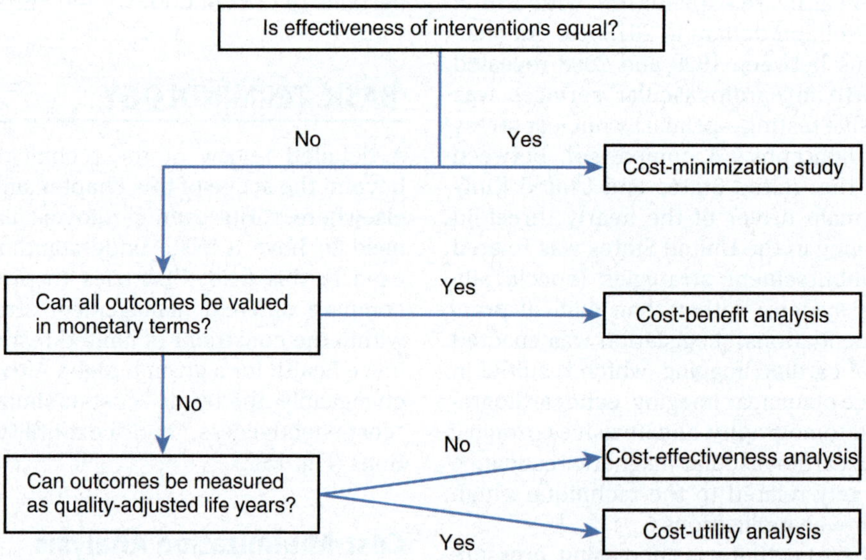

FIG. 15.2 Cost-effectiveness plane. Most new treatments or technologies lie in the upper right corner.

systems, placing a direct monetary value on human health and life extension can be difficult to estimate in practice.

Cost-Effectiveness Analysis

Due to the difficulty of assigning a dollar value to human health, many health economists prefer cost effectiveness, which describes the relationship between cost and a measure of health relevant to the intervention being analyzed—such as life-years gained, disease-free survival in a cancer treatment study, or reductions in blood pressure in a trial of an antihypertensive. The central metric of cost effectiveness is the cost-effectiveness ratio, with cost in the numerator (in dollars, euros, etc.) and effectiveness in the denominator.[9,10] In the context of a CEA, the cost of a particular therapy is the net sum of all resources consumed. This may include the direct cost of care (e.g., hospital, drugs, treatments, diagnostic tests, physician fees, all of which can include potential cost savings from averted disease) and indirect costs (e.g., lost productivity from work, travel, day care). Other more intangible costs (e.g., patient preferences related to certain elements of treatments that are not captured in health outcome measure) could also be included, but caution should be taking against double-counting effects in the numerator and denominator of the cost-effectiveness ratio. Effectiveness is often estimated using a disease simulation such as a Markov model, in which a hypothetical cohort of patients moves between different health states. In the evaluation of CAD, for instance, patients are assigned to different states such as true positive for patients who were correctly identified and revascularized, true negative for those without significant stenosis, and false negative for patients who were misidentified and not revascularized or who died as a result of the mortality risks associated with CAD. The proportion of patients in each state is dependent on the sensitivities and specificities of the various tests in the diagnostic strategy, and each state is then linked to subsequent cardiovascular events, which can be linked to short- and long-term health and cost outcomes.

For a particular treatment or test, the cost-effectiveness ratio in isolation is of little value unless compared with an alternative treatment/test (or no treatment/test). CEA may therefore be better characterized as an incremental cost-effectiveness ("comparative effectiveness") ratio (ICER), as detailed in the formula below:

$$\text{Incremental cost} - \text{effectiveness ratio} = \frac{\text{Cost}_{\text{new strategy}} - \text{Cost}_{\text{current practice}}}{\text{Effect}_{\text{new strategy}} - \text{Effect}_{\text{current practice}}}$$

Quality-Adjusted Life Year

In its most basic form, the "effectiveness" of a treatment can be represented as the years of life gained. However, for most interventions, improvements in quality of life are more prominent, giving rise to a quality-adjusted life year (QALY). The QALY applies a weighting factor to account for varying degrees of health for each year of life gained or lost. By convention, perfect health is assigned a value of 1, and death a value of 0. For all the health states in between, there is a deduction in QALY.

Cost-Utility Analysis

A cost-utility analysis is a type of cost-effective analysis that uses QALY to measure treatment effect. It therefore allows for the comparison of different treatments across different diseases such as dialysis in end-stage kidney disease versus transcatheter aortic valve replacement for aortic stenosis. Cost-utility analyses are important from a public health policy and societal standpoint.

Societal Perspective

Depending on the specific healthcare system, there are many different stakeholders: governments, insurance companies, hospitals, physicians, employers, and patients. Each participant has a different perspective with regard to cost and effect. It is important to recognize that what may be cost effective from a societal standpoint may not be from the perspective of an individual hospital, medical practice, or institution. The societal perspective attempts to look at the aggregate costs and effects on all members and is the one most often employed in CEA.[11]

Time Horizon

The analytic time horizon is the period of time for which the analysis is conducted. It has significant impact on both costs and effects, because over time the costs of an intervention may change and the effectiveness provided may have limited longevity. Short-term (e.g., limited to the follow-up time in a clinical trial) versus long-term (e.g., lifetime time horizon, which is often estimated using simulation models) costs/effects may be very different and thus can alter the cost-effectiveness ratio of a given therapy depending on the analytic time horizon used in the analysis.[12] Discounting in CEA studies refers to the concept that costs and health outcomes that occur at different times have different values, (i.e., the delay in achieving a positive outcome or incurring a cost must be accounted for). Typically, a discount rate of 3% per year is applied.[9]

Cost-Effectiveness Thresholds

There are several commonly used thresholds seen in the literature, which are sometimes used to define the boundaries of a cost-effective therapy. For example, in the United States, $100K/QALY is a commonly cited threshold, as compared with £20–30K/QALY in the United Kingdom.[13] Such thresholds are somewhat arbitrary and do not necessarily reflect a society's willingness to pay, leading some to suggest alternative methods to determine what is cost effective—such as using annual average income.[14] These threshold values are therefore highly dependent on regional economic and cultural forces. In the United States, the American College of Cardiology/American Heart Association statement on cost/value methodology has suggested that ICERs of <$50K/QALY be considered high value, whereas ICERs of >$150K/QALY be considered low value.[15]

CHALLENGES IN CONDUCTING COST-EFFECTIVENESS ANALYSIS IN CARDIOVASCULAR IMAGING

CEAs for diagnostic technologies differ from the evaluation of therapeutic interventions in many respects.[16] One of the most important and challenging differences is the indirect relationship between the results of a diagnostic test and health outcomes. Diagnostic tests only provide intermediate results, often a surrogate of a disease state, which may influence treatment decisions but not directly alter hard clinical health outcomes.

Many factors can alter the chain of events between diagnostic test performance and clinical outcome. For example, the diagnostic test may be technically inadequate, or it may be technically adequate, but the reader may fail to correctly interpret the images. The correct interpretation may not be accurately transmitted or received by the referring physicians, or the referring physicians may vary in their treatment decisions based on their clinical practice pattern. In addition, the patient may choose not to comply with the recommended treatments. Most importantly, outcomes are ultimately driven by the effectiveness of the downstream treatment. Therefore, consideration needs to be given not only to the diagnostic imaging study, but also to the cost effectiveness of any subsequent therapies instituted as a result of imaging. Another approach is to solely examine the outcome of the diagnostic strategy by presenting the results as cost per correct diagnosis (instead of costs per QALY gained).

Although imaging procedures share many of the features of other diagnostic tests, there are several issues that may be unique to imaging: (1) imaging results are often multidimensional (e.g., presence or absence, location, size) rather than one-dimensional (e.g., plasma creatinine level), (2) clear quantitative cut-off points are often not established (i.e., results are presented in terms such as "mild," "moderate," or "severe"), and (3) images can incidentally reveal other diseases (e.g., an unsuspected lung mass). Analogous to interventions and treatments, imaging procedures may be associated with side effects and increased risk of harm (e.g., radiation exposure or renal dysfunction).

Finally, it should be noted that disease prevalence in the study population plays an important role in any assessment of cost effectiveness because it affects diagnostic performance through Bayesian principles. For example, CEA of CMR in symptomatic patients with CAD cannot be applied to a broad population of asymptomatic patients without known CAD.

COST-EFFECTIVE ANALYSES OF CARDIOVASCULAR MAGNETIC RESONANCE

Differences in healthcare systems across the world greatly impact CEAs. To a large extent, the assumptions and conclusions of these studies are limited to the country or region and the time period in which they were performed. Therefore, in the following sections of this chapter we will separately review studies performed in the United States and Europe/UK. Most of the CEA studies have focused on the diagnosis of stable CAD.

US Perspective

Compared to many countries with universal health care systems, it is more difficult to accurately assess actual costs in the US healthcare system. In many instances, there is complex and opaque accounting—with varying cost-to-charge ratios resulting in differences between what is charged or billed and actual payments or costs received. The "charge" is the price the consumer is billed by the healthcare facility for the service. This charge is highly variable depending on the hospital and other local factors, which can be very unclear. The actual payment received may be a small fraction of the charge, and varies widely among hospitals, states, and third-party payers. Consequently, investigators frequently use cost estimates derived from average US Centers for Medicare and Medicaid Services reimbursements. They can be accessed online using the Healthcare Common Procedure Coding System or Current Procedural Technology codes of the procedures (http://www.cms.gov/apps/physician-fee-schedule/search/search-criteria.aspx). Despite these challenges, reports of CEA of CMR in the Untied States are increasing. Major cost studies of CMR within the US healthcare system are summarized below (Table 15.1).

Genders et al. examined the cost effectiveness of various combinations of imaging strategies in patients presenting with stable chest pain and an intermediate pretest probability (30%) of CAD in the US, UK, and Dutch healthcare systems.[17] Five sets of diagnostic strategies were modeled, namely: no imaging, coronary computed tomographic angiography (CCTA), cardiac stress imaging, CCTA with positive results followed by cardiac stress imaging, and immediate invasive coronary angiography. The authors also analyzed an aggressive and conservative approach to CAD management, whereby either all abnormal studies or only those with severe CAD on CCTA and more than

TABLE 15.1 Summary of major cost-effectiveness studies for cardiovascular magnetic resonance performed in the United States.

AUTHOR	DESIGN	COUNTRY	STUDY AND METHODS	STUDY CONCLUSIONS
Genders et al.[17]	Cost effectiveness	US, UK, Netherlands	Comparison between combination of strategies involving CCTA, stress CMR, stress echocardiogram, SPECT, and ICA in an intermediate CAD prevalence population (30%).	CCTA-based strategies are most cost effective.
Stojanovic et al.[41]	Cost-projection analysis	US	Comparison of the costs of dobutamine stress CMR versus SPECT in a low CAD prevalence population (11.7%).	Stress CMR is less costly than SPECT when considering total direct and indirect costs of testing.
Ge et al.[18]	Cost effectiveness	US	Comparison between CCTA, stress CMR, SPECT, and ICA in an intermediate CAD prevalence population (32.4%).	Stress CMR was cost effective, with ICER of $52,000/QALY versus no imaging.
Moschetti et al.[27]	Cost minimization	Norway, UK, Belgium, Germany, France, Switzerland, Italy, Greece, US, Mexico, Brazil, Beijing (China)	Comparison of the costs of a CMR-guided strategy versus two invasive strategies in the EuroCMR and SPINS registry population.	A CMR+ICA strategy for patients with suspected CAD provides cost reduction compared with a hypothetical ICA+FFR strategy in patients with low-to-intermediate disease prevalence in all twelve countries.

CCTA, Coronary computed tomography angiography; *CMR,* cardiovascular magnetic resonance; *ICA,* invasive coronary angiography; *ICER,* incremental cost-effectiveness ratio; *SPECT,* single photon emission computed tomography; *US,* United States.

moderate ischemia on stress testing underwent coronary angiography. The authors concluded that CCTA-based strategies were the most cost effective. In the US system, a strategy combining CCTA as the initial test, stress echocardiogram in abnormal CCTA, and finally invasive coronary angiogram demonstrated an ICER of $21,000–22,000/QALY versus no imaging, whereas other strategies were dominated. Similar conclusions were reached in the Dutch healthcare system, whereas in the UK, such a strategy would not be cost effective unless one increased the willingness-to-pay threshold to £32,000 and £53,000/QALY for males and females, respectively.

In contrast, an analysis by Ge et al. found stress CMR to be cost effective[18] using coronary angiography with fractional flow reserve (FFR) as the gold standard to guide revascularization.[19] The authors used data from the contemporary, multicenter Stress CMR Perfusion Imaging in the United States (SPINS) study to build their base-case cohort, and compared stress CMR to coronary angiography with FFR, single-photon emission computed tomography (SPECT), CCTA with CT-FFR, and no imaging. The authors concluded that stress CMR provided an ICER of $52,000/QALY over no imaging and dominated other noninvasive strategies. The authors also modeled a conservative approach to coronary angiography, whereby only patients with two or more ischemic segments underwent invasive testing. In this scenario, stress CMR remained the most cost-effective strategy, with an ICER of $60,000/QALY compared with no imaging. Importantly, the model results were not sensitive to the proportion of patients undergoing FFR assessment (either with CCTA or during coronary angiography). Despite lower upfront CCTA imaging costs compared to CMR, the latter results in less downstream invasive angiography. Only when the prevalence of CAD exceeded 60% did immediate coronary angiography become more cost effective.

TABLE 15.2 Summary of major cost-effectiveness studies for cardiovascular magnetic resonance performed in Europe.

AUTHOR	DESIGN	COUNTRY	STUDY AND METHODS	STUDY CONCLUSIONS
Walker et al.[29]	Cost effectiveness	UK	Comparison between eight strategies involving exercise treadmill testing, SPECT, stress CMR, and ICA for the diagnosis of CAD in an intermediate CAD prevalence population (39.5%), based on CE-MARC data.	Two strategies incorporating stress CMR are cost effective at thresholds of £20,000/QALY and £30,000/QALY.
Boldt et al.[20]	Cost effectiveness	Germany	Stress CMR was compared to SPECT and ICA in patients across spectrum of CAD prevalence (base case 50%).	Stress CMR is more cost effective than SPECT. ICA as first test is cost effective at CAD prevalence >60%.
Thom et al.[34]	Cost effectiveness	UK	Comparison of stress CMR with SPECT, stress echocardiogram, and ICA in an intermediate CAD prevalence population (revascularization in 34%).	SPECT is more cost effective. Majority of noninvasive patients underwent ICA (75%–80%).
Genders et al.[17]	Cost effectiveness	US, UK, Netherlands	Comparison between combination of strategies involving CCTA, stress CMR, stress echocardiogram, SPECT, and ICA in an intermediate CAD prevalence population (30%).	CCTA-based strategies are most cost effective.
Pletscher et al.[31]	Cost effectiveness	Switzerland	Comparison between eight strategies involving exercise treadmill testing, SPECT, stress CMR, and ICA for the diagnosis of CAD in an intermediate CAD prevalence population (39.5%), based on CE-MARC data.	A strategy incorporating stress CMR was dominant (lower cost/highest QALY): Exercise treadmill testing, followed by ICA in positive cases, and by stress CMR in inconclusive cases with subsequent ICA if stress CMR was positive or inconclusive.
Walker et al.[32]	Cost effectiveness	UK	Cost-effectiveness analysis comparing three strategies for the diagnosis of CAD based on CE-MARC 2 data in a low CAD prevalence population (overall revascularization rate ~10%).	Stress CMR dominated SPECT and NICE guidelines–based strategies.
Moschetti et al.[27]	Cost minimization	Norway, UK, Belgium, Germany, France, Switzerland, Italy, Greece, US, Mexico, Brazil, Beijing (China)	Comparison of the costs of a CMR-guided strategy versus two invasive strategies in the EuroCMR and SPINS registry population.	A CMR+ICA strategy for patients with suspected CAD provides cost reduction compared with a hypothetical ICA+FFR strategy in patients with low to intermediate disease prevalence in all twelve countries.
Nazir et al.[33]	Cost effectiveness	UK	Comparison between combination of 17 strategies involving CCTA, stress CMR, stress echocardiogram, SPECT, PET, and ICA for the diagnosis of CAD in an intermediate CAD prevalence population (37.6%).	Stress CMR, either followed by CCTA or ICA+FFR was most cost effective, from a range of £3,000–£22,000 per correct diagnosis.

CAD, Coronary artery disease; *CE-MARC,* clinical evaluation of magnetic resonance imaging in coronary heart disease; *CMR,* cardiovascular magnetic resonance imaging; *FFR,* fractional flow reserve; *ICA,* invasive coronary angiography; *PET,* positron emission tomography; *QALY,* quality-adjusted life years; *SPECT,* single photon emission computed tomography; *UK,* United Kingdom; *US,* United States.

European Perspective

There are more published data regarding the cost effectiveness of CMR in the European context—predominantly from Switzerland, Germany, and the United Kingdom (Table 15.2). However, it is important to realize that there are significant differences between different European countries in terms of healthcare economics and delivery. Thus, studies in one country cannot necessarily be extrapolated to other countries in Europe.

Boldt et al. compared cost effectiveness and the utility of stress CMR and SPECT versus invasive coronary angiography as the standard of reference in a German population with CAD prevalence rates ranging from 0% to 100%, with base case set at 50%.[20] From a third-payer perspective, stress CMR was more cost effective than SPECT at any CAD prevalence, which was true for costs per correct diagnosis of CAD as well as for costs per QALY gained (€2,246/QALY). However, this rank order changed in favor of invasive coronary angiography when CAD prevalence was above 60%. The authors concluded that, from an economic point of view, first-line invasive coronary angiography is a reasonable alternative to stress CMR for patients with a pretest likelihood greater than 60%.

Moschetti et al. provided a series of cost-related studies using stress CMR. Using data modeled from real-life performance of CMR in the European CMR registry (EuroCMR), the authors compared downstream cost with invasive coronary angiography.[21] In this registry population with a CAD prevalence of 21%, stress CMR yielded the correct diagnosis of CAD at lower costs than invasive coronary angiography when calculated for the German healthcare system—which is consistent with the earlier findings of Boldt et al.[20] Costs were also calculated for the UK, Swiss, and US healthcare systems, with similar results demonstrating reduced costs of CMR in patient diagnosis and management. In a subsequent study, Moschetti et al. compared ischemia detection by stress CMR with coronary angiography + FFR.[22] In the CMR arm, all patients with ischemia on CMR were investigated by additional invasive coronary angiography, whereas in the coronary angiography arm, all patients underwent first-line invasive coronary angiography and those with >50% diameter stenosis were further investigated via FFR. The CMR strategy was more cost effective than the coronary angiography + FFR strategy below a CAD prevalence of 62%, 65%, 83%, and 82% for the Swiss, German, UK, and US healthcare systems, respectively. These numbers have important implications, given the low pretest probability of CAD for patients undergoing elective coronary angiography, which has ranged from approximately 30%–40% in healthcare systems around the world.[22–25] These numbers are considerably below the calculated thresholds needed for cost effectiveness of the angiography + FFR strategy.

Two cost-minimization studies were performed on the assumption that a CMR-guided strategy is clinically equivalent to an angiography-guided strategy,[26,27] which is now well supported by a randomized trial.[28] In the updated analysis, Moschetti et al. compared (1) CMR + coronary angiography and revascularization at the treating physician's discretion, (2) coronary angiography + FFR, and (3) coronary angiography and revascularization of all stenoses ≥50%. Costs were calculated across 12 different healthcare systems, including the United States, 8 European countries, Mexico, Brazil, and Beijing (China). Compared to coronary angiography + FFR, the CMR strategy resulted in savings in all healthcare setting studied, ranging from 42% ± 20% and 52% ± 15% in low-risk EuroCMR and SPINS patients with atypical chest pain, to 31% ± 16% in high-risk SPINS patients with known CAD. Cost savings were even more substantial when compared to coronary angiography alone. The authors offer a calculator, as used in that study, which allows users to input the costs of their healthcare system to assess potential cost savings associated with the use of CMR (available at www.herz-mri.ch).

Walker et al. compared eight different diagnostic pathways applying exercise treadmill testing, SPECT, or CMR in various combinations using patients from the UK Clinical Evaluation of MAgnetic Resonance imaging in Coronary heart disease (CE-MARC) study.[29,30] The CE-MARC study was a diagnostic accuracy study that compared stress CMR with SPECT, with all patients subsequently undergoing coronary angiography. In the CEA study, the authors modeled the base case as a 60-year-old male with Canadian Cardiovascular Society (CCS) class 2 angina and a 39.5% likelihood of significant stenosis based on CE-MARC data. They found only two strategies to be cost effective for the diagnosis of CAD, both of which included CMR. In the first strategy, CMR followed a positive or inconclusive exercise treadmill test, followed by coronary angiography if CMR was positive or inconclusive. In the second strategy, coronary angiography followed a positive or inconclusive CMR. The optimal strategy depended upon the cost-effectiveness threshold used, as the first strategy had an ICER of £7,779/QALY gained in males and £3,650/QALY gained in females, whereas the second provided an ICER of £26,858/QALY and £20,914/QALY in males and females, respectively. Using the same cohort, Pletscher et al. applied a CEA model to the Swiss healthcare system.[31] In this study, a strategy of exercise treadmill testing followed by coronary angiography in positive cases, and by stress CMR in inconclusive cases with subsequent coronary angiography if stress CMR was positive or inconclusive dominated the other diagnostic pathways (i.e., provided the highest QALY at the lowest cost). Interestingly, considering the lifetime costs for CAD management (including costs for diagnosis, revascularization if needed, and drug treatment post revascularization), the costs for diagnostic workup of eight different strategies accounted for only 8.8% to 13.0% of the total costs. Walker et al. performed another CEA study within the UK system using data from CE-MARC 2.[32] In this study, the authors compared a stress CMR strategy to a SPECT strategy and National Institute for Health & Care Excellence (NICE) guidelines–based strategy (low pretest likelihood underwent CCTA, intermediate pretest likelihood underwent SPECT, high pretest likelihood underwent coronary angiography). Stress CMR dominated the other two strategies. Nazir et al. compared 17 strategies using a combination of CTCA, stress echocardiography, CT-based FFR, SPECT, stress CMR, positron emission tomography, coronary angiography, and coronary angiography + FFR.[33]

In the base case scenario, for which disease prevalence was set at 37.6%, stress CMR, either followed by CCTA or invasive coronary angiography + FFR, was most cost effective, ranging from £3,000–£22,000 per correct diagnosis.

Not all studies have found stress CMR to be the most cost-effective strategy. In the Cost Effectiveness of noninvasive Cardiac Testing (CECaT) trial, UK patients were randomized to coronary angiography, SPECT, stress CMR, or stress echocardiogram.[34] SPECT was found to be the most cost-effective strategy; however, this study is limited due to its relatively short time horizon of 3 years. Furthermore, a large portion of patients (75%–80%) undergoing noninvasive testing ultimately underwent coronary angiography, raising questions about the utility of any noninvasive testing in this cohort.

FUTURE DIRECTIONS

Thus far, studies have mostly focused on stable CAD, but interest is growing, and CEA studies are emerging for conditions for which CMR plays a crucial role. In patients with ischemic cardiomyopathy undergoing revascularization, Campbell et al. compared the cost effectiveness of CMR to stress echocardiogram, SPECT, PET, and no testing for viability assessment.[35] Testing with CMR was the most cost-effective strategy at a threshold of £20,000/QALY; however, if the assumptions were modified such that both viable and nonviable patients benefited from revascularization, then a no-testing (i.e., revascularize all) strategy became more cost effective. CEA studies on CAD patients in other settings (symptomatic revascularized patients and acute CAD patients in observation or emergency care units) and on heart failure and arrhythmia patients are summarized elsewhere.[36]

In patients with suspected transthyretin amyloid cardiomyopathy (ATTR-CMP), Ge et al. modeled seven diagnostic pathways involving a combination of technetium-99m pyrophosphate (PYP), CMR, and endomyocardial biopsy.[37] With the contemporary pricing of tafamidis, no strategies were cost effective. However, once drug pricing was removed as a factor, a PYP-only strategy to diagnose ATTR-CMP was cost effective at a threshold of $100,000/QALY, whereas PYP followed by CMR was cost effective at a threshold of $150,000/QALY. However, the ability of CMR to detect other etiologies underlying concentric left ventricular hypertrophy also has to be considered.

Another interesting approach is the development of a meta-model, which is a simple version of a full disease simulation model (e.g., Markov model) that can be used to approximate the results of the full model instantly. Pandya et al. performed a systematic review of cost-effectiveness studies using stress CMR.[38] In the 15 studies included, stress CMR was cost effective in the majority (10 studies), with three studies reporting equivocal results, and two studies showing that CCTA was optimal. More importantly, the authors built a calculator that allows users to input and evaluate key model parameters, such as disease prevalence, cost of imaging/procedures, and test sensitivity specificity, and determine their impact on cost effectiveness. The meta-model can therefore be used not only to test cost effectiveness in hypothetical health scenarios, but it also allows investigators to easily explain and explore discrepancies when these arise between two different CEA studies.

CONCLUSIONS

The field of CMR has developed over recent years on the basis of a large and growing body of published evidence showing excellent diagnostic and prognostic performance across a wide range of cardiovascular conditions. However, given the rising costs of imaging, there is increasing pressure worldwide from government agencies, insurance companies, and other stakeholders to demonstrate proof of value for all medical expenditures. Therefore, demonstrating the cost effectiveness of CMR across a spectrum of disease will be critical to ensure continued growth and appropriate utilization. Of course, it is possible to directly ascertain downstream costs, as some have done within either observation cohorts[39] or randomized trials,[40] but such endeavors are limited by the length of downstream follow-up and sample size. CEA modeling studies have the potential to overcome these limitations and will be pivotal in demonstrating the value of CMR and its impact on patient outcomes.

REFERENCES

1. Tsao CW, Aday AW, Almarzooq ZI, et al. Heart Disease and Stroke Statistics-2023 Update: A Report From the American Heart Association. *Circulation*. 2023;147:e93–e621. https://doi.org/10.1161/CIR.0000000000001123.
2. Andrus BW, Welch HG. Medicare services provided by cardiologists in the United States: 1999-2008. *Circ Cardiovasc Qual Outcomes*. 2012;5:31–36. https://doi.org/10.1161/CIRCOUTCOMES.111.961813.
3. Petersen SE, Friebel R, Ferrari V, et al. Recent Trends and Potential Drivers of Non-invasive Cardiovascular Imaging Use in the United States of America and England. *Front Cardiovasc Med*. 2020;7:617771. https://doi.org/10.3389/fcvm.2020.617771.
4. Ferrari VA, Whitman B, Blankenship JC, et al. Cardiovascular imaging payment and reimbursement systems: understanding the past and present in order to guide the future. *JACC Cardiovasc Imaging*. 2014;7:324–332. https://doi.org/10.1016/j.jcmg.2014.01.008.
5. Francis SA, Daly C, Heydari B, Abbasi S, Shah RV, Kwong RY. Cost-effectiveness analysis for imaging techniques with a focus on cardiovascular magnetic resonance. *J Cardiovasc Magn Reson*. 2013;15:52. https://doi.org/10.1186/1532-429X-15-52.
6. Weinstein MC, Stason WB. Foundations of cost-effectiveness analysis for health and medical practices. *N Engl J Med*. 1977;296:716–721. https://doi.org/10.1056/NEJM197703312961304.
7. Torrance GW. Measurement of health state utilities for economic appraisal. *J Health Econ*. 1986;5:1–30. https://doi.org/10.1016/0167-6296(86)90020-2.
8. Diamond GA, Kaul S. Cost, effectiveness, and cost-effectiveness. *Circ Cardiovasc Qual Outcomes*. 2009;2:49–54. https://doi.org/10.1161/CIRCOUTCOMES.108.793406.
9. Weinstein MC, Siegel JE, Gold MR, Kamlet MS, Russell LB. Recommendations of the Panel on Cost-effectiveness in Health and Medicine. *JAMA*. 1996;276:1253–1258.
10. Siegel JE, Weinstein MC, Russell LB, Gold MR. Recommendations for reporting cost-effectiveness analyses. Panel on Cost-Effectiveness in Health and Medicine. *JAMA*. 1996;276:1339–1341. https://doi.org/10.1001/jama.276.16.1339.
11. Russell LB, Gold MR, Siegel JE, Daniels N, Weinstein MC. The role of cost-effectiveness analysis in health and medicine. Panel on Cost-Effectiveness in Health and Medicine. *JAMA*. 1996;276:1172–1177.
12. Kim DD, Wilkinson CL, Pope EF, Chambers JD, Cohen JT, Neumann PJ. The influence of time horizon on results of cost-effectiveness analyses. *Expert Rev Pharmacoecon Outcomes Res*. 2017;17:615–623. https://doi.org/10.1080/14737167.2017.1331432.
13. Neumann PJ, Kim DD. Cost-effectiveness Thresholds Used by Study Authors, 1990-2021. *JAMA*. 2023;329:1312–1314. https://doi.org/10.1001/jama.2023.1792.
14. Garber AM, Phelps CE. Economic foundations of cost-effectiveness analysis. *J Health Econ*. 1997;16:1–31. https://doi.org/10.1016/s0167-6296(96)00506-1.

15. Anderson JL, Heidenreich PA, Barnett PG, et al. ACC/AHA statement on cost/value methodology in clinical practice guidelines and performance measures: a report of the American College of Cardiology/American Heart Association Task Force on Performance Measures and Task Force on Practice Guidelines. *J Am Coll Cardiol*. 2014;63:2304–2322. https://doi.org/10.1016/j.jacc.2014.03.016.
16. Gazelle GS, McMahon PM, Siebert U, Beinfeld MT. Cost-effectiveness analysis in the assessment of diagnostic imaging technologies. *Radiology*. 2005;235:361–370. https://doi.org/10.1148/radiol.2352040330.
17. Genders TS, Petersen SE, Pugliese F, et al. The optimal imaging strategy for patients with stable chest pain: a cost-effectiveness analysis. *Ann Intern Med*. 2015;162:474–484. https://doi.org/10.7326/M14-0027.
18. Ge Y, Pandya A, Steel K, et al. Cost-effectiveness analysis of stress cardiovascular magnetic resonance imaging for stable chest pain syndromes. *JACC Cardiovasc Imaging*. 2020;13:1505–1517. https://doi.org/10.1016/j.jcmg.2020.02.029.
19. Tonino PA, De Bruyne B, Pijls NH, et al. Fractional flow reserve versus angiography for guiding percutaneous coronary intervention. *N Engl J Med*. 2009;360:213–224. https://doi.org/10.1056/NEJMoa0807611.
20. Boldt J, Leber AW, Bonaventura K, et al. Cost-effectiveness of cardiovascular magnetic resonance and single-photon emission computed tomography for diagnosis of coronary artery disease in Germany. *J Cardiovasc Magn Reson*. 2013;15:30. https://doi.org/10.1186/1532-429X-15-30.
21. Moschetti K, Muzzarelli S, Pinget C, et al. Cost evaluation of cardiovascular magnetic resonance versus coronary angiography for the diagnostic work-up of coronary artery disease: application of the European Cardiovascular Magnetic Resonance registry data to the German, United Kingdom, Swiss, and United States health care systems. *J Cardiovasc Magn Reson*. 2012;14:35. https://doi.org/10.1186/1532-429X-14-35.
22. Moschetti K, Favre D, Pinget C, et al. Comparative cost-effectiveness analyses of cardiovascular magnetic resonance and coronary angiography combined with fractional flow reserve for the diagnosis of coronary artery disease. *J Cardiovasc Magn Reson*. 2014;16:13. https://doi.org/10.1186/1532-429X-16-13.
23. Horstkotte D, Wiemer M, van Buuren F. Performance figures of invasive cardiology in Germany 2006 and 2007 focussing on coronary artery disease. *Clin Res Cardiol*. 2011;100:187–190. https://doi.org/10.1007/s00392-010-0244-5.
24. Patel MR, Peterson ED, Dai D, et al. Low diagnostic yield of elective coronary angiography. *N Engl J Med*. 2010;362:886–895. https://doi.org/10.1056/NEJMoa0907272.
25. Ko DT, Tu JV, Austin PC, et al. Prevalence and extent of obstructive coronary artery disease among patients undergoing elective coronary catheterization in New York State and Ontario. *JAMA*. 2013;310:163–169. https://doi.org/10.1001/jama.2013.7834.
26. Moschetti K, Petersen SE, Pilz G, et al. Cost-minimization analysis of three decision strategies for cardiac revascularization: results of the "suspected CAD" cohort of the european cardiovascular magnetic resonance registry. *J Cardiovasc Magn Reson*. 2016;18:3. https://doi.org/10.1186/s12968-015-0222-1.
27. Moschetti K, Kwong RY, Petersen SE, et al. Cost-Minimization Analysis for Cardiac Revascularization in 12 Health Care Systems Based on the Euro-CMR/SPINS Registries. *JACC Cardiovasc Imaging*. 2022;15:607–625. https://doi.org/10.1016/j.jcmg.2021.11.008.
28. Nagel E, Greenwood JP, McCann GP, et al. Magnetic resonance perfusion or fractional flow reserve in coronary disease. *N Engl J Med*. 2019;380:2418–2428. https://doi.org/10.1056/NEJMoa1716734.
29. Walker S, Girardin F, McKenna C, et al. Cost-effectiveness of cardiovascular magnetic resonance in the diagnosis of coronary heart disease: an economic evaluation using data from the CE-MARC study. *Heart*. 2013;99:873–881. https://doi.org/10.1136/heartjnl-2013-303624.
30. Greenwood JP, Maredia N, Younger JF, et al. Cardiovascular magnetic resonance and single-photon emission computed tomography for diagnosis of coronary heart disease (CE-MARC): a prospective trial. *Lancet*. 2012;379:453–460. https://doi.org/10.1016/S0140-6736(11)61335-4.
31. Pletscher M, Walker S, Moschetti K, et al. Cost-effectiveness of functional cardiac imaging in the diagnostic work-up of coronary heart disease. *Eur Heart J Qual Care Clin Outcomes*. 2016;2:201–207. https://doi.org/10.1093/ehjqcco/qcw008.
32. Walker S, Cox E, Rothwell B, et al. Cost-effectiveness of cardiovascular imaging for stable coronary heart disease. *Heart*. 2021;107:381–388. https://doi.org/10.1136/heartjnl-2020-316990.
33. Nazir MS, Rodriguez-Guadarrama Y, Rua T, et al. Cost-effectiveness in diagnosis of stable angina patients: a decision-analytical modelling approach. *Open Heart*. 2022;9:e001700. https://doi.org/10.1136/openhrt-2021-001700.
34. Thom H, West NE, Hughes V, et al. Cost-effectiveness of initial stress cardiovascular MR, stress SPECT or stress echocardiography as a gate-keeper test, compared with upfront invasive coronary angiography in the investigation and management of patients with stable chest pain: mid-term outcomes from the CECaT randomised controlled trial. *BMJ Open*. 2014;4:e003419. https://doi.org/10.1136/bmjopen-2013-003419.
35. Campbell F, Thokala P, Uttley LC, et al. Systematic review and modelling of the cost-effectiveness of cardiac magnetic resonance imaging compared with current existing testing pathways in ischaemic cardiomyopathy. *Health Technol Assess*. 2014;18:1–120. https://doi.org/10.3310/hta18590.
36. Murphy T, Schwitter J, Petersen S. Economy – Cost effectiveness. In: *CMR-Update*. 3rd edition. ; 2020.
37. Ge Y, Pandya A, Cuddy SAM, Singh A, Singh A, Dorbala S. Modeling the cost and health impacts of diagnostic strategies in patients with suspected transthyretin cardiac amyloidosis. *J Am Heart Assoc*. 2022;11:e026308. https://doi.org/10.1161/JAHA.122.026308.
38. Pandya A, Yu YJ, Ge Y, et al. Evidence-based cardiovascular magnetic resonance cost-effectiveness calculator for the detection of significant coronary artery disease. *J Cardiovasc Magn Reson*. 2022;24:1. https://doi.org/10.1186/s12968-021-00833-1.
39. Pontone G, Andreini D, Guaricci AI, et al. The STRATEGY Study (Stress Cardiac Magnetic Resonance Versus Computed Tomography Coronary Angiography for the Management of Symptomatic Revascularized Patients): Resources and Outcomes Impact. *Circ Cardiovasc Imaging*. 2016;9:e005171. https://doi.org/10.1161/CIRCIMAGING.116.005171.
40. Miller CD, Hwang W, Case D, et al. Stress CMR imaging observation unit in the emergency department reduces 1-year medical care costs in patients with acute chest pain: a randomized study for comparison with inpatient care. *JACC Cardiovasc Imaging*. 2011;4:862–870. https://doi.org/10.1016/j.jcmg.2011.04.016.
41. Stojanovic I, Schneider JE, Cooper J. Cost-impact of cardiac magnetic resonance imaging with Fast-SENC compared to SPECT in the diagnosis of coronary artery disease in the U.S. *J Med Econ*. 2019;22:430–438. https://doi.org/10.1080/13696998.2019.1580713.

16 Normal Values in Cardiovascular Magnetic Resonance Imaging

DAVID A. BLUEMKE AND NADINE KAWEL-BOEHM

INTRODUCTION

Magnetic resonance imaging (MRI) is widely considered to be the most accurate imaging modality for the assessment of myocardial function and structure. Clinically important measurements such as ejection fraction, myocardial wall thickness, and chamber volumes are readily available using MRI. In addition, MRI offers the opportunity for tissue characterization using both noncontrast and contrast-enhanced techniques.

MRI cardiac parameters are routinely quantified; by comparison, echocardiography assessment may be visual or semiquantitative. The use of MRI instead of echocardiography may be needed when there is limited echocardiography assessment due to poor acoustic windows. Although technical limitations also occur with MRI, its limitations (e.g., pacemakers, metal implants) usually do not overlap with those of echocardiography. Thus, patients with technically limited echocardiographic examinations are likely to have interpretable MRI combined with the advantage of quantitative evaluation.

The list of quantitative parameters available from cardiovascular MRI is vast, involving almost every possible element of cardiovascular structure, function, and tissue analysis. An encyclopedic listing of such parameters is available online.[1] In this chapter, our purpose is to present a summary of the most common parameters that are routinely used for clinical patient care using cardiovascular MRI. Major considerations regarding the use of normal values for cardiovascular disease are also presented.

BACKGROUND

The relatively recent proliferation of the study of normal or reference values for cardiovascular MRI extends from the earlier efforts to standardize reference values for echocardiography. Each echocardiographic report contains a list of reference values for comparison to an individual patient's cardiac parameters. Cardiac MRI has followed this pattern with reference values that are provided alongside a patient's cardiac MRI analysis. Comparison of a patient's values to the reference values is expected to calibrate to a "normal" patient. Patient values that deviate from the reference values are "abnormal." The numerical summary in the clinical report is typically superior to qualitative assessments, such as mild, moderate, or marked abnormalities.

Typically, normal values are calculated based on a reference population free of cardiovascular risk factors. Assuming a Gaussian distribution, the normal range of the reference population is taken as the mean value ± two times the standard deviation.

It is critical that the reference population is relevant to the patient in question. The reference population should be of sufficient size (generally at least 40 subjects) to allow estimates of the distribution.[2] Ethnicity, sex, and common cardiovascular risk factors and conditions are well known to result in alterations in cardiac size and function. A healthy sex and ideally ethnicity-matched reference population is optimal for comparison to the individual patient.

IMPACT OF BODY SIZE ON HEART SIZE AND FUNCTION

For clinical use, most cardiovascular reference values are adjusted for body size. For pediatric patients, age must also be considered. Adjustments for age are uncommon for adult patients but may be useful for some situations (discussed further below). The most common method for body size adjustment is dividing the cardiac parameter by body surface area. Body surface area is used for body size standardization because it is a better indicator of metabolic mass than, for example, body weight. Cardiac parameters divided by body surface area results in an "indexed" value (e.g., end-diastolic volume divided by body surface area is equal to the end-diastolic index).

The clinician needs to be aware that multiple formulas have been developed to calculate body surface area. The most common formula used for calculation of body surface area that is used clinically was published in 1916 by Du Bois and Du Bois as:

$$\text{Body surface area} = 0.007184 \times \text{Height}\ 0.725 \times \text{Weight}\ 0.425$$ [3,4]

where body surface area is in square meters, height is in centimeters, and weight is in kilograms. Du Bois and Du Bois estimated the errors in their formula at 1.5% for "average body" shapes.

Limitations of the Du Bois and Du Bois formula have been discussed at length.[5] In particular, the original experiments of Du Bois and Du Bois were conducted on only nine individuals. Different exponents and formulas derived from somewhat larger populations have resulted in different estimates of body surface area. However, most formulas are within 10% of the original Du Bois and Du Bois formula. Web-based body surface area calculators frequently have the option of using different formulas, including those optimized for specific populations (e.g.,[6]). Body surface area formulas have been reviewed by Burton.[5] Although Burton identified formulas that may result in improved body surface estimates, he states "there is no strong reason to abandon the form of equation introduced by Du Bois and Du Bois". In particular, "no one formula can fit all shapes of people."

Alternatives to Body Surface Area

The concept of normalizing cardiac parameters by body surface area is frequently challenged in the published literature. The goal of such studies is to find improved cutoff values above which cardiovascular risk is substantially increased and below which individuals are classified as "normal." As discussed above, the use of body size adjustment as a ratio follows the general formula:

$$S = x / y$$

where S is the adjusted parameter, x the measured parameter, and y is body surface area. This is termed the ratiometric scaling approach and assumes a linear relationship between the cardiovascular variable and body size. However, there is good evidence that a nonlinear relationship exists. Allometric scaling divides the cardiovascular parameter by a body size variable raised to a scalar exponent, as:

$$S = x / y^b$$

where b is termed the allometric scaling exponent.[7] The exponent b can be derived empirically and may differ for different cardiovascular parameters. For example, left ventricular mass is a three-dimensional variable, whereas left ventricular wall diameter is a unidimensional variable. As a result, the allometric parameter b would be expected to be different since the mass and wall diameters are not expected to scale in the same fashion with body size.

In the allometric approach, even the ideal choice of the body size parameter y may vary depending on the patient population and goal of the research. Dewey et al.[7] have tabulated multiple studies of body size adjustment of left ventricular mass from four different literature studies. When y was set to represent body surface area, the parameter b varied in the literature from 1.44 to 1.67 for populations ranging from normotensive individuals to trained athletes.

The scaling of left ventricular mass by body size may be used to illustrate the challenges. In a group of 444 normotensive children and 241 adults studied by echocardiography, the optimum scaling parameter was found to be left ventricle (LV) mass/height$^{2.7}$.[7] However, a subsequent analysis of the Asklepios and MESA studies (7528 total individuals) found that LV mass/height$^{1.7}$ was better at identifying obesity-related left ventricular hypertrophy and better predicted cardiovascular events and death.[8]

To summarize, many alternatives exist to the common clinical approach of adjustment for body size using body surface area normalization. These more specialized formulas are typically optimized for specific populations, such as children or adults undergoing athletic training. Such formulas may also be optimized to predict specific types of cardiovascular events or to account for common cardiovascular risk factors such as diabetes. One such example is the MESA generalized prediction equation for LV mass, a particularly powerful predictor of cardiovascular events.[9] Nevertheless, specialized normalization equations remain uncommon for routine clinical application.

IMPACT OF SEX

Investigators have long identified functional and structural differences between the male and female human heart that are not accounted for by body size. Differences have been extensively reviewed by St Pierre et al.[10] Overall, the left ventricular mass of the female heart is 34% less than the male heart, while the right ventricular mass is 25% less.[11] The left ventricular wall thickness of the septum is approximately 11% less in females versus males. The mean cardiac output in females is 5.6 L/min versus 6.7 L/min in males,[12] with corresponding mean heart rates of 79 and 74 beats per minute for females and males, respectively.[13]

Regarding function, the ejection fraction is 7% and 11% larger for the left and right ventricle, respectively for females compared to males. Similarly, circumferential strain is 11% greater and longitudinal strain is 14% greater in the left ventricle in females compared to males.[14]

Although tables of normal values reflect the above differences, the determination of pathologic significance used in common clinical conditions may not reflect the relevant physiology. For example, hypertrophic cardiomyopathy is defined by left ventricular wall thickness greater than or equal to 15 mm for both males and females.[15] Heart failure with preserved ejection fraction is considered as an ejection fraction greater than or equal to 50% for both males and females[16] (despite females having a higher baseline ejection fraction than males).

ETHNICITY VARIATION

Differences in cardiovascular outcome by ethnicity are well known. Excess risk of certain ethnic groups may be explained by different exposures (e.g., through environmental or socioeconomic differences) leading to the accumulation of risk factors. In addition, there may be different susceptibilities of some ethnic groups to certain exposures, such that risk factors have a stronger effect on certain ethnic groups.[17]

For example, in the National Health and Nutrition Examination Survey in the United States, Mexican Americans and non-Hispanic Blacks had elevated rates of cardiovascular risk factors compared to non-Hispanic Whites and non-Hispanic Asians.[18] However, in a large healthcare survey of 34,621 patients, Black patients had a 20% lower rate of death than Whites even after extensive adjustment for multiple healthcare characteristics and cardiovascular risk factors.[19] Thus, further understanding of the interaction between ethnicity and cardiovascular disease is warranted.

Techniques to measure cardiac size and structure have become more precise using cardiac MRI compared to echocardiography. Therefore, small differences between ethnic groups are more likely to be identified using MRI. In most populations, differences in cardiac size due to ethnicity may be obscured by structural and functional changes due to common cardiovascular risk factors. Therefore, large population samples of multiple ethnicities are needed to select only individuals without traditional cardiovascular risk factors. After removal of individuals with known risk factors, the remaining variation between ethnic groups has been ascribed to "ethnic variation."

The MESA study was the first large population study using cardiac MRI and had the aim of evaluating cardiovascular risk by ethnicity in the United States.[20] In this study, White, Hispanic, Asian, and African American individuals in the United States were evaluated. Only individuals without clinical cardiovascular disease were included. Natori et al. compared cardiac size and structure in 400 males and 400 females aged 45–84 years.[21] Individuals with traditional cardiovascular risk factors were excluded.

In MESA, the absolute values of cardiac size were similar for all groups with the exception of Asian Americans. Asian Americans had substantially smaller hearts than other groups for both males and females. For example, left ventricular volume for White males was 148 mL, but only 117 mL for Asian males (21% less). Left ventricular mass for Whites was 170 and 129 g for Asians (24% less). After indexing by body surface area, significant differences between Whites and Asians remained but were of lower magnitude. For example, the left ventricular end diastolic volume index for White males was 75 mL/m^2 and for Asian males was 68 mL/m^2 (9% less, $P < .05$). Left ventricular mass for White males was 86 g/m^2 and for Asian males was 76 g/m^2 (11% less, $P < .05$). Similar trends were noted in females. Further differences in cardiac parameters between various ethnic groups are increasingly being reported.[22–24]

Cardiac function is usually evaluated by ejection fraction, which is the difference between end diastolic and end systolic volume normalized by (divided by) end diastolic volume. In MESA, differences in ejection fraction by ethnicity were small (e.g., 66% for White males vs. 69% for Asian males). In addition, ejection fraction varies widely in the normal population and the reproducibility of measurement of ejection fraction is relatively low compared to other cardiac parameters. Thus, it is likely that differences in ejection fraction require less adjustment for ethnicity than other parameters. Compared to ejection fraction, myocardial strain is a sensitive measure of absolute values of myocardial contraction. In the MESA study, African Americans had 11% less circumferential myocardial strain than Chinese Americans.[25]

In summary, mean differences in cardiovascular structural parameters measured by MRI may vary by 10% to 20% between some ethnic groups. Cardiovascular function as measured by ejection fraction shows less variation by ethnicity. However, newer myocardial strain measures readily detect differences in function as a function of ethnicity. In recent years, gaps in the literature regarding cardiovascular parameters for individual ethnic groups are gradually being filled. In the coming years, it seems likely that imaging physicians will need to adapt normal reference values for cardiovascular structure and function to more closely match the ethnic characteristics of the local hospital population.

VARIATION WITH AGE

In adults, variation with age was demonstrated for some quantitative cardiovascular magnetic resonance parameters. In several studies it has been shown that absolute and indexed parameters of left and right ventricular volume are lower in older compared to younger males and females.[26–28] For left ventricular mass normalized to body surface area, no significant difference with age has been found.[28,29]

MAGNETIC RESONANCE IMAGING SCANNER AND PULSE SEQUENCE

The majority of clinical MRI scanners operate at either 1.5 or 3.0 T. Field strength as well as MRI scanner manufacturer are not expected to substantially affect normal cardiovascular parameters. Cardiac function and size are measured based on cine MRI. There are two cine methods that are used. The most common MRI cine pulse sequence is termed balanced steady-state free precession (bSSFP). This pulse sequence is preferred because blood and myocardial signal is relatively high and constant throughout the cardiac cycle. No exogenous contrast agent is needed. The bSSFP pulse sequence provides better contrast between the myocardial wall and blood pool relative to the previously used method for cardiac MRI cine, termed the fast gradient echo (FGRE) pulse sequence.

Today, the FGRE pulse sequence is primarily used for patients with implanted cardiac devices. This is because FGRE has less artifact around cardiac leads and generators compared to bSSFP. In addition, less interaction of FGRE versus bSSFP pulse sequences with implanted devices is expected. FGRE cine MRI may also be used for 3.0 T MRI when image quality is otherwise poor with bSSFP. Using FGRE, contrast between the myocardium and blood is derived from moving blood flowing into the imaging plane of interest. Particularly for long-axis views of the ventricles, blood is flowing within rather than through the plane of interest. As a result, myocardial blood pool contrast is highly variable on FGRE cine MRI.

Due to differences in spatial and contrast resolution, normal cardiac parameters will differ when derived from bSSFP versus FGRE cine MRI. Although FGRE normal values are available,[21] the remainder of this review will focus on bSSFP cine MRI, which is predominantly used for clinical cardiac MRI.

MAGNETIC RESONANCE IMAGING ANALYSIS METHODS AND SOFTWARE

Cine MRI using bSSFP pulse sequences shows relatively high signal in the myocardial cavity, compared to lower signal in the myocardial wall. This allows excellent depiction of intracavitary structures such as the papillary muscles, trabecula, and moderator band. However, the spatial resolution (1.5–2 mm in plane) is relatively low compared to the size of these structures. In addition, the bSSFP pulse sequence is associated with the so-called "India ink"artifact. This appears as a dark band (i.e., no signal) at any water-fat interface.[30] In the heart, the myocardium contains water; the fat interface is due to epicardial fat. The India ink artifact occurs when a single voxel contains both fat and water. In that circumstance, the signal cancels and is replaced by a black signal void.

Both the India ink artifact and somewhat low spatial resolution of cardiac cine MRI contribute to interobserver variation in defining the epicardial and endocardial contours. Most software for cardiac analysis is considered semiautomated: the software provides initial identification of myocardial contours with the human reader providing corrections. Substantial interobserver variation in cardiac volumes and function (10%–30%) will result unless strict training regimens are undertaken for the cardiac analyst to define myocardial borders.

Newer software increasingly uses artificial intelligence algorithms for contouring the epi and endocardial surfaces of the myocardium. Such software has been trained to mimic one or more human observers and has the advantage of consistency in defining the myocardial contours. However, different software packages use extremely different algorithms for defining myocardial contours. Normal cardiac values are expected to have different biases for quantifying myocardial volumes and mass depending on the software that is used. Algorithms are available for correcting differences between various software[31] but are not clinically used. The magnitude of differences between different cardiac software packages is generally unknown, but is likely to be on the order of 5% to 10%. Therefore, consistent use of the same cardiac software package is advised. When possible, published normal values that have been analyzed using the same individual site software package is preferred.

Cardiac Magnetic Resonance Imaging Analysis of the Ventricles

LEFT VENTRICLE

In general, analysis of the left ventricle is performed by evaluating a stack of short-axis slices extending from above the mitral valve to the cardiac apex. Cine MRI shows a generally smooth contour of the outer ventricular border: the epicardium. The endocardial border of the left ventricle is trabeculated most prominently in the mid and apical regions, sparing the septum. In addition, the anterior and posterior papillary muscles are identified (Fig. 16.1). Depending on the analysis software, the user has the option of two analysis approaches: (1) a smooth endocardial tracing resulting in papillary muscle volume being included as part of the left ventricular volume, and (2) an irregular endocardial tracing of major trabeculations with separate identification of the papillary muscles. In this model, the papillary muscles will be part of the left ventricular mass rather than the left ventricle volume (Fig. 16.1). The Society of Cardiovascular Magnetic Resonance indicates that either approach is acceptable[32] and that the choice of methods will depend on the available software. However, the Society standards also recommend that, ideally, the papillary muscles and trabeculation should be a component of left ventricular mass.[32] Finally, some centers have published a combination of these methods using a smooth endocardial contour with separate identification of papillary muscle mass.

As expected, the choice of segmentation method of the left ventricle has a substantial influence on the resulting normal values. For example, in the MESA study, the papillary muscles accounted for 9% of total left ventricular mass.[33] A proportional reduction in left ventricular volume will be obtained. Thus, each imaging center needs to be aware of the methods used for segmentation of the left ventricle and be certain to identify normal values that correspond with that method (i.e., as given in[1]). Normal values for the function and structure of the left ventricle are given in Tables 16.1–16.5.

MYOCARDIAL STRAIN

Myocardial strain is a general term used to describe deformation of the myocardial wall during contraction or relaxation. The most clinically used strain measurement (Lagrangian strain) is defined as (L1-L0)/L0, where L0 is the initial tissue position (typically at end diastole) and L1 is the final tissue position (at end systole). Thus, strain is expressed as a percentage. By convention, shortening of the myocardium (as in systole) is a negative strain. MRI-derived strain is analogous to echocardiography speckle tracking and is seeing increasing use for the evaluation of both ischemic and nonischemic heart disease.

There are two general methods for determining strain with cardiac MRI.[34] The original approach uses special MRI pulse sequences to allow tracking of myocardial motion. This approach is termed tagged MRI.[35] Tagged MRI is implemented clinically as a spatial modulation of magnetization pulse sequence.[36] While it is considered the standard of reference, the tagged MRI approach is used infrequently due to the requirement for additional MRI scan time and complex postprocessing.

A more recent development for extracting myocardial strain values from cardiac cine MRI is the use of so-called "feature-tracking" software. This software approach identifies the movement of endocardial and epicardial features during the cardiac cycle, allowing rapid calculation of myocardial strain from standard cine images. The calculations can be applied to any cardiac chamber; strain values can be regional (e.g., over the septum only) or over the entire heart chamber (e.g., left ventricular global strain). For MRI, the most common strain measures include assessment of longitudinal and circumferential shortening. Shortening in the radial direction may also be reported but is less accurate due to the relatively thin ventricular wall.

Myocardial strain measured by feature-tracking software is dependent on the sophistication and internal calculations of each specific software package.[37] In addition, strain calculations will vary depending on the MRI cine pulse sequence parameters. A guide to normal left ventricular myocardial strain values is given in Table 16.6.

RIGHT VENTRICLE

Segmentation of the right ventricle is usually performed based on short-axis views.[1] Unfortunately, standard short-axis images are oblique to the right ventricular outflow tract. Identification of the boundary between the right

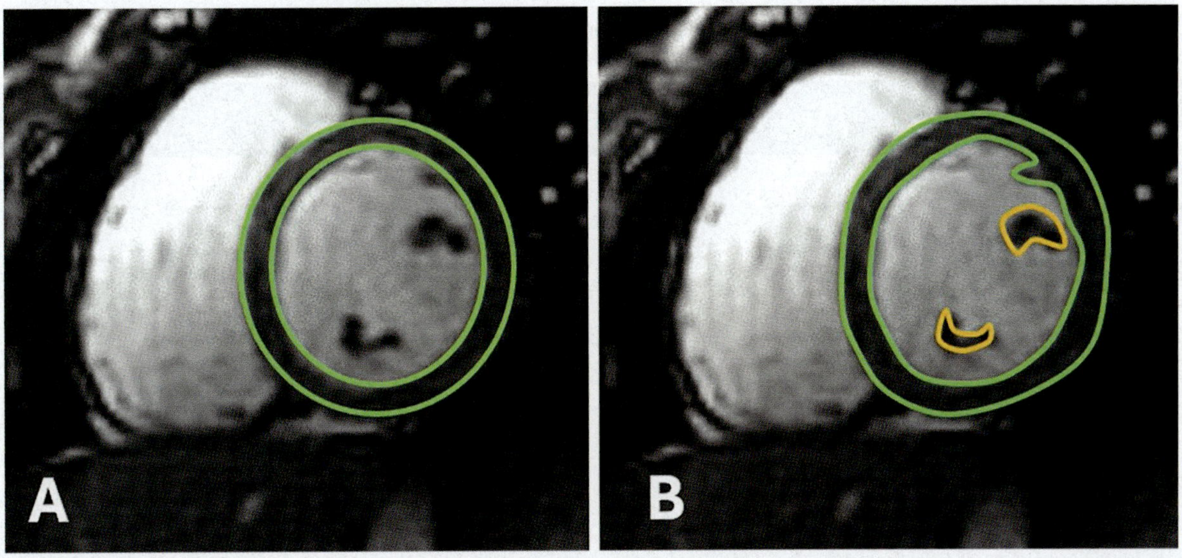

FIG. 16.1 Comparison of two contouring methods according to the Society for Cardiac Magnetic Resonance.[32] (A) Smooth endocardial contour (*green*) without consideration of trabeculation or papillary muscles. (B) Endocardial contour (*green*) that accounts for trabeculation as well as papillary muscles (*orange*). In this method, the left ventricular mass includes papillary muscle mass and trabecular mass.

TABLE 16.1 Left ventricular parameters for adult males and females (age 18–83), papillary muscles included in the left ventricular mass.

	MALES		FEMALES	
PARAMETER	MEAN	LL–UL	MEAN	LL–UL
LVEDV (mL)	155	95–215	123	78–167
LVEDV/BSA (mL/m²)	79	50–108	73	50–96
LVESV (mL)	55	25–85	43	21–64
LVESV/BSA (mL/m²)	29	11–47	25	10–40
LVSV (mL)	103	61–145	83	52–114
LVSV/BSA (mL/m²)	52	33–72	49	33–64
LVEF (%)	64	49–79	66	52–79
LVM (g)	121	66–176	83	41–125
LVM/BSA (g/m²)	62	39–85	49	30–68
LVCO (L/min)	5.6	3.4–7.8	4.5	2.7–6.3
LVCI (L/min/m²)	3	1.8–4.2	2.9	1.9–3.9
LVM/LVEDV (g/mL)	0.7	0.4–0.9	0.6	0.3–0.8

BSA, body surface area; *CI*, cardiac index; *CO*, cardiac output; *EDV*, end-diastolic volume; *EF*, ejection fraction; *ESV*, end-systolic volume; *LL*, lower limit; *LV*, left ventricular; *LVM*, left ventricular mass; *SV*, stroke volume; *UL*, upper limit.

From Kawel-Boehm, N. et al., Reference ranges ("normal values") for cardiovascular magnetic resonance (CMR) in adults and children: 2020 update. *J Cardiovasc Magn Reson*. 2020. 22(1): p. 87.

atrium and right ventricle is difficult. The right ventricle is also highly trabeculated, with similar considerations for tracing endocardial contours as discussed previously for the left ventricle. The greatest variability between observers has been found to be in the tricuspid zone and the right ventricular outflow tract.[38] This can result in substantial interobserver variation in right ventricular volumes of 10% to 15% unless substantial training is undertaken. While this interobserver variation can be substantially reduced for core laboratory research studies,[39] variability is likely to be higher for clinical studies.

An alternative approach is the use of a stack of transaxially oriented slices for segmentation of the right ventricle. This method has been shown to substantially reduce segmentation errors compared to short-axis right ventricle segmentation (e.g., ejection fraction error 1.7% for transaxial images vs. 10.5% for short-axis images).[40] In addition, reader reproducibility is much better when transaxial images are used for right ventricle segmentation (e.g., intraclass correlation, 0.67 transaxial images vs. 0.42 for short-axis images). Cardiac MRI physicians may consider the use of transaxial image acquisition and analysis for particularly critical cases, such as congenital heart disease. This method, however, can require 8 to 10 minutes of additional imaging time. Therefore, for unstable infants, additional imaging time must be weighed relative to potential negative consequences of longer MRI scan time.

TABLE 16.2 Left ventricular parameters for adult males and females (age 18–83), papillary muscles included in the left ventricular volume.

	MALES		FEMALES	
PARAMETER	MEAN	LL–UL	MEAN	LL–UL
LVEDV (mL)	145	83–207	112	70–155
LVEDV/BSA (mL/m²)	77	47–107	69	45–93
LVESV (mL)	53	19–88	39	15–64
LVESV/BSA (mL/m²)	29	11–47	24	10–38
LVSV (mL)	91	55–127	73	47–99
LVSV/BSA (mL/m²)	48	30–66	45	30–59
LVEF (%)	63	51–76	66	52–79
LVM (g)	105	57–152	73	43–103
LVM/BSA (g/m²)	56	36–75	45	30–59
LVCO (L/min)	6.1	3.9–8.3	4.9	3.0–6.9
LVCI (L/min/m²)	3.2	2.1–4.3	2.9	1.9–4.0
LVM/LVEDV (g/mL)	0.7	0.3–1.2	0.7	0.4–1.0

BSA, Body surface area *CI*, cardiac index; *CO*, cardiac output; *EDV*, end-diastolic volume; *EF*, ejection fraction; *ESV*, end-systolic volume; *LL*, lower limit; *LV*, left ventricular; *LVM*, left ventricular mass; *SV*, stroke volume; *UL*, upper limit.
From Kawel-Boehm, N. et al., Reference ranges ("normal values") for cardiovascular magnetic resonance (CMR) in adults and children: 2020 update. *J Cardiovasc Magn Reson*, 2020. 22(1): p. 87.

TABLE 16.3 Left ventricular diameters in adult males and females.

	MALES		FEMALES	
PARAMETER	MEAN	LL–UL	MEAN	LL–UL
LV end-diastolic diameter 4Ch (mm)	52	42–62	49	39–59
LV end-diastolic diameter SAx (mm)	53	44–62	49	41–57
LV end-systolic diameter 4Ch (mm)	32	26–38	28	16–40
LV end-systolic diameter SAx (mm)	34	28–40	31	23–39

4Ch, 4-Chamber view; *BSA*, body surface area; *CI*, cardiac index; *LL*, lower limit; *LV*, left ventricular; *SAx*, short-axis cardiac output; *UL*, upper limit.
From Kawel-Boehm, N. et al., Reference ranges ("normal values") for cardiovascular magnetic resonance (CMR) in adults and children: 2020 update. *J Cardiovasc Magn Reson*. 2020. 22(1): p. 87.

Normal values for the function and structure of the right ventricle are given in Table 16.7.

Cardiovascular Magnetic Resonance Analysis of the Atria

Atrial volumes and function are most commonly assessed using the biplane or monoplane area-length formulas adapted from echocardiography.[41] An alternative approach uses the Simpson method (sum of the cross-sectional areas) based on short-axis cine images of the ventricles.

For the monoplane and biplane methods, the left atrium is modeled as an ellipse. For the biplane method, the left atrial volume is calculated as $[8/3\pi] * [(A1 * A2)/(L)]$, where A1 and A2 are the areas of the left atrium in the four-chamber and two-chamber views (Fig. 16.2). In this formula, L is the shortest length of either A1 or A2. Atrial volume can also be estimated from a single view, typically the 4-chamber view, by assuming A1 = A2. In this case, the monoplane area-length formula is $8(A^2/3\pi L)$, where A is the area of the atrium and L is the long-axis dimension of the atria in the same view. Most prior research recommends the biplane method.[41] For normal values determined using the biplane and monoplane approaches, the left atrial appendage and the confluence of the pulmonary veins are excluded from the atrial areas.

A complete segmentation of the atria at end systole and end diastole can also be performed without assumption of an ellipsoidal volume using a stack of short-axis slices (Simpson's rule, sum of the cross-sectional areas). This approach is theoretically the most accurate approach. In this method, atrial appendage volume is included in the total atrial volume. The method, however, requires additional short-axis acquisitions through the atria that are otherwise omitted in a routine cardiac acquisition. Further, due to their small size, thinner slices are more accurate than the relatively thick (6–8 mm) slices used to image the ventricles. Nacif et al. compared the biplane and Simpson's method. While both methods were found to be reproducible, the resulting volumes were not interchangeable.[42]

Normal values for the left and right atria are given in Tables 16.8–16.11.

TABLE 16.4 Left ventricular wall thickness for males and females.

IMAGING PLANE: SHORT AXIS						IMAGING PLANE: LONG AXIS					
		MALES		FEMALES				MALES		FEMALES	
LEVEL	SEGMENT	MEAN (MM)	LL–UL	MEAN (MM)	LL–UL	LEVEL	SEGMENT	MEAN (MM)	LL–UL	MEAN (MM)	LL–UL
Basal	1	7.8	5–10	6.4	4–9	Basal	Anterior	8.2	6–11	7	5–9
	2	9	6–12	7.6	5–10		Inferior	8.2	6–10	6.7	5–9
	3	8.8	6–11	7.3	5–9		Septal	9.1	7–12	7.3	5–10
	4	7.9	6–10	6.4	4–8		Lateral	7.6	5–10	6	4–8
	5	7.7	5–10	6.3	4–9		Mean	8.3	6–10	6.8	5–9
	6	7.5	5–10	6.1	4–8	Midcavity	Anterior	6	3–9	4.9	3–7
Midcavity	7	6.7	4–9	5.6	4–8		Inferior	7.7	5–10	6.5	4–9
	8	7.4	5–10	6.1	4–8		Septal	8.3	6–11	6.8	5–9
	9	7.9	6–10	6.6	5–9		Lateral	6.6	4–9	5.3	3–8
	10	7	5–9	5.8	4–8		Mean	7.2	5–9	6	4–8
	11	6.5	4–9	5.3	3–7	Apical	Anterior	5.1	3–8	4.2	2–6
	12	6.6	4–9	5.5	4–8		Inferior	5.8	3–8	5	3–7
Apical	13	6.5	4–9	5.9	3–9		Septal	5.8	3–8	5	3–7
	14	6.8	4–9	5.8	4–8		Lateral	5.5	3–8	4.6	2–7
	15	6.1	4–8	5.2	3–7		Mean	5.6	4–8	4.7	3–7
	16	6.2	4–8	5.6	4–8						

LL, lower limits; *SD,* standard deviation; *UL,* upper limits.
Segments: 1: basal anterior, 2: basal anteroseptal, 3: basal inferoseptal, 4: basal inferior, 5: basal inferolateral, 6: basal anterolateral, 7: midanterior, 8: midanteroseptal, 9: midinferoseptal, 10: midinferior, 11: midinferolateral, 12: midanterolateral, 13: apical anterior, 14: apical septal, 15: apical inferior, 16: apical lateral.
From Kawel-Boehm, N. et al., Reference ranges ("normal values") for cardiovascular magnetic resonance (CMR) in adults and children: 2020 update. *J Cardiovasc Magn Reson.* 2020. 22(1): p. 87.

TABLE 16.5 Left ventricular end-diastolic wall thickness (short-axis measurement).

		MALES		FEMALES	
LEVEL	SEGMENT	MEAN (MM)	LL–UL	MEAN (MM)	LL–UL
Basal	1	7.8	5–10	6.4	4–9
	2	9	6–12	7.6	5–10
	3	8.8	6–11	7.3	5–9
	4	7.9	6–10	6.4	4–8
	5	7.7	5–10	6.3	4–9
	6	7.5	5–10	6.1	4–8
Midcavity	7	6.7	4–9	5.6	4–8
	8	7.4	5–10	6.1	4–8
	9	7.9	6–10	6.6	5–9
	10	7	5–9	5.8	4–8
	11	6.5	4–9	5.3	3–7
	12	6.6	4–9	5.5	4–8
Apical*	13	6.5	4–9	5.9	3–9
	14	6.8	4–9	5.8	4–8
	15	6.1	4–8	5.2	3–7
	16	6.2	4–8	5.6	4–8

*Due to nonorthogonal image slices at the apex, the measured apical wall thickness may be greater on short-axis images versus long-axis images. Orthogonal long-axis images should be checked to confirm wall thickness.
Segments: 1: basal anterior, 2: basal anteroseptal, 3: basal inferoseptal, 4: basal inferior, 5: basal inferolateral, 6: basal anterolateral, 7: midanterior, 8: midanteroseptal, 9: midinferoseptal, 10: midinferior, 11: midinferolateral, 12: midanterolateral, 13: apical anterior, 14: apical septal, 15: apical inferior, 16: apical lateral
LL, Lower limits; *UL,* upper limits.
From Kawel-Boehm, N. et al., Reference ranges ("normal values") for cardiovascular magnetic resonance (CMR) in adults and children: 2020 update. *J Cardiovasc Magn Reson,* 2020. 22(1): p. 87.

TABLE 16.6 Left ventricular global peak circumferential and longitudinal strain in adults, 2D feature tracking.

	MALES		FEMALES	
PARAMETER	MEAN	LL–UL	MEAN	LL–UL
Circumferential strain (%)	−20.9	−27.2 to −14.6	−22.7	−29.2 to −16.2
Longitudinal strain (%)	−19.4	−26.1 to −12.7	−21.4	−28.7 to −14.2

LL, lower limit; *UL*, upper limit.

From Kawel-Boehm, N. et al., Reference ranges ("normal values") for cardiovascular magnetic resonance (CMR) in adults and children: 2020 update. *J Cardiovasc Magn Reson*. 2020. 22(1): p. 87.

TABLE 16.7 Right ventricular parameters in adult males and females (age 20–83); papillary muscles included in the right ventricular volume.

	MALES		FEMALES	
PARAMETER	MEAN	LL–UL	MEAN	LL–UL
RVEDV (mL)	166	87–244	122	68–176
RVEDV/BSA (mL/m²)	88	53–123	76	48–104
RVESV (mL)	73	29–117	50	20–80
RVESV/BSA (mL/m²)	38	17–59	30	13–48
RVSV (mL)	95	43–146	74	39–109
RVSV/BSA (mL/m²)	52	28–75	48	29–66
RVEF (%)	57	42–72	60	46–74
RVM (g)	36	17–54	30	13–48
RVM/BSA (g/m²)	19	10–28	17	7–28
RVCO (L/min)	5.6	2.8–8.3	4.4	2.4–6.4
RVCI (L/min/m²)	3	1.5–4.5	2.8	1.6–4.0

BSA, body surface area; *CI*, cardiac index; *CO*, cardiac output; *EDV*, end-diastolic volume; *EF*, ejection fraction; *ESV*, end-systolic volume; *LL*, lower limit; *RV*, right ventricular; *RVM*, right ventricular mass; *SV*, stroke volume; *UL*, upper limit.

From Kawel-Boehm, N. et al., Reference ranges ("normal values") for cardiovascular magnetic resonance (CMR) in adults and children: 2020 update. *J Cardiovasc Magn Reson*. 2020. 22(1): p. 87.

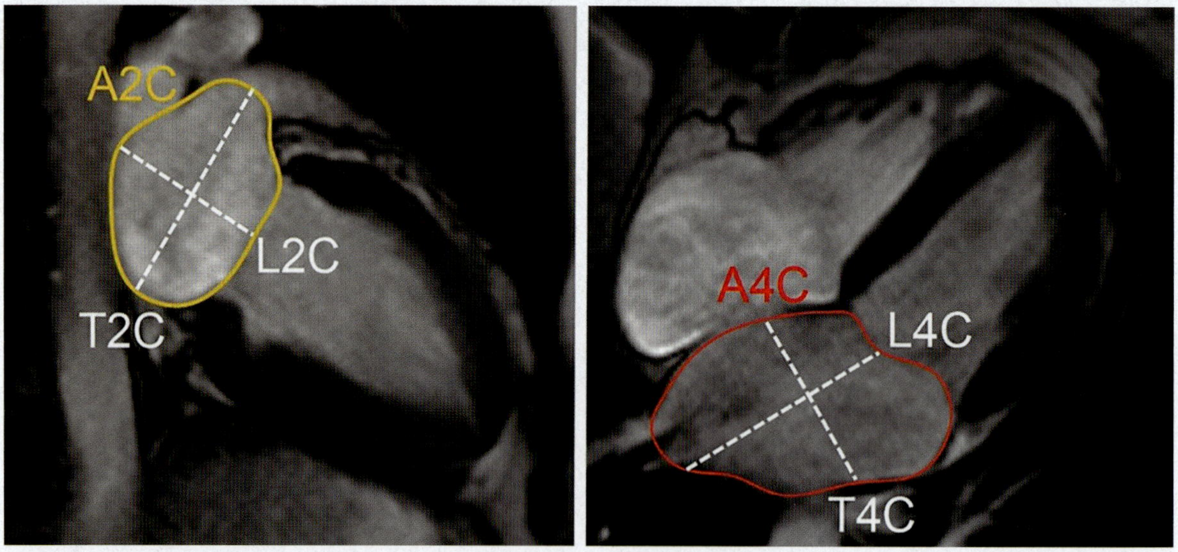

FIG. 16.2 Measurement of left atrial dimensions using the biplanar method. Measurement of left atrial area on 2- and 4-chamber views. (A2Ch, A4Ch—atrial area on 2- and 4-chamber views respectively) (L2Ch, L4Ch—longitudinal diameters on 2- and 4-chamber views) (T2Ch, T4Ch—transverse diameters on 2- and 4-chamber views). (From Maceira AM, Cosin-Sales J, Roughton M, et. al., Reference left atrial dimensions and volumes by steady state free precession cardiovascular magnetic resonance. *J Cardiovasc Magn Reson*, 2010; 12(1):65)

CONSIDERATIONS FOR ATHLETES

Due to cardiovascular adaptation and training, normal cardiovascular structure and function in athletes need separate consideration from nonathletes. The primary concern is competitive rather than recreational athletes: in competitive athletes, physiologic adaptation of the heart can overlap with pathologic conditions on imaging studies.

Physical activity is classified by the level of intensity (low, medium, or high) in addition to the type of exercise being performed. Two extremes of exercise category can be defined as "dynamic" or "static" activity.[43] Dynamic

TABLE 16.8 Left atrial volumes and function in the adult, biplane area-length method (left atrial appendage excluded (Fig. 16.2)).

	MALES		FEMALES	
PARAMETER	MEAN	LL–UL	MEAN	LL–UL
Max. LA volume (mL)	72	31–112	64	28–100
Max. LA volume/BSA (mL/m^2)	38	17–59	39	17–61
Min. LA volume (mL)	25	6–44	22	7–38
Min. LA volume/BSA (mL/m^2)	14	3–24	13	4–23
LA stroke volume (mL)	44	21–67	42	21–62
LA stroke volume/BSA (mL/m^2)	22	10–34	22	10–34
LA ejection fraction (%)	62	46–77	63	48–78

BSA, body surface area; *LA*, left atrial; *LL*, lower limit; *Max*, maximal; *Min*, minimal; *UL*, upper limit.
From Kawel-Boehm, N. et al., Reference ranges ("normal values") for cardiovascular magnetic resonance (CMR) in adults and children: 2020 update. *J Cardiovasc Magn Reson*. 2020. 22(1): p. 87.

TABLE 16.9 Left atrial diameters in the adult.

	MALES		FEMALES	
PARAMETER	MEAN	LL–UL	MEAN	LL–UL
Max. LA longitudinal diameter 2Ch (cm)	4.9	3.5–6.2	4.6	3.3–5.9
Max. LA transverse diameter 2Ch (cm)	4.4	3.2–5.6	4.3	3.3–5.2
Max. LA longitudinal diameter 3Ch (cm)	5.5	4.2–6.8	5.4	4.0–6.7
Max. LA antero-posterior diameter 3Ch (cm)	3	2.0–4.0	3	2.0–4.0
Max. LA longitudinal diameter 4Ch (cm)	5.8	4.6–7.1	5.5	4.2–6.8
Max. LA transverse diameter 4Ch (cm)	4.3	3.3–5.3	4.1	3.1–5.1

2Ch, 2-chamber view; *3Ch*, 3-chamber view; *4Ch*, 4-chamber view; *LA*, left atrial; *LL*, lower limit; *Max*, maximal; *UL*, upper limit.
From Kawel-Boehm, N. et al., Reference ranges ("normal values") for cardiovascular magnetic resonance (CMR) in adults and children: 2020 update. *J Cardiovasc Magn Reson*. 2020. 22(1): p. 87.

TABLE 16.10 Right atrial volumes and function in the adult, biplane area-length method (right atrial appendage excluded).

	MALES		FEMALES	
PARAMETER	MEAN	LL–UL	MEAN	LL–UL
Max. RA volume (mL)	20	69	14	24–81
Max. RA volume/BSA (mL/m^2)	12	69	10	16–54
Min. RA volume (mL)	12	69	7	9–37
Min. RA volume/BSA (mL/m^2)	7	69	5	6–24
RA ejection fraction (%)	9	69	9	38–74

BSA, body surface area; *LL*, lower limit; *Max*, maximal; *Min*, minimal; *RA*, right atrial; *UL*, upper limit.
From Kawel-Boehm, N. et al., Reference ranges ("normal values") for cardiovascular magnetic resonance (CMR) in adults and children: 2020 update. *J Cardiovasc Magn Reson*. 2020. 22(1): p. 87.

exercise involves contraction of large muscle groups and maximal aerobic activity. Examples of primarily dynamic exercise include long-distance running, badminton, cross-country skiing, and soccer. Static exercise refers to exercise with sustained muscular contraction, often repetitive, with maximum voluntary contraction. Examples of primarily static exercise include martial arts, weightlifting, and gymnastics. However, many types of exercise are a combination of both dynamic and static types (e.g., boxing, kayaking, cycling, triathlon).

The distinction between dynamic and static exercise types corresponds to an observed pattern of exercise-induced cardiac remodeling (Fig 16.3). Athletes who engage primarily in dynamic exercise, such as endurance athletes, display a pattern of eccentric left ventricular remodeling; this is frequently accompanied by dilatation of the right ventricle and both atria. Athletes who engage primarily in static exercise, such as weightlifters, display concentric left ventricular remodeling with minimal effects on the other three chambers. Activities with both dynamic and static exercise, or simply more modern exercise programs involving combination-type training, show intermediate patterns between these two extremes.

Exercise-induced cardiac remodeling with concentric hypertrophy (11–13 mm wall thickness) in athletes has the potential to overlap with the normal values of nonathletes for cardiac chamber size.[44] For example, thickening of the left ventricular chamber wall of more

TABLE 16.11 Right atrial diameters in the adult.

	MALES		FEMALES	
PARAMETER	MEAN	LL–UL	MEAN	LL–UL
Max. RA area 2Ch (cm^2)	23	15–31	21	13–29
Max. RA area 4Ch (cm^2)	21	13–30	19	12–26
Max. RA longitudinal diameter 2Ch (cm)	5.5	4.2–6.7	5.1	3.9–6.3
Max. RA transverse diameter 2Ch (cm)	4.2	2.4–6.0	4.1	2.4–5.9
Max. RA longitudinal diameter 4Ch (cm)	5.3	4.0–6.6	5.1	4.0–6.3
Max. RA transverse diameter 4Ch (cm)	4.8	3.7–5.9	4.3	3.2–5.4

2Ch, 2-Chamber view; *3Ch*, 3-chamber view; *4Ch*, 4-chamber view; *LL*, lower limit; *Max*, maximal; *RA*, right atrial; *UL*, upper limit.
From Kawel-Boehm, N. et al., Reference ranges ("normal values") for cardiovascular magnetic resonance (CMR) in adults and children: 2020 update. *J Cardiovasc Magn Reson*. 2020. 22(1): p. 87.

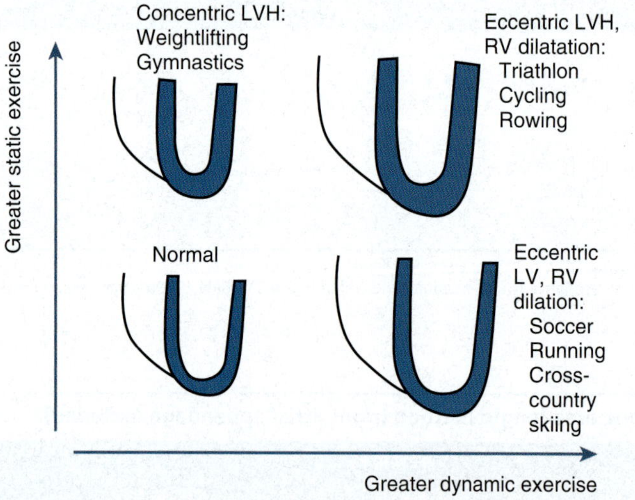

FIG. 16.3 The relationship between exercise-induced cardiac remodeling and type of exercise. Dynamic exercise involves contraction of large muscle groups and maximal aerobic activity. Static exercise refers to exercise with sustained muscular contraction, often repetitive, with maximum voluntary contraction. (Adapted from Baggish, A.L. et al., Sports Cardiology: Core Curriculum for Providing Cardiovascular Care to Competitive Athletes and Highly Active People. *J Am Coll Cardiol*. 2017. **70**(15): p. 1902–1918.)

than 12mm may result in a diagnosis of left ventricular hypertrophy. Hypertrophic cardiomyopathy is a potential diagnostic consideration when left ventricular wall thickness is greater than or equal to 15mm. This level of hypertrophy is felt to be uncommon in athletes and warrants individualized evaluation.[43]

Overlap between chamber size normal values and physiological adaptation from exercise has been described as the "gray zone."[45] Three patterns of gray zone overlap between athlete and nonathlete normal values are described:[43]

1) Thickened left ventricular wall. This category is associated with static exercise. In the athlete's heart (vs. pathologic thickening), wall thickness is usually less than 15mm; right ventricular dimensions are normal. Valves are normal.
2) Dilatation of the left ventricle. This category is associated with dynamic exercise. In the athlete's heart, associated findings include mild right ventricular dilatation and mild left ventricular wall thickening. The atria are within normal limits or mildly enlarged. Valves are normal. Ejection fraction is normal or low normal.
3) Dilation of the right ventricle. This category is also associated with dynamic exercise. In the athlete's heart, the left ventricle may also be mildly dilated. The right ventricle has normal morphology, and atrial size is within normal limits or mildly enlarged. Valves are normal. Ejection fraction is normal or low normal.

Normal values for the right and left ventricle for athletes are given in Table 16.12.

EVALUATION OF VALVULAR DISEASE AND FLOW BY CARDIAC MAGNETIC RESONANCE IMAGING

Methods for flow evaluation by MRI use phase-contrast MRI techniques to determine blood flow, velocity, and direction. Both two-dimensional and three-dimensional pulse sequences are available using cine phase-contrast MRI.[46,47] Normal flow values and criteria for assessment of valvular stenosis or insufficiency are based on American Heart Association guidelines.[48] Cut-off values for normal and criteria for various valvular disease states are shown in Table 16.13. These cut-off values are based on echocardiography, as cardiac MRI–based values have not been published to date.

AORTA AND PULMONARY ARTERIES

Aortic and pulmonary artery evaluation is relatively routine and rapid using cardiac magnetic resonance angiography (MRA). Three-dimensional MRA methods are available for single breath-hold (approximately 20seconds) evaluation. However, breath-hold MRA lacks the spatial and temporal resolution generally required for evaluation of aortic root size (e.g., for transcatheter aortic valve replacement). Evaluation of the aortic root during systole is performed using electrocardiographic- and

TABLE 16.12 Ventricular parameters for adult elite athletes >18 hours sports activity per week (papillary muscles included in the left ventricular volume).

	MEAN ± SD (LL–UL)			MEAN ± SD (LL–UL)	
LEFT VENTRICLE	MALES	FEMALES	RIGHT VENTRICLE	MALES	FEMALES
LVEDV (mL)	261 ± 39 (183–339)	199 ± 31 (137–261)	RVEDV (mL)	291 ± 48 (195–387)	219 ± 35 (149–289)
LVEDV/BSA (mL/m²)	129 ± 17 (95–163)	107 ± 14 (79–135)	RVEDV/BSA (mL/m²)	144 ± 20 (104–184)	118 ± 17 (84–152)
LVESV (mL)	117 ± 24 (69–165)	85 ± 20 (45–125)	RVESV (mL)	148 ± 30 (88–208)	103 ± 24 (55–151)
LVESV/BSA (mL/m²)	58 ± 11 (36–80)	46 ± 11 (24–68)	RVESV/BSA (mL/m²)	73 ± 13 (47–99)	56 ± 13 (30–82)
LVM (g)	139 ± 28 (83–195)	92 ± 15 (62–122)	RVM (g)	30 ± 6 (18–42)	25 ± 5 (15–35)
LVM/BSA (g/m²)	69 ± 13 (43–95)	50 ± 8 (34–66)	RVM/BSA (g/m²)	15 ± 2 (11–19)	14 ± 3 (8–20)
LVEF (%)	55 ± 5 (45–65)	58 ± 7 (44–72)	RVEF (%)	50 ± 4 (42–58)	53 ± 7 (39–67)
Max. IVS (mm)	11 ± 1 (9–13)	9 ± 1 (7–11)			

BSA, Body surface area; *EDV*, end-diastolic volume; *EF*, ejection fraction; *ESV*, end-systolic volume; *LL*, lower limit; *LV*, left ventricular; *LVM*, left ventricular mass; *max. IVS*, maximal thickness of the interventricular septum; *RV*, right ventricular; *RVM*, right ventricular mass; *SD*, standard deviation; *UL*, upper limit.
From Kawel-Boehm, N. et al., Reference ranges ("normal values") for cardiovascular magnetic resonance (CMR) in adults and children: 2020 update. *J Cardiovasc Magn Reson*. 2020. 22(1): p. 87.

TABLE 16.13 Assessment of valvular heart disease in the adult.

		STAGE	
VALVE DISEASE	PARAMETER	PROGRESSIVE	SEVERE
Aortic stenosis	Maximum velocity (m/s)	Mild: 2.0–2.9	Severe: ≥4
		Moderate: 3.0–3.9	Very severe: ≥5
			Low-flow/low-gradient: <4 m/s (at rest)
	Orifice area (cm²)		≤1.0
	Orifice area/BSA (cm²/m²)		≤0.6
Aortic regurgitation	Regurgitant volume (ml/beat)	Mild: <30	≥60
		Moderate: 30–59	
	Regurgitant fraction (%)	Mild: <30	≥50
		Moderate: 30–49	
	Effective regurgitant orifice (cm2)	Mild: <0.10	≥0.30
		Moderate: 0.10–0.29	
Mitral stenosis	Transmitral flow velocity (m/s)	Increased	
	Orifice area (cm²)	>1.5	Severe: ≤1.5
			Very severe: ≤1.0
Primary mitral regurgitation	Regurgitant volume (ml/beat)	<60	≥60
	Regurgitant fraction (%)	<50	≥50
	Effective regurgitant orifice (cm²)	<0.40	≥0.40
Secondary mitral regurgitation	Regurgitant volume (ml/beat)	<60	≥60
	Regurgitant fraction (%)	<50	≥50
	Effective regurgitant orifice (cm²)	<0.40	≥0.40
Pulmonic stenosis	Peak velocity (m/s)		>4
Tricuspid stenosis	Orifice area (cm²)		<1.0

BSA, body surface area
From Kawel-Boehm, N. et al., Reference ranges ("normal values") for cardiovascular magnetic resonance (CMR) in adults and children: 2020 update. *J Cardiovasc Magn Reson*. 2020. 22(1): p. 87.

respiratory-gated three-dimensional MRA, which requires longer scan times of several minutes. Two-dimensional flow images are less attractive for this purpose due to difficulty in obtaining multiple imaging planes exactly orthogonal to the valve and aorta. Normal values for MRI of the thoracic aorta and pulmonary arteries are shown in Tables 16.14 and 16.15.

MYOCARDIAL TISSUE CHARACTERIZATION

An important use of cardiac MRI is for the evaluation of infiltrative or inflammatory changes in the myocardium. The most frequently detected myocardial abnormality by MRI is myocardial scar using late gadolinium enhancement (LGE) MRI methods. This well-known

TABLE 16.14 Normal diameter of the thoracic aortic lumen for adults.

LEVEL	MALES MEAN ± SD (LL–UL)	FEMALES MEAN ± SD (LL–UL)
Ascending aorta diameter	27 ± 4 (19–34) mm	26 ± 4 (18–33) mm
Proximal descending aorta diameter	21 ± 3 (15–26) mm	19 ± 2 (15–23) mm
Distal descending aorta diameter	18 ± 3 (13–23) mm	16 ± 2 (12–20) mm
Aortic sinus diameter (cusp-commissure)	34 ± 3 (27–40) mm	30 ± 3 (25–35) mm
Aortic sinus diameter (cusp-cusp)	36 ± 4 (28–44) mm	32 ± 3 (26–38) mm
Aortic sinus area	9.2 ± 2.1 (5.0–13.4) cm^2	7.1 ± 1.4 (4.3–9.9) cm^2

Diameters measured on balanced steady-state free precession images.
LL, lower limit; *SD*, standard deviation; *UL*, upper limit.
Aortic sinus measurements at systole.
From Kawel-Boehm, N. et al., Reference ranges ("normal values") for cardiovascular magnetic resonance (CMR) in adults and children: 2020 update. *J Cardiovasc Magn Reson*. 2020. 22(1): p. 87.

TABLE 16.15 Normal diameter of the pulmonary arteries in adults.

VESSEL	PARAMETER	MALES MEAN	MALES LL–UL	FEMALES MEAN	FEMALES LL–UL
MPA	Systolic diameter (mm)	27.4	21–33	25.3	19–31
	Systolic area (cm^2)	5.9	3.7–8.1	5	3.0–7.0
RPA	Systolic diameter (mm)	20.2	14–26	17.8	14–22
	Systolic area (cm^2)	3.3	1.3–5.3	2.6	1.2–4.0
LPA	Systolic diameter (mm)	20.1	16–24	18.4	14–22
	Systolic area (cm^2)	3.3	1.7–4.9	2.8	1.6–4.0

LL, lower limit; *LPA*, left pulmonary artery; *MPA*, main pulmonary artery; *RPA*, right pulmonary artery; *UL*, upper limit.
From Kawel-Boehm, N. et al., Reference ranges ("normal values") for cardiovascular magnetic resonance (CMR) in adults and children: 2020 update. *J Cardiovasc Magn Reson*. 2020. 22(1): p. 87.

method identifies collagen deposition in dense myocardial scar. The general method of LGE MRI involves qualitative/visual evaluation of myocardial tissue with enhancing (bright) regions after the administration of a gadolinium-based contrast agent. Because it is a qualitative method, normal values are not applicable to the LGE technique.

For quantitative analysis, measurement of MRI signal over the entire myocardium is termed MRI tissue "mapping". The MRI parameters that are "mapped" are the T1, T2, and T2* relaxation times of the myocardium. In brief, the T1 relaxation time measures the longitudinal relaxation rate of the myocardium while T2 reflects the transverse magnetization. The T2* time reflects rapid decay of the T2 relaxation time due to local magnetic field inhomogeneities associated with iron deposition. More complete descriptions of MRI relaxation times can be found in standard texts and descriptions.[30]

At present, the most frequent use of the T1 relaxation time is for diagnosis of deposition disease (e.g., amyloidosis, Fabry disease). For deposition disease, a range of normal T1 relaxation times needs to be identified; very high or low values are due to abnormal tissue deposition within the myocardium. Both T1 and T2 relaxation times have special utility for identification of myocarditis.[49] T2* times are evaluated when iron deposition disease is a diagnostic consideration.

Normal values for quantitative MRI parameters are influenced by multiple factors, including MRI field strength, MRI manufacturer, and pulse sequence. The Society for Cardiac Magnetic Resonance suggests that each MRI site develop local normative standards for MRI tissue mapping.[50] This involves scanning 50 or more normal volunteers on each MRI scanner.[51] Caution is advised when using published normal values for diagnostic purposes for T1 and T2 relaxation times; cardiac imaging physicians must ensure that similar pulse sequence parameters and field strengths are comparable to the published values. Tables 16.16 and 16.17 show representative combinations for MRI field strengths, pulse sequences, and manufacturer. T2* times are not expected to show large variation by manufacturer or pulse sequence. Cut-off values for normal and abnormal T2* times are shown in Table 16.18.

The usefulness of the T1 mapping technique in clinical routine is limited by a large overlap between the normal reference range and various cardiomyopathies and infiltrative cardiopathies. Furthermore, a change in myocardial T1 time is not specific for a particular substrate. An increase in the native T1 time can be due to, for example, fibrosis, amyloid, or edema, a shortening due to fat or iron. The parallel deposition of fibrosis and fat, for example, can result in a pseudonormalization of myocardial T1 time. An increase in myocardial T2 relaxation time is more specific and usually related to edema.

TABLE 16.16 Native myocardial T1 relaxation time and extracellular volume fraction in adults.

PARAMETER	FS (T)	VENDOR	TECHNIQUE	MEAN (MS)	SD (MS)	LL–UL (MS)
Native T1 time (ms)	1.5	Siemens	MOLLI	972	43	885–1059
	1.5	Siemens	ShMOLLI	960	29	903–1017
	1.5	Philips	MOLLI	989	42	905–1073
	3	Siemens	MOLLI	1196	47	1103–1290
	3	Siemens	ShMOLLI	1130	55	1021–1240
	3	Philips	MOLLI	1097	66	964–1230
ECV (%)	1.5	Siemens	MOLLI	26	3	20–32
	1.5	Siemens	ShMOLLI	27	3	21–33
	1.5	Philips	MOLLI	23	3	17–29
	3	Siemens	MOLLI	26	3	20–32
	3	Siemens	ShMOLLI	25	2	20–29
	3	Philips	MOLLI	26	5	16–36

ECV, extracellular volume fraction; *FS,* field strength; *LL,* lower limit; *MOLLI,* modified Look-Locker inversion recovery; *SD,* standard deviation; *ShMOLLI,* short MOLLI; *Siemens,* Siemens Medical Solutions, Erlangen, Germany, Philips Philips Healthcare, Best, The Netherlands; *T,* Tesla; *UL,* upper limit.
From Kawel-Boehm, N. et al., Reference ranges ("normal values") for cardiovascular magnetic resonance (CMR) in adults and children: 2020 update. *J Cardiovasc Magn Reson.* 2020. 22(1): p. 87.

TABLE 16.17 Myocardial T2 relaxation time in adults.

FS (T)	VENDOR	TECHNIQUE	MEAN (MS)	SD (MS)	LL–UL (MS)
1.5	Siemens	FLASH	52	5	42–62
1.5	Siemens	T2P bSSFP	51	3	45–57
1.5	Philips	GSE	56	3	50–62
3	Philips	GSE	52	3	46–58

bSSFP, balanced steady-state free precession; *FLASH,* fast low angle shot; *FS,* field strength; *GSE,* gradient spin echo; *LL,* lower limit; *SD,* standard deviation; *T,* Tesla; *T2P,* T2 preparation; *Siemens,* Siemens Medical Solutions, Erlangen, Germany, Philips Philips Healthcare, Best, The Netherlands; *UL,* upper limit.
From Kawel-Boehm, N. et al., Reference ranges ("normal values") for cardiovascular magnetic resonance (CMR) in adults and children: 2020 update. *J Cardiovasc Magn Reson.* 2020. 22(1): p. 87.

CARDIOVASCULAR PARAMETERS IN CHILDREN AND ADOLESCENTS

The evaluation of normal cardiovascular function and structure is assessed differently in children compared to adults due to the variation in these parameters in relationship to body size as well as age. Two methods for normalization of cardiac parameters by body size are in common use. The *z*-score (standard deviation) method is given as:

$$\text{z - score} = (\text{patient measurement} - \text{mean of the population}) / \text{standard deviation of the population}$$

where the standard deviation of the population will vary by age. For the z-score method, online calculators are available that incorporate age, weight, height, and sex for determination of the appropriate normal values.[52]

The second method for determining appropriate body size adjustments for pediatric patients is termed the Lambda-Mu-Sigma (LMS) method. While the z-score method assumes a linear correlation between ventricular volumes and body surface area, the LMS method recognizes that growth rate is unlikely to be linear with age during child development. In the LMS approach, a power transformation is used to transform skewness into normality; trends are summarized in a smooth curve (L). Trends in the mean (M) and coefficient of variation (S) are similarly smoothed. LMS curves can be readily applied in daily practice and can account for nonlinear relationships between body, cardiac size, and age, even with relatively small sample sizes.[53] A resource for application of LMS curves for the right and left ventricles is available.[54]

TABLE 16.18 Grading of myocardial iron content on T2* measurements at 1.5 T.

IRON AMOUNT	T2* (MS)
Normal	>20
Iron overload	10–20
Severe iron overload	<10

From Kawel-Boehm, N. et al., Reference ranges ("normal values") for cardiovascular magnetic resonance (CMR) in adults and children: 2020 update. *J Cardiovasc Magn Reson.* 2020. 22(1): p. 87.

SUMMARY

There is increasing emphasis on quantitative imaging using cardiac MRI. With the advent of artificial intelligence algorithms incorporated into software analysis tools, quantitative imaging will become easier to implement with better reproducibility. Such tools should ultimately improve the ability of the cardiovascular physician to identify abnormal cardiac function at an early stage of disease when treatment is more likely to be effective. The identification of more sophisticated cardiac MRI quantitative metrics will also likely lead to greater use of normal values in cardiac MRI.

REFERENCES

1. Kawel-Boehm N, et al. Reference ranges ("normal values") for cardiovascular magnetic resonance (CMR) in adults and children: 2020 update. *J Cardiovasc Magn Reson*. 2020;22(1):87.
2. Horowitz GL. Estimating reference intervals. *Am J Clin Pathol*. 2010;133(2):175–177.
3. Burton RF. Estimating body surface area from mass and height: theory and the formula of Du Bois and Du Bois. *Ann Hum Biol*. 2008;35(2):170–184.
4. Body surface area calculator. [cited 2024 March 12]; Available from: https://www.calculator.net/body-surface-area-calculator.html.
5. Dewey FE, et al. Does size matter? Clinical applications of scaling cardiac size and function for body size. *Circulation*. 2008;117(17):2279–2287.
6. Chirinos JA, et al. Left ventricular mass: allometric scaling, normative values, effect of obesity, and prognostic performance. *Hypertension*. 2010;56(1):91–98.
7. MESA LV mass calculator. [cited 2024 March 12]; Available from: https://internal.mesa-nhlbi.org/about/procedures/tools/lv-mass-calculator.
8. St Pierre SR, Peirlinck M, Kuhl E. Sex matters: a comprehensive comparison of female and male hearts. *Front Physiol*. 2022;13:831179.
9. Sandstede J, et al. Age- and gender-specific differences in left and right ventricular cardiac function and mass determined by cine magnetic resonance imaging. *Eur Radiol*. 2000;10(3):438–442.
10. Argiento P, et al. Exercise stress echocardiography of the pulmonary circulation: limits of normal and sex differences. *Chest*. 2012;142(5):1158–1165.
11. Ramaekers D, et al. Heart rate variability and heart rate in healthy volunteers. Is the female autonomic nervous system cardioprotective? *Eur Heart J*. 1998;19(9):1334–1341.
12. Lawton JS, et al. Magnetic resonance imaging detects significant sex differences in human myocardial strain. *Biomed Eng Online*. 2011;10:76.
13. Gersh BJ, et al. 2011 ACCF/AHA guideline for the diagnosis and treatment of hypertrophic cardiomyopathy: executive summary: a report of the American College of Cardiology Foundation/American eart ssociation Task Force on practice guidelines. *Circulation*. 2011;124(24):2761–2796.
14. Ponikowski P, et al. 2016 ESC guidelines for the diagnosis and treatment of acute and chronic heart failure: the Task Force for the diagnosis and treatment of acute and chronic heart failure of the European Society of Cardiology (ESC)Developed with the special contribution of the Heart Failure Association (HFA) of the ESC. *Eur Heart J*. 2016;37(27):2129–2200.
15. Diderichsen F, Hallqvist J, Whitehead M. Differential vulnerability and susceptibility: how to make use of recent development in our understanding of mediation and interaction to tackle health inequalities. *Int J Epidemiol*. 2019;48(1):268–274.
16. Lopez-Neyman SM, et al. Racial disparities and prevalence of cardiovascular disease risk factors, cardiometabolic risk factors, and cardiovascular health metrics among US adults: NHANES 2011-2018. *Sci Rep*. 2022;12(1):19475.
17. Savitz ST, et al. Contemporary reevaluation of race and ethnicity with outcomes in heart failure. *J Am Heart Assoc*. 2021;10(3):e016601.
18. Bild DE, et al. Multi-ethnic study of atherosclerosis: objectives and design. *Am J Epidemiol*. 2002;156(9):871–881.
19. Natori S, et al. Cardiovascular function in multi-ethnic study of atherosclerosis: normal values by age, sex, and ethnicity. *AJR Am J Roentgenol*. 2006;186(6 Suppl 2):S357–S365.
20. Parke KS, et al. Ethnic differences in cardiac structure and function assessed by MRI in healthy South Asian and White European people: a UK Biobank Study. *J Cardiovasc Magn Reson*. 2024;26(1):100001.
21. Freedman BI, et al. The impact of ethnicity and sex on subclinical cardiovascular disease: the Diabetes Heart Study. *Diabetologia*. 2005;48(12):2511–2518.
22. Chandra A, et al. Race- and gender-based differences in cardiac structure and function and risk of heart failure. *J Am Coll Cardiol*. 2022;79(4):355–368.
23. Fernandes VR, et al. Racial and ethnic differences in subclinical myocardial function: the Multi-Ethnic Study of Atherosclerosis. *Heart*. 2011;97(5):405–410.
24. Bulow R, et al. Reference ranges of left ventricular structure and function assessed by contrast-enhanced cardiac MR and changes related to ageing and hypertension in a population-based study. *Eur Radiol*. 2018;28(9):3996–4005.
25. Luu JM, et al. Normal sex and age-specific parameters in a multi-ethnic population: a cardiovascular magnetic resonance study of the Canadian Alliance for Healthy Hearts and Minds cohort. *J Cardiovasc Magn Reson*. 2022;24(1):2.
26. Petersen SE, et al. Reference ranges for cardiac structure and function using cardiovascular magnetic resonance (CMR) in Caucasians from the UK Biobank population cohort. *J Cardiovasc Magn Reson*. 2017;19(1):18.
27. Le Ven F, et al. Cardiac morphology and function reference values derived from a large subset of healthy young Caucasian adults by magnetic resonance imaging. *Eur Heart J Cardiovasc Imaging*. 2016;17(9):981–990.
28. Elster AD. Questions and Answers in MRI. [cited 2024 March 12]; Available from: https://mriquestions.com/chemical-shift-2nd-kind.html; 2024.
29. Zhao D, et al. Correcting bias in cardiac geometries derived from multimodal images using spatiotemporal mapping. *Sci Rep*. 2023;13(1):8118.
30. Schulz-Menger J, et al. Standardized image interpretation and post-processing in cardiovascular magnetic resonance - 2020 update : Society for Cardiovascular Magnetic Resonance (SCMR): Board of Trustees Task Force on standardized post-processing. *J Cardiovasc Magn Reson*. 2020;22(1):19.
31. Vogel-Claussen J, et al. Left ventricular papillary muscle mass: relationship to left ventricular mass and volumes by magnetic resonance imaging. *J Comput Assist Tomogr*. 2006;30(3):426–432.
32. Rajiah PS, et al. Myocardial strain evaluation with cardiovascular MRI: physics, principles, and clinical applications. *Radiographics*. 2022;42(4):968–990.
33. Zerhouni EA, et al. Human heart: tagging with MR imaging-a method for noninvasive assessment of myocardial motion. *Radiology*. 1988;169(1):59–63.
34. Axel L, Dougherty L. Heart wall motion: improved method of spatial modulation of magnetization for MR imaging. *Radiology*. 1989;172(2):349–350.
35. Bourfiss M, et al. Feature tracking CMR reveals abnormal strain in preclinical arrhythmogenic right ventricular dysplasia/cardiomyopathy: a multisoftware feasibility and clinical implementation study. *J Cardiovasc Magn Reson*. 2017;19(1):66.
36. Bonnemains L, et al. Assessment of right ventricle volumes and function by cardiac MRI: quantification of the regional and global interobserver variability. *Magn Reson Med*. 2012;67(6):1740–1746.
37. Kawut SM, et al. Sex and race differences in right ventricular structure and function: the multi-ethnic study of atherosclerosis-right ventricle study. *Circulation*. 2011;123(22):2542–2551.
38. Atalay MK, et al. The transaxial orientation is superior to both the short axis and horizontal long axis orientations for determining right ventricular volume and ejection fraction using Simpson's method with cardiac magnetic resonance. *ISRN Cardiol*. 2013;2013:268697.
39. Lang RM, et al. Recommendations for chamber quantification: a report from the American Society of Echocardiography's Guidelines and Standards Committee and the Chamber Quantification Writing Group, developed in conjunction with the European Association of Echocardiography, a branch of the European Society of Cardiology. *J Am Soc Echocardiogr*. 2005;18(12):1440–1463.
40. Nacif MS, et al. Left atrial volume quantification using cardiac MRI in atrial fibrillation: comparison of the Simpson's method with biplane area-length, ellipse, and three-dimensional methods. *Diagn Interv Radiol*. 2013;19(3):213–220.
41. Baggish AL, et al. Sports Cardiology: core Curriculum for providing cardiovascular care to competitive athletes and highly active people. *J Am Coll Cardiol*. 2017;70(15):1902–1918.
42. Sharma S, et al. Physiologic limits of left ventricular hypertrophy in elite junior athletes: relevance to differential diagnosis of athlete's heart and hypertrophic cardiomyopathy. *J Am Coll Cardiol*. 2002;40(8):1431–1436.
43. Maron BJ. Structural features of the athlete heart as defined by echocardiography. *J Am Coll Cardiol*. 1986;7(1):190–203.
44. Azarine A, et al. Four-dimensional flow MRI: principles and cardiovascular applications. *Radiographics*. 2019;39(3):632–648.
45. Lotz J, et al. Cardiovascular flow measurement with phase-contrast MR imaging: basic facts and implementation. *Radiographics*. 2002;22(3):651–671.
46. Nishimura RA, et al. 2017 AHA/ACC focused update of the 2014 AHA/ACC guideline for the management of patients with valvular heart disease: a report of the American College of Cardiology/American Heart Association Task Force on Clinical Practice Guidelines. *J Am Coll Cardiol*. 2017;70(2):252–289.
47. Ferreira VM, et al. Cardiovascular magnetic resonance in nonischemic myocardial inflammation: expert recommendations. *J Am Coll Cardiol*. 2018;72(24):3158–3176.
48. Moon JC, et al. Myocardial T1 mapping and extracellular volume quantification: a Society for Cardiovascular Magnetic Resonance (SCMR) and CMR Working Group of the European Society of Cardiology consensus statement. *J Cardiovasc Magn Reson*. 2013;15(1):92.
49. Messroghli DR, et al. Clinical recommendations for cardiovascular magnetic resonance mapping of T1, T2, T2* and extracellular volume: a consensus statement by the Society for Cardiovascular Magnetic Resonance (SCMR) endorsed by the European Association for Cardiovascular Imaging (EACVI). *J Cardiovasc Magn Reson*. 2017;19(1):75.
50. Parameter. [cited 2024 March 14]; Available from. https://www.rchsd.org/zscore/.
51. Cole TJ. The LMS method for constructing normalized growth standards. *Eur J Clin Nutr*. 1990;44(1):45–60.
52. van der Ven JPG, et al. Multicentre reference values for cardiac magnetic resonance imaging derived ventricular size and function for children aged 0-18 years. *Eur Heart J Cardiovasc Imaging*. 2020;21(1):102–113.
53. Du Bois D, Du Bois EF. A formula to estimate the approximate surface area if height and weight be known. *1916. Nutrition*. 1989;5(5):303–311.
54. de Simone G, et al. Left ventricular mass and body size in normotensive children and adults: assessment of allometric relations and impact of overweight. *J Am Coll Cardiol*. 1992;20(5):1251–1260.

17 Left Ventricular Structure and Function

AFSHIN FARZANEH-FAR

INTRODUCTION

The accurate and reproducible measurement of cardiac function is a fundamental aim of cardiac imaging. It forms the foundation upon which much of the assessment and management of cardiovascular disease is built. Evaluations of ventricular size, geometry, and performance are critical for evaluating processes such as ischemia, viability, remodeling, and valvular disease. In this chapter, we discuss the role of cardiovascular magnetic resonance (CMR) for assessing left ventricular systolic and diastolic function and provide a brief overview of left ventricular myocardial fiber structure. In addition, we will describe the key value of measuring global left ventricular longitudinal function in assessing cardiac performance and provide an overview of CMR techniques to quantitate this.

VENTRICULAR VOLUMES AND SYSTOLIC FUNCTION

CMR has some fundamental advantages over other imaging techniques, which have fueled the growing enthusiasm for its use in clinical practice and research. CMR offers accurate and reproducible tomographic, static, or cine images of high spatial resolution in any desired plane without exposure to contrast agents or ionizing radiation. As such, true two-, three-, four-chamber, and short-axis views can be easily and rapidly acquired to allow a visual, qualitative assessment of ventricular size, geometry, and function qualitatively similar to echocardiography. The main advantage of CMR, however, lies in its quantitative accuracy and reproducibility in conjunction with independence from the availability of optimal acoustic windows.

Ventricular volumes and function are measured by the use of Simpson's rule. A stack of contiguous tomographic slices are acquired that encompass the entire left ventricle. The ventricular volume is equal to the sum of the endocardial areas multiplied by the distance between the centers of each slice (Figs. 17.1 and 17.2).[1] The volumes that are obtained by this method are independent of geometric assumptions and dimensionally accurate.[2] Of note, papillary muscles and endocardial trabeculae should be excluded from the LV volume and included in the LV mass.

ACCURACY, REPRODUCIBILITY, AND APPLICATION TO CLINICAL TRIALS

It is now widely accepted that CMR is the reference standard for the noninvasive assessment of cardiac function, being both accurate (Figs. 17.3–17.5)[3,4] and reproducible in normal as well as abnormal ventricles, both with nonbreath-hold[5] and breath-hold techniques.[6]

CMR has been shown to have higher reproducibility than two-dimensional echocardiography (2DE) for LV end-systolic volume (4.4% to 9.2% vs. 13.7% to 20.3%, $P < .001$), left ventricular ejection fraction (LVEF) (2.4% to 7.3% vs. 8.6% to 19.4%, $P < .001$), and LV mass measurements (2.8% to 4.8% vs. 11.6% to 15.7%, $P < .001$), and this higher reproducibility allows for sample size reductions of 55% to 93% in clinical trials using these variables as endpoints.[7] The excellent reproducibility of CMR versus 2DE can be illustrated by considering the sample sizes required for a drug trial designed to show prespecified changes in LV mass, LV volumes, or LVEF following a specific treatment (Fig. 17.6).[6] A direct comparison of CMR with 2DE for reproducibility has shown that for an 80% power and a P value of .05, the sample size required would be 505 patients with 2DE but only 14 patients with CMR.[7] Equally, it has been demonstrated that to show a 5% difference in LVEF with a 90% power and a P value of .05 would require only seven normal subjects or five patients with dilated ventricles.[8]

DIASTOLIC FUNCTION

For diastolic function, phase-contrast CMR can be applied to measure, analogous to 2DE, both mitral inflow at the tip of the mitral valve leaflets and pulmonary venous flow (Fig. 17.7).[9] This technique is fast and reproducible, with good agreement with Doppler echocardiography.[10] Typically, these sequences are electrocardiographically gated in a retrospective manner (i.e., they capture the entire cardiac cycle) and can be performed within a single breath hold. Phase-contrast CMR directly measures blood flow through an en-face image of the orifice with through-plane velocity encoding (unlike Doppler echocardiography, which quantifies flows using in-plane imaging and assumes a flat blood flow profile). An encoding velocity should be optimized to match the peak velocity as closely as possible without aliasing, typically 100–150 cm/s for the mitral and pulmonary venous inflow. Ideally, a mitral valve tracking

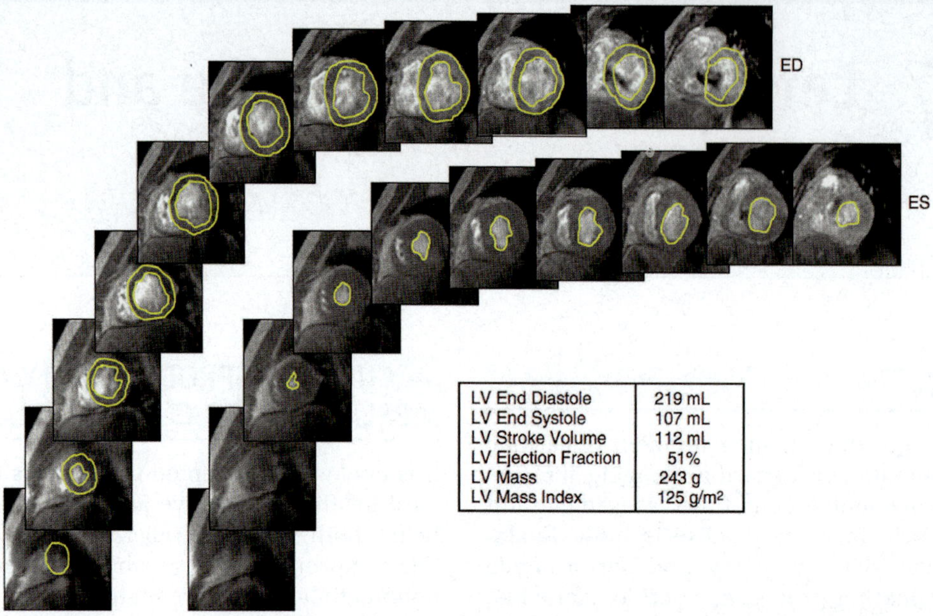

FIG. 17.1 The end-diastolic (*ED*) and end-systolic (*ES*) slices from multiple contiguous short-axis cines that encompass the left ventricle (*LV*), from base to apex, in a patient with ventricular dilatation and hypertrophy from chronic aortic regurgitation. The epicardial and endocardial borders are traced, and the summation values are shown. Note that there is one more image at end-diastole 11 than at end-systole 10, reflecting the need to allow for the systolic descent of the atrioventricular ring, as described in the text. Note also the ingress of the LV outflow tract in the most basal end-diastolic image, where there is no ventricular mass, and the open ends of the LV myocardial horseshoe are joined together to form the appropriate volume.

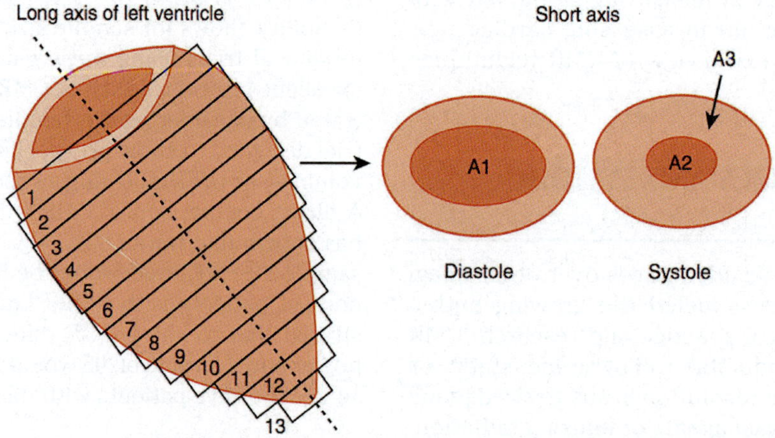

FIG. 17.2 Schematic of the left ventricular short-axis slices that encompass the entire left ventricle. Each slice is acquired as a cine. (*A1*) End-diastolic endocardial area; (*A2*) end-systolic endocardial area; (*A3*) myocardium.

technique should be implemented to overcome the limitation of not measuring velocities at the same level throughout the cardiac cycle.

Left atrial dilatation is an excellent marker of diastolic dysfunction. Left atrial volumes are easy to obtain with CMR,[11,12] and can be derived from the area–length method or Simpson's biplane method in the two-chamber and four-chamber views. LA volume is measured at end ventricular systole immediately before mitral valve opening. CMR-derived LA volumes are typically larger than echocardiography-derived volumes because of better alignment and visualization of the atrium.[9] Additional functional parameters, such as LA ejection fraction and strain, can also be obtained, although their additional value is unclear.[9] With current analysis software it is also possible to measure volumes over a complete cardiac cycle, obtaining a volume–time curve whose first derivative is the flow curve.[13]

Cine CMR also allows direct visualization of the abnormal diastolic filling in dilated ventricles with inflow directed not toward the apex but toward the free wall, giving rise to a well-developed circular flow pattern turning back toward the septum and outflow tract, persisting through diastole.[14]

Other techniques such as tagging or elastography have been used to assess myocardial relaxation and/or stiffness in the research setting but are cumbersome and currently do not have widespread clinical use.[9,15]

LEFT VENTRICULAR STRUCTURE

Cardiomyocytes measure approximately 150 × 20 µm, and each one intercalates with several other cardiomyocytes.[16] Although their branching nature means that cardiomyocytes do not strictly align in fibers, there is a directional grain to their appearance.[16,17] This has led

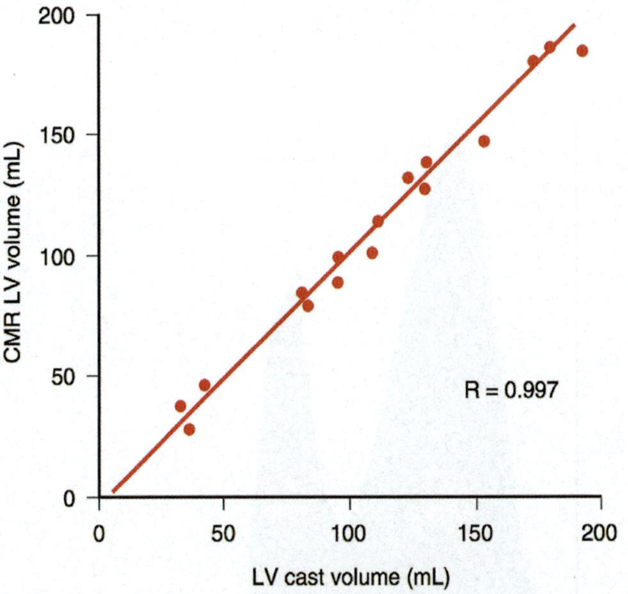

FIG. 17.3 Validation of left ventricular (*LV*) volume measurements by cardiovascular magnetic resonance (*CMR*). CMR-derived volume (vertical scale) is compared with the displacement volume of the LV casts from human postmortem hearts. There is excellent accuracy, and the regression line slope is close to identity. (Data from Rehr RB, Malloy CR, Filipchuk NG, et al. Left ventricular volumes measured by MR imaging. *Radiology*. 1985;156:717–719.)

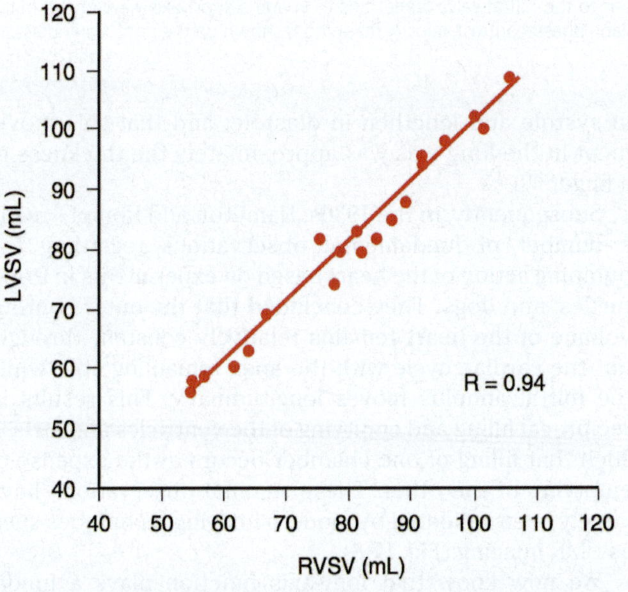

FIG. 17.4 Validation of right and left ventricular stroke volumes (*RVSV* and *LVSV*, respectively) in vivo using cardiovascular magnetic resonance (CMR) ventricular volume analysis. There is an excellent agreement between the stroke volumes of both ventricles, which is strong evidence that both measurements are accurate, because they are equivalent in vivo in the absence of valve regurgitation or shunting. (From Longmore DB, Klipstein RH, Underwood SR, et al. Dimensional accuracy of magnetic resonance in studies of the heart. *Lancet*. 1985; 1:1360–1362.)

to variable terminology, when some use "fiber" to mean cardiomyocytes or groups of cardiomyocytes. Here, the phrase "cardiomyocyte orientation" is used to avoid confusion.[18] Furthermore, cardiomyocytes aggregate into secondary structures called "sheetlets," each about four cardiomyocytes thick, surrounded and interconnected by collagenous perimysium.[18] This arrangement allows shear between neighboring sheetlets during cardiac contraction.

Gross dissection reveals that the left ventricular wall is comprised of three layers based on cardiomyocyte orientation: superficial (subepicardial), middle (mid-myocardial), and deep (subendocardial). Importantly, these layers represent changes in the orientation of myocardial strands transmurally and are not separated by cleavage planes or fibrous tissue, as strands of one layer interconnect with those of the next in a continuum.[17]

Cardiomyocyte orientation follows a specific pattern. The superficial (subepicardial) layer occupies approximately 25% of the wall thickness and runs obliquely. The mid-myocardial layer, thicker in the elderly, occupies about 53%–59% of the wall thickness and is arranged circumferentially nearly parallel to the mitral orifice. The subendocardial layer, less than 20% of the wall thickness, radiates longitudinally and forms a meshwork determined by trabeculations and muscle bundles. This complex fiber architecture is vital for normal cardiac function and

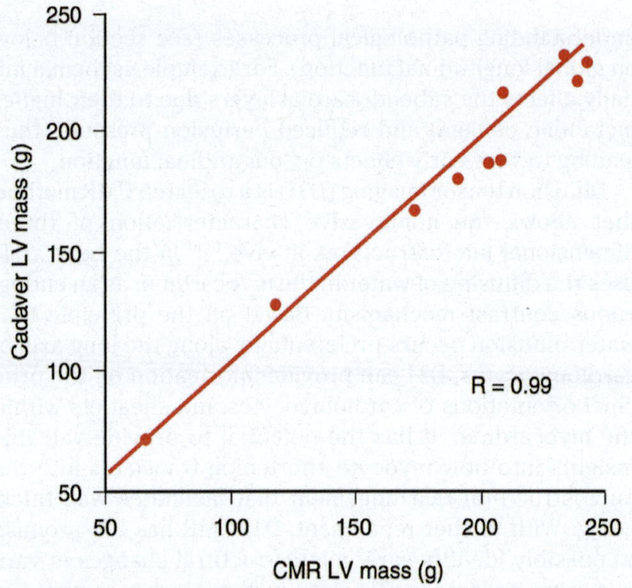

FIG. 17.5 Validation of left ventricular (*LV*) mass with comparison of cardiovascular magnetic resonance (*CMR*)-derived mass against human cadaver hearts. (Data from Katz J, Millikem MC, Stray-Gunderson J, et al. Estimation of human myocardial mass with MR imaging. *Radiology*. 1988;169:495–498.)

Clinical Change	Echo		CMR		% Reduction in Sample Size
	SD	*N*	SD	*N*	
EDV, 10 ml	23.8	121	7.4	12	90
ESV, 10 ml	15.8	53	6.5	10	81
EF, 3% (abs)	6.6	102	2.5	15	85
Mass, 10 g	36.4	273	6.4	9	97

FIG. 17.6 Sample size required to detect the same change by echo and cardiovascular magnetic resonance (*CMR*) with a power of 90% and $P<.05$.

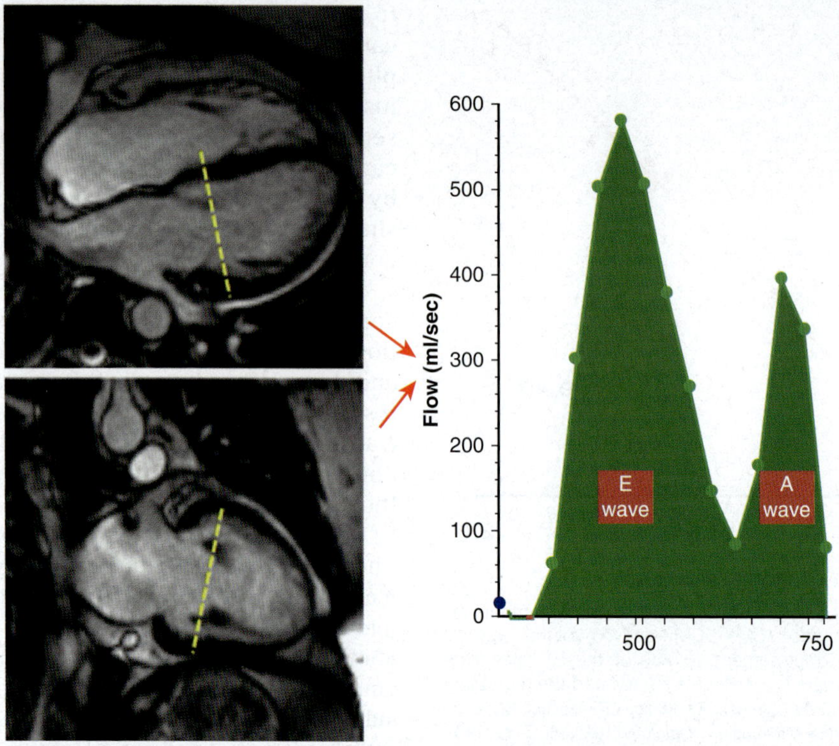

FIG. 17.7 Phase-contrast cardiovascular magnetic resonance (PC-CMR) sequence for estimating velocities across mitral valve inflow. Cine-CMR sequence in four-chamber and two-chamber views showing a slice prescribed perpendicular to the mitral valve leaflet tips to image a short-axis view of the mitral valve on PC-CMR. The transmitral flow-time graph generated by CMR through-plane phase-contrast velocity mapping is shown on the right. Early-diastolic (*E*) and late-diastolic (*A*) waves are depicted.

understanding pathological processes (see section below on global longitudinal function). For example, ischemia initially affects the subendocardial layers due to their higher metabolic demand and reduced perfusion pressure, thus leading to very early effects on longitudinal function.

Diffusion tensor imaging (DTI) is a research CMR method that allows the noninvasive characterization of three-dimensional microstructures in vivo.[18,19] In the heart, DTI uses the diffusion of water in the myocardium as an endogenous contrast mechanism. Based on the principle that water diffusion occurs preferentially along the long axis of cardiomyocytes, DTI can provide information on the principal orientations of cardiomyocytes and sheetlets within the myocardium. It has the potential to provide valuable insights into how myocyte shortening translates into the microstructural rearrangement that facilitates wall thickening. With further refinement, DTI CMR has the promise to possibly identify early microstructural changes in various cardiac diseases. However, further work is required to broaden its applicability and to provide clinical value for the technique.

LONGITUDINAL VENTRICULAR FUNCTION

It was Leonardo da Vinci who first described the importance of longitudinal ventricular function in cardiac mechanics.[20] In a well-known experiment, he observed peasants slaughtering pigs in Tuscany using an instrument called a "spillo" when it penetrated the chest wall and heart. By noting the direction of movement of the "spillo" handle, he concluded that the ventricles shorten in systole and lengthen in diastole; and that this movement in the long axis was approximately the thickness of a finger.[20]

Subsequently, in the 1930s, Hamilton and Rompf[21] made a number of fundamental observations regarding the pumping action of the heart based on experiments in frogs, turtles, and dogs. They concluded that the outer contour volume of the heart remains relatively constant throughout the cardiac cycle with the apex remaining still, while the mitral annulus moves longitudinally. This results in reciprocal filling and emptying of the ventricles and atria—such that filling of one chamber occurs at the expense of emptying of the other. These seminal observations have largely been validated by modern imaging techniques such as CMR imaging (Fig. 17.8).

We now know that long-axis function plays a fundamental role in cardiac mechanics. Longitudinal movement of the mitral annulus is the major driver of ventricular ejection and atrial filling. Since the outer contour of the heart remains relatively constant, movement of the annulus in systole results not just in shortening of ventricular length but also an increase in wall thickness due to conservation of myocardial volume.[22] CMR has been used to measure the contribution of longitudinal mitral plane displacement to overall stroke volume in normal subjects, elite athletes, and patients with dilated cardiomyopathy.[22] These studies suggest that as much as 60% of stroke volume may be explained by longitudinal mitral annular motion. In diastole, the mitral annulus springs back to its equilibrium position, moving around the column of blood passing through the mitral valve, thus aiding ventricular filling. Possibly because of their subendocardial location,

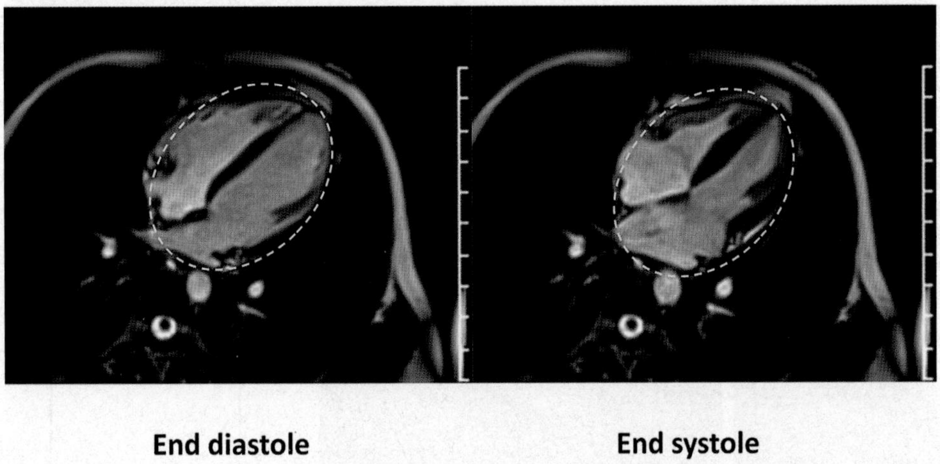

FIG. 17.8 CMR imaging shows that the outer contour of the heart remains relatively constant throughout the cardiac cycle with the apex remaining still, while the mitral annulus moves longitudinally. There is reciprocal filling and emptying of the ventricles and atria—such that filling of one chamber occurs at the expense of emptying of the other.

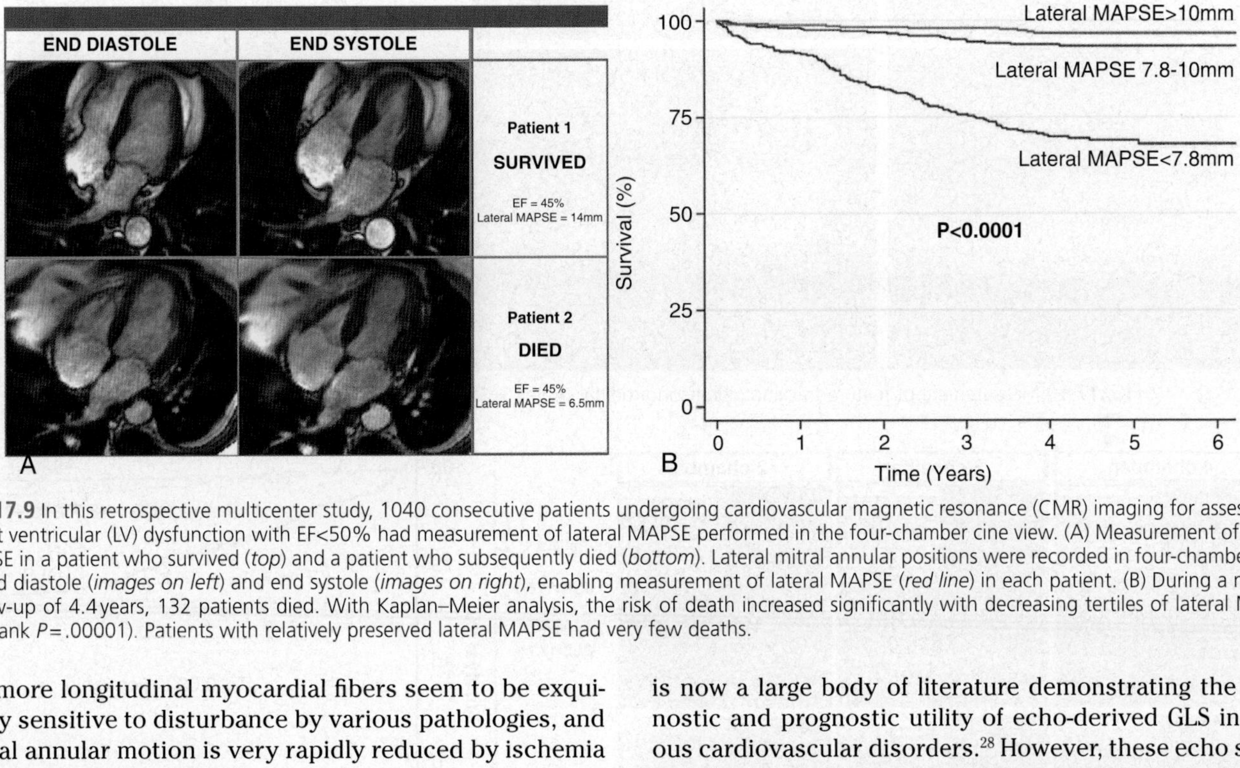

FIG. 17.9 In this retrospective multicenter study, 1040 consecutive patients undergoing cardiovascular magnetic resonance (CMR) imaging for assessment of left ventricular (LV) dysfunction with EF<50% had measurement of lateral MAPSE performed in the four-chamber cine view. (A) Measurement of lateral MAPSE in a patient who survived (*top*) and a patient who subsequently died (*bottom*). Lateral mitral annular positions were recorded in four-chamber view at end diastole (*images on left*) and end systole (*images on right*), enabling measurement of lateral MAPSE (*red line*) in each patient. (B) During a median follow-up of 4.4years, 132 patients died. With Kaplan–Meier analysis, the risk of death increased significantly with decreasing tertiles of lateral MAPSE (log-rank *P*=.00001). Patients with relatively preserved lateral MAPSE had very few deaths.

the more longitudinal myocardial fibers seem to be exquisitely sensitive to disturbance by various pathologies, and mitral annular motion is very rapidly reduced by ischemia in experimental models.[23]

Since the cardiac apex is fixed with respect to the chest wall, long-axis function was initially assessed by measuring changes in the position of the mitral annulus. These studies used M-mode echocardiography, and more recently CMR, to directly follow the position of the mitral annulus and measure mitral annular plane systolic excursion (MAPSE).[24–27] CMR-derived MAPSE has been shown to be an independent predictor of adverse events in many patient groups including ischemic and nonischemic cardiomyopathy, as well as hypertension (Fig. 17.9).[25,26]

However, over the last few years, enormous interest has been generated by the development of echocardiographic 2D speckle tracking techniques to assess long-axis function by measuring global longitudinal strain (GLS).[28] There is now a large body of literature demonstrating the diagnostic and prognostic utility of echo-derived GLS in various cardiovascular disorders.[28] However, these echo strain techniques are highly dependent on attainment of good-quality imaging, and there are significant intervendor measurement differences.[28] More recently, the development of CMR feature-tracking technology allows measurement of GLS with proprietary software by recognition of "patterns of features" or "irregularities" in the endocardial border that are tracked and followed in successive frames. Importantly, this approach can be applied to routine cine CMR acquisitions, thus avoiding the need for dedicated pulse sequences, which are required for other specialized CMR strain techniques such as tagging, HARP (harmonic phase), DENSE (displacement encoding with stimulated echoes), and SENC (strain-encoded CMR). Feature-tracking-derived GLS has been shown to be an independent predictor of adverse events in many patient groups including ischemic and nonischemic cardiomyopathy, hypertension,

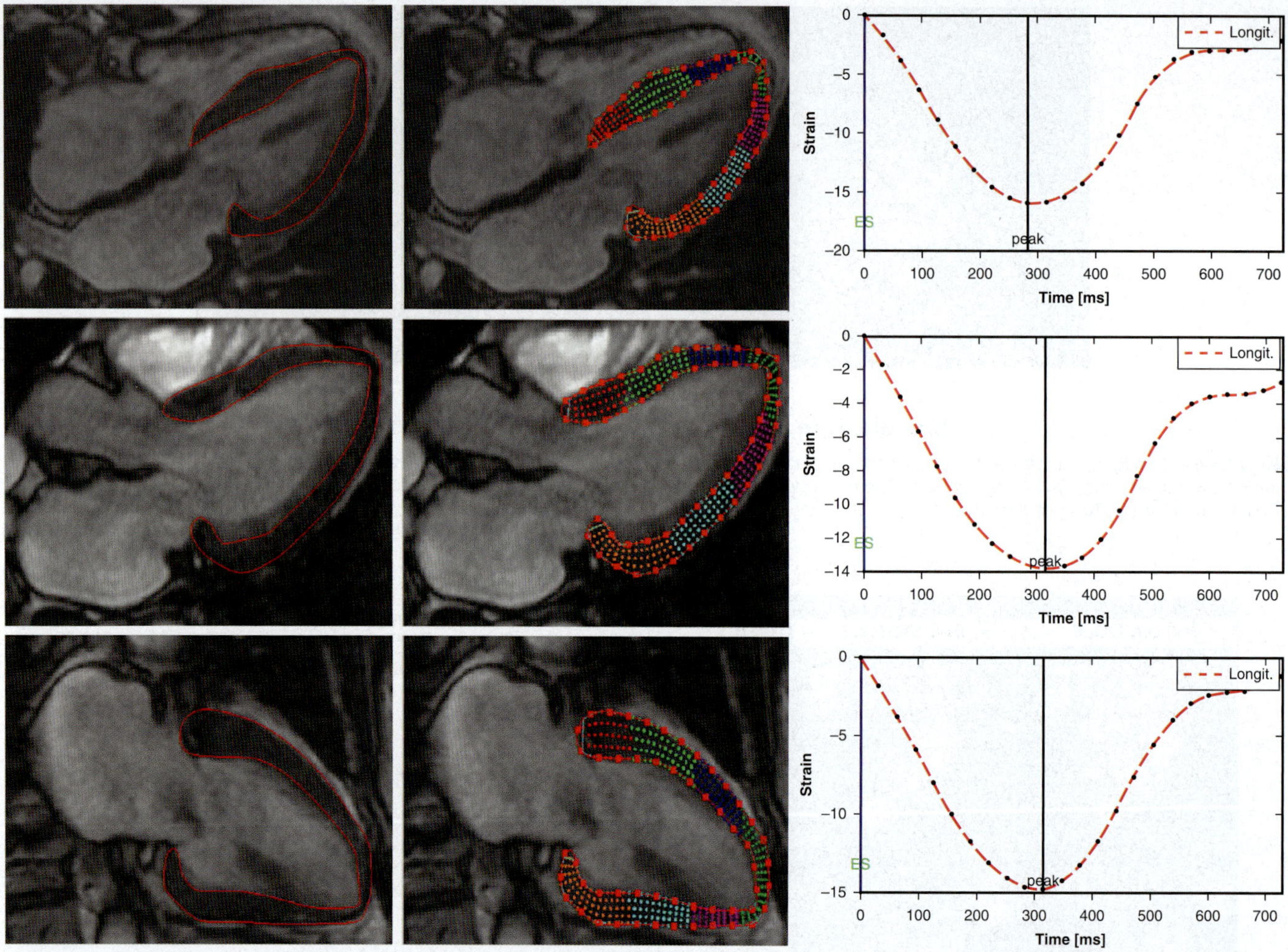

FIG. 17.10 Measurement of feature-tracking global longitudinal strain (GLS) from three standard long-axis cine views.

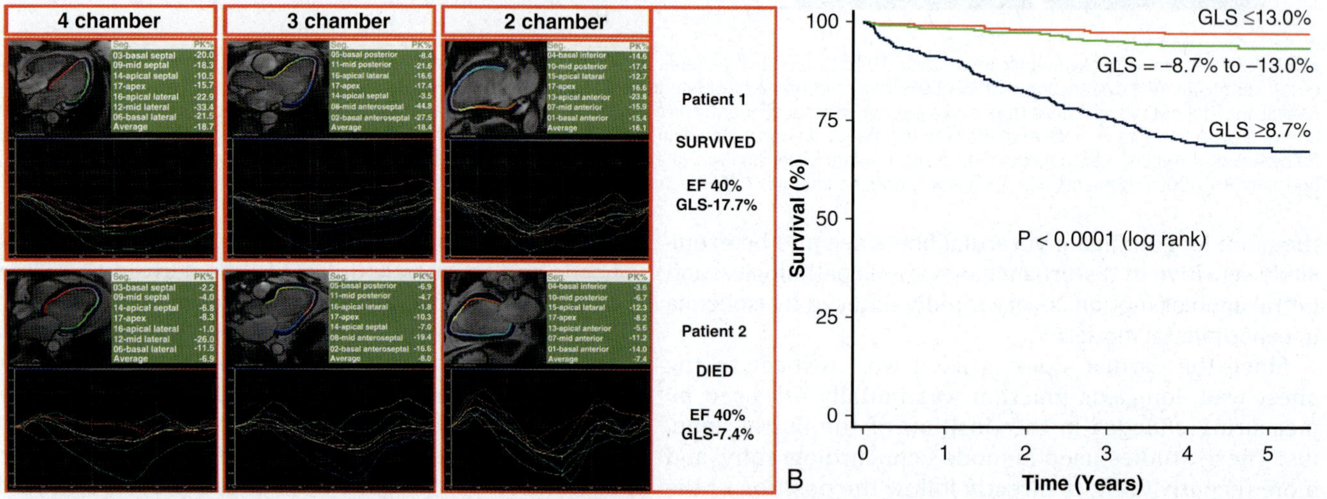

FIG. 17.11 In this retrospective multicenter study, 1012 consecutive patients undergoing cardiovascular magnetic resonance (CMR) imaging for assessment of left ventricular (LV) dysfunction with EF<50% had measurement of feature-tracking GLS performed. (A) Measurement of lateral MAPSE in a patient who survived (*top*) and a patient who subsequently died (*bottom*). (B) During a median follow-up of 4.4 years, 133 patients died. With Kaplan–Meier analysis, the risk of death increased significantly with worsening tertiles of GLS (log-rank $P = .0001$). Patients with relatively preserved GLS had very few deaths.

postmyocardial infarction (MI), postmyocarditis, post-heart transplantation, and during stress perfusion imaging (Figs. 17.10 and 17.11).[29–35]

The precise mechanism underlying the association between impaired longitudinal motion (measured by GLS or MAPSE) and adverse outcomes is unclear. It has been suggested that the subendocardial myocardial fibers (which are more longitudinally aligned) are extremely sensitive to disturbance because of greater compressive forces and higher oxygen consumption.[17,36–39] The subendocardial fibers are therefore more vulnerable to increased wall stress and imbalances between oxygen supply and

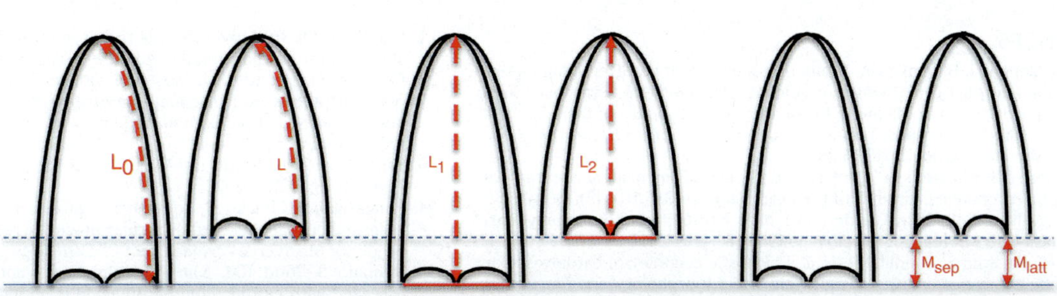

	GLS	LAS	MAPSE
Definition	$\frac{(L-L_0)}{L_0}$ *	$\frac{(L_2-L_1)}{L_1}$	$\frac{(M_{sep}+M_{lat})}{2}$ or M_{lat}
Pulse Sequence	SSFP cine	SSFP cine	SSFP cine
Special Analysis Software	✓	×	×
Inter-Vendor Variability	✓	×	×
Image Quality Dependent	+++	++	+
Foreshortening Errors	✓	✓	×
Simplicity	+	++	+++
Prognostic Data	+++	+	++

FIG. 17.12 Comparison of cardiovascular magnetic resonance methods for assessment of global longitudinal function.

demand, which may be seen in the early stages of many cardiovascular conditions, including atherosclerosis and heart failure.

Recently Schuster et al.[40] used global long-axis strain (LAS) measured by CMR as a measure of global longitudinal function and demonstrated that it is independently associated with MACE incremental to clinical and imaging variables. LAS was defined as the change in length of a line drawn between the apex and the middle of the mitral annulus corrected to its end-diastolic length (Fig. 17.12). The mean values from standard two- and four-chamber cine steady state free precession (SSFP) views were used. They also reported no significant difference between the incremental prognostic value of LAS compared with GLS when added to clinical and imaging predictors.

Compared with GLS, LAS is faster to measure and requires no proprietary software. However, MAPSE is an even simpler measure of longitudinal function and has a much larger body of prognostic literature both by CMR and echocardiography.[24–27] Moreover, there is strong evidence that MAPSE assessment can be simplified even further by measuring only at the lateral annulus in the four-chamber view.[24–26] Lateral MAPSE has shown powerful independent prognostic value in large multicenter CMR studies of patients with reduced ejection fraction as well as hypertension, incremental to late gadolinium enhancement, and ejection fraction.[25,26] It has been shown that the mitral annulus moves as a unified structure such that a similar global MAPSE decrease is seen regardless of MI location—explaining the strong prognostic value of simply measuring MAPSE at the lateral position. Moreover, in a recent echocardiographic study of normal subjects, Stoylen et al.[42] found that normalizing LV shortening to ventricular length (as in GLS or LAS) results in a systematic bias, increasing dependency of the measurement to body size, which is not the case for MAPSE. Given these and other advantages of MAPSE (Fig. 17.12), it remains to be seen if LAS is able to provide additive diagnostic or prognostic value beyond this simple measure.

In conclusion, CMR techniques measuring longitudinal function allow better identification of high-risk patients than current clinical approaches, in many different patient groups. Of particular future interest is the potential value of long-axis function for better risk stratification of sudden cardiac death in primary prevention, which currently relies exclusively on the ejection fraction to decide defibrillator placement. In addition, long-axis function assessment may hold promise in early identification of patients at risk of cancer-related cardiotoxicity.[43] However, the manner in which measurement of long-axis function will affect patient care requires careful further investigation. Future studies will need to demonstrate that such imaging-driven strategies improve outcomes before these techniques can be advocated and included in guideline recommendations.

REFERENCES

1. Schulz-Menger J, Bluemke DA, Bremerich J, et al. Standardized image interpretation and post processing in cardiovascular magnetic resonance: Society for Cardiovascular Magnetic Resonance (SCMR) board of trustees task force on standardized post processing. *J Cardiovasc Magn Reson : Off J Soc Cardiovasc Magn Reson*. 2013;15:35.
2. Longmore DB, Klipstein RH, Underwood SR, et al. Dimensional accuracy of magnetic resonance in studies of the heart. *Lancet*. 1985;1(8442):1360–1362.
3. Katz J, Milliken MC, Stray-Gunderson J, et al. Estimation of human myocardial mass with MR imaging. *Radiology*. 1988;169:495–498.
4. Swift AJ, Rajaram S, Condliffe R, et al. Diagnostic accuracy of cardiovascular magnetic resonance imaging of right ventricular morphology and function in the assessment of suspected pulmonary hypertension results from the ASPIRE registry. *J Cardiovasc Magn Reson : Off J Soc Cardiovasc Magn Reson*. 2012;14:40.
5. Lorenz CH, Walker ES, Morgan VL, Graham TP, Klein SS. Normal human right and left ventricular mass, systolic function and gender differences by cine magnetic resonance imaging. *J Cardiovasc Magn Reson: Off J Soc Cardiovasc Magn Reson*. 1999;1:7–21.
6. Bellenger NG, Davies LC, Francis JM, Marcus NJ, Pennell DJ. Reduction in sample size for studies of remodelling in heart failure by the use of cardiovascular magnetic resonance. *J Cardiovasc Magn Reson: Off J Soc Cardiovasc Magn Reson*. 2000;2:271–278.
7. Grothues F, Smith GC, Moon JCC, et al. Comparison of interstudy reproducibility of cardiovascular magnetic resonance with two-dimensional echocardiography in normal subjects and in patients with heart failure or left ventricular hypertrophy. *Am J Cardiol*. 2002;90:29–34.
8. Bottini PB, Carr AA, Prisant M, Flickinger FW, Allison JD, Gottdiener JS. Magnetic resonance imaging compared to echocardiography to assess left ventricular mass in the hypertensive patient. *Am J Hypertension*. 1995;8:221–228.
9. Chamsi-Pasha MA, Zhan Y, Debs D, Shah DJ. CMR in the Evaluation of Diastolic Dysfunction and Phenotyping of HFpEF: Current Role and Future Perspectives. *JACC, Cardiovasc Imaging*. 2020;13:283–296.
10. Bollache E, Redheuil A, Clément-Guinaudeau S, et al. Automated left ventricular diastolic function evaluation from phase-contrast cardiovascular magnetic resonance and comparison with Doppler echocardiography. *J Cardiovasc Magn Reson : Off J Soc Cardiovasc Magn Reson*. 2010;12(1):63.
11. Maceira AM, Cosín-Sales J, Roughton M, Prasad SK, Pennell DJ. Reference left atrial dimensions and volumes by steady state free precession cardiovascular magnetic resonance. *J Cardiovasc Magn Reson: Off J Soc Cardiovasc Magn Reson*. 2010;12:65.
12. Farzaneh-Far A, Ariyarajah V, Shenoy C, et al. Left atrial passive emptying function during dobutamine stress MR imaging is a predictor of cardiac events in patients with suspected myocardial ischemia. *JACC, Cardiovasc Imaging*. 2011;4(4):378–388.
13. Maceira AM, Prasad SK, Khan M, Pennell DP. Normalized left ventricular systolic and diastolic function by steady state free precession cardiovascular magnetic resonance. *J Cardiovasc Magn Reson*. 2006;8:417–426.
14. Mohiaddin R, Hasegawa M. Flow pattern in the dilated ischaemic left ventricle studied by MRI in healthy volunteers and in patients with myocardial infarction. *J Magn Reson Imaging*. 1995;5:493–498.
15. Rajiah PS, Kalisz K, Broncano J, et al. Myocardial Strain Evaluation with Cardiovascular MRI: Physics, Principles, and Clinical Applications. *Radiographics*. 2022;42:968–990.
16. Sengupta PP, Korinek J, Belohlavek M, Narula J. Left ventricular structure and function: basic science for cardiac imaging. *J Am Coll Cardiol*. 2006;48:1988–2001.
17. Ho SY. Anatomy and myoarchitecture of the left ventricular wall in normal and in disease. *Eur J Echocardiogr*. 2009;10(8):iii3–iii7.
18. Khalique Z, Ferreira PF, Scott AD, Nielles-Vallespin S, Firmin DN, Pennell DJ. Diffusion tensor cardiovascular magnetic resonance imaging: a clinical perspective. *JACC Cardiovasc Imaging*. 2020;13(5):1235–1255.
19. Nielles-Vallespin S, Khalique Z, Ferreira PF, de Silva R. Assessment of myocardial microstructural dynamics by in vivo diffusion tensor cardiac magnetic resonance. *J Am Coll Cardiol*. 2020;69:661–676.
20. Wandt B. Long-axis contraction of the ventricles: a modern approach, but described already by Leonardo da Vinci. *J Am Soc Echocardiogr*. 2000;13(7):699–706.
21. Hamilton Wfr JH. Movements of the base of the ventricle and relative constancy of the cardiac volume. *Am J Physiol*. 1932;102(3):559–565.
22. Carlsson M, Ugander M, Mosen H, Buhre T, Arheden H. Atrioventricular plane displacement is the major contributor to left ventricular pumping in healthy adults, athletes, and patients with dilated cardiomyopathy. *Am J Physiol Heart Circ Physiol*. 2007;292(3):H1452–H1459.
23. Sanderson JE. Left and right ventricular long-axis function and prognosis. *Heart*. 2008;94(3):262–263.
24. Rangarajan V, Chacko SJ, Romano S, et al. Left ventricular long axis function assessed during cine-cardiovascular magnetic resonance is an independent predictor of adverse cardiac events. *J Cardiovasc Magn Reson*. 2016;18(1):35.
25. Romano S, Judd RM, Kim RJ, et al. Left ventricular long-axis function assessed with cardiac cine MR imaging is an independent predictor of all-cause mortality in patients with reduced ejection fraction: a multicenter study. *Radiology*. 2018;286(2):452–460.
26. Romano S, Judd RM, Kim RJ, et al. Prognostic Implications of Mitral Annular Plane Systolic Excursion in Patients with Hypertension and a Clinical Indication for Cardiac Magnetic Resonance Imaging: A Multicenter Study. *JACC, Cardiovasc Imaging*. 2019;12(9):1769–1779.
27. Hu K, Liu D, Herrmann S, et al. Clinical implication of mitral annular plane systolic excursion for patients with cardiovascular disease. *Eur Heart J Cardiovasc Imaging*. 2013;14(3):205–212.
28. Kalam K, Otahal P, Marwick TH. Prognostic implications of global LV dysfunction: a systematic review and meta-analysis of global longitudinal strain and ejection fraction. *Heart*. 2014;100(21):1673–1680.
29. Romano S, Judd RM, Kim RJ, et al. Association of feature-tracking cardiac magnetic resonance imaging left ventricular global longitudinal strain with all-cause mortality in patients with reduced left ventricular ejection fraction. *Circulation*. 2017;135(23):2313–2315.
30. Romano S, Judd RM, Kim RJ, et al. Feature-tracking global longitudinal strain predicts death in a multicenter population of patients with ischemic and nonischemic dilated cardiomyopathy incremental to ejection fraction and late gadolinium enhancement. *JACC, Cardiovasc Imaging*. 2018;11(10):1419–1429.
31. Romano S, Romer B, Evans K, Trybula M, Shenoy C, Kwong RY, et al. Prognostic implications of blunted feature-tracking global longitudinal strain during vasodilator cardiovascular magnetic resonance stress imaging. *JACC, Cardiovasc Imaging*. 2020;13(1 Pt 1):58–65.
32. Romano S, Judd RM, Kim RJ, et al. Feature-tracking global longitudinal strain predicts mortality in patients with preserved ejection fraction: a multicenter study. *JACC, Cardiovasc Imaging*. 2020;13(4):940–947.
33. Farzaneh-Far A, Romano S. Imaging and impact of myocardial strain in myocarditis. *JACC, Cardiovasc Imaging*. 2020;13:1902–1905.
34. Shenoy C, Romano S, Hughes A, et al. Cardiac magnetic resonance feature tracking global longitudinal strain and prognosis after heart transplantation. *JACC, Cardiovasc Imaging*. 2020;13(9):1934–1942.
35. Romano S, Kitkungvan D, Nguyen DT, et al. Implications of myocardial strain in primary mitral regurgitation - a cardiovascular magnetic resonance study. *Eur Heart J Cardiovasc Imaging*. 2024;26(1):126–134.
36. Henein MY, Gibson DG. Long axis function in disease. *Heart*. 1999;81(3):229–231.
37. Henein MY, Gibson DG. Normal long axis function. *Heart*. 1999;81(2):111–113.
38. Chilian WM. Microvascular pressures and resistances in the left ventricular subepicardium and subendocardium. *Circ Res*. 1991;69(3):561–570.
39. Greenbaum RA, Ho SY, Gibson DG, Becker AE, Anderson RH. Left ventricular fibre architecture in man. *Br Heart J*. 1981;45(3):248–263.
40. Schuster A, Backhaus SJ, Stiermaier T, et al. Fast manual long axis strain assessment provides optimized cardiovascular event prediction following myocardial infarction. *Eur Heart J Cardiovasc Imaging*. 2019;20(11):1262–1270.
41. Pahlm U, Seemann F, Engblom H, et al. Longitudinal left ventricular function is globally depressed within a week of STEMI. *Clin Physiol Funct Imaging*. 2018. https://doi.org/10.1111/cpf.12521.
42. Stoylen A, Molmen HE, Dalen H. Relation between Mitral Annular Plane Systolic Excursion and Global longitudinal strain in normal subjects: The HUNT study. *Echocardiography*. 2018;35(5):603–610.
43. Marwick TH, Dewar E, Nolan M, et al. Strain surveillance during chemotherapy to improve cardiovascular outcomes: the SUCCOUR-MRI trial. *Eur Heart J*. 2024;45(41):4414–4424. https://doi.org/10.1093/eurheartj/ehae574.

motion abnormalities in the infundibular part of the RV. Abnormal hemodynamic interaction of the LV and RV can be assessed using free breathing real-time cine images in mid-ventricular short-axis orientation by the presence of increased respiratory shifting of the septum during normal and increased breathing effort as an indicator for constrictive pericarditis.

IMAGE ANALYSIS

Visual Analysis

The initial step includes visual assessment of the RV long-axis and short-axis views to determine if RV size and global function are normal or abnormal, and if abnormal, an initial broad categorization as mild, moderate, or severe is sufficient. In addition, the presence of RV hypertrophy is determined, which is not only manifested as an increase in absolute wall thickness but also in increased volume and thickness of RV trabeculations. This first step requires expertise of the reader as well as high-quality images, and serves as the basis for subsequent quantitative analysis. Visual segmental analysis is the next step, whereby the RV is typically segmented in basal, mid-, and apical levels, with the basal section further subdivided into an anterior and inferior/diaphragmatic segment. Each segment is scored visually as normokinetic/hyperkinetic, mild/moderately hypokinetic, severely hypokinetic, akinetic, and dyskinetic, similarly to LV segmental interpretation. The septum should be assessed for evidence of abnormal hemodynamic interaction of the LV and RV, or RV pressure/volume overload states recognized by flattened and D-shaped septum bowing into the LV.

Quantitative Analysis

The dataset used for RV volumetric analysis is the stack of contiguous short-axis images. There is a number of

software tools ava
ally the myocardia
algorithms to sepa
automatically or s
culated by adding
the Simpson meth
The endocardial c
the end-diastolic ar
result in data on
ume, stroke volume
There are a few
reproducible volum
Key point 1. *De*
first step is to defi
frames correctly. T
with the largest (e
blood pool area. Th
same for LV and RV
indicators of end-sy
valve leaflets seen c
is typically the last
triggered by the R v
triggered acquisitic
rhythm).
Key point 2. *Th*
ventricular from atr
long-axis RV views t
define the most ba
volume (Fig. 18.3B)
and identify the v
has thicker walls c
Similarly, the pu
border between th
the area of the basa
be included in the

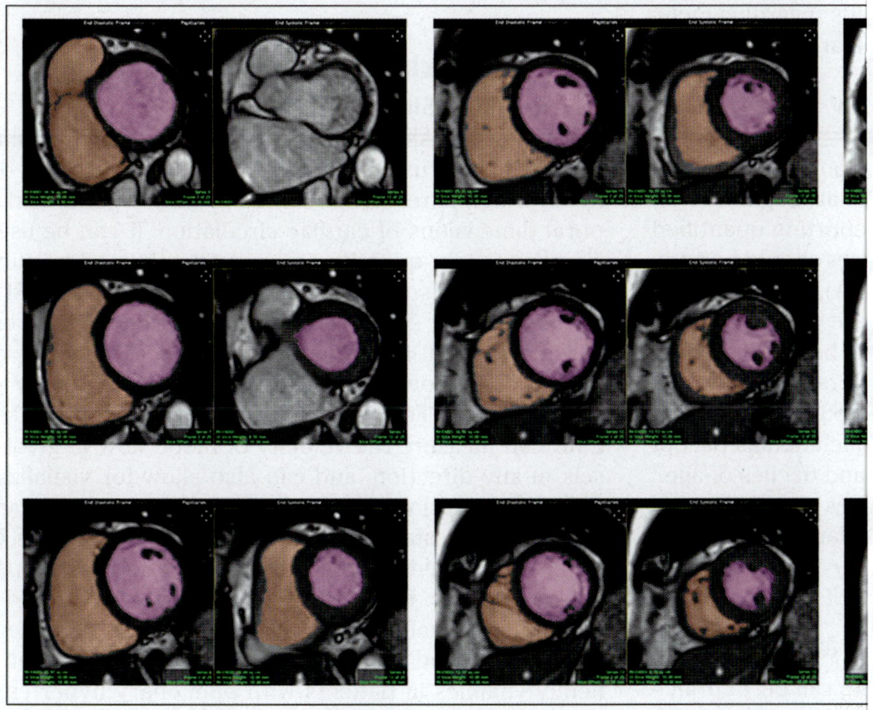

FIG. 18.2 Planimetry of LV and RV volumes on short axis cine

18 Right Ventricular Cardiovascular Magnetic Resonance Imaging

FAWAZ ALENEZI AND IGOR KLEM

INTRODUCTION

Right ventricular (RV) function is crucial for evaluating outcomes in various pulmonary and cardiac conditions. Identifying sensitive functional and structural markers of RV dysfunction is vital for enhancing daily clinical practice and patient management, enabling earlier detection and more effective treatment strategies. However, assessing RV structure and function presents challenges due to its complex geometry, the presence of comorbid pulmonary diseases, and the overlap of hemodynamic abnormalities with the left ventricle (LV). While transthoracic echocardiography (TTE) is commonly recommended as the initial imaging modality for RV assessment, its diagnostic capabilities are limited. The thin walls, unique morphology, and anterior position of the RV in the chest can hinder accurate evaluation using TTE. The complex geometry of the RV poses challenges for reliably measuring RV volume, making TTE often suboptimal for RV assessment. These limitations underscore the need for advanced imaging techniques and more refined assessment methods to better evaluate RV function in clinical practice. Recent advancements in computed tomography (CT) technology have improved temporal and spatial resolution, allowing for better evaluation of RV volume and function. However, studies comparing cardiac CT measurements with cardiac magnetic resonance (CMR) imaging as the reference standard have shown variable agreement. These discrepancies may stem from differences in RV segmentation methods between cardiac CT and CMR. Additionally, the use of CT for evaluating the RV, particularly in congenital heart disease, is limited due to concerns about high radiation exposure and the lack of tissue characterization. Nuclear imaging techniques, such as single-photon emission computed tomography (SPECT) and positron emission tomography (PET), can assess RV perfusion and metabolism, as well as determine the RV ejection fraction (RVEF). However, these techniques have low temporal resolution and carry a high risk of radiation exposure. Right heart catheterization (RHC) provides valuable insights into RV hemodynamics, including cardiac output, contractility, and RV–pulmonary artery coupling. However, its invasive nature restricts its application to a limited number of patients requiring RV assessment. These limitations highlight the need for more accessible and less invasive methods to evaluate RV effectively in clinical practice.

CMR imaging is ideally suited for assessing the RV due to its ability to provide a comprehensive evaluation of cardiovascular morphology and physiology without many limitations faced by other imaging modalities. CMR does not rely on acoustic windows, body size, or postoperative changes, and it avoids exposure to harmful ionizing radiation. Additionally, it eliminates the morbidity associated with invasive diagnostic catheterization. With high-resolution, time-resolved three-dimensional (3D) visualization, CMR enables detailed depiction and quantification of blood flow, measurement of valve regurgitation, and assessment of tissue characteristics, such as scar tissue. Currently, no other imaging modality offers such extensive and reproducible information in a clinical context. This chapter will demonstrate the practical application of CMR in both normal and various pathological conditions of the RV, highlighting its critical role in diagnosing and managing RV-related issues effectively.

RV STRUCTURE AND FUNCTION

The right and left ventricles have a number of morphological differences. Embryologically, the RV is derived from the secondary heart field, whereas the LV is derived from the primary heart field. The RV can be described in terms of morphology into three components: (1) the inlet, which consists of the tricuspid valve, chordae tendineae, and papillary muscles; (2) the trabeculated apical myocardium; and (3) the infundibulum, or conus, which corresponds to the outlet. The RV has three to eight papillary muscles, a moderator band which incorporates the right bundle branch, septo-marginal trabeculations, and a myocardial fold called the crista supraventricularis. RV myocardial fibers are arranged circumferentially in the superficial (epicardial layer) and longitudinally in the deep layers (endocardial layer) leading to a contraction from the inlet to the outlet and from the free wall to the septum. The blood supply of the RV varies according to the dominance of the coronary system. In a right-dominant system, which is found in ≈80% of the population, the right coronary artery (RCA) supplies most of the RV. Normal to the RV coronary perfusion occurs during both systole and diastole in contrast with the LV which is perfused mainly in diastole.

The RV is uniquely adapted for its role in the circulatory system, primarily due to its thin-walled, crescent-shaped structure. This design allows the RV to handle volume overload effectively but makes it less efficient under pressure overload. In contrast to the systemic circulation, the pulmonary vascular system is characterized by low impedance and high distensibility, resulting in lower vascular resistance. The RV and LV are interdependent, sharing the interventricular septum and encased within the same pericardium. The RV's muscle mass is approximately one-sixth that of the LV, reflecting its need to pump against much lower resistance. The contraction of the RV is sequential and peristaltic, starting at the inlet and progressing toward the outlet, whereas the LV contracts uniformly with a torsional motion.

When the RV experiences volume or pressure overload, its contraction pattern becomes more uniform. The RV employs three mechanisms for contraction:

1. Free wall inward movement (the "bellows-like" effect), which relies on the position of the moderator band and septo-marginal trabeculation.
2. Contraction of longitudinal fibers, which shortens the long axis toward the apex.
3. Traction of the free wall during septal contraction.

Approximately 25% of the RV's stroke volume results from the interventricular septum's motion, demonstrating "systolic ventricular interdependence." However, the RV primarily relies on longitudinal shortening for stroke volume generation, accounting for about 75%, with less emphasis on twisting or rotational movements. The RV's high surface-to-volume ratio allows it to eject an equivalent stroke volume with less free wall inward motion compared to the LV. Additionally, because of the low diastolic pressures in the pulmonary artery, the RV's isovolumetric contraction and relaxation times are shorter than those of the LV. This efficiency is crucial for the RV's role in maintaining adequate pulmonary circulation.

CMR IMAGIN

Assessment o

IMAGE ACQUI

CMR imaging of
tocol showing b
RV images. Rou
covering both t
beyond the atric
diac core exam.
1 cm to provide a
images through
set for volumetri
orientation can b
umetry, however
mize the scan ti
specific situatior
motion abnorma
arrhythmogenic
is being conside
RV inflow view,
four-chamber vi
phragmatic RV
plane rotated in
axis image (Fig.
(Fig. 18.1D). By p
tract, the RV out
used to separate
in volume anal

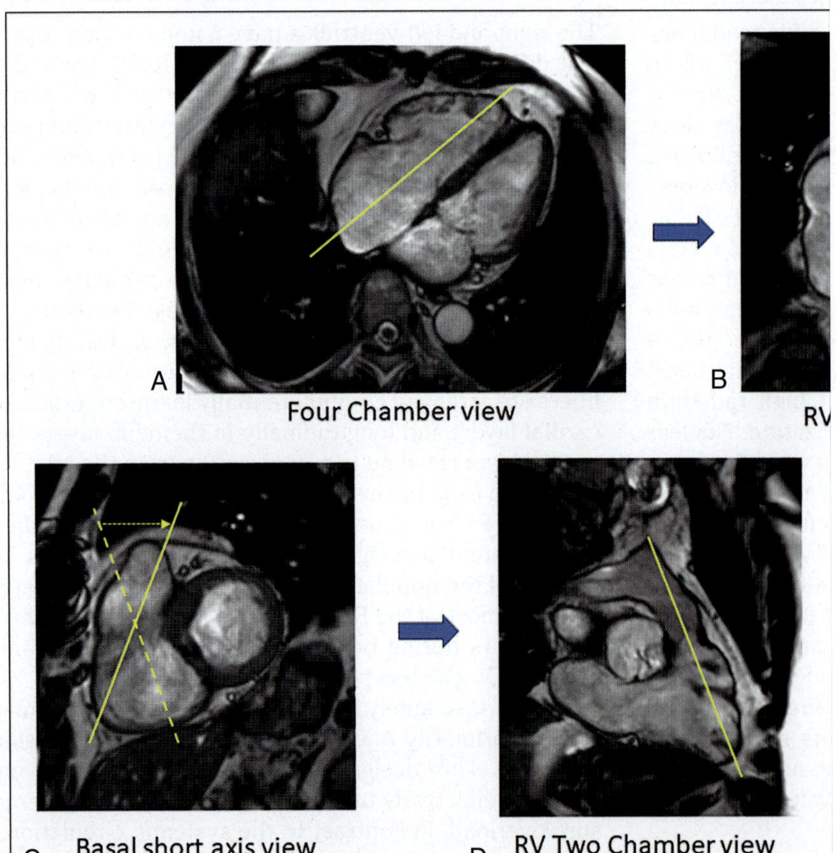

FIG. 18.1 Specific RV images. Based on the apical horizontal view, the RV inflow view (B), RV two-ch
(see text for detail).

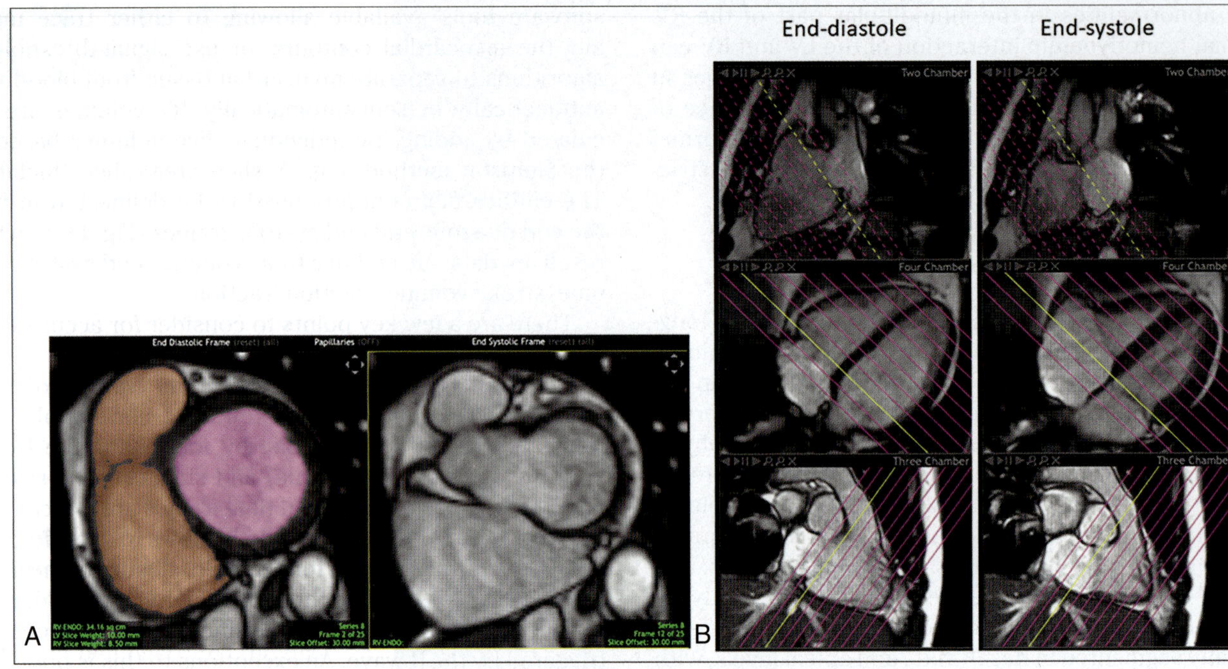

FIG. 18.3 Long-axis RV views to determine RV volumes at the base.

note that the basal slice showing ventricular volume in end-diastole will likely not be the same for end-systole due to the apical shift of the cardiac base during systole (Fig. 18.3A).

Key point 3*. Trabeculations and papillary muscles*: These represent myocardium and hence should be included in the myocardial volume and excluded from RV cavity volume. However, manual tracing of all trabeculations and papillary muscles that are detached from the compact RV wall is time consuming and reduces reproducibility. Most image analysis software solutions offer semiautomatic contouring tools, which allow faster and more reproducible analysis. However, it is important to reference normal values from publications using the same methods regarding inclusion or exclusion of trabeculations/papillary muscles.[1]

REFERENCE VALUES FOR NORMAL RV VOLUMES AND FUNCTION

Normal values for RV volumes, mass, and function are published by the Society of Cardiovascular Magnetic Resonance[1] summarizing several studies reporting quantified volumes of healthy volunteers. RV volumes should be compared indexed to body surface area (BSA), and are larger in men compared to women and decrease with age (Table 18.1). Therefore, normal values should be compared to appropriate gender- and age-based reference values. In one study, steady-state free precession (SSFP) techniques were used, the papillary muscles were included as part of LV mass, and reported by both gender and deciles of age.[2] Other studies have reported normal values used older gradient echo techniques, or included papillary muscles into the blood pool.

Tissue Characterization of the RV Myocardium

Tissue characterization of RV myocardium can be, in principle, performed similar to LV tissue characterization, however, due to thinner walls, the confounding effect of partial-volume effects from adjacent blood pool and fat will be significantly higher. In CMR in the case of right ventrcile delayed enhancemnet (RV-DE) suspicion, it is necessary to carefully adjust the inversion time to maximize the contrast between remote and fibrotic myocardium. In some patients, RV fibrosis could be visualized in the absence of ECG or echocardiographic signs. In addition, RV involvement in patients with acute LV myocardial infarction (MI) is an independent prognostic indicator for major adverse cardiovascular events (MACE) and that CMR is superior to ECG and echocardiography for the detection of RV involvement.[3]

Emerging Techniques for RV Assessment

FOUR-DIMENSIONAL FLOW

MRI four-dimensional (4D) flow is a type of phase-contrast (PC) MRI that uses blood flow encoded in three directions, which is resolved relative to three spatial and temporal dimensions of cardiac circulation. It can be used to simultaneously quantify and visualize hemodynamics or morphology disorders. Four-dimensional flow MRI can retrospectively evaluate flow information for the entire vascular system from any image plane, as both the anatomy and the flow information are applied to every pixel in a 3D volume. Four-dimensional phase-contrast (4D flow) CMR can measure the velocity of blood flow in great vessels in any direction, and can also allow for visualization and quantification of the multidimensional intracardiac hemodynamic status and kinetic energy, as well as functional assessment without breath-hold and/or the use of contrast agents. Research has showed that RV blood flow components qualified with 4D flow CMR is a valuable non-invasive method for the assessment of RV function and hemodynamics in patients with pulmonary hypertension. However, this is still not ready for clinical use.[4]

TABLE 18.1 Reference values for normal RV volumes and function stratified by gender[1].

Age (years)	20–29	30–39	40–49	50–59	60–69	70–79
Males: RV volumes, systolic function, and mass (absolute and normalized to BSA) by age decile (mean, 95% confidence interval)						
Absolute values						
EDV (mL) SD 25.4	177 (127, 227)	171 (121, 221)	166 (116, 216)	160 (111, 210)	155 (105, 205)	150 (100, 200)
ESV (mL) SD 15.2	68 (38, 98)	64 (34, 94)	59 (29, 89)	55 (25, 85)	50 (20, 80)	46 (16, 76)
SV (mL) SD 17.4	108 (74, 143)	108 (74, 142)	107 (73, 141)	106 (72, 140)	105 (71, 139)	104 (70, 138)
EF (%) SD 6.5	61 (48, 74)	63 (50, 76)	65 (52, 77)	66 (53, 79)	68 (55, 81)	70 (57, 83)
Mass (g) SD 14.4	70 (42, 99)	69 (40, 97)	67 (39, 95)	65 (37, 94)	63 (35, 92)	62 (33, 90)
Normalized to BSA						
EDV/BSA (mL/m^2) SD 11.7	91 (68, 114)	88 (65, 111)	85 (62, 108)	82 (59, 105)	79 (56, 101)	75 (52, 98)
ESV/BSA (mL/m^2) SD 7,4	35 (21, 50)	33 (IS, 47)	30 (16, 45)	28 (13, 42)	25 (11, 40)	23 (8, 37)
SV/BSA (mL/m^2) SD 8.2	56 (40, 72)	55 (39, 71)	55 (39, 71)	54 (38, 70)	53 (37, 69)	52 (36, 69)
EF/BSA (%/m^2) SD 4	32 (24, 40)	32 (25, 40)	33 (25, 41)	34 (26, 42)	35 (27, 42)	35 (27, 43)
Mass/BSA (g/m^2) SD 6.8	36 (23, 50)	35 (22, 49)	34 (21, 48)	33 (20, 46)	32 (19, 45)	31 (18, 44)
Females: RV volumes, systolic function, and mass (absolute and normalized to BSA) by age decile (mean, 95% confidence interval)						
Age (years)	**20–29**	**30–39**	**40–49**	**50–59**	**60–69**	**70–79**
Absolute values						
EDV (mL) SD 21.6	142 (100, 184)	136 (94, 178)	130 (87, 172)	124 (81, 166)	117 (75, 160)	111 (69, 153)
ESV (mL) SD 13.3	55 (29, 82)	51 (25, 77)	46 (20, 72)	42 (15, 58)	37 (11, 63)	32 (6, 58)
SV (mL) SD 13.1	87 (61, 112)	85 (59, 111)	84 (58, 109)	82 (56, 108)	80 (55, 106)	79 (53, 105)
EF (%) SD 6	61 (49, 73)	63 (51, 75)	65 (53, 77)	67 (55, 79)	69 (57, 81)	71 (59, 83)
Mass (g) SD 10.6	54 (33, 74)	51 (31, 72)	49 (28, 70)	47 (26, 68)	45 (24, 66)	43 (22, 63)
Normalized to BSA						
EDV/BSA (mL/m^2) SD 9.4	84 (65, 102)	80 (61, 98)	76 (57, 94)	72 (53, 90)	68 (49, 86)	64 (45, 82)
ESV/BSA (mL/m^2) SD 6.6	32 (20, 45)	30 (17, 43)	27 (14, 40)	24 (11, 37)	21 (8, 34)	19 (6, 32)
SV/BSA (mL/m^2) SD 6.1	51 (39, 63)	50 (38, 62)	49 (37, 61)	48 (36, 60)	46 (34, 58)	45 (33, 57)
EF/BSA (%/m^2) SD 5.2	37 (27, 47)	38 (27, 48)	38 (28, 49)	39 (29, 49)	40 (30, 50)	41 (31, 51)
Mass/BSA (g/m^2) SD 5.2	32 (22, 42)	30 (20, 40)	29 (19, 39)	27 (17, 37)	26 (16, 36)	24 (14, 35)

XENON MRI

^{129}Xe gas-exchange magnetic resonance imaging/MR spectroscopy (^{129}Xe MRI/MRS) is an emerging functional lung-imaging technology that has the potential to provide a "one-stop shop" for precise, spatial, and quantitative measurement for pulmonary ventilation, gas exchange and hemodynamics. ^{129}Xe MRI methods have an excellent safety profile in patients with respiratory disease. ^{29}Xe MRI is particularly invaluable for longitudinal monitoring of disease progression, disease phenotypes, and/or treatment response (in and outside of clinical trials) because it poses no radiation burden on patients. The lack of ionizing radiation is particularly needed for examinations in vulnerable populations, such as children with chronic lung disease. It is sensitive to functional and structural changes in early lung disease and can be used in longitudinal studies of disease progression and therapy response.[5]

CONDITIONS ASSOCIATED WITH ABNORMAL RV STRUCTURE AND FUNCTION

Changes in RV structure and function are seen in conditions associated with volume overload, pressure overload, or intrinsic right ventricular myocardial disease, which can cause dilation, global and/or regional systolic dysfunction, hypertrophy, and abnormal tissue characteristics (late gadolinium enhancement [LGE]) (Table 18.2). Given its relatively thin walls and a low-pressure condition, the RV can accommodate volume overload states by continued dilation while remaining compensated over prolonged periods of

TABLE 18.2 RV remodeling/adaptation in response to different cardiopulmonary diseases.

	DILATATION	GLOBAL DYSFUNCTION	REGIONAL DYSFUNCTION	HYPERTROPHY	ABNORMAL LGE
Cardiac shunts (ASD, PAPV)	xxx	xx			
Valvular heart disease (primary TR, PR)	xx	xx			
Pressure overload (PH)	xx	xx		xxx	
ARVC	xx	xx	xxx		xx
CAD	xx	x	xx		xx
DCM	xx	xx			
Sarcoidosis		x	x		xx

time, before it eventually decompensates with a reduction in systolic function. Conditions associated with RV volume overload are left-to-right shunts (e.g., atrial septal defects or anomalous pulmonary venous returns), and valvular heart disease such as primary tricuspid regurgitation, or pulmonic insufficiency which is often seen in complex congenital heart disease (surgically corrected right ventricular outflow tract [RVOT] obstruction in tetralogy of Fallot). The RV is very sensitive to changes in afterload, with the stroke volume decreasing rapidly when pulmonary artery pressure increases in experimental studies, and RV dysfunction in patients with increased transpulmonary gradient.[6] With gradually increasing afterload, a compensatory increase in RV muscle mass and hypertrophy occurs and ultimately results in global RV dysfunction. Intrinsic myocardial disease from cardiomyopathies (ARVC, dilated cardiomyopathy [DCM]) or ischemic events (RV infarcts) results in isolated regional dysfunction (ARVC, MI) and subsequently disease progression with global dysfunction and dilatation.

Volume Overload States

LEFT-TO-RIGHT SHUNTS

In adults with isolated atrial septal defects and functional impairment, the demonstration of right atrial and/or ventricular RV enlargement and a net left-to-right shunt sufficiently large to cause physiologic sequelae (e.g., pulmonary–systemic blood flow ratio [Qp:Qs] ≥1.5:1) determines that closure of the atrial septal defect (ASD) is indicated. A typical indication for CMR is to confirm the presence of an ASD if suspected with either Doppler or bubble study during transthoracic echocardiography. Beyond confirming the presence of an ASD, the CMR exam is expected to determine the type of ASD (primum-secundum-sinus venosus), assess RV volumes and function, quantify noninvasively the Qp:Qs with volumetric analysis and flow velocity mapping, and exclude the presence of partial anomalous venous return or other congenital malformations.

Similar criteria are applied for the timing of repair of partial anomalous venous return, and the CMR protocol is identical to the ASD protocol. Given these malformations can occur at the same time, it is advisable to assess routinely the pulmonary venous return in a patient scanned for ASD for closure planning, for example. If an enlarged RV is noted incidentally during a study performed for other indications, a shunt should be considered and appropriate images obtained to assess for a shunt. Obtaining the Qp:Qs allows very quickly to determine the presence of a shunt, and imaging the atrial septum with long- and short-axis cine images often allows to identify an ASD on morphological images (Fig. 18.4).

VALVE PATHOLOGY

Tricuspid Regurgitation

Tricuspid regurgitation (TR), often trivial or mild, is frequently seen on cardiac exams in patients without significant symptoms. Moderate or severe primary TR is seen in rheumatic heart disease, infectious endocarditis, along RV leads, congenital deformities such as Ebstein's anomaly, or carcinoid. Secondary TR is more frequent than primary TR, accompanying pulmonary hypertension with RV remodeling, DCM, annular dilation with atrial fibrillation, and RV volume overload states. A common indication for CMR assessment of the tricuspid valve is in patients with congenital heart disease such as Ebstein's anomaly. More often TR is noted in patients with other indications, for example for the assessment of cardiomyopathies or pre-ablation for atrial fibrillation. The severity of TR should be determined both visually and using velocity flow mapping to determine the regurgitant fraction (planimetric stroke volume = pulmonic flow/planimetric stroke volume). If significant TR (regurgitant volume >45 mL, regurgitant orifice ≥0.40 cm^2) is noted, the imaging protocol should include assessment of valve morphology to determine the etiology and mechanism of TR. Measurements of RV volumes and ejection fraction (EF) are important to identify the hemodynamic significance or TR, which is a key criterion for surgical repair and is performed before RV dysfunction of heart failure ensues. Left heart disease or imaging signs of pulmonary hypertension (PH) such as right ventricle hypertrophy (RVH), dilated pulmonary artery (PA), and flattened D-shaped septum may provide additional information about the etiology.

Pulmonic Insufficiency

Pulmonic insufficiency is often encountered after surgical repair of tetralogy of Fallot, which typically encompasses relief of RVOT obstruction by infundibulotomy, and a patch to enlarged the pathway between the RV and pulmonary artery. The most common sequelae of surgical repair are severe pulmonic insufficiency with RV dilatation and dysfunction. The optimal timing for pulmonic valve repair in this situation has been linked to preoperative RV volumes that would result in normalization of RV volumes and function postoperatively. CMR is considered the test of choice for quantification of RV volumes, and mild or

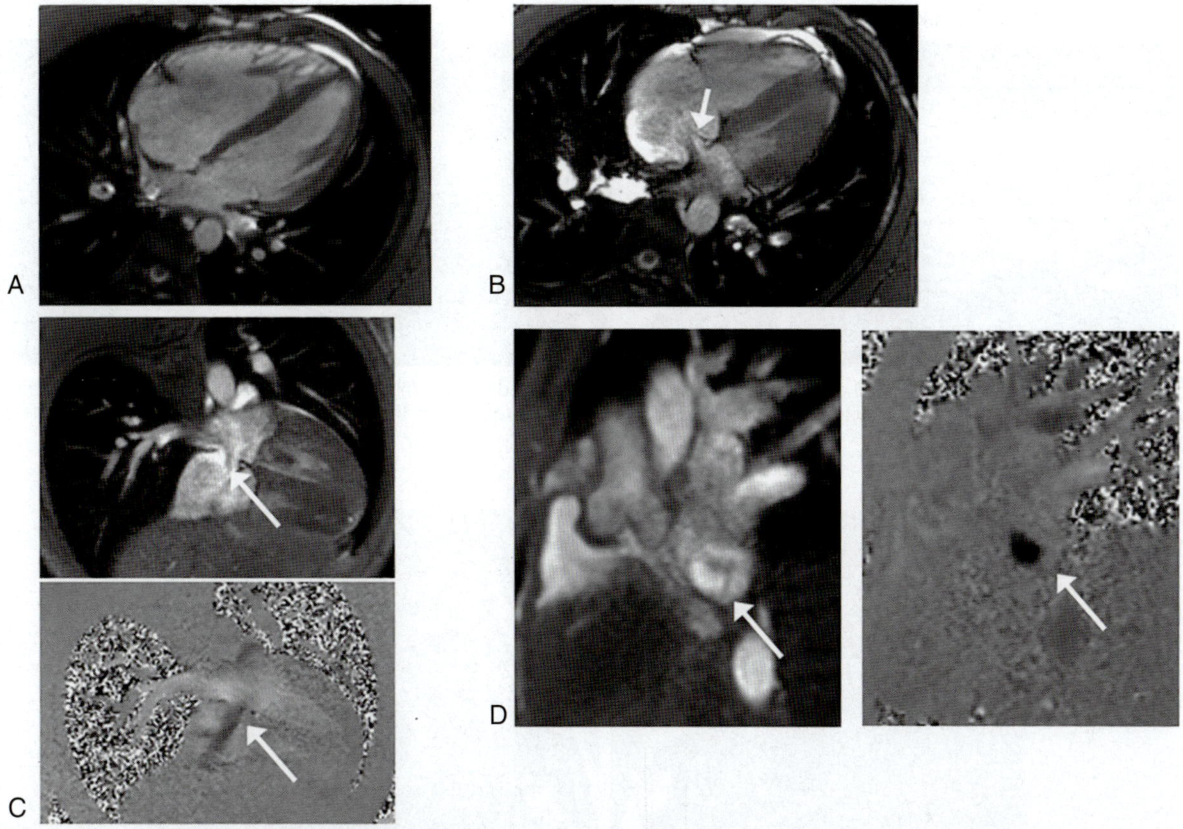

FIG. 18.4 A 20-year-old varsity basketball player with abnormal preparticipation ECG. On 4CV enlarged RV and RA were noted, prompting imaging tailored for intracardiac shunt (atrial septal defect) which includes a stack of axial cine images. This revealed concern for a low-seated atrial septal defect (B). Flow velocity imaging confirms left-to-right shunting with a Qp:Qs = 1.9 and direct flow across the ASD of 5.6 L/min across a 2.0 × 1.3 cm secundum atrial septal defect.

moderate RV dysfunction and severe RV dilatation defined as RV end-diastolic volume index ≥160 mL/m², or RV end-systolic volume index ≥80 mL/m² are current criteria used for decisions on timing. The CMR protocol in patients with tetralogy of Fallot includes imaging of the cardiac chamber volumes and function, regional RV function, and pulmonic valve morphology including assessment of stenosis and grade of insufficiency, but is also aimed at assessing for associated lesions such as branch pulmonary artery stenosis, residual atrial or ventricular septal defects, tricuspid valve regurgitation, aortic dilatation, aortic valve insufficiency, and LV dysfunction.

Pressure Overload States

Pulmonary hypertension (PH) is characterized by a progressive rise in pulmonary artery (PA) pressure and can eventually lead to RV dysfunction in advanced stages. CMR offers simultaneous morphologic and functional evaluation. Several cardiac MRI markers are identified as important prognostic factors, including RV end-diastolic volume (RVEDV), RV systolic volume (RVSV), and interventricular septal bowing. Cardiac MRI is an ideal method for analyzing RV morphology and function, evaluating the RV-PA functional unit, risk stratification, and obtaining important prognostic information. During RV remodeling secondary to long-standing altered afterload, the RV compensates with eccentric remodeling and dilatation. The presence and extent of LGE have been related to RV performance and pulmonary hemodynamics. PH patients with LGE show significantly higher mean PA pressure (obtained with right heart catheterization) and lower RV ejection fraction than patients without LGE. The indexed RV mass is the main predictor of total LGE mass, indicating that the amount of LGE at the RV attachment sites is directly related to the degree of RV remodeling.

Arrhythmogenic Right Ventricular Cardiomyopathy

Regional akinesia, dyskinesia, or bulging plus either global RV dilatation (increase in RV-EDV according to reference values) or global RV systolic dysfunction (reduced RVEF EDV according to reference values) remains a major CMR criterion of ARVC.[7] These revised 2020 International (Padua) criteria include a number of changes compared to the 2010 revised Task-Force criteria for ARVC.[8]

- To increase sensitivity, a minor criterion of regional akinesia, dyskinesia, or bulging even without global RV enlargement and/or dysfunction was added.
- The reference values for RVEDV (up to 110 mL/m² in men and 100 mL/m² in women) were based on healthy controls from the multiethnic study of atherosclerosis (MESA) and determined using older fast gradient echo CMR cine techniques. The revised criteria refer to more recent published normal values using SSFP techniques.[1]
- Transmural LGE affecting ≥1 RV region (inlet, outlet, and apex in two orthogonal views), with or without fat signal on dedicated fat-saturation sequences, is considered a major structural criterion (Fig. 18.5).

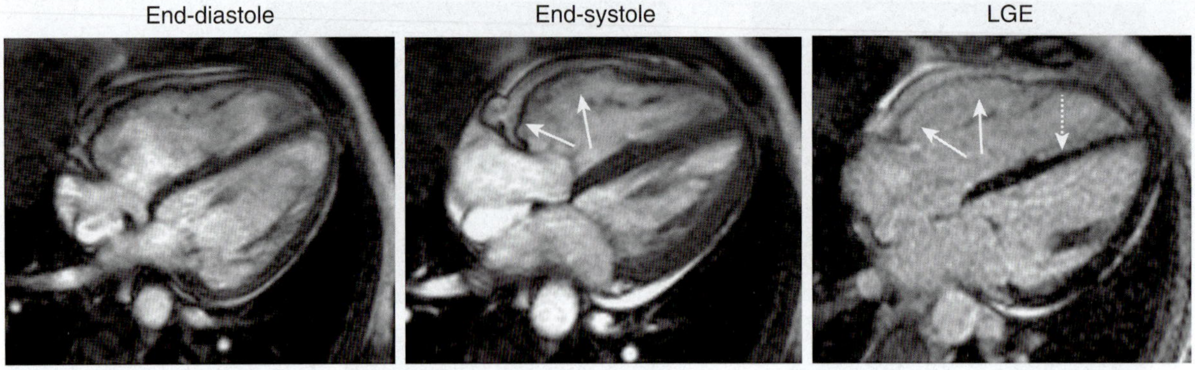

FIG. 18.5 A 50-year old F w NSVT, PVCs, ECG criteria for ARVC. CMR shows enlarged RV (125 mL/m^2), reduced RVEF 34%, with akinesia and dyskinesia of the basal free wall consistent with major criterion for ARVC. LGE images demonstrate scar in the RV free wall (*white arrows*) and RV side of the basal inferoseptum (*white dashed arrow*).

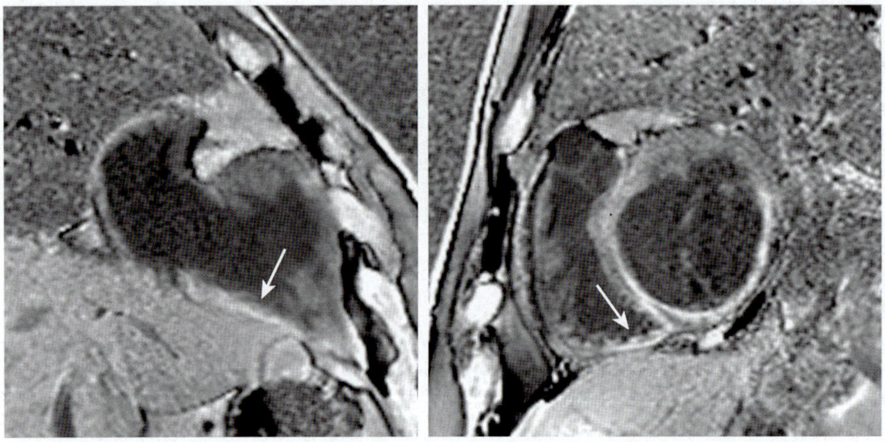

FIG. 18.6 RV infarct example seen in the RV two-chamber and short-axis inferior wall.

Ischemic Heart Disease (RV Infarcts)

Involvement of the RV in acute myocardial infarction (AMI) has prognostic value in regard to complications and mortality. It ranges from 20% to 60% of inferior wall infarcts, and is rare to be isolated. ECG is less sensitive for RV myocardial infarction detection, and can hardly delineate RV infraction in the presence of an LV infarction. However, detection of an RV myocardial fibrosis pattern is fundamental for differential diagnosis of RV pathology. Compared to the LV, there is a large discrepancy in the literature regarding fibrosis detection in the RV. It has been suggested that, in LGE images, accurate RV assessment needs a shorter inversion time compared to the LV. Previous studies demonstrated that early postinfarction RV injury is common and is characterized by the presence of myocardial edema, DE, and functional abnormalities (Fig. 18.6). RV injury typically occurs with infarction of the LV inferior wall. However, to date, there is no systematic evaluation of the clinical prognostic value of RV injury assessed by CMR in a large ST-elevation MI population.[9]

Nonischemic Dilated Cardiomyopathies

In one study of 423 patients with DCM, only about 20% were found to have RV dysfunction.[6] In this study, RV dysfunction was defined as an RVEF ≤35% and was determined based on the associated cardiac mortality risk (Fig. 18.7), whereby an incremental cardiac mortality risk was observed with RVEF ≤45%, albeit a statistically significant risk was seen with RVEF ≤35%. This provides some data on grading severity of RV dysfunction based on the associated mortality risk (rather than the deviation from a normal population), with an RVEF >45% being normal (similar HR to RVEF >55%), mildly reduced with RVEF >35% and ≤45%, moderately reduced RVEF >25% and ≤35%, and severe RV dysfunction as RVEF ≤25% (Fig. 18.8). Determinants of RV dysfunction were LVEF, which may be secondary to the intrinsic cardiomyopathy process, impaired contraction of the septal myocardium and mutually encircling epicardial muscle-fiber layers, or hemodynamic sequelae of a failing LV, with upward shift of the RV diastolic pressure–volume relationship due to pericardial constraints and result in RV impairment through diastolic ventricular interdependence. In addition, LV failure may result in increased RV afterload (mean pulmonary artery pressure).

Cardiac Sarcoidosis

With clinical criteria used as the reference and nonischemic LGE patterns used as the definition of a positive case, CMR had a high sensitivity (95%) and specificity (85%) for the diagnosis of CS in a meta-analysis of 17 studies and 1031 individuals. It is important to note that myocardial LGE also carries significant prognostic value as the

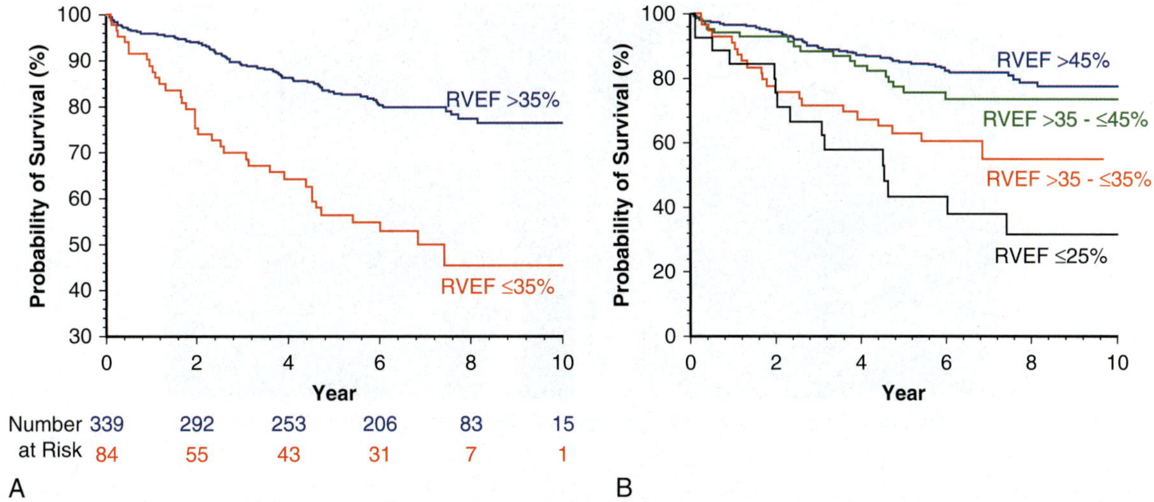

FIG. 18.7 Kaplan–Meier estimates of survival according to RVEF. The difference in cardiac survival between patients with an RVEF ≤35% and >35% was significant (*P*<.0001, by the log rank test) (A). The Kaplan–Meier estimates of cardiac death-free survival stratified by RVEF is shown in (B). Both subgroups with an RVEF ≤25% and RVEF >25% and ≤35% had significantly lower probability of survival compared to those with RVEF >45% (*P*<.001 for both), whereas those with an RVEF >35% and ≤45% had a similar probability of survival compared to those with an RVEF >45% (*P*=.09). (JACC Cardiovasc Imaging. 2017;10(10 Pt B):1225–1236.)

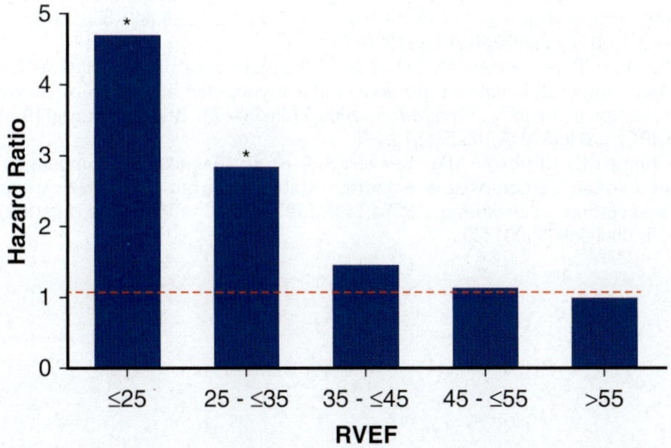

FIG. 18.8 The hazard ratios for cardiac mortality are shown according to different levels of right ventricular ejection fraction (*RVEF*). The red dashed line displays the hazard ratio of 1 of the reference group with RVEF >55%. Patients with an RVEF ≤35% had a significantly higher event risk compared to the reference group. Patients with an RVEF >35 and ≤45%, as well as those >45 and ≤55% had similar risk to the group with RVEF >55%. **P*<.001.

strongest predictor for all-cause mortality and sustained VA among individuals with known or suspected CS. There are no patterns of LGE that are sufficient for the diagnosis CS. However, the features seen in more than 90% of cases were LV subepicardial, LV multifocal, septal, and RV free-wall involvement, while infrequent features included the absence of gross myocardial involvement, isolated LV midmyocardial involvement, isolated LV subendocardial involvement, and the absence of septal involvement (Fig. 18.9).[10]

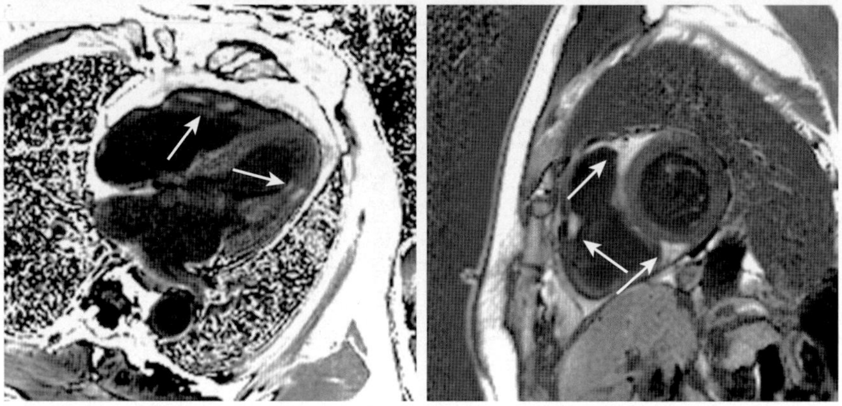

FIG. 18.9 Cardiac sarcoidosis (CS) example with multifocal DE involving LV and RV.

REFERENCES

1. Kawel-Boehm N, Hetzel SJ, Ambale-Venkatesh B, et al. Reference ranges ("normal values") for cardiovascular magnetic resonance (CMR) in adults and children: 2020 update. *J Cardiovasc Magn Reson*. 2020;22:87. https://doi.org/10.1186/s12968-020-00683-3.
2. Maceira AM, Prasad SK, Khan M, Pennell DJ. Reference right ventricular systolic and diastolic function normalized to age, gender and body surface area from steady-state free precession cardiovascular magnetic resonance. *Eur Heart J*. 2006;27:2879–2888. https://doi.org/10.1093/eurheartj/ehl336.
3. Karamitsos TD, Arvanitaki A, Karvounis H, Neubauer S, Ferreira VM. Myocardial tissue characterization and fibrosis by imaging. *JACC Cardiovasc Imaging*. 2020;13:1221–1234. https://doi.org/10.1016/j.jcmg.2019.06.030.
4. Wang L, Liu M, Zhang PY, et al. Analysis of right ventricular flow with 4-dimensional flow cardiovascular magnetic resonance imaging in patients with pulmonary arterial hypertension. *Quant Imaging Med Surg*. 2021;11:3655–3665. https://doi.org/10.21037/qims-20-1267.
5. Alenezi F, Covington TA, Mukherjee M, Mathai SC, Yu PB, Rajagopal S. Novel approaches to imaging the pulmonary vasculature and right heart. *Circ Res*. 2022;130:1445–1465. https://doi.org/10.1161/CIRCRESAHA.121.319990.
6. Pueschner A, Chattranukulchai P, Heitner JF, et al. The prevalence, correlates, and impact on cardiac mortality of right ventricular dysfunction in nonischemic cardiomyopathy. *JACC Cardiovasc Imaging*. 2017;10:1225–1236. https://doi.org/10.1016/j.jcmg.2017.06.013.
7. Corrado D, Zorzi A, Cipriani A, et al. Evolving diagnostic criteria for arrhythmogenic cardiomyopathy. *J Am Heart Assoc*. 2021;10:e021987. https://doi.org/10.1161/JAHA.121.021987.
8. Peters MN, Katz MJ, Alkadri ME. Diagnosis of arrhythmogenic right ventricular cardiomyopathy. *Proc (Bayl Univ Med Cent)*. 2012;25:349–353. https://doi.org/10.1080/08998280.2012.11928874.
9. Ibrahim T, Schwaiger M, Schomig A. Images in cardiovascular medicine. Assessment of isolated right ventricular myocardial infarction by magnetic resonance imaging. *Circulation*. 2006;113:e78–e79. https://doi.org/10.1161/CIRCULATIONAHA.105.536615.
10. Cheng RK, Kittleson MM, Beavers CJ, et al. Diagnosis and management of cardiac sarcoidosis: a scientific statement from the american heart association. *Circulation*. 2024;149:e1197–e1216. https://doi.org/10.1161/CIR.0000000000001240.

19 Atrial Structure and Function

ANDREAS SCHUSTER AND INGO EITEL

INTRODUCTION

Cardiac magnetic resonance (CMR) imaging has revolutionized the way we assess and understand cardiovascular health. It has enabled the exploration of various facets of cardiovascular health and disease that were not previously feasible with other imaging techniques, including the assessment of atrial structure and function.

As essential components of the heart, the atria play a critical role in managing hemodynamics and ensuring efficient blood flow from the veins to the ventricles. The complex dynamics of atrial physiology underscore their importance, as they function not only as reservoirs for incoming blood but also as facilitators of effective ventricular filling through conduit and contractile mechanisms. A thorough understanding of atrial structure is equally vital. The anatomical features of the atria, including their volume, wall thickness, and chamber architecture and tissue composition, are pivotal in influencing their mechanical properties and overall function. Pathological changes, such as atrial enlargement or fibrotic changes, can significantly impair atrial performance, potentially leading to adverse clinical outcomes.

Advances in imaging techniques, particularly CMR, facilitate detailed visualization and measurement of these structural attributes, enabling a deeper understanding of atrial health and pathologies. Furthermore, the assessment of atrial function encompasses the intricate patterns of contraction and relaxation that occur during the cardiac cycle. These dynamic processes are affected by various factors, including loading conditions and heart rate, which can alter the efficacy of atrial mechanics. Understanding these aspects is crucial for identifying patients at risk for atrial-related disorders, such as atrial fibrillation (AF) or heart failure. In addition, the ability to evaluate atrial structure and function under different physiological conditions, such as during exercise stress, offers valuable insights into the adaptive responses of the atria. This information can enhance our understanding of cardiovascular function in both healthy individuals and those with existing heart conditions.

Ultimately, a comprehensive evaluation of atrial structure and function through CMR has significant clinical implications, providing essential information for diagnosing and managing various cardiovascular diseases. By fostering a deeper understanding of the underlying physiological concepts, we can improve patient care and outcomes, ensuring a more effective approach to cardiovascular health. However, access to CMR technology and expertise is often still restricted to larger hospitals, academic centers, and university hospitals, which may limit patient access and the overall adoption of this valuable diagnostic tool.[1] This chapter aims to provide a comprehensive overview of atrial structure and function through advanced imaging techniques, while also highlighting the clinical significance of these assessments; finally, we will discuss future developments and novel approaches in CMR that promise to further enhance our understanding and management of atrial conditions.

ATRIAL PHYSIOLOGY

The heart operates as a synchronized, multichambered pump that relies on the coordinated actions of both the atria and ventricles to ensure efficient blood flow throughout the body. Atrial physiology is critical, particularly in understanding how the left and right atria function during the cardiac cycle, which is composed of distinct phases: diastole and systole. For this chapter, we will specifically refer to atrial and ventricular systole, as well as atrial and ventricular diastole, when using the terms systole and diastole, since they represent opposing phases between the chambers.

The atria perform three essential functional roles (reservoir function, conduit function, and contractile booster pump function) each contributing uniquely to the mechanics of the cardiac cycle. Atrial physiology and its different phases can be measured with different imaging technologies and all specific phases of that physiology can be individually targeted.[2] Fig. 19.1 provides an overview of these phases and how they can be measured throughout the cardiac cycle.

The atrial cardiac cycle is normally quantified beginning with atrial diastole (during ventricular systole), a phase wherein the atrial heart muscle relaxes while the ventricular heart muscle contracts and blood fills the atria. The right atrium (RA) receives deoxygenated blood from the systemic circulation via the superior and inferior vena cavae, while the left atrium (LA) collects oxygenated blood from the pulmonary circulation through the pulmonary veins. During this phase, the atria serve as reservoirs, collecting pulmonary venous return with gradually increasing atrial pressure due to the influx of blood. This reservoir function is essential for preventing congestion and ensures that there is a steady flow of blood into the ventricles later during ventricular diastole. The effectiveness of the reservoir function can be assessed using global

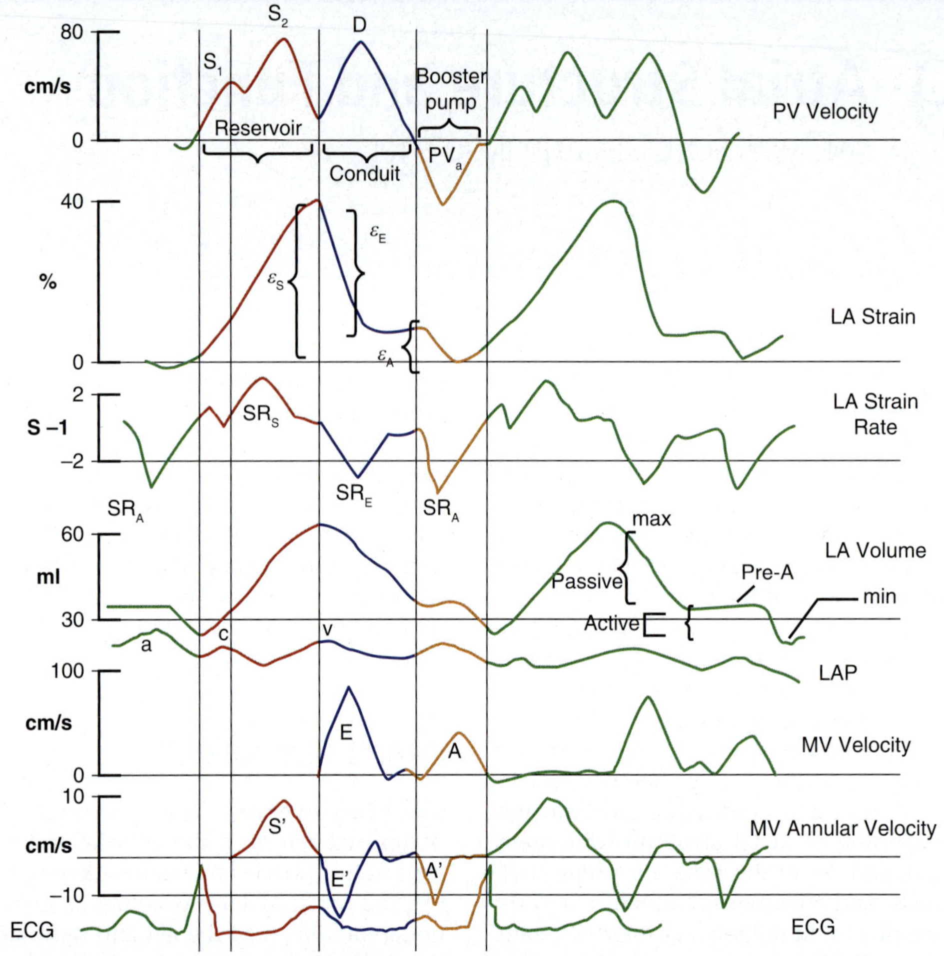

FIG. 19.1 Atrial physiology and its color-coded connection to the cardiac cycle. This figure provides an overview of atrial physiology and its different components in relation to the electrocardiogram (ECG) and the different phases of the atrial cardiac cycle including reservoir, conduit, and booster pump function. The following parameters are presented in the figure: Pulmonary venous (PV) velocity, left atrial (LA) strain (ε), LA strain rate (SR), LA volume, LA pressure (LAP), as well as mitral valve (MV) spectral and tissue Doppler data. The functions of the left atrium are categorized using colored lines: Reservoir function is shown in red, conduit function in blue, and booster pump function in yellow. Figure illustration by Craig Skaggs.

peak longitudinal strain (εs) and global peak positive strain rate (SRs), which measure the atrial deformation during this phase (Fig. 19.2). Furthermore, it can be estimated by assessing the total ejection or emptying fraction of the LA (LAEF total, corresponding to atrial reservoir function).[3]

As the atria keep filling, they stretch, and the pressure rises sufficiently to overcome that in the ventricles. At around the end of ventricular systole, the AV valves open, allowing blood to flow into the ventricles during early ventricular diastole. This passive filling phase is crucial for maintaining optimal preload, influencing the Frank–Starling relationship and ultimately affecting stroke volume. The atria facilitate the passage of blood into the ventricles, functioning as conduits. This conduit function is crucial for rapid ventricular filling and can be evaluated using global passive longitudinal strain (εe), global peak early negative strain rate (SRe) and passive LA emptying fraction (LAEF passive, incorporating the atrial volume preatrial contraction), which assess the blood flow dynamics during this initial filling period (Fig. 19.2).[3]

Following passive filling, the atria contract in a phase known as atrial systole, which corresponds with the end-diastolic phase of the ventricles. This action increases atrial pressure, driving additional blood into the ventricles. Atrial contraction contributes approximately 20%–30% of the ventricular filling in a healthy heart, especially under conditions of increased demand, such as during exercise. The signaling for atrial contraction is initiated by the electrical impulse from the sinoatrial (SA) node, establishing atrial depolarization. This phase is particularly significant in individuals with certain pathologies, where impaired ventricular filling can lead to reliance on atrial contraction for adequate blood volume (e.g., hypertrophic cardiomyopathy [HCM]). The end of atrial systole coincides with the augmentation of ventricular filling during late ventricular diastole. This booster pump function occurs through active contraction of the atrium, enhancing ventricular filling and optimizing cardiac output (Fig. 19.2). The effectiveness of this function is typically assessed using global longitudinal strain during atrial contraction (εa), global peak late negative strain rate (SRa), and LA active emptying fraction (LAEF booster).[3] Following these atrial functions, the onset of ventricular systole occurs, after the AV valves have closed to prevent backflow into the atria. This marks the beginning of isovolumetric contraction of the ventricles. During this phase, the ventricles contract without a

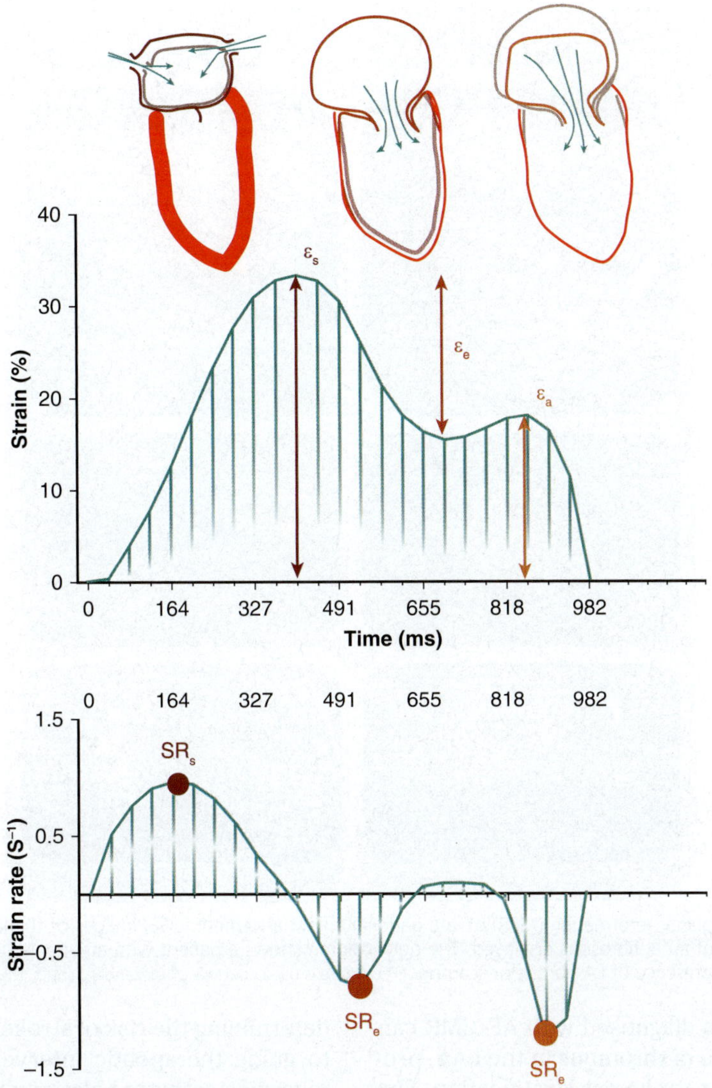

FIG. 19.2 Assessing atrial physiology using strain and strain rate (SR) imaging. The measurements for atrial function include reservoir function (assessed using global peak longitudinal strain, εs, and global peak positive strain rate, SRs), conduit function (assessed using global passive longitudinal strain, εe, and global peak early negative strain rate, SRe), and booster pump function (assessed using global longitudinal strain during atrial contraction, εa, and global peak late negative strain rate, SRa). (This figure is used courtesy of Alexander Schulz, MD, Harvard Medical School.)

change in volume as pressure builds until it exceeds that in the pulmonary artery and aorta, leading to the ejection of blood.

The understanding of atrial physiology is crucial in various pathological states. Conditions such as heart failure, atrial enlargement, and arrhythmias can significantly impact the functions of the atria, leading to compromised cardiac output and increased risk of thromboembolic events such as stroke. For example, in atrial fibrillation (AF), the loss of coordinated atrial contraction diminishes ventricular filling and increases the likelihood of stasis in the left atrial appendage (LAA), a common site for thrombus formation. In summary, atrial physiology plays an essential role in the overall mechanics of the cardiac cycle. The coordinated actions of the atria ensure effective filling and optimal ventricular function, which is paramount for maintaining hemodynamic stability. The integration of reservoir, conduit, and contractile booster pump functions emphasizes the atria's critical role in cardiac performance. A deeper understanding of these processes aids in the management of cardiovascular diseases and the development of targeted therapies.

ATRIAL STRUCTURE

In addition to the described complex physiological functions there are many aspects of atrial structure that are important and unique. This structure allows the atrium to provide adequate physiologic function, playing a pivotal role in the heart's overall efficiency. Understanding the anatomy of the LA, which is positioned posteriorly and superiorly to the left ventricle (LV), is critical, particularly when evaluating different cardiovascular conditions. Advances in CMR have enhanced our ability to visualize this anatomy and changes in atrial size and structure, allowing a better diagnosis and management of various cardiac conditions. The anatomy comprises of the interatrial septum and features the fossa ovalis, a remnant of the fetal foramen ovale, which opposes the LAA a site predisposed to thrombus

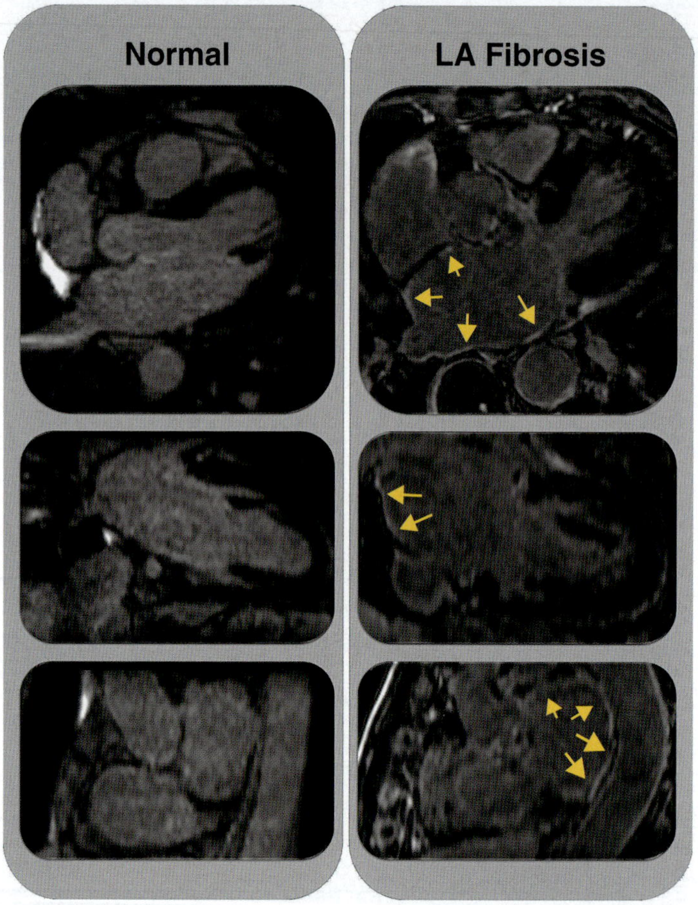

FIG. 19.3 This figure shows a multiplanar reformation (MPR) of late gadolinium enhancement (LGE) images of the left atrium (LA). In the left column an example of a healthy subject without atrial fibrosis is displayed. The right column shows a patient with atrial enlargement and a longstanding history of paroxysmal AF. *Arrows* indicate the presence of LA fibrosis or scarring. (This figure is used courtesy of Alexander Schulz, MD, Harvard Medical School.)

formation in AF. For patients diagnosed with AF, CMR can aid in assessing the presence of thrombus in the LAA, providing critical information for stroke risk stratification. The LA is also subject to age-related changes and the impact of chronic conditions. Hypertension, valvular disease, and AF can lead to LA enlargement, compromising its function. The most established global parameter to estimate LA size is the left atrial volume index (LAVI), which is calculated by normalizing the LA volume to body surface area. CMR imaging provides precise and reproducible measurements of LA volume, allowing for accurate assessment of LAVI and enhanced risk stratification in patients with cardiovascular conditions.[4] On a more regional level the LA anatomy is complex, with a thin (2–3 mm) muscular wall and a smooth main body with pectinate muscles that aid contraction. High-resolution CMR provides precise assessment of these structural details, aiding the diagnosis and management of various conditions. Fibrosis and remodeling may occur as a response to sustained elevated pressures or atrial stretch, leading to increased likelihood of AF, which is characterized by disorganized electrical activity in the atria and can further exacerbate structural changes. One of the key advantages of CMR in general is the ability to assess not only the size and volume of myocardial chambers but also tissue characteristics. Through techniques such as late gadolinium enhancement (LGE), CMR can identify areas of fibrosis within the LA wall, which may predispose patients to arrhythmias (Fig. 19.3). This information is crucial for determining the risk of stroke and other complications and to guide therapeutic interventions and inform decisions regarding catheter ablation procedures or surgical options to mitigate risks. In addition, there has been an extensive debate regarding the existence of atrial cardiomyopathy as a distinct entity. Whether intrinsic atrial dysfunction, independent of hemodynamic factors, can lead to atrial remodeling and impaired function, or atrial abnormalities are largely a response to chronic volume or pressure overload cannot be answered by CMR; however, the functional consequences of these alterations can be studied in great detail.

Notwithstanding, the determination of the exact amount of LA fibrosis is challenging due to spatial resolution of the available CMR sequences within the range of the very thin-layered LA wall. Furthermore, a prospective advantage of a CMR-guided pulmonary vein isolation procedure has not yet been demonstrated in AF.[5] As a result, atrial scar imaging is not widely adopted in clinical CMR imaging. Novel approaches use holistic three-dimensional (3D) LA shape analyses to determine morphological changes without employing tissue characteristics at the atrial level.[6] The heart failure with preserved ejection fraction (HFpEF) stress trial demonstrated that changes in LA anatomy can predict future events, including AF. Moving beyond simple volume assessments, this study identified LA roof dilation as a crucial early indicator of HFpEF, preceding global LA enlargement (and potentially scarring). This novel finding forms the basis of an LA HFpEF shape score, a biomarker that effectively discriminates HFpEF from noncardiac dyspnea and predicts both AF and cardiovascular hospitalization.[6] The complex LA structure and anatomy and changes in response to various conditions underscore the necessity of thorough evaluation. CMR imaging stands out as a transformative tool for visualizing both the anatomy and functional dynamics of the LA. As our comprehension of the LA continues to evolve with advancements in imaging technology and clinical research, it becomes increasingly vital to integrate these insights into practiced cardiology, enhancing diagnostic accuracy and optimizing treatment strategies.

COMPREHENSIVE ASSESSMENT OF ATRIAL FUNCTION AT REST AND DURING EXERCISE STRESS

Atrial function and the three phases of atrial physiology can be assessed using different CMR techniques including volumetric approaches and deformation imaging techniques. This offers a more nuanced understanding of atrial function and allows for cross-validation of results within a single study.[3] By integrating these methodologies, healthcare providers can discern how different aspects of atrial function contribute to overall cardiovascular health. This is crucial for identifying patients at risk of adverse cardiac events and developing effective intervention strategies. Atrial strain and SR imaging, using techniques like speckle tracking echocardiography or CMR feature tracking (FT), offers the potential to differentiate various cardiac diseases. CMR-FT is a postprocessing technique based on optical flow used to analyze CMR steady-state free precession (SSFP) images. It automatically tracks the movement of anatomical structures (like the endocardium) throughout the cardiac cycle. This allows for the quantitative assessment of myocardial deformation, providing measures such as strain (the change in length relative to the original length) and SR (the speed of deformation).[7] These quantitative measures provide more detailed information about myocardial function compared to traditional visual or volumetric assessments of CMR images. This allows precise differentiation of different pathologies that affect atrial mechanics in unique ways. For example, atrial fibrosis in conditions like heart failure alters strain patterns differently than the effects of pressure overload or valvular disease. By quantifying these subtle differences in deformation, atrial strain and strain rate imaging can provide valuable insights into disease mechanisms and potentially improve diagnostic accuracy. Fig. 19.4 provides examples of different pathologies and how they affect CMR-FT strain measurements.

Considering abnormalities in conditions with impaired systolic function (Fig. 19.4), there are also conditions without systolic impairment such as HFpEF, which are best studied during exercise because the characteristic abnormalities in diastolic filling and overall cardiac function often only become apparent under increased hemodynamic stress.[8] Exercise testing allows for the assessment of functional limitations and reveals subtle cardiac dysfunction not easily detectable at rest, thereby providing valuable insights into disease pathophysiology. While physiological exercise testing has been well established during cardiac catheterization or echocardiographic studies, CMR has been a challenge due to limited space in the imaging bore and the magnetic environment. The HFpEF-Stress trial demonstrated the feasibility of real-time cardiac magnetic resonance (RT-CMR) imaging during exercise stress in HFpEF patients. Furthermore RT-exercise CMR provided superior diagnostic accuracy compared to both standard echocardiographic parameters (including E/E′ and LAVI) and biomarkers like NT-proBNP. Specifically, LA manual long-axis strain during exercise (LA LAS), as measured by RT-CMR, emerged as the strongest independent predictor of HFpEF (Fig. 19.5).[9] The significant increase in the area under the curve (AUC) from 0.82 at rest to 0.93 during stress testing demonstrates the enhanced diagnostic accuracy of LA LAS during exercise-induced conditions for differentiating HFpEF from other cardiac conditions. This CMR approach demonstrates significant potential in improving the early diagnosis and management of HFpEF, especially during stress conditions where traditional parameters may be insufficient.

CLINICAL IMPLICATIONS

CMR has the capability to assess atrial structure and function. Efforts have partly moved toward establishing parameters that assess chamber coupling by incorporating LA information and their relation to LV performance such as the Left Atrioventricular Coupling Index (LACI).[10] This novel parameter offers additional prognostically important insights since LACI reflects both atrial and ventricular pathology by using the ratio of LA end-diastolic volume (EDV) to LV EDV.[10] A higher LACI reflects a disproportionately enlarged LA relative to the LV, indicating impaired atrioventricular coupling. This imbalance can stem from both structural changes (increased LA size) and functional abnormalities (reduced LV function affecting filling dynamics). Following acute myocardial infarction (AMI), LACI's incorporation provides a more comprehensive assessment of cardiac function beyond LVEF alone, improving risk stratification and prognostication of adverse events.[10] Beyond LV function and chamber coupling, LA function plays a key role in prognostication following AMI. Specifically, LA εs provided independent prognostic information, even after adjusting for established risk factors and other CMR parameters (LVEF, LV global longitudinal strain (LV-GLS), infarct size, microvascular obstruction). The addition of LA εs to these parameters further improved the accuracy of MACE prediction. This highlights the potential of LA strain analysis via CMR-FT as a valuable tool for risk stratification and patient management following AMI.[11] Similar observations were made in different cardiomyopathies including dilated cardiomyopathy (DCM). A recent study highlights the prognostic value of LA εe, measured by CMR-FT, in patients with DCM.[12] LA εe proved to be a stronger predictor of adverse cardiac events (death, hospitalization, or life-threatening arrhythmias) than standard measures like LVEF, LAVI, and LV-GLS. Furthermore, LA εe provided

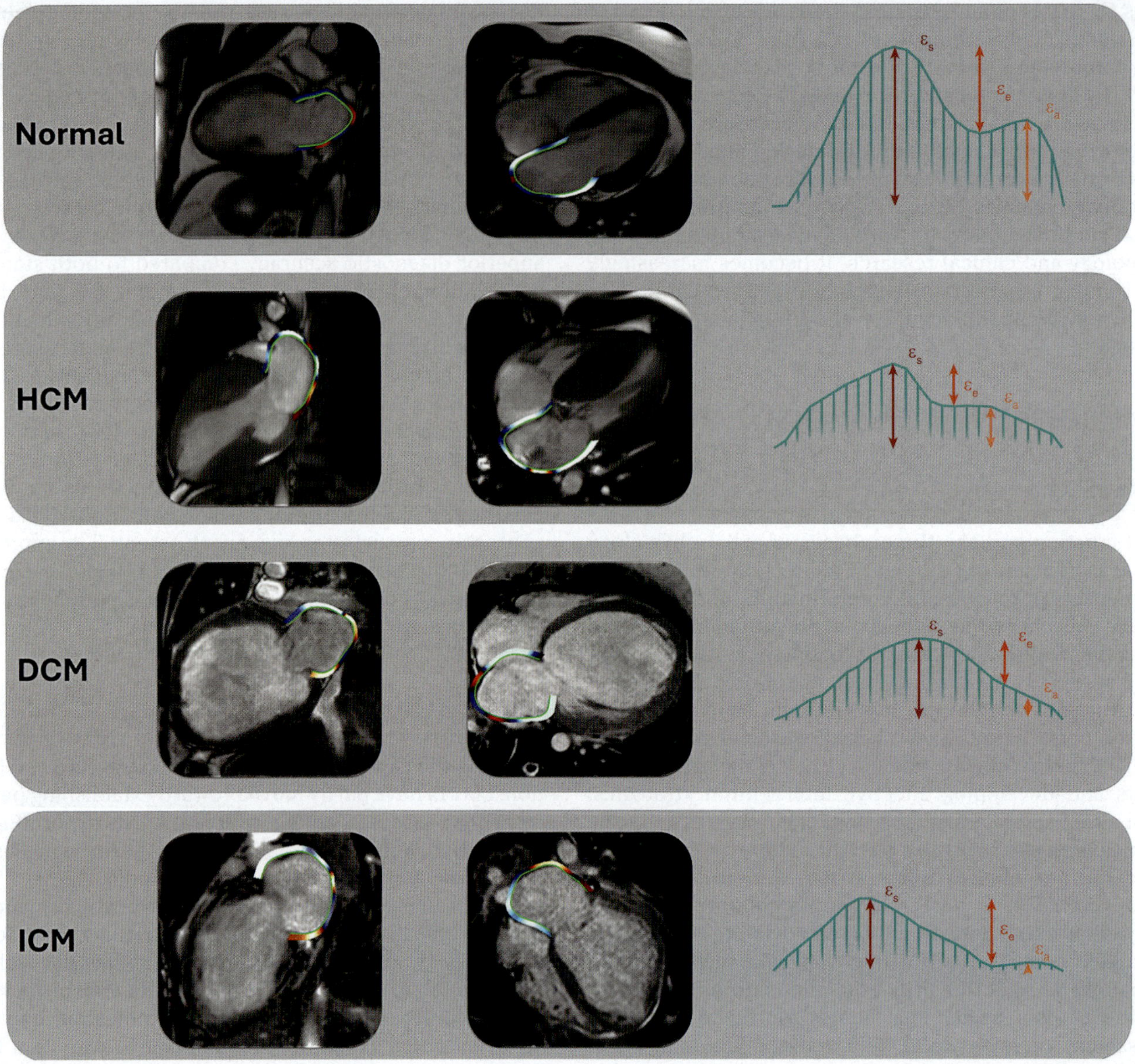

FIG. 19.4 Impact of cardiac pathologies on myocardial strain. Examples of CMR-FT strain patterns in different cardiomyopathies compared to a normal subject. The figure illustrates how hypertrophic cardiomyopathy (*HCM*), dilated cardiomyopathy (*DCM*), and ischemic cardiomyopathy (*ICM*) each produce distinct alterations in myocardial strain compared to a healthy heart. These differences in strain patterns reflect the unique pathophysiological mechanisms underlying each condition and highlight the potential of CMR-FT strain analyses for differential diagnoses. (This figure is used courtesy of Alexander Schulz, MD, Harvard Medical School.)

incremental prognostic value even when considering established risk factors like LGE and New York Heart Association (NYHA) functional class. This suggests LA εe, easily obtainable from standard CMR, could significantly improve risk stratification and patient management in DCM.[12] Furthermore, LA function is valuable in predicting the response to cardiac resynchronization therapy (CRT) as it provides an insight into LA mechanics that correlate with overall cardiac performance. In addition, LA structural and functional parameters serve as important prognostic indicators, with the absence of specific LA criteria significantly increasing the risk of adverse clinical outcomes, such as death or heart failure hospitalization, in CRT recipients with significantly reduced systolic function.[13] Significant prognostic value of LA LAS and strain was also observed in preserved systolic function. LA LAS, assessed both at rest and during exercise using CMR, emerged as a strong predictor of cardiovascular events over a 4-year follow-up in HFpEF patients.[14] In particular, impaired LA LAS at rest was independently associated with a higher risk of cardiovascular events, even when considering other factors like AF. The study highlights the importance of evaluating LA function, particularly LA LAS, for improved diagnostic accuracy and prognostic stratification in HFpEF patients. This noninvasive approach offers a valuable tool for risk assessment and potentially guiding treatment strategies such as placement of an interatrial shunt device (IASD) in this challenging patient population.[14] Importantly, patients that potentially benefit from an IASD can be identified using exercise stress CMR without the need for an invasive catheterization.[15] Lastly, LA function is also useful in healthy subjects as it helps detect subtle cardiac changes that may not be apparent through traditional measures like LVEF. Additionally, impaired LA mechanics have prognostic significance, as they are associated with a higher risk of incident major adverse cardiovascular events (MACEs)

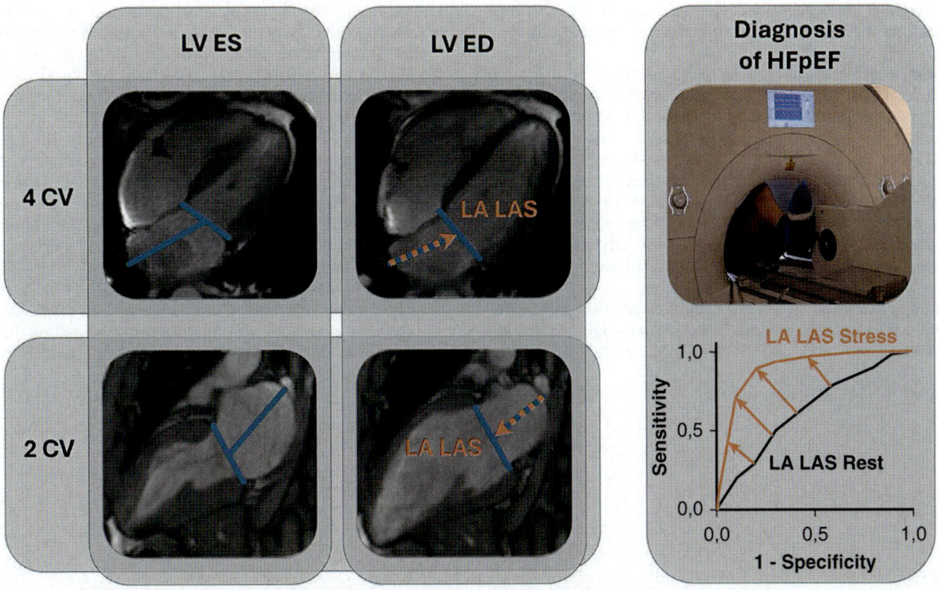

FIG. 19.5 Left atrial manual long-axis strain (*LA LAS*) quantification in four-chamber (*4 CV*) and two-chamber (*2 CV*) orientations for the diagnosis of heart failure with preserved ejection fraction (*HFpEF*). This figure illustrates the assessment of LA dimensions and LA LAS in both four-chamber and two-chamber CMR views. In the upper row the four-chamber orientation is displayed at left ventricular (*LV*) end-systole (*ES*) and end-diastole (*ED*). The lower row shows the two-chamber orientation, respectively. LA LAS was measured from the midpoint of a line connecting the mitral leaflet origins to a line to the most distant point on the posterior atrial wall. By assessing changes in length between the end of ventricular systole and diastole a quantitative percent LA LAS can be obtained. This can be measured during physiological exercise (*upper right*) providing a significant increase in diagnostic accuracy for HFpEF detection compared to obtaining LA LAS at rest (*bottom right*). The enhanced diagnostic accuracy of these measures during stress testing showcases how exercise-induced changes in LA LAS parameters can assist in differentiating HFpEF from other cardiac conditions. (This figure is used courtesy of Alexander Schulz, MD, Harvard Medical School.)

and heart failure or death, even in individuals without a history of cardiovascular disease.[16]

SUMMARY AND FUTURE OUTLOOK

Atrial structure and function carry crucial importance in cardiovascular health and disease and can be comprehensively assessed using advanced CMR studies. CMR allows detailed visualization of atrial anatomy (volume, wall thickness, chamber architecture) and the quantification of atrial physiology's three key functions: reservoir, conduit, and booster pump. These functions, assessed via strain and SR imaging, are vital for efficient ventricular filling. Pathological changes affecting atrial structure and function have significant clinical implications in cardiovascular diseases including HFpEF, DCM, and AMI. CMR, including exercise stress CMR, allows diagnosis and management of these conditions, and demonstrates the prognostic value of atrial parameters in predicting adverse events.

Future research should prioritize several key areas to improve our understanding and management of atrial conditions. This includes developing and validating novel CMR sequences and analysis methods, potentially incorporating artificial intelligence, to enhance both the precision of atrial function, including strain and strain rate measurements, and atrial structure, predominantly atrial tissue characterization. Integrating CMR data with other imaging modalities and clinical data will create more comprehensive assessments, improving diagnostic accuracy and risk stratification. Addressing limitations in access to CMR technology and expertise as well as technical limitations such as spatial resolution is crucial, and might involve developing more accessible CMR systems, expanding training programs, and sequence development. Finally, exploring and testing new therapeutic strategies based on detailed CMR assessments of atrial structure and function is necessary to improve treatments and patient outcomes for atrial-related disorders. By focusing on these key areas, future research will advance the field of atrial assessment in cardiovascular health and disease, leading to improved diagnostic accuracy, prognostic stratification, and therapeutic interventions.

REFERENCES

1. Westwood M, Almeida AG, Barbato E, et al. Competency-based cardiac imaging for patient-centred care. A statement of the European Society of Cardiology (ESC). With the contribution of the European Association of Cardiovascular Imaging (EACVI), and the support of the Association of Cardiovascular Nursing & Allied Professions (ACNAP), the Association for Acute Cardiovascular Care (ACVC), the European Association of Preventive Cardiology (EAPC), the European Association of Percutaneous Cardiovascular Interventions (EAPCI), the European Heart Rhythm Association (EHRA), and the Heart Failure Association (HFA) of the ESC. *Eur Heart J.* 2023;44:4771–4780.
2. Hoit BD. Left atrial size and function: role in prognosis. *J Am Coll Cardiol.* 2014;63:493–505.
3. Kowallick JT, Kutty S, Edelmann F, et al. Quantification of left atrial strain and strain rate using cardiovascular magnetic resonance myocardial feature tracking: a feasibility study. *J Cardiovasc Magn Reson: Off J Soc Cardiovasc Magn Reson.* 2014;16:60.
4. Khan MA, Yang EY, Zhan Y, et al. Association of left atrial volume index and all-cause mortality in patients referred for routine cardiovascular magnetic resonance: a multicenter study. *J Cardiovasc Magn Reson.* 2019;21:4.
5. Marrouche NF, Wazni O, McGann C, et al. Effect of MRI-guided fibrosis ablation vs conventional catheter ablation on atrial arrhythmia recurrence in patients with persistent atrial fibrillation: the DECAAF II randomized clinical trial. *JAMA.* 2022;327:2296–2305.
6. Backhaus SJ, Nasopoulou A, Lange T, et al. Left atrial roof enlargement is a distinct feature of heart failure with preserved ejection fraction. *Circ: Cardiovasc Imaging.* 2024;17:e016424.

7. Schuster A, Hor KN, Kowallick JT, Beerbaum P, Kutty S. Cardiovascular magnetic resonance myocardial feature tracking: concepts and clinical applications. *Circ Cardiovasc Imaging*. 2016;9.
8. Pieske B, Tschöpe C, de Boer RA, et al. How to diagnose heart failure with preserved ejection fraction: the HFA–PEFF diagnostic algorithm: a consensus recommendation from the heart failure association (HFA) of the European society of cardiology (ESC). *Eur Heart J*. 2019;40:3297–3317.
9. Backhaus SJ, Lange T, George EF, et al. Exercise stress real-time cardiac magnetic resonance imaging for noninvasive characterization of heart failure with preserved ejection fraction. *Circulation*. 2021;143:1484–1498.
10. Lange T, Backhaus SJ, Schulz A, et al. Cardiovascular magnetic resonance-derived left atrioventricular coupling index and major adverse cardiac events in patients following acute myocardial infarction. *J Cardiovasc Magn Reson*. 2023;25:24.
11. Schuster A, Backhaus SJ, Stiermaier T, et al. Left atrial function with MRI enables prediction of cardiovascular events after myocardial infarction: insights from the AIDA STEMI and TATORT NSTEMI trials. *Radiology*. 2019;293:292–302.
12. Raafs AG, Vos JL, Henkens MTHM, et al. Left atrial strain has superior prognostic value to ventricular function and delayed-enhancement in dilated cardiomyopathy. *JACC, Cardiovasc Imaging*. 2022;15:1015–1026.
13. Ma X, Chen Z, Song Y, et al. CMR feature tracking–based left atrial mechanics predicts response to cardiac resynchronization therapy and adverse outcomes. *Heart Rhythm*. 2024;21:1354–1362.
14. Backhaus SJ, Schulz A, Lange T, et al. Real-time cardiovascular magnetic resonance imaging for non-invasive characterisation of heart failure with preserved ejection fraction: final outcomes of the HFpEF stress trial. *Clin Res Cardiol*. 2024;113:496–508.
15. Schuster A, Schulz A, Lange T, et al. Concomitant latent pulmonary vascular disease leads to impaired global cardiac performance in heart failure with preserved ejection fraction. *Eur J Heart Fail*. 2023;25:322–331.
16. Subramanian V, Keshvani N, Segar MW, et al. Association of global longitudinal strain by feature tracking cardiac magnetic resonance imaging with adverse outcomes among community-dwelling adults without cardiovascular disease: the Dallas heart study. *Eur J Heart Fail*. 2024;26:208–215.

20 Stress Cardiovascular Magnetic Resonance: Myocardial Perfusion Imaging

EIKE NAGEL, LAURA PAPPAS, AND ANDREW ARAI

OPTIONS FOR INDUCING STRESS IN CARDIAC PERFUSION STUDIES

The various options for inducing stress are discussed in Chapter 7. In clinical practice, the decision is usually determined by cost and equipment. Currently, most centers use vasodilation with adenosine or regadenoson, and less frequently adenosine triphosphate or dipyridamole.[1,2] Dobutamine is used less frequently for two main reasons: First, it is a positive chronotropic resulting in high heart rates, making imaging more challenging; second, dobutamine induces true ischemia, which increases the likelihood of side effects. Reasons to perform inotropic stress with dobutamine are mainly as an add-on to late gadolinium enhancement for viability studies or in patients with suspected vasospastic angina or a myocardial bridge. This chapter will focus on vasodilator stress.

WALL MOTION VERSUS PERFUSION IMAGING

CMR stress imaging may focus on wall motion imaging, assessing myocardial contractility, or focus on perfusion imaging, where myocardial perfusion is visualized by a contrast agent after induction of hyperemia. The concept of wall motion imaging during dobutamine stress was developed based on two main observations. First, high-dose dobutamine stress echocardiography is a robust clinical method to detect stress-induced myocardial ischemia but frequently suffers from suboptimal image quality. CMR can be an excellent alternative, using the same concept of stress-induced wall motion abnormalities in patients with stress-induced ischemia while offering higher-quality images and lower interobserver variability.[3] Second, wall motion imaging with CMR is robust and very close to physiological stress, allowing to assess hibernating myocardium simultaneously.[4] In a direct comparison of dobutamine stress CMR and dobutamine stress echocardiography, CMR was shown to be superior to echocardiography in terms of accuracy due to its better image quality.[5] Since those observations, the image quality of CMR perfusion imaging has significantly improved due to better sequences and faster hardware. This has led to a change of clinical practice toward direct perfusion assessment. Perfusion imaging has several advantages, such as better spatial resolution, allowing to determine the coronary artery territory and the extent of the ischemia, easier (semi-)quantification, and—most importantly—higher sensitivity, as perfusion defects precede wall motion abnormalities in the ischemic cascade.[6] This chapter will focus on stress perfusion imaging.

CLINICAL PERFORMANCE OF PERFUSION CARDIOVASCULAR MAGNETIC RESONANCE

Reference Standard

A key issue in evaluating CAD is determining the appropriate reference standard that enables a veritable comparison of technologies. Historically, stenosis severity (e.g., >50% or >70% lumen reduction) was the accepted standard. However, it is now recognized that flow reduction is not directly proportional to anatomical stenosis severity. Clinical significance is better assessed by measuring flow or pressure reduction distal to a stenosis, rather than merely identifying or quantifying the stenosis itself. Studies using fractional flow reserve (FFR) to detect pressure drops in the coronary arteries have shown that revascularization without a significant pressure drop leads to a higher number of adverse events than conservative therapy, i.e., harming the patient.[7] As such, international guidelines require proof of ischemia before revascularization. However, FFR also has its limitations, as it is invasive and does not consider the size of the territory subtended by the respective coronary artery. Interestingly, the original validation of FFR was performed against positron emission tomography (PET) in 22 patients with isolated proximal or mid left anterior descending coronary artery stenosis.[8] The strongest reference standard for scientific validation is patient outcome, and a good diagnostic test should be able to separate patients with high likelihood for a cardiac event from those with event-free survival. Such analyses, however, are burdened by duration and—if not done in a strict prospective setting—frequently influenced by medical interventions after the test, especially revascularization by percutaneous coronary intervention (PCI) or bypass surgery. Since the severity of an anatomical stenosis is a weak comparator, we mainly refer to fractional flow reserve and outcome as the reference standards for assessing the accuracy of a stress test in this chapter.

Accuracy of Stress Perfusion CMR

Based on more than 30 large (>50 patients) single-center studies and summarized in several meta-analyses,[9–13] stress perfusion CMR and PET have the highest diagnostic accuracy for the noninvasive assessment of suspected CAD with sensitivities between 86% and 90% and specificities between 76% and 94%. Notably, the diagnostic accuracy reported in single-center studies has recently been confirmed in the GadaCAD (Gadobutrol-Enhanced Cardiac Magnetic Resonance Imaging for Detection of Coronary Artery Disease) I and II studies.[14] For GadaCAD, 764 patients were recruited from 47 international centers, and six fully blinded readers. The blinded read yielded excellent interobserver reproducibility, underlining the robustness of the test.[14] In a systematic comparison of various imaging modalities versus FFR, stress CMR reached the highest accuracy both per patient (sensitivity: 90%, specificity: 94%) and per vessel (sensitivity: 91%, specificity: 85%).[11]

The high diagnostic accuracy of stress perfusion CMR is due to a favorable combination of factors. This includes a high spatial resolution (about 2 × 2–3 × 3 mm in-plane), providing sufficient voxels in the myocardium to visualize subendocardial perfusion defects, as well as a high temporal resolution, allowing visualization of the wash-in of contrast agent through the myocardium to appreciate microvascular disease and diffuse perfusion defects, as in triple vessel disease. Moreover, its accuracy is only minimally affected by body weight or composition, making it especially valuable in more complex patients, such as those with known CAD,[15,16] previous myocardial infarction, previous revascularization, left ventricular dysfunction, or autoimmune/inflammatory disorders. Its robust image quality has been confirmed in patients with atrial fibrillation, obesity, or women, who frequently have a limited echocardiographic window.[17,18]

CMR STUDIES ON PERFUSION AND ISCHEMIC HEART DISEASE

The tables summarize key studies on perfusion CMR and ischemic heart disease, including diagnostic accuracy (Table 20.1), prognostic value (Table 20.2), specific subgroups such as patients with ischemia without obstructive coronary artery disease (INOCA), microvascular disease, and obesity (Table 20.3). Table 20.4 summarizes studies connected to revascularization therapy.

Perfusion Cardiovascular Magnetic Resonance and Prediction of Outcome

Myocardial ischemia is a strong predictor of outcome, and the amount of ischemia is highly relevant for the prediction of major adverse cardiac events. Based on outcome studies, the presence of ≥10% of ischemic myocardium (or ≥4 out of 32 segments) was regarded as a criterion for moderate to severe ischemia in the ISCHEMIA trial.[38] Patients with no ischemia have a low event rate ranging between 0.3%–1.4% per year.[39] In the large (2349 patients) multicenter SPINS study, patients without evidence of ischemia or scar had a yearly event rate of 0.7% per year over the next 5.5 years.[25] Data from meta-analyses similarly show an event rate of <2% within 25 months of a negative CMR study.[15,40] The prognostic power of perfusion CMR has been confirmed in specific subgroups, such as patients with pacemakers,[29] previous myocardial infarction,[41] reduced left ventricular ejection fraction,[33] obesity,[18] previous bypass surgery,[31,32] or atrial fibrillation.[30]

Importantly, highlighting one of the major strengths of CMR, the combination of ischemia and scar tissue as detected by late gadolinium enhancement (LGE) pertains to a significantly higher event rate. The presence of LGE without ischemia is also relevant to predict prognosis.[15] Given the high number of unrecognized myocardial infarctions in the elderly population, the use of CMR as an early technique to assess cardiovascular prognosis has the

TABLE 20.1 Diagnostic accuracy.

STUDY	AUTHOR, DATE	SUMMARY OF FINDINGS	NUMBER OF PATIENTS
GadaCAD I + II[14] (Gadobutrol-enhanced cardiac magnetic resonance imaging for detection of coronary artery disease)	Arai et al., 2020	Phase III trials to assess diagnostic accuracy of gadobutrol-enhanced stress perfusion CMR and LGE with invasive coronary angiography as a reference standard. CMR reached the highest accuracy per patient and per vessel as well as excellent interobserver variability in six blinded readers	764
MR-IMPACT[19] (Comparison of perfusion cardiac magnetic resonance with single-photon emission computed tomography for the detection of coronary artery disease)	Schwitter et al., 2008	Comparison of perfusion CMR to SPECT, with superior performance of CMR	241
CE-MARC[20] (Cardiovascular magnetic resonance and single-photon emission computed tomography for diagnosis of coronary heart disease)	Greenwood et al., 2012	Comparison of perfusion CMR to SPECT with angiography as a reference standard in a prospective trial. CMR showed better sensitivity and negative predictive value. In addition to diagnostic findings, long-term follow-up showed that CMR-derived data had strong prognostic value, with CMR-negative patients showing favorable outcomes	752

TABLE 20.2 Prognosis.

STUDY	AUTHOR, DATE	SUMMARY OF FINDINGS	NUMBER OF PATIENTS	YEARS OF FOLLOW-UP (MEAN)
Prognostic role of CMR and conventional risk factors in myocardial infarction with nonobstructed coronary arteries[21]	Dastidar et al., 2019	CMR added significant prognostic value in predicting cardiovascular outcomes in patients with MINOCA, outperforming traditional risk factors like age and cholesterol levels	388	3.5
Safety and prognostic value of vasodilator stress perfusion cardiovascular magnetic resonance in patients with heart failure[22]	Pezel et al., 2020	Stress perfusion CMR was found to predict heart failure-related outcomes, including hospitalization and cardiovascular death, with high accuracy in patients with heart failure with reduced ejection fraction (HFrEF)	1053	5.6
Stress perfusion CMR in patients with known and suspected CAD: Prognostic value and optimal ischemic threshold for revascularization[23]	Vincenti et al., 2017	Demonstrated that stress perfusion CMR is useful in both known and suspected CAD patients, showing significant prognostic relevance for future ischemic events	1024	2.5
Prognostic value of vasodilator stress cardiac magnetic resonance imaging[24]	Heitner et al., 2019	Shows that clinical vasodilator stress CMR is associated with patient mortality in a large, diverse population of patients with known or suspected CAD	9151	5
SPINS[25] (Stress perfusion imaging in the United States)	Kwong et al., 2019	Multicenter evaluation of US patients with stable chest pain and intermediate- to high-risk chest pain syndromes showed that patients with negative CMR criteria for ischemia had a low event rate and lower costs on further cardiac testing	2349	5.4
The prognostic significance of quantitative myocardial perfusion: An artificial intelligence–based approach using perfusion mapping[26]	Knott et al., 2020	The two-center study using AI-based perfusion CMR analysis showed that reduced myocardial blood flow or myocardial perfusion reserve provide strong independent predictors of adverse cardiovascular outcomes	1049	1.7

TABLE 20.3 Specific subgroups.

STUDY	AUTHOR, DATE	SUMMARY OF FINDINGS	NUMBER OF PATIENTS	YEARS OF FOLLOW-UP (MEAN)
Stress CMR in patients with obesity: Insights from the stress CMR perfusion imaging in the United States (**SPINS**) registry[18]	Ge et al., 2021	Stress perfusion CMR was shown to be effective in assessing ischemia in **obese patients**, offering insights into myocardial perfusion without the limitations seen in other modalities	1177	5.4
Stratified medical therapy using invasive coronary function testing in angina: The **CorMicA** (coronary microvascular angina) trial[27]	Ford et al., 2018	In patients with **INOCA and microvascular dysfunction**, stress perfusion CMR was used to guide therapy and improve outcomes. CMR-based detection of microvascular disease led to significant changes in management	391	0.5
WISE (Women's ischemia syndrome evaluation)[28]	Bairey Merz et al., 2006	CMR demonstrated its utility in detecting **microvascular disease and INOCA in women**, showing improved identification of ischemia in the absence of obstructive CAD	456	5
Diagnostic accuracy of stress perfusion CMR for risk stratification in patients with MR-conditional pacemakers[29]	Pezel et al., 2021	This study evaluated the diagnostic accuracy of stress perfusion CMR for patients with **MR-conditional devices**. The study highlighted CMR's effectiveness in this subgroup	224	7
Long-term prognostic value of vasodilator stress cardiac magnetic resonance in patients with atrial fibrillation[30]	Weiss et al., 2022	CMR stress perfusion was predictive of long-term cardiovascular outcomes in patients with **atrial fibrillation**, including stroke and heart failure	164	6.6
Quantitative myocardial perfusion predicts outcomes in patients with prior surgical revascularization[31]	Seraphim et al., 2022	Quantitative myocardial perfusion derived from CMR was an important predictor of outcomes in patients **post-revascularization surgery**	341	1.7
Prognostic value of vasodilator stress perfusion CMR in patients with previous coronary artery bypass graft[32]	Kinnel et al., 2021	This study evaluated CMR's ability to predict long-term outcomes in patients with **prior CABG**. Stress perfusion CMR showed a strong prognostic signal for future ischemic events	866	4.2
Prognostic value of stress cardiac magnetic resonance in patients with known coronary artery disease[16]	Antiochos et al., 2022	CMR stress perfusion demonstrated high prognostic value in patients with **established CAD**, identifying those at higher risk of adverse cardiovascular events	755	5.3
Prognostic value of stress CMR perfusion imaging in patients with reduced left ventricular function[33]	Ge et al., 2020	Stress perfusion CMR was shown to have substantial prognostic value in patients with **reduced LV function**, helping predict adverse outcomes	582	5.0

TABLE 20.4 **Management guidance.**

STUDY	AUTHOR, DATE	SUMMARY OF FINDINGS	NUMBER OF PATIENTS	YEARS OF FOLLOW-UP (MEAN)
MR-INFORM[34] (Magnetic resonance perfusion or fractional flow reserve in coronary disease)	Nagel et al., 2019	In patients with stable angina, MRI stress perfusion imaging was found to lead to less coronary revascularization than FFR-guided therapy, as well as being noninferior concerning major adverse cardiac events	916	1
CE-MARC 2[35] (Clinical evaluation of magnetic resonance imaging in coronary heart disease 2)	Greenwood et al., 2016	CE-MARC 2 trial found that CMR-guided management significantly reduced unnecessary angiography and provided superior diagnostic and prognostic performance over nuclear testing in patients with suspected coronary artery disease	1202	1
ISCHEMIA[36] (Initial invasive or conservative strategy for stable coronary disease)	Maron et al., 2020	While primarily focusing on ischemic heart disease, stress CMR was only performed in 5% of patients, raising questions about whether CMR would have been a superior guide for therapy	5179	3.2[a]

[a]The ISCHEMIA-EXTEND[37] study is evaluating longer follow-up.

potential for improved (secondary) prevention and therapy guidance.[25,42,63]

A summary of the specific features of perfusion CMR is provided in Fig. 20.1.

Perfusion CMR and Therapy Guidance

It is imperative for both patients and their healthcare providers to accurately diagnose symptoms and relate them to a specific diagnosis. However, the primary objective of conducting imaging tests lies in directing treatment and enhancing patient outcomes. The Magnetic Resonance Perfusion or Fractional Flow Reserve in Coronary Disease (MR-INFORM) trial[34] showcased the utility of perfusion CMR in guiding patient care. In this multinational trial involving 918 patients with stable angina and multiple risk factors, participants were randomly assigned to either an FFR-guided or an MR-guided approach. All patients received guideline-directed medical therapy. In the FFR-guided group, invasive angiography was standard practice for all patients, with revascularization carried out only in cases of coronary artery stenosis exceeding 95% or an FFR below 0.8. Conversely, patients in the MR-informed group underwent invasive angiography solely if significant ischemia was detected in the perfusion CMR study. The primary endpoint was 1-year outcome. Despite a median ischemic burden of 18%, indicating moderate to severe ischemia in many patients, only 49% of the patients exhibited positive findings on perfusion CMR, allowing a significant reduction of invasive angiographies in this group despite the high pretest likelihood. Similarly, revascularization was required significantly less frequently in the MR-guided group compared to the invasively guided arm (36% vs. 45% $P<.005$). At 1-year follow-up, both groups demonstrated comparable outcomes, with a low incidence of adverse events (3.6% vs. 3.7%, ns) and freedom from angina (49.2% vs. 43.8%, ns), affirming the safety and efficacy of using noninvasive stress perfusion CMR to guide the management of patients with stable chest pain. In a comparison of CMR, SPECT, and CCTA in terms of the number of unnecessary invasive coronary angiographies within a year after testing in 1202 symptomatic patients, those guided by CMR required 7.5% unnecessary invasive procedures versus 28.8% in those guided by Coronary Computed Tomography Angiography (CCTA).[35] Similarly, a comparison of CMR and CCTA in 600 previously revascularized patients[43] demonstrated a lower utilization of resources post CMR compared to post CCTA after 2 years (downstream noninvasive testing: 17 vs. 28%; invasive testing: 20 vs. 31%; and revascularization 16 vs. 24%; all $P<.01$), while reducing the number of adverse cardiac events (5% vs. 10%, $P<.01$) and improving cost-effectiveness.

These studies affirm the benefit of using CMR in stable CAD, reducing unnecessary intervention (and iatrogenic procedural complications) without compromising patient safety.

Perfusion CMR in the Guidelines

CHRONIC CORONARY SYNDROMES OR STABLE CHEST PAIN

The latest European and US guidelines underscore the importance of stress perfusion CMR for patients experiencing chronic chest pain, assigning it a class I recommendation with robust evidence from randomized controlled trials.[44–47] These guidelines universally emphasize the necessity of employing a noninvasive test prior to resorting to invasive angiography in cases of stable chest pain. They further stress that revascularization should not be undertaken without prior evidence of myocardial ischemia, ideally established through noninvasive means. The central value of a diagnostic test, however, is not merely in confirming a very high or very low pretest likelihood, but rather in furnishing a clear and dependable diagnosis for patients with intermediate pretest likelihoods—those for whom the diagnosis is uncertain prior to testing. Data outlined in the ESC guidelines illustrate that coronary CTA, PET, and stress CMR are the most accurate tests for ruling in or ruling out CAD in patients with intermediate pretest likelihoods. Crucially, their efficacy was demonstrated not only against invasive coronary angiography but also against fractional flow reserve as the reference standard.

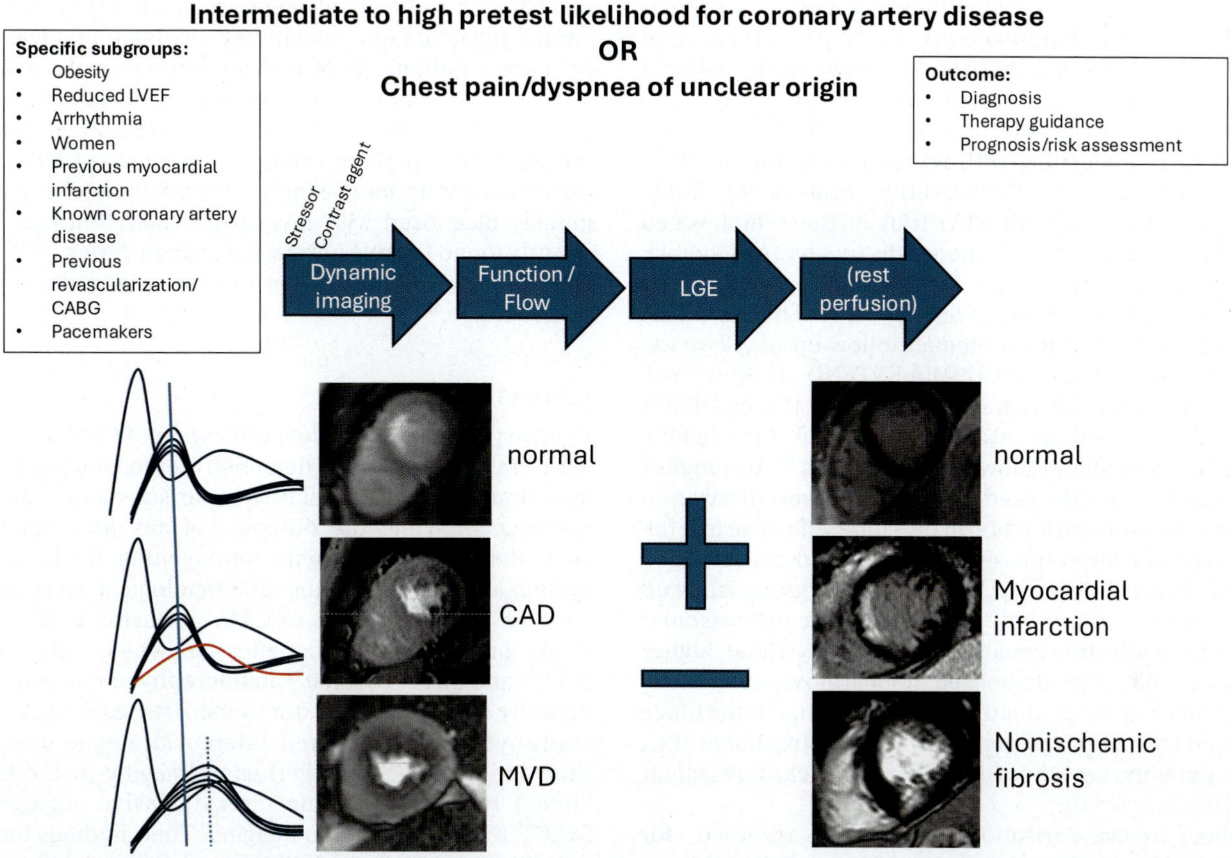

FIG. 20.1 Diagnostic workup of patients with intermediate-to-high pretest likelihood for coronary artery disease (*CAD*) or chest pain/dyspnea of unclear origin with CMR. Dynamic stress perfusion with contrast agent provides information on normal, regional ischemia (*CAD*) or diffuse subendocardial ischemia (microvascular disease, *MVD*). Additional late gadolinium enhancement imaging (*LGE*) adds information on previous myocardial infarction or nonischemic fibrosis. Usually, a function and flow module is added between stress perfusion and LGE to allow interstitial contrast agent distribution. Rest perfusion may be added for full quantification but is not routinely done in clinical practice. Diagnostic accuracy has been shown in a large variety of subgroups including highly complex patients, and results frequently clarify the diagnosis and origin of the chest pain beyond the coronary arteries and provide strong prognostic markers.

While coronary CTA excels in ruling out disease, PET and stress CMR are particularly advantageous in patients with intermediate or higher pretest likelihoods. Both the ESC and ACC/AHA guidelines on stable chest pain advocate for CTA as the preferred modality to rule out CAD, owing to its exceptionally high negative predictive value, while stress testing is favored over anatomical imaging to rule in CAD. This preference stems from the recognition that the extent of ischemia, rather than the mere confirmation of disease, is paramount for subsequent management.[48]

Nevertheless, it remains important to remember that patients and their doctors want to understand the underlying reason for chest pain or shortness of breath, rather than only excluding disease. CMR is uniquely positioned to answer these additional questions (see below).

PERFUSION CMR IN ACUTE CHEST PAIN

Following the integration of high-sensitivity troponin into the guidelines, the role of imaging in patients with acute chest pain or acute coronary syndromes underwent a reassessment, leading to a perceived downgrade. However, recent developments have highlighted specific scenarios where imaging remains crucial for achieving a diagnosis.

Patients deemed to be at intermediate risk following initial evaluation through established clinical decision pathways may benefit from undergoing assessment with stress perfusion CMR, particularly if they lack a history of known CAD or prior coronary arterial bypass grafting (as indicated by Class I in ACC guidelines[44]). Additionally, CMR imaging is recommended for patients presenting with acute chest pain when myopericarditis is suspected. However, in cases of myocardial injury, characterized by elevated troponin levels, the primary objective is to rule out obstructive CAD before considering further diagnostic or therapeutic steps.

Additional Considerations

OVERESTIMATION OF THE IMPORTANCE OF REVASCULARIZATION

In recent decades, there has been an overestimation of the beneficial impact of revascularization on patient outcome. Emerging evidence suggests, however, that revascularization may not improve outcome for the majority of cases. The Clinical Outcomes Utilizing Revascularization and Aggressive Drug Evaluation (COURAGE) trial failed to demonstrate the superiority of revascularization over conservative therapy, albeit this trial did not specifically target patients with moderate or severe ischemia.[49,50] The Fractional Flow Reserve versus Angiography for Guiding Percutaneous Coronary Intervention (FAME) trials revealed that revascularization in patients without ischemia could potentially lead to adverse outcomes, underscoring the necessity for confirming ischemia before proceeding with revascularization.[7] In 2021, the Initial Invasive or Conservative Strategy for Stable Coronary Disease (ISCHEMIA) trial further emphasized that even in patients with moderate to severe ischemia, revascularization primarily alleviates symptoms rather than significantly improving outcomes.[36,51] The ISCHEMIA trial evaluated data for a median follow-up of 3.2 years. Currently, the ongoing ISCHEMIA-EXTEND study is evaluating long-term (10 years) mortality for the ISCHEMIA trial patients,[37] with an interim report in 2023 publishing results for a median follow-up of 5.7 years.[52] Although it was initially hypothesized that initial revascularization may at least improve long-term outcome, all-cause mortality proved similar in the revascularized and conservative groups. Interestingly, the revascularized group showed less cardiovascular, but increased noncardiovascular mortality, while the conservative group yielded higher cardiovascular, but decreased noncardiovascular mortality. These findings illustrate the increasing importance of selecting the right patients for invasive treatment (i.e., those patients for whom the decreased cardiovascular mortality is crucial).

Hence, revascularization should be reserved for patients experiencing severe symptoms attributable to proven myocardial ischemia, with testing for CAD primarily aimed at guiding therapy rather than solely confirming or excluding a specific diagnosis.

OVERESTIMATION OF THE PREVALENCE OF ISCHEMIC HEART DISEASE

Despite the significant impact of CAD on outcome, recent guidelines have lowered the pretest likelihoods for the presence of CAD considerably. According to the European Society of Cardiology (ESC) guidelines, even a 70-year-old male with typical chest pain only reaches a pretest likelihood of 52%, a woman 27%.

These aspects underscore that the diagnostic approach in patients with stable chest pain should not merely focus on confirming or ruling out CAD but should also provide insights into the presence and severity of ischemia to evaluate the potential benefit of revascularization. Additionally, it should offer information on the underlying pathophysiology of the disease. Merely visualizing the coronary arteries may suffice to exclude CAD but may fail to assess the severity of ischemia and other underlying issues such as myocardial inflammation, infiltration, or microvascular disease (INOCA).

ASSESSMENT OF OTHER CAUSES OF CHEST PAIN

A standard perfusion CMR examination enables routine assessment of alternative causes of chest pain. Myocardial damage or infiltration can be effectively evaluated using late gadolinium enhancement (LGE), which is a component of any perfusion CMR scan. LGE has been extensively validated for its diagnostic accuracy and strong prognostic value in nonischemic heart disease.[53,54] Similarly, pericardial effusion and enhancement provide indications of pericardial inflammation, which may elucidate atypical chest pain presentations. Moreover, microvascular disease manifests as a circumferential reduction of subendocardial blood flow, which can be readily assessed due to the high temporal and spatial resolution of perfusion CMR. Consequently, CMR is increasingly recommended for patients initially diagnosed with myocardial infarction but subsequently found to have normal coronary arteries (MINOCA), where it aids in determining the underlying cause of the troponin rise.[55,56]

Cost-Effectiveness

Contrary to common belief, utilization of CMR in patients with stable chest pain demonstrates cost-effectiveness in various imaging modality comparisons and healthcare systems.[57,58] While the outcome of any assessment for cost-effectiveness is heavily contingent on the healthcare system and the underlying epidemiological assumptions, such as the prevalence of CAD, perfusion CMR consistently proved to be cost-effective when compared to SPECT and direct coronary angiography or coronary angiography combined with fractional flow reserve. A recent study by Ge et al. compared different strategies using data from the SPINS (Stress Perfusion Imaging in the United States) registry, including direct invasive angiography, SPECT, CTA, CMR, and no imaging. Their findings indicate that CMR outperforms SPECT and CTA, yielding lower costs and more quality-of-life years. Furthermore, CMR demonstrates a favorable incremental cost-effectiveness ratio compared to no imaging and immediate invasive angiography.[59]

PERSPECTIVES

Even though the significance of stress perfusion CMR is increasingly recognized, it has not reached its full potential yet. In current clinical routine, applications using several 2D slices with visual assessment already prove to be highly accurate, predictive of outcome, and as a guidance for therapy—safely and cost-effectively. Several advanced innovations are starting to further enhance the potential of stress perfusion CMR. First, the use of faster image acquisition schemes based on artificial intelligence or compressed sensing will allow an improvement of spatial resolution or coverage (e.g., 3D imaging[60]). Second, the use of quantification techniques will further improve the differentiation of multivessel disease and microvascular dysfunction, and thus provide a better measure of therapy-induced changes. Third, the increased research focus on inflammatory diseases that cause cardiovascular events not only by themselves, but also by reducing myocardial perfusion, will require a noninvasive radiation-free technique to phenotype patients and guide their therapy.[61] Finally, the assessment of periinfarct ischemia as a strong risk factor for subsequent events will further improve secondary prevention in this high-risk population.[62]

REFERENCES

1. Monmeneu Menadas JV, García Gonzalez MP, Lopez-Lereu MP, Higueras Ortega L, Maceira Gonzalez AM. Safety and tolerability of regadenoson in comparison with adenosine stress cardiovascular magnetic resonance: data from a multicentre prospective registry. *Int J Cardiovasc Imaging.* 2022;38(1):195–209. https://doi.org/10.1007/s10554-021-02363-4.
2. Kotecha T, Monteagudo JM, Martinez-Naharro A, et al. Quantitative cardiovascular magnetic resonance myocardial perfusion mapping to assess hyperaemic response to adenosine stress. *Eur Heart J Cardiovasc Imaging.* 2021;22(3):273–281. https://doi.org/10.1093/ehjci/jeaa252.
3. Nagel E, Lehmkuhl HB, Bocksch W, et al. Noninvasive diagnosis of ischemia-induced wall motion abnormalities with the use of high-dose dobutamine stress MRI: comparison with dobutamine stress echocardiography. *Circulation.* 1999;99(6):763–770. https://doi.org/10.1161/01.cir.99.6.763.
4. Nagel E, Klein C, Paetsch I, et al. Magnetic resonance perfusion measurements for the noninvasive detection of coronary artery disease. *Circulation.* 2003;108(4):432–437. https://doi.org/10.1161/01.CIR.0000080915.35024.A9.
5. Baer FM, Voth E, LaRosée K, et al. Comparison of dobutamine transesophageal echocardiography and dobutamine magnetic resonance imaging for detection of residual myocardial viability. *Am J Cardiol.* 1996;78(4):415–419. https://doi.org/10.1016/s0002-9149(96)00329-3.
6. Haberkorn SM, Haberkorn SI, Bönner F, Kelm M, Hopkin G, Petersen SE. Vasodilator myocardial perfusion cardiac magnetic resonance imaging is superior to dobutamine stress echocardiography in the detection of relevant coronary artery stenosis: a systematic review and meta-analysis on their diagnostic accuracy. *Front Cardiovasc Med.* 2021;8:630846. https://doi.org/10.3389/fcvm.2021.630846.
7. Tonino PAL, De Bruyne B, Pijls NHJ, et al. Fractional flow reserve versus angiography for guiding percutaneous coronary intervention. *N Engl J Med.* 2009;360(3):213–224. https://doi.org/10.1056/NEJMoa0807611.
8. De Bruyne B, Baudhuin T, Melin JA, et al. Coronary flow reserve calculated from pressure measurements in humans. Validation with positron emission tomography. *Circulation.* 1994;89(3):1013–1022. https://doi.org/10.1161/01.CIR.89.3.1013.
9. Ullah W, Roomi S, Abdullah HM, et al. Diagnostic accuracy of cardiac magnetic resonance versus fractional flow reserve: a systematic review and meta-analysis. *Cardiol Res.* 2020;11(3):145–154. https://doi.org/10.14740/cr1028.
10. Danad I, Szymonifka J, Twisk JWR, et al. Diagnostic performance of cardiac imaging methods to diagnose ischaemia-causing coronary artery disease when directly compared with fractional flow reserve as a reference standard: a meta-analysis. *Eur Heart J.* 2017;38(13):991–998. https://doi.org/10.1093/eurheartj/ehw095.
11. Takx RAP, Blomberg BA, El Aidi H, et al. Diagnostic accuracy of stress myocardial perfusion imaging compared to invasive coronary angiography with fractional flow reserve meta-analysis. *Circ Cardiovasc Imaging.* 2015;8(1):e002666. https://doi.org/10.1161/CIRCIMAGING.114.002666.
12. Jaarsma C, Leiner T, Bekkers SC, et al. Diagnostic performance of noninvasive myocardial perfusion imaging using single-photon emission computed tomography, cardiac magnetic resonance, and positron emission tomography imaging for the detection of obstructive coronary artery disease: a meta-analysis. *J Am Coll Cardiol.* 2012;59(19):1719–1728. https://doi.org/10.1016/j.jacc.2011.12.040.
13. Xu J, Cai F, Geng C, Wang Z, Tang X. Diagnostic performance of CMR, SPECT, and PET imaging for the identification of coronary artery disease: a meta-analysis. *Front Cardiovasc Med.* 2021;8:621389. https://doi.org/10.3389/fcvm.2021.621389.
14. Arai AE, Schulz-Menger J, Berman D, et al. Gadobutrol-enhanced cardiac magnetic resonance imaging for detection of coronary artery disease. *J Am Coll Cardiol.* 2020;76(13):1536–1547. https://doi.org/10.1016/j.jacc.2020.07.060.
15. Ricci F, Khanji MY, Bisaccia G, et al. Diagnostic and prognostic value of stress cardiovascular magnetic resonance imaging in patients with known or suspected coronary artery disease: a systematic review and meta-analysis. *JAMA Cardiol.* 2023;8(7):662–673. https://doi.org/10.1001/jamacardio.2023.1290.
16. Antiochos P, Ge Y, Heydari B, et al. Prognostic value of stress cardiac magnetic resonance in patients with known coronary artery disease. *JACC, Cardiovasc Imaging.* 2022;15(1):60–71. https://doi.org/10.1016/j.jcmg.2021.06.025.
17. Greenwood JP, Motwani M, Maredia N, et al. Comparison of cardiovascular magnetic resonance and single-photon emission computed tomography in women with suspected coronary artery disease from the clinical evaluation of magnetic resonance imaging in coronary heart disease (CE-MARC) trial. *Circulation.* 2014;129(10):1129–1138. https://doi.org/10.1161/CIRCULATIONAHA.112.000071.
18. Ge Y, Steel K, Antiochos P, et al. Stress CMR in patients with obesity: insights from the stress CMR perfusion imaging in the United States (SPINS) registry. *Eur Heart J Cardiovasc Imaging.* 2021;22(5):518–527. https://doi.org/10.1093/ehjci/jeaa281.
19. Schwitter J, Wacker CM, van Rossum AC, et al. MR-IMPACT: comparison of perfusion-cardiac magnetic resonance with single-photon emission computed tomography for the detection of coronary artery disease in a multicentre, multivendor, randomized trial. *Eur Heart J.* 2008;29(4):480–489. https://doi.org/10.1093/eurheartj/ehm617.
20. Greenwood JP, Maredia N, Younger JF, et al. Cardiovascular magnetic resonance and single-photon emission computed tomography for diagnosis of coronary heart disease (CE-MARC): a prospective trial. *Lancet.* 2012;379(9814):453–460. https://doi.org/10.1016/S0140-6736(11)61335-4.
21. Dastidar AG, Baritussio A, De Garate E, et al. Prognostic role of CMR and conventional risk factors in myocardial infarction with nonobstructed coronary arteries. *JACC, Cardiovasc Imaging.* 2019;12(10):1973–1982. https://doi.org/10.1016/j.jcmg.2018.12.023.
22. Pezel T, Sanguineti F, Kinnel M, et al. Safety and prognostic value of vasodilator stress cardiovascular magnetic resonance in patients with heart failure and reduced ejection fraction. *Circ: Cardiovasc Imaging.* 2020;13(9):e010599. https://doi.org/10.1161/CIRCIMAGING.120.010599.
23. Vincenti G, Masci PG, Monney P, et al. Stress perfusion CMR in patients with known and suspected CAD: prognostic value and optimal ischemic threshold for revascularization. *JACC Cardiovasc Imaging.* 2017;10(5):526–537. https://doi.org/10.1016/j.jcmg.2017.02.006.
24. Heitner JF, Kim RJ, Kim HW, et al. Prognostic value of vasodilator stress cardiac magnetic resonance imaging: a multicenter study with 48 000 patient-years of follow-up. *JAMA Cardiol.* 2019;4(3):256–264. https://doi.org/10.1001/jamacardio.2019.0035.
25. Kwong RY, Ge Y, Steel K, et al. Cardiac magnetic resonance stress perfusion imaging for evaluation of patients with chest pain. *J Am Coll Cardiol.* 2019;74(14):1741–1755. https://doi.org/10.1016/j.jacc.2019.07.074.
26. Knott KD, Seraphim A, Augusto JB, et al. The prognostic significance of quantitative myocardial perfusion. *Circulation.* 2020;21(141):1282–1291.
27. Ford TJ, Stanley B, Good R, et al. Stratified medical therapy using invasive coronary function testing in angina: the CorMicA trial. *J Am Coll Cardiol.* 2018;72(23, Part A):2841–2855. https://doi.org/10.1016/j.jacc.2018.09.006.
28. Bairey Merz CN, Shaw LJ, Reis SE, et al. Insights from the NHLBI-sponsored women's ischemia syndrome evaluation (WISE) study. *J Am Coll Cardiol.* 2006;47(3):S21–S29. https://doi.org/10.1016/j.jacc.2004.12.084.
29. Pezel T, Lacotte J, Toupin S, et al. Diagnostic accuracy of stress perfusion CMR for risk stratification in patients with MR-conditional pacemakers. *JACC, Cardiovasc Imaging.* 2021;14(10):2053–2054. https://doi.org/10.1016/j.jcmg.2021.06.014.
30. Weiss KJ, Nasser SB, Bigvava T, et al. Long-term prognostic value of vasodilator stress cardiac magnetic resonance in patients with atrial fibrillation. *ESC Heart Fail.* 2022;9(1):110–121. https://doi.org/10.1002/ehf2.13736.
31. Seraphim A, Dowsing B, Rathod KS, et al. Quantitative myocardial perfusion predicts outcomes in patients with prior surgical revascularization. *J Am Coll Cardiol.* 2022;79(12):1141–1151. https://doi.org/10.1016/j.jacc.2021.12.037.
32. Kinnel M, Sanguineti F, Pezel T, et al. Prognostic value of vasodilator stress perfusion CMR in patients with previous coronary artery bypass graft. *Eur Heart J Cardiovasc Imaging.* 2021;22(11):1264–1272. https://doi.org/10.1093/ehjci/jeaa316.
33. Ge Y, Antiochos P, Steel K, et al. Prognostic value of stress CMR perfusion imaging in patients with reduced left ventricular function. *JACC, Cardiovasc Imaging.* 2020;13(10):2132–2145. https://doi.org/10.1016/j.jcmg.2020.05.034.
34. Nagel E, Greenwood JP, McCann GP, et al. Magnetic resonance perfusion or fractional flow reserve in coronary disease. *N Engl J Med.* 2019;380(25):2418–2428. https://doi.org/10.1056/NEJMoa1716734.
35. Greenwood JP, Ripley DP, Berry C, et al. Effect of care guided by cardiovascular magnetic resonance, myocardial perfusion scintigraphy, or NICE guidelines on subsequent unnecessary angiography rates: the CE-MARC 2 randomized clinical trial. *JAMA.* 2016;316(10):1051. https://doi.org/10.1001/jama.2016.12680.
36. Maron DJ, Hochman JS, Reynolds HR, et al. Initial invasive or conservative strategy for stable coronary disease. *N Engl J Med.* 2020;382(15):1395–1407. https://doi.org/10.1056/NEJMoa1915922.
37. Anthopolos R, Maron DJ, Bangalore S, et al. ISCHEMIA-EXTEND studies: rationale and design. *Am Heart J.* 2022;254:228–233. https://doi.org/10.1016/j.ahj.2022.09.009.
38. Shaw LJ, Berman DS, Picard MH, et al. Comparative definitions for moderate-severe ischemia in stress nuclear, echocardiography, and magnetic resonance imaging. *JACC Cardiovasc Imaging.* 2014;7(6):593–604. https://doi.org/10.1016/j.jcmg.2013.10.021.
39. Heydari B, Juan YH, Liu H, et al. Stress perfusion cardiac magnetic resonance imaging effectively risk stratifies diabetic patients with suspected myocardial ischemia. *Circ Cardiovasc Imaging.* 2016;9(4):e004136. https://doi.org/10.1161/CIRCIMAGING.115.004136.
40. Gargiulo P, Dellegrottaglie S, Bruzzese D, et al. The prognostic value of normal stress cardiac magnetic resonance in patients with known or suspected coronary artery disease. *Circ: Cardiovasc Imaging.* 2013;6(4):574–582. https://doi.org/10.1161/CIRCIMAGING.113.000035.
41. Pezel T, Garot P, Kinnel M, et al. Prognostic value of vasodilator stress perfusion cardiovascular magnetic resonance in patients with prior myocardial infarction. *JACC, Cardiovasc Imaging.* 2021;14(11):2138–2151. https://doi.org/10.1016/j.jcmg.2021.04.021.
42. Fu Q, Alabed S, Hoole SP, Abraham G, Weir-McCall JR. Prognostic value of stress perfusion cardiac MRI in cardiovascular disease: a systematic review and meta-analysis of the effects of the scanner, stress agent, and analysis technique. *Radiol Cardiothorac Imaging.* 2024;6(3):e230382. https://doi.org/10.1148/ryct.230382.
43. Pontone G, Andreini D, Guaricci AI, et al. The STRATEGY study (stress cardiac magnetic resonance versus computed tomography coronary angiography for the management of symptomatic revascularized patients). *Circ: Cardiovasc Imaging.* 2016;9(10):e005171. https://doi.org/10.1161/CIRCIMAGING.116.005171.
44. Gulati M, Levy PD, Mukherjee D, et al. 2021 AHA/ACC/ASE/CHEST/SAEM/SCCT/SCMR guideline for the evaluation and diagnosis of chest pain: a report of the American college of cardiology/American heart association joint committee on clinical practice guidelines. *Circulation.* 2021;144(22):e368–e454. https://doi.org/10.1161/CIR.0000000000001029.

45. Knuuti J, Wijns W, Saraste A, et al. 2019 ESC guidelines for the diagnosis and management of chronic coronary syndromes: the task force for the diagnosis and management of chronic coronary syndromes of the European society of cardiology (ESC). *Eur Heart J.* 2020;41(3):407–477. https://doi.org/10.1093/eurheartj/ehz425.
46. Arai AE, Kwong RY, Salerno M, Greenwood JP, Bucciarelli-Ducci C. Society for cardiovascular magnetic resonance perspective on the 2021 AHA/ACC chest pain guidelines. *J Cardiovasc Magn Reson.* 2022;24(1):8. https://doi.org/10.1186/s12968-021-00835-z.
47. Vrints C, Andreotti F, Koskinas KC, et al. 2024 ESC guidelines for the management of chronic coronary syndromes: developed by the task force for the management of chronic coronary syndromes of the European society of cardiology (ESC) endorsed by the European association for cardio-thoracic surgery (EACTS). *Eur Heart J.* 2024;45(36):3415–3537. https://doi.org/10.1093/eurheartj/ehae177.
48. Knuuti J, Ballo H, Juarez-Orozco LE, et al. The performance of non-invasive tests to rule-in and rule-out significant coronary artery stenosis in patients with stable angina: a meta-analysis focused on post-test disease probability. *Eur Heart J.* 2018;39(35):3322–3330. https://doi.org/10.1093/eurheartj/ehy267.
49. Boden WE, O'Rourke RA, Teo KK, et al. Optimal medical therapy with or without PCI for stable coronary disease. *N Engl J Med.* 2007;356(15):1503–1516. https://doi.org/10.1056/NEJMoa070829.
50. Boden WE, O'rourke RA, Teo KK, et al. The evolving pattern of symptomatic coronary artery disease in the United States and Canada: baseline characteristics of the clinical outcomes utilizing revascularization and aggressive DruG evaluation (COURAGE) trial. *Am J Cardiol.* 2007;99(2):208–212. https://doi.org/10.1016/j.amjcard.2006.07.082.
51. Nagel E, Carerj ML, Arendt CT, Puntmann VO. After ISCHEMIA: Is cardiac MRI a reliable gatekeeper for invasive angiography and myocardial revascularization? *Herz.* 2020;45(5):446–452. https://doi.org/10.1007/s00059-020-04936-w.
52. Hochman JS, Anthopolos R, Reynolds HR, et al. Survival after invasive or conservative management of stable coronary disease. *Circulation.* 2023;147(1):8–19. https://doi.org/10.1161/CIRCULATIONAHA.122.062714.
53. Yang Z, Fu H, Li H, et al. Late gadolinium enhancement is a risk factor for major adverse cardiac events in unrecognised myocardial infarction without apparent symptoms: a meta-analysis. *Clin Radiol.* 2021;76(1):79.e1–79.e11. https://doi.org/10.1016/j.crad.2020.07.038.
54. Gaztanaga J, Paruchuri V, Elias E, et al. Prognostic value of late gadolinium enhancement in nonischemic cardiomyopathy. *Am J Cardiol.* 2016;118(7):1063–1068. https://doi.org/10.1016/j.amjcard.2016.06.059.
55. Hausvater A, Smilowitz NR, Li B, et al. Myocarditis in relation to angiographic findings in patients with provisional diagnoses of MINOCA. *JACC Cardiovasc Imaging.* 2020;13(9):1906–1913. https://doi.org/10.1016/j.jcmg.2020.02.037.
56. Mileva N, Paolisso P, Gallinoro E, et al. Diagnostic and prognostic role of cardiac magnetic resonance in MINOCA: systematic review and meta-analysis. *JACC Cardiovasc Imaging.* 2023;16(3):376–389. https://doi.org/10.1016/j.jcmg.2022.12.029.
57. Moschetti K, Petersen SE, Pilz G, et al. Cost-minimization analysis of three decision strategies for cardiac revascularization: results of the "suspected CAD" cohort of the european cardiovascular magnetic resonance registry. *J Cardiovasc Magn Reson.* 2016;18:3. https://doi.org/10.1186/s12968-015-0222-1.
58. Kozor R, Walker S, Parkinson B, et al. Cost-effectiveness of cardiovascular magnetic resonance in diagnosing coronary artery disease in the Australian health care system. *Heart Lung Circ.* 2021;30(3):380–387. https://doi.org/10.1016/j.hlc.2020.07.008.
59. Ge Y, Pandya A, Steel K, et al. Cost-effectiveness analysis of stress cardiovascular magnetic resonance imaging for stable chest pain syndromes. *JACC, Cardiovasc Imaging.* 2020;13(7):1505–1517. https://doi.org/10.1016/j.jcmg.2020.02.029.
60. Manka R, Wissmann L, Gebker R, et al. Multicenter evaluation of dynamic three-dimensional magnetic resonance myocardial perfusion imaging for the detection of coronary artery disease defined by fractional flow reserve. *Circ Cardiovasc Imaging.* 2015;8(5):e003061. https://doi.org/10.1161/CIRCIMAGING.114.003061.
61. Mavrogeni SI, Kitas GD, Dimitroulas T, et al. Cardiovascular magnetic resonance in rheumatology: current status and recommendations for use. *Int J Cardiol.* 2016;217:135–148. https://doi.org/10.1016/j.ijcard.2016.04.158.
62. Bernhard B, Ge Y, Antiochos P, et al. Association of adverse clinical outcomes with peri-infarct ischemia detected by stress cardiac magnetic imaging. *J Am Coll Cardiol.* 2024;84(5):417–429. https://doi.org/10.1016/j.jacc.2024.04.062.
63. Schelbert Erik, Cao Jie, Sigurdsson Sigurdur, et al. Prevalence and prognosis of unrecognized myocardial infarction determined by cardiac magnetic resonance in older adults. *JAMA.* 2012;308(9):890–896. https://doi.org/10.1001/2012.jama.11089.

21 Technical Foundation and Clinical Utility of Coronary MRI

SHIRO NAKAMORI, MASAKI ISHIDA, KAORU DOHI, HAJIME SAKUMA, RENE BOTNAR, WARREN J. MANNING, AND REZA NEZAFAT

INTRODUCTION

Despite advances in its prevention and management, coronary artery disease (CAD) remains the leading cause of death in the Western world. CMR is a promising noninvasive tool for comprehensive early risk assessment, guidance of therapy, and treatment monitoring of CAD. Coronary MRI is a noninvasive diagnotic alternative to catheter-based x-ray angiography among patients with suspected anomalous coronary artery disease and coronary artery aneurysms. Coronary MRI is recommended and deemed appropriate in patients suspected of anomalous coronary artery disease by the American College of Cardiology and the American Heart Association.[1,2] Despite ongoing technical advances, CMR assessment of coronary lumen integrity and plaque burden/activity remains technically challenging. Therefore, coronary MRI is not currently clinically recommended for assessing anatomical stenosis. This chapter will review the imaging strategies for assessing coronary artery anatomy and its potential clinical utility.

Technical Foundation of Coronary MRI

The coronary MRI sequences consist of two major components: (a) magnetization preparation sequences and (b) imaging sequences. Other considerations include image prescription (e.g., targeting a single vessel or whole heart), cardiac and respiratory motion correction (free-breathing, navigator-gated, or self-gating), and MRI contrast agents. This section provides an overview of the technical foundation of coronary MRI sequences.

The early approaches to coronary MRI were based on two-dimensional (2D) breath-hold electrocardiogram (ECG) triggered segmented sequences.[3,4] Three-dimensional (3D) approaches have largely replaced 2D sequences, enabling greater anatomical coverage and a higher signal-to-noise ratio (SNR). Three-dimensional coronary MRI can be acquired with a targeted coronary or whole-heart coverage of the coronary anatomy. The targeted technique acquires a double-oblique 3D volume aligned along the major axis of the left main (LM) or right coronary artery (RCA).[5–7] For the visualization, the imaging plane passing through the proximal, mid, and distal RCA, and the targeted 3D coronary sequence is acquired in this orientation (typically the AV groove), typically with a 30-mm slab with 20 slices.[6,7] For imaging the LM, left anterior descending artery (LAD), and proximal left circumflex (LCX) coronary arteries, a 3D volume is interactively prescribed in the axial plane centered about the LM coronary artery.[7,8] In the whole-heart coronary MRI technique (Fig. 21.1),[9–23] an axial (or coronal) 3D volume encompassing the entire heart is sampled in a single acquisition. This facilitates the imaging setup via a more straightforward slab prescription and provides a more complete anatomical coverage, positioned ~1 cm above the LM and extending to the inferior cardiac border.

Targeted thin-slab 3D acquisitions have been acquired using spoiled gradient echo (GRE) and balanced steady-state free precession (bSSFP) sequences.[24] A thin-slab 3D targeted acquisition with a GRE sequence results in a more homogeneous blood pool signal but heavily depends on the inflow of unsaturated protons.[25] Saturation effects will cause a local signal loss if the coronary flow is slow

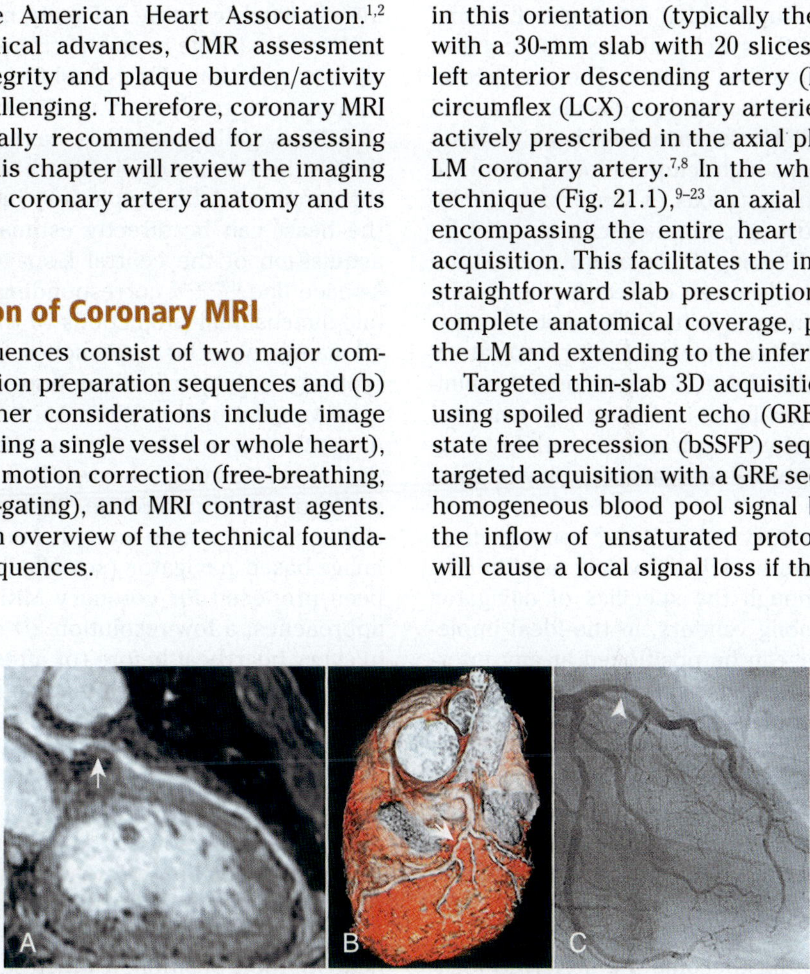

FIG. 21.1 Whole-heart coronary MRI. (A) A stenosis in the LAD is visualized using a curved multiplanar reconstruction (*white arrow*). (B) A three-dimensional view of LAD with stenosis is depicted in the volume-rendered image. (C) X-ray coronary angiography confirms proximal LAD stenosis (*arrowhead*). (Adapted from Sakuma H, Ichikawa Y, Chino S, Hirano T, Makino K, Takeda K. Detection of coronary artery stenosis with whole-heart coronary magnetic resonance angiography. *J Am Coll Cardiol* 2006;48:1946–1950. https://doi.org/10.1016/j.jacc.2006.07.055.)

or stagnant. This is often relatively exaggerated as compared with lumen stenosis. Compared to GRE sequences, bSSFP provides intrinsically higher SNR due to its balanced gradients and improved blood–myocardium contrast due to its T_2/T_1 weighting[26] with reduced sensitivity to inflow effects. Both GRE and bSSFP have been used for targeted 3D coronary MRI, showing similar diagnostic accuracy for CAD.[26,27] For whole-heart noncontrast coronary MRI at 1.5 T, bSSFP appears to be the sequence of choice due to its higher blood–myocardium contrast and superior inflow properties.[25] A T_2 magnetization preparation pulse is often used in coronary MRI sequences immediately before image acquisition to enhance blood–myocardium contrast.[28] If imaging is performed postgadolinium, an inversion preparation pulse, instead of T_2 magnetization preparation, is applied to reduce the signal from myocardial tissue. Coronary arteries are usually surrounded by epicardial fat. Therefore, fat saturation is essential in both targeted and whole-heart imaging.[29]

Bulk epicardial motion is a major impediment to coronary MRI. It can be separated into motions related to cardiac contraction/relaxation during the cardiac cycle and motion due to superimposed diaphragmatic and chest wall motion from respiration. The magnitude of motion from each component may greatly exceed the coronary artery diameter, thereby leading to blurring artifacts in the absence of motion-suppressive methods. External electrocardiographic (ECG) synchronization is required to compensate for bulk cardiac motion. The acquisition interval is adapted to the heart rate/diastasis interval using a patient-specific diastasis period. This can be readily identified by acquiring a high temporal resolution cine dataset orthogonal to the long axis of the proximal/mid-RCA and the LAD. The use of patient-specific acquisition windows reduces image blurring.[30,31] An adaptive real-time arrhythmia rejection algorithm can correct for heart rate variability and improve image quality.[32] The second major challenge for coronary MRI is compensation for respiratory motion. Several approaches have been proposed to minimize respiratory motion artifacts, including supplemental oxygen-assisted sustained end-expiratory breath-holding, chest wall bellows, respiratory navigators, fat navigators, and self-gating methods.

Diaphragmatic respiratory navigators[33] enable free-breathing acquisitions and have been widely used in coronary MRI studies. Although the specifics of navigator implementation vary among vendors, in the ideal implementation, the navigator can be positioned at any interface that accurately reflects respiratory motion, including the dome of the right hemidiaphragm,[34,35] the left hemidiaphragm, the anterior chest wall, or the anterior free wall of the left ventricle.[35,36] The navigator should ideally not cause an image artifact and should be temporally located immediately preceding the imaging portion of the sequence with data accepted (used for image reconstruction) only when the navigator indicates that the "interface" (e.g., diaphragm position) falls within a user-defined window. The dome of the right hemidiaphragm has become the preferred location[6,36] due to the simplicity and ease of set-up, where the motion of the right hemidiaphragm in the superior–inferior direction can be tracked. CMR studies of cardiac border position during the respiratory cycle showed that the ratio between cardiac and diaphragmatic displacement is ~0.6 for the RCA and ~0.7 for the left coronary artery at the end-expiration.[37] However, there is variability among subjects[38–40] and position (e.g., supine vs. prone imaging).[41] This rule-of-thumb offers the opportunity for prospective navigator gating with real-time tracking,[35,39] in which the position of the interface (diaphragm) is determined, and the slice position coordinates can then be shifted in real time (before the data collection) to adjust spatial coordinates appropriately.[42] This technique allows wider gating windows and increased navigator efficiency, leading to shorter scan times. Several refinements to the navigator method have been proposed. While a "fixed" foot–head correction factor of 0.6 (with no left–right or anterior–posterior correction)[42,43] is commonly used, significant individual variability has been observed.[38] A subject-specific tracking factor has been studied and shown to improve image quality when the subject-specific tracking factor differs from 0.6.[44] Multiple navigator locations, leading and trailing navigators, and navigators that guide affine transformations, that is, 3D translations and rotations, of the slice prescription for each heartbeat have also been proposed.[17,36,45,46] The affine transformation permits a larger navigator window and higher navigator efficiency. A navigator with fixed scan efficiency has also been introduced, resulting in imaging at a fixed scan time.[47] Finally, novel k-space trajectories and various image reconstruction-based methods, such as cross-correlation of low-resolution images, have also been proposed for respiratory motion compensation.[22,48–50]

Self-navigation methods have also been proposed to derive the respiratory-induced motion of the heart from the acquired data. Respiratory-induced displacements of the heart can be directly estimated from the repetitive acquisition of the central k-space point[51] or the central k-space line,[13,22,52,53] corresponding to zero-dimensional or one-dimensional projections of the field of view. Like the 1D navigator echo approaches, self-navigation methods typically only perform motion correction in the foot–head translational motion. Another drawback of the self-navigation approach is the inclusion of static structures in the field of view (e.g., chest wall), which can degrade motion estimation and correction. To overcome these problems and account for more complex motion, several 2D and 3D image-based navigator (so-called iNAV) approaches have been proposed for coronary MRI (Fig. 21.2).[54–62] In these approaches, a low-resolution 2D or 3D image is acquired in every heartbeat before (or after) the acquisition of coronary MRI data. The main advantage of this approach is that the moving heart can be spatially isolated from surrounding static tissues, and the respiratory-induced cardiac motion can be directly estimated via (rigid or affine) image registration of iNAVs at different respiratory positions. Self-navigation and image-based navigator methods can be used to gate the acquisition and correct for motion within a small gating window as described for 1D navigator echoes. Furthermore, since these methods directly track heart motion/position, a much larger gating window can be used or removed entirely if combined with 3D nonrigid motion correction, thereby increasing the scan efficiency to or close to 100%.[63,64]

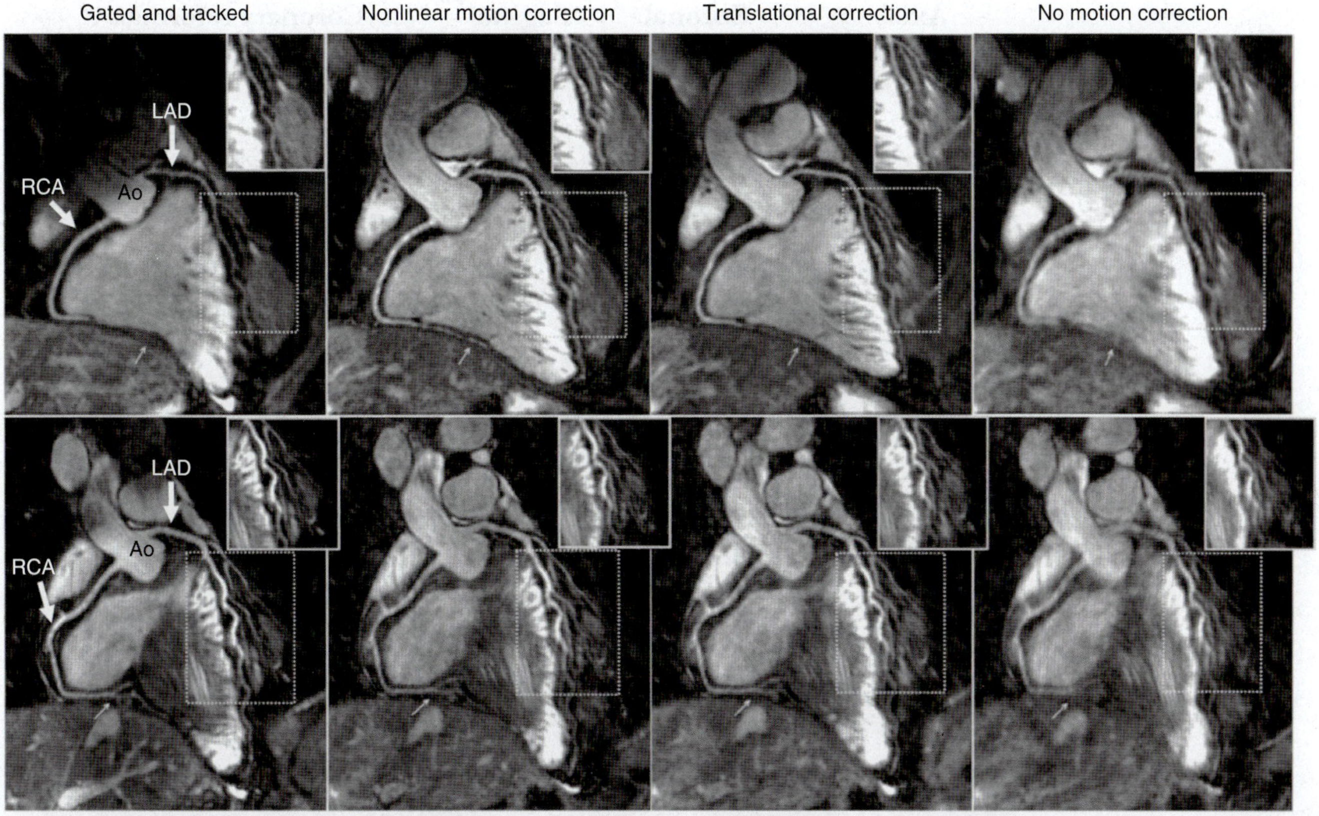

FIG. 21.2 Coronary MRI images acquired with nearly 100% scan efficiency using nonrigid motion correction. This approach is based on beat-to-beat translation correction followed by respiratory bin-to-bin nonlinear motion correction. Reformatted images are shown for conventional navigator gated and tracked acquisition, nonrigid motion correction, translation correction only, and no motion correction for two subjects. Blurring in the no-motion correction images is reduced with translation correction, and sharpness is further increased with the nonlinear motion correction approach (*boxes*). The distal parts of both the RCA and the LAD are particularly affected by motion (*arrows*). The nonlinear motion correction approach has similar image quality to the conventional navigator-gated and tracked acquisition; however, the latter requires significantly longer scan times (~2–3 times longer).

Non-Cartesian acquisitions provide efficient k-space sampling, leading to incoherent or less visually significant artifacts. Spiral acquisitions are advantageous to Cartesian acquisitions in several respects, including a more efficient sampling of k-space, enhanced SNR, and favorable flow properties.[65,66] However, there are also drawbacks associated with spiral trajectories, such as increased sensitivity to magnetic field inhomogeneity. Radial trajectories also enable more rapid acquisitions while decreasing sensitivity to motion.[22] Other non-Cartesian k-space trajectories, such as 3D cones or spiral phyllotaxis, have also been investigated to improve image acquisition efficiency and reduce image artifacts.[67–70]

One of the challenges of coronary MRI scans is their relatively long acquisition time. Therefore, image acceleration is frequently used to reduce scan time. Parallel imaging techniques[71,72] are the most commonly used to reduce the scan time by two to four factors. These techniques are available from all vendors and are now part of any coronary MRI protocol. Compressed sensing (CS) is an alternative acceleration technique that exploits the sparsity of the image in a transform domain[73] to reduce the scan time. CS can reduce the scan time beyond what can be achieved with parallel imaging.[74,75] Other iterative image reconstruction methods successfully employed to accelerate coronary MRI include low-rank-based image reconstructions, which enable acceleration factors of up to 5.[74,76] However, lengthy reconstruction time and limited availability of CS reconstruction algorithms by vendors have contributed to the low adoption of CS-based image acceleration in coronary MRI. New advances in artificial intelligence and deep learning (DL)-based image acceleration in CMR[77] could also be exploited for coronary MRI. DL image-acceleration methods have also been demonstrated to reduce the imaging time of coronary MRI.[78–80] Fig. 21.3 shows coronary MRI images reconstructed using a super-resolution DL model, which is trained to enhance image sharpness of low-resolution images, demonstrating the DL potential in reducing the scan time with rapid postprocessing of images.

One of the limitations of coronary MRI is its relatively coarse spatial resolution. The spatial resolution could be increased with a longer scan time; however, there is a trade-off between spatial resolution and imaging SNR. Therefore, coronary MRI may benefit from enhanced SNR, available at 3 T.[81] The SNR gain can be used to achieve higher spatial resolution (as high as 0.35 mm^2) at 3 T in coronary MRI;[82] however, imaging at 3 T is more susceptible to imaging artifacts due to higher field inhomogeneity. Field inhomogeneity could manifest as banding artifacts or signal loss (shading) in images. It could be associated with image preparation (such as T_2 magnetization preparation) or imaging

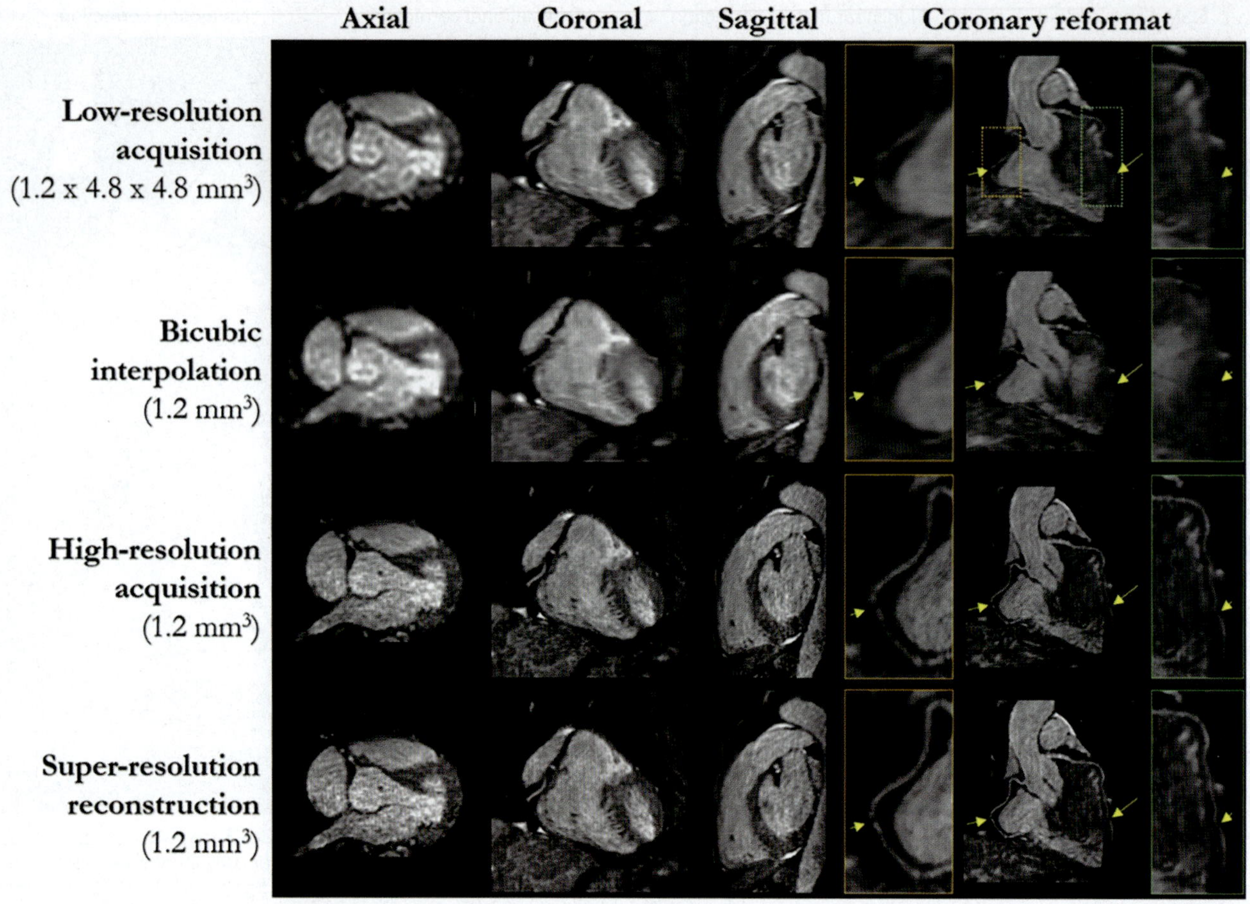

FIG. 21.3 A deep learning-based super-resolution coronary MRI image acquisition. The deep learning model reconstructs low-resolution image ($1.2 \times 4.8 \times 4.8\,mm^3$) in ~50s to $1.2\,mm^3$ resolution. In contrast, high HR acquisition ($1.2\,mm^3$) images are acquired in ~7min. Axial, sagittal, and coronal images of the 3D CMRA are depicted. Coronary reformat magnified RCA with moderate (50%–69%) stenosis and magnified LAD with mild (25%–49%) stenosis, as indicated by the arrows. (Adapted from Küstner T, Munoz C, Psenicny A et al. Deep-learning based super-resolution for 3D isotropic coronary MR angiography in less than a minute. *Magn Reson Med* 2021;86:2837-2852. https://doi.org/10.1002/mrm.28911.)

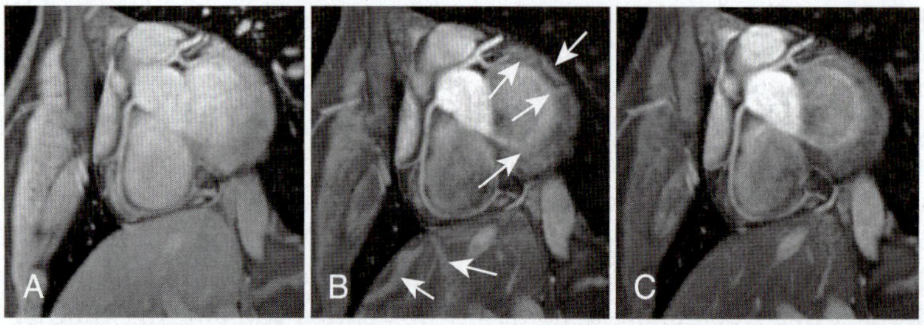

FIG. 21.4 Example reformatted 3D coronary MRI of the right coronary artery at 3T (A) acquired with no T_2-prep; (B) with T_2-prep; (C) with adiabatic T_2-prep. *Arrows* in (B) point to the artifacts resulting from T_2-prep sequence. The banding artifacts are suppressed in (C), where the homogeneity of the signal is also improved.

sequence (e.g., bSSFP banding artifacts). Various solutions have been proposed to mitigate these issues, including more robust radio-frequency pulses and advanced shimming algorithms. To reduce the impact of B_1 inhomogeneity at higher field strengths, improved preparation sequences such as adiabatic T_2 magnetization preparation[83,84] and adiabatic fat saturation have been utilized. Fig. 21.4 shows an example of coronary MRI acquired at 3T using adiabatic T_2 magnetization preparation, suppressing the banding artifact resulting from conventional T_2 magnetization preparation. Conventional spectrally selective fat suppression may not also be effective at 3T. Therefore, water–fat separation techniques such as Dixon or improved fat suppression radio-frequency pulses were investigated.[85–88] The feasibility of coronary MRI at high magnetic fields of 5T and 7T has also been demonstrated, but numerous technical challenges still limit their clinical utility.[89,90] Another technique to improve SNR in coronary MRI is the administration of vasodilators since the increased coronary blood flow secondary to vasodilatation reduces the inflow saturation effects.[91,92] Fig. 21.5 demonstrates the impact of sublingual isosorbide dinitrate administration on coronary MRI up to 30min after drug administration. Ferumoxytol, a novel iron-based contrast agent, has also been used to enhance the SNR and CNR of coronary MRI with promising diagnostic accuracy (Fig. 21.6).[93,94]

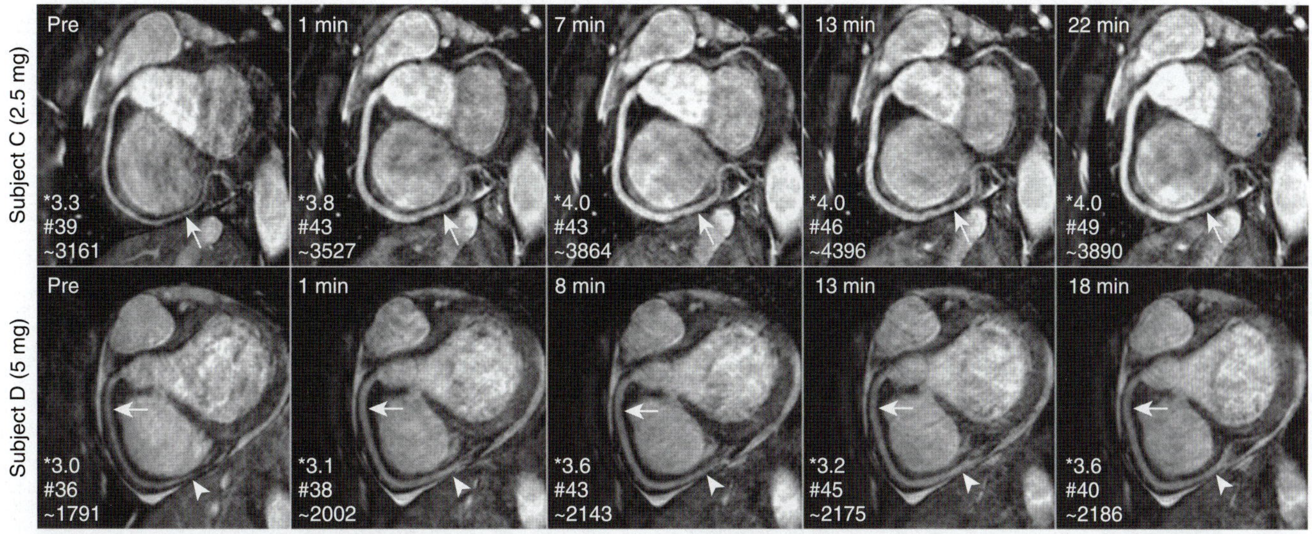

FIG. 21.5 Reformatted images from a targeted 3D coronary MRI of the RCA acquired before and after sublingual isosorbide dinitrate administration on two healthy subjects using a 3D free-breathing SSFP with 2.5 mg (*top row*) and 5 mg doses (*bottom row*) as a function of time. Improved RCA vasodilation and signal enhancement can be observed in all images postisosorbide dinitrate (*arrows in top and bottom rows*). The enhanced SNR with isosorbide dinitrate also allows for improved visualization of the distal segments.

In summary, ongoing technical advances have been used to overcome challenges in successful coronary anatomy imaging, including improved cardiac and respiratory motion methods and enhanced spatial resolution, SNR, and CNR.

Imaging of Anomalous Coronary Arteries

Using current whole-heart imaging with or without gadolinium contrast agent, the native proximal coronary arteries can be reliably visualized in nearly all subjects. Although unusual (<1% of the general population[95,96] and most often benign), congenital coronary anomalies in which the anomalous segment courses anterior to the aorta and posterior to the pulmonary artery are well-recognized causes of myocardial ischemia and sudden cardiac death in children and young adults.[97,98] These adverse events typically occur during or immediately after intense exercise and are believed to be related to compression of the anomalous segment, vessel kinking, or coexistent eccentric ostial stenoses.[97] The ability of CMR to reliably identify the major coronary arteries and their relationship to the ascending aorta and pulmonary artery immediately provides for its application for the identification and characterization of anomalous coronary artery disease. The spatial resolution requirements for identifying anomalous coronary vessels are less stringent than for defining native vessel stenoses, allowing for lower resolution and faster CMR imaging.

Invasive coronary angiography had traditionally been the imaging test of choice for diagnosing and characterizing these anomalies. However, the presence of an anomalous vessel is sometimes suspected only after the procedure, particularly in a situation in which there was unsuccessful engagement of a coronary artery. In addition, the infrequent use of a pulmonary artery catheter has made characterization of the anterior or posterior trajectory of the anomalous vessels more difficult to appreciate on projection x-ray angiography.

CMR has several advantages over coronary CTA and invasive coronary angiography in diagnosing coronary anomalies. It is noninvasive, does not require ionizing radiation or iodinated contrast agents, and provides a definitive 3D "road map" of the mediastinum (Fig. 21.7). Several studies[70,99–106] of patients who underwent a comparison of CMR with invasive coronary angiography for suspected anomalous coronary artery disease have shown excellent accuracy, including several instances in which CMR was determined to be superior to invasive coronary angiography (Table 21.1).

Data also suggest that CMR evidence of an anomalous coronary provides important prognostic information,[107] identifying the anomalous segment originating from the opposite sinus of Valsalva (Fig. 21.7) as conveying an adverse prognosis. As a result, CMR is considered a class I indication for suspected anomalous coronary artery disease.[108] At experienced CMR centers, clinical coronary MRI is the preferred test for patients in whom anomalous disease is suspected, those with known anomalous disease that must be further clarified, and those with coronary anomalies associated with other cardiac anomalies (e.g., tetralogy of Fallot). Although coronary CTA has also been shown to be efficacious for this indication,[109–111] coronary MRI is often preferred in younger patients because it does not require ionizing radiation or intravenous contrast.

Coronary artery aneurysms are relatively uncommon but have been receiving more attention due to their occurrence in pediatric and young adult patients with a history of mucocutaneous lymph node syndrome, also known as Kawasaki disease. This disease is a generalized vasculitis of unknown etiology, usually occurring in children under five. The highest prevalence of Kawasaki disease is found in East Asian countries, especially in Japan.[112] Infants and children with this syndrome may show evidence of myocarditis or pericarditis, with nearly 20% having coronary artery aneurysms. These aneurysms (Fig. 21.8) are the source of both short- and long-term morbidity and mortality.[113] Fortunately, half of the children with coronary

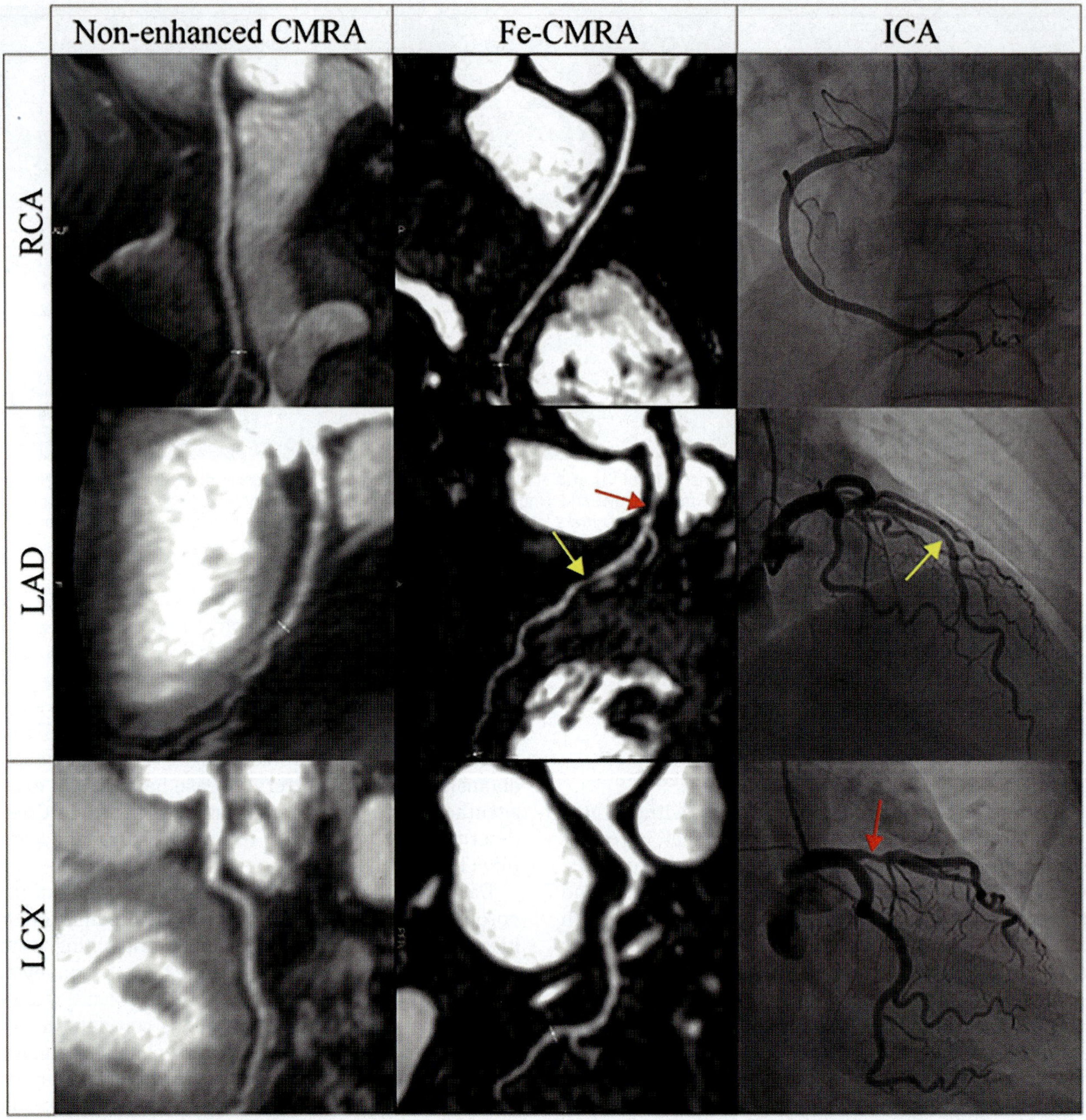

FIG. 21.6 Ferumoxytol-enhanced coronary magnetic resonance angiography (Fe-CMRA) in a 67-year-old female patient whose invasive coronary angiography showed a significant stenosis (*red arrow*) in proximal left anterior descending coronary artery (*LAD*), and an intermediate stenosis (*yellow arrow*) in middle LAD. (Adapted from Dong Z, Si G, Zhu X et al. Diagnostic Performance and Safety of a Novel Ferumoxytol-Enhanced Coronary Magnetic Resonance Angiography. *Circ Cardiovasc Imaging* 2023;16:580–590. https://doi.org/10.1161/circimaging.123.015404).

aneurysms during the acute phase of the disease have a normal-appearing coronary lumen on catheter-based x-ray angiography 2 years later.[113,114] Transthoracic echocardiography is often used to diagnose and monitor these proximal and mid-vessel aneurysms in very young children, but it is not as effective for adolescents and obese children. These young adults are, therefore, often referred for serial catheter-based x-ray coronary angiography or coronary CTA, which can lead to significant radiation exposure over time. Coronary MRI data from two series of adolescents and young adults with coronary artery aneurysms have shown that coronary MRI is highly accurate in identifying and characterizing these aneurysms, including their size and length[115–119] with the addition of cine ventricular function and LGE for a comprehensive cardiac assessment.[117] Although not specifically examined in long-term follow-up studies, these data suggest coronary aneurysms can be effectively followed with serial CMR studies, including vessel wall inflammation.[118,119]

Native Vessel Coronary Artery Stenosis

The available data support a broad clinical role for coronary MRI in the assessment of suspected anomalous coronary artery disease (and coronary artery bypass graft patency) (Fig. 21.9), but there is not sufficient evidence to recommend the routine use of clinical coronary MRI for

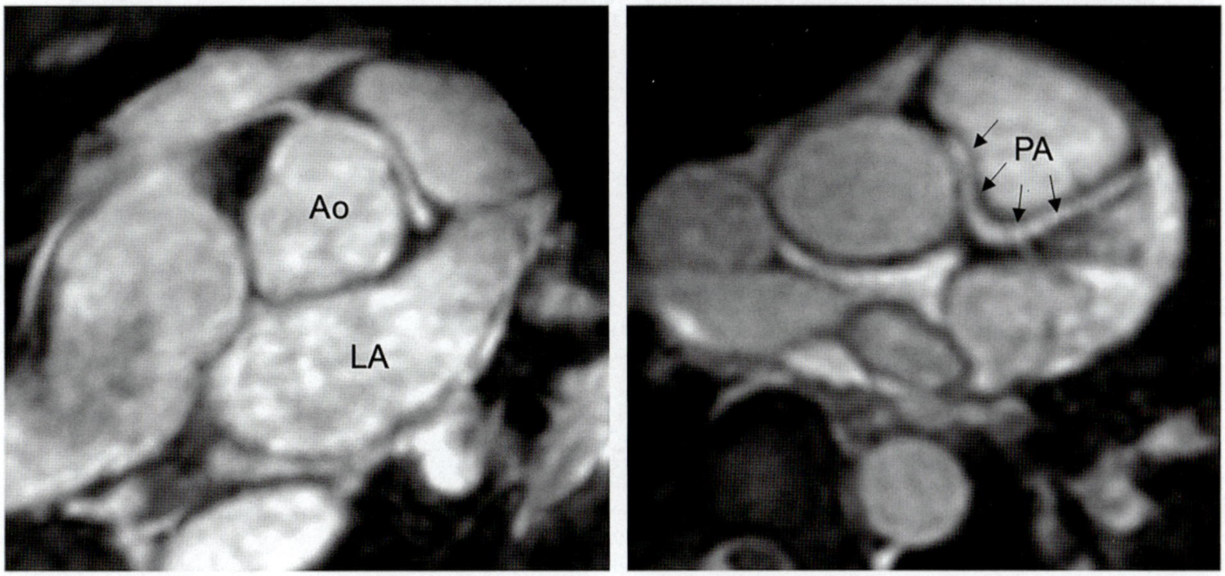

FIG. 21.7 Noncontrast whole-heart 3 T coronary MRI in a patient with an anomalous left coronary artery (*arrow*) from the right sinus of Valsalva. This is the malignant form of this anomalous disease in which the anomalous segment courses between the anterior right ventricular outflow tract/pulmonary artery (PA) and posterior aorta (Ao). LA, left atrium.

TABLE 21.1 Coronary MRI for anomalous coronary artery disease.

	# PATIENTS	CORRECTLY CLASSIFIED VESSELS
McConnell[99]	15	14 (93%)
Post[100]	19	19 (100%)[a]
Vliegen[101]	12	11 (92%)[b]
Taylor[102]	25	24 (96%)
Bunce et al.[103]	26	26 (100%)[c]
Razmi et al.[104]	12	12 (100%)
Tangcharoen et al.[106]	46	46 (100%)
Piccini[70]	16	15 (94%)

[a]Three patients originally misclassified by invasive coronary angiography.
[b]Five patients unable to be classified by invasive coronary.
[c]Eleven patients unable to be classified by invasive coronary angiography.

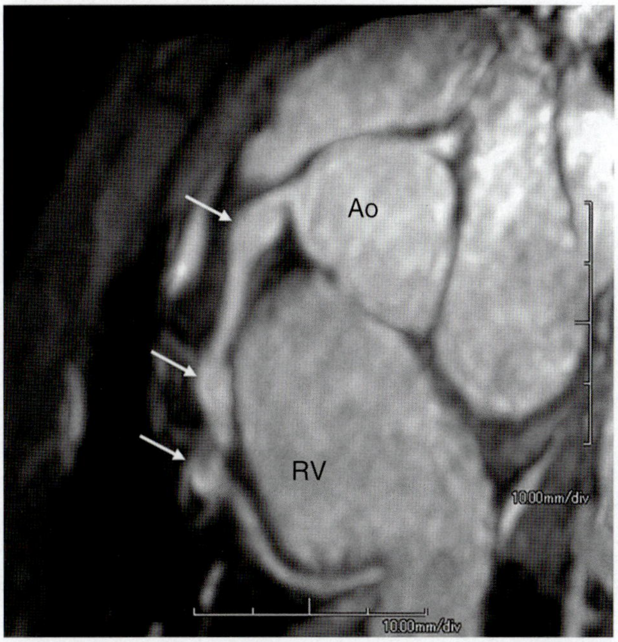

FIG. 21.8 Noncontrast whole-heart coronary MRI in a child with Kawasaki disease and serial coronary artery aneurysms (*white arrows*) involving the right coronary artery. *Ao*, aorta; *RV*, right ventricle.

identifying coronary artery stenoses among patients presenting with chest pain or for screening purposes, even in high-risk patients.

Numerous single-center studies have used 3D GRE or bSSFP coronary MRI with targeted 3D or whole-heart approaches with or without contrast agents at 1.5 and 3 T (Table 21.2).[20,21,26,27,81,120–128,130–133,135,137] Although the sensitivity assessment of coronary artery stenosis is similar for both source and projection images,[138] it is recommended to make diagnoses through a review of the source images and use the projection images to visually convey findings to the referring physician. An international, multicenter, free-breathing, noncontrast 3D targeted coronary MRI study of 109 patients without previous invasive coronary angiography showed high sensitivity (although only modest specificity) and negative predictive value of coronary MRI for the identification of coronary artery disease (>50% diameter stenosis by quantitative coronary angiography) (Table 21.3).[139] The sensitivity and negative predictive value were sufficient for identifying left main or multivessel disease. Accordingly, coronary MRI was especially valuable for patients with dilated cardiomyopathy in the absence of clinical myocardial infarction.

The role of contrast-enhanced coronary MRI for disease detection has also been studied. Paetsch and associates[129] compared noncontrast 3D targeted coronary MRI with an investigational intravascular agent using an inversion recovery prepulse and found that contrast improved specificity. As expected, multicenter coronary MRI data (Table 21.3) are less favorable than those reported in single centers.[139–141] A systematic review and meta-analysis of coronary MRI[142] involving 24 reports and 1638 patients showed a pooled sensitivity of 89% (95% CI 86%–92%) and specificity of 72% (95% CI 63%–79%). The sensitivity of contrast-enhanced coronary MRI was higher (95%

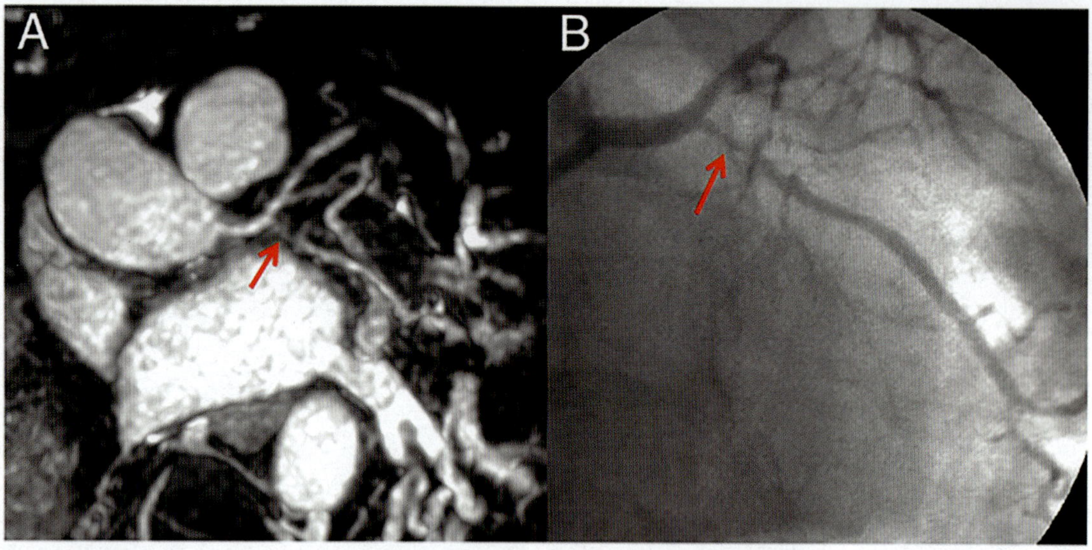

FIG. 21.9 (A) Noncontrast 3D coronary MRA in a patient with significant stenosis (*arrow*) of the left anterior descending coronary artery with (B) comparative projection x-ray angiogram. (With permission from Yoon YE, Kitagawa K, Kato S et al. Prognostic value of coronary magnetic resonance angiography for prediction of cardiac events in patients with suspected coronary artery disease. *J Am Coll Cardiol.* 2012;60:2316–2322.)

TABLE 21.2 Free-breathing 3D coronary MRI to identify focal coronary stenoses 50% or more in diameter.

	#SUBJECTS	TECHNIQUE	SENSITIVITY	SPECIFICITY
1.5 T prospective navigator coronary MRI with targeted 3D approach				
Regenfus[120]	50	GRE	94%	57%
Bunce[121]	34	GRE	88%	72%
Moustapha[122]	25	GRE	92%	55%
			90% (proximal)	92% (proximal)
Sommer[123]	112	GRE	74%	63%
			88% (good quality)	91% (good quality)
Bogaert[124]	19	GRE	85%–92%	50%–83%
Plein[125]	10	GRE	75%	85%
Ozgun[126]	14	GRE	91%	57%
		bSSFP	76%	85%
Dewey[127]	15[a]	bSSFP	86%	98%
Maintz[26]	12	GRE	92%	67%
		bSSFP	81%	82%
Ozgun[27]	20	bSSFP	82%	82%
Jahnke[128]	21	bSSFP	79%	91%
Paetsch[129]	18	bSSFP	83%	77%
	18	+Gd	86%	95%
Sommer[81]	18	GRE	82%	88%
1.5 T prospective navigator coronary MRI with whole-heart approach				
Sakuma[21]	39	bSSFP	82%	91%
Jahnke[130]	55	bSSFP	78%	91%
Sakuma[20]	113	bSSFP	82%	90%
Nagata[131]	62	bSSFP	83%	93%
Klein[132]	46	bSSFP	91%	54%
Pouleur[133]	77	bSSFP	100%	72%
Greenwood[134]	598	bSSFP	72% (M)/67%(F)	90%(M)/88%(F)
Nagata[135]	67	bSSFP	87%	86%
Heer[136]	59	bSSFP	86.7%	79.3%
1.5 T self-gated contrast-enhanced coronary MRI with whole-heart approach				
Piccini[70]	40	bSSFP + Gd	71%	63%
3 T prospective navigator coronary MRI				
Sommer[81]	18	GRE	82%	89%
Yang[137]	69	GRE + Gd	94%	82%

[a]Based on 60% of patients with good free-breathing images.
bSSFP, balanced steady-state free precession; *GRE*, gradient recalled echo sequence.

TABLE 21.3 Multicenter coronary MRI trials.

		# PATIENTS	SENSITIVITY (%)	SPECIFICITY (%)	PPV (%)	NPV (%)
Kim[139]	1.5 T	109	93	42	70	81
Kato[140]	1.5 T	138	88	72	71	88
Yang[141]	3.0 T	272	91	80		

TABLE 21.4 Comparison of different components of the CMR examination for detection of significant coronary artery disease.

CMR COMPONENT	N (SEX)	SENSITIVITY (%)	SPECIFICITY (%)
Greenwood[147]			
LV function	393 (M)	49.2	92.9
	235 (F)	39.6	95.1
Perfusion	388 (M)	75.4	92.9
	229 (F)	81.1	89.2
LGE	392 (M)	41.2	94.4
	235 (F)	34.0	97.8
Coronary MRI	349 (M)	72.3	90.3
	208 (F)	66.7	87.7
Heer et al.[148]			
Coronary MRI	59	86.7	79.3
Coronary MRI with perfusion	59	95.7	88.9

vs. 87% for noncontrast). The specificity of 3T coronary MRI, particularly with whole-heart imaging, was superior (83% vs. 68% for 1.5T), and 78% versus 57% for whole-heart versus targeted methods. Another meta-analysis involving 1899 patients from 34 reports demonstrated that contrast-enhanced coronary MRI at 3.0 T had significantly higher specificity than noncontrast coronary MRI at 1.5 T on a patient-based analysis (0.87, 95% CI 0.80–0.92 vs. 0.74, 95% CI 0.64–0.82, $P = .02$). Additionally, there were no differences in diagnostic performance using vasodilators or beta-blockers between Asian and Western countries.[143]

Over the years, there have been significant advances in other CMR sequences. With a shift toward assessing the functional significance of stenosis instead of merely focusing on anatomical stenosis, there has been a growing interest in myocardial perfusion imaging. Late gadolinium imaging has also become essential to any CMR protocol for assessing coronary disease. The multicenter Clinical Evaluation of Magnetic Resonance Imaging in Coronary heart disease (CE-MARC) study offered the unique opportunity to examine different components of the CMR, such as left ventricular function, myocardial perfusion, LGE, and coronary artery imaging for the detection of coronary artery disease (Table 21.4),[134] and suggests that coronary MRI images acquisition had the *lowest* technical success and offered no additional benefit for the detection of angiographic disease. However, a single-center study by Heer et al.[136] found that combining coronary MRI with adenosine stress perfusion improved overall accuracy from 78% to 92% for detecting angiographically significant coronary artery disease. A 3 T study by Zhang et al. involving 46 patients found the addition of contrast-enhanced coronary MRI resulted in higher sensitivity (100% vs. 76.5%) and accuracy (89% vs. 74%) with no change in specificity.[146] Further rigorous studies utilizing the latest coronary MRI sequences are required to evaluate the incremental value of coronary MRI in a comprehensive CMR exam.

There have been numerous recent advances in both coronary MRI and CTA technologies. However, existing data comparing the two modalities are relatively outdated and use old technologies. The recent introduction of photon-counting CT has ignited renewed interest in using CT in CAD detection, demonstrating high accuracy with ultrahigh-resolution imaging,[147] but there are currently no data comparing photon-counting CT vs. coronary MRI in CAD detection.

Coronary MRI for Coronary Artery Bypass Graft Assessment

Assessment of coronary artery bypass graft patency is a common clinical issue.[144,148] Compared with the native coronary arteries, reverse saphenous vein and internal mammary artery grafts are relatively easy to image because of their minimal motion during the cardiac and respiratory cycle and the larger lumen of reverse saphenous vein grafts (Fig. 21.10). Furthermore, their predictable and less convoluted course has allowed imaging of bypass grafts, even with less sophisticated CMR methods. The assessment of coronary artery bypass grafts using CMR imaging has limitations due to difficulties related to local signal loss and artifacts caused by implanted metallic objects such as hemostatic clips, stainless steel graft markers, sternal wires, prosthetic valves, supporting struts or rings, and graft stents (Fig. 21.11, Table 21.5).[145,149–157] The inability to identify severely diseased yet patent grafts is also a hindrance to clinical utility and acceptance. Langerak and colleagues[158] found that free-breathing navigator 3D coronary MRI was accurate for assessing saphenous vein graft stenoses, showing good agreement with quantitative invasive angiography for both graft occlusion and graft stenoses. This group has also advocated the assessment of rest and adenosine stress coronary artery flow assessment using the phase contrast MRI technique,[159,160] suggesting superior results for flow assessment.

Coronary Artery Wall Imaging

As with coronary lumen CMR, the first in vivo CMR demonstrating the coronary vessel wall was obtained using 2D fat-saturated fast-spin echo techniques.[161,162] A double-inversion recovery preparation pulse was applied to obtain black-blood images and improved contrast between the blood and

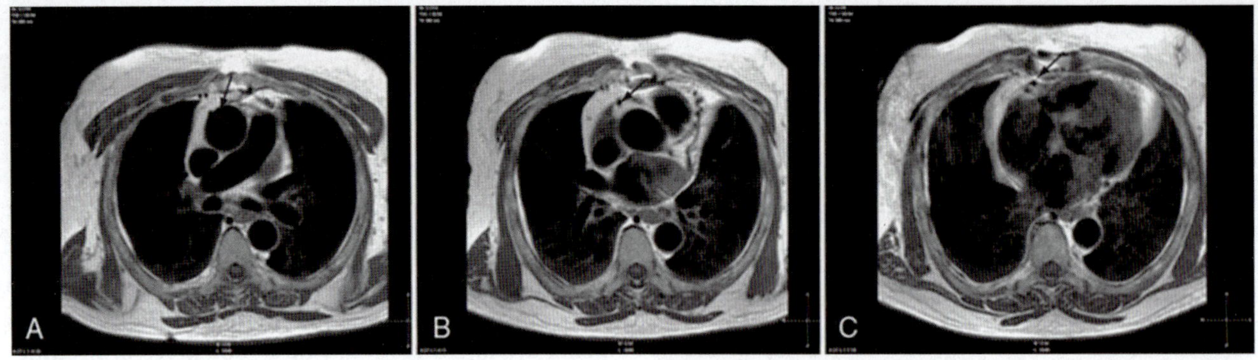

FIG. 21.10 Transverse fast-spin echo images in a patient with previous coronary artery bypass grafting. (A) The proximal graft is identified (*arrow*), with subsequent inferior sections (B) and (C) showing a patent graft (*arrows*).

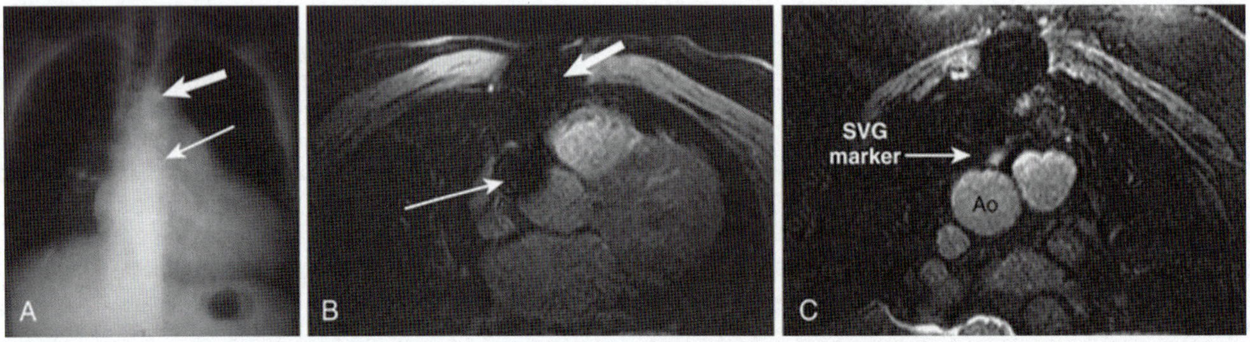

FIG. 21.11 (A) Posterior–anterior chest radiograph in a patient with coronary artery bypass grafts. Note the sternal wires (*thick arrow*) and the coronary artery bypass markers (*thin arrow*). (B) Transverse coronary cardiovascular magnetic resonance in the same patient. Note the large local artifacts (signal voids) related to sternal wires (*thick arrow*) and bypass graft markers (*thin arrow*). (C) Barium and tantalum markers (*arrow*) result in the smallest artifacts. The size of the artifacts is reduced somewhat with spin echo and black-blood cardiovascular magnetic resonance.

TABLE 21.5 Sensitivity, specificity, and accuracy of coronary MRI for assessment of coronary artery bypass graft patency.

	TECHNIQUE	# GRAFTS	PATENCY (%)	SENSITIVITY (%)	SPECIFICITY (%)	ACCURACY (%)
White[145]	2D SE	72	69	86	59	78
Rubinstein[149]	2D SE	47	62	90	72	83
Jenkins[150]	2D SE	41	63	89	73	83
Galjee[151]	2D SE	98	74	98	85	89
White[152]	2D GRE	28	50	93	86	89
Aurigemma[153]	2D GRE	45	73	88	100	91
Galjee[151]	2D GRE	98	74	98	88	96
Molinari[154]	3D GRE	51	76.5	91	97	96
Engelmann[155]	GRE + Gd	96 SVG	66	92	85	89
		37 IMA	100	100	100	
Wintersperger[156]	GRE + Gd	39	87	97	100	97
Vrachliotis[157]	CE-	45	67	93	97	95

SE, spin echo; *GRE*, gradient recalled echo; 2D, two-dimensional; 3D, three-dimensional; *Gd*, gadolinium contrast; *GRE*, gradient recalled echo; *IMA*, internal mammary artery graft; *SVG*, saphenous vein graft.

the vessel wall.[163] Further developments of the technique include combining the double-inversion recovery preparation with fast gradient echo readout techniques,[164] including spiral[165] and radial[166] acquisition trajectories. An example of coronary vessel wall images with double-inversion recovery preparation and radial acquisition is shown in Fig. 21.12. Clinical studies demonstrated outward positive remodeling with lumen preservation in patients with established CAD and increased vessel wall thickness in patients with type I diabetes and renal dysfunction.[167,168]

One limitation of black-blood approaches for coronary vessel wall imaging is that these techniques rely on blood flow, which may be insufficient in patients with very low coronary flow or heavily calcified coronary plaque.

Furthermore, these acquisitions are limited in coverage to 2D acquisitions or targeted 3D scans, and because the coronary arteries have a tortuous course, complicated scan planning is required. A 3D flow-independent approach for vessel wall imaging was proposed based on an interleaved acquisition and subtraction of bSSFP data with and without a T_2 preparation pulse.[169] This allows suppressing arterial blood signals while maintaining myocardial and vessel wall signals. A combination of this approach with iNAV-based navigation, nonrigid motion corrected undersampled reconstruction, and optimized magnetization preparation (IR-T_2 preparation in odd heartbeats and no preparation in even heartbeats) enabled obtaining a coronary MR angiogram in odd heartbeats (IR-T_2 preparation) and a black blood 3D vessel wall dataset by direct subtraction of even and odd heartbeats.[170] The feasibility of this approach to detect coronary thrombus and plaque has been validated in 41 patients with suspected non-ST elevation myocardial infarction. Comparison with invasive x-ray coronary angiography, intravascular ultrasound, and optical coherence tomography demonstrated that the plaque-to-muscle ratio of vulnerable plaque and thrombus measured of black blood vessel wall images was significantly higher than that of stable plaque or normal vessel wall.[171]

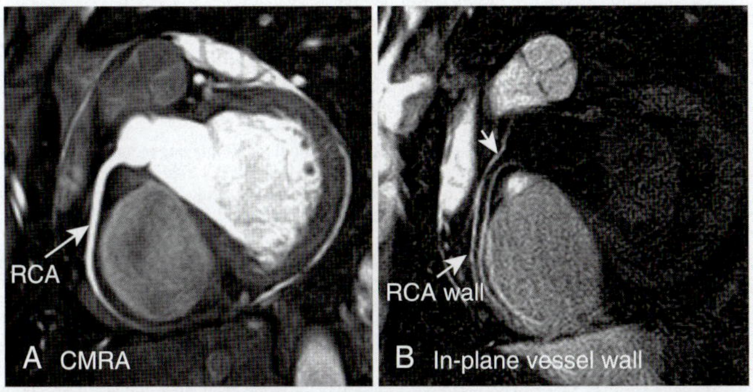

FIG. 21.12 (A) Coronary MRI, (B) 3D in-plane coronary vessel wall imaging using a local inversion preparation pulse and a 3D stack-of-stars (radial) scan with an in-plane spatial resolution of 0.9 × 0.9 mm and a slice thickness of 2.4 mm.

Coronary MRI and Prognosis

The validation of cardiac imaging is increasingly focused on the impact on outcomes. There are limited data on the prognostic value of coronary MRI. Yoon and colleagues[172] studied 207 consecutive patients without known CAD using whole-heart bSSFP free-breathing coronary MRI at 1.5 T. Follow-up was available for a median of 25 months, and 41% of the patients had CAD on coronary MRI (Fig. 21.13). The presence of stenosis on coronary MRI had a univariate hazard ratio of 20.8 (multivariate 18)/12% risk of cardiac death (1.2%), unstable angina (4.8%), or late revascularization (8.3%). In comparison, the absence of stenosis was associated with late revascularization in <1% of subjects. In another study by Nakamura and colleagues,[173] 506 patients without known CAD were assessed using a 1.5 T or 3 T CMR scanner. Over a median follow-up of 5.6 years, 31 cardiac events, including cardiac death, nonfatal myocardial infarction, and unstable angina, occurred. Not only the presence but also the severity of obstructive CAD detected by coronary MRI was associated with a worse prognosis, with annualized event rates in patients with different degrees of CAD severity (0.6% for patients with no obstructive CAD, 1.5% for those with one-vessel disease 2.3% for two-vessel disease, and 3.6% for left main or three-vessel disease).

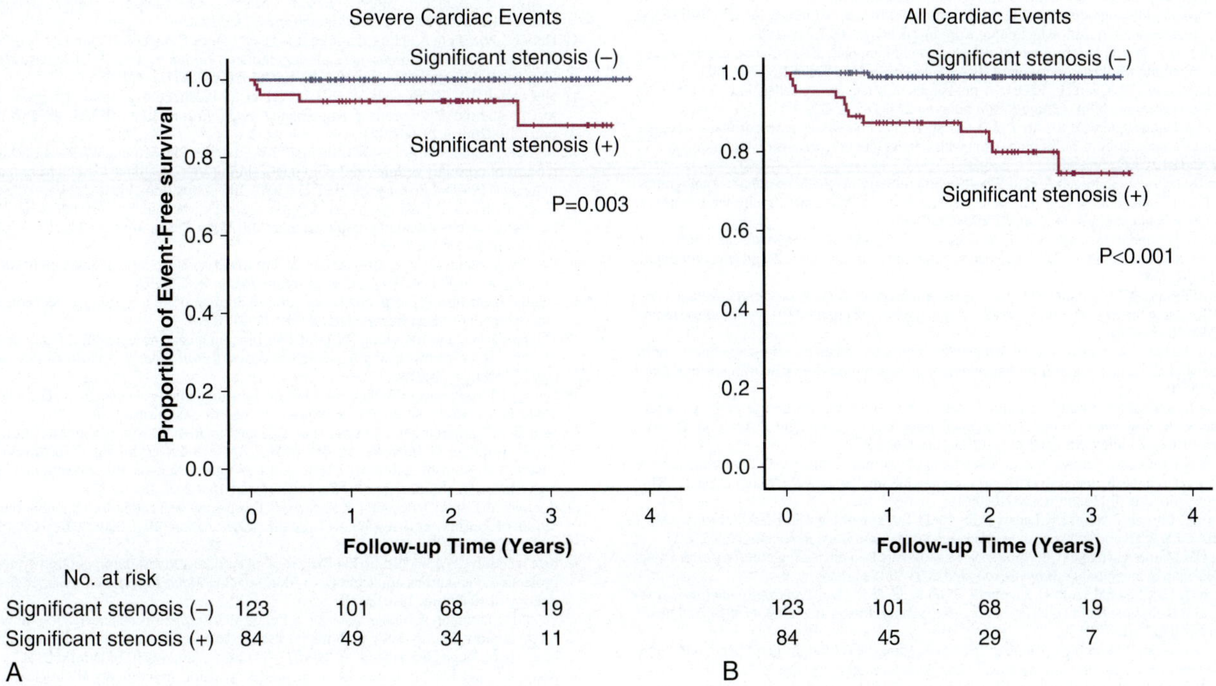

FIG. 21.13 Kaplan–Meier event-free survival curves based on noncontrast 3D whole-heart coronary MRI for (A) severe cardiac events and (B) all cardiac events. (With permission from Yoon YE, Kitagawa K, Kato S et al. Prognostic value of coronary magnetic resonance angiography for prediction of cardiac events in patients with suspected coronary artery disease. *J Am Coll Cardiol.* 2012;60:2316–2322.)

Conclusions

CMR has become integral to the noninvasive assessment of patients with known or suspected CAD. Coronary MRI can identify and characterize coronary anomalies, assess aneurysms, and determine the patency of coronary artery bypass grafts. Due to lower spatial resolution and inferior image quality compared to coronary CTA, coronary MRI for assessing native vessel integrity remains a research tool and has not been clinically adopted. Normal results on coronary MRI strongly suggest the absence of left main or multivessel disease and also convey an excellent prognosis. CMR is more effective in patients with prominent epicardial calcium and avoids ionizing radiation and iodinated contrast. Further technical improvements are still needed to address challenges for robust imaging of coronary stenosis with CMR.

REFERENCES

1. Hendel RC, Patel MR, Kramer CM, et al. ACCF/ACR/SCCT/SCMR/ASNC/NASCI/SCAI/SIR 2006 appropriateness criteria for cardiac computed tomography and cardiac magnetic resonance imaging: a report of the American College of Cardiology Foundation Quality Strategic Directions Committee Appropriateness Criteria Working Group, American College of Radiology, Society of Cardiovascular Computed Tomography, Society for Cardiovascular Magnetic Resonance, American Society of Nuclear Cardiology, North American Society for Cardiac Imaging, Society for Cardiovascular Angiography and Interventions, and Society of Interventional Radiology. *J Am Coll Cardiol*. 2006;48:1475–1497. https://doi.org/10.1016/j.jacc.2006.07.003.
2. Hundley WG, Bluemke DA, Finn JP, et al. ACCF/ACR/AHA/NASCI/SCMR 2010 Expert Consensus Document on Cardiovascular Magnetic Resonance. A Report of the American College of Cardiology Foundation Task Force on Expert Consensus Documents. *Circulation*. 2010;121(22):2462–2508.
3. Manning WJ, Edelman RR. Magnetic resonance coronary angiography. *Magn ResonQ*. 1993;9:131–151.
4. Manning WJ, Li W, Edelman RR. A preliminary report comparing magnetic resonance coronary angiography with conventional angiography. *New Engl J Med*. 1993;328:828.
5. Stuber M, Botnar RM, Danias PG, Kissinger KV, Manning WJ. Breathhold three-dimensional coronary magnetic resonance angiography using real-time navigator technology. *J Cardiovasc Magn Reson*. 1999;1:233–238.
6. Stuber M, Botnar RM, Danias PG, Kissinger KV, Manning WJ. Submillimeter three-dimensional coronary MR angiography with real-time navigator correction: comparison of navigator locations. *Radiology*. 1999;212:579–587.
7. Stuber M, Botnar RM, Danias PG, et al. Double-oblique free-breathing high resolution three-dimensional coronary magnetic resonance angiography. *J Am Coll Cardiol*. 1999;34:524–531. https://doi.org/10.1016/s0735-1097(99)00223-5.
8. Botnar RM, Stuber M, Danias PG, Kissinger KV, Manning WJ. Improved coronary artery definition with T2-weighted, free-breathing, three-dimensional coronary MRA. *Circulation*. 1999;99:3139–3148. https://doi.org/10.1161/01.cir.99.24.3139.
9. Bhat H, Zuehlsdorff S, Bi X, Li D. Whole-heart contrast-enhanced coronary magnetic resonance angiography using gradient echo interleaved EPI. *Magn Reson Med*. 2009;61:1388–1395.
10. Bi X, Carr JC, Li D. Whole-heart coronary magnetic resonance angiography at 3 Tesla in 5 minutes with slow infusion of Gd-BOPTA, a high-relaxivity clinical contrast agent. *Magn Reson Med*. 2007;58:1–7. https://doi.org/10.1002/mrm.21224.
11. Bi X, Deshpande V, Carr J, Li D. Coronary artery magnetic resonance angiography (MRA): a comparison between the whole-heart and volume-targeted methods using a T2-prepared SSFP sequence. *J Cardiovasc Magn Reson*. 2006;8:703–707. https://doi.org/10.1080/10976640600723706.
12. Kim YJ, Seo JS, Choi BW, Choe KO, Jang Y, Ko YG. Feasibility and diagnostic accuracy of whole heart coronary MR angiography using free-breathing 3D balanced turbo-field-echo with SENSE and the half-fourier acquisition technique. *Korean J Radiol*. 2006;7:235–242.
13. Lai P, Bi X, Jerecic R, Li D. A respiratory self-gating technique with 3D-translation compensation for free-breathing whole-heart coronary MRA. *Magn Reson Med*. 2009;62(3):731–738.
14. Lai P, Larson AC, Bi X, Jerecic R, Li D. A dual-projection respiratory self-gating technique for whole-heart coronary MRA. *J Magn Reson Imaging*. 2008;28:612–620.
15. Liu X, Bi X, Huang J, Jerecic R, Carr J, Li D. Contrast-enhanced whole-heart coronary magnetic resonance angiography at 3.0 T: comparison with steady-state free precession technique at 1.5 T. *Invest Radiol*. 2008;43:663–668.
16. Maintz D, Ozgun M, Hoffmeier A, et al. Whole-heart coronary magnetic resonance angiography: value for the detection of coronary artery stenoses in comparison to multislice computed tomography angiography. *Acta Radiol*. 2007;48:967–973.
17. Nehrke K, Bornert P, Mazurkewitz P, Winkelmann R, Grasslin I. Free-breathing whole-heart coronary MR angiography on a clinical scanner in four minutes. *JMagn ResonImaging*. 2006;23:752–756.
18. Niendorf T, Hardy CJ, Giaquinto RO, et al. Toward single breath-hold whole-heart coverage coronary MRA using highly accelerated parallel imaging with a 32-channel MR system. *Magn Reson Med*. 2006;56:167–176.
19. Okada T, Kanao S, Ninomiya A, et al. Whole-heart coronary magnetic resonance angiography with parallel imaging: comparison of acceleration in one-dimension vs. two-dimensions. *Eur J Radiol*. 2008.
20. Sakuma H, Ichikawa Y, Chino S, Hirano T, Makino K, Takeda K. Detection of coronary artery stenosis with whole-heart coronary magnetic resonance angiography. *J Am Coll Cardiol*. 2006;48:1946–1950. https://doi.org/10.1016/j.jacc.2006.07.055.
21. Sakuma H, Ichikawa Y, Suzawa N, et al. Assessment of coronary arteries with total study time of less than 30 minutes by using whole-heart coronary MR angiography. *Radiology*. 2005;237:316–321. https://doi.org/10.1148/radiol.2371040830.
22. Stehning C, Bornert P, Nehrke K, Eggers H, Stuber M. Free-breathing whole-heart coronary MRA with 3D radial SSFP and self-navigated image reconstruction. *Magn Reson Med*. 2005;54.
23. Weber OM, Martin AJ, Higgins CB. Whole-heart steady-state free precession coronary artery magnetic resonance angiography. *Magn Reson Med*. 2003;50:1223–1228.
24. Deshpande VS, Shea SM, Laub G, Simonetti OP, Finn JP, Li D. 3D magnetization-prepared true-FISP: a new technique for imaging coronary arteries. *Magn Reson Med*. 2001;46:494–502. https://doi.org/10.1002/mrm.1219.
25. Nezafat R, Herzka D, Stehning C, Peters DC, Nehrke K, Manning WJ. Inflow quantification in three-dimensional cardiovascular MR imaging. *J Magn Reson Imaging*. 2008;28:1273–1279.
26. Maintz D, Aepfelbacher FC, Kissinger KV, et al. Coronary MR angiography: comparison of quantitative and qualitative data from four techniques. *AJR AmJRoentgenol*. 2004;182:515–521.
27. Ozgun M, Hoffmeier A, Kouwenhoven M, et al. Comparison of 3D segmented gradient-echo and steady-state free precession coronary MRI sequences in patients with coronary artery disease. *AJR Am J Roentgenol*. 2005;185:103–109.
28. Brittain JH, Hu BS, Wright GA, Meyer CH, Macovski A, Nishimura DG. Coronary angiography with magnetization-prepared T2 contrast. *Magn Reson Med*. 1995;33:689–696. https://doi.org/10.1002/mrm.1910330515.
29. Manning WJ, Li W, Boyle NG, Edelman RR. Fat-suppressed breath-hold magnetic resonance coronary angiography. *Circulation*. 1993;87:94–104. https://doi.org/10.1161/01.cir.87.1.94.
30. Jahnke CPI, Gebker R, Schnackenburg B, Bornstedt A, Fleck E, et al. Comparison of individually adapted breath-hold and free-breathing coronary MRA using steady state free precession [abstr]. *J Cardiovasc Magn Reson*. 2004;6:166–167.
31. Plein S, Jones TR, Ridgway JP, Sivananthan MU. Three-dimensional coronary MR angiography performed with subject-specific cardiac acquisition windows and motion-adapted respiratory gating. *AJR Am J Roentgenol*. 2003;180:505–512. https://doi.org/10.2214/ajr.180.2.1800505.
32. Leiner T, Katsimaglis G, Yeh EN, et al. Correction for heart rate variability improves coronary magnetic resonance angiography. *J Magn Reson Imaging*. 2005;22:577–582. https://doi.org/10.1002/jmri.20399.
33. Ehman RL, Felmlee JP. Adaptive technique for high-definition MR imaging of moving structures. *Radiology*. 1989;173:255–263. https://doi.org/10.1148/radiology.173.1.2781017.
34. Oshinski JN, Hofland L, Mukundan Jr S, Dixon WT, Parks WJ, Pettigrew RI. Two-dimensional coronary MR angiography without breath holding. *Radiology*. 1996;201:737–743. https://doi.org/10.1148/radiology.201.3.8939224.
35. Sachs TS, Meyer CH, Hu BS, Kohli J, Nishimura DG, Macovski A. Real-time motion detection in spiral MRI using navigators. *Magn Reson Med*. 1994;32:639–645. https://doi.org/10.1002/mrm.1910320513.
36. McConnell MV, Khasgiwala VC, Savord BJ, et al. Comparison of respiratory suppression methods and navigator locations for MR coronary angiography. *AJR Am J Roentgenol*. 1997;168:1369–1375. https://doi.org/10.2214/ajr.168.5.9129447.
37. Wang Y, Riederer SJ, Ehman RL. Respiratory motion of the heart: kinematics and the implications for the spatial resolution in coronary imaging. *Magn Reson Med*. 1995;33:713–719. https://doi.org/10.1002/mrm.1910330517.
38. Taylor AM, Jhooti P, Wiesmann F, Keegan J, Firmin DN, Pennell DJ. MR navigator-echo monitoring of temporal changes in diaphragm position: implications for MR coronary angiography. *J Magn Reson Imaging*. 1997;7:629–636. https://doi.org/10.1002/jmri.1880070404.
39. Danias PG, McConnell MV, Khasgiwala VC, Chuang ML, Edelman RR, Manning WJ. Prospective navigator correction of image position for coronary MR angiography. *Radiology*. 1997;203:733–736. https://doi.org/10.1148/radiology.203.3.9169696.
40. Nagel E, Bornstedt A, Schnackenburg B, Hug J, Oswald H, Fleck E. Optimization of realtime adaptive navigator correction for 3D magnetic resonance coronary angiography. *Magn Reson Med*. 1999;42:408–411. https://doi.org/10.1002/(sici)1522-2594(199908)42:2<408::aid-mrm24>3.0.co;2-u.
41. Huber S, Bornstedt A, Schnackenburg B, Paetsch I, Fleck E, Nagel E. The impact of different positions and thoracial restrains on respiratory induced cardiac motion. *J Cardiovasc Magn Reson*. 2006;8:483–488. https://doi.org/10.1080/10976640600572871.
42. McConnell MV, Khasgiwala VC, Savord BJ, et al. Prospective adaptive navigator correction for breath-hold MR coronary angiography. *Magn Reson Med*. 1997;37:148–152. https://doi.org/10.1002/mrm.1910370121.
43. Danias PG, Stuber M, Botnar RM, Kissinger KV, Edelman RR, Manning WJ. Relationship between motion of coronary arteries and diaphragm during free breathing: lessons from real-time MR imaging. *AJR Am J Roentgenol*. 1999;172:1061–1065. https://doi.org/10.2214/ajr.172.4.10587147.
44. Moghari MH, Hu P, Kissinger KV, et al. Subject-specific estimation of respiratory navigator tracking factor for free-breathing cardiovascular MR. *Magn Reson Med*. 2012;67:1665–1672. https://doi.org/10.1002/mrm.23158.
45. Nezafat R, Stehning C, Gharib AM, et al. Improved spatial-temporal resolution MR coronary blood flow imaging at 3T. *J Cardiovasc Magn Reson*. 2005;7:199.
46. Nehrke K, Bornert P. Prospective correction of affine motion for arbitrary MR sequences on a clinical scanner. *Magn Reson Med*. 2005;54:1130–1138.
47. Moghari MH, Chan RH, Hong SN, et al. Free-breathing cardiac MR with a fixed navigator efficiency using adaptive gating window size. *Magn Reson Med*. 2012;68:1866–1875. https://doi.org/10.1002/mrm.24210.
48. Gurney PT, Hargreaves BA, Nishimura DG. Design and analysis of a practical 3D cones trajectory. *Magn Reson Med*. 2006;55:575–582. https://doi.org/10.1002/mrm.20796.
49. Santos JM, Cunningham CH, Lustig M, et al. Single breath-hold whole-heart MRA using variable-density spirals at 3T. *Magn Reson Med*. 2006;55:371–379. https://doi.org/10.1002/mrm.20765.
50. Sussman M, Stainsby J, Robert N, Merchant N, Wright G. Variable-density adaptive imaging for high-resolution coronary artery MRI. *Magn Reson Med*. 2002;48:753–764.
51. Buehrer M, Curcic J, Boesiger P, Kozerke S. Prospective self-gating for simultaneous compensation of cardiac and respiratory motion. *Magn Reson Med*. 2008;60:683–690. https://doi.org/10.1002/mrm.21697.
52. Kim WS, Mun CW, Kim DJ, Cho ZH. Extraction of cardiac and respiratory motion cycles by use of projection data and its applications to NMR imaging. *Magn Reson Med*. 1990;13:25–37. https://doi.org/10.1002/mrm.1910130105.
53. Piccini D, Littmann A, Nielles-Vallespin S, Zenge MO. Respiratory self-navigation for whole-heart bright-blood coronary MRI: methods for robust isolation and automatic segmentation of the blood pool. *Magn Reson Med*. 2012;68:571–579. https://doi.org/10.1002/mrm.23247.
54. Addy NO, Ingle RR, Luo J, et al. 3D image-based navigators for coronary MR angiography. *Magnc Reson Med*. 2016;77:1874–1883. https://doi.org/10.1002/mrm.26269.
55. Henningsson M, Koken P, Stehning C, Razavi R, Prieto C, Botnar RM. Whole-heart coronary MR angiography with 2D self-navigated image reconstruction. *Magn Reson Med*. 2012;67:437–445. https://doi.org/10.1002/mrm.23027.

56. Henningsson M, Smink J, Razavi R, Botnar RM. Prospective respiratory motion correction for coronary MR angiography using a 2D image navigator. *Magn Reson Med*. 2013;69:486–494. https://doi.org/10.1002/mrm.24280.
57. Kawaji K, Spincemaille P, Nguyen TD, et al. Direct coronary motion extraction from a 2D fat image navigator for prospectively gated coronary MR angiography. *Magn Reson Med*. 2014;71:599–607. https://doi.org/10.1002/mrm.24698.
58. Luo J, Addy NO, Ingle RR, et al. Nonrigid motion correction with 3D image-based navigators for coronary MR angiography. *Magnetic Resonance in Medicine*. 2016;77:1884. https://doi.org/10.1002/mrm.26273.
59. Moghari MH, Annese D, Geva T, Powell AJ. Three-dimensional heart locator and compressed sensing for whole-heart MR angiography. *Magn Reson Med*. 2016;75:2086–2093. https://doi.org/10.1002/mrm.25800.
60. Moghari MH, Roujol S, Henningsson M, et al. Three-dimensional heart locator for whole-heart coronary magnetic resonance angiography. *Magn Reson Med*. 2014;71:2118–2126. https://doi.org/10.1002/mrm.24881.
61. Wu HH, Gurney PT, Hu BS, Nishimura DG, McConnell MV. Free-breathing multiphase whole-heart coronary MR angiography using image-based navigators and three-dimensional cones imaging. *Magn Reson Med*. 2013;69:1083–1093. https://doi.org/10.1002/mrm.24346.
62. Wood G, Hajhosseiny R, Pedersen AU, et al. iNav-based, automated coronary magnetic resonance angiography for the detection of coronary artery stenosis (iNav-AUTO CMRA). *J Cardiovasc Magn Reson*. 2024;26:101097. https://doi.org/10.1016/j.jocmr.2024.101097.
63. Bustin A, Rashid I, Cruz G, et al. 3D whole-heart isotropic sub-millimeter resolution coronary magnetic resonance angiography with non-rigid motion-compensated PROST. *J Cardiovasc Magn Reson*. 2020;22:24. https://doi.org/10.1186/s12968-020-00611-5.
64. Cruz G, Atkinson D, Henningsson M, Botnar RM, Prieto C. Highly efficient nonrigid motion-corrected 3D whole-heart coronary vessel wall imaging. *Magn Reson Med*. 2017;77:1894–1908. https://doi.org/10.1002/mrm.26274.
65. Meyer CH, Hu BS, Nishimura DG, Macovski A. Fast spiral coronary artery imaging. *Magn Reson Med*. 1992;28:202–213. https://doi.org/10.1002/mrm.1910280204.
66. Börnert P, Stuber M, Botnar RM, et al. Direct comparison of 3D spiral vs. Cartesian gradient-echo coronary magnetic resonance angiography. *Magn Reson Med*. 2001;46:789–794. https://doi.org/10.1002/mrm.1258.
67. Ingle RR, Wu HH, Addy NO, et al. Nonrigid autofocus motion correction for coronary MR angiography with a 3D cones trajectory. *Magn Reson Med*. 2014;72:347–361. https://doi.org/10.1002/mrm.24924.
68. Addy NO, Ingle RR, Wu HH, Hu BS, Nishimura DG. High-resolution variable-density 3D cones coronary MRA. *Magn Reson Med*. 2015;74:614–621. https://doi.org/10.1002/mrm.25803.
69. Piccini D, Littmann A, Nielles-Vallespin S, Zenge MO. Spiral phyllotaxis: the natural way to construct a 3D radial trajectory in MRI. *Magn Reson Med*. 2011;66:1049–1056. https://doi.org/10.1002/mrm.22898.
70. Piccini D, Monney P, Sierro C, et al. Respiratory self-navigated postcontrast whole-heart coronary MR angiography: initial experience in patients. *Radiology*. 2014;270:378–386. https://doi.org/10.1148/radiol.13132045.
71. Griswold MA, Jakob PM, Heidemann RM, et al. Generalized autocalibrating partially parallel acquisitions (GRAPPA). *Magn Reson Med*. 2002;47:1202–1210. https://doi.org/10.1002/mrm.10171.
72. Pruessmann KP, Weiger M, Börnert P, Boesiger P. Advances in sensitivity encoding with arbitrary k-space trajectories. *Magn Reson Med*. 2001;46:638–651. https://doi.org/10.1002/mrm.1241.
73. Lustig M, Donoho DL, Pauly JM. Sparse MRI: the application of compressed sensing for rapid MR imaging. *Magn Reson Med*. 2007;58:1182–1195. https://doi.org/10.1002/mrm.21391.
74. Akçakaya M, Basha TA, Goddu B, et al. Low-dimensional-structure self-learning and thresholding: regularization beyond compressed sensing for MRI reconstruction. *Magn Reson Med*. 2011;66:756–767. https://doi.org/10.1002/mrm.22841.
75. Akçakaya M, Basha TA, Chan RH, et al. Accelerated contrast-enhanced whole-heart coronary MRI using low-dimensional-structure self-learning and thresholding. *Magn Reson Med*. 2012;67:1434–1443. https://doi.org/10.1002/mrm.24242.
76. Bustin A, Ginami G, Cruz G, et al. Five-minute whole-heart coronary MRA with sub-millimeter isotropic resolution, 100% respiratory scan efficiency, and 3D-PROST reconstruction. *Magn Reson Med*. 2019;81:102–115. https://doi.org/10.1002/mrm.27354.
77. Morales MA, Manning WJ, Nezafat R. Present and future innovations in AI and cardiac MRI. *Radiology*. 2024;310:e231269. https://doi.org/10.1148/radiol.231269.
78. Küstner T, Munoz C, Psenicny A, et al. Deep-learning based super-resolution for 3D isotropic coronary MR angiography in less than a minute. *Magn Reson Med*. 2021;86:2837–2852. https://doi.org/10.1002/mrm.28911.
79. Wu X, Deng L, Li W, et al. Deep learning-based acceleration of compressed sensing for noncontrast-enhanced coronary magnetic resonance angiography in patients with suspected coronary artery disease. *J Magn Reson Imaging*. 2023;58:1521–1530. https://doi.org/10.1002/jmri.28653.
80. Wu X, Tang L, Li W, et al. Feasibility of accelerated non-contrast-enhanced whole-heart bSSFP coronary MR angiography by deep learning-constrained compressed sensing. *Eur Radiol*. 2023;33:8180–8190. https://doi.org/10.1007/s00330-023-09740-8.
81. Sommer T, Hackenbroch M, Hofer U, et al. Coronary MR angiography at 3.0 T versus that at 1.5 T: initial results in patients suspected of having coronary artery disease. *Radiology*. 2005;234:718–725. https://doi.org/10.1148/radiol.2343031784.
82. Gharib AM, Abd-Elmoniem KZ, Ho VB, et al. The feasibility of 350 mum spatial resolution coronary magnetic resonance angiography at 3 T in humans. *Invest Radiol*. 2012;47:339–345. https://doi.org/10.1097/RLI.0b013e3182479ec4.
83. Nezafat R, Ouwerkerk R, Derbyshire AJ, Stuber M, McVeigh ER. Spectrally selective B1-insensitive T2 magnetization preparation sequence. *Magn Reson Med*. 2009;61:1326–1335. https://doi.org/10.1002/mrm.21742.
84. Nezafat R, Stuber M, Ouwerkerk R, Gharib AM, Desai MY, Pettigrew RI. B1-insensitive T2 preparation for improved coronary magnetic resonance angiography at 3 T. *Magn Reson Med*. 2006;55:858–864.
85. Börnert P, Koken P, Nehrke K, Eggers H, Ostendorf P. Water/fat-resolved whole-heart Dixon coronary MRA: an initial comparison. *Magn Reson Med*. 2014;71:156–163. https://doi.org/10.1002/mrm.24648.
86. Nezafat M, Henningsson M, Ripley DP, et al. Coronary MR angiography at 3T: fat suppression versus water-fat separation. *Magma*. 2016;29:733–738. https://doi.org/10.1007/s10334-016-0550-7.
87. Coristine AJ, van Heeswijk RB, Stuber M. Fat signal suppression for coronary MRA at 3T using a water-selective adiabatic T2 -preparation technique. *Magn Reson Med*. 2014;72:763–769. https://doi.org/10.1002/mrm.24961.
88. Bastiaansen JAM, van Heeswijk RB, Stuber M, Piccini D. Noncontrast free-breathing respiratory self-navigated coronary artery cardiovascular magnetic resonance angiography at 3 T using lipid insensitive binomial off-resonant excitation (LIBRE). *J Cardiovasc Magn Reson*. 2019;21:38. https://doi.org/10.1186/s12968-019-0543-6.
89. Lu H, Miao X, Wang D, et al. Feasibility and clinical application of 5-T noncontrast dixon whole-heart coronary mr angiography: a prospective study. *Radiology*. 2024;313:e240389. https://doi.org/10.1148/radiol.240389.
90. van Elderen SG, Versluis MJ, Westenberg JJ, et al. Right coronary MR angiography at 7 T: a direct quantitative and qualitative comparison with 3 T in young healthy volunteers. *Radiology*. 2010;257:254–259. https://doi.org/10.1148/radiol.100615.
91. Terashima M, Meyer CH, Keeffe BG, et al. Noninvasive assessment of coronary vasodilation using magnetic resonance angiography. *J Am Coll Cardiol*. 2005;45:104–110.
92. Hu P, Chuang ML, Ngo LH, et al. Coronary MR imaging: effect of timing and dose of isosorbide dinitrate administration. *Radiology*. 2010;254:401–409. https://doi.org/10.1148/radiol.09090483.
93. Dong Z, Si G, Zhu X, et al. Diagnostic performance and safety of a novel ferumoxytol-enhanced coronary magnetic resonance angiography. *Circ Cardiovasc Imaging*. 2023;16:580–590. https://doi.org/10.1161/circimaging.123.015404.
94. Roy CW, Di Sopra L, Whitehead KK, et al. Free-running cardiac and respiratory motion-resolved 5D whole-heart coronary cardiovascular magnetic resonance angiography in pediatric cardiac patients using ferumoxytol. *J Cardiovasc Magn Reson*. 2022;24:39. https://doi.org/10.1186/s12968-022-00871-3.
95. Engel HJ, Torres C, Page Jr HL. Major variations in anatomical origin of the coronary arteries: angiographic observations in 4,250 patients without associated congenital heart disease. *Cathet Cardiovasc Diagn*. 1975;1:157–169. https://doi.org/10.1002/ccd.1810010205.
96. Chaitman BR, Lespérance J, Saltiel J, Bourassa MG. Clinical, angiographic, and hemodynamic findings in patients with anomalous origin of the coronary arteries. *Circulation*. 1976;53:122–131. https://doi.org/10.1161/01.cir.53.1.122.
97. Cheitlin MD, De Castro CM, McAllister HA. Sudden death as a complication of anomalous left coronary origin from the anterior sinus of Valsalva, A not-so-minor congenital anomaly. *Circulation*. 1974;50:780–787. https://doi.org/10.1161/01.cir.50.4.780.
98. Maron BJ, Doerer JJ, Haas TS, Tierney DM, Mueller FO. Sudden deaths in young competitive athletes: analysis of 1866 deaths in the United States, 1980-2006. *Circulation*. 2009;119:1085–1092. https://doi.org/10.1161/circulationaha.108.804617.
99. McConnell MV, Ganz P, Selwyn AP, Li W, Edelman RR, Manning WJ. Identification of anomalous coronary arteries and their anatomic course by magnetic resonance coronary angiography. *Circulation*. 1995;92:3158–3162. https://doi.org/10.1161/01.cir.92.11.3158.
100. Post JC, van Rossum AC, Bronzwaer JG, et al. Magnetic resonance angiography of anomalous coronary arteries. A new gold standard for delineating the proximal course? *Circulation*. 1995;92:3163–3171. https://doi.org/10.1161/01.cir.92.11.3163.
101. Vliegen HW, Doornbos J, de Roos A, Jukema JW, Bekedam MA, van der Wall EE. Value of fast gradient echo magnetic resonance angiography as an adjunct to coronary arteriography in detecting and confirming the course of clinically significant coronary artery anomalies. *Am J Cardiol*. 1997;79:773–776. https://doi.org/10.1016/s0002-9149(96)00866-1.
102. Taylor AM, Thorne SA, Rubens MB, et al. Coronary artery imaging in grown up congenital heart disease: complementary role of magnetic resonance and x-ray coronary angiography. *Circulation*. 2000;101:1670–1678. https://doi.org/10.1161/01.cir.101.14.1670.
103. Bunce NH, Lorenz CH, Keegan J, et al. Coronary artery anomalies: assessment with free-breathing three-dimensional coronary MR angiography. *Radiology*. 2003;227:201–208. https://doi.org/10.1148/radiol.2271020316.
104. Razmi RMCW, Rathi VK, Pohost GM. Coronary magnetic resonance angiography (CMRA): the gold standard for determining the proximal course of anomalous coronary arteries. *J Am Coll Cardiol*. 2001;380. [abstract].
105. Setser RMAJ, Weaver JA, et al. Exclusion of coronary artery anomalies in patients with congenital cardiovascular abnormalities using whole heart approach [abstract]. *J Cardiovasc Magn Reson*. 2007;9:128–129.
106. Tangcharoen T, Bell A, Hegde S, et al. Detection of coronary artery anomalies in infants and young children with congenital heart disease by using MR imaging. *Radiology*. 2011;259:240–247. https://doi.org/10.1148/radiol.10100828.
107. Ripley DP, Saha A, Teis A, et al. The distribution and prognosis of anomalous coronary arteries identified by cardiovascular magnetic resonance: 15 year experience from two tertiary centres. *J Cardiovasc Magn Reson*. 2014;16:34. https://doi.org/10.1186/1532-429x-16-34.
108. Hundley WG, Bluemke DA, Finn JP, et al. ACCF/ACR/AHA/NASCI/SCMR 2010 expert consensus document on cardiovascular magnetic resonance: a report of the American college of cardiology foundation task force on expert consensus documents. *J Am Coll Cardiol*. 2010;55:2614–2662. https://doi.org/10.1016/j.jacc.2009.11.011.
109. Schmid M, Achenbach S, Ludwig J, et al. Visualization of coronary artery anomalies by contrast-enhanced multi-detector row spiral computed tomography. *Int J Cardiol*. 2006;111:430–435. https://doi.org/10.1016/j.ijcard.2005.08.027.
110. Deibler AR, Kuzo RS, Vöhringer M, et al. Imaging of congenital coronary anomalies with multislice computed tomography. *Mayo Clin Proc*. 2004;79:1017–1023. https://doi.org/10.4065/79.8.1017.
111. Budoff MJ, Ahmed V, Gul KM, Mao SS, Gopal A. Coronary anomalies by cardiac computed tomographic angiography. *Clin Cardiol*. 2006;29:489–493. https://doi.org/10.1002/clc.4960291104.
112. Makino N, Nakamura Y, Yashiro M, et al. Descriptive epidemiology of kawasaki disease in Japan, 2011-2012: from the results of the 22nd nationwide survey. *J Epidemiol*. 2015;25:239–245. https://doi.org/10.2188/jea.JE20140089.
113. Akagi T, Rose V, Benson LN, Newman A, Freedom RM. Outcome of coronary artery aneurysms after Kawasaki disease. *J Pediatr*. 1992;121:689–694. https://doi.org/10.1016/s0022-3476(05)81894-3.
114. Kato H, Ichinose E, Yoshioka F, et al. Fate of coronary aneurysms in kawasaki disease: serial coronary angiography and long-term follow-up study. *Am J Cardiol*. 1982;49:1758–1766. https://doi.org/10.1016/0002-9149(82)90256-9.
115. Greil GF, Stuber M, Botnar RM, et al. Coronary magnetic resonance angiography in adolescents and young adults with kawasaki disease. *Circulation*. 2002;105:908–911. https://doi.org/10.1161/hc0802.105563.
116. Mavrogeni S, Papadopoulos G, Douskou M, et al. Magnetic resonance angiography is equivalent to X-ray coronary angiography for the evaluation of coronary arteries in kawasaki disease. *J Am Coll Cardiol*. 2004;43:649–652. https://doi.org/10.1016/j.jacc.2003.08.052.
117. Mavrogeni S, Papadopoulos G, Douskou M, et al. Magnetic resonance angiography, function and viability evaluation in patients with kawasaki disease. *J Cardiovasc Magn Reson*. 2006;8:493–498. https://doi.org/10.1080/10976640600604773.
118. Greil GF, Seeger A, Miller S, et al. Coronary magnetic resonance angiography and vessel wall imaging in children with kawasaki disease. *Pediatr Radiol*. 2007;37:666–673. https://doi.org/10.1007/s00247-007-0498-x.
119. Mavrogeni S, Bratis K, Karanasios E, et al. CMR evaluation of cardiac involvement during the convalescence of kawasaki disease. *JACC Cardiovasc Imaging*. 2011;4:1140–1141. https://doi.org/10.1016/j.jcmg.2011.04.021.
120. Regenfus M, Ropers D, Achenbach S, et al. Noninvasive detection of coronary artery stenosis using contrast-enhanced three-dimensional breath-hold magnetic resonance coronary angiography. *J Am Coll Cardiol*. 2000;36:44–50. https://doi.org/10.1016/s0735-1097(00)00672-0.
121. Bunce NRSJP, Lorenz C, Pennell D. The assessment of coronary artery disease by combined magnetic resonance coronary arteriography and perfusion. *J Cardiovasc Magn Reson*. 2001;3:118. [abstract].
122. Moustapha AIMR, Wilson J, Flamm SD. Coronary magnetic resonance angiography using a free breathing, T2 weighted, three-dimensional gradient echo sequence with navigator respiratory and ECG gating can be used to detect coronary artery disease. *J Am Coll Cardiol*. 2001;37(supp):380. [abstract].

123. Sommer THU, Meyer C, et al. Submillimeter 3D coronary MR angiography with real-time navigator correction in 112 patients with suspected coronary artery disease. *J Cardiovasc Magn Reson*. 2002;4:28. [abstract].
124. Bogaert J, Kuzo R, Dymarkowski S, Beckers R, Piessens J, Rademakers FE. Coronary artery imaging with real-time navigator three-dimensional turbo-field-echo MR coronary angiography: initial experience. *Radiology*. 2003;226:707–716. https://doi.org/10.1148/radiol.2263011750.
125. Plein S, Ridgway JP, Jones TR, Bloomer TN, Sivananthan MU. Coronary artery disease: assessment with a comprehensive MR imaging protocol-initial results. *Radiology*. 2002;225:300–307. https://doi.org/10.1148/radiol.2243011436.
126. Ozgun MQM, Kouwenhoven M, et al. Comparison of spoiled TFE and BalancedTFE coronary MR angiography [abstract]. *J Cardiovasc Magn Reson*. 2004;6:268–269.
127. Dewey M, Teige F, Schnapauff D, et al. Combination of free-breathing and breathhold steady-state free precession magnetic resonance angiography for detection of coronary artery stenoses. *J Magn Reson Imaging*. 2006;23:674–681. https://doi.org/10.1002/jmri.20568.
128. Jahnke C, Paetsch I, Schnackenburg B, et al. Coronary MR angiography with steady-state free precession: individually adapted breath-hold technique versus free-breathing technique. *Radiology*. 2004;232:669–676. https://doi.org/10.1148/radiol.2323031225.
129. Paetsch I, Jahnke C, Barkhausen J, et al. Detection of coronary stenoses with contrast enhanced, three-dimensional free breathing coronary MR angiography using the gadolinium-based intravascular contrast agent gadocoletic acid (B-22956). *J Cardiovasc Magn Reson*. 2006;8:509–516. https://doi.org/10.1080/10976640600604922.
130. Jahnke C, Paetsch I, Nehrke K, et al. Rapid and complete coronary arterial tree visualization with magnetic resonance imaging: feasibility and diagnostic performance. *Eur Heart J*. 2005;26:2313–2319. https://doi.org/10.1093/eurheartj/ehi391.
131. Nagata MSH, Ishida N, et al. Whole heart coronary magnetic resonance angiography using 32-channel cardiac coils and high parallel imaging factor. *Circulation*. 2008;118:S778. [abstract].
132. Klein C, Gebker R, Kokocinski T, et al. Combined magnetic resonance coronary artery imaging, myocardial perfusion and late gadolinium enhancement in patients with suspected coronary artery disease. *J Cardiovasc Magn Reson*. 2008;10:45. https://doi.org/10.1186/1532-429x-10-45.
133. Pouleur AC, le Polain de Waroux JB, Kefer J, Pasquet A, Vanoverschelde JL, Gerber BL. Direct comparison of whole-heart navigator-gated magnetic resonance coronary angiography and 40- and 64-slice multidetector row computed tomography to detect the coronary artery stenosis in patients scheduled for conventional coronary angiography. *Circ Cardiovasc Imaging*. 2008;1:114–121. https://doi.org/10.1161/circimaging.107.756304.
134. Greenwood JP, Motwani M, Maredia N, et al. Comparison of cardiovascular magnetic resonance and single-photon emission computed tomography in women with suspected coronary artery disease from the clinical evaluation of magnetic resonance imaging in coronary heart disease (CE-MARC) trial. *Circulation*. 2014;129:1129–1138. https://doi.org/10.1161/circulationaha.112.000071.
135. Nagata M, Kato S, Kitagawa K, et al. Diagnostic accuracy of 1.5-T unenhanced whole-heart coronary MR angiography performed with 32-channel cardiac coils: initial single-center experience. *Radiology*. 2011;259:384–392. https://doi.org/10.1148/radiol.11101323.
136. Heer T, Reiter S, Höfling B, Pilz G. Diagnostic performance of non-contrast-enhanced whole-heart magnetic resonance coronary angiography in combination with adenosine stress perfusion cardiac magnetic resonance imaging. *Am Heart J*. 2013;166:999–1009. https://doi.org/10.1016/j.ahj.2013.08.018.
137. Yang Q, Li K, Liu X, et al. Contrast-enhanced whole-heart coronary magnetic resonance angiography at 3.0-T: a comparative study with X-ray angiography in a single center. *J Am Coll Cardiol*. 2009;54:69–76. https://doi.org/10.1016/j.jacc.2009.03.016.
138. van Geuns RJ, de Bruin HG, Rensing BJ, et al. Magnetic resonance imaging of the coronary arteries: clinical results from three dimensional evaluation of a respiratory gated technique. *Heart*. 1999;82:515–519. https://doi.org/10.1136/hrt.82.4.515.
139. Kim WY, Danias PG, Stuber M, et al. Coronary magnetic resonance angiography for the detection of coronary stenoses. *N Engl J Med*. 2001;345:1863–1869. https://doi.org/10.1056/NEJMoa010866.
140. Kato S, Kitagawa K, Ishida N, et al. Assessment of coronary artery disease using magnetic resonance coronary angiography: a national multicenter trial. *J Am Coll Cardiol*. 2010;56:983–991. https://doi.org/10.1016/j.jacc.2010.01.071.
141. Yang QLK, Sun B, et al. Assessment of coronary artery disease using 3.0 T magnetic resonance coronary angiography: a national multicenter trial. *J Cardiovasc Magn Reson*. 2013;15(Appl 1):E5.
142. Di Leo G, Fisci E, Secchi F, et al. Diagnostic accuracy of magnetic resonance angiography for detection of coronary artery disease: a systematic review and meta-analysis. *Eur Radiol*. 2016;26:3706–3718. https://doi.org/10.1007/s00330-015-4134-0.
143. Kato S, Azuma M, Nakayama N, et al. Diagnostic accuracy of whole heart coronary magnetic resonance angiography: a systematic review and meta-analysis. *J Cardiovasc Magn Reson*. 2023;25:36. https://doi.org/10.1186/s12968-023-00949-6.
144. Lopes RD, Hafley GE, Allen KB, et al. Endoscopic versus open vein-graft harvesting in coronary-artery bypass surgery. *N Engl J Med*. 2009;361:235–244. https://doi.org/10.1056/NEJMoa0900708.
145. White RD, Caputo GR, Mark AS, Modin GW, Higgins CB. Coronary artery bypass graft patency: noninvasive evaluation with MR imaging. *Radiology*. 1987;164:681–686. https://doi.org/10.1148/radiology.164.3.3497409.
146. Zhang L, Song X, Dong L, et al. Additive value of 3T cardiovascular magnetic resonance coronary angiography for detecting coronary artery disease. *J Cardiovasc Magn Reson*. 2018;20:29. https://doi.org/10.1186/s12968-018-0450-2.
147. Hagar MT, Soschynski M, Saffar R, et al. Accuracy of ultrahigh-resolution photon-counting CT for detecting coronary artery disease in a high-risk population. *Radiology*. 2023;307:e223305. https://doi.org/10.1148/radiol.223305.
148. Shroyer AL, Grover FL, Hattler B, et al. On-pump versus off-pump coronary-artery bypass surgery. *N Engl J Med*. 2009;361:1827–1837. https://doi.org/10.1056/NEJMoa0902905.
149. Rubinstein RI, Askenase AD, Thickman D, Feldman MS, Agarwal JB, Helfant RH. Magnetic resonance imaging to evaluate patency of aortocoronary bypass grafts. *Circulation*. 1987;76:786–791. https://doi.org/10.1161/01.cir.76.4.786.
150. Jenkins JP, Love HG, Foster CJ, Isherwood I, Rowlands DJ. Detection of coronary artery bypass graft patency as assessed by magnetic resonance imaging. *Br J Radiol*. 1988;61:2–4. https://doi.org/10.1259/0007-1285-61-721-2.
151. Galjee MA, van Rossum AC, Doesburg T, van Eenige MJ, Visser CA. Value of magnetic resonance imaging in assessing patency and function of coronary artery bypass grafts. An angiographically controlled study. *Circulation*. 1996;93:660–666. https://doi.org/10.1161/01.cir.93.4.660.
152. White RD, Pflugfelder PW, Lipton MJ, Higgins CB. Coronary artery bypass grafts: evaluation of patency with cine MR imaging. *AJR Am J Roentgenol*. 1988;150:1271–1274. https://doi.org/10.2214/ajr.150.6.1271.
153. Aurigemma GP, Reichek N, Axel L, Schiebler M, Harris C, Kressel HY. Noninvasive determination of coronary artery bypass graft patency by cine magnetic resonance imaging. *Circulation*. 1989;80:1595–1602. https://doi.org/10.1161/01.cir.80.6.1595.
154. Molinari G, Sardanelli F, Zandrino F, Balbi M, Masperone MA. Value of navigator echo magnetic resonance angiography in detecting occlusion/patency of arterial and venous, single and sequential coronary bypass grafts. *Int J Card Imaging*. 2000;16:149–160. https://doi.org/10.1023/a:1006432027712.
155. Engelmann MG, Knez A, von Smekal A, et al. Non-invasive coronary bypass graft imaging after multivessel revascularisation. *Int J Cardiol*. 2000;76:65–74. https://doi.org/10.1016/s0167-5273(00)00371-5.
156. Wintersperger BJ, Engelmann MG, von Smekal A, et al. Patency of coronary bypass grafts: assessment with breath-hold contrast-enhanced MR angiography-value of a non-electrocardiographically triggered technique. *Radiology*. 1998;208:345–351. https://doi.org/10.1148/radiology.208.2.9680557.
157. Vrachliotis TG, Bis KG, Aliabadi D, Shetty AN, Safian R, Simonetti O. Contrast-enhanced breath-hold MR angiography for evaluating patency of coronary artery bypass grafts. *AJR Am J Roentgenol*. 1997;168:1073–1080. https://doi.org/10.2214/ajr.168.4.9124118.
158. Langerak SEVH, de Roos A, Zwinderman AH, et al. Detection of vein graft disease using high-resolution magnetic resonance angiography. *Circulation*. 2002;105:328–333.
159. Langerak SE, Kunz P, Vliegen HW, et al. MR flow mapping in coronary artery bypass grafts: a validation study with Doppler flow measurements. *Radiology*. 2002;222:127–135. https://doi.org/10.1148/radiol.2221010560.
160. Langerak SE, Vliegen HW, Jukema JW, et al. Value of magnetic resonance imaging for the noninvasive detection of stenosis in coronary artery bypass grafts and recipient coronary arteries. *Circulation*. 2003;107:1502–1508. https://doi.org/10.1161/01.cir.0000056107.05724.40.
161. Botnar RM, Stuber M, Kissinger KV, Kim WY, Spuentrup E, Manning WJ. Noninvasive coronary vessel wall and plaque imaging with magnetic resonance imaging. *Circulation*. 2000;102:2582–2587. https://doi.org/10.1161/01.cir.102.21.2582.
162. Fayad ZA, Fuster V, Fallon JT, et al. Noninvasive in vivo human coronary artery lumen and wall imaging using black-blood magnetic resonance imaging. *Circulation*. 2000;102:506–510. https://doi.org/10.1161/01.cir.102.5.506.
163. Edelman RR, Chien D, Kim D. Fast selective black blood MR imaging. *Radiology*. 1991;181:655–660.
164. Botnar RM, Stuber M, Lamerichs R, et al. Initial experiences with in vivo right coronary artery human MR vessel wall imaging at 3 tesla. *J Cardiovasc Magn Reson*. 2003;5:589–594. https://doi.org/10.1081/jcmr-120025232.
165. Botnar RM, Kim WY, Börnert P, Stuber M, Spuentrup E, Manning WJ. 3D coronary vessel wall imaging utilizing a local inversion technique with spiral image acquisition. *Magn Reson Med*. 2001;46:848–854. https://doi.org/10.1002/mrm.1268.
166. Katoh M, Spuentrup E, Buecker A, Manning WJ, Günther RW, Botnar RM. MR coronary vessel wall imaging: comparison between radial and spiral k-space sampling. *J Magn Reson Imaging*. 2006;23:757–762. https://doi.org/10.1002/jmri.20569.
167. Kim WY, Astrup AS, Stuber M, et al. Subclinical coronary and aortic atherosclerosis detected by magnetic resonance imaging in type 1 diabetes with and without diabetic nephropathy. *Circulation*. 2007;115:228–235. https://doi.org/10.1161/circulationaha.106.633339.
168. Kim WY, Stuber M, Börnert P, Kissinger KV, Manning WJ, Botnar RM. Three-dimensional black-blood cardiac magnetic resonance coronary vessel wall imaging detects positive arterial remodeling in patients with nonsignificant coronary artery disease. *Circulation*. 2002;106:296–299. https://doi.org/10.1161/01.cir.0000025629.85631.1e.
169. Andia ME, Henningsson M, Hussain T, et al. Flow-independent 3D whole-heart vessel wall imaging using an interleaved T2-preparation acquisition. *Magn Reson Med*. 2013;69:150–157. https://doi.org/10.1002/mrm.24231.
170. Milotta G, Ginami G, Cruz G, Neji R, Prieto C, Botnar RM. Simultaneous 3D whole-heart bright-blood and black blood imaging for cardiovascular anatomy and wall assessment with interleaved T(2) prep-IR. *Magn Reson Med*. 2019;82:312–325. https://doi.org/10.1002/mrm.27734.
171. Hajhosseiny R, Hartley A, Cole G, et al. Simultaneous, free-breathing, non-contrast 3D whole-heart coronary magnetic resonance angiography and vulnerable plaque imaging in patients with suspected acute coronary syndrome. *Eur Heart J*. 2023;44:1386.
172. Yoon YE, Kitagawa K, Kato S, et al. Prognostic value of coronary magnetic resonance angiography for prediction of cardiac events in patients with suspected coronary artery disease. *J Am Coll Cardiol*. 2012;60:2316–2322. https://doi.org/10.1016/j.jacc.2012.07.060.
173. Nakamura S, Ishida M, Nakata K, et al. Long-term prognostic value of whole-heart coronary magnetic resonance angiography. *J Cardiovasc Magn Reson*. 2021;23:56. https://doi.org/10.1186/s12968-021-00749-w.

22 Acute Myocardial Infarction

YODYING KAOLAWANICH, HAN W. KIM, AND RAYMOND J. KIM

INTRODUCTION

Myocardial infarction (MI) is a leading cause of death worldwide.[1] Accordingly, numerous preventative and therapeutic strategies are aimed at reducing its occurrence and adverse consequences. The development of increasingly sensitive biomarkers of myocardial necrosis, such as high-sensitivity troponin assays, has radically improved the diagnosis of MI and enabled the recognition of a group of patients with small infarcts, many of whom would not have been identified in earlier eras.[2] Reclassifying this group as patients with MI has significant implications.[2–4] From an epidemiological perspective, a substantial increase in the number of patients diagnosed with MI creates difficulties in comparing the results of new trials to older ones and confounds efforts to monitor the impact of public health measures and treatments. In some clinical trials the results may be significantly altered, since the diagnosis of MI can be used as an entry criterion, an endpoint, or both. For individual patients, the "label" of MI can affect a wide range of issues including employment, disability claims, insurance, and psychological well-being. Importantly, the diagnosis of MI also impacts clinical management, and all the available data indicates that even small infarcts with slight troponin elevations portend worse short- and long-term prognosis.[5]

Despite the use of high-sensitivity biomarkers, in practice, the diagnosis of MI can still be difficult. There is marked heterogeneity in the clinical presentation of MI and significant overlap with other cardiac disorders that result in myocardial injury, such as myocarditis and takotsubo cardiomyopathy. In this context, it is noteworthy that the latest consensus guidelines defining MI include noninvasive imaging, as it may be helpful in cases of uncertainty.[2] The new criteria that incorporate imaging evidence of MI involve echocardiography, radionuclide imaging, cardiac computed tomography, and cardiovascular magnetic resonance (CMR). CMR with delayed contrast-enhancement imaging (DE-CMR) appears to offer advantages in detecting small or subendocardial infarcts with high accuracy as well as improvements in specificity in differentiating ischemic from nonischemic causes of myocardial necrosis.[6–11] In this chapter, we will discuss the pathophysiology of acute MI with a focus on utilizing physiological concepts as a basis for correct image interpretation. We will also examine the clinical value of CMR in patients with known or suspected MI with an emphasis on the additive information it may provide. Finally, there is growing interest in using the infarct size measured by DE-CMR (also known as late gadolinium enhancement or LGE imaging) as an endpoint for clinical trials, and we will discuss operational and other relevant issues with this application.

PATHOPHYSIOLOGIC CONCEPTS AS A BASIS FOR IMAGE INTERPRETATION

The "Area-at-Risk" Concept

The myocardium that becomes ischemic after occlusion of its supplying coronary artery defines the myocardium that is at risk of death, the so-called area at risk (AAR).[12] The portion of the AAR that survives, if any, represents myocardium that has been salvaged by treatment during acute MI. Thus, in the setting of acute MI, the AAR may include both infarcted (nonviable) and salvaged (viable) myocardium depending upon the timeliness of reperfusion therapy.

Modern percutaneous revascularization techniques and pharmacological therapies aim to salvage areas of acutely ischemic (but reversibly injured) myocardium and have proven to limit myocardial infarct size and reduce mortality. Although infarct size provides a rough (inverse) estimate of myocardial salvage, the extent of the AAR is highly variable and dependent on the location of the culprit lesion and the caliber and branching of the infarct-related coronary artery. Thus, a better measure of therapeutic efficacy would be the proportion of the AAR that is infarcted rather than absolute infarct size. The rationale is that for two infarcts of the same size, the infarct that represents a larger proportion of the AAR corresponds to a greater amount of ischemic injury (Fig. 22.1).[13] Accordingly, imaging methods that could delineate the AAR (in combination with that of infarction) have the potential to offer an improved measure of the efficacy of acute MI therapies and could provide a better endpoint in clinical trials than indirect metrics such as left ventricular ejection fraction and absolute infarct size.

The "Wavefront" Phenomenon and its Borders

In the late 1960s, myocardial necrosis was believed to expand in concentric rings, with a core lesion progressing concentrically into the surrounding ischemic tissue and an acute mismatch between myocardial demand and supply.[14] In the late 1970s, Reimer and Jennings corrected this misconception by showing in canine experiments that necrosis actually ensues as a "wavefront" from the subendocardium to the subepicardium, following a transmural gradient of collateral flow within the AAR (Fig. 22.2A).[12] In their pioneering study, Reimer and Jennings also described

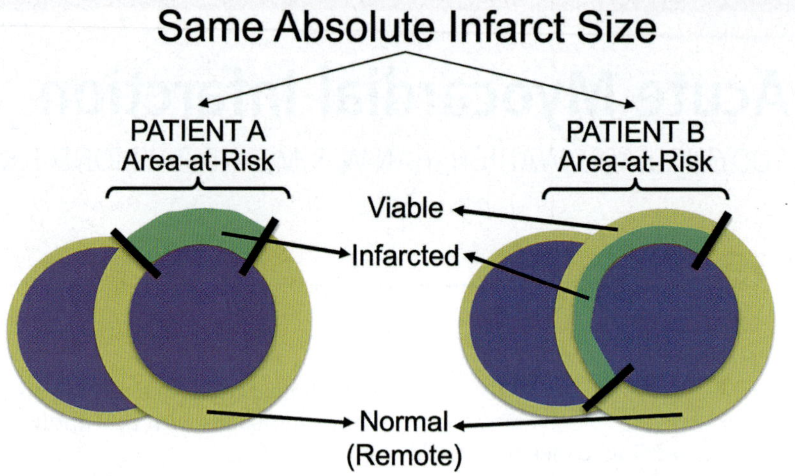

FIG. 22.1 Diagram showing importance of determining area at risk. Two patients with the same absolute infarct size may have different amounts of salvage. In patient A, the entire area at risk is transmurally infarcted, indicating prolonged ischemia with no salvage. In patient B, subendocardial infarction is present, suggesting shorter ischemia duration and substantial salvage.

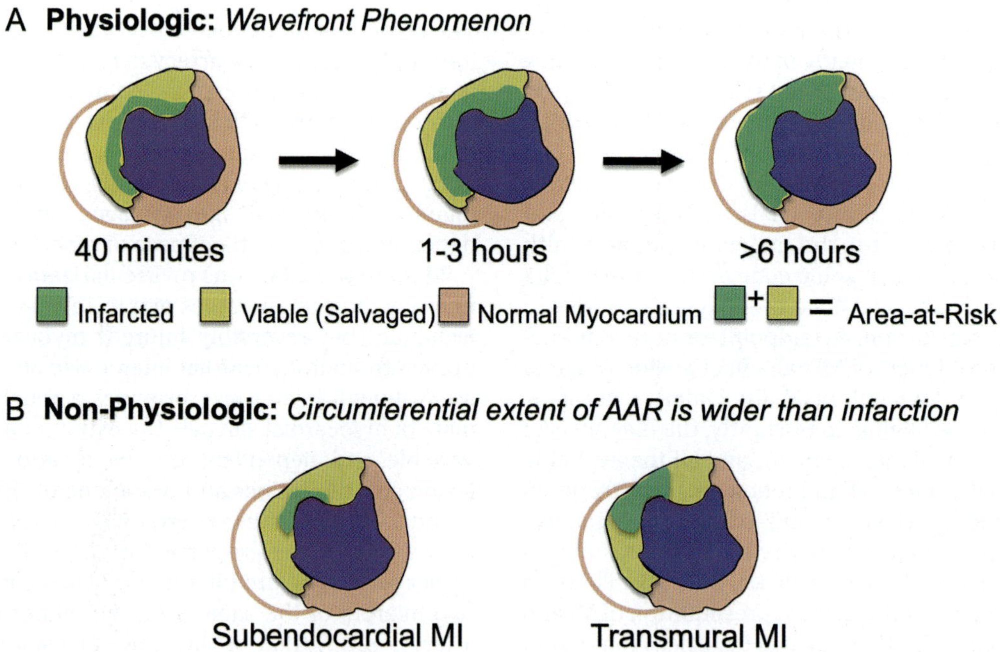

FIG. 22.2 (A) With increasing duration of ischemia, a "wavefront" of cell death moves from the subendocardium to the epicardium. In contrast, the lateral margins in the subendocardial region of the infarct are established as early as 40 minutes after occlusion and are sharply defined by the anatomic boundaries of the ischemic bed. (B) A "bull's eye" pattern of ischemia, in which the lateral borders of the area at risk (*AAR*) extend far beyond those of the infarct, is incompatible with the wavefront phenomenon and has no physiological basis. *MI*, Myocardial infarction.

a corollary principle—that is, there is no wavefront circumferentially since there is no perfusion gradient in that direction. Reperfusion after only 40 minutes of ischemia resulted in a confluent subendocardial infarct that already extended to within 1–2 mm of the lateral edge of the AAR. Although some investigators initially suggested the existence of a wide lateral "border zone" of intermediate-level perfusion, later studies showed this was a partial volume artifact due to the limited resolution of the techniques used, and indeed, with progressively higher levels of sampling resolution, investigators have concluded that there is no zone of intermediate perfusion (or injury) at the lateral border of the AAR.[15,16] Although intramural and epicardial collateral anastomoses have been described in various species, detailed anatomical studies have shown "end-capillary loops" without microvascular connections between adjacent vascular beds in both dogs and man.[17,18] These data indicate there is no anatomic basis for a lateral border zone, and demonstrate that a "bull's-eye" pattern of centrally severe ischemia—with gradients of increasing collateral flow in transmural and circumferential directions toward the edges of the AAR—is incorrect (Fig. 22.2B).

At the infarct border in the epicardial direction, histologic sections can show apparent isolated islands of surviving myocardium within areas of necrotic tissue, as well as isolated islands of necrosis within areas of viable tissue.[19] Early descriptions considered this "periinfarct" border zone to be a distinct region of tissue that is jeopardized but receives just the right level of oxygen to survive in a precarious "twilight zone".[20] Later studies employing three-dimensional reconstructions of MI, however, demonstrated that the infarct border is remarkably discrete, albeit irregular, and that isolated islands of either necrotic or viable tissue are merely artifacts of sectioning peninsulas of necrotic or viable tissue in a two-dimensional plane.[19] Hence, the periinfarct zone should not be considered to represent a special pathophysiology resulting from an intermediate level of ischemia. Apparent intermediate levels of damage—either biochemical, electrophysiologic, or imaging based—should be interpreted with the knowledge that the infarct border is complex but sharp and that any methodology with limited spatial resolution will result in an admixture of necrotic and viable myocardium at the infarct border.

The described pathophysiology presents multiple implications for imaging ischemic injury. These include the following: (1) A method that consistently measures similar amounts of salvage for both transmural versus nontransmural infarcts should be considered erroneous. This is based on the fact that a relatively transmural infarct should not have a significantly larger AAR, hence there should be little salvage compared with a nontransmural infarct. (2) In the setting of a confluent but subendocardial infarction, a technique that consistently depicts the AAR as circumferentially larger than the infarct is erroneous. This is because the lateral borders of a confluent infarct should nearly match that of the AAR. One caveat is if the infarct is small and patchy with discontinuous foci, in which case the infarct may not have yet reached the circumferential extent of the ischemic bed (i.e., the infarct is not yet confluent). (3) Descriptions of a "periinfarct zone" at the infarct border in the epicardial direction should be avoided, since the so-called periinfarct zone does not represent a distinct or special pathophysiology.

Edema in Irreversible Versus Reversible Ischemic Injury

Given that the AAR is defined as the perfusion territory of the infarct-related-artery, imaging methods that directly provide an assessment of myocardial perfusion can reliably depict the AAR in an acute setting. However, perfusion methods do not allow retrospective depiction of the AAR after successful reperfusion of the infarct-related-artery, and a variety of nonperfusion-based CMR methods have been proposed to delineate the AAR. These methods invariably image sequelae of ischemic injury—such as myocardial edema—which are only indirectly related to the anatomical definition of the AAR as a vascular bed. Hence, many of these methods do not have a sound pathophysiological basis.

Consider T2-weighted imaging or T2 mapping, which have been promulgated as techniques to depict the AAR.[13] While T2 imaging appears sensitive to increased myocardial water content,[21] the underlying assumption that T2 imaging depicts the AAR because of its sensitivity to edema is flawed. The experimental evidence points to substantial edema occurring in the infarcted region, with minimal or no edema occurring in the portion of the AAR suffering reversible injury. Specifically, Whalen et al. observed a 44% increase in water content (expressed as [wet—dry]/dry weight) in myocardium exposed to ischemia, sufficient to result in infarction of half of the tissue.[22] From this, one can calculate that a pure sample of infarcted (irreversibly injured) myocardium would have an 88% increase in water content. A shorter period of ischemia leading to reversible injury did not lead to significant changes in water content. In a separate study, Jennings et al. reported a 9.6% increase in water content in myocardium reversibly injured by 15 minutes of ischemia followed by 20 minutes of reperfusion.[23] However, up to 40% of the increase in tissue water may have been secondary to reactive hyperemia, which would be expected to resolve in a few hours. Thus, reversible injury leads to minimal edema. The range in increased water content is 0% to 10%, with the upper range expected to occur only for a brief period (<1–2 hours) following an ischemic event. Accordingly, the difference in edema between infarcted and salvaged (reversibly injured) myocardium should be large, and at a minimum the ratio should be at least ninefold (88%/9.6% = 9.2).

As an aside, it should be mentioned that in the literature there are two ways in which % tissue water content is expressed: (1) as percent *wet* weight: (100 × [wet weight—dry weight]/wet weight), or (2) as percent *dry* weight: (100 × [wet weight—dry weight]/dry weight), where dry weight represents the weight of the tissue sample following desiccation. The first definition has the disadvantage that edema (an increase in water content) affects both the numerator (the water mass) and the denominator (the tissue wet weight). Hence, the same increase in absolute water content may result in different increases in % tissue water content depending on the starting % tissue water content. One implication of using the first definition is that if the starting % tissue water content is high, then small changes in % tissue water content can actually reflect large changes in absolute water content and substantial tissue swelling. As an extreme example, a 1% increase in tissue water content from 98% to 99% actually reflects a doubling in absolute water content (i.e., a 100% increase relative to dry weight). Additionally, for any given tissue, T2 relaxation time is generally more related to the proportion of water to protein content (i.e., ratio defined as water weight divided by dry weight) than it is to the proportion of water to the total weight of tissue (i.e., the ratio defined as water weight divided by tissue wet weight). For these reasons, it is important to express % tissue water content as a percentage of the dry weight.

Returning back to the large difference in edema between acutely infarcted tissue and salvaged myocardium, this pathophysiology is why several investigators have found that regional end-diastolic wall thickness can double in the setting of transmural MI, but is unchanged following shorter periods of ischemia with complete salvage.[24–26] Indeed, Haendchen et al. found that end-diastolic wall thickness early after ischemia and reperfusion correlates directly with the transmural extent of infarction, and they proposed that an acute increase in end-diastolic wall thickness might be used as an (inverse) index of salvage.[24] Fully transmural infarcts were associated with a 100% increase in wall thickness, which is consistent with the 88% increase in water content calculated earlier.[22,23]

Therefore, if T2 imaging truly tracked edema, image intensity differences (or T2 relaxation times) between infarcted and reversibly injured myocardium should be far greater than between reversibly injured and normal myocardium. The changes in edema are mirrored by a host of other biological changes including tissue electrolyte levels, high-energy phosphate levels, fine structure at light and electron microscopy, and sodium-23 magnetic resonance imaging (MRI) data.[11,23,27–30] Specifically, there are large changes in all of these characteristics in irreversibly injured tissue compared with minimal to no changes in reversibly injured tissue (Fig. 22.3). Given the consistency of these findings, it is perplexing that many investigators have proposed that T2 imaging or mapping delineates the AAR, which would mean greater changes between normal and reversibly injured tissue (i.e., outside vs. inside the AAR) than between reversibly injured and infarcted tissue (both inside the AAR). A more recent investigation indicated that T2 imaging delineates acutely infarcted tissue, not the AAR, once motion artifacts and arbitrary thresholds are taken into account.[31] Specifically, there was no relationship between the transmural extent of T2-hyperintense regions and that of the AAR; instead, there was a strong correlation with that of infarction, where both the AAR and infarction were defined by gold-standard pathology methods (fluorescent microspheres and triphenyl tetrazolium chloride staining, respectively), which were performed immediately following CMR.

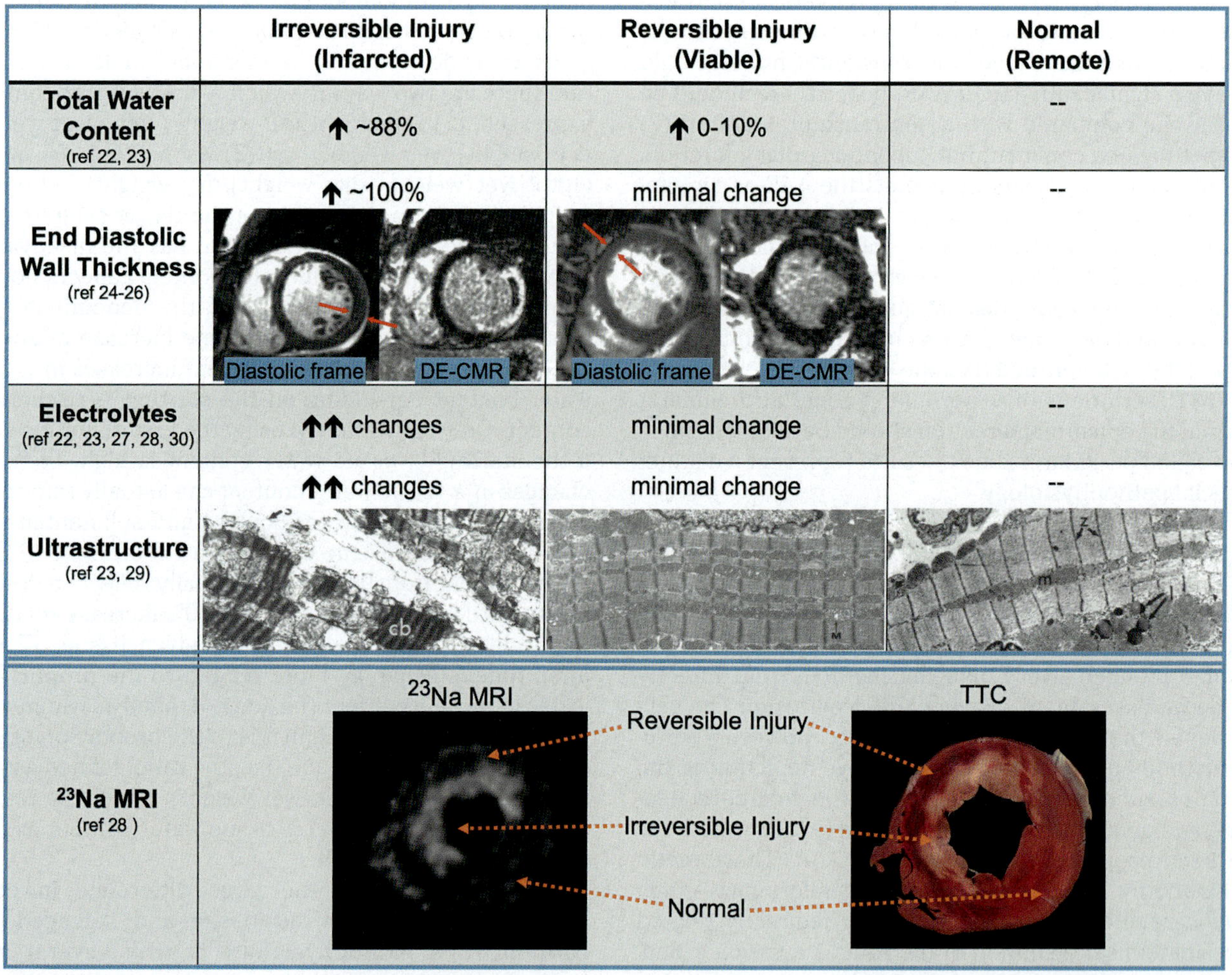

FIG. 22.3 Expected changes in several biological characteristics in myocardium following ischemic injury and reperfusion are summarized with comparisons between irreversibly injured, reversibly injured, and normal tissue. *Red arrows* point to regions that are akinetic on cine magnetic resonance imaging (*MRI*) from temporary occlusion to the left circumflex and left anterior descending artery (LAD) coronaries, respectively. Note, near doubling of end-diastolic wall thickness in the patient with transmural infarction. Irreversibly injured tissue shows greatly distorted ultrastructure with formation of vacuoles, large subsarcolemmal blebs, contraction bands (*cb*), and swollen mitochondria containing dense bodies. In reversibly injured tissue, ultrastructure is virtually indistinguishable from control, normal tissue. Total myocardial sodium content as reflected by 23Na MRI is substantially elevated in infarcted regions but not in salvaged myocardium at-risk, which is consistent with changes in total water content measured in pathology studies. Given these findings, if T2-MRI tracked edema, it should delineate between infarcted and reversibly injured myocardium (both within the area at risk [AAR]), and not between reversibly injured tissue and normal myocardium (i.e., inside vs. outside the AAR). *DE-CMR*, Delayed contrast-enhancement cardiovascular magnetic resonance; *TTC*, triphenyltetrazolium chloride.

(Electron microscopy images were reproduced from references Jennings RB, Schaper J, Hill ML, Steenbergen C, Jr., Reimer KA. Effect of reperfusion late in the phase of reversible ischemic injury. Changes in cell volume, electrolytes, metabolites, and ultrastructure. *Circ Res*. 1985;56(2):262–278 and Kloner RA, Ganote CE, Whalen DA, Jr., Jennings RB. Effect of a transient period of ischemia on myocardial cells. II. Fine structure during the first few minutes of reflow. *Am J Pathol*. 1974;74(3):399–422 with permission. Adapted with permission from reference Kim RJ, Lima JA, Chen EL, Reeder SB, Klocke FJ, Zerhouni EA, et al. Fast 23Na magnetic resonance imaging of acute reperfused myocardial infarction. Potential to assess myocardial viability. *Circulation*. 1997;95(7):1877–1885.[91] Adapted with permission from reference Croisille P, Kim HW, Kim RJ. Controversies in cardiovascular MR imaging: T2-weighted imaging should not be used to delineate the area at risk in ischemic myocardial injury. *Radiology*. 2012;265(1):12–22.)

Effects of Infarct Size Dynamics and Partial Volume on Delayed Contrast-Enhancement Cardiac Magnetic Resonance Imaging Interpretation

The infarcted region is highly dynamic in size following acute MI. In their landmark study, Reimer and Jennings demonstrated that infarct volume can nearly double over the first few days of acute MI—even in the absence of additional myocyte death via lethal reperfusion injury or infarct extension—primarily because of edema.[22] Subsequently, infarct involution during healing—as edema resolves and necrotic tissue is replaced by collagenous scar—resulted in 28-day-old infarcts that were on average only 25% their size at 4 days.[32] This was demonstrated through a clever use of the microsphere technique to measure tissue blood flow at baseline before occluding the infarct-related-artery (Fig. 22.4).

The fact that apparently "dead" (e.g., necrotic) myocardium is highly dynamic in size is often neglected in the interpretation of studies that employ delayed-enhancement imaging. The shrinkage in hyperenhancement or late gadolinium enhancement (LGE) size between a scan performed in the early days after acute MI and a repeat scan performed days to weeks later is frequently misconstrued as evidence that LGE represents both viable and nonviable myocardium acutely, whereas LGE represents only nonviable myocardium chronically. This interpretation does not account for the known physiological changes in infarct size that occur during infarct healing, and overlooks validation studies that have shown that the shape and size of LGE match those of infarction defined by pathology throughout a range of infarct ages (from 4 hours to 8 weeks), and are independent of wall motion and reperfusion status (Fig. 22.5).[8,33] It is important to note that the pathology assessment in these validation studies immediately followed delayed-enhancement imaging. In the acute setting, given the rapid dynamics in infarct size, it is not valid to compare LGE size with infarct size by pathology or other comparator methods if both are not performed on the same day.

Infarct involution during healing can also interact with partial volume effects to accentuate changes that might occur in LGE size from the acute to the chronic setting. Voxels containing islands or peninsulas of necrosis at the infarct border are often partially "bright" on delayed-enhancement imaging and may be above the arbitrary threshold used to define abnormal myocardium (e.g., "n" standard deviations above remote or greater than 50% of maximum using the full-width-at-half-maximum algorithm). But at a later time point, shrinkage of these islands leads to a changed partial volume effect and voxels at the infarct border may no longer be considered hyperenhanced since they are now below the cutoff threshold (Fig. 22.6).

For certain types of injuries, the combination of infarct shrinkage and partial volume effect can lead to DE-CMR findings that are particularly prone to misinterpretation. If there is patchy necrosis—for instance due to aborted MI or myocarditis—hyperenhancement in the acute setting may completely disappear in the chronic setting (Fig. 22.7). Again, many consider this finding evidence that LGE "overestimates" the infarcted region in the acute setting, even when there is elevated troponins confirming irreversible injury, and it is clear that, if anything, the chronic scan is incorrect since it indicates an infarct size of zero. Fig. 22.8 demonstrates how this scenario can occur and is still consistent with the concept that hyperenhanced myocardium in the acute setting accurately delineates the region of irreversible injury. The only mechanisms that are necessary to explain these findings are the precept that acute infarct size is dynamic and partial volume effect.

Given the dynamics of acutely infarcted myocardium, there are several implications to the design and interpretation of CMR studies that evaluate methods to depict MI, salvage, or the AAR. *Size differences in abnormal myocardium delineated by the same or different imaging techniques performed on separate days should not be considered to*

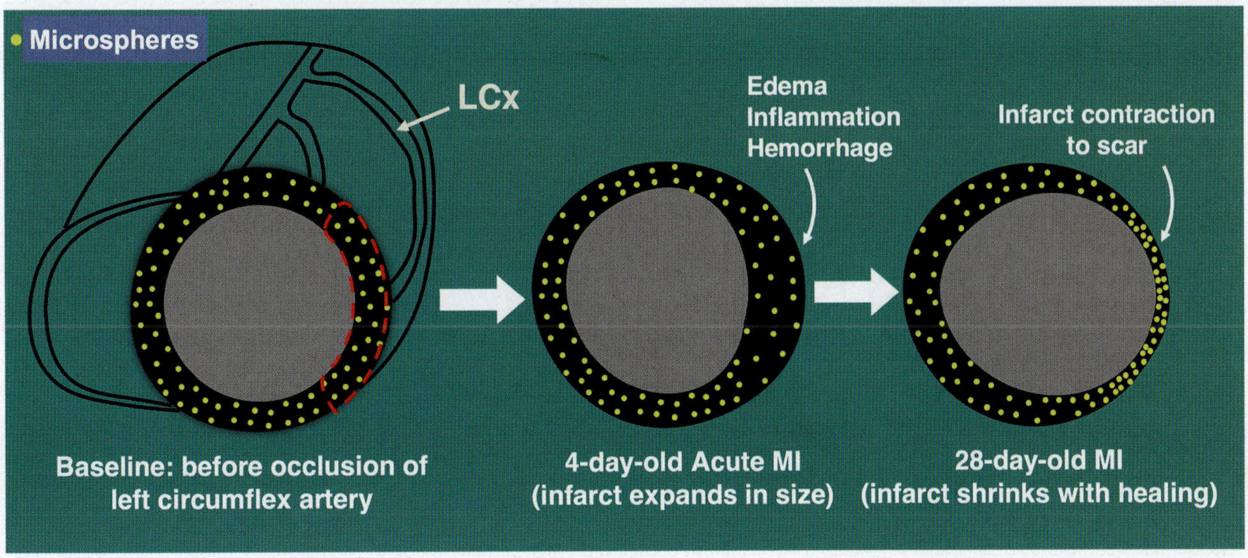

FIG. 22.4 Changes in microsphere-measured myocardial blood flow can be used to measure expansion of infarct volume in the acute setting and infarct involution in the chronic setting. Microspheres administered prior to occlusion of the infarct-related artery should have homogeneous density throughout the left ventricle (*left panel*). At 4 days, there is rarefaction of microsphere density in the lateral wall due to near doubling of infarct volume (*middle panel*). At 28 days, microsphere density is increased due to infarct healing, which shrinks the infarct to one-fourth its size at 4 days. *MI*, Myocardial infarction; *LCx*, left circumflex artery.

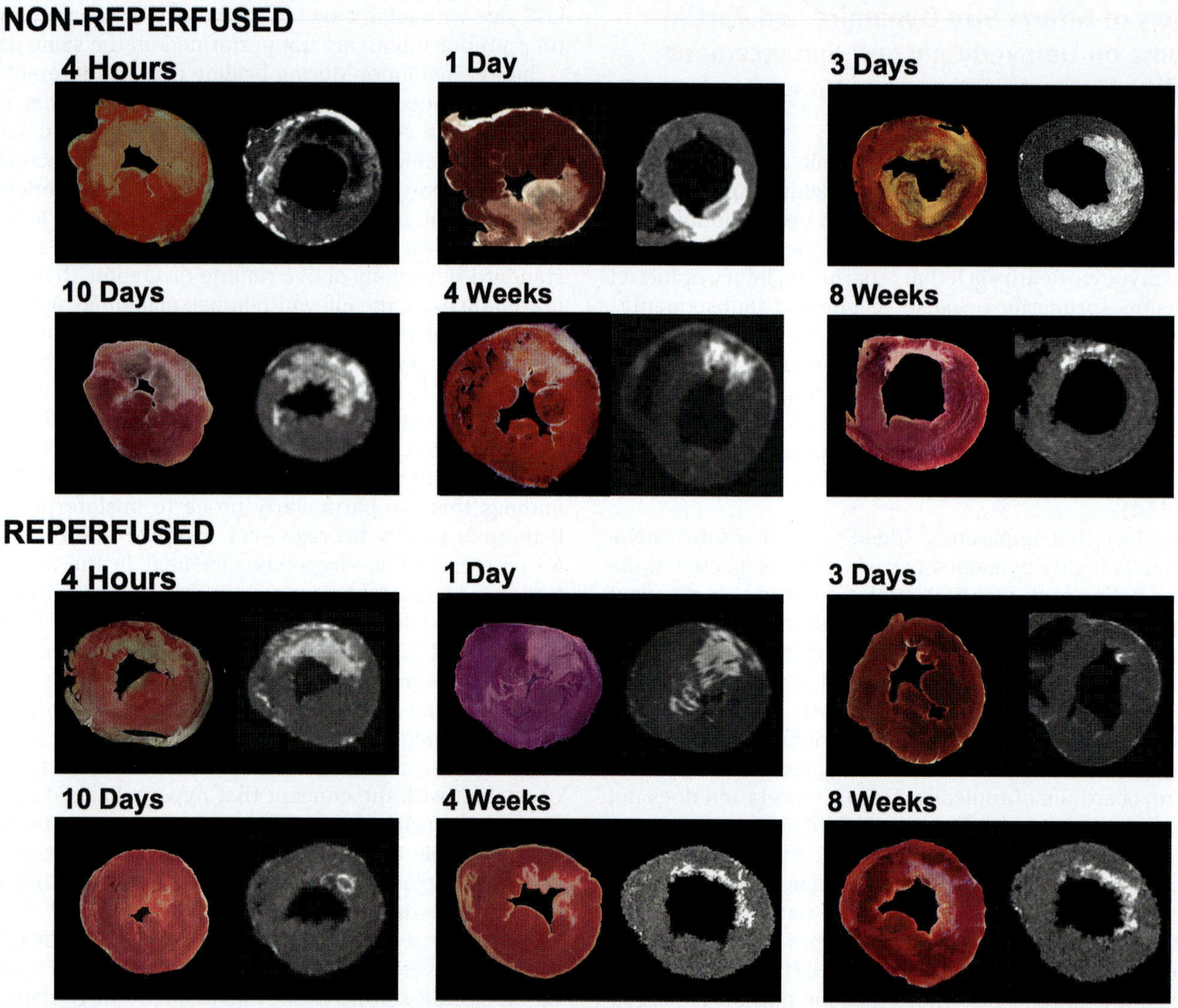

FIG. 22.5 The size and shape of hyperenhanced regions by magnetic resonance imaging matches the irreversible injury defined by pathology (triphenyltetrazolium chloride [TTC] staining) throughout infarct healing (from 4 hours to 8 weeks after acute myocardial infarction) and independent of reperfusion status.

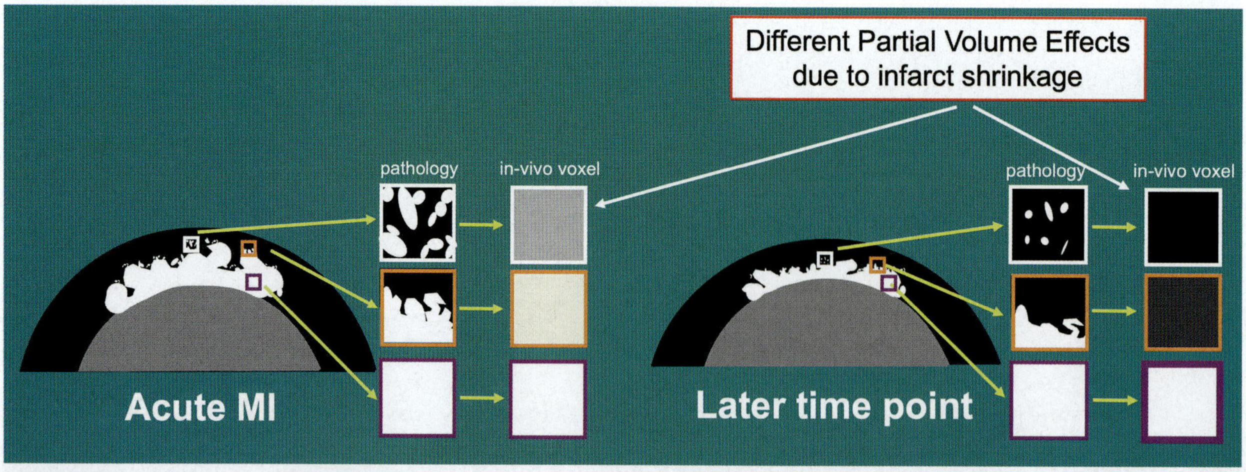

FIG. 22.6 The epicardial border of an acute infarct can be highly irregular with apparent islands and peninsulas of necrosis. This can lead to small regions of tissue that are only partially infarcted but, on the scale of a voxel on late gadolinium enhancement imaging, of sufficient extent to render the voxel gray enough to be considered "bright". At a later time point, infarct shrinkage will occur both in the infarct core and periphery. Islands of infarction at the border may no longer be of sufficient size to render a voxel of tissue as bright on delayed-enhancement imaging. See text for details. *MI*, Myocardial infarction.

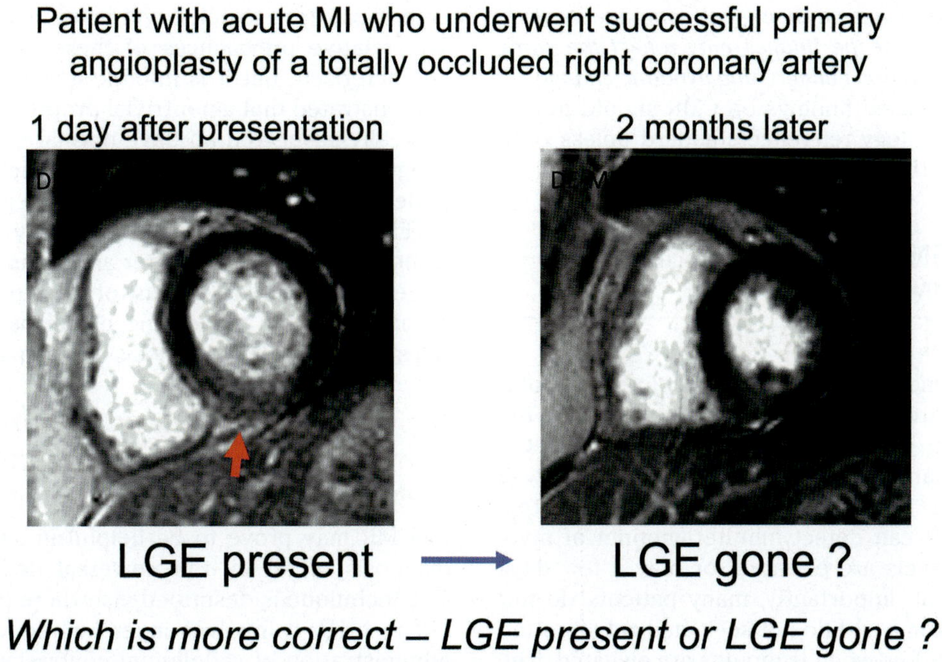

FIG. 22.7 Forty-seven-year-old male with chest pain and ECG changes consistent with an acute myocardial infarction (*MI*). He underwent successful primary angioplasty of a totally occluded right coronary artery. Cardiac troponin levels were abnormal but only moderately elevated, consistent with a small amount of necrosis. Delayed-enhancement imaging at 1 day shows patchy hyperenhancement of the inferior wall, which is not readily visible 2 months later. Cases such as these are often touted as evidence that hyperenhancement or late gadolinium enhancement (*LGE*) "overestimates" infarct size acutely and may include reversibly injured myocardium since it disappears at a chronic time point. However, the elevated troponins confirm irreversible injury and, if anything, the chronic—not the acute—scan is incorrect since it indicates an infarct size of zero. See text for details.

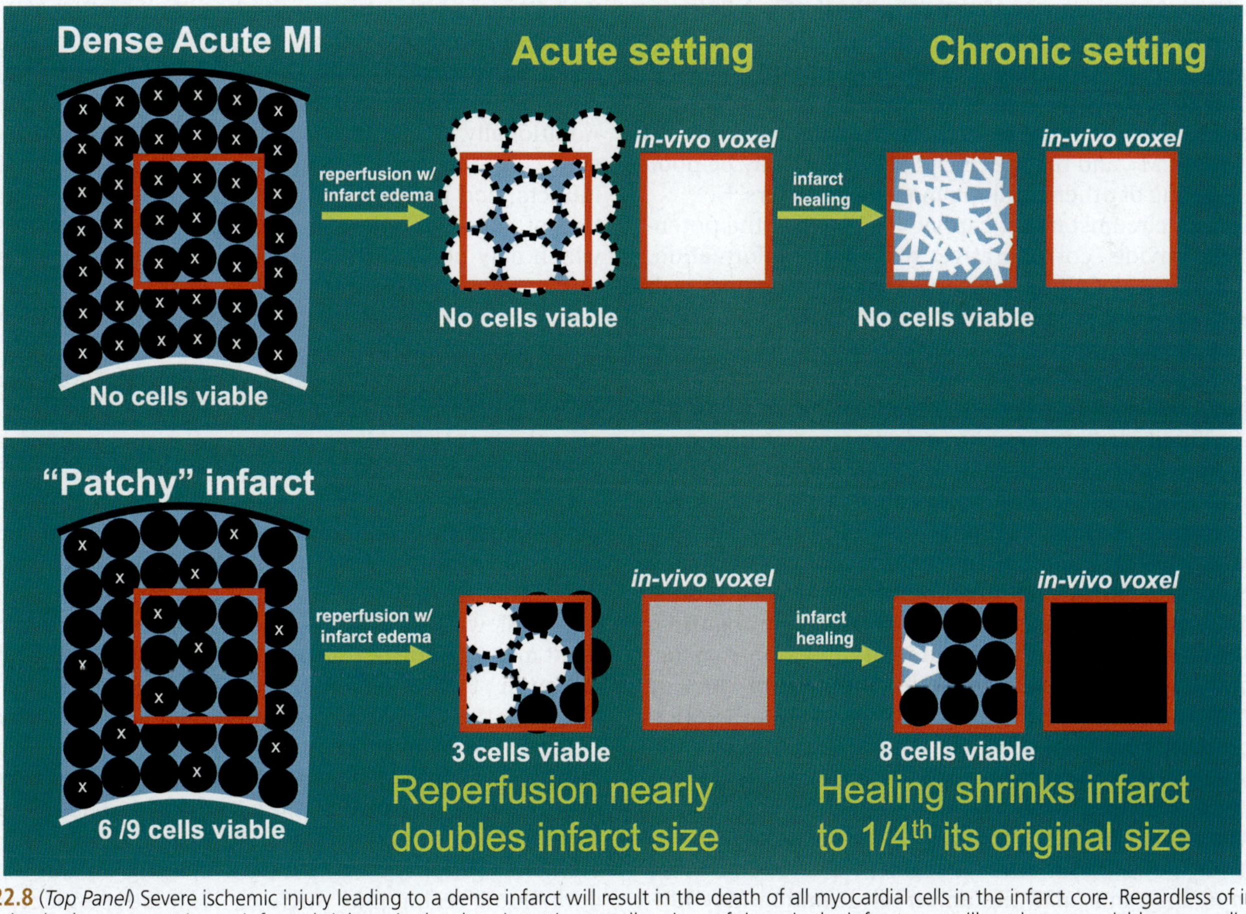

FIG. 22.8 (*Top Panel*) Severe ischemic injury leading to a dense infarct will result in the death of all myocardial cells in the infarct core. Regardless of infarct expansion in the acute setting or infarct shrinkage in the chronic setting, small regions of tissue in the infarct core will not have any viable myocardial cells and representative voxels on delayed-enhancement imaging will be "bright" at both time points. (*Bottom Panel*) Conversely, patchy necrosis can lead to hyperenhancement in the acute setting that disappears in the chronic setting. In the example shown for illustrative purposes, we assume that nine viable cells fit into a voxel (*red box*) and three are killed during ischemia. Reperfusion with infarct edema can double the size of the infarcted portion within the voxel, leading to room for only three viable cells. Since the majority of the voxel (two-thirds) is nonviable, the voxel will appear gray enough to be considered "bright" on delayed contrast-enhancement cardiovascular magnetic resonance imaging. After infarct healing, when the infarcted portion shrinks to 25% of its original size, the majority of the voxel will now be viable and hence will appear black on delayed-enhancement imaging. *MI*, Myocardial infarction.

*reflect different underlying physiological components without first considering that the images may reflect the same component (*e.g., *infarction) undergoing dynamic changes in size*. Similarly, size-based findings on CMR should not be compared to a pathology reference standard unless both were performed on the same day.

CLINICAL DIAGNOSIS AND ASSESSMENT OF MYOCARDIAL INFARCTION

Issues in Clinical Diagnosis

According to the American College of Cardiology and European Society of Cardiology consensus document on the universal definition of MI, the cornerstone tests for the diagnosis are biomarkers such as troponin I and T as well as the 12-lead ECG.[2] Although troponin assays are exquisitely sensitive and can detect minute amounts of myocardial necrosis, levels are elevated for only a few days after an acute event. Importantly, many patients do not have classic symptoms and do not seek medical attention within the time window when troponins are elevated. The consequence is that many acute MIs will not be identified by troponins. The ECG is helpful in this situation, and incident Q waves have been the basis for diagnosing "silent" or clinically "unrecognized" MI in population studies.[34] These surveys have shown that unrecognized MIs are common, accounting for as many as 40%–60% of all MIs. By definition, however, all unrecognized infarcts that are non-Q wave will be missed[34] and even if Q waves are present initially, up to 25% may disappear at a later time point.[35] Additionally, Q waves often occur in the setting of nonischemic cardiomyopathy (NICM), and the specificity of the ECG may be poor in the setting of other cardiopulmonary disorders.[36]

In these circumstances, cardiac imaging has the potential to provide corroborative diagnostic information. The universal definition indicates that new regional wall motion abnormalities or a loss of viable myocardium could be considered evidence of MI.[2] It should be noted, however, that wall motion abnormalities may not occur unless the infarcted region exceeds 20%–50% of the myocardial wall.[37,38] Similarly, scintigraphic defects may not be apparent until >10g of myocardial tissue is infarcted.[38] Thus, because a sizable threshold of damage is required, echocardiography or radionuclide imaging may miss MI, particularly when small or subendocardial. Conversely, when abnormalities in regional function or perfusion are present, they do not always indicate MI. Both may be abnormal in the setting of ischemia without infarction. Nonischemic conditions such as cardiomyopathy and inflammatory or infiltrative diseases can also lead to regional wall motion abnormalities or loss of viable myocardium. Hence, the positive predictive value of these imaging findings are not high unless these conditions can be excluded.

Even some patients who have all the classical features of MI (e.g., chest pain, new ST-segment changes, and rise in troponins) and fulfill the universal definition may ultimately prove not to have had an MI. For instance, it is well known that ST-segment changes and elevated troponins can occur in the setting of many disorders including myocarditis, takotsubo cardiomyopathy, trauma, pulmonary embolism, drug toxicity, and acute neurological disease.[2] The relative prevalences of these disorders are poorly characterized, but it is notable that several studies have demonstrated that a nontrivial proportion of patients with clinically suspected MI have normal coronary arteries or insignificant disease at angiography, including up to 10% of patients initially diagnosed with ST-segment elevation MI (STEMI) and 32% with acute coronary syndrome (ACS).[39] Although recanalization after an occlusive coronary event is well documented,[40,41] many of these patients are unlikely to have had an MI, leaving clinicians with unanswered questions regarding diagnosis and management.

Improving the Diagnosis With Delayed Contrast-Enhancement Cardiovascular Magnetic Resonance Imaging

DE-CMR may prove to be helpful in situations when the diagnosis of MI by the universal definition is difficult. The technique is described elsewhere (Chapters 1, 6, 14), but in brief, it involves inversion-recovery imaging after administration of gadolinium contrast and a 5–10-minute delay.[42,43] When run properly, normal myocardium appears black or "nulled," whereas nonviable regions appear bright or "hyperenhanced". Although gadolinium contrast media is inert, hyperenhancement appears to be quite specific for nonviable tissue; the mechanism is elucidated in Fig. 22.9. Earlier in this chapter, we described pathology-based validation studies demonstrating that DE-CMR can distinguish between reversible and irreversible injury independent of infarct age, wall motion, and reperfusion status.[8,33] Additionally, DE-CMR is superior to single-photon emission computed tomography in detecting subendocardial infarcts, and its high spatial resolution enables visualization of microinfarctions involving as little as 1g of tissue, which may occur during otherwise successful percutaneous coronary interventions (Fig. 22.10). Finally, the performance of DE-CMR for the detection of MI was tested in an international multicenter trial.[7] In that study, conducted in 26 centers throughout the United States, Europe, and South America, 282 patients with acute and 284 with chronic first-time MI were scanned using commercially available scanners and sequences from a variety of different manufacturers,. The sensitivity of DE-CMR increased with increasing gadolinium dose, reaching 99% and 94% in acute and chronic MI, respectively, with the 0.3-mmol/kg dose. Furthermore, with doses of 0.2 mmol/kg or higher, when MI was identified, the location of hyperenhancement matched the perfusion territory of the infarct-related artery in >97% of patients. It should be emphasized that although the study demonstrated high sensitivity for the detection of chronic MI overall, it is often more difficult to detect than acute MI because substantial infarct shrinkage may occur during healing. In particular, smaller subendocardial chronic infarcts may be difficult to detect with conventional (bright-blood) DE-CMR imaging; in this cohort dark-blood techniques such as Flow-Independent Dark-blood DeLayed Enhancement (FIDDLE)[44] may be especially helpful (see Chapter 6).

One emerging application has been the identification of unrecognized MI. Kwong et al. found that the prevalence

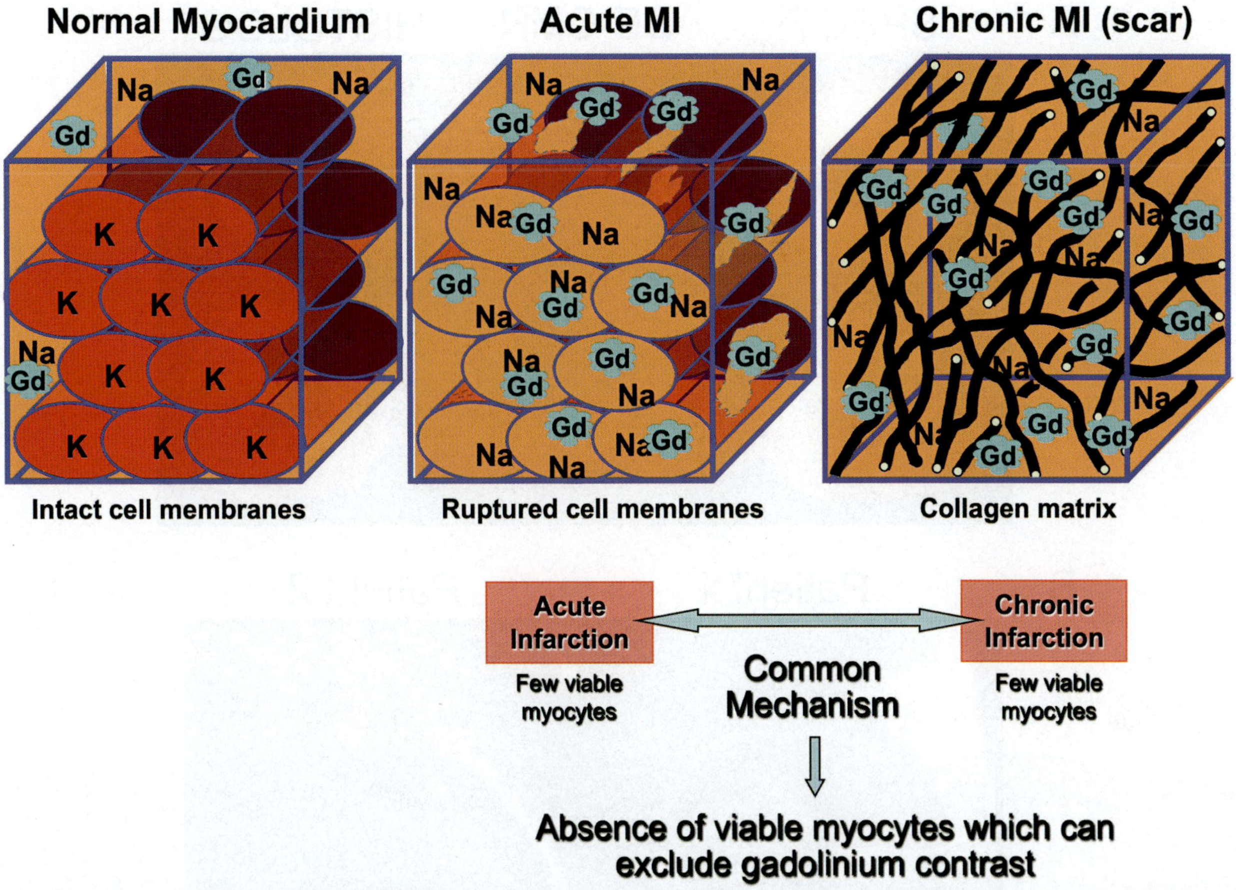

FIG. 22.9 The mechanism of myocardial hyperenhancement in nonviable myocardium is based on two physiological facts: (1) in normal myocardium, tissue volume is predominantly intracellular and (2) extracellular gadolinium (*Gd*) contrast media are inert and cannot cross intact sarcolemmal membranes. Hence, gadolinium distribution volume is small and tissue concentration is low in a typical voxel of normal myocardium. With acute necrosis (acute myocardial infarction [*MI*], myocarditis, etc.), there is membrane rupture, which allows gadolinium to diffuse into irreversibly injured myocytes. This results in increased gadolinium concentration, shortened T1 relaxation time, and thus hyperenhancement. In the chronic setting, scar has replaced necrotic tissue and the interstitial space is expanded. This again leads to increased gadolinium concentration and hyperenhancement. In both acute and chronic settings (and all stages in between) one can consider viable myocytes as actively excluding gadolinium contrast. Thus, the unifying mechanism of hyperenhancement appears to be the absence of viable myocytes rather than any inherent properties that are specific for acute necrosis, collagenous scar, or other forms of nonviable myocardium. *Na*, high sodium content consistent with extracellular fluid; *K*, high potassium content consistent with intracellular fluid.

of unrecognized MI by DE-CMR was 76% higher than by ECG.[45] Kim et al.[46] and Barbier et al.[47] reported, respectively, that the prevalence was 313% and 390% higher. In all three studies, several patients with Q waves (unrecognized MI by ECG) did not have hyperenhancement, which reflects the limited specificity of electrocardiography for diagnosing MI. From a public health standpoint, the implications of these studies may be considerable. It has been estimated that 190,000 patients in the United States and perhaps as many as 300,000 in Europe suffer from unrecognized MI annually.[48,49] Since these estimates reflect only patients with electrocardiographic Q waves, the DE-CMR studies suggest that the actual incidence may be threefold higher. However, in general, infarct size is larger and LVEF is lower in patients with unrecognized MI with Q-waves than those without,[46] and overall one might suspect that the prognosis of individuals with unrecognized MI by DE-CMR is relatively benign. On this point, it is important to note that Kwong et al. reported that the presence of unrecognized MI on DE-CMR conferred a nearly sixfold increased risk for major adverse cardiac events. Likewise, Kim et al. reported that the presence of unrecognized non-Q-wave MI predicted an 11-fold higher risk of all-cause mortality than in those without MI.

Similar to troponins, the detection of injury by DE-CMR is specific for irreversible myocardial damage but is not specific for MI. One potential advantage of DE-CMR is that the pattern of hyperenhancement, rather than simply the presence or extent, may offer important information regarding the etiology of myocardial damage.[50] For this purpose, the concept that ischemic myonecrosis proceeds as a "wavefront"[12] from the subendocardium to the epicardium with increasing coronary occlusion time is crucial. Correspondingly, hyperenhancement patterns that spare the subendocardium and are limited to the middle or epicardial portion of the LV wall are invariably nonischemic in origin since damage in the setting of coronary artery disease almost always involves the subendocardium.[50] Moreover, certain nonischemic disorders such as myocarditis have characteristic hyperenhancement patterns that may suggest a specific diagnosis, and a systematic approach to interpreting DE-CMR images in patients with cardiomyopathy has been proposed.[50,51] This topic is discussed in detail in Chapter 25.

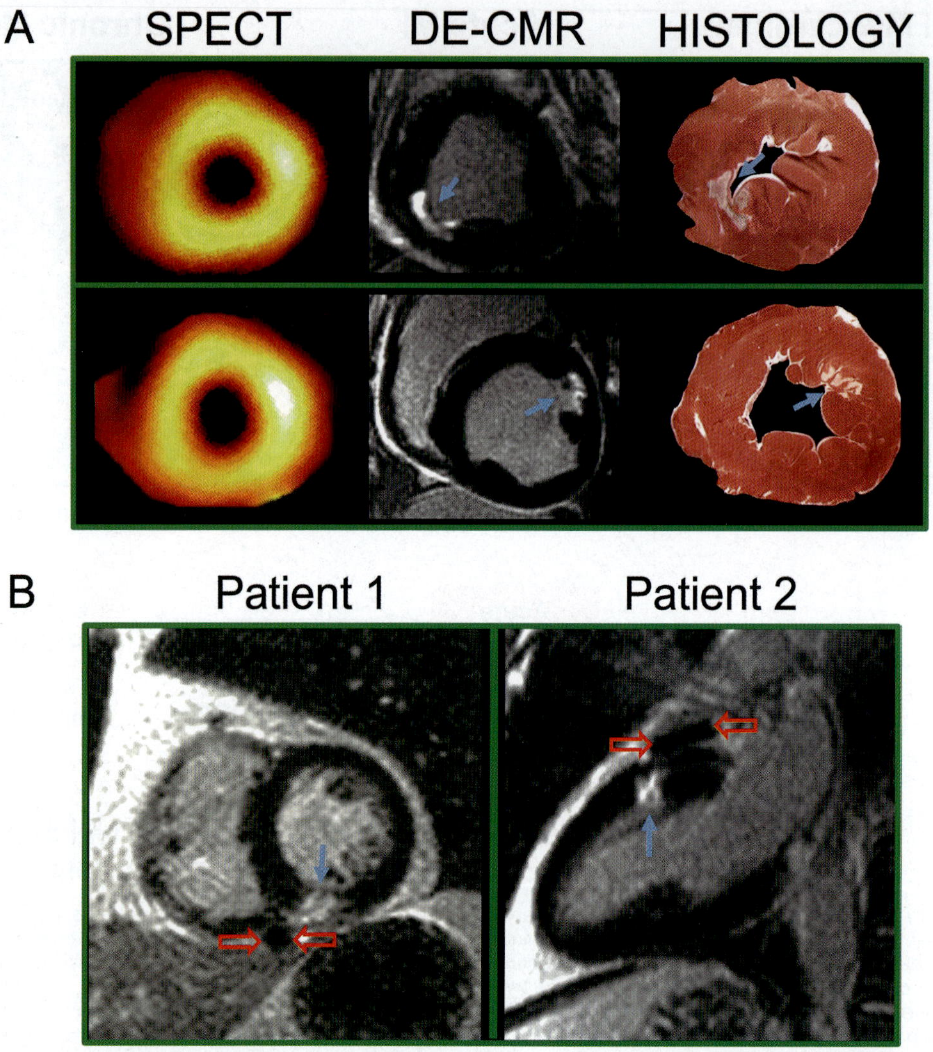

FIG. 22.10 (A) Comparison of delayed contrast-enhancement cardiovascular magnetic resonance (*DE-CMR*) with histopathology and single-photon emission tomography (*SPECT*) in two animals with subendocardial myocardial infarction. Note that the size, shape, and location of hyperenhanced regions by DE-CMR (*blue arrows*) match that of infarction delineated by histological vital staining. No infarcts are evident by SPECT. (B) Microinfarction (*blue arrows*) associated with successful percutaneous coronary intervention is demonstrated in two patients. *Red arrows* point to the coronary stents. (Adapted with permission from reference Wagner A, Mahrholdt H, Holly TA, Elliott MD, Regenfus M, Parker M, et al. Contrast-enhanced MRI and routine single photon emission computed tomography (SPECT) perfusion imaging for detection of subendocardial myocardial infarcts: an imaging study. *Lancet*. 2003;361(9355):374–379. Adapted with permission from reference Ricciardi MJ, Wu E, Davidson CJ, Choi KM, Klocke FJ, Bonow RO, et al. Visualization of discrete microinfarction after percutaneous coronary intervention associated with mild creatine kinase-MB elevation. *Circulation*. 2001;103(23):2780–2783.)

In patients presenting with acute MI and unobstructed coronary arteries (MINOCA), society guidelines emphasize that the diagnosis of MINOCA is inherently descriptive and is just a *working* diagnosis that should prompt physicians to seek the underlying cause.[52] This is because rational treatment follows from the etiologic diagnosis, and therapy that may be appropriate for one cause (e.g., anticoagulation for thromboembolism or calcium channel blockers for vasospasm) will be inappropriate for others. Society guidelines also emphasize that this diagnosis should be reserved solely for those suspected to have an ischemic cause. Although many investigations have demonstrated the diagnostic value of CMR in patients with elevated cardiac biomarkers and unobstructed coronary arteries, most studies included patients suspected to have nonischemic disorders such as myocarditis, hence they were not strict in including only patients with a true working diagnosis of MINOCA. A recent study confirmed CMR as a key test in the contemporary diagnosis of MINOCA.[53] There were several important findings. First, CMR allowed a final diagnosis of true MINOCA to be ruled out in over half the patients (e.g., non-coronary artery disease (CAD)-type hyperenhancement patterns were detected on delayed-enhancement imaging). Second, over a follow-up time of up to 10 years, CMR provided incremental prognostic value over conventional clinical factors (e.g., age, sex, CAD risk factors, presentation with ST elevation, and peak troponin). Third, the specific CMR diagnoses of acute MI, myocarditis, and NICM were independently associated with adverse outcome (Fig. 22.11). Finally, a normal CMR examination portended a benign prognosis. Indeed, the 10-year event rate of major adverse cardiac events was 3.5% and, in line with age-matched population-based cohorts, completely free of clinical cardiovascular disease. The exceptionally low event rate raises questions about the underlying mechanism of MINOCA in these patients. Current guidelines stipulate that patients with normal CMR examinations remain categorized as unclassified MINOCA patients, since it is

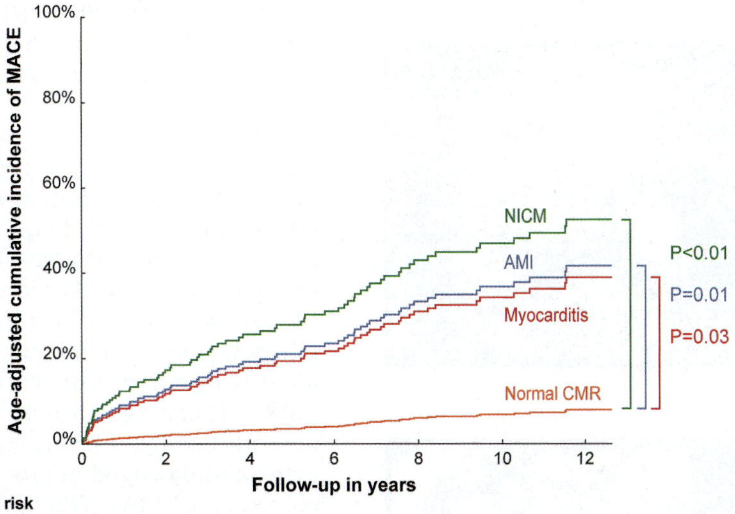

No. at risk							
AMI	63	46	35	31	24	17	11
Myocarditis	33	27	21	20	18	17	10
NICM	111	80	65	57	44	37	28
Normal CMR	37	33	27	25	17	15	9

FIG. 22.11 Curves show the age-adjusted cumulative incidence of major adverse cardiac events (*MACEs*) during follow-up, according to the prespecified cardiovascular magnetic resonance (*CMR*) diagnostic categories. Patients with nonischemic cardiomyopathy (*NICM*), acute myocardial infarction (*AMI*), and myocarditis all have higher age-adjusted rates of MACEs compared to patients with a normal CMR study.

possible that these patients had a true acute MI but the extent of necrosis was below the CMR detection threshold. However, the results of this study indicate that patients with normal examinations have a very different clinical profile (younger, less often female, and fewer CAD risk factors) than patients with a visible acute MI on CMR and raise the possibility that the majority of patients with normal CMR examinations do not have true MINOCA (i.e., an ischemic etiology). This suggests that the classification of normal CMR examination patients as MINOCA patients could be reconsidered. Fig. 22.12 shows representative examples of how DE-CMR may be clinically useful in three patients presenting with a working diagnosis of MINOCA.

In many patients with non-ST-segment elevation MI (NSTEMI), compared with those with STEMI, identification of the infarct-related artery (IRA) can be challenging because patients are more likely to present with either insignificant CAD or multivessel CAD (i.e., no culprit/IRA is seen or more than one culprit/IRA is possible).[54] The ability of CMR to detect even small MIs and determine alternative diagnoses makes it an appealing technique for the evaluation of patients presenting with NSTEMI. A recent study of patients with NSTEMI undergoing x-ray coronary angiography and CMR found that in over half the patients the IRA either could not be identified (37%) or was incorrectly assigned by coronary angiography (14%).[55] In addition, 15% of the patients had a noncoronary diagnosis made by CMR. Importantly, of the patients undergoing revascularization based on angiography, 27% had revascularization solely of nonculprit arteries, which presumably was not the operator's intent. From this and other studies of patients with NSTEMI, it is apparent that correct assignment of the IRA can be challenging, and that CMR can supply useful information aiding in this determination and in differentiation from noncoronary etiologies. In this regard, it is important to note that the CARMENTA study, which compared a CMR-first strategy to a standard evaluation with invasive coronary angiography showed that the CMR-first approach was safe in NSTEMI patients, with no deleterious change in outcomes while reducing the number of negative invasive coronary angiograms.[56] In this study, both CMR and coronary computed tomographic angiography (CTA) served as effective gatekeepers, with a greater reduction in invasive catheterizations in the CTA arm; nonetheless, those with negative anatomic imaging (coronary computed tomography or invasive angiography) frequently proceeded to CMR (67% of cases) in order to establish a definitive diagnosis.

Infarct Age, Characterization, and Sequelae

In cases where the acuity of an infarction is uncertain or there are multiple infarcts, possibly with different infarct ages, T2-weighted imaging and/or mapping can be useful in demonstrating the edema characteristically seen in the acute phase of MI (Fig. 22.13). These sequences are generally performed prior to the administration of IV contrast, as the presence of contrast may complicate image interpretation. These can be obtained via a double or triple inversion fast spin-echo black-blood sequence or with a T2-preparation steady-state free precession (SSFP) bright-blood sequence. The T2-preparation bright-blood sequence, which is also used for T2 mapping, is far more resistant to artifacts than the black-blood sequence. However, the bright-blood sequence may be less sensitive for detecting regions with more moderate levels of edema, particularly if limited to the subendocardium. Regarding the timeframe for detecting "acute" changes, however, it is important to recognize that infarct zone T2 hyperintensity and elevated T2 relaxation times are often present for subacute, intermediate-aged infarcts that are 1–6 months old, and occasionally even persist 6–12 months following acute MI.[57,58] Native T1 mapping is equally sensitive to T2 mapping in detecting myocardial edema,[58] however, it is less specific in that there are multiple causes of elevated T1, including artifactual T1-mapping bias due to intramyocardial fat.[59]

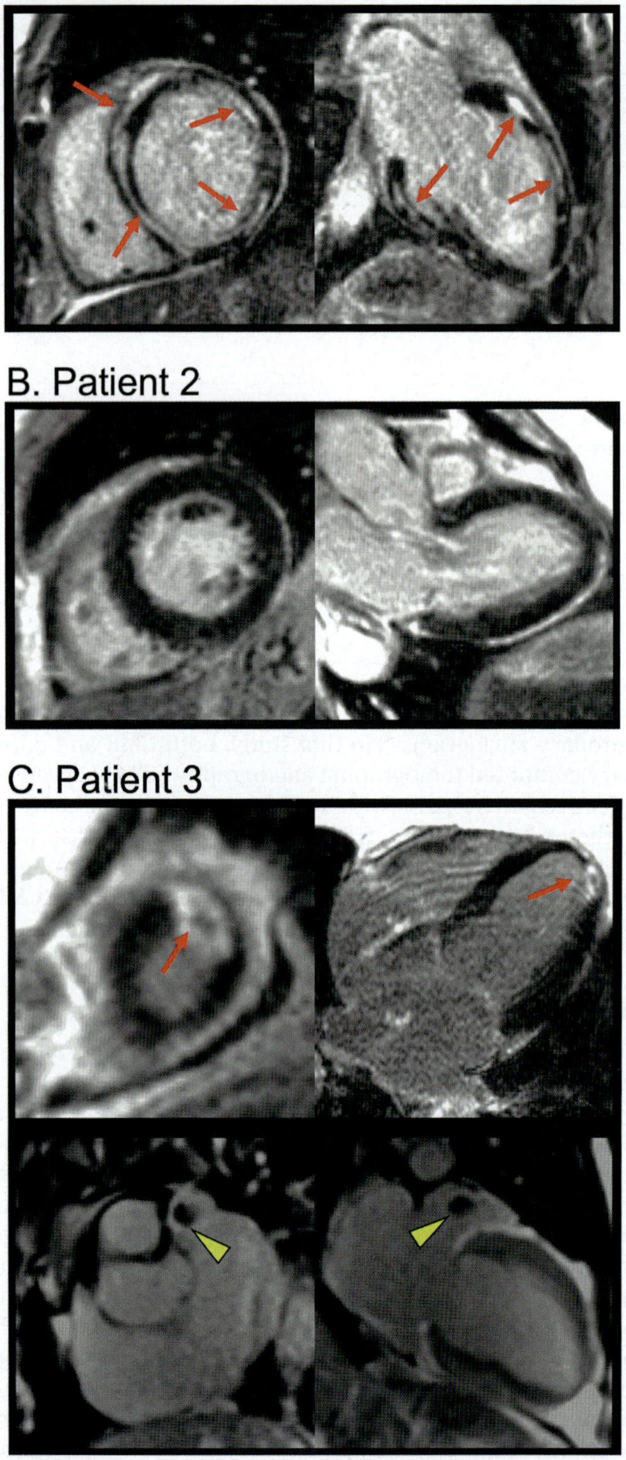

FIG. 22.12 Typical delayed contrast-enhancement cardiovascular magnetic resonance (DE-CMR) images in three patients with an initial diagnosis of ST-segment elevation myocardial infarction (MI) but then with normal coronary arteries found at angiography. DE-CMR was performed in these patients with a working diagnosis of MI and unobstructed coronary arteries, and in each case provided additional information to clarify the underlying etiology. (A) Linear, midmyocardial hyperenhancement is present, particularly in the septum, and is indicative of myocarditis. (B) In the setting of sudden emotional stress and apical ballooning, the absence of hyperenhancement is consistent with takotsubo cardiomyopathy. (C) Focal, but transmural hyperenhancement involving the lateral apex is present and indicative of MI due to temporary occlusion of a small diagonal branch off the distal left anterior descending coronary artery (*top row*). DE-CMR with a long inversion time (~600 ms) demonstrates a thrombus in the left atrial appendage (*bottom panel*), suggesting that an embolus led to the MI.

Even when the diagnosis of acute MI is certain, it is often useful to further characterize the infarct and identify sequelae. Infarct size can be measured accurately and with a high level of reproducibility in both the acute and chronic settings.[60–62] Additionally, the high spatial resolution of DE-CMR allows determination of the transmural extent of infarction, which provides supplemental information on infarct size for the prediction of regional and global improvement in contractile function with mechanical revascularization and medical therapy.[63–67] DE-CMR may also allow the assessment of gradations of injury within acute MI. For instance, rather than simply identifying a region of acute infarction as nonviable, DE-CMR can distinguish between acute infarcts with only necrotic myocytes from acute infarcts with necrotic myocytes and damaged microvasculature within the infarct core (Fig. 22.14A). The latter—known as microvascular obstruction or the "no-reflow" phenomenon—signifies more severe ischemic injury and results in compromised myocardial perfusion even after restoration of epicardial coronary flow.[68] Tissue hypoperfusion is due to obstruction at the capillary level rather than in large epicardial vessels and is associated with capillaries plugged by erythrocytes and loss of microvascular integrity (Fig. 22.14B).[68–70] The severe tissue hypoperfusion that characterizes myocardial no-reflow can be detected by first-pass perfusion imaging; however, delayed-enhancement imaging provides better image quality, complete ventricular coverage (i.e., complete short-axis stack and multiple long-axis images), and higher diagnostic specificity in that the contrast-devoid hypoenhanced area should be completely surrounded (in 3D space) by bright, hyperenhancement myocardium or bright ventricular cavity blood pool. The latter is an important consideration for image interpretation, since both viable myocardium and nonviable no-reflow zones will be dark on conventional delayed-enhancement imaging. If there is any remaining diagnostic uncertainty, then a useful technique is "long-TI" imaging in which the inversion time is set to null native (precontrast) normal myocardial tissue (approximately 500–550 ms at 1.5 T and 850–900 ms at 3 T). Since there is little uptake of gadolinium contrast in no-reflow zones, these regions will remain dark on long-TI imaging whereas normal myocardial tissue will become gray (Fig. 22.14C). One complicating factor is that mural thrombus will also remain dark on long-TI imaging since it is avascular and there is no gadolinium contrast uptake. In this situation, it is helpful to remember that while no-reflow zones have very low perfusion, the level of perfusion is not zero (unlike thrombus). Additionally, a longer interval between contrast media administration and image acquisition enables more gadolinium to slowly wash into the no-reflow zone via diffusion (Fig. 22.14D). This means that over time (5–10 minutes) the size of no-reflow zones will shrink whereas the size of thrombus will not.

Myocardial no-reflow is important to detect since it is associated with adverse ventricular remodeling and poor clinical outcome.[71–74] However, no-reflow is a transient phenomenon and disappears with infarct healing. This feature can be beneficial in that in combination

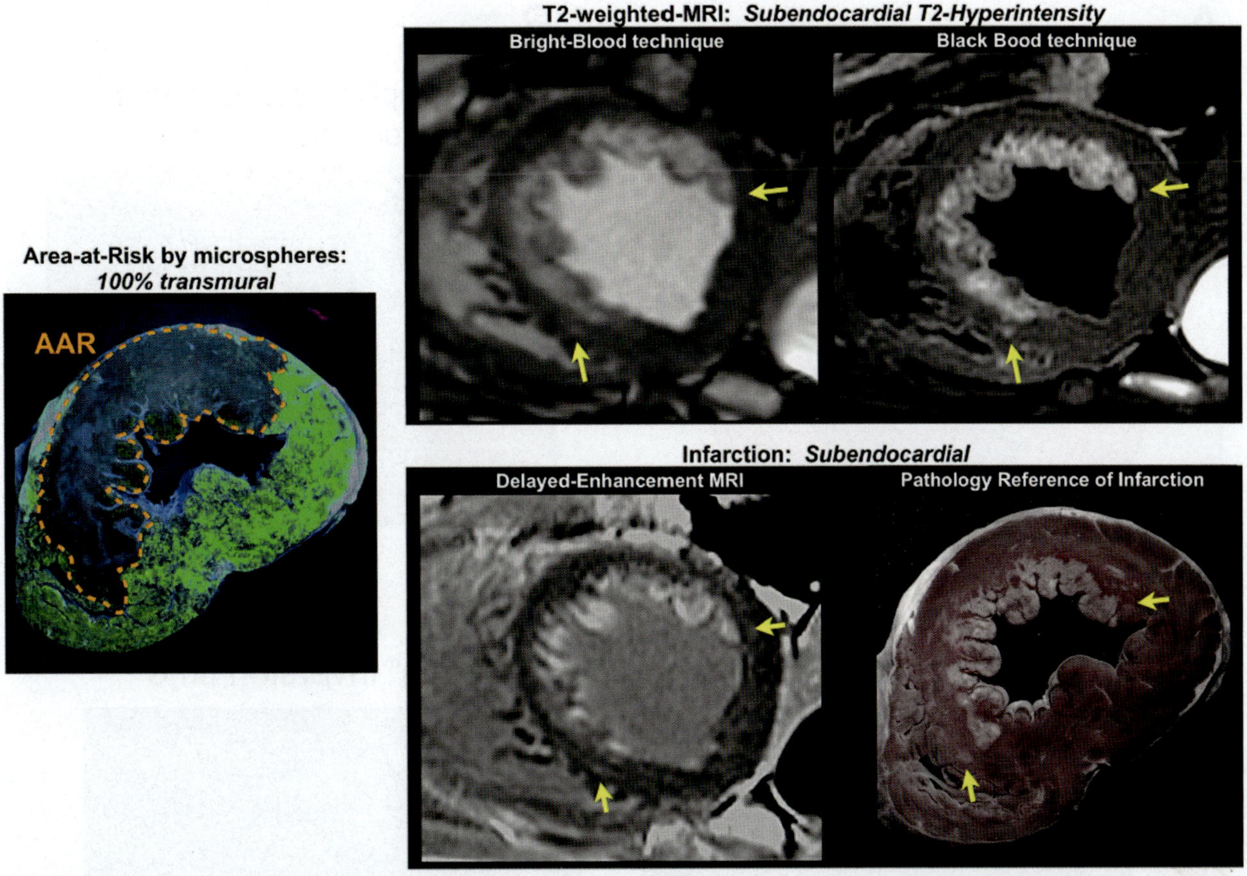

FIG. 22.13 The area at risk (*AAR*) by histopathology (*left panel, orange outline* depicting absence of fluorescent microspheres) is nearly 100% transmural, whereas T2-hyperintense (*top row*) and infarcted regions (*bottom row*) are clearly nontransmural (*yellow arrows*). The T2-hyperintense region closely resembles the shape of infarction, not the AAR. Additionally, the intricate contour and shape of the infarcted region by delayed-enhancement magnetic resonance imaging (*MRI*) is matched by the contour of T2 hyperintensity on both bright-blood and black-blood images. (Based on data by Reimer and Jennings. Whalen DA, Jr., Hamilton DG, Ganote CE, Jennings RB. Effect of a transient period of ischemia on myocardial cells. I. Effects on cell volume regulation. *Am J Pathol*. 1974;74(3):381–397. Reimer KA, Jennings RB. The changing anatomic reference base of evolving myocardial infarction. Underestimation of myocardial collateral blood flow and overestimation of experimental anatomic infarct size due to tissue edema, hemorrhage, and acute inflammation. *Circulation*. 1979;60(4):866–876.)

with other CMR markers it can lead to a more precise assessment of infarct age than T2 imaging alone.[57] However, conversely, if CMR is not performed in the acute setting—which can occur because acute MI is often clinically unrecognized—the absence of no-reflow may not reflect a benign prognosis since it may simply reflect its resolution. In effect, the transient nature of no-reflow provides only a limited time window of a pathophysiological process with long-term implications for prognosis. In this regard, it is of interest that a recent investigation has introduced a novel index of infarction—the epicardial surface area of full-thickness infarction (EpiSA)—which can be assessed with conventional DE-CMR and appears to be strongly associated with no-reflow in the acute setting, but is stable over time and does not disappear with infarct healing.[75] A greater EpiSA extent in the acute setting was predictive of adverse ventricular remodeling and worse clinical outcome during follow-up.

Intramyocardial hemorrhage (IMH) represents erythrocyte extravasation from damaged capillaries and is closely related to the no-reflow phenomenon (Fig. 22.15). It is considered a subset of no-reflow since in one direction the presence of IMH guarantees microvascular damage. In the other direction, there are mechanisms of microvascular dysfunction that could result in no-reflow without IMH such as swollen myocytes, which could compress adjacent capillaries. However, this is likely only a theoretical consideration since pathology studies of acute MI show IMH occurring concurrently with microvascular damage/destruction with close anatomic correlation.[70] Hence, any differences between the presence and/or extent of IMH in comparison to no-reflow in a given patient or patient cohort are more likely related to differences in the sensitivity and accuracy of the techniques used to detect the disorders rather than any special distinctions in physiology. IMH can be detected by native T2* or T2 imaging; paramagnetic effects from hemoglobin breakdown products results in shortening of T2* and T2 relaxation times. An advantage over the assessment of no-reflow is that these parameters are independent of contrast media kinetics since contrast is not needed. Disadvantages, however, are sizable and include lower image quality (T2* and T2 are more susceptible to magnetic field inhomogeneity and off-resonance effects), competing effects from other physiological changes (edema results in directionally opposite increases in T2* and T2 relaxation times), and increased scan time

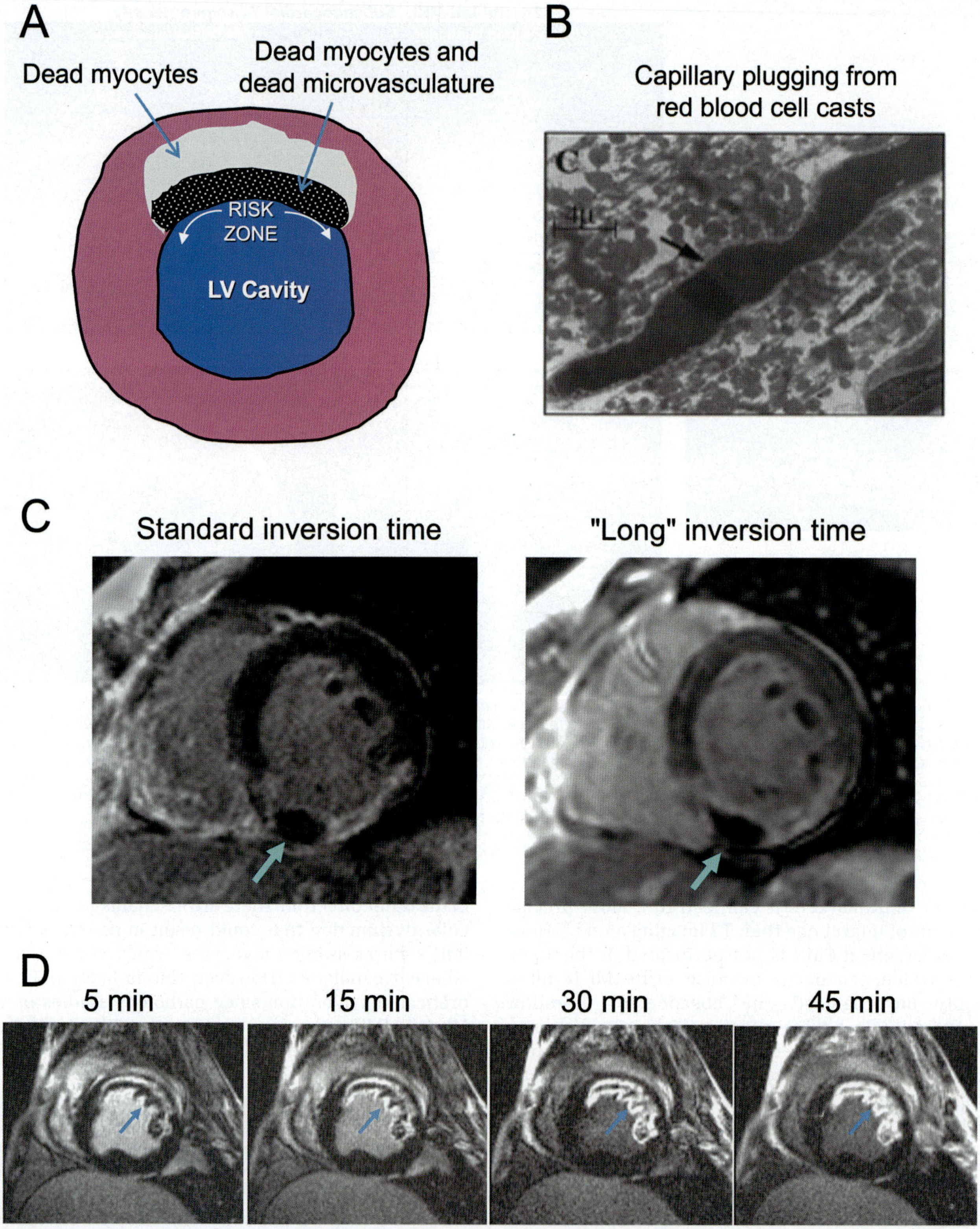

FIG. 22.14 (A) If ischemic injury is severe, the infarct core (subendocardial portion that suffers more extreme hypoperfusion) can exhibit microvascular damage in addition to necrotic myocytes. (B) Electron micrograph (×4500) from the infarct core showing capillary plugging with red blood cell stasis (*arrow*). Microvascular damage could lead to prolonged wash-in/washout gadolinium kinetics in infarcted tissue. (C) Patient with an inferior wall acute myocardial infarction. Note that both the no-reflow zone (*arrow*) in the infarct core and remote normal myocardium are both dark on conventional delayed contrast-enhancement cardiovascular magnetic resonance imaging using a standard inversion time that nulls normal myocardium postcontrast. Repeating the image using a "long TI" will result in normal myocardium becoming gray whereas the no-reflow zone will remain dark. (D) Another way to differentiate a no-reflow zone from normal myocardium (and also from thrombus) is to repeat imaging after 5–10 minutes. A longer time interval between contrast material administration and image acquisition enables wash-in of gadolinium contrast into the no-reflow zone. Listed times represent minutes following gadolinium administration. See text for details. *LV*, left ventricular (Adapted from Higgins CB, de Roos A (eds). Cardiovascular MRI & MRA. Philadelphia: Lippincott Williams & Wilkins; 2003:209-237.)

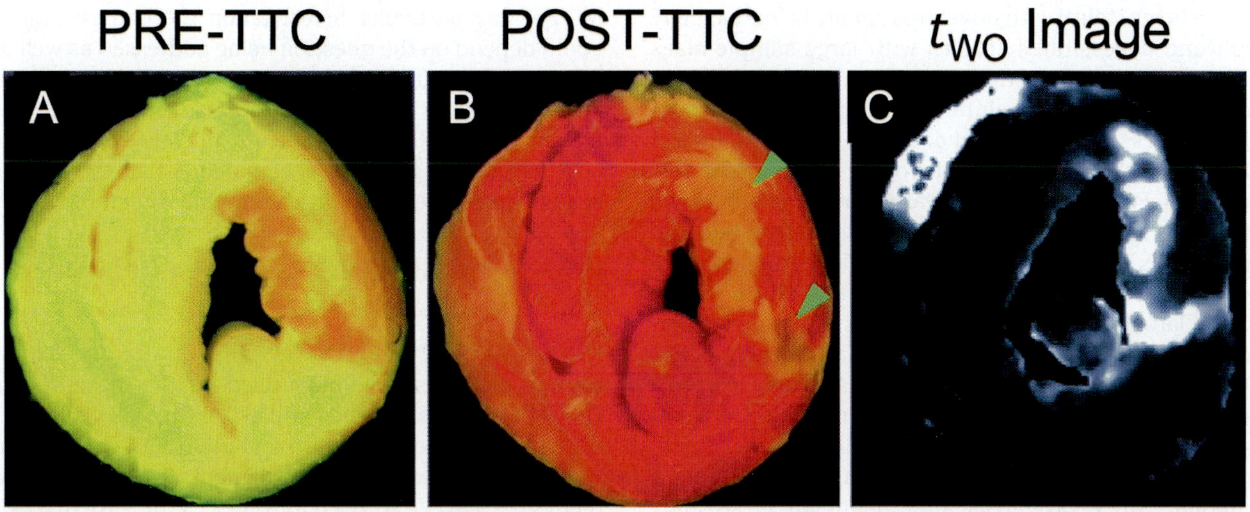

FIG. 22.15 The position and extent of gross intramyocardial hemorrhage (IMH) shown on the unstained myocardial slice (A) is within and smaller than the infarcted area (*green arrows*) shown after triphenyl tetrazolium chloride (*TTC*) staining of the same myocardial slice (B). The area of infarction has elevated gadolinium washout time as depicted by pixels with high image intensity on the two parametric maps (C). Note, however, that areas of hemorrhage have extremely abnormal washout kinetics, indicating a direct link between IMH and microvascular damage. (Adapted with permission from reference Kim RJ, Chen EL, Lima JA, Judd RM. Myocardial Gd-DTPA kinetics determine MRI contrast enhancement and reflect the extent and severity of myocardial injury after acute reperfused infarction. *Circulation*. 1996;94(12):3318–3326.)

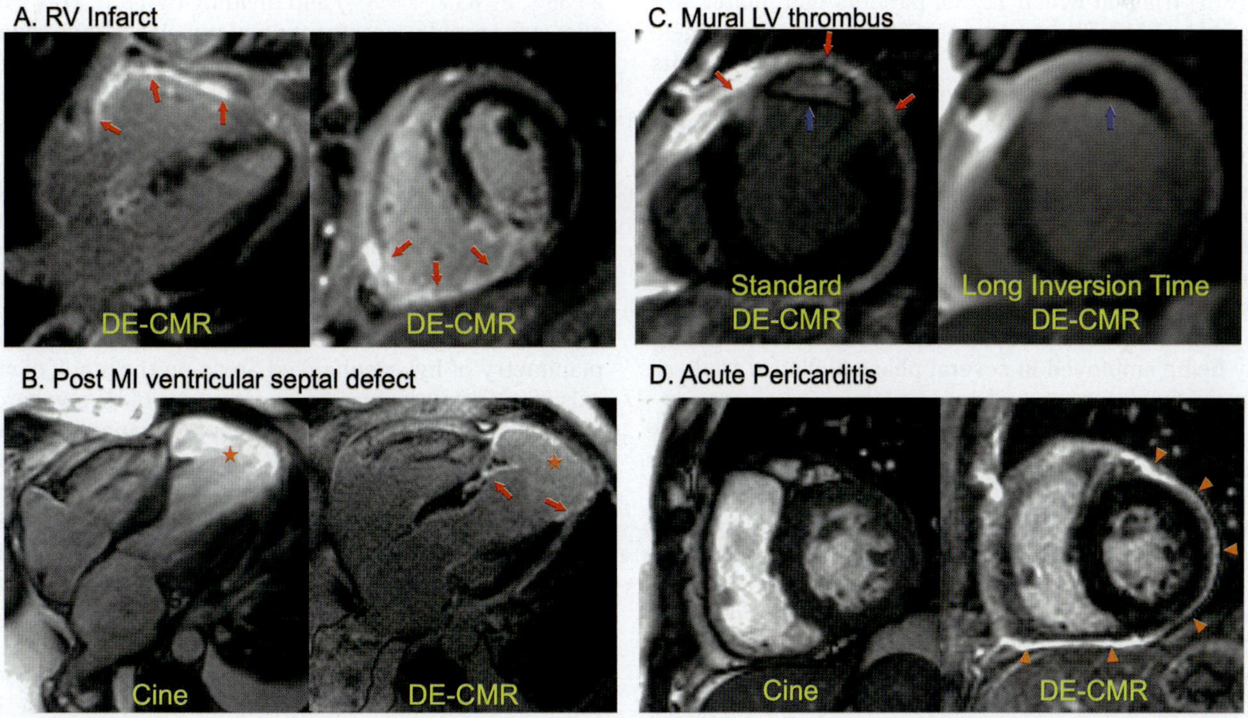

FIG. 22.16 Examples are shown of patients with myocardial infarction (*MI*) complicated by (A) right ventricular (*RV*) involvement and (B) post-MI (*red arrows*) ventricular septal defect (*orange star*). (C) Mural left ventricular (*LV*) thrombus (*blue arrow*) immediately adjacent to MI (*red arrows*) can be identified by both standard and "long inversion" time delayed contrast-enhancement cardiovascular magnetic resonance (*DE-CMR*). (D) Acute pericarditis can be diagnosed by the presence of hyperenhanced pericardium (*orange arrowheads*).

given the need for additional native T2* or T2 image acquisition.

Increasing experience with CMR has led to the development of new applications that may be used to diagnose post-MI complications and other sequelae such as intracardiac thrombus and pericarditis. Fig. 22.16 demonstrates a few typical examples; these disorders are described in detail in other chapters.

CARDIOVASCULAR MAGNETIC RESONANCE INFARCT SIZE AS A SURROGATE ENDPOINT FOR CLINICAL TRIALS

The ultimate goal of a new therapy for acute MI is a reduction in mortality. In the current era, treatment of acute MI is quite effective; therefore, demonstrating a further reduction in mortality with novel treatments is increasingly difficult and necessitates studies with large sample sizes and corresponding logistical and financial barriers. As such, there is considerable interest in using surrogate endpoints to assess the efficacy of acute MI therapies. Infarct size is a particularly attractive surrogate endpoint for several reasons. First, it is useful in early screening studies to test whether a new therapy is biologically active. Second, it can serve as an endpoint for phase II dose-ranging studies to test treatment efficacy and/or safety. Third, it may indicate a late mortality benefit, and thus rationale for performing a longer-term study, even if an early benefit is not seen. For instance, a reduction in infarct size may lead to a long-term improvement in ventricular remodeling, a benefit that may not manifest in 30-day mortality rates. Fourth, it can provide a physiological mechanism for improvement in outcome, since prognosis after acute MI is strongly determined by the extent of myocardial injury.[76,77]

Specifically concerning CMR studies, several investigations have reported that infarct size measured by DE-CMR is a stronger predictor of outcomes than LVEF and left ventricular (LV) volumes.[78–80] Stone et al. performed a pooled analysis of 10 primary percutaneous coronary intervention (PCI) trials in which 72% of patients had infarct size assessed by CMR. The study reported that infarct size (generally measured within the first week after PCI in patients undergoing CMR) was strongly associated with all-cause mortality and hospitalization for heart failure at 1 year.[81] Every 5% increase in infarct size contributed to a 19% and 20% increase in the relative hazard for mortality and hospitalization for heart failure, respectively. The authors concluded, therefore, that infarct size may be useful as an endpoint in clinical trials and as an important prognostic measure when caring for patients with STEMI. Based on data such as these, infarct size measured by CMR is currently being employed in several phase 3 clinical trials as a primary endpoint.

When to Measure Infarct Size

Earlier in this chapter we described how the pioneering pathology studies by Reimer and Jennings demonstrated *the changing anatomic reference base of evolving myocardial infarction*.[32] That is, the infarcted region is highly dynamic in size following acute MI. Using DE-CMR, similar findings have been observed in-vivo in a canine model (Fig. 22.17).[82,83] Fieno et al. demonstrated that terminal infarct size at 4 to 8 weeks averaged 24% of that found at 3 days, and reperfusion accelerated infarct resorption.[82] Moreover, the mass of viable myocardium increased systematically with time, although the time course of hypertrophy was different from the time course of infarct resorption. Importantly, measurements of total LV mass did not reflect the changes occurring separately in infarcted and viable regions. These results highlight the capability of DE-CMR to improve the assessment of post-infarction ventricular remodeling by allowing the evaluation of concurrent changes such as resorption of infarcted tissue and hypertrophy of viable myocardium at an early time point before measurements of total mass have changed. Given the dynamics of acutely infarcted myocardium, care should be taken in planning the timing of infarct size measurement after MI. For any particular investigation the chosen time point could depend on the question being addressed as well as the logistics of the trial, however, the advantages of measuring infarct size early (vs. late) after MI usually outweigh the disadvantages (Table 22.1). For acute MI clinical trials, our CMR core laboratory generally recommends that the index CMR scan be performed 4 ± 2 days after admission for MI.

How to Measure Infarct Size on Delayed Contrast-Enhancement Cardiovascular Magnetic Resonance Images

Several methods have been used for the measurement of DE-CMR infarct size. The simplest of these is visual scoring of hyperenhanced tissue on a standard 17-segment model with a 5-point scale for each segment (0, no hyperenhancement; 1, 1% to 25%; 2, 26% to 50%; 3, 51% to 75%; 4, 76% to 100%).[66,85] Dark regions entirely encompassed within hyperenhanced myocardium are interpreted as regions of microvascular damage and included as part of the infarct. Infarct size as a percentage of LV myocardium is calculated by summing the regional scores, each weighted by the midpoint of the range of hyperenhancement (i.e., 1 = 13%, 2 = 38%, 3 = 63%, 4 = 88%) and dividing by 17.[7,84] This system allows for rapid assessment of infarct size in increments of approximately 1.2% of LV mass (100% ÷ 85 possible scores) without the need for planimetry of endocardial/epicardial borders. More generally, the presence, location, and extent of hyperenhancement can be quickly assessed on the 17-segment model regardless of whether hyperenhancement represents acute MI, chronic MI, or nonischemic scarring. The ease and simplicity of this approach is the reason why visual scoring is used by our clinical service for standard CMR reporting and documentation.

Alternatively, infarct size can be quantified by manual planimetry of hyperenhanced areas on the stack of short-axis images. Infarct size as a percentage of LV myocardium is calculated as total volume of hyperenhanced regions on all slices divided by total LV myocardial cross-sectional volume. This is the standard method used by our core laboratory for clinical trials. For visual scoring and manual planimetry, reproducibility is improved by explicitly defining how to treat intermediate signal intensities (e.g., "gray" zones) due to partial volume. One simple approach is to include 50% of regions with intermediate signal intensity as part of the infarct.[85] Given that manual planimetry requires visual assessment, a standard practice in our core laboratory is to first perform visual scoring (on a 17-segment model as described above) before undertaking manual planimetry. The visual scores provide a quality assessment check to guide manual planimetry and can be useful in explaining any intra- and interobserver differences in planimetered infarct size measurements.

In an attempt to be more standardized and objective, a number of "automatic" methods have been proposed to delineate the infarct border. However, these methods are not as objective or automatic as one might assume. For example, the n-SD technique requires user input to manually select a "remote" zone region of interest (ROI) to define the reference signal intensity (mean and standard deviation [SD]). This subjective selection can greatly affect

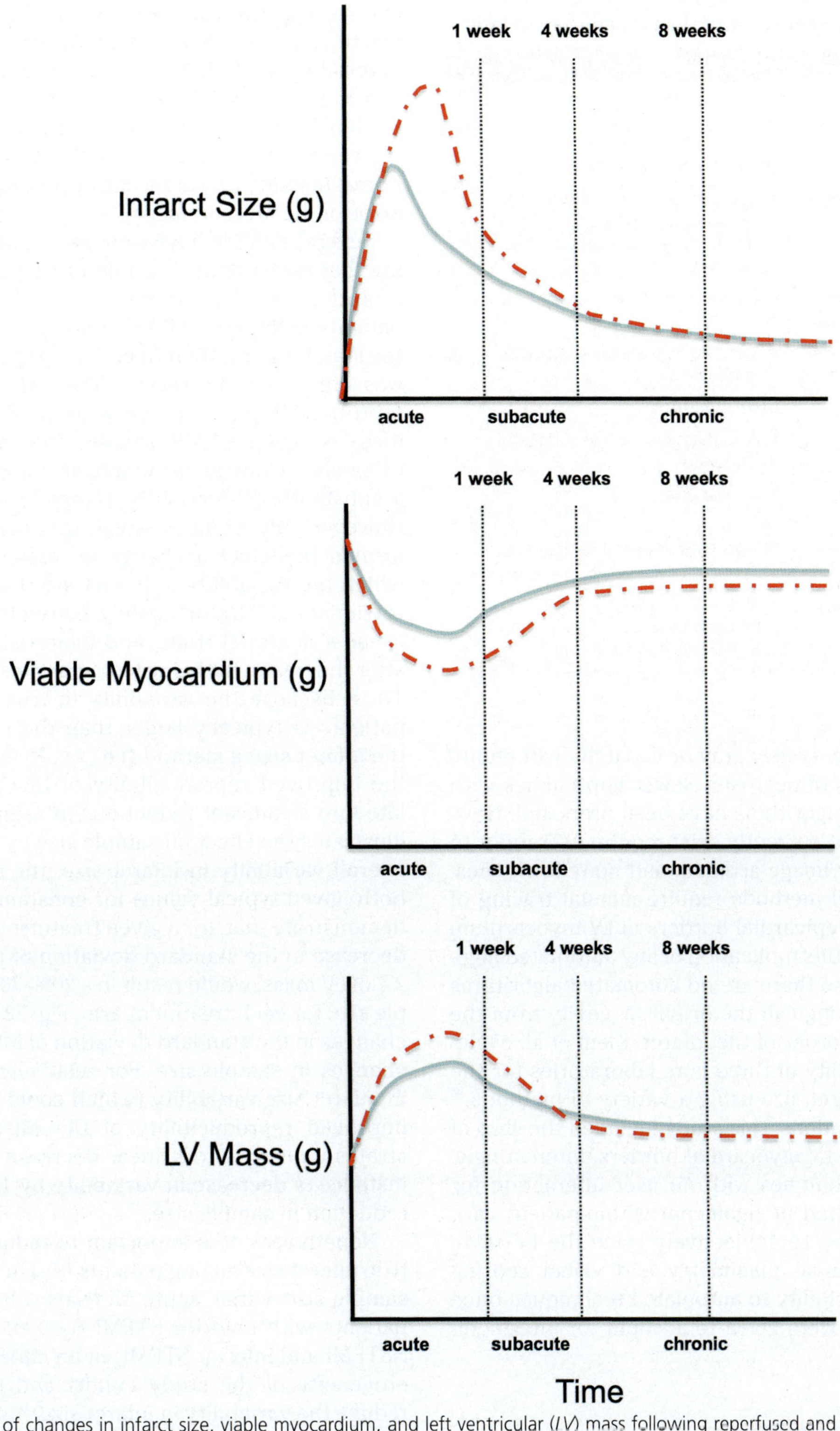

FIG. 22.17 Time course of changes in infarct size, viable myocardium, and left ventricular (*LV*) mass following reperfused and nonreperfused myocardial infarction (*MI*). The top (*infarct size*), middle (*viable myocardium*), and bottom (LV mass) panels demonstrate idealized curves based on data from multiple sources.[82,83] *Blue lines* denote reperfused MI, *dashed red lines* nonreperfused MI. Within the first few days post-MI, infarct size can substantially increase because of the addition of edema and cellular elements within the necrotic zone. Thereafter, infarct volume can shrink to ~25% of its initial size over the next 4–6 weeks as edema is resorbed and necrotic myocytes are replaced by scar tissue. After ~6 weeks, infarct size is relatively stable. The volume of viable myocardium (e.g., noninfarcted LV mass) correspondingly declines initially, but may increase over the course of infarct healing due to myocyte hypertrophy. Changes in total LV mass reflect the sum of changes occurring in infarcted and viable myocardium.

measurements. An alternative method that uses a threshold value of 50% of the maximum intensity within the infarct (full-width at half-maximum [FWHM]) may be more resistant to surface-coil intensity variations and provide improved reproducibility. However, FWHM requires visual determination of whether hyperenhancement is present or not, and if present, manual selection of an ROI that includes the region of "maximum" signal. This subjective selection can affect measurements. Additionally, FWHM assumes a bright infarct core and may not be accurate if

TABLE 22.1 Measurement of infarct size: early versus late.

EARLY (≤7 DAYS)	LATE (>4 WEEKS)
ADVANTAGES	*ADVANTAGES*
• Larger infarct size	• Infarct size is stable
Higher detection rate	Imaging time frame can be wide
May reduce required sample size	• Can also assess left ventricular ejection fraction (LVEF), which is stable (stunning, if present, has resolved)
• Can also assess presence and extent of "no-reflow"	• Can also assess recovery of function
• Can also assess presence and extent of stunning	• Can also assess early ventricular remodeling
DISADVANTAGES	*DISADVANTAGES*
• Infarct size is dynamic	• Presumes survival and successful follow-up
Imaging time window must be narrow	• Smaller infarct size
Recommend imaging 4±2 days after MI	May increase required sample size
• Requires patient stability	Infarct healing (shrinkage) may preclude detection of very small myocardial infarction (MI)

the infarct is homogeneously gray or is patchy with multiple, separate islands of necrosis. Newer approaches with more sophisticated algorithms have been proposed. However, all methods that currently exist require user input to manually correct for image artifacts and no-reflow zones. Most importantly, all methods require manual tracing of the endocardial and epicardial borders of LV myocardium as a first step before the application of any automated algorithm. This is because there are no automated algorithms that can reliably distinguish the bright LV cavity from the bright endocardial border of the infarct. Klem et al. evaluated the reproducibility of three core laboratories for the measurement of infarct size using a variety of methods.[85] Unlike prior investigations, this study included the step of manually tracing the LV myocardial borders. Interestingly, even automated techniques with no user interaction for infarct borders resulted in significant within-patient variability given the need to subjectively trace the LV myocardial borders. Manual planimetry and visual scoring had similar reproducibility to automated techniques once explicit instructions were given to account for intermediate signal intensities.

Sample Size Considerations

When testing new therapies using infarct size as a surrogate endpoint, sample size (n) calculations are based on the following formula:

$$n = \frac{2\left(\sigma^2\right)\left(z_{\frac{\alpha}{2}} + z_{\beta}\right)^2}{\delta^2}$$

where σ is the standard deviation of infarct size, δ is the expected reduction in infarct size due to the new therapy, and z is the value of the z-statistic depending on the alpha and beta levels set by the study design. Thus, sample size is determined by both the expected effect of the therapy (δ) and the variability of measured infarct size within a population (σ).[86] The latter is comprised of two components: the variability in infarct size between patients (σ_T) and the reproducibility (σ_e) of the sizing method (e.g., the standard error of the measurement).

Several studies have now been published demonstrating that measurement of infarct size by DE-CMR is highly reproducible. For example, in a three-center study of patients with acute MI undergoing paired DE-CMR scans, the standard deviation (e.g., σ_e) in repeated measurements was only 1% of LV mass.[61] The implication of improved reproducibility (compared with non-CMR imaging modalities) is that DE-CMR enables the systematic detection of smaller changes in infarct size and potentially allows a substantial reduction in sample size for clinical trials. However, this might presume that paired imaging is performed to detect a change in infarct size over time, in which the variability in infarct size between patients (σ_T) is eliminated.[87] Unfortunately, paired testing is not feasible in most acute MI trials, and infarct size is only assessed after the treatment being tested has been given (unpaired). Thus, because the variability in true infarct size among patients is typically larger than the variability added by the infarct sizing method (i.e., $\sigma_T > \sigma_e$), it is possible that the improved reproducibility of DE-CMR may not translate into significant reductions in sample size. Fig. 22.18A illustrates the effect on sample size by changing either the overall variability in infarct size, the treatment effect, or both, given typical values for constants. The calculations demonstrate that, for a given treatment effect, even a small decrease in the standard deviation of infarct size, such as 2% of LV mass, would result in a 20%–30% reduction in sample size for each treatment arm. Fig. 22.18B relates percent changes in the standard deviation of infarct size to percent changes in sample size. For relatively modest decreases in infarct size variability (which could be procured by the improved reproducibility of DE-CMR), the plot demonstrates a nearly 2-to-1 linear decrease in sample size. For instance, a decrease in variability by 10% results in a 19% reduction in sample size.

Nonetheless, it is important to reduce the variability in true infarct size among patients (σ_T) in order to reduce the sample size. Often, acute MI trials will limit enrollment to patients with anterior STEMI (i.e., exclude patients with NSTEMI and inferior STEMI) in an effort to reduce the heterogeneity of the study cohort and thereby potentially reduce the variability in infarct size. A major portion of the variability in absolute infarct size is due to variability in the size of the AAR. Hence, as discussed earlier in this chapter, a much better measure of the efficacy of an acute MI therapy would be the proportion of the AAR that is infarcted—which directly indexes salvage—rather than infarct size as a percentage of LV mass or absolute infarct size. But to obtain infarct size as a percentage of the AAR, one needs to know the size of the AAR. We have described the problems with using edema as a surrogate for the AAR. Ortiz-Perez et al. proposed that the infarct endocardial surface area (ESA) could be used to measure the size of the AAR.[88] This

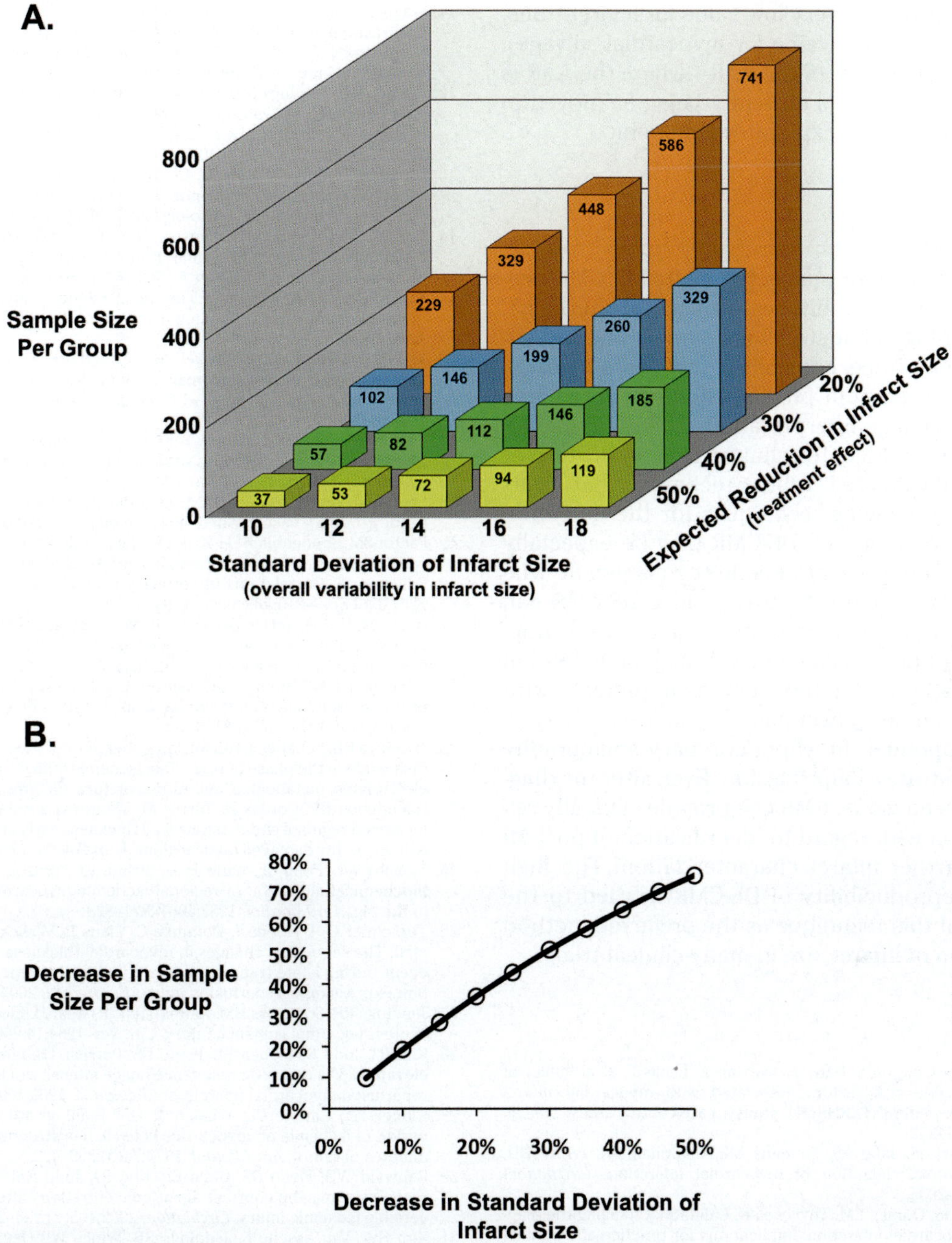

FIG. 22.18 Sample size calculations. (A) Sample size per group depending on the expected standard deviation of infarct size and expected changes in treatment effect. Even small decreases in infarct size variability result in appreciable reductions in sample size. Calculations assume mean infarct size of 13.1% of left ventricular (*LV*) myocardium, $\alpha = 0.05$, and $\beta = 0.2$. (B) Percent decrease in sample size associated with percent decrease in standard deviation of infarct size. The relationship is relatively linear (with slope = 2) for modest decreases in infarct size variability. Calculations assume mean infarct size of 13.1% of LV myocardium, a constant treatment effect, $\alpha = 0.05$, and $\beta = 0.2$. See text for further details.

method leverages the physiologic principle that the lateral boundaries of the AAR nearly equal the lateral boundaries of the infarction starting relatively early in the process of evolving MI.[12] Versteylen et al. demonstrated that infarct-ESA was superior to electrocardiographic (Aldrich), angiographic (BARI, APPROACH), and T2-weighted imaging methods for measuring AAR size when using established physiological concepts to provide a reference standard.[89] A significant advantage of infarct-ESA for delineating the AAR is that it offers full LV coverage without any additional scan time since the data are acquired with conventional DE-CMR imaging. A disadvantage is that the lateral boundaries of the AAR cannot be established unless there is at least a confluent subendocardial infarct. If there is minimal or no necrosis, such as from aborted MI, the AAR borders cannot be determined. That said, it should be recognized that expressing infarct size as a percentage of the AAR is equivalent to the calculation of mean infarct transmurality, and if infarct size is zero, it is not much of a stretch to argue that mean infarct transmurality is also zero.[90] In other words, if there is minimal or no necrosis, a practical solution is to use a nominal value for the denominator, such as the median or lower quartile value of infarct-ESA for the population studied. Note that since the problem only occurs when the numerator is zero or very small, even a conservatively small value for the denominator (such as the lower quartile value) will yield a very low value for infarct transmurality (e.g., a very high value for myocardial salvage). Infarct size as a percentage of the AAR—where the AAR is estimated by infarct-ESA—is currently being employed in several clinical trials as an exploratory endpoint.

SUMMARY

In patients with known or suspected acute MI, CMR provides a comprehensive, multifaceted view of the heart. The pathophysiology of acute MI is complex but important to understand since physiologic concepts such as the AAR and the wavefront phenomenon can serve as a basis for correct image interpretation. The data, including from a recent multicenter clinical trial, indicate that DE-CMR is a well-validated, robust technique that rivals the best available imaging techniques for the detection and assessment of acute MI. DE-CMR may be especially useful when patients present outside the diagnostic window of cardiac troponins. Moreover, since DE-CMR can uniquely differentiate between ischemic and various nonischemic forms of myocardial injury, it may be helpful in cases of diagnostic uncertainty such as in patients with classical features of MI (chest pain, ST-segment changes, and elevated troponins) in whom coronary angiography does not demonstrate a culprit lesion. Even after the diagnosis of MI has been made, CMR can provide clinically relevant information with regard to identification of post-MI sequelae and further infarct characterization. The high accuracy and reproducibility of DE-CMR has led to the increasing use of this technique as the preferred method for quantification of infarct size in many clinical trials.

REFERENCES

1. Yusuf S, Hawken S, Ounpuu S, Dans T, Avezum A, Lanas F, et al. Effect of potentially modifiable risk factors associated with myocardial infarction in 52 countries (the INTERHEART study): case-control study. *Lancet.* 2004;364(9438):937–952.
2. Thygesen K, Alpert JS, Jaffe AS, Simoons ML, Chaitman BR, White HD, et al. Third universal definition of myocardial infarction. *Circulation.* 2012;126(16):2020–2035.
3. Newby LK, Alpert JS, Ohman EM, Thygesen K, Califf RM. Changing the diagnosis of acute myocardial infarction: implications for practice and clinical investigations. *Am Heart J.* 2002;144(6):957–980.
4. White HD. Things ain't what they used to be: impact of a new definition of myocardial infarction. *Am Heart J.* 2002;144(6):933–937.
5. Hochholzer W, Buettner HJ, Trenk D, Laule K, Christ M, Neumann FJ, et al. New definition of myocardial infarction: impact on long-term mortality. *Am J Med.* 2008;121(5):399–405.
6. Ibrahim T, Bülow HP, Hackl T, Hörnke M, Nekolla SG, Breuer M, et al. Diagnostic value of contrast-enhanced magnetic resonance imaging and single-photon emission computed tomography for detection of myocardial necrosis early after acute myocardial infarction. *J Am Coll Cardiol.* 2007;49(2):208–216.
7. Kim RJ, Albert TS, Wible JH, Elliott MD, Allen JC, Lee JC, et al. Performance of delayed-enhancement magnetic resonance imaging with gadoversetamide contrast for the detection and assessment of myocardial infarction: an international, multicenter, double-blinded, randomized trial. *Circulation.* 2008;117(5):629–637.
8. Kim RJ, Fieno DS, Parrish TB, Harris K, Chen EL, Simonetti O, et al. Relationship of MRI delayed contrast enhancement to irreversible injury, infarct age, and contractile function. *Circulation.* 1999;100(19):1992–2002.
9. Ricciardi MJ, Wu E, Davidson CJ, Choi KM, Klocke FJ, Bonow RO, et al. Visualization of discrete microinfarction after percutaneous coronary intervention associated with mild creatine kinase-MB elevation. *Circulation.* 2001;103(23):2780–2783.
10. Selvanayagam JB, Porto I, Channon K, Petersen SE, Francis JM, Neubauer S, et al. Troponin elevation after percutaneous coronary intervention directly represents the extent of irreversible myocardial injury: insights from cardiovascular magnetic resonance imaging. *Circulation.* 2005;111(8):1027–1032.
11. Wagner A, Mahrholdt H, Holly TA, Elliott MD, Regenfus M, Parker M, et al. Contrast-enhanced MRI and routine single photon emission computed tomography (SPECT) perfusion imaging for detection of subendocardial myocardial infarcts: an imaging study. *Lancet.* 2003;361(9355):374–379.
12. Reimer KA, Jennings RB. The "wavefront phenomenon" of myocardial ischemic cell death. II. Transmural progression of necrosis within the framework of ischemic bed size (myocardium at risk) and collateral flow. *Lab Investig; J Tech Methods Pathol.* 1979;40(6):633–644.
13. Croisille P, Kim HW, Kim RJ. Controversies in cardiovascular MR imaging: T2-weighted imaging should not be used to delineate the area at risk in ischemic myocardial injury. *Radiology.* 2012;265(1):12–22.
14. Cox JL, McLaughlin VW, Flowers NC, Horan LG. The ischemic zone surrounding acute myocardial infarction. Its morphology as detected by dehydrogenase staining. *Am Heart J.* 1968;76(5):650–659.
15. Axford-Gatley RA, Wilson GJ. The "border zone" in myocardial infarction. An ultrastructural study in the dog using an electron-dense blood flow marker. *Am J Pathol.* 1988;131(3):452–464.
16. Yellon DM, Hearse DJ, Maxwell MP, Chambers DE, Downey JM. Sustained limitation of myocardial necrosis 24 hours after coronary artery occlusion: verapamil infusion in dogs with small myocardial infarcts. *Am J Cardiol.* 1983;51(8):1409–1413.
17. Factor SM, Okun EM, Minase T, Kirk ES. The microcirculation of the human heart: end-capillary loops with discrete perfusion fields. *Circulation.* 1982;66(6):1241–1248.
18. Lee JT, Ideker RE, Reimer KA. Myocardial infarct size and location in relation to the coronary vascular bed at risk in man. *Circulation.* 1981;64(3):526–534.
19. Factor SM, Sonnenblick EH, Kirk ES. The histologic border zone of acute myocardial infarction-islands or peninsulas? *Am J Pathol.* 1978;92(1):111–124.
20. Edwards JE. Correlations in coronary arterial disease. *Bull N Y Acad Med.* 1957;33(3):199–210. discussion, 1-7.
21. Boxt LM, Hsu D, Katz J, Detweiler P, McLaughlin S, Kolb TJ, et al. Estimation of myocardial water content using transverse relaxation time from dual spin-echo magnetic resonance imaging. *Magn Reson Imaging.* 1993;11(3):375–383.
22. Whalen Jr DA, Hamilton DG, Ganote CE, Jennings RB. Effect of a transient period of ischemia on myocardial cells. I. effects on cell volume regulation. *Am J Pathol.* 1974;74(3):381–397.
23. Jennings RB, Schaper J, Hill ML, Steenbergen Jr C, Reimer KA. Effect of reperfusion late in the phase of reversible ischemic injury. Changes in cell volume, electrolytes, metabolites, and ultrastructure. *Circ Res.* 1985;56(2):262–278.
24. Haendchen RV, Corday E, Torres M, Maurer G, Fishbein MC, Meerbaum S. Increased regional end-diastolic wall thickness early after reperfusion: a sign of irreversibly damaged myocardium. *J Am Coll Cardiol.* 1984;3(6):1444–1453.
25. Murphy ML, Peng CF, Kane Jr JJ, Straub KD. Ventricular performance and biochemical alteration of regional ischemic myocardium after reperfusion in the pig. *Am J Cardiol.* 1982;50(4):821–828.
26. Turschner O, D'Hooge J, Dommke C, Claus P, Verbeken E, De Scheerder I, et al. The sequential changes in myocardial thickness and thickening which occur during acute transmural infarction, infarct reperfusion and the resultant expression of reperfusion injury. *Eur Heart J.* 2004;25(9):794–803.
27. Jennings RB, Sommers HM, Kaltenbach JP, West JJ. Electrolyte alterations in acute myocardial ischemic injury. *Circ Res.* 1964;14:260–269.
28. Kim RJ, Judd RM, Chen EL, Fieno DS, Parrish TB, Lima JA. Relationship of elevated 23Na magnetic resonance image intensity to infarct size after acute reperfused myocardial infarction. *Circulation.* 1999;100(2):185–192.
29. Kloner RA, Ganote CE, Whalen Jr DA, Jennings RB. Effect of a transient period of ischemia on myocardial cells. II. fine structure during the first few minutes of reflow. *Am J Pathol.* 1974;74(3):399–422.
30. Rehwald WG, Fieno DS, Chen EL, Kim RJ, Judd RM. Myocardial magnetic resonance imaging contrast agent concentrations after reversible and irreversible ischemic injury. *Circulation.* 2002;105(2):224–229.
31. Kim HW, Van Assche L, Jennings RB, Wince WB, Jensen CJ, Rehwald WG, et al. Relationship of T2-weighted MRI myocardial hyperintensity and the ischemic area-at-risk. *Circ Res.* 2015;117(3):254–265.
32. Reimer KA, Jennings RB. The changing anatomic reference base of evolving myocardial infarction. Underestimation of myocardial collateral blood flow and overestimation of experimental anatomic infarct size due to tissue edema, hemorrhage and acute inflammation. *Circulation.* 1979;60(4):866–876.
33. Fieno DS, Kim RJ, Chen EL, Lomasney JW, Klocke FJ, Judd RM. Contrast-enhanced magnetic resonance imaging of myocardium at risk: distinction between reversible and irreversible injury throughout infarct healing. *J Am Coll Cardiol.* 2000;36(6):1985–1991.
34. Kannel WB, Abbott RD. Incidence and prognosis of unrecognized myocardial infarction. An update on the framingham study. *N Engl J Med.* 1984;311(18):1144–1147.
35. Cox CJ. Return to normal of the electrocardiogram after myocardial infarction. *Lancet.* 1967;1(7501):1194–1197.
36. Uusitupa M, Pyörälä K, Raunio H, Rissanen V, Lampainen E. Sensitivity and specificity of minnesota Code Q-QS abnormalities in the diagnosis of myocardial infarction verified at autopsy. *Am Heart J.* 1983;106(4 Pt 1):753–757.
37. Mahrholdt H, Wagner A, Parker M, Regenfus M, Fieno DS, Bonow RO, et al. Relationship of contractile function to transmural extent of infarction in patients with chronic coronary artery disease. *J Am Coll Cardiol.* 2003;42(3):505–512.
38. Alpert JS, Thygesen K, Antman E, Bassand JP. Myocardial infarction redefined-a consensus document of the joint European society of cardiology/American college of cardiology committee for the redefinition of myocardial infarction. *J Am Coll Cardiol.* 2000;36(3):959–969.
39. Kim HW, Farzaneh-Far A, Kim RJ. Cardiovascular magnetic resonance in patients with myocardial infarction. *J Am Coll Cardiol.* 2009;55(1):1–16.

40. Arroyo LH, Lee RT. Mechanisms of plaque rupture: mechanical and biologic interactions. *Cardiovasc Res*. 1999;41(2):369–375.
41. Topol EJ, Yadav JS. Recognition of the importance of embolization in atherosclerotic vascular disease. *Circulation*. 2000;101(5):570–580.
42. Kim RJ, Shah DJ, Judd RM. How we perform delayed enhancement imaging. *J Cardiovasc Magn Reson*. 2003;5(3):505–514.
43. Simonetti OP, Kim RJ, Fieno DS, Hillenbrand HB, Wu E, Bundy JM, et al. An improved MR imaging technique for the visualization of myocardial infarction. *Radiology*. 2001;218(1):215–223.
44. Kim HW, Rehwald WG, Jenista ER, Wendell DC, Filev P, van Assche L, et al. Dark-blood delayed enhancement cardiac magnetic resonance of myocardial infarction. *JACC Cardiovasc Imaging*. 2018;11(12):1758–1769.
45. Kwong RY, Chan AK, Brown KA, Chan CW, Reynolds HG, Tsang S, et al. Impact of unrecognized myocardial scar detected by cardiac magnetic resonance imaging on event-free survival in patients presenting with signs or symptoms of coronary artery disease. *Circulation*. 2006;113(23):2733–2743.
46. Kim HW, Klem I, Shah DJ, Wu E, Meyers SN, Parker MA, et al. Unrecognized non-Q-wave myocardial infarction: prevalence and prognostic significance in patients with suspected coronary disease. *PLoS Med*. 2009;6(4):e1000057.
47. Barbier CE, Bjerner T, Johansson L, Lind L, Ahlström H. Myocardial scars more frequent than expected: magnetic resonance imaging detects potential risk group. *J Am Coll Cardiol*. 2006;48(4):765–771.
48. Camm AJ, Lüscher TF, Maurer G, Serruys PW. *The ESC Textbook of Cardiovascular Medicine*. Oxford University Press; 2018.
49. Tsao CW, Aday AW, Almarzooq ZI, Anderson CAM, Arora P, Avery CL, et al. Heart disease and stroke statistics-2023 update: a report from the American heart association. *Circulation*. 2023;147(8):e93–e621.
50. Mahrholdt H, Wagner A, Judd RM, Sechtem U, Kim RJ. Delayed enhancement cardiovascular magnetic resonance assessment of non-ischaemic cardiomyopathies. *Eur Heart J*. 2005;26(15):1461–1474.
51. Senthilkumar A, Majmudar MD, Shenoy C, Kim HW, Kim RJ. Identifying the etiology: a systematic approach using delayed-enhancement cardiovascular magnetic resonance. *Heart Fail Clin*. 2009;5(3):349–367. vi.
52. Tamis-Holland JE, Jneid H, Reynolds HR, Agewall S, Brilakis ES, Brown TM, et al. Contemporary diagnosis and management of patients with myocardial infarction in the absence of obstructive coronary artery disease: a scientific statement from the American heart association. *Circulation*. 2019;139(18):e891–e908.
53. Konst RE, Parker M, Bhatti L, Kaolawanich Y, Alenezi F, Elias-Smale SE, et al. Prognostic value of cardiac magnetic resonance imaging in patients with a working diagnosis of MINOCA—an outcome study with up to 10 years of follow-up. *Circulation: Cardiovas Imaging*. 2023;16(8):e014454.
54. Kerensky RA, Wade M, Deedwania P, Boden WE, Pepine CJ. Revisiting the culprit lesion in non-Q-wave myocardial infarction. Results from the VANQWISH trial angiographic core laboratory. *J Am Coll Cardiol*. 2002;39(9):1456–1463.
55. Heitner JF, Senthilkumar A, Harrison JK, Klem I, Sketch Jr MH, Ivanov A, et al. Identifying the infarct-related artery in patients with non-ST-segment-elevation myocardial infarction. *Circ Cardiovasc Interv*. 2019;12(5):e007305.
56. Smulders MW, Kietselaer B, Wildberger JE, Dagnelie PC, Brunner-La Rocca HP, Mingels AMA, et al. Initial imaging-guided strategy versus routine care in patients with non-ST-segment elevation myocardial infarction. *J Am Coll Cardiol*. 2019;74(20):2466–2477.
57. Smulders MW, Bekkers SC, Kim HW, Van Assche LM, Parker MA, Kim RJ. Performance of CMR methods for differentiating acute from chronic MI. *JACC Cardiovasc Imaging*. 2015;8(6):669–679.
58. Tahir E, Sinn M, Bohnen S, Avanesov M, Säring D, Stehning C, et al. Acute versus chronic myocardial infarction: diagnostic accuracy of quantitative native T1 and T2 mapping versus assessment of edema on standard T2-weighted cardiovascular MR images for differentiation. *Radiology*. 2017;285(1):83–91.
59. Kaolawanich Y, Azevedo CF, Kim HW, Jenista ER, Wendell DC, Chen EL, et al. Native T1 mapping for the diagnosis of myocardial fibrosis in patients with chronic myocardial infarction. *JACC, Cardiovasc Imaging*. 2022;15(12):2069–2079.
60. Mahrholdt H, Wagner A, Holly TA, Elliott MD, Bonow RO, Kim RJ, et al. Reproducibility of chronic infarct size measurement by contrast-enhanced magnetic resonance imaging. *Circulation*. 2002;106(18):2322–2327.
61. Wagner A, Mahrholdt H, Thomson L, Hager S, Meinhardt G, Rehwald W, et al. Effects of time, dose, and inversion time for acute myocardial infarct size measurements based on magnetic resonance imaging-delayed contrast enhancement. *J Am Coll Cardiol*. 2006;47(10):2027–2033.
62. Thiele H, Kappl MJ, Conradi S, Niebauer J, Hambrecht R, Schuler G. Reproducibility of chronic and acute infarct size measurement by delayed enhancement-magnetic resonance imaging. *J Am Coll Cardiol*. 2006;47(8):1641–1645.
63. Choi KM, Kim RJ, Gubernikoff G, Vargas JD, Parker M, Judd RM. Transmural extent of acute myocardial infarction predicts long-term improvement in contractile function. *Circulation*. 2001;104(10):1101–1107.
64. Gerber BL, Garot J, Bluemke DA, Wu KC, Lima JA. Accuracy of contrast-enhanced magnetic resonance imaging in predicting improvement of regional myocardial function in patients after acute myocardial infarction. *Circulation*. 2002;106(9):1083–1089.
65. Kim RJ, Wu E, Rafael A, Chen EL, Parker MA, Simonetti O, et al. The use of contrast-enhanced magnetic resonance imaging to identify reversible myocardial dysfunction. *N Engl J Med*. 2000;343(20):1445–1453.
66. Kühl HP, Lipke CS, Krombach GA, Katoh M, Battenberg TF, Nowak B, et al. Assessment of reversible myocardial dysfunction in chronic ischaemic heart disease: comparison of contrast-enhanced cardiovascular magnetic resonance and a combined positron emission tomography-single photon emission computed tomography imaging protocol. *Eur Heart J*. 2006;27(7):846–853.
67. Bello D, Shah DJ, Farah GM, Di Luzio S, Parker M, Johnson MR, et al. Gadolinium cardiovascular magnetic resonance predicts reversible myocardial dysfunction and remodeling in patients with heart failure undergoing beta-blocker therapy. *Circulation*. 2003;108(16):1945–1953.
68. Kloner RA, Ganote CE, Jennings RB. The "no-reflow" phenomenon after temporary coronary occlusion in the dog. *J Clin Investig*. 1974;54(6):1496–1508.
69. Kim RJ, Chen EL, Lima JA, Judd RM. Myocardial Gd-DTPA kinetics determine MRI contrast enhancement and reflect the extent and severity of myocardial injury after acute reperfused infarction. *Circulation*. 1996;94(12):3318–3326.
70. Robbers LF, Eerenberg ES, Teunissen PF, Jansen MF, Hollander MR, Horrevoets AJ, et al. Magnetic resonance imaging-defined areas of microvascular obstruction after acute myocardial infarction represent microvascular destruction and haemorrhage. *Eur Heart J*. 2013;34(30):2346–2353.
71. Ito H, Maruyama A, Iwakura K, Takiuchi S, Masuyama T, Hori M, et al. Clinical implications of the 'no reflow' phenomenon. A predictor of complications and left ventricular remodeling in reperfused anterior wall myocardial infarction. *Circulation*. 1996;93(2):223–228.
72. Morishima I, Sone T, Okumura K, Tsuboi H, Kondo J, Mukawa H, et al. Angiographic no-reflow phenomenon as a predictor of adverse long-term outcome in patients treated with percutaneous transluminal coronary angioplasty for first acute myocardial infarction. *J Am Coll Cardiol*. 2000;36(4):1202–1209.
73. Wu KC, Zerhouni EA, Judd RM, Lugo-Olivieri CH, Barouch LA, Schulman SP, et al. Prognostic significance of microvascular obstruction by magnetic resonance imaging in patients with acute myocardial infarction. *Circulation*. 1998;97(8):765–772.
74. Hombach V, Grebe O, Merkle N, Waldenmaier S, Höher M, Kochs M, et al. Sequelae of acute myocardial infarction regarding cardiac structure and function and their prognostic significance as assessed by magnetic resonance imaging. *Eur Heart J*. 2005;26(6):549–557.
75. Smulders MW, Van Assche LMR, Bekkers SCAM, Nijveldt R, Beijnink CWH, Kim HW, et al. Epicardial surface area of infarction: a stable surrogate of microvascular obstruction in acute myocardial infarction. *Circulation: Cardiovasc Imaging*. 2021:152–162.
76. Multicenter Postinfarction Research Group. Risk stratification and survival after myocardial infarction. *N Engl J Med*. 1983;309(6):331–336.
77. Burns RJ, Gibbons RJ, Yi Q, Roberts RS, Miller TD, Schaer GL, et al. The relationships of left ventricular ejection fraction, end-systolic volume index and infarct size to six-month mortality after hospital discharge following myocardial infarction treated by thrombolysis. *J Am Coll Cardiol*. 2002;39(1):30–36.
78. Roes SD, Kelle S, Kaandorp TA, Kokocinski T, Poldermans D, Lamb HJ, et al. Comparison of myocardial infarct size assessed with contrast-enhanced magnetic resonance imaging and left ventricular function and volumes to predict mortality in patients with healed myocardial infarction. *Am J Cardiol*. 2007;100(6):930–936.
79. Wu E, Ortiz JT, Tejedor P, Lee DC, Bucciarelli-Ducci C, Kansal P, et al. Infarct size by contrast enhanced cardiac magnetic resonance is a stronger predictor of outcomes than left ventricular ejection fraction or end-systolic volume index: prospective cohort study. *Heart*. 2008;94(6):730–736.
80. Kwon DH, Halley CM, Carrigan TP, Zysek V, Popovic ZB, Setser R, et al. Extent of left ventricular scar predicts outcomes in ischemic cardiomyopathy patients with significantly reduced systolic function: a delayed hyperenhancement cardiac magnetic resonance study. *JACC Cardiovasc Imaging*. 2009;2(1):34–44.
81. Stone GW, Selker HP, Thiele H, Patel MR, Udelson JE, Ohman EM, et al. Relationship between infarct size and outcomes following primary PCI: patient-level analysis from 10 randomized trials. *J Am Coll Cardiol*. 2016;67(14):1674–1683.
82. Fieno DS, Hillenbrand HB, Rehwald WG, Harris KR, Decker RS, Parker MA, et al. Infarct resorption, compensatory hypertrophy, and differing patterns of ventricular remodeling following myocardial infarctions of varying size. *J Am Coll Cardiol*. 2004;43(11):2124–2131.
83. Rochitte CE, Lima JA, Bluemke DA, Reeder SB, McVeigh ER, Furuta T, et al. Magnitude and time course of microvascular obstruction and tissue injury after acute myocardial infarction. *Circulation*. 1998;98(10):1006–1014.
84. Sievers B, Elliott MD, Hurwitz LM, Albert TS, Klem I, Rehwald WG, et al. Rapid detection of myocardial infarction by subsecond, free-breathing delayed contrast-enhancement cardiovascular magnetic resonance. *Circulation*. 2007;115(2):236–244.
85. Klem I, Heiberg E, Van Assche L, Parker MA, Kim HW, Grizzard JD, et al. Sources of variability in quantification of cardiovascular magnetic resonance infarct size - reproducibility among three core laboratories. *J Cardiovasc Magn Reson*. 2017;19(1):62.
86. Fleiss JL. *The Design and Analysis of Clinical Experiments*. Wiley; 1986:432. xiv.
87. Gibbons RJ, Valeti US, Araoz PA, Jaffe AS. The quantification of infarct size. *J Am Coll Cardiol*. 2004;44(8):1533–1542.
88. Ortiz-Pérez JT, Meyers SN, Lee DC, Kansal P, Klocke FJ, Holly TA, et al. Angiographic estimates of myocardium at risk during acute myocardial infarction: validation study using cardiac magnetic resonance imaging. *Eur Heart J*. 2007;28(14):1750–1758.
89. Versteylen MO, Bekkers SC, Smulders MW, Winkens B, Mihl C, Winkens MH, et al. Performance of angiographic, electrocardiographic and MRI methods to assess the area at risk in acute myocardial infarction. *Heart*. 2012;98(2):109–115.
90. Kapur NK, Alkhouli MA, DeMartini TJ, Faraz H, George ZH, Goodwin MJ, et al. Unloading the left ventricle before reperfusion in patients with anterior ST-segment–elevation myocardial infarction. *Circulation*. 2019;139(3):337–346.
91. Kim RJ, Lima JA, Chen EL, Reeder SB, Klocke FJ, Zerhouni EA, et al. Fast 23Na magnetic resonance imaging of acute reperfused myocardial infarction. Potential to assess myocardial viability. *Circulation*. 1997;95(7):1877–1885.

23 Myocardial Viability

CÉLESTE CHEVALIER, YODYING KAOLAWANICH, AND RAYMOND J. KIM

BACKGROUND

Dysfunctional Myocardium May Be Viable

The concept that myocardium with impaired contractile function may be viable has been known for decades. Specific physiologic states that can result in dysfunctional, yet viable myocardium are stunning and hibernation. "Myocardial stunning" describes the state of postischemic myocardial dysfunction in the presence of relatively normal blood flow.[1] On light microscopy, stunned myocardium appears normal. However, there is decreased adenosine triphosphate and subtle ultrastructural abnormalities.[2] The mechanism underlying stunning is not completely understood but has been proposed to involve myofilament desensitization to calcium, possibly by initial calcium overload during reperfusion, leading to troponin I proteolysis and/or oxygen radical formation during ischemia–reperfusion damaging the contractile cell membranes. In general, stunned myocardium has been shown to recover function within hours to days, and recovery may take longer in cases of longer ischemic episodes prior to revascularization.[3]

The term "myocardial hibernation" describes the state of chronic myocardial dysfunction at rest that can be partially or completely restored to normal either by improving blood flow and/or by reducing demand.[4] This physiology was first noted when ventricular wall motion abnormalities improved after coronary artery bypass grafting.[5–7] Biopsy specimens from regions of dysfunctional myocardium that recovered function after coronary artery bypass grafting showed that ~90% of the volume consisted of viable cells.[8,9] However, increased glycogen is seen in areas previously occupied by myofilaments, and small mitochondria are present.[10] The mechanism underlying hibernating myocardium is not completely understood but many investigators believe it is due to a chronic reduction in resting coronary blood flow. Others suggest that blood flow is normal in hibernating myocardium, and that the dysfunction results from repetitive episodes of stunning.[10] In contrast to the relatively early recovery of function seen with myocardial stunning, recovery of function has been shown to take up to 1 year after revascularization in myocardial hibernation.[3] Thus, myocardial stunning and hibernation both represent myocardium that is alive (or viable), rather than dead (or nonviable).

Mechanistic Basis of Viability Imaging

The concept that dysfunctional myocardium may be viable is only one of several concepts that connect to form the basis for the clinical use of "viability imaging" (Fig. 23.1). The chain of concepts is straightforward and appears obvious, but it is worthwhile reviewing because—as we will see later in the chapter—many presumed issues with viability imaging are problems that arise because one or more individual concepts are mistakenly assumed to be unimportant. The first concept in the mechanistic basis is that myocardial ischemia from large conduit coronary artery disease (CAD) is the root cause of the problem. The second is that ischemia then leads to resting systolic dysfunction of which, third, much of the dysfunction is secondary to hibernating myocardium rather than infarction. Identification of each of these steps, usually with diagnostic imaging tests, then leads to treatment with revascularization. For this step, revascularization is hopefully complete and sustained, and leads to the final step in which prognosis is improved, usually concomitant with improved symptoms and LV function.

Current Recommendations for Viability Assessment

Guidelines for revascularization are provided by the American College of Cardiology Foundation, American Heart Association (ACCF/AHA), and European Society of Cardiology (ESC).[11,12] In patients with stable ischemic heart disease (SIHD) and poor LV function (LVEF <35%), surgical revascularization is given a Class I recommendation (evidence/agreement that treatment is useful/efficacious) for patients with the following coronary anatomy: (1) significant left main stenosis or (2) multivessel disease.[11] These recommendations are based largely upon data from older randomized trials that focused primarily on the angiographic appearance of CAD and showed benefit in cohorts with anatomically severe disease. These recommendations are essentially unchanged from those published 20 years earlier.[13] However, the older guidelines included other factors such as myocardial viability as part of their recommendations. For example, the ACC/AHA guidelines on coronary artery bypass graft surgery from 2004 and the diagnosis and management of heart failure from 2009 stated that coronary artery bypass graft (CABG) may be performed in SIHD patients with poor LV function and obstructive CAD—in addition to those with the coronary anatomy described above—*if* there is significant viable myocardium (Class IIa recommendation [weight of evidence/opinion is in favor of usefulness/efficacy]).[13,14] Furthermore, CABG was discouraged in patients without evidence of intermittent ischemia and significant viable myocardium (Class III

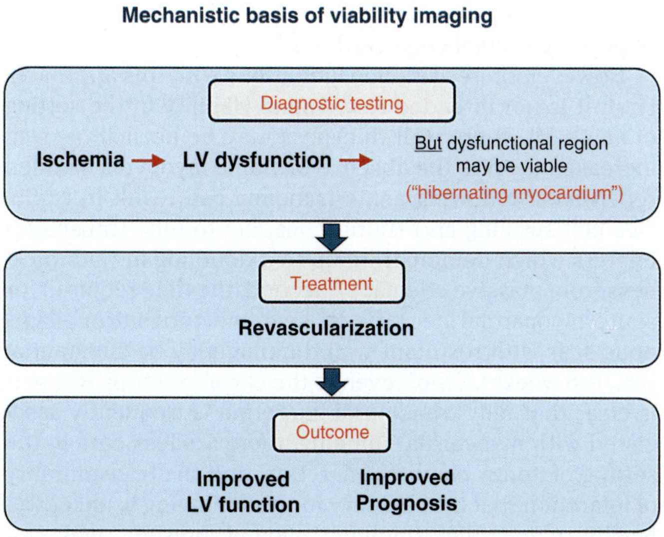

FIG. 23.1 Several concepts connect to form the mechanistic basis of viability imaging. The first concept is that myocardial ischemia, presumably from large conduit vessels, is the root cause of the problem. Second, ischemia results in resting systolic dysfunction. Third, the dysfunction reflects "hibernating myocardium," which is viable rather than infarcted. Treatment with revascularization, which is hopefully complete and sustained, then leads to improved prognosis, typically with improved symptoms and LV function.

recommendation [evidence/agreement that treatment is not useful/efficacious or may be harmful]). As part of a marked change in the guidelines regarding diagnostic imaging, the current versions of these documents from 2021 and 2022 have removed myocardial viability as a factor for consideration in treatment decisions regarding coronary revascularization.

From a mechanistic point-of-view (as described in Fig. 23.1), one would expect that additional information, such as the presence or absence of extensive viable myocardium, could improve patient risk stratification for revascularization. Indeed, multiple observational studies demonstrated improved survival in patients with viability undergoing revascularization compared to those not undergoing revascularization.[15] Allman et al., in a meta-analysis of these older studies involving 3088 patients, concluded that in patients with significant viability (as determined by thallium perfusion imaging, F-18 fluorodeoxyglucose metabolic imaging, or dobutamine echocardiography), revascularization was associated with a 79.6% reduction in annual mortality compared with medical treatment (3.2% vs. 16%, $P<.0001$).[16] Conversely, in patients without viability, mortality rates were similar for revascularization and medical therapy (7.7% vs. 6.2%, P=NS). This meta-analysis, however, has some limitations. First, the individual studies that were included were small, not randomized, and retrospective, leading to potential patient selection bias. Second, the methodology and criteria for defining viability, as well as the treatment regimens, were not standardized among the different studies. Finally, the success and completeness of myocardial revascularization was not investigated by follow-up angiography or stress imaging data in most studies.[15] In part, due to these limitations, the Surgical Treatment for Heart Disease Trial (STICH) was undertaken.[17]

STICH was a randomized, multicenter, nonblinded trial funded by the National Heart, Lung, and Blood Institute.[17] Patients with angiographic documentation of coronary artery disease amenable to surgical revascularization and left ventricular systolic dysfunction (ejection fraction ≤35%) were eligible for enrollment. Exclusion criteria were left main stenosis >50%, cardiogenic shock, myocardial infarction within 3 months, and need for aortic valve surgery. In hypothesis 1, enrolled patients were randomly assigned to receive medical therapy alone or medical therapy plus CABG. In hypothesis 2, enrolled patients were randomly assigned to CABG or CABG and surgical ventricular reconstruction. Between 2002 and 2007, 1212 patients from 99 centers in 22 countries were enrolled in hypothesis 1. The primary endpoint was death from any cause. In the initial design of the STICH trial, viability testing with single-photon emission computed tomography (SPECT) was required. However, this requirement proved to be an impediment to study enrollment. Therefore, the protocol was revised in 2004 to make viability testing optional and the decision to perform the test was left up to the recruiting investigators. In addition, the viability test options were expanded to include SPECT (four separate protocols), dobutamine stress echocardiography (DSE), or both.[18]

Initially, at a median of 4.7 years of follow-up, there was no significant difference in the primary end-point of all-cause mortality between patients with CABG versus medical therapy alone. A subsequent report evaluating long-term outcome at 10 years, however, did show a survival benefit in patients with CABG compared with medical therapy alone.[19] Since CABG was associated with a risk of death within the initial 30 days after randomization that was triple that for medical therapy alone, the authors speculated that the operative risk associated with CABG was offset by a durable effect that translated into increasing clinical benefit to at least 10 years. In the cohort who underwent viability testing (601 patients), however, in contrast to the prior literature the assessment of myocardial viability did not identify patients with a differential survival benefit from CABG either initially[18] or at 10 years of follow-up.[20]

The authors point out that conclusions drawn from the STICH viability substudy are limited by a number of factors.[18] First, slightly less than half of the 1212 patients enrolled in the hypothesis 1 comparison underwent viability testing. Second, patients were not randomized to viability testing, and third, testing could have been performed prior to, on the day of, or after study enrollment. These factors may have led to patient selection/enrollment bias and influenced subsequent clinical decision-making. Additionally, only a small percentage of patients were deemed not to have viable myocardium (19%) which limited the power of the analysis to detect a differential effect of CABG versus medical therapy alone in patients with viability as compared to those without viability. Lastly, the viability testing was limited to SPECT and DSE imaging, and extrapolating these results to other imaging modalities that were not tested in STICH could be problematic.

The REVIVED-BCIS2 (Randomized Evaluation of Vascular Infarction and Ventricular Dysfunction) trial published in 2022 addresses some of the limitations of STICH.[21] It evaluated whether revascularization by percutaneous coronary intervention (PCI) could improve survival in patients with severe ischemic left ventricular systolic dysfunction (LVEF ≤35%) compared with medical therapy alone. The trial enrolled 700 patients with extensive CAD (defined as a British Cardiovascular Intervention Society jeopardy score of ≥6), all of whom were required to demonstrate myocardial viability in at least four dysfunctional myocardial segments (on DSE, CMR, SPECT, or PET). Despite a more selective study design including only patients with viability as defined by protocol and allowing other imaging modalities, the findings were similar to STICH: revascularization in patients with myocardial viability did not reduce the primary endpoint (composite of all-cause mortality or hospitalization for heart failure).

As with STICH, the design of REVIVED has some important limitations which will be discussed later in this chapter. However, STICH and REVIVED are landmark investigations which appear to have answered the question whether viability testing is clinically useful; and it is on the basis of these two trials that the guidelines have removed viability testing as a factor in clinical decision-making. Nonetheless, it is worthwhile to reconsider the question and step through the ramifications of the results of the clinical trials. Do the results of STICH and REVIVED actually mean that the mechanistic basis of viability imaging (Fig. 23.1) is fatally flawed? Is it possible that revascularization of nonviable myocardium provides the same benefit as revascularization of viable myocardium? Or that distinguishing alive from dead myocardium is of no consequence? From a physiological perspective—despite the findings of STICH and REVIVED—these implications appear illogical. Hence, this conundrum shows a clear need to reassess how viability tests are assumed to work and are interpreted. In the following sections we will describe the current techniques used to image myocardial viability and their underlying pathophysiological foundations. We will examine fundamental concepts in viability assessment, and explore what might constitute an "ideal" technique. Based on these considerations we then discuss the possibility that *some* form of viability imaging with *some* form of revascularization in the *correct* cohort may indeed improve patient risk stratification and prognosis.

PHYSIOLOGICAL BASIS OF VIABILITY TESTING

Morphology

Simple morphological characteristics of the left ventricle may provide useful information about viability. For instance, ventricular wall thinning has been used as a marker for the absence of viability based on the hypothesis that a thinned region represents scar tissue and chronic myocardial infarction (MI). Cwajg et al.[22] studied 45 patients with stable CAD and LV dysfunction using echocardiography and concluded that "a simple measurement of end-diastolic wall thickness less than or equal to 6 mm virtually excludes the potential for recovery of function." Similarly, Baer et al.[23] studied 43 patients with chronic MI and LV dysfunction with CMR and concluded that "the depiction of significantly reduced end-diastolic wall thickness [<5.5 mm] excludes a clinically relevant amount of persistent viable myocardium."

However, there are some limitations with this approach. First, it is not intended to examine viability in the setting of acute MI where wall thickness may be normal or even increased despite the absence of viable myocytes. Sudden reperfusion following acute ischemia can result in explosive cell swelling and rupture, leading to fully transmural infarcts which demonstrate up to a doubling in wall thickness from massive edema.[24,25] Second, the time required for acute myocardial necrosis to heal and turn into collagenous scar with resultant wall thinning may be substantial (i.e., 6–8 weeks). Third, even in the chronic setting where it is clear that fully transmural infarction is frequently associated with myocardial thinning, there are less data in the setting of nontransmural infarction, and the transmurality of infarction that is necessary for wall thinning is unknown. Finally, myocardial thinning, even if present, may not always reflect underlying scar tissue. Animal models of acute MI have demonstrated that side-to-side slippage of myocytes plays a fundamental role in infarct expansion, remodeling, and ultimately wall thinning.[26,27] Whether chronic ischemia without infarction might also result in myocyte slippage was not evaluated in these experimental studies. A recent investigation of SIHD patients, however, has shown that up to 20% of regions with myocardial wall thinning have substantial viability (<50% scar) as determined by DE-CMR.[28] Moreover, revascularization of these territories resulted in disappearance of regional wall thinning with a possible mechanism suggested by the documentation that reverse remodeling following revascularization was not accompanied by any change in total LV myocardial mass. The authors postulated that myocyte slippage can also occur in the setting of chronic ischemia without infarction and that this process is reversible following coronary revascularization.

Function

By definition, the presence of contraction or systolic wall thickening in a region demonstrates substantial viable myocardium. However, the converse may not be true. Absent resting contraction does not necessarily mean that the myocardium is dead. Obvious examples of this include the phenomena of myocardial "stunning" and "hibernation," as described earlier in this chapter.

Clinically, dysfunctional but viable myocardium may be differentiated from infarction by assessing contractile reserve, as only viable myocardium will respond to inotropic stimulation by demonstrating enhanced contraction and systolic thickening. Based on this principle, both echocardiography and CMR with dobutamine stimulation have been used to assess contractile reserve and thus viability. In general, both dobutamine stress echocardiography and CMR demonstrate lower sensitivity than specificity for predicting functional improvement.[23,29,30]

The observation that contractile reserve may have relatively modest sensitivity for predicting functional improvement underlines the indirect relationship between contractile reserve and viability. Experimental studies of chronic low-flow ischemia have shown that some viable

Low-dose dobutamine echocardiography for predicting functional recovery after revascularization?

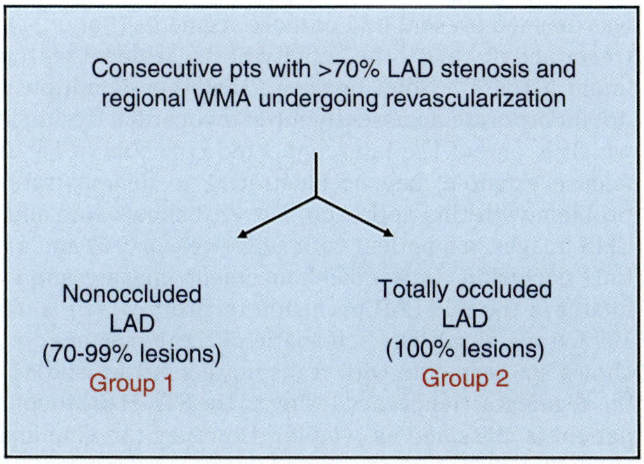

HK and AK segments

	LDDE	
	Group 1	Group 2
Sensitivity	87% (55/63)	52% (36/69) **
Specificity	68% (57/83)	74% (60/81)
Accuracy	77% (112/146)	64% (96/150)*

AK segments

	LDDE	
	Group 1	Group 2
Sensitivity	72% (13/18)	26% (9/34) **
Specificity	94% (46/49)	93% (52/56)
Accuracy	88% (59/67)	68% (61/90)*

*p≤0.01, **p<0.001 Heart 2001;86:679-86

FIG. 23.2 Relationship between limited coronary flow reserve and reduced sensitivity of contractile reserve for predicting functional recovery after coronary revascularization. See text for details. (Table results are adapted from Piscione F, Perrone-Filardi P, De Luca G, et al. Low dose dobutamine echocardiography for predicting functional recovery after coronary revascularisation. *Heart*. 2001;86:679–686.)

regions are so delicately balanced between reductions in flow and function, with exhausted coronary flow reserve, that any inotropic stimulation merely results in ischemia and precludes the ability to enhance contractility.[31] A study by Piscione et al. highlights the importance of this pathophysiology (Fig. 23.2). Consecutive patients with high-grade stenosis (≥70%) of the left anterior descending coronary artery (LAD) and regional ventricular dysfunction were divided into two groups. Group I involved patients with nonoccluded LADs (70%–99% lesions), and group II patients with totally occluded LADs (100% lesions). The authors demonstrated that contractile reserve (as determined by low-dose dobutamine echo) had a much lower sensitivity for predicting functional recovery after revascularization in group II compared with group I patients (52% vs. 87%; $P<.001$). The difference in sensitivity was even greater if the analysis was limited to segments that were akinetic at baseline (26% vs. 72%, $P<.001$), presumably due to worse baseline function reflecting even lower residual coronary flow reserve.[32] These results show that patients who would benefit the most from revascularization—those with the most limited coronary flow reserve subtending viable but dysfunctional myocardium—are, paradoxically, the candidates in whom contractile reserve is most prone to be insensitive in detecting viability.

Perfusion

Myocardial perfusion is related to myocardial viability in that chronic absence of blood flow, of course, is incompatible with viability. However, it is important to recognize that perfusion does not have a direct one-to-one relationship with viability. For example, myocardial ischemia is caused by reduced perfusion, but this pathophysiological state, by definition, requires viable myocardium. Reperfused acute infarction is another pathophysiological state where perfusion and viability are dissociated. The entire infarcted region is by definition nonviable, however, tissue perfusion may range from nearly zero in central regions of the infarct with profound microvascular damage to nearly normal in other regions in which the microvasculature is intact.[33] The heterogeneity of perfusion in reperfused infarction has been demonstrated in humans using contrast echocardiography[34] and measured in animal models using radioactive microspheres.[35] Additionally, the pathophysiology of hibernating myocardium itself suggests a discordance. Although there are some conflicting data, hibernating myocardium, which represents viable tissue, is believed to be due to chronically reduced perfusion. These discrepancies in the relationship between perfusion and viability underscore the potential limitations in utilizing a technique that measures perfusion for assessing viability.

Metabolism and Cell Membrane Integrity

Techniques that examine the metabolic activity or cell membrane integrity of myocytes should provide, at least theoretically, the most direct means for determining whether myocytes are alive or dead. Scintigraphic techniques using positron emission tomography (PET) or single-photon emission computed tomography (SPECT) are examples of such methods.[36] Specifically, preserved glucose metabolism can be examined by F18-fluorodeoxyglucose (FDG) PET, cell membrane integrity by thallium-201 SPECT, and intact mitochondria by technetium-99m sestamibi SPECT. For the latter two techniques, however, myocardial perfusion probably also affects tracer activity to some degree.

Overall, radionuclide techniques demonstrate moderate to good sensitivity (81%–93%) but poor specificity (50%–66%) for predicting functional improvement.[29] In general, SPECT has lower diagnostic accuracy than PET and is more prone to underestimate viability,[37] most likely because of technical limitations such as lower spatial resolution, use of lower energy tracers, and lack of built-in attenuation correction. The poor specificity of both techniques may also relate to technical limitations, however, the use of functional improvement after revascularization as the truth standard for viability may result in an artificially low specificity, as will be discussed later in the chapter.

Delayed-enhancement CMR (DE-CMR) is another technique that can index cell membrane integrity. Although the gadolinium-based contrast media used for DE-CMR is inert and active transport processes across cell membranes such as for thallium are not present, there appears to be a direct but inverse relationship between gadolinium concentration and the percentage of viable myocytes within any given region of myocardial tissue.[38] The mechanism is likely based on the following: first, tissue volume in normal myocardium is predominantly intracellular (75%–80% of the water space[39]); and second, currently available gadolinium contrast media are "extracellular" agents since they do not cross cell membranes.[40] Thus, the volume of distribution of gadolinium contrast in normal myocardium is quite small (~20% of water space), and one can consider viable myocytes as actively excluding contrast media.[41] Pathophysiological states which result in a reduced density of viable myocytes will then have increased volume of distribution of gadolinium and higher concentration.[38] Note that this mechanism is independent of the cause or etiology for nonviable myocardium. Whether the tissue consists of contraction-band necrosis in the setting of acute MI, collagenous scar in chronic MI, or fibrosis in various nonischemic cardiomyopathies, the region will have increased gadolinium concentration if there is a reduced density of viable myocytes.[41] DE-CMR has been shown to be highly effective in identifying the presence, location, and extent of myocardial infarction in both the acute and chronic settings in both animal and human studies.[38,42–45] Additionally, it has been used to predict reversible myocardial dysfunction in those undergoing revascularization procedures.[46–48]

Recently the delayed-enhancement concept has been extended to MDCT. The interpretation of contrast-enhancement patterns on MDCT appears quite similar to that for DE-CMR, and is likely based on the same underlying mechanism since the iodinated contrast media used for MDCT has nearly identical pharmacokinetics as that of "extracellular" gadolinium contrast.[49] Likewise, in animal models, delayed-enhancement MDCT assessment of acute and chronic MI has been shown to accurately reflect true infarct size and morphology as determined by histopathology.[50] Although currently there are few studies in humans,[49,51] these initial studies have demonstrated an excellent agreement between delayed-enhancement MDCT and CMR, albeit with reduced contrast-to-noise ratio and image quality for MDCT.[49]

PROBLEMS WITH CLINICAL DEFINITIONS OF VIABILITY

Viability Without Dysfunction

We have discussed the mechanistic basis of viability imaging which depends on several interconnected concepts (Fig. 23.1). Unfortunately, however, clinical trials utilizing viability imaging often apply simplified criteria for determining "viability" and disregard one or more individual concepts. Consider the STICH viability substudy in which nuclear imaging accounted for the majority of viability scans (471 patients, 78%). On a per-patient basis, viability was deemed present if 11 or more segments (out of 17) had tracer activity ≥50% the activity of the segment with maximum activity.[18] Note, however, that this definition does not incorporate an assessment of myocardial dysfunction, which is one of the interconnected concepts in Fig. 23.1. A case example may be illustrative to demonstrate the problem with this approach. Fig. 23.3 shows cine and DE-CMR images in a patient with single-vessel CAD and a mid-LAD occlusion. Delayed-enhancement imaging shows an infarct in the mid-LAD perfusion territory which is nearly 100% transmural. The schematic of the 17-segment model shows six segments with transmural scarring and 11 viable segments. Hence, according to the STICH protocol, this patient is classified as "viable." However, the cine images show that all viable regions had normal wall motion, which means that there were *zero* dysfunctional but viable segments. Consequently, following revascularization there was no improvement in wall motion because all dysfunctional segments are not viable and all viable segments are not dysfunctional. Additionally, we would expect no improvement in prognosis because in addition to no change in contractile function there were no myocardial regions with ischemia that were alleviated in this patient. To summarize the problem, the fact that this patient is labeled as "viable" and follow-up shows no benefit with revascularization should not be used as evidence that viability imaging in general doesn't work, but rather that simplified definitions of viability can be highly problematic.

Intermediate Levels of Viability

Viability testing is thought to be less helpful when intermediate levels of viability are measured (i.e., levels of viability that result in only approximately 50% of these regions recovering function after revascularization). This view is a result of two misconceptions regarding functional recovery. First, it is important to distinguish between what would be desirable clinically from what can actually occur physiologically. While we may ask for an improved technique with better predictive value, perhaps in reality we are asking for a different physiological relationship—an abrupt threshold of viability, below which there is virtually no chance for functional recovery, and above which nearly all have functional recovery. Fig. 23.4A demonstrates that with an abrupt threshold, the problem of predicting an intermediate likelihood for functional recovery is greatly minimized. Unfortunately, this relationship is physiologically implausible. There is no reason to suspect that a small change in the level of viability from just above to just below the threshold (e.g., going from 51% to 49%) would result in the chance of functional recovery abruptly changing from nearly 100% to nearly zero. Far more physiologic would be a smooth linear relationship between the amount of viability and the likelihood of functional recovery.

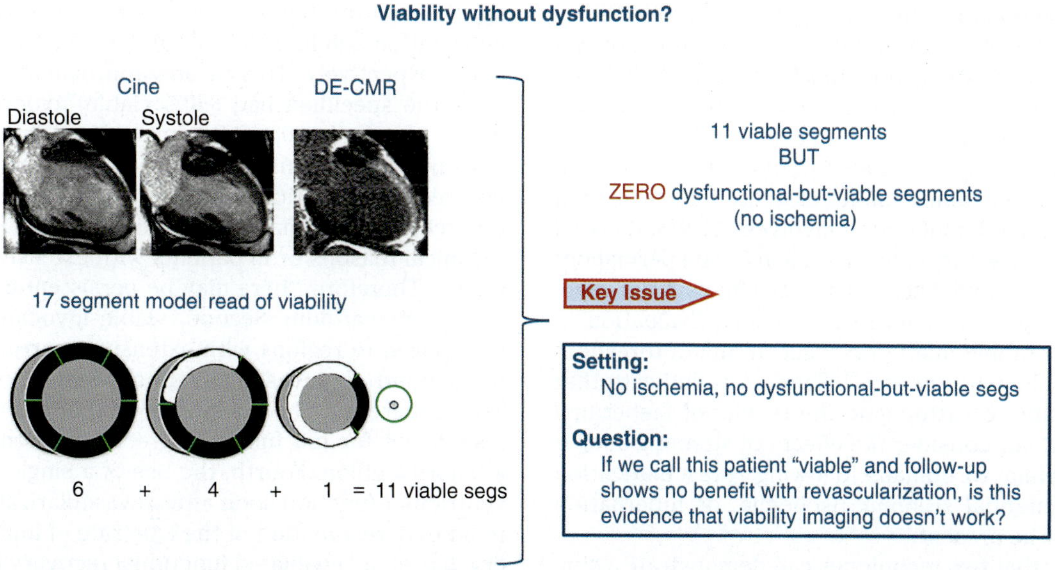

FIG. 23.3 Case example demonstrating the problem with a simplified definition of viability that does not incorporate an assessment of myocardial dysfunction. Cine and DE-CMR images in a patient with single-vessel CAD and a mid-LAD occlusion. Delayed-enhancement imaging shows an infarct in the mid-LAD perfusion territory which is nearly 100% transmural. The schematic of the 17-segment model shows six segments with transmural scarring (*white*) and 11 viable (*black*) segments. See text for details.

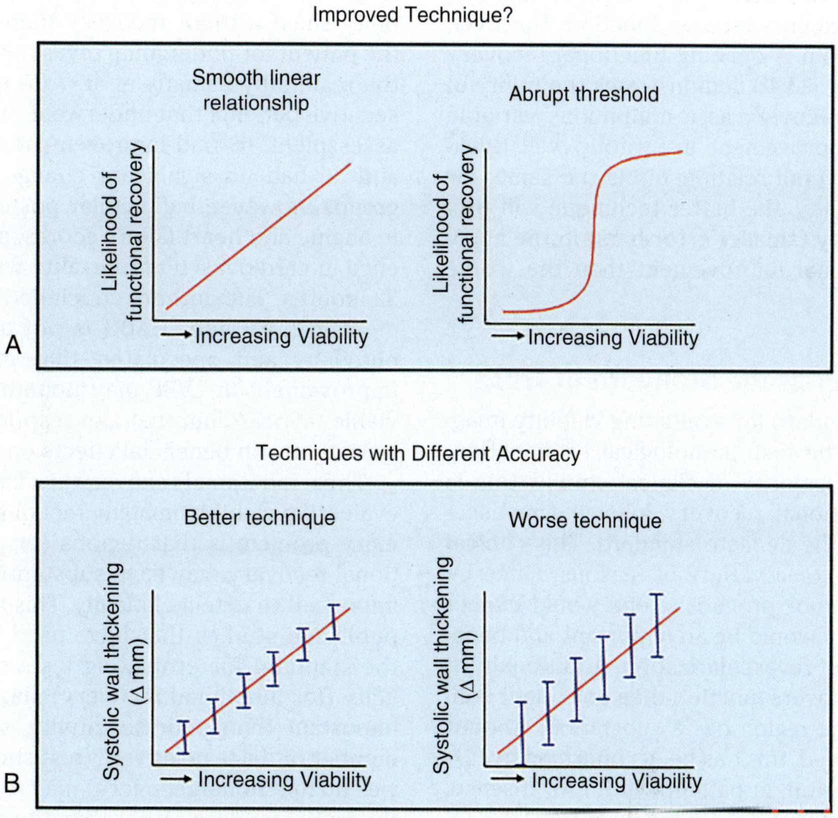

FIG. 23.4 Assumptions in evaluating viability techniques. (A) A technique that demonstrates a smooth linear relationship between viability and functional recovery may be considered limited in that intermediate levels of viability predict intermediate likelihood for functional recovery. With an abrupt threshold relationship between viability and functional recovery, the problem of predicting intermediate likelihood for functional recovery is greatly minimized. See text for details. (B) Two techniques with different diagnostic capability may show a similar overall relationship between viability and functional improvement. However, if functional improvement is expressed as a continuous rather than binary variable, the better technique may reduce the variability (*smaller error bars*) in predicting the absolute amount of functional improvement.

Second, it is essential to remember that functional recovery is a continuum (as is viability itself), and not simply a binary—yes or no—function. Thus, part of the problem with intermediate levels of viability is expecting that these regions will or will not have functional recovery in this binary fashion. Since it more closely reflects reality, it would be better to consider most regions with *intermediate* levels of viability as having a high chance for an *intermediate* amount of improvement rather than 50% likely to have complete recovery and the other 50% no improvement whatsoever. Complicating this issue is the belief that a threshold phenomenon exists between the transmural extent of infarction and systolic thickening. This assumption is based primarily on results by Lieberman et al.[52] who demonstrated in a canine model of acute infarction that akinesia is expected if infarction involves ≥20% of the wall thickness. However, the animal model involved permanent coronary ligation and likely included effects from myocardial stunning and/or ongoing ischemia. Evaluation in humans with chronic infarction suggests that a threshold phenomenon does not exist.[53,54] These data indicate that it is problematic to extrapolate the results of Lieberman et al., who did not consider the effects of stunning and/or ongoing ischemia, to humans following revascularization in whom substantial stunning, ischemia, or hibernation may no longer be present.

The finding that two techniques can demonstrate a similar linear relationship between the amount of viability and the likelihood of functional recovery does not mean that the techniques have the same diagnostic capability. For example, both an accurate and a less accurate technique may show that for a given intermediate level of viability, on average, 50% of segments recover function. However, part of the problem again is defining functional recovery as a binary variable. Fig. 23.4B demonstrates the utility of expressing functional recovery as a continuous variable (e.g., millimeters of improvement in systolic wall thickening). Although the overall relationship is the same, for any given level of viability, the better technique will provide a smaller variability (smaller error bars) in the absolute amount of functional improvement than the worse technique.

Functional Recovery as the Standard of Truth

The ideal reference standard for evaluating viability imaging techniques would be histopathological examination. However, for the vast majority of clinical studies this is not feasible, and functional recovery following revascularization has become the de facto standard. This clinical endpoint makes sense for a variety of reasons. Since LV dysfunction portends poor prognosis, one would expect that functional recovery would be an important and beneficial clinical outcome of revascularization. Additionally, if a myocardial region recovers function then one might confidently assume that the region has a substantial amount of viable myocytes. Indeed, this has been confirmed by histopathological examination. In patients with LAD disease, Maes et al.[9] took transmural needle biopsies from the LV anterior wall during CABG. The biopsies from regions that were dysfunctional prior to revascularization but recovered afterwards showed that 89 ± 6% of the volume consisted of viable cells. Similarly, Dakik et al.[8] reported that among biopsied dyssynergic myocardial segments, those which recovered function after CABG had 93 ± 4% viability by volume.

However, a common misconception is that if a region does not have functional improvement then this region is nonviable. In fact, Maes[9] and Dakik[8] observed that biopsy specimens from regions that did not improve after revascularization still had 65 ± 25% and 69 ± 21% viability by volume, respectively. This means approximately 70% of the time, the specimen had >50% viable myocytes, and 16% of the time had >90% viable myocytes. There are several reasons why regions that are predominantly viable may not recover function following revascularization. First, revascularization may often be incomplete, either due to technical reasons or in patients with extensive atherosclerosis.[55] Therefore, there may be persistent areas of hibernating myocardium. Second, viable myocardium may be juxtaposed to regions with extensive scarring and unable to respond to revascularization because of tethering.[56] Third, there may be substantial viability but the level is insufficient for full functional recovery as determined in a binary fashion. Fourth, the use of a single evaluation of ventricular function soon after revascularization may lead to an underestimation of the true rate of functional recovery. Bax et al.[3] evaluated functional recovery in 26 patients at 3 and 14 months following CABG. At 3 months, only 31% of hibernating segments recovered, whereas at 14 months an additional 61% recovered.

Even with these limitations, one could argue that functional recovery is an appropriate truth standard for viability since without recovery there may be no benefit to the patient for undergoing revascularization. On this point, the results by Samady et al.[57] are instructive. Of 104 consecutive patients that underwent pre- and post-CABG LVEF assessment, 68 had improvement in LVEF (>5% increase) and 36 had no significant change. Surprisingly, the two groups, however, had similar postoperative improvement in angina and heart failure scores, and there was no difference in cardiovascular mortality with a mean follow-up of 32 months. The authors concluded that a lack of improvement in LVEF after CABG is not associated with poorer outcome, and speculated that many patients without improvement in LVEF may nonetheless have substantial viable myocardium that can respond to effective revascularization with beneficial effects on prognosis.

Thus, functional recovery is a flawed truth standard for evaluating viability imaging techniques (Fig. 23.5). The primary problem is that regions (or patients) without functional recovery may have substantial viability that may be important to detect clinically. This has implications for the published studies that have used functional recovery as the standard for evaluating tests of viability. Poor specificity (for functional recovery) should be considered less important than poor sensitivity, since for the former, a number of "false positives" (test showed viability but there was no functional recovery) may represent a problem with the truth standard rather than the technique.

THE "IDEAL" TECHNIQUE

Knowing How Much is Alive is Not Enough

A useful exercise is to consider what might constitute an "ideal" technique for assessing viability. Certainly, it would be important for the technique to be fast, safe, and provide reproducible results. However, what might not be so apparent is that even if a technique were available that could

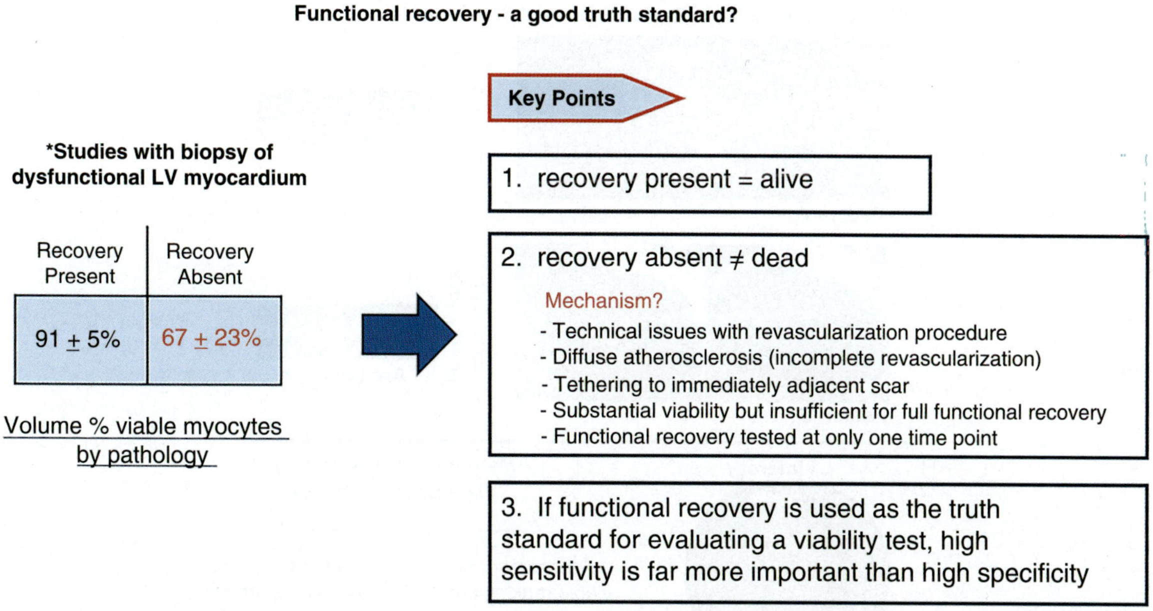

FIG. 23.5 Functional recovery is a flawed truth standard for defining myocardial viability. Pathology data show that myocardial biopsy specimens from regions that do not improve after revascularization can often have substantial viability. A variety of potential mechanisms for why viable regions do not recover function have been postulated. See text for further details. (*Data from Maes, A, et al., Histological alterations in chronically hypoperfused myocardium. Correlation with PET findings. *Circulation*. 1994;90(2):735–745 and Dakik, H.A, et al., Assessment of myocardial viability with ^{99m}Tc-Sestamibi tomography before coronary bypass graft surgery. *Circulation*. 1997:96(9):2892–2898.)

offer precise quantification of viability without technical limitations (infinite spatial resolution, no artifacts, etc.), this would still be insufficient to provide a complete characterization of viability and thus insufficient to provide the highest accuracy in predicting wall motion improvement or clinical benefit after coronary revascularization.[58] Certainly, there are additional factors that are not related to limitations in noninvasive testing that could reduce accuracy in predicting functional improvement. These have been well described and include peri- or postoperative occult MI,[59] and incomplete revascularization as a result of diffuse disease.[55] For the purposes of this section we will not consider these clinical factors, but instead focus on issues related to the noninvasive assessment of viability and examine the concept that "*knowing how much is alive is not enough*."

A central tenet of this concept is that a technique that offers even a perfect assessment of what is alive (viable) has substantial and practical limitations compared with a technique that offers both an assessment of what is alive *and* what is dead (nonviable). This tenet may be counterintuitive, since it would seem that by knowing exactly how much is alive, by deductive logic, one should know how much is dead. However, this is incorrect, and the patient examples in Fig. 23.6A may be illustrative.

The left panel in the top row (Patient A) shows a midventricular, short-axis DE-CMR image of a normal heart in diastole. With DE-CMR, nonviable regions such as infarction appear bright (hyperenhanced), whereas viable regions appear black. First, consider only a "nonviability" or bright region assessment. A quick visual inspection shows no evidence of myocardial bright regions, thus one rapidly concludes that no infarction is present. In comparison, now consider only a "viability" or black region assessment. One can trace the endocardial and epicardial borders of viable myocardium (center panel), and then plot the transmural extent of viability as a function of position starting from the anterior wall at 12 o'clock and moving counterclockwise around the LV (right panel). From the plot, it is obvious that there is marked heterogeneity in the transmural extent of viability, with as much as 12 mm of viable myocardium in the portion of the inferior wall adjacent to the posterior papillary muscle and as little as 7 mm in the anteroseptal wall at the RV insertion site. Concerning this finding, it is important to note that it has been long known that there can be significant variation in diastolic wall thickness at different points around the LV, even if papillary muscles are excluded and healthy volunteers are studied.[60] This observation then naturally proceeds to the conclusion that there can be significant variability in the transmural extent of viable myocardium at different locations of the normal LV, as was found in Patient A.

The principle that normal hearts can have significant heterogeneity in the extent of viable myocardium has direct clinical implications. For example, a region with 70% the viability of the region with the maximum amount of viability may represent either a normal region with 70% the wall thickness of the thickest region or a region with a subendocardial MI. The images from Patient B (Fig. 23.6A) underscore this concept. This particular patient had a clinically documented MI due to occlusion of the right coronary artery (RCA) which was reopened during primary angioplasty. Again, consider first only a "nonviability" assessment. From a quick visual perusal (left panel), one can determine that there is a subendocardial bright region in the inferoseptal wall consistent with the patient's prior MI in the RCA perfusion territory. Next, consider only a "viability" assessment, similar to that performed in Patient A. Again, endocardial and epicardial contours are traced (center panel), however, one difference should be noted. The

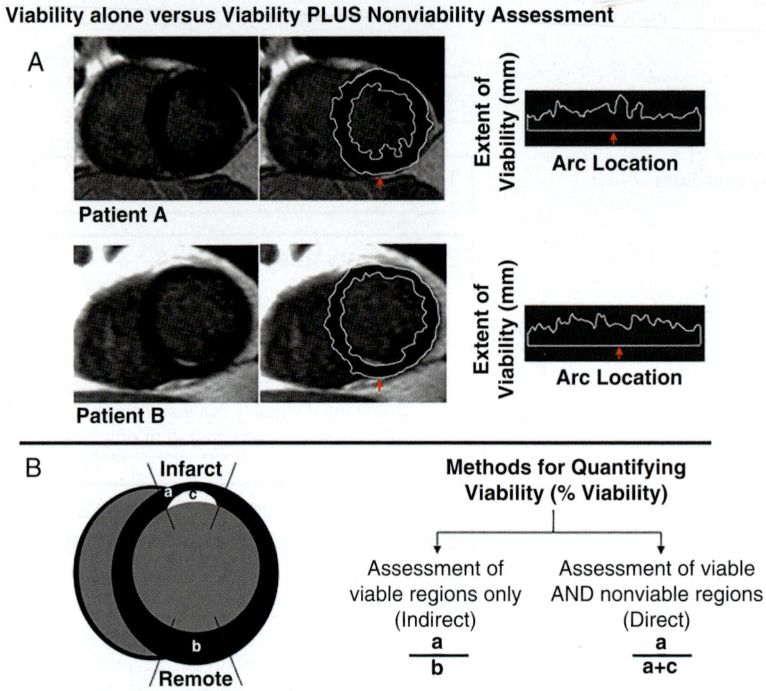

FIG. 23.6 (A) Left panels show delayed-enhancement images of a normal subject (Patient A) and a patient with a subendocardial, inferior wall MI (Patient B). The center panels show tracing of the borders of viable myocardium. The right panels plot the extent of viability (*thickness*) as a function of LV location. Note that there is significant regional variation in the extent of viable myocardium. See text for details. (B) Cartoon highlighting differences between an indirect and direct method of quantifying regional viability. The indirect method is based on assessment of viable regions only. The direct method is based on assessment of viable and nonviable regions. Viable myocardium is black, and infarct is white. "Remote" zone represents segment with maximum amount of viability. (Adapted from Kim, R.J. and D.J. Shah, Fundamental concepts in myocardial viability assessment revisited: when knowing how much is "alive" is not enough. *Heart*. 2004;90(2):137–140.)

endocardial contour is along the border of viable (black) myocardium, and the infarcted region is not included. The plot showing the extent of viable myocardium (right panel) once more shows marked regional variability, and from this assessment the presence and location of infarction are not evident. Thus, in this patient, the intrinsic variation in the extent of viable myocardium for noninfarcted regions is greater than the reduction in viable myocardium for the region with subendocardial infarction. This renders the subendocardial infarction "invisible" for any technique that can assess only viable myocardium, even if the technique has perfect accuracy and infinite spatial resolution.

These two patient examples highlight the differences between techniques that can visualize only viable myocardium as opposed to techniques that can visualize viable and nonviable myocardium. Additionally, it is important to recognize that the use of different techniques often lead to differences in the way in which viability is quantified although the nomenclature used may be the same. For instance, when only viable myocardium can be visualized, the percentage of viability in any given segment is assessed indirectly and generally refers to the amount of viability in the segment normalized to the segment with the maximum amount of viability or to data from a gender-specific database of controls. Conversely, when both viable and nonviable myocardium can be visualized, the percentage of viability can be assessed directly and expressed as the amount of viability in the segment normalized to the amount of viability plus infarction in the same segment (Fig. 23.6B). These differences in the way in which viability is measured can alter the clinical interpretation. For the normal heart in Patient A, the indirect method would show that there is significant regional variability in the extent of viable myocardium: 60%–100% of maximum viability; whereas, the direct method would show essentially no variability since all segments would be classified as 100% viable. Likewise for Patient B, the indirect method would not be able to identify the region of subendocardial infarction since the extent of viable myocardium in this sector is within the normal variation; whereas, the direct method would clearly identify the region with subendocardial infarction since this region would be the only region with less than 100% viable myocardium.

These patient examples also clarify the mechanism by which subendocardial infarcts are routinely missed by techniques such as SPECT and PET (Fig. 23.7).[61–63] Although it is often reported that limited spatial resolution is the reason, it should be evident that even infinite spatial resolution would not improve the detection of subendocardial infarction by these or other methodologies based on assessing only viable myocardium. Conversely, a methodology with poor spatial resolution (e.g., a single voxel across the LV wall) would still be able to detect subendocardial infarction if it had the ability to assess both alive and dead tissue.

Is "Thinned" Myocardium Always Dead?

As discussed earlier in the chapter, prior studies report that in patients with coronary disease and LV dysfunction, regions with thinned myocardium represent scar tissue and cannot improve in contractile function after

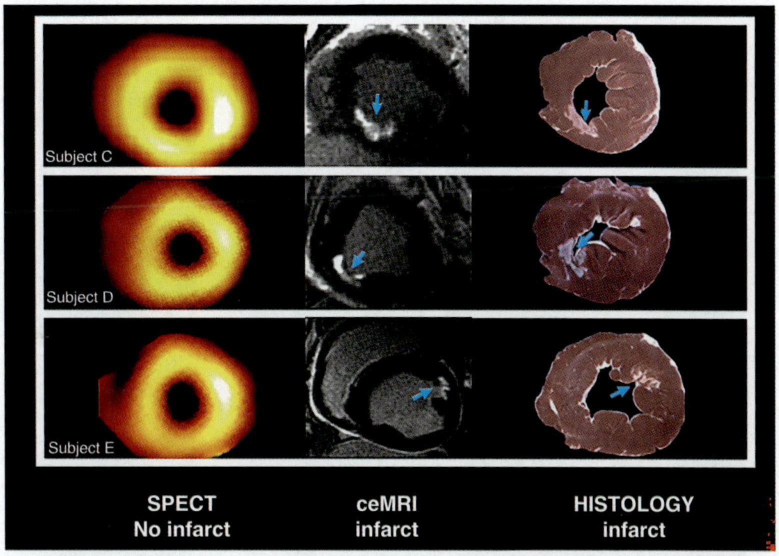

FIG. 23.7 Comparison of a method that indexes cell membrane integrity and detects only viable myocardium (SPECT) and a method that indexes cell membrane integrity and detects both viable and nonviable myocardium (DE-CMR) with histology in three canines with subendocardial infarcts (*arrows*). Note that the infarcts are not evident on SPECT. (Reprinted with permission from Elsevier, Wagner A., et al., Contrast-enhanced MRI and routine single photon emission computed tomography (SPECT) perfusion imaging for detection of subendocardial myocardial infarcts: an imaging study. *Lancet*. 2003;361(9355):374–379.)

revascularization.[22] Some recent observations refute this concept.[28] Fig. 23.8 shows CMR images of two patients (C and D) who have severe CAD and chronic LV dysfunction. The left panels represent long-axis views acquired before coronary revascularization, and two points should be noted on the cine images. First, both patients have severe contractile dysfunction of the anterior wall. Second, Patient D has associated thinning of the anterior wall (diastolic wall thickness, 5.0 mm) while Patient C does not (diastolic wall thickness, 8.0 mm). Based on these cine images and the existing literature, one might expect that there is more viable myocardium in the anterior wall of Patient C than in Patient D, and in fact, question the need for viability testing at all in Patient D since the thinned, akinetic anterior wall must undoubtedly be scar tissue and thus nonviable. The DE-CMR images acquired before revascularization, however, indicate a different clinical interpretation. In Patient C, there is a bright endocardial rim of hyperenhancement (infarction) that measures on average 4.5 mm in thickness. The remaining epicardial rim of tissue, which is black (viable), measures 3.5 mm in thickness (total thickness, 8 mm). In Patient D, there is also an endocardial rim of hyperenhancement, however, it measures on average only 1.5 mm in thickness. The epicardial rim, which is viable, measures 3.5 mm in thickness (total thickness, 5 mm). Note that in both patients the absolute amount of viable myocardium is the same (3.5 mm), however, when the extent of viability is expressed as a percentage of the total amount of myocardium in the segment, Patient C has less than 50% viable myocardium (3.5/8 = 44%), whereas Patient D has greater than 50% viable myocardium (3.5/5 = 70%). The right-most panels represent cine images acquired 2 months after coronary revascularization. Patient C exhibits no improvement in contractile function in the anterior wall and in fact develops diastolic wall thinning in this region. Conversely, Patient D exhibits not only a significant improvement in anterior wall contractile function, but also recovery of diastolic wall thickness in this region (from 5 to 9 mm).

Three fundamental points are raised by these patient examples. First, it is apparent that a method that can quantify only viable myocardium, even if technically flawless (infinite spatial resolution, no artifacts, etc.), provides insufficient information to allow a comprehensive assessment of myocardial viability. Since both patients had the same, reduced amount of viable myocardium (3.5 mm thick) we would have predicted, incorrectly as it turns out, that both patients would not improve in contractile function following revascularization. Second, it is evident that the absolute amount of viable myocardium in a given region is dynamic and can increase or decrease as a result of ventricular remodeling. Whereas it is common knowledge that myocardial viability can decrease, for example, due to MI with associated wall thinning, the reverse process in which regions of thin myocardium become thick with an absolute increase in the transmural extent of viability (as in patient D) has only recently been described. Third, it appears that quantification of nonviable in addition to viable myocardium is important in predicting contractile improvement following revascularization. For instance, incorporating information regarding nonviable myocardium into a ratio of viable to total myocardium (viable plus nonviable) within the same region would lead to the conclusion that the anterior wall of Patient D has a higher percentage of viable myocardium (70%) than Patient C (44%) and thus is more likely to improve in contractile function. The follow-up cine images in Fig. 23.4 demonstrate that this prediction is correct. Patient example D indicates that wall thinning should not be equated with the absence of viability. In some patients, such as Patient D, these regions can improve after revascularization. An investigation systematically evaluating these concepts has recently been reported. Shah et al. studied 1055 patients with CAD referred for DE-CMR at three sites and found that 201 (19%) had regional wall thinning. Limited scar burden was present in 18% of thinned regions and was

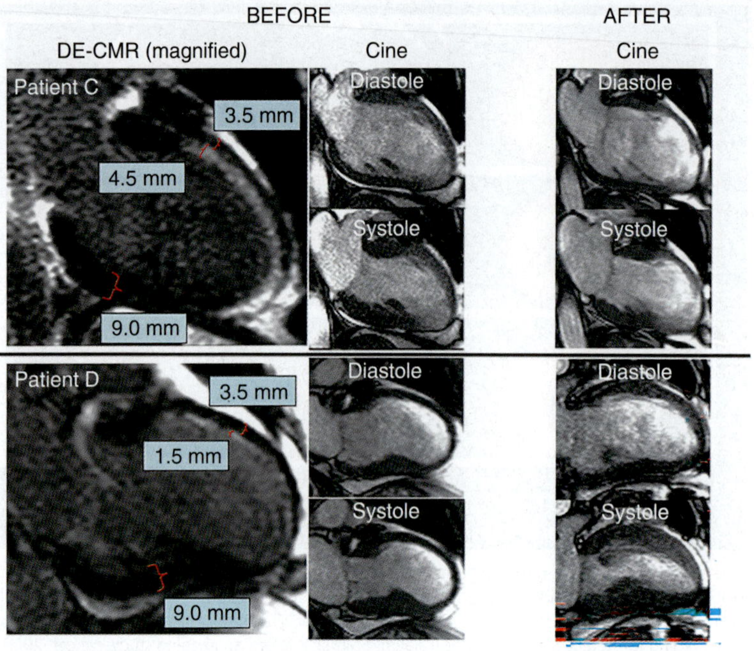

FIG. 23.8 Delayed-enhancement and cine CMR images of two patients (C and D) before coronary revascularization and cine images 2 months after revascularization. See text for details. (From Kim, R.J. and D.J. Shah, Fundamental concepts in myocardial viability assessment revisited: when knowing how much is "alive" is not enough. *Heart*. 2004;90(2):137–140.)

associated with improved contractility and resolution of wall thinning after revascularization.[28]

Viability Without Ischemia

The first concept in the chain of concepts that form the mechanistic basis of viability imaging is that myocardial ischemia is the root cause of the problem (Fig. 23.1). The presence of coronary lesions does not mean that ischemia is present, and of course without ischemia, there is no need for revascularization. For the STICH viability substudy, we have discussed that patients underwent nuclear imaging or DSE. For nuclear imaging, four separate protocols were allowed—thallium imaging using a rest–redistribution or stress–rest–reinjection protocol, rest–redistribution thallium imaging as part of a dual-isotope protocol with a technetium-99m perfusion tracer, or imaging with a technetium-99m tracer at rest after the administration of nitroglycerin[18]—of which three did not involve the detection of ischemia. For DSE, there are responses to incremental doses of dobutamine that are consistent with the interpretation of ischemia (i.e., biphasic response, worsening contractility) as opposed to demonstrating viability without ischemia (i.e., sustained improvement). In STICH, the interpretation of DSE did not require the presence of ischemia to classify a patient as "viable," similar to that for nuclear imaging. Fig. 23.9 shows a case example which illustrates the problem with this approach. The patient presented with chest pain and had a 70% mid-LAD lesion on x-ray coronary angiography, along with global LV dysfunction (LVEF of 30%) on echocardiography. DSE demonstrated sustained contractile improvement globally throughout the LV, hence the patient was deemed "viable." DE-CMR also revealed substantial viability throughout the LV. However, in addition, there was a thin striae of midwall scarring in the basal septum. This is a non-CAD-type scar pattern that is typically found in idiopathic dilated cardiomyopathy. Therefore, the LV dysfunction found in this patient was likely nonischemic in etiology and the CAD found on coronary angiography incidental. This case raises the following question: If we classify this patient as "viable" based on DSE, and follow-up shows no improvement in LV function (or clinical status) after revascularization, does that mean that viability imaging doesn't work? Or rather that in many patients, the initial step of assessment for ischemia may be a required component of "viability imaging."

VIABILITY TESTING AND PROGNOSIS

STICH Revisited

As discussed earlier, the results from recent multicenter clinical trials do not support the use of viability assessment to guide revascularization. While the STICH trial reported better outcomes with CABG than with medical therapy, the advantage of CABG over medical therapy was independent of the results of viability testing. We have shown that the definitions of viability used by STICH—which are simplistic and incomplete (see Figs. 23.4 and 23.9)—are possibly a mitigating factor. In this section, we underscore another important issue related to the statistical design of the STICH viability substudy. Commentators have often remarked that the group of patients deemed as "nonviable" was especially small (114 patients), which may limit the power of the study.[64] However, the sample size alone does not portray the full extent of the problem. In this situation, it is important to examine what might be expected in patients *with* viability separately from those *without* viability. In the Allman et al. meta-analysis of studies performed pre-STICH, revascularization reduced the

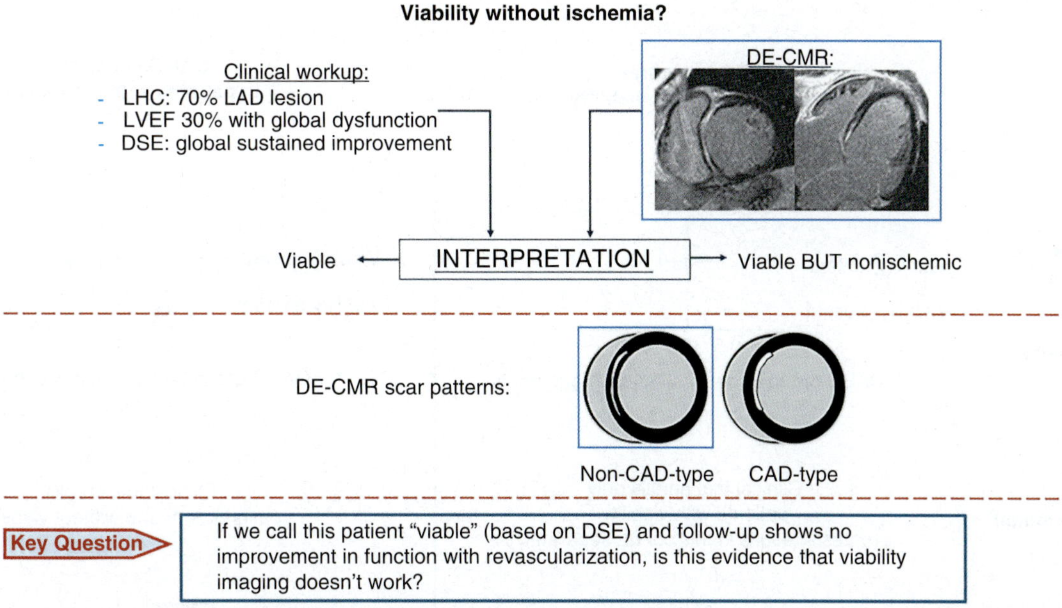

FIG. 23.9 Case example demonstrating the problem with a simplified definition of viability that does not incorporate an assessment of myocardial ischemia. Patient presented with chest pain and a 70% mid-LAD lesion found on x-ray coronary angiography. Dobutamine stress echocardiography (DSE) demonstrated sustained contractile improvement globally throughout the LV, hence the patient is deemed "viable." DE-CMR confirmed substantial viability (black myocardium), but also demonstrated a non-CAD-type scar pattern (midwall scarring in the basal septum). Hence, this patient has nonischemic cardiomyopathy and revascularization is unlikely to improve function.

death rate in patients with viable myocardium by 79.6% ($P<.0001$), whereas there was no significant difference in mortality in patients without viable myocardium ($P=.23$). The expectation then is that for viability testing to be shown as useful, a large clinical trial needs to show that revascularization improves outcome in patients with viable myocardium. If this is demonstrated, what happens in "nonviable" patients is partially a separate issue. Whether revascularization is neutral (which is expected from the results of Allman et al.[16]) or harmful in "nonviable" patients should not be used to affect the value of viability imaging in patients deemed to be "viable."

Fig. 23.10A reiterates the expected findings of viability testing from the pre-STICH historical data. Namely, in patients with viability, CABG should result in better outcome compared with medical therapy alone (i.e., mean hazard ratio [HR] with 95% confidence intervals [CI] all less than 1.0), whereas in patients without viability, CABG should be neutral compared with medical therapy (i.e., HR 95% CI includes 1.0). Accordingly, a clinical trial assessing the utility of viability imaging should only enroll patients with viability (or test the results in this cohort separately), and the statistical model would be simple, with CABG as the single independent variable (Fig. 23.10B).

Revisiting the 10-year results of STICH (Fig. 23.11), we highlight that the findings appear to match what would be expected based on the pre-STICH data, namely that CABG was beneficial in patients with viability while it was neutral for those without. Specifically, for the primary endpoint of all-cause mortality (left-most panel), in patients with viability, the mean HR with 95% CI were all less than 1.0 (HR 0.70 CI [0.56–0.88]), and in patients without viability, the HR 95% CI included 1.0 (HR 0.81 CI [0.50–1.31]). For the secondary endpoints of cardiovascular mortality and a composite of all-cause mortality or hospitalization for cardiovascular causes, the results were identical: CABG was beneficial in patients with viability while it was neutral in those without.

So why was the final conclusion of the study that viable myocardium is not associated with a long-term beneficial effect of CABG? To answer this question, it is helpful to explore the statistical model employed by STICH.[18,20] They used a Cox regression model testing the interaction between treatment assignment (CABG vs. medical therapy) and viability status (Fig. 23.10B shows a logistic regression model, excluding the effects of time, for simplicity). The interaction quantifies the "difference-in-differences" in outcome among the four groups. This means that whether CABG was neutral versus harmful in patients without viability affects the strength of the interaction. Specifically, if CABG is neutral, the significance of the interaction is appreciably reduced. Additionally, testing for an interaction is known to severely reduce statistical power. For instance, the sample size required to detect an interaction is estimated to be 16 times that needed to detect a main effect of the same magnitude.[65] Consequently, by using an interaction to evaluate the utility of viability imaging the chance of a false-negative result becomes very high. Unfortunately, the authors of STICH state, "the tests of interaction between myocardial viability and treatment effect of CABG were not significant for any of the three end points. Therefore, we must conclude that there is no statistical evidence of association between myocardial viability and benefit from CABG."[20]

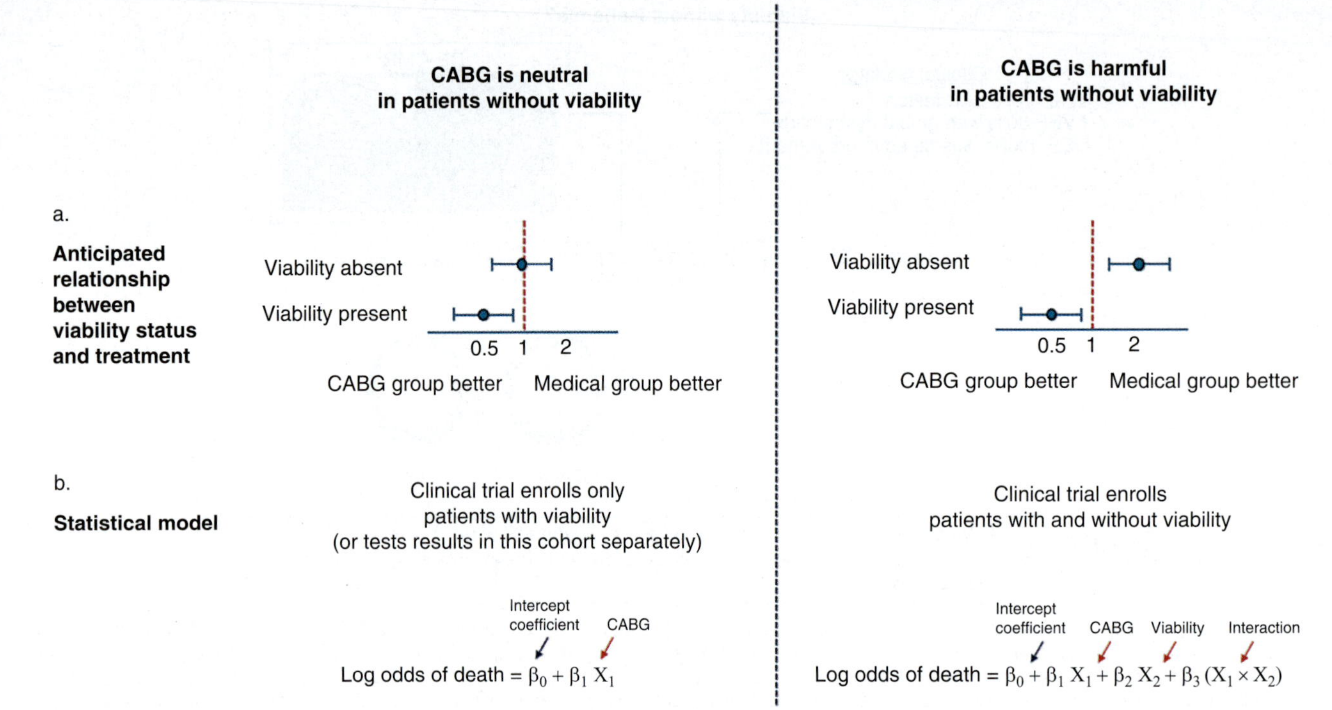

FIG. 23.10 (A) Anticipated relationship between viability status and treatment based on pre-STICH historical data. In patients with viability, the mean hazard ratio (*HR*) with 95% confidence interval are all expected to be less than 1.0 (i.e., CABG is better), whereas in patients without viability, the HR 95% confidence interval should include 1.0 (i.e., CABG is neutral). There is no expectation that CABG is worse in patients without viability (*right panel*). (B) The statistical model testing the benefit of CABG in patients with viability is far simpler than the model testing the interaction between treatment assignment and viability status (*right panel*). For the latter model, whether CABG is neutral versus harmful in patients without viability affects the strength of the interaction. Note: for simplicity, logistic regression (rather than Cox regression models as in the original STICH analysis) are shown for the probability of a binary outcome (e.g., death, yes/no) excluding the effect of time.

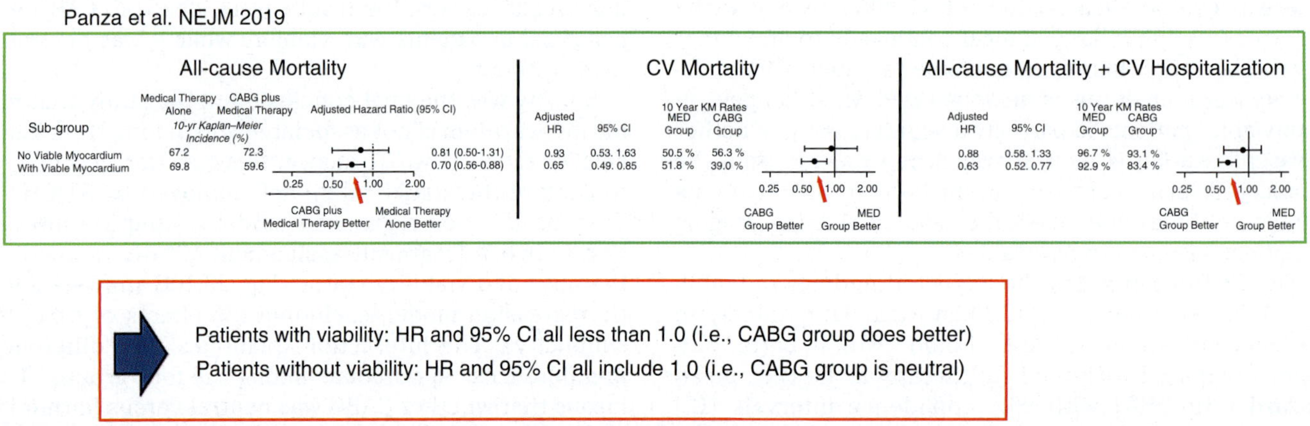

FIG. 23.11 Ten-year outcome data of the STICH viability substudy. Hazard ratios (*HR*) and 95% confidence intervals (*CI*) are shown for the primary endpoint of all-cause mortality (*left*) and for the secondary endpoints of cardiovascular (*CV*) mortality (*middle*) and a composite of all-cause mortality or hospitalization for cardiovascular causes (*right*). In patients with viability, the HR and 95% CI are all less than 1.0 (i.e., CABG group does better), while in patients without viability, the HR and 95% CI all include 1.0 (i.e., CABG group is neutral). See text for details. (Adapted from Panza JA, et al. Myocardial viability and long-term outcomes in Ischemic cardiomyopathy. *N Engl J Med.* 2019;381(8):739–748.)

The REVIVED-BCIS2 Trial

The REVIVED-BCIS2 trial evaluated whether revascularization by percutaneous coronary intervention (PCI) could improve outcome in patients with severe ischemic left ventricular systolic dysfunction, as compared with optimal medical therapy alone.[21] Contrary to the STICH 10-year follow-up report, the study found that revascularization had no benefit on outcome, as PCI did not result in a lower incidence of the primary endpoint, which was a composite of death from any cause or hospitalization for heart failure. While the REVIVED-BCIS2 trial addresses some aforementioned limitations with STICH (e.g., the presence of viability was required for enrollment in REVIVED), other shortcomings complicate the interpretation of the trial's results. First, there is PCI as the revascularization strategy. Society guidelines emphasize that PCI is not equivalent to CABG, given that they "are inherently different in the mechanisms by which they improve blood flow to the jeopardized myocardium. PCI will directly relieve a discrete obstruction and increase the arterial lumen in the stented area but will have no effect on preventing plaque progression or rupture in other diseased segments within the artery. In contrast, bypass of a coronary artery will improve blood flow to the jeopardized myocardium supplied by the diseased artery and will also protect the distal myocardial beds from future ischemic insult caused by proximal plaque progression or rupture."[11] Hence, while CABG is given a Class I recommendation in patients with LV dysfunction and left main stenosis or multivessel disease, the guidelines state that "there are insufficient data to make recommendations for using PCI in patients with multivessel CAD and LV dysfunction."[11] Even in the backdrop of remarkable advances in PCI, CABG techniques and postoperative care have also improved dramatically. In terms of contemporary care, it is noteworthy that FAME (Fractional flow reserve vs. Angiography for Multivessel Evaluation) 3, a multicenter, noninferiority trial, randomizing patients with three-vessel CAD to undergo CABG or FFR-guided PCI, did not meet the criterion set for noninferiority of PCI. CABG resulted in a lower incidence of major adverse cardiovascular events at 1 year.[66]

A second issue with REVIVED is the choice of adverse events that were used to form the primary composite endpoint. As background, we note that following STEMI, the amount of nonviable myocardium (i.e., infarct size) is known to be strongly associated with all-cause mortality. Additionally, a recent meta-analysis of the relationship between infarct size and outcomes following primary PCI has shown that infarct size is also associated with hospitalization for heart failure (presumably because of a mechanistic link between infarct size and adverse ventricular remodeling) but not with subsequent re-infarction.[67] On the other hand, the guiding hypothesis of the series of FAME[66,68,69] investigations is that eliminating myocardial ischemia through coronary revascularization can improve patient outcome. Hence, in these studies, the primary endpoint was a composite that included ischemia-related events such as spontaneous MI and subsequent unplanned revascularization. Concerning viability imaging for the guidance of revascularization, we reiterate that the first step in its mechanistic basis is myocardial ischemia (Fig. 23.1). It seems intuitive, therefore, that the primary endpoint for a viability revascularization trial should include ischemia-related events. Presumably, successful revascularization of viable (and ischemic) myocardium would reduce ischemia-related events, and hence, improve outcome. Conversely, the pathway between successful revascularization of viable myocardium and a reduction in hospitalization for heart failure is less intuitive. Indeed, it would seem that the amount of nonviable, rather than viable, myocardium would be more directly related to future heart failure events, as suggested by the primary PCI trials.

Given this discussion regarding the appropriate choice of endpoints, it may be worthwhile to point out that if REVIVED had included ischemia-related events as part of its primary endpoint, it may well have shown a significant reduction in adverse events. Patients undergoing PCI had a markedly lower rate of spontaneous MI (48.7% vs. 86.8%) and subsequent unplanned revascularization (2.9% vs.10.5%) compared with patients receiving medical therapy.[21] To first order, we can estimate the effect of adding these two event types to the primary endpoint. REVIVED showed the primary endpoint occurred in 129 patients in the PCI group and 134 in the medical therapy group, a benefit of five patients, which was not statistically significant (HR 0.99, $P = .96$). But adding spontaneous MI and unplanned revascularization to the primary outcome would result in the primary endpoint occurring in 157 and 204 patients, respectively; a benefit of 47 fewer patients in the PCI group, which is nearly 10-fold higher than that reported.

Finally, a recent follow-up analysis of REVIVED appears to bolster evidence that there is a stronger link between nonviable, rather than viable, myocardium and future heart failure events. Perera et al. demonstrated that the extent of nonviable myocardium, but not the extent of viable myocardium, was associated with the primary endpoint of all-cause mortality or hospitalization for heart failure (HR 1.07).[70] Fig. 23.12 summarizes potential limitations in STICH and REVIVED with regards to viability imaging.

In summary, these data indicate that choosing the appropriate endpoint is crucial, and our recommendation is that studies evaluating viability-guided revascularization should prespecify ischemic outcomes (spontaneous MI and unplanned revascularization) as primary and consider heart failure outcomes as secondary or mechanistically indirect. REVIVED does not prove that viability testing or revascularization are futile. Rather it shows that determining the "value" of viability imaging is multifactorial and complex, and foremost requires careful consideration of its mechanistic basis.

Limitations in 'Viability Imaging' Clinical Trials

	STICH	REVIVED
➤ Viability testing required for patient enrollment	No	Yes
➤ Direct testing of revascularization versus medical therapy in only viable patients (e.g., no interaction term required)	No	Yes
➤ Core lab assessment of viability blinded to patient details	Yes	No*
➤ Viability paradigm depends on most efficacious form of revascularization *PCI is NOT the same as CABG*	Yes	No
➤ Suitable composite endpoint ➤ Composite should include ischemia related events (e.g., spontaneous MI, need for urgent revascularization, etc.) rather than HF related events	No#	No

* Post-hoc implementation of core lab analysis
# Composite endpoint of all-cause mortality or hospitalization for cardiovascular causes was a secondary endpoint

FIG. 23.12 Potential limitations in clinical trials utilizing viability imaging. The STICH (Surgical Treatment for Ischemic Heart Failure) and REVIVED (Revascularization for Ischemic Ventricular Dysfunction) trials are compared.

REFERENCES

1. Braunwald E, Kloner RA. The stunned myocardium: prolonged, postischemic ventricular dysfunction. *Circulation*. 1982;66(6):1146–1149.
2. Kloner RA, et al. Medical and cellular implications of stunning, hibernation, and preconditioning. *Circulation*. 1998;97(18):1848–1867.
3. Bax JJ, et al. Time course of functional recovery of stunned and hibernating segments after surgical revascularization. *Circulation*. 2001;104(suppl_1):1314–1318.
4. Rahimtoola SH. The hibernating myocardium. *Am Heart J*. 1989;117(1):211–221.
5. Alderman EL, et al. Results of coronary artery surgery in patients with poor left ventricular function (CASS). *Circulation*. 1983;68(4):785–795.
6. Chatterjee K, et al. Influence of direct myocardial revascularization on left ventricular asynergy and function in patients with coronary heart disease. *Circulation*. 1973;47(2):276–286.
7. Rees G, et al. Influence of aortocoronary bypass surgery on left ventricular performance. *N Engl J Med*. 1971;284(20):1116–1120.
8. Dakik HA, et al. Assessment of myocardial viability with ^{99m}Tc-Sestamibi tomography before coronary bypass graft surgery. *Circulation*. 1997;96(9):2892–2898.
9. Maes A, et al. Histological alterations in chronically hypoperfused myocardium. Correlation with PET findings. *Circulation*. 1994;90(2):735–745.
10. Wijns W, Vatner SF, Camici PG. Hibernating myocardium. *N Engl J Med*. 1998;339(3):173–181.
11. Lawton JS, et al. 2021 ACC/AHA/SCAI guideline for coronary artery revascularization: a report of the American college of cardiology/American heart association joint committee on clinical practice guidelines. *Circulation*. 2022;145(3):e18–e114.
12. Windecker S,KP, Alfonso F, et al. 2014 ESC/EACTS guidelines on myocardial revascularization. *Eur Heart J*. 2014;35(37):2541–2619.
13. Committee M, et al. ACC/AHA 2004 guideline update for coronary artery bypass graft surgery: summary article. *Circulation*. 2004;110(9):1168–1176.
14. Writing Group To Review, New E, et al. 2009 Focused update: ACCF/AHA guidelines for the diagnosis and management of heart failure in adults. *Circulation*. 2009;119(14):1977–2016.
15. Bonow RO. Myocardial viability and prognosis in patients with ischemic left ventricular dysfunction. *J Am Coll Cardiol*. 2002;39(7):1159–1162.
16. Allman KC, et al. Myocardial viability testing and impact of revascularization on prognosis in patients with coronary artery disease and left ventricular dysfunction: a meta-analysis. *J Am Coll Cardiol*. 2002;39(7):1151–1158.
17. Velazquez EJ,LKL, Deja MA, et al. Coronary-artery bypass surgery in patients with left ventricular dysfunction. *N Engl J Med*. 2011;365(5):468–471.
18. Bonow RO, et al. Myocardial viability and survival in ischemic left ventricular dysfunction. *N Engl J Med*. 2011;364(17):1617–1625.
19. Velazquez EJ, et al. Coronary-artery bypass surgery in patients with ischemic cardiomyopathy. *N Engl J Med*. 2016;374(16):1511–1520.
20. Panza JA, et al. Myocardial viability and long-term outcomes in ischemic cardiomyopathy. *N Engl J Med*. 2019;381(8):739–748.
21. Perera D, et al. Percutaneous revascularization for ischemic left ventricular dysfunction. *N Engl J Med*. 2022;387(15):1351–1360.
22. Cwajg JM,CE, Nagueh SF, et al. End-diastolic wall thickness as a predictor of recovery of function in myocardial hibernation: relation to rest redistribution Tl-201 tomography and dobutamine stress echocardiography. *ACC Curr J Rev*. 2001;10(2):35.
23. Baer FM, et al. Dobutamine magnetic resonance imaging predicts contractile recovery of chronically dysfunctional myocardium after successful revascularization. *J Am Coll Cardiol*. 1998;31(5):1040–1048.
24. Reimer KA, Jennings RB. The changing anatomic reference base of evolving myocardial infarction. Underestimation of myocardial collateral blood flow and overestimation of experimental anatomic infarct size due to tissue edema, hemorrhage and acute inflammation. *Circulation*. 1979;60(4):866–876.
25. Whalen Jr DA, et al. Effect of a transient period of ischemia on myocardial cells. I. effects on cell volume regulation. *Am J Pathol*. 1974;74(3):381–397.
26. Olivetti G, et al. Side-to-side slippage of myocytes participates in ventricular wall remodeling acutely after myocardial infarction in rats. *Circ Res*. 1990;67(1):23–34.
27. Weisman HF, et al. Cellular mechanisms of myocardial infarct expansion. *Circulation*. 1988;78(1):186–201.
28. Shah DJ, et al. Prevalence of regional myocardial thinning and relationship with myocardial scarring in patients with coronary artery disease. *Jama*. 2013;309(9):909–918.
29. Bax JJ, et al. Sensitivity, specificity, and predictive accuracies of various noninvasive techniques for detecting hibernating myocardium. *Curr Probl Cardiol*. 2001;26(2):147–181.
30. Gunning MG, et al. Comparison of ^{201}Tl, ^{99m}Tc-Tetrofosmin, and dobutamine magnetic resonance imaging for identifying hibernating myocardium. *Circulation*. 1998;98(18):1869–1874.
31. Sansoy V, et al. Comparison of thallium-201 resting redistribution with technetium-99m–sestamibi uptake and functional response to dobutamine for assessment of myocardial viability. *Circulation*. 1995;92(4):994–1004.
32. Piscione F, et al. Late reopening of an occluded infarct related artery improves left ventricular function and long term clinical outcome. *Heart*. 2005;91(5):646–651.
33. Ambrosio G, et al. Progressive impairment of regional myocardial perfusion after initial restoration of postischemic blood flow. *Circulation*. 1989;80(6):1846–1861.
34. Ito H, et al. Lack of myocardial perfusion immediately after successful thrombolysis. A predictor of poor recovery of left ventricular function in anterior myocardial infarction. *Circulation*. 1992;85(5):1699–1705.
35. Judd RM, et al. Physiological basis of myocardial contrast enhancement in fast magnetic resonance images of 2-day-old reperfused canine infarcts. *Circulation*. 1995;92(7):1902–1910.
36. Dilsizian V, Bonow RO. Current diagnostic techniques of assessing myocardial viability in patients with hibernating and stunned myocardium. *Circulation*. 1993;87(1):1–20.
37. Brunken RC, et al. Positron emission tomography detects metabolic viability in myocardium with persistent 24-hour single-photon emission computed tomography ^{201}Tl defects. *Circulation*. 1992;86(5):1357–1369.
38. Rehwald WG, et al. Myocardial magnetic resonance imaging contrast agent concentrations after reversible and irreversible ischemic injury. *Circulation*. 2002;105(2):224–229.
39. Polimeni PI. Extracellular space and ionic distribution in rat ventricle. *Am J Physiol*. 1974;227(3):676–683.
40. Weinmann HJ, et al. Characteristics of gadolinium-DTPA complex: a potential NMR contrast agent. *Am J Roentgenol*. 1984;142(3):619–624.

41. Shah DJ, Jones KR. Magnetic resonance of myocardial viability. In: Edelman RR, ed. *Clinical Magnetic Resonance Imaging*. Elsevier; 2005.
42. Choi KM, et al. Transmural extent of acute myocardial infarction predicts long-term improvement in contractile function. *Circulation*. 2001;104(10):1101–1107.
43. Fieno DS, et al. Contrast-enhanced magnetic resonance imaging of myocardium at risk. *J Am Coll Cardiol*. 2000;36(6):1985–1991.
44. Kim RJ, et al. Relationship of MRI delayed contrast enhancement to irreversible injury, infarct age, and contractile function. *Circulation*. 1999;100(19):1992–2002.
45. Wu E, et al. Visualisation of presence, location, and transmural extent of healed Q-wave and non-Q-wave myocardial infarction. *The Lancet*. 2001;357(9249):21–28.
46. Kim RJ, et al. The use of contrast-enhanced magnetic resonance imaging to identify reversible myocardial dysfunction. *N Engl J Med*. 2000;343(20):1445–1453.
47. Schvartzman PR, et al. Nonstress delayed-enhancement magnetic resonance imaging of the myocardium predicts improvement of function after revascularization for chronic ischemic heart disease with left ventricular dysfunction. *Am Heart J*. 2003;146(3):535–541.
48. Wellnhofer E, et al. Magnetic resonance low-dose dobutamine test is superior to scar quantification for the prediction of functional recovery. *Circulation*. 2004;109(18):2172–2174.
49. Gerber BL, et al. Characterization of acute and chronic myocardial infarcts by multidetector computed tomography. *Circulation*. 2006;113(6):823–833.
50. Lardo AC, et al. Contrast-enhanced multidetector computed tomography viability imaging after myocardial infarction. *Circulation*. 2006;113(3):394–404.
51. Mahnken AH, et al. Assessment of myocardial viability in reperfused acute myocardial infarction using 16-slice computed tomography in comparison to magnetic resonance imaging. *J Am Coll Cardiol*. 2005;45(12):2042–2047.
52. Lieberman AN, et al. Two-dimensional echocardiography and infarct size: relationship of regional wall motion and thickening to the extent of myocardial infarction in the dog. *Circulation*. 1981;63(4):739–746.
53. Mahrholdt H, et al. Relationship of contractile function to transmural extent of infarction in patients with chronic coronary artery disease. *J Am Coll Cardiol*. 2003;42(3):505–512.
54. Nelson C, et al. Impact of scar thickness on the assessment of viability using dobutamine echocardiography and thallium single-photon emission computed tomography. *J Am Coll Cardiol*. 2004;43(7):1248–1256.
55. Ragosta M, et al. Quantitative planar rest-redistribution ^{201}Tl imaging in detection of myocardial viability and prediction of improvement in left ventricular function after coronary bypass surgery in patients with severely depressed left ventricular function. *Circulation*. 1993;87(5):1630–1641.
56. Force T, et al. Overestimation of infarct size by quantitative two-dimensional echocardiography: the role of tethering and of analytic procedures. *Circulation*. 1986;73(6):1360–1368.
57. Samady H, et al. Failure to improve left ventricular function after coronary revascularization for ischemic cardiomyopathy is not associated with worse outcome. *Circulation*. 1999;100(12):1298–1304.
58. Kim RJ, Shah DJ. Fundamental concepts in myocardial viability assessment revisited: when knowing how much is "alive" is not enough. *Heart*. 2004;90(2):137–140.
59. Selvanayagam JB, et al. Value of delayed-enhancement cardiovascular magnetic resonance imaging in predicting myocardial viability after surgical revascularization. *Circulation*. 2004;110(12):1535–1541.
60. Helak JW, Reichek N. Quantitation of human left ventricular mass and volume by two-dimensional echocardiography: in vitro anatomic validation. *Circulation*. 1981;63(6):1398–1407.
61. Ibrahim T, et al. Diagnostic value of contrast-enhanced magnetic resonance imaging and single-photon emission computed tomography for detection of myocardial necrosis early after acute myocardial infarction. *J Am Coll Cardiol*. 2007;49(2):208–216.
62. Klein C, Nekolla SG, Bengel FM. Assessment of myocardial viability with contrast-enhanced magnetic resonance imaging. Comparison with positron emission tomography. *ACC Curr J Rev*. 2002;11(4):54.
63. Wagner A, et al. Contrast-enhanced MRI and routine single photon emission computed tomography (SPECT) perfusion imaging for detection of subendocardial myocardial infarcts: an imaging study. *Lancet*. 2003;361(9355):374–379.
64. Heidenreich PA, et al. 2022 AHA/ACC/HFSA guideline for the management of heart failure: a report of the American college of cardiology/American heart association joint committee on clinical practice guidelines. *Circulation*. 2022;145(18):e895–e1032.
65. Gelman A, Hill J, Vehtari A. *Regression and Other Stories*. Cambridge University Press; 2020.
66. Fearon WF, et al. Fractional flow reserve–guided PCI as compared with coronary bypass surgery. *N Engl J Med*. 2022;386(2):128–137.
67. Zhang L, et al. Cardiovascular magnetic resonance in immune checkpoint inhibitor-associated myocarditis. *Eur Heart J*. 2020;41(18):1733–1743.
68. Tonino PA, et al. Fractional flow reserve versus angiography for guiding percutaneous coronary intervention. *N Engl J Med*. 2009;360(3):213–224.
69. De Bruyne B, et al. Fractional flow reserve-guided PCI versus medical therapy in stable coronary disease. *N Engl J Med*. 2012;367(11):991–1001.
70. Perera D, et al. Viability and outcomes with revascularization or medical therapy in ischemic ventricular dysfunction: a prespecified secondary analysis of the REVIVED-BCIS2 trial. *JAMA Cardiol*. 2023;8(12):1154–1161.

24 Identifying the Etiology: A Systematic Approach to Differentiating Ischemic From Nonischemic Disease

CÉLESTE CHEVALIER, ROBIN NIJVELDT, AND RAYMOND J. KIM

INTRODUCTION

In patients presenting with myocardial dysfunction or injury, a practical first step is to assess whether the patient has ischemic or nonischemic heart disease. This simple classification is important because it can directly impact patient management. If ischemic disease is identified, there are clearly defined treatment strategies that have proven survival benefit, such as coronary artery bypass grafting in patients with left main or three-vessel disease.[1,2] This classification also provides an insight into patient prognosis; ischemic cardiomyopathy is associated with reduced survival compared with nonischemic cardiomyopathy (Fig. 24.1).[3,4] Within the broad category of nonischemic cardiomyopathy (CM), a second step is to determine the specific etiology. Again, the importance of determining the etiology is related to patient treatment and survival. For instance, beta-blockers are beneficial in some forms of nonischemic CM (e.g., idiopathic dilated CM) but not others (e.g., cardiac amyloidosis),[5] and the prognosis is quite variable depending on the underlying disease. Patients with peripartum CM have significantly better survival than those with idiopathic dilated CM, who in turn have better survival than those with infiltrative myocardial disorders.[6] Similarly, in patients with a working diagnosis of myocardial infarction with unobstructed coronary arteries (MINOCA), specific final diagnoses such as myocardial infarction (MI), myocarditis, and nonischemic CM are associated with varied prognoses (Fig. 24.1).[7]

Clinically, identifying the presence or absence of obstructive epicardial coronary artery disease (CAD), via coronary angiography or stress testing, has been the cornerstone in differentiating ischemic from nonischemic disease. DE-CMR provides a novel approach to determining the etiology by allowing a direct assessment of myopathic processes. Comparative studies with histopathology have shown that the presence, extent, and location of hyperenhancement (HE) by DE-CMR is a precise indicator of nonviable myocardium in both ischemic[8] and nonischemic disorders.[9,10] Although nonviable myocardium can be identified by several imaging modalities, DE-CMR may be particularly suited to evaluating the diverse myopathic processes in different cardiomyopathies. DE-CMR offers significantly higher spatial resolution (40-fold greater than radionuclide imaging[11]), can systematically detect subendocardial infarcts that are missed by SPECT,[12] and may even identify microscars that cannot be detected by other imaging techniques (Fig. 24.2).[13]

In this chapter, we present an overall imaging approach for differentiating ischemic from nonischemic disease, which is fundamentally based on DE-CMR. We describe how this approach is based on the underlying myocardial pathophysiology that is present, and we discuss how a DE-CMR-based approach may provide insight into the conundrums that can occur when CAD may coexist with nonischemic disorders.

TRADITIONAL APPROACH TO ETIOLOGY

Ischemic CM is usually diagnosed by identifying the presence of obstructive CAD. The coronary anatomy can be assessed either directly, e.g., x-ray coronary angiography, or indirectly via stress testing, depending on the pretest probability of disease. An individual with few risk factors and atypical symptoms may undergo stress testing (or simple reassurance if the risk is deemed particularly low), whereas an individual with multiple risk factors and classic symptoms of angina may proceed directly to the catheterization laboratory. Likewise, the broad diagnosis of nonischemic CM is usually also made by assessing the coronary anatomy, either directly or indirectly. Once significant CAD has been excluded, a comprehensive evaluation including possibly endomyocardial biopsy may allow a specific etiology to be determined.

However, there are several drawbacks to the traditional approach. For one, it appears that many patients do not undergo definitive testing (invasive coronary angiography), and the accuracy of diagnosing CAD indirectly is only moderate. Autopsy data from patients enrolled in the ATLAS (Assessment of Treatment with Lisinopril and Survival) trial,[14] a large multicenter randomized trial of patients with moderate to severe heart failure, underscores this concern. Of the 171 patients who had autopsy, 70% (n = 120) were diagnosed in life as having ischemic CM and 30% (n = 51) as having nonischemic CM. Autopsy documented that 17% of those diagnosed with ischemic CM did not have CAD, whereas 31% of those diagnosed with nonischemic CM had significant CAD. Overall, 21% had an incorrect clinical diagnosis.

One possible reason for the high rate of misdiagnosis may be an overreliance on certain findings from noninvasive imaging. Initially, it was thought that ventricular dysfunction due to nonischemic CM was primarily global

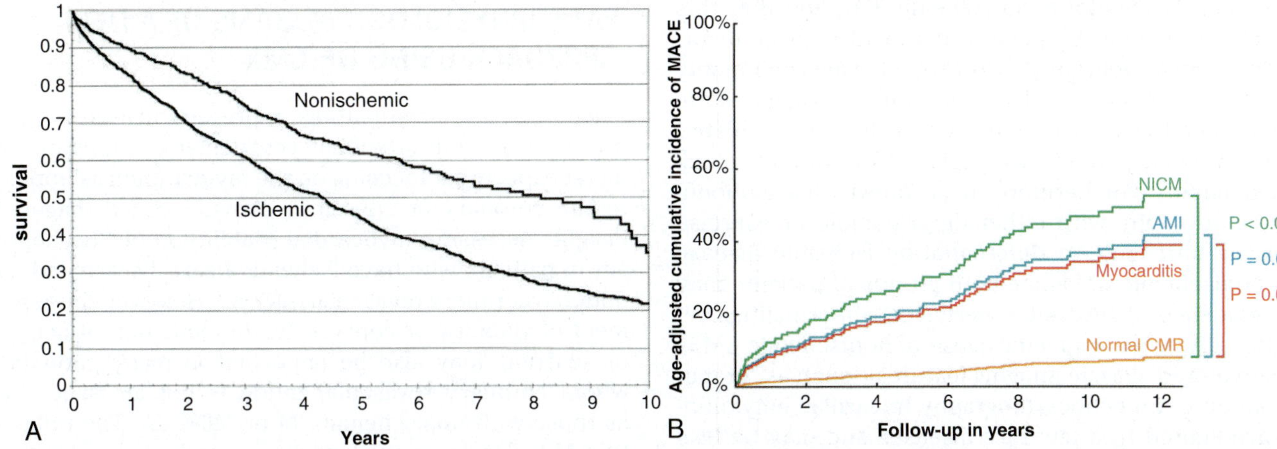

FIG. 24.1 (A) Kaplan–Meier survival curves for ischemic versus nonischemic cardiomyopathy. (B) Cumulative incidence of major adverse cardiac event (MACE) according to cardiac magnetic resonance diagnosis. ((A) Reproduced with permission from Felker GM, LK Shaw, and CM O'Connor, A standardized definition of ischemic cardiomyopathy for use in clinical research. *J Am Coll Cardiol*. 2002;39(2):210–218. (B) Reproduced with permission from Konst RE, et al., Prognostic value of cardiac magnetic resonance imaging in patients with a working diagnosis of MINOCA-An outcome study with up to 10 years of follow-up. *Circ Cardiovasc Imaging*. 2023;16(8):e014454.)

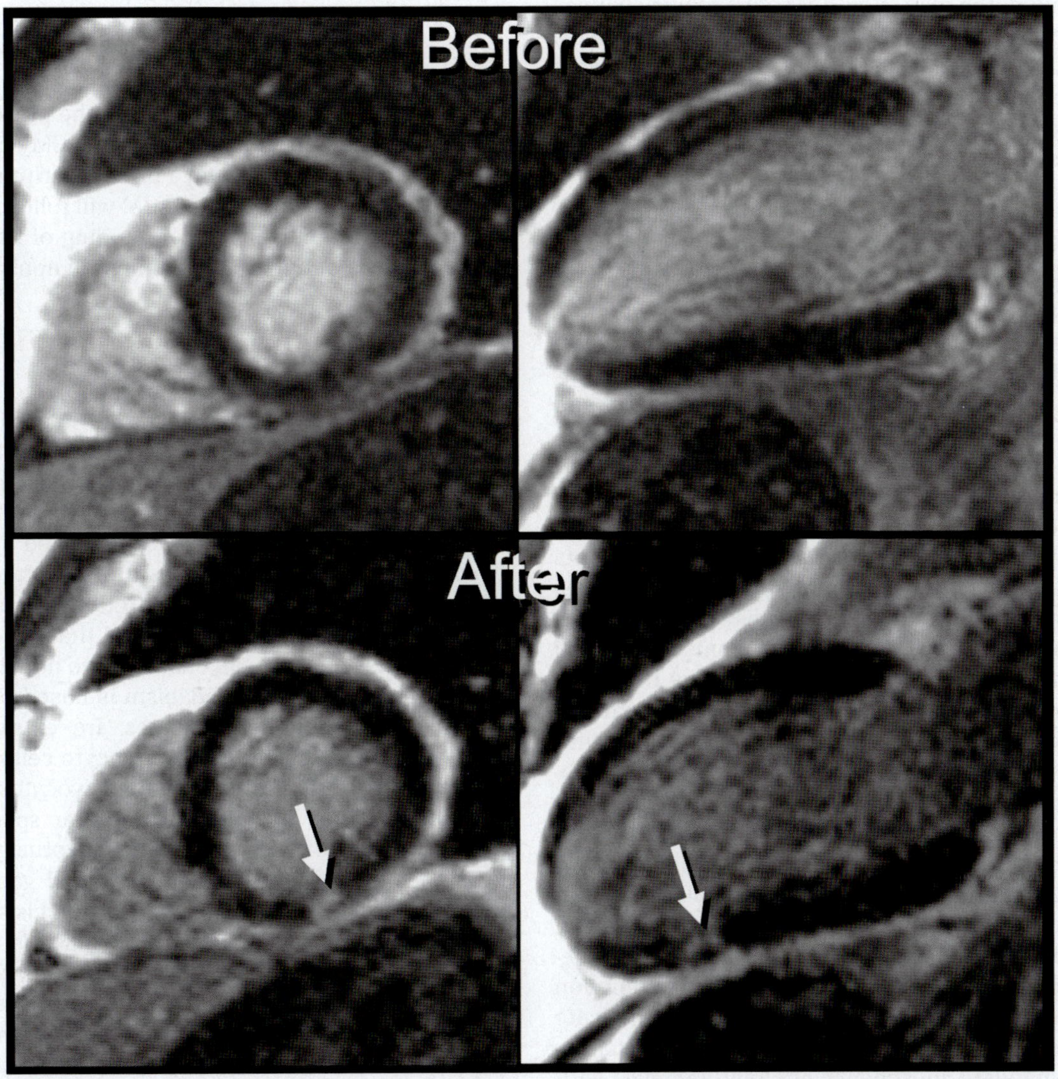

FIG. 24.2 Images before and after coronary stenting demonstrate the ability of delayed enhancement cardiac magnetic resonance to identify microinfarcts. *Arrows* point to new discrete regions of hyperenhancement in the inferior wall related to the procedure. (Adapted with permission from. Ricciardi M.J., et al., Visualization of discrete microinfarction after percutaneous coronary intervention associated with mild creatine kinase-MB elevation. *Circulation*. 2001;103(23):2780–2783.)

rather than segmental as in ischemic CM, and that this characteristic could be used to distinguish these disorders by echocardiography.[15] However, it is now commonly recognized that segmental wall motion abnormalities are evident in up to 60% of patients with nonischemic dilated CM, even when patients with left bundle branch block are excluded.[16] Furthermore, it is known that radionuclide scintigraphy with either dipyridamole or exercise testing is unreliable in differentiating ischemic disease from nonischemic CM since both groups of patients may have evidence of reversible perfusion abnormalities.[17,18] Additionally, when a specific cause of nonischemic CM is being explored, classic imaging features—such as "granular sparkling" on echocardiography in cardiac amyloidosis—are limited to a few rare diseases and may be less accurate than first reported. In fact, in a study of 196 patients clinically suspected to have cardiac amyloidosis, this finding had a sensitivity of only 26%.[19] Endomyocardial biopsy, the presumed gold standard, has limitations as well. Because of sampling error, test sensitivity may be low,[20] and especially in the chronic setting, many patients with cardiomyopathy may show only nonspecific changes on biopsy (e.g., cell loss and fibrosis). Not surprisingly, Felker et al.[6] reported that among 1230 patients that underwent endomyocardial biopsy as part of an evaluation for unexplained cardiomyopathy, a specific histologic diagnosis was provided by the biopsy in only 15% of patients.

Finally, simple distinctions between cardiomyopathies based on the presence or absence of CAD can be problematic. For instance, it is possible that a patient with nonischemic CM may also have CAD, but which is incidental and is not causing ischemia or contributing to contractile dysfunction. The quandary is that coronary atherosclerosis is common, especially in the elderly and those with diabetes mellitus, even if patients are asymptomatic and do not have myocardial dysfunction.[21] A study in 1921 patients with symptomatic heart failure and LV dysfunction (LVEF <40%) undergoing diagnostic coronary angiography highlights this issue.[3] Among patients with LV dysfunction "out of proportion" to their degree of CAD (i.e., those with single-vessel disease), the prognosis was more similar to those with nonischemic CM than the remaining group with more extensive CAD (i.e., those with multivessel disease). The authors concluded that even though obstructive CAD is present, those with single-vessel disease should be reclassified as nonischemic for prognostic purposes.

Another problem with the traditional approach is the inherent assumption that ischemic and nonischemic cardiomyopathy cannot coexist. However, it is plausible that both ischemic and nonischemic myopathic processes can be present simultaneously and may be contributing independently or synergistically toward systolic dysfunction (mixed cardiomyopathy). Thus, these limitations indicate that the presence of obstructive coronary atherosclerosis does not mandate an ischemic etiology, and even with objective information such as from invasive coronary angiography, the appropriate classification for a given patient is not always clear.

PATHOPHYSIOLOGICAL BASIS OF A NEW APPROACH USING DE-CMR

Since the cardiomyopathies represent diseases of the myocardium with attendant ventricular dysfunction, one might expect that focusing on the myocardium as opposed to the coronary arteries may provide added diagnostic insight. Assessing myocardial viability could be important in patients who have ischemic heart disease and may undergo coronary revascularization.[22] However, the assessment of viability, or conversely, the detection of necrosis or scarring, may also be important in many patients in whom coronary revascularization is not an issue, such as those with nonischemic CM or MINOCA. The utility of DE-CMR in the setting of cardiomyopathy is based on the understanding that rather than simply measuring viability, the presence and pattern of hyperenhancement (nonviable myocardium) holds additional information. In this section, we will first explore the mechanism of myocardial hyperenhancement in the setting of acute and chronic myocardial infarction and review the spatial progression of cell death that occurs over time following coronary occlusion. These will set the basis for understanding the DE-CMR findings that can occur in the setting of ischemic CM. Next, we will review the initial studies comparing the presence and pattern of hyperenhancement in ischemic CM to that found in idiopathic dilated CM. Then, a brief description of findings in other forms of nonischemic CM will follow, along with a summary of the current understanding of the pathophysiological basis of hyperenhancement in nonischemic CM.

Mechanism of Hyperenhancement in Myocardial Infarction

Both acute and chronic myocardial infarction are accurately depicted by DE-CMR as hyperenhanced regions, independent of wall motion and reperfusion status.[8] The gadolinium chelates that are used for DE-CMR are biologically inert and are not actively transported by any cells or tissues. Although the mechanism of myocardial hyperenhancement in the setting of infarction has not been fully elucidated, one has been proposed that accounts for the variety of tissues that can characterize nonviable myocardium.[23] The proposed mechanism is based on two simple facts. First, gadolinium chelates are extracellular contrast agents that cannot cross myocyte cell membranes.[24] Secondly, in normal myocardium, myocytes are densely packed, and thus myocyte intracellular space forms the majority (78%) of the volume.[25] Conceptually, it then follows that the volume of distribution of gadolinium in a hypothetical voxel of normal myocardium is small, and the overall number of gadolinium molecules is low. In acute MI, there is myocyte membrane rupture, which allows additional gadolinium to diffuse into what was previously intracellular space. This, in turn, results in increased gadolinium concentration.[26] In chronic MI, myocytes have been replaced with collagenous scar tissue. In this situation, the interstitial space is expanded, which again leads to increased gadolinium concentration and hyperenhancement.[26] In both acute and chronic MI (and all stages in-between) one can consider viable myocytes as actively excluding gadolinium contrast media. Thus, the unifying mechanism for the hyperenhancement of nonviable myocardium may then be the absence of viable myocytes rather than any inherent properties that are specific for acutely necrotic tissue, collagenous scar, or other forms of nonviable tissue.

The "Wavefront" of Ischemic Necrosis

The typical pattern of hyperenhancement that occurs in patients with prior MI, and thus in those with ischemic CM, can be explained by the pathophysiology of ischemia. Following a coronary occlusion, myocardial contractility falls within seconds throughout the "area at risk," which is the ischemic zone with reduced perfusion. Although blood begins to flow by way of preexisting collaterals—vascular channels that interconnect ordinary arteries—collateral flow is lowest and myocardial oxygen consumption is highest in the subendocardium. As a consequence, ischemia is most severe and necrosis begins first in the subendocardium starting about 15–20 minutes after total occlusion.[27] Necrosis then progresses as a "wavefront" toward the epicardium over the next few hours. During this period the size of the "area at risk" remains the same, but the size of the infarcted region within the "area at risk" increases continuously toward a transmural infarction (Fig. 24.3). Another facet of the wavefront phenomenon is that increasing the time or severity of ischemic injury generally increases the transmurality of infarction, whereas the circumferential extent of infarction does not increase appreciably since the lateral margins are established relatively early in the ischemic period.[27] Therefore, an "ischemic-type" or "CAD-type" pattern of hyperenhancement should always involve the subendocardium (i.e., subendocardial or transmural) and be located in a region, which is consistent with the perfusion territory of an epicardial coronary artery. Conversely, a "non-CAD-type" pattern of hyperenhancement is one that spares the subendocardium and is secondary to nonischemic disorders.

Ischemic Versus Idiopathic Dilated Cardiomyopathy

Several studies have compared the presence and pattern of hyperenhancement on DE-CMR among patients with various forms of cardiomyopathy. Wu et al.[11] were the first to report that DE-CMR may hold promise in differentiating ischemic from nonischemic, idiopathic dilated CM. In this study, nearly all patients with CAD and prior MI had myocardial hyperenhancement, whereas none of the patients with idiopathic dilated CM or the normal volunteers had hyperenhancement. In another study, Bello et al.[28] evaluated a cohort of patients with severe LV systolic dysfunction; hyperenhancement was found in 100% of patients with ischemic CM, but in only 12% with idiopathic dilated CM. From these data we can conclude that myocardial

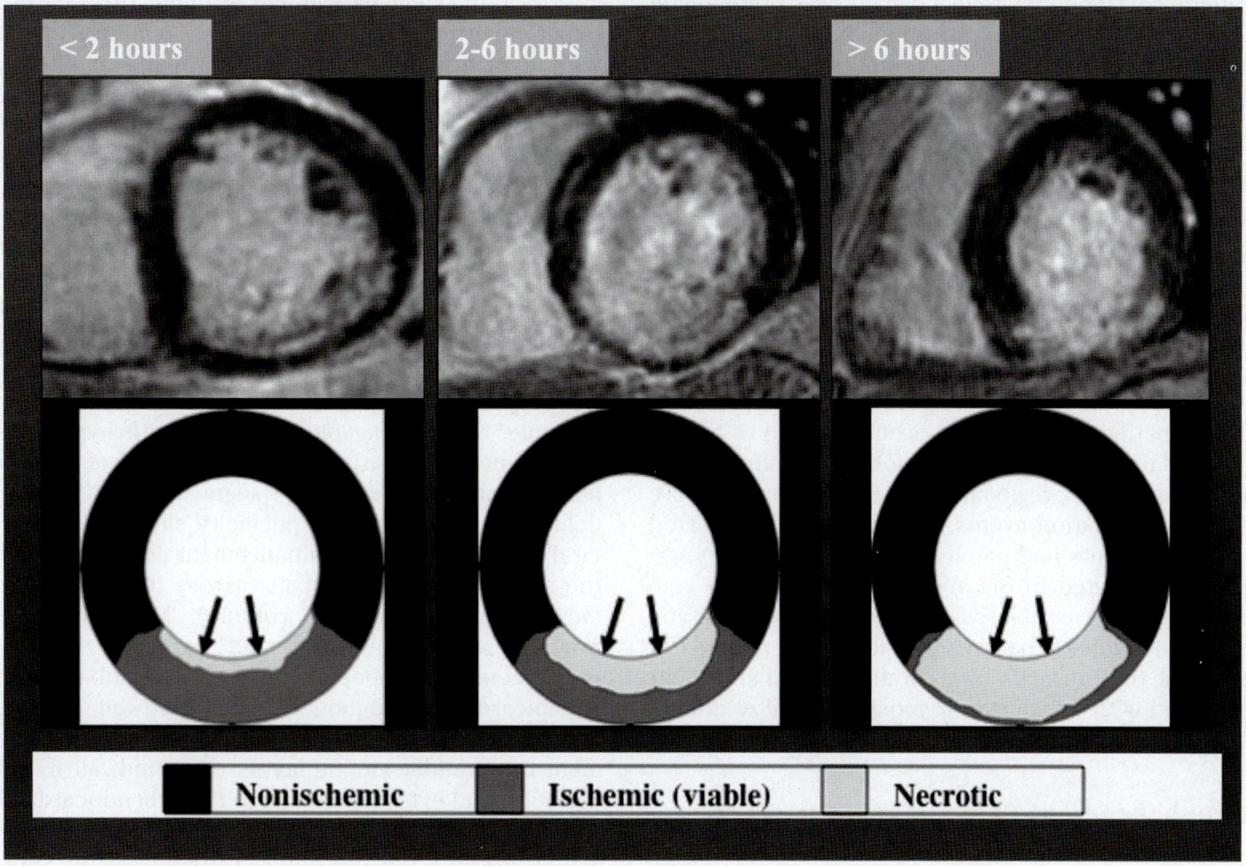

FIG. 24.3 The wavefront phenomenon of ischemic necrosis. The transmurality of infarction increases with increased duration of ischemia. (Reproduced with permission from. Mahrholdt H. et al., Delayed enhancement cardiovascular magnetic resonance assessment of nonischemic cardiomyopathies. *Eur Heart J.* 2005;26(15):1461–1474.)

hyperenhancement consistent with gross myocardial scarring is virtually always present in patients with chronic ischemic CM, whereas it is relatively rare in patients with idiopathic dilated CM. This conclusion is consistent with previous pathology studies.[29,30] Schuster and Bulkley[29] demonstrated that virtually all patients with congestive heart failure and significant CAD have gross myocardial scarring at autopsy, even in those without a clinical history of myocardial infarction, angina, or Q-waves. Conversely, Roberts et al.[31] found visible scars at necropsy in only 14% of patients with idiopathic dilated CM.

McCrohon et al.[32] performed DE-CMR in 90 patients diagnosed with ischemic ($n = 27$) or idiopathic dilated CM ($n = 63$) on the basis of coronary angiography. Whereas all patients with ischemic CM had myocardial hyperenhancement, 41% of patients with idiopathic dilated CM also had hyperenhancement. Although the prevalence of hyperenhancement in patients with idiopathic dilated CM in this study appears to be significantly higher than that reported by Wu et al.[11] and Bello et al.,[28] it is important to note that there were differences in how hyperenhancement was defined in these studies. For instance, in the earlier studies only hyperenhancement patterns consistent with regions of prior myocardial infarction were included in the analysis. Taking into account the pattern of hyperenhancement (CAD-type vs. non-CAD-type), McCrohon et al. found that 13% of patients with idiopathic dilated CM had CAD-type hyperenhancement, whereas 28% had non-CAD-type. These findings are now consistent with those of Bello et al.[28] in that among patients with idiopathic dilated CM the rate of CAD-type hyperenhancement was quite low in both studies (13% vs. 12%). Additionally, these rates are nearly identical to the rate of chronic infarcts found at autopsy in patients with idiopathic dilated CM by Roberts et al.[31] and in the ATLAS substudy by Uretsky et al.[14] (14% and 12%, respectively).

The clinical interpretation of CAD-type hyperenhancement in patients with idiopathic dilated CM is unclear. Certainly the occurrence of recanalization after an occlusive coronary event or embolization from minimally stenotic but unstable plaque is well documented.[33,34] Therefore, McCrohon et al. believed that these patients were incorrectly diagnosed by coronary angiography as patients with idiopathic dilated CM. However, this interpretation (i.e., these patients should have been classified as having CAD) would not explain relatively global LV dysfunction in the setting of a small, regional MI, since this would require multiple recanalization events. McCrohon et al. reported that 28% of patients had patchy or linear striae of hyperenhancement limited to the mid-myocardium of the ventricular wall, and were classified as having non-CAD-type scar. Current studies in patients with idiopathic dilated CM suggest that the presence of midwall hyperenhancement is associated with worsened prognosis, even after adjustment for left ventricular ejection fraction.[35,36]

Hyperenhancement Patterns in Nonischemic CM

In the studies above, only patients with ischemic or idiopathic dilated CM were evaluated. Patients with hypertrophic cardiomyopathy, myocarditis, infiltrative disorders, or other forms of nonischemic CM were excluded. Many of these diseases will be addressed in detail in other chapters, but a brief summary of DE-CMR findings in several cardiomyopathies is listed in Table 24.1.

The location and pattern of scarring on DE-CMR are often quite distinct, and a pattern recognition approach based on the visualization of hyperenhancement will provide useful diagnostic information as to the likely etiology. In this context, the most recent ESC Guidelines for the management of cardiomyopathies give a Class I Level B recommendation for contrast-enhanced CMR at initial evaluation.[132] Fig. 24.4 illustrates potential hyperenhancement patterns that may be encountered in clinical practice with a partial list of their differential diagnoses. Importantly, there are data that indicate that certain nonischemic cardiomyopathies have a predilection for specific scar patterns. For instance, in the setting of LV hypertrophy, the presence of mid-wall hyperenhancement in one or both junctions of the interventricular septum and right ventricular free wall is highly suggestive of hypertrophic cardiomyopathy,[50] whereas mid-wall or subepicardial hyperenhancement in the inferolateral wall is consistent with Anderson–Fabry disease.[63] Likewise, in a patient with the appropriate demographic profile, involvement of both the LV basal lateral wall and apex appears to be relatively specific for Chagas disease.[87] Moreover, instead of an infinite variety of patterns, a general classification into a limited number of common hyperenhancement phenotypes seems to be possible. In some disorders, however, more than one pattern can occur or coexist in the same patient. For example, three patterns of hyperenhancement are commonly encountered in patients with myocarditis (Fig. 24.5). Certain patterns of hyperenhancement appear to be related to the type of virus causing myocarditis, and importantly, to the clinical course.[79,80] A similar variety of patterns have been observed for myocarditis associated with mRNA COVID-19 vaccination.[133]

Genetic testing has identified pathogenic variants in a number of DCM-associated genes that may constitute an "arrhythmogenic DCM" phenotype. This phenotype often demonstrates a "ring-like" pattern of hyperenhancement, for which there are at least three contiguous segments with subepicardial or midmyocardial LGE in the same short-axis slice.[134] However, this definition is somewhat unclear. For example, three *contiguous* segments with hyperenhancement is not necessarily the same as *continuous* hyperenhancement that spans three segments. Additionally, the definition appears to lack specificity, since in patients with viral myocarditis, hyperenhancement commonly involves the subepicardium and spans across three or more segments (Fig. 24.5 middle column). Moreover, whereas previous studies have suggested that if the ring of hyperenhancement is subepicardial in one location, it remains subepicardial throughout[40] (or if midwall, is midwall throughout), we have found that the ring of hyperenhancement can wander among layers (e.g., midwall to subepicardium) and even sometimes to the subendocardial layer (Fig. 24.6). The ring-like pattern has also been described in arrhythmogenic left ventricular cardiomyopathy (ALVC), a diagnosis and/or clinical phenotype that appears to have overlap with arrhythmogenic DCM. A more specific feature

TABLE 24.1 Left ventricular scar characteristics in nonischemic cardiomyopathies.

DISEASE	HYPERENHANCEMENT PATTERNS/ADDITIONAL CHARACTERISTICS	REPORTED PREVALENCE	REFERENCES
Idiopathic dilated CM	Linear mid-wall HE, typically in the basal septum	10%–35%	32,35,37–39
Arrhythmogenic dilated CM (overlap with arrhythmogenic left ventricular CM [ALVC] with or without LV dilatation)	Ring-like HE pattern (midwall or epicardial HE extending three or more contiguous segments in the same short-axis slice) • Some pathogenic genotypes include variants in Desmoplakin (DSP) and Filamin-C (FLNC), which are particularly associated with ALVC; a component of HE may be due to fatty infiltration (Fig. 24.7) Other pathogenic genotypes which may present with or without ring-like HE include: • Titin (TTN): often septal midwall striae • Lamin A/C (LMNA): often septal midwall striae (perhaps more diffuse and broader than Titin); occasionally presents with ring-like pattern • Desmin (DES)/primary desminopathies: midwall HE which is septal or ring-like	21%–84% (depending on study cohort and genetic variants evaluated); highest for variants in DSP 26%–47% 16%–75% 36% (4 of 11 patients)	40–43 40,43 40,43–46 47–49
Other genetic (with or without dilatation)			
Hypertrophic CM	Patchy, multifocal, predominantly midwall, with end-stage disease also transmural More common in hypertrophied areas If HE is present, RV insertion sites of the septum are almost always involved	42%–89%; higher prevalence in patients with severe hypertrophy (wall thickness >30 mm)	38,50–62
Anderson–Fabry	HE in the basal inferolateral wall, often subepicardial or intramural	31%–50% (prevalence dependent on hypertrophy and sex)	63–66
Muscular dystrophies	Subepicardial or midwall HE which is septal, lateral, or ring-like	21%–75%	67–70
Infiltrative			
Amyloidosis	Diffuse HE often with global subendocardial involvement HE may also be localized (for early disease)	66%–100% (depending on type of amyloid deposition and disease stage)	71–77
Sarcoidosis	May have CAD-type (subendocardial and/or transmural) and/or non-CAD-type (midwall or subepicardial) HE Involvement of RV side of the basal septum appears to be relatively specific for sarcoidosis Involvement of RV free wall can occur, but may be difficult to diagnose with conventional bright blood DE	13%–70%; almost 100% in known cardiac sarcoidosis	78
Infectious/Inflammatory			
Viral myocarditis	Three different patterns: (1) linear midwall striae in the basal septum; (2) lateral subepicardial HE; and (3) multiple, focal midwall HE globally More than one pattern can coexist in the same patient (Fig. 24.5)	75%–100%	9,79–83
Immune checkpoint inhibitor-induced myocarditis	Midwall or subepicardial, less frequently diffuse or transmural	22%–82% (depending on acuteness of presentation and LV function)	84–86
Chagas disease	Preferentially affects basal lateral wall and apex Involvement of both areas concomitantly is relatively specific for Chagas disease May be CAD-type (subendocardial and/or transmural) and/or non-CAD-type (midwall or subepicardial)	7%–20% in seropositive asymptomatic patients; 52%–100% in clinical Chagas disease; 100% in those with VT	87–91
Miscellaneous			
SLE	Usually midwall in septum but occasionally can be CAD-type and affect the LV free wall	20%–53%	92–96
Systemic sclerosis	Can be poorly defined/patchy or diffuse	15%–66%	97–100
Takotsubo CM	HE typically absent		101,102
Uremic CM	CAD-type HE in patients with CAD risk factors Diffuse, near global HE, possibly in patients with prior exposure to gadolinium	14%–32% 14%–37%	103,104
Aortic stenosis	May be CAD-type or non-CAD-type (patchy midwall)	27%–74% (depending on severity of aortic stenosis and/or LVH)	105–109
ANCA-associated vasculitis (AAV)	Predominantly subendocardial, but midwall or subepicardial can also occur	39%–93% (depending on subtype of AAV)	110–113

Continued

TABLE 24.1 Left ventricular scar characteristics in nonischemic cardiomyopathies.—cont'd

DISEASE	HYPERENHANCEMENT PATTERNS/ADDITIONAL CHARACTERISTICS	REPORTED PREVALENCE	REFERENCES
HIV positive	Asymptomatic HIV+ patients reportedly often have small amounts of epicardial HE in the inferolateral wall; however, the specificity of this finding is suspect	5%–84%	114–116
Pulmonary hypertension (PH)	Right ventricular insertion sites of the interventricular septum, may additionally involve septal midwall	27%–97% (depending on clinical classification of PH)	117–120
Peripartum CM	HE absent Often absent, but when present is usually midwall or epicardial	0%–55% (depending on presence or absence of LV recovery, higher border in nonrecovered cases)	121–124
Post-chemotherapy CM	Pattern is ill-defined	0%–35% (treatment with anthracyclines and/or trastuzumab is unlikely to be associated with HE)	125
Endomyocardial fibrosis (EMF)			
Tropical EMF	HE in the endocardium, most prominent in the apex LV and/or RV involvement "V sign" (three-layer appearance with inner layer of thrombus, middle layer of HE reflecting EMF, and an outer layer of normal myocardium)	100% (33%–36% for biventricular HE, 15%–50% for LV involvement only, 14%–50% for RV involvement only)	126–128
EMF associated with Loeffler's endocarditis	Cardiac manifestation of hypereosinophilic syndrome with HE in the fibrotic stage similar to that seen in tropical EMF		129–131

CAD, coronary artery disease; *CM*, cardiomyopathy; *ESRD*, end-stage renal disease; *HE*, hyperenhancement; *HIV*, human immunodeficiency virus; *LV*, left ventricle; *MI*, myocardial infarction; *RV*, right ventricle; *SLE*, systemic lupus erythematosus; *VT*, ventricular tachycardia.

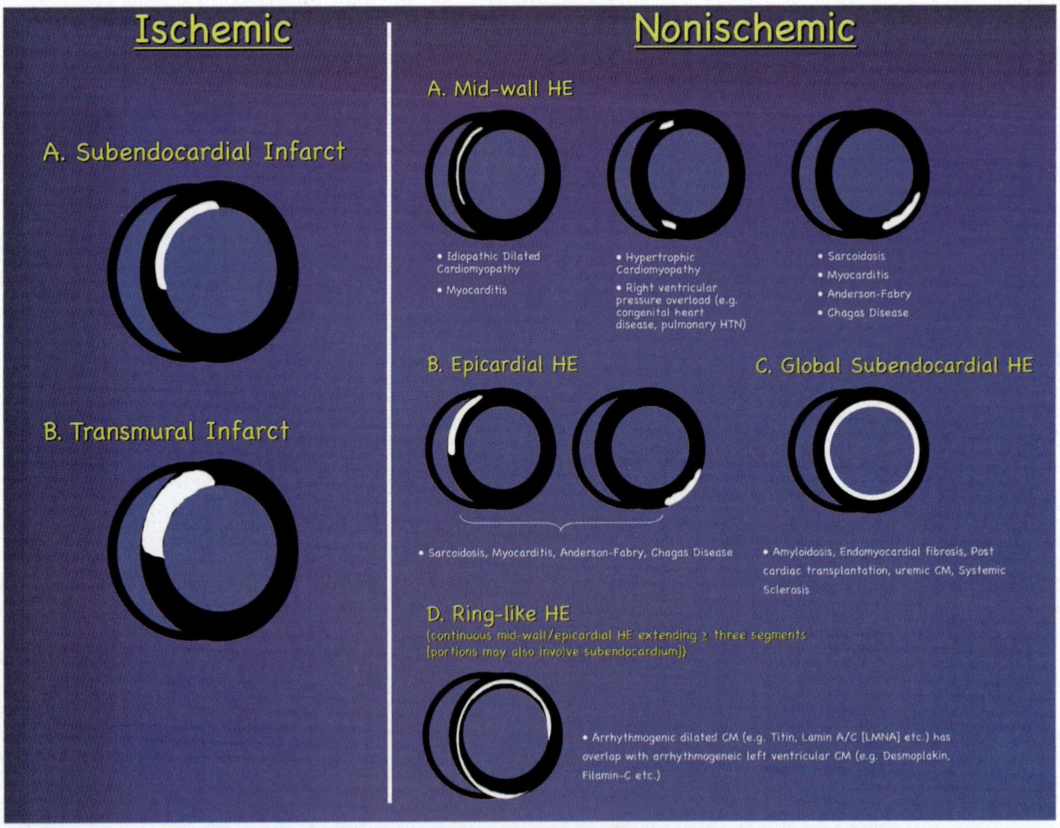

FIG. 24.4 Hyperenhancement (*HE*) patterns encountered in clinical practice. If hyperenhancement is present, the endocardium should be involved in patients with ischemic disease. Isolated midwall or epicardial hyperenhancement strongly suggests a nonischemic etiology. Text includes additional details.

to characterize ALVC may be the presence of fat, similar to arrhythmogenic right ventricular cardiomyopathy (ARVC) (Fig. 24.7). However, this aspect was not included in the 2020 international diagnostic criteria for arrhythmogenic cardiomyopathy ("Padua criteria"), as fatty infiltration identified by CMR—using dark-blood TSE sequences—was not considered a robust parameter that could be consistently reproduced in different laboratories.[135]

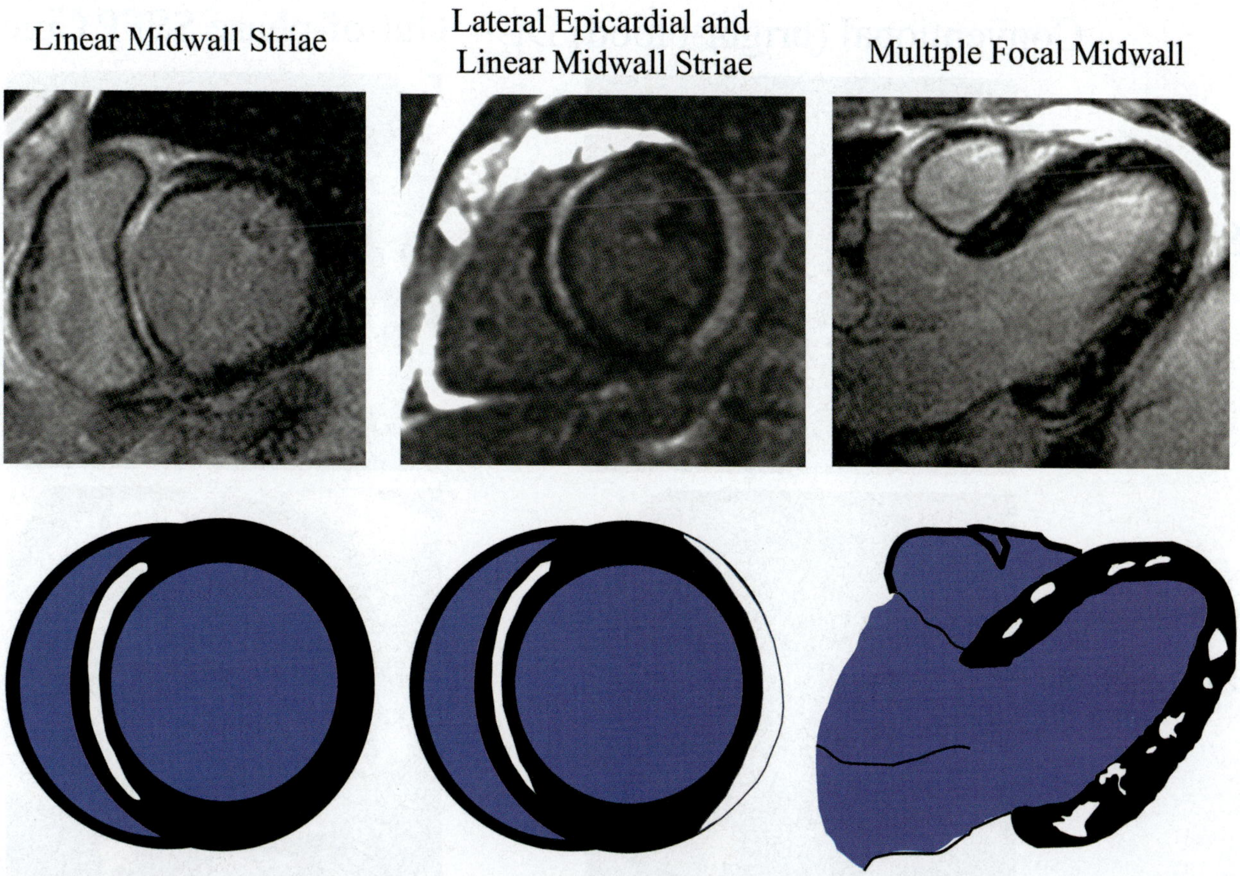

FIG. 24.5 Delayed enhancement images in patients with myocarditis with schematic representations. There are three commonly encountered patterns of hyperenhancement in patients with myocarditis (note that in the middle patient two patterns coexist).

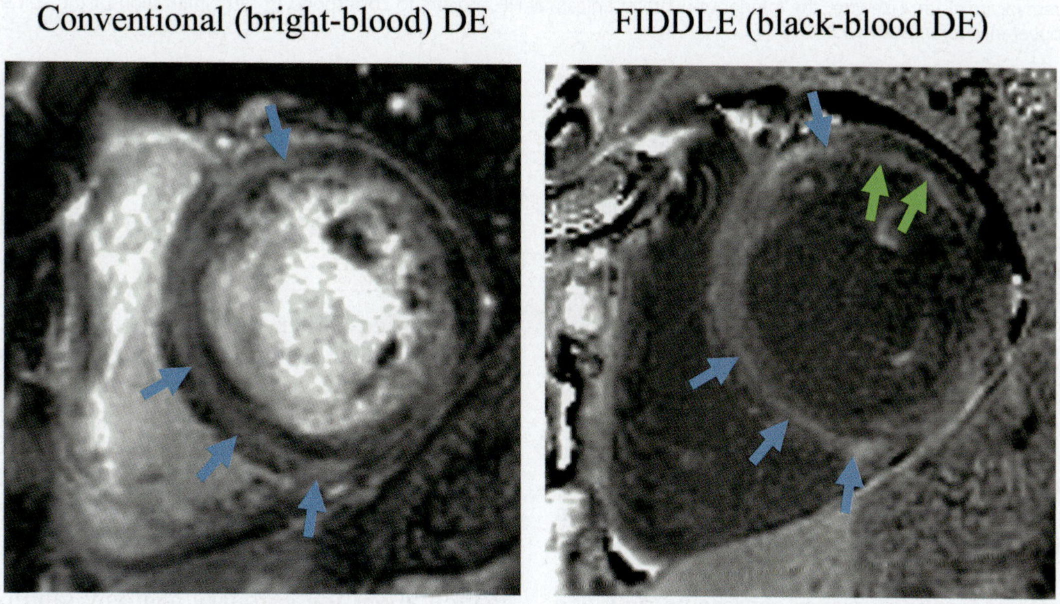

FIG. 24.6 Ring-like hyperenhancement. The conventional delayed enhancement image (*left*) shows a continuous midwall ring of hyperenhancement in the septum (*blue arrows*). The flow-independent dark blood delayed enhancement image (*FIDDLE*) shows continuation of the ring to the subendocardial layer (*green arrows*), which is not visible on the conventional DE image.

Pathophysiological Basis of Hyperenhancement in Nonischemic Cardiomyopathy

Currently, two lines of evidence indicate that areas of gadolinium hyperenhancement represent regions of nonviable myocardium. First, the locations and patterns of hyperenhancement seen in vivo in patients with various forms of nonischemic CM appear to match the locations and patterns of scarred or necrotic myocardium seen in gross pathology specimens of autopsy studies of those forms of nonischemic CM. For example, in patients with

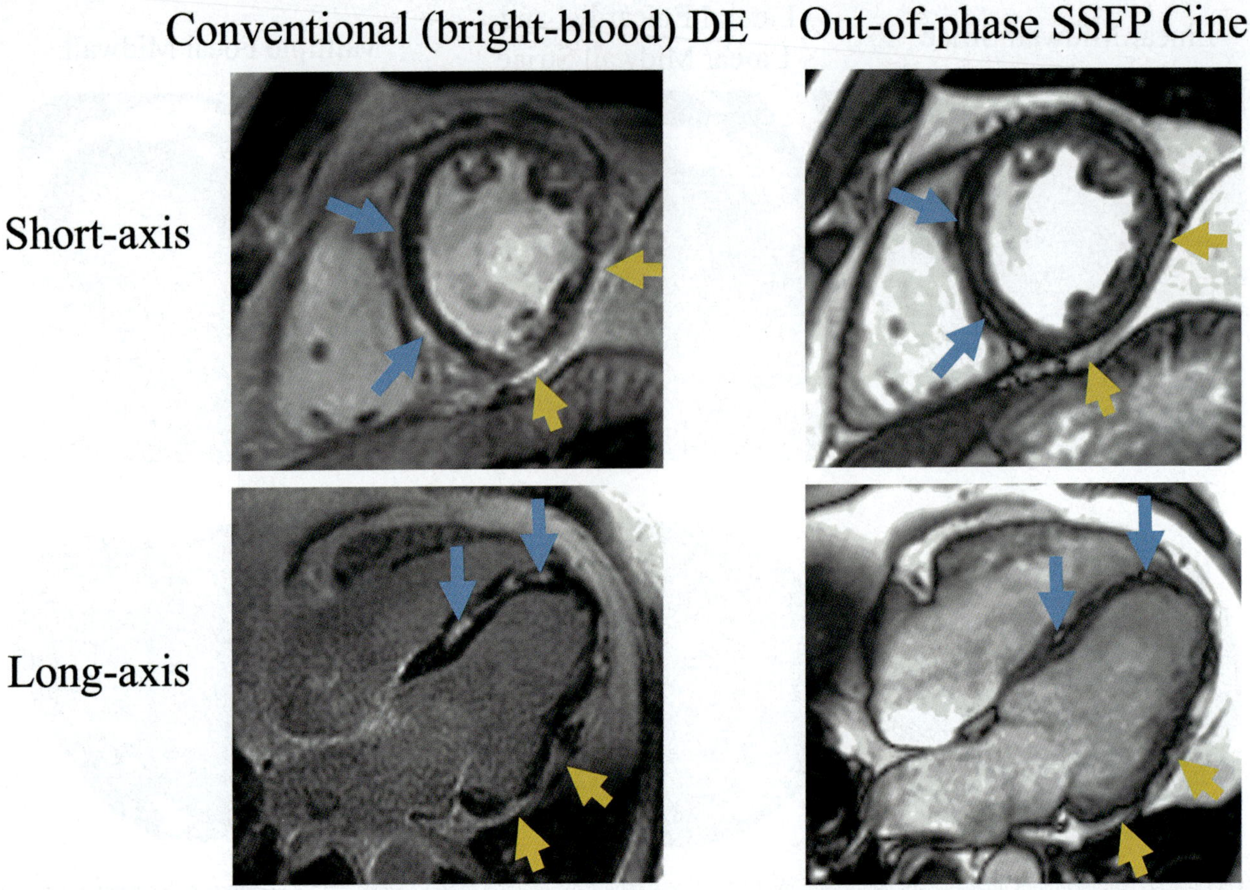

FIG. 24.7 A patient with a clinical diagnosis of arrhythmogenic left ventricular cardiomyopathy (ALVC). The DE images show a midwall ring of hyperenhancement in the septum (*blue arrows*) as well as epicardial hyperenhancement in the inferior and lateral walls (*orange arrows*). The corresponding "out-of-phase" cine images, which are sensitive to detecting fatty metaplasia (see Chapter 6), demonstrate that the septal midwall ring of HE is predominantly secondary to intramyocardial fat. Likewise, the inferior and lateral epicardial HE appears to correspond to fatty infiltration of the epicardial layer with a "moth-eaten" appearance (*orange arrows*).

hypertrophic cardiomyopathy, the common pattern of hyperenhancement at the RV insertion sites into the ventricular septum neatly matches the scarring that is often prominent at these sites in separate pathology studies.[136] Second, there are now data, although limited, comparing in vivo hyperenhancement patterns with gross pathology findings in the same patients. In a study of 19 patients who underwent heart transplantation or myomectomy, there was a direct relationship between the presence and location of hyperenhancement on DE-CMR and the presence and location of replacement scarring on pathology, and a high correlation was observed between the extent of hyperenhancement and histological fibrosis measured on the explanted heart specimens.[137] Similarly, a study of patients with sarcoidosis also showed that antemortem DE-CMR findings closely matched postmortem pathology findings.[138]

Grossly visible scarring, however, represents only one type of myocardial fibrosis. Diffuse fine interstitial fibrosis is common in many cardiomyopathies, including idiopathic dilated CM,[31] and this form of fibrosis is unlikely to lead to focal hyperenhancement. One should remember that the voxel resolution of DE-CMR is approximately $1.8 \times 1.3 \times 6$ mm. A region of hyperenhancement that is visible on DE-CMR will comprise several voxels, and the pathology analog would be a macroscopic scar that is visible to the naked eye. Thus, DE-CMR depicts regions of replacement scarring in vivo that previously could only be detected at autopsy, but currently, it is unable to identify the presence of diffuse reticular interstitial fibrosis.

A STEPWISE APPROACH INCORPORATING DE-CMR

As discussed earlier, the traditional approach of differentiating ischemic from nonischemic CM by identifying (or excluding) the presence of obstructive CAD is problematic. However, rather than simply examining the coronary anatomy to obtain a binary diagnosis of cardiomyopathy, we can leverage new information that is provided by DE-CMR—which is the presence (or absence) of myocardial damage that is specifically caused by a nonischemic disorder. It is with this information in combination with information about the coronary anatomy (and/or myocardial ischemia) that allows a nonbinary diagnosis of CM by adding the possibility of mixed CM or nonischemic CM with incidental CAD (Fig. 24.8).

A systematic approach to interpreting DE-CMR images in patients with heart failure or cardiomyopathy has been proposed.[23,139] In clinical practice, DE-CMR is almost never performed or interpreted in isolation, and a slightly modified approach to determining the etiology of cardiomyopathy is shown in Fig. 24.9. Cine imaging is always part

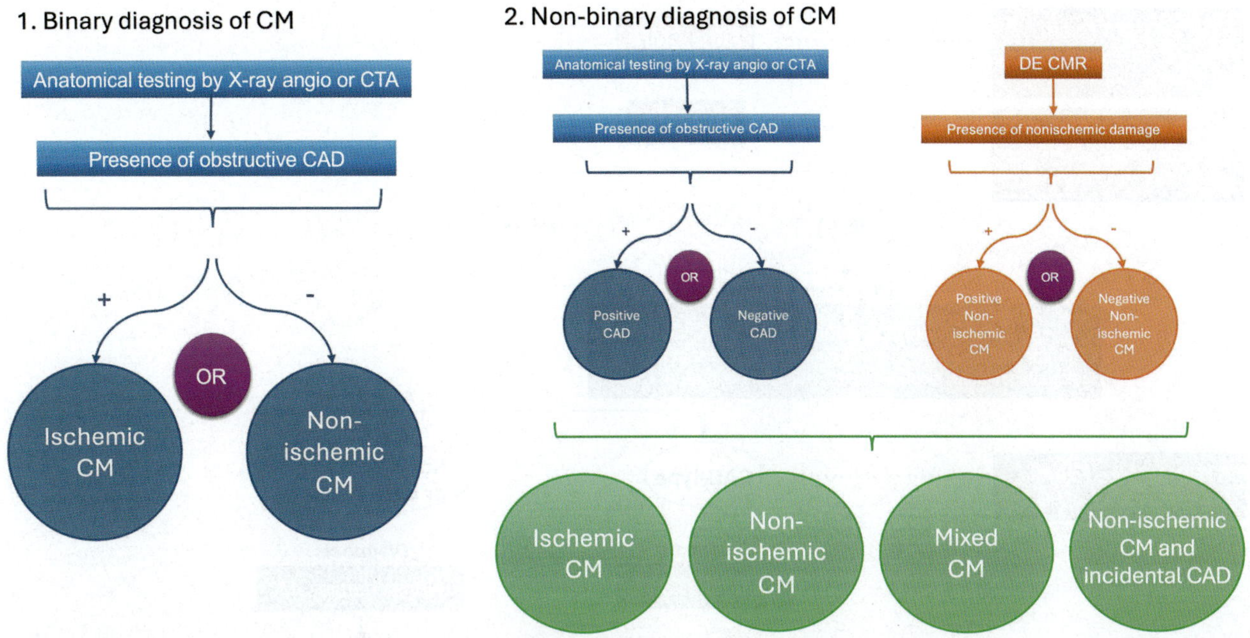

FIG. 24.8 Comparison of a traditional pathway versus a new approach incorporating DE-CMR to determine the underlying etiology of cardiomyopathy. The traditional approach only allows a binary diagnosis of CM, for example, ischemic or nonischemic CM. By leveraging the information provided by DE-CMR—which is the presence (or absence) of nonischemic damage—the new approach allows a nonbinary diagnosis of CM by adding the possibility of mixed CM or nonischemic CM with incidental CAD.

of an initial evaluation of heart failure and is part of the core CMR examination. As discussed elsewhere in other chapters, cine CMR is the "gold standard" technique for the evaluation of myocardial structure and function. Thus, **Step 1** is to assess the severity and regionality of LV dysfunction, along with an assessment of chamber sizes, wall thickness, and valvular function, using cine CMR. **Step 2** is to determine the presence or absence of hyperenhancement on DE-CMR. In patients with longstanding ischemic CM, virtually all patients have evidence of prior MI (as discussed above). The implication is that in patients with longstanding, severe cardiomyopathy but without hyperenhancement, the diagnosis of nonischemic CM should be strongly considered. Common etiologies in which hyperenhancement is frequently absent include idiopathic dilated, alcoholic, Takotsubo, and peripartum cardiomyopathy (Table 24.1).

If hyperenhancement is present, **Step 3** is to classify the location and distribution of hyperenhancement as CAD-type or non-CAD-type. For this determination, the concept that ischemic injury progresses as a "wavefront" from the subendocardium to the epicardium is crucial. Correspondingly, hyperenhancement patterns that spare the subendocardium and are limited to the middle or epicardial portion of the LV wall are clearly non-CAD-type. For a given patient, however, it is important to note that both CAD-type and non-CAD-type hyperenhancement may be present. This does not necessarily indicate a mixed cardiomyopathy, since both patterns are commonly present in certain nonischemic cardiomyopathies (e.g., cardiac sarcoidosis). As a second part of this step, further classification should be considered if hyperenhancement is present in a non-CAD pattern. Depending on the clinical history and associated data, a specific etiology may be entertained as described in Table 24.1 and Fig. 24.4.

In some patients, additional testing might aid in the interpretation of DE-CMR findings (**Step 4**). These may be acquired during the same CMR imaging session (e.g., coronary MRA, stress perfusion CMR), or via other modalities prior or subsequent to CMR. In a patient with an ischemic myopathic process (CAD-type scarring), knowledge of the coronary anatomy and/or presence of ischemia will be valuable for decisions regarding treatment including revascularization. However, in a patient with a nonischemic myopathic process (non-CAD-type scarring), additional testing may hone the precise etiology or etiologies of cardiomyopathy. If coronary angiography demonstrates no atherosclerosis, the ventricular dysfunction is solely due to nonischemic CM (see Potential Complexities section below). If there is anatomic evidence of coronary atherosclerosis, but no evidence of ischemia on functional testing, this suggests the presence of nonischemic CM with incidental CAD. On the other hand, if there are coronary lesions and inducible ischemia, this patient is likely to have a mixed disorder and have ischemic as well as nonischemic cardiomyopathy concomitantly.

Potential Complexities

Several issues may complicate the clinical interpretation of DE-CMR. Although the absence of hyperenhancement suggests a nonischemic process, this presumes long-standing, chronic cardiomyopathy and severe ventricular dysfunction. If the LV ejection fraction is only mildly reduced (e.g., LVEF >40%) or if the cardiomyopathy is of recent onset, then an ischemic process may be operative and dysfunctional regions without hyperenhancement may represent areas of stunned or hibernating myocardium.

Occasionally, CAD-type hyperenhancement may be present along with normal-appearing coronary arteries on

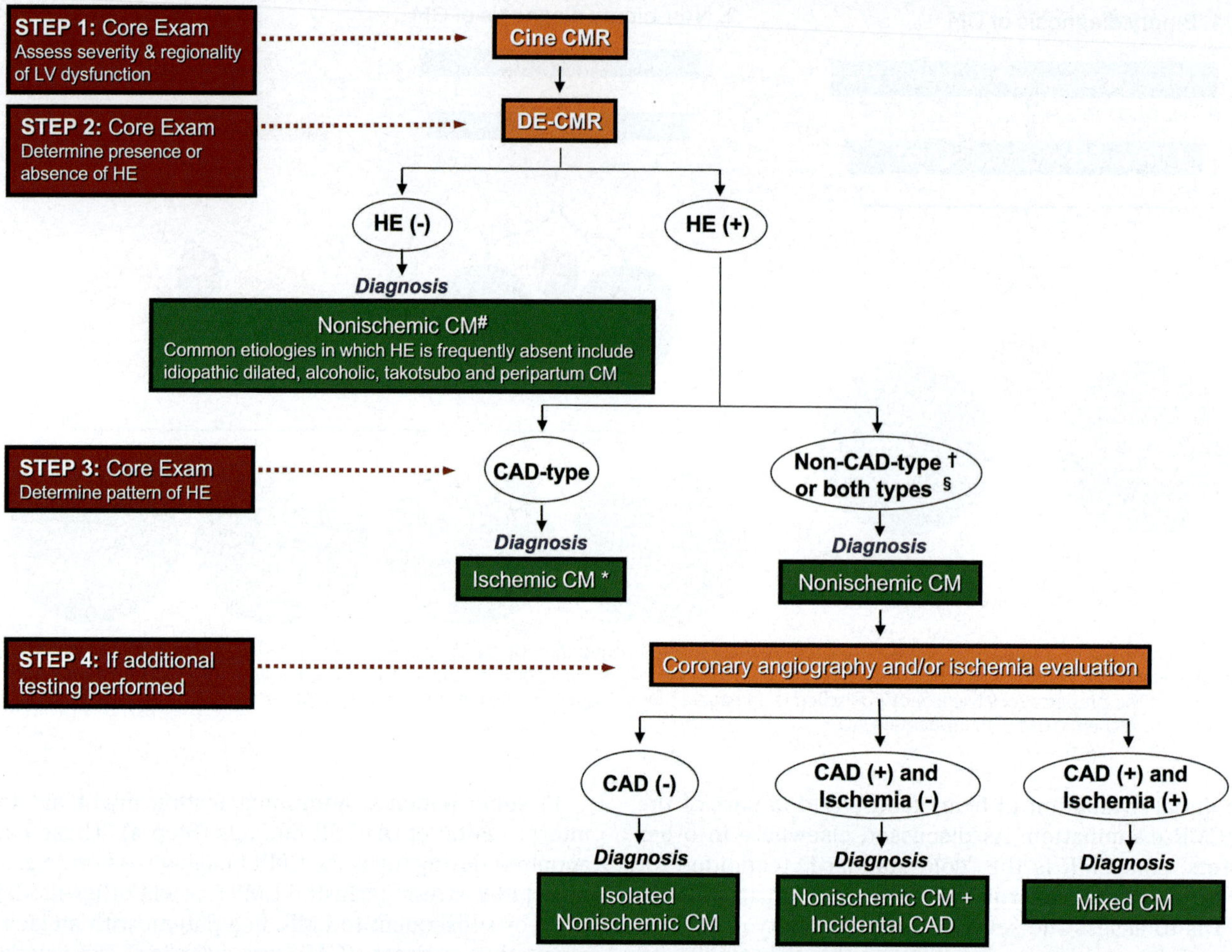

FIG. 24.9 A proposed stepwise approach for evaluating patients with heart failure incorporating DE-CMR. #Presumes long-standing, chronic cardiomyopathy and severe ventricular dysfunction. *Occasionally CAD-type HE may be present along with nonobstructive CAD on x-ray angiography. There are several possible explanations for this scenario (see text section, *Potential Complexities*). †See Table 24.1 and Fig. 24.4 for details of non-CAD-type patterns of HE in various nonischemic cardiomyopathies. §Often patients with nonischemic CM can have both non-CAD and CAD type HE (e.g., sarcoidosis).

x-ray angiography. There are several possible explanations for this scenario: (1) Coronary artery disease is present but was missed by angiography. In our experience this is rare but can occur when there is a flush, ostial occlusion of a secondary coronary branch. The infarct-related artery is usually small and, correspondingly, the size of hyperenhancement is also small. (2) Coronary artery disease is present but represents a dynamic process and a ruptured plaque with acute thrombotic occlusion—while leading to acute MI—may have healed without residual stenosis.[140] In this case, intravascular ultrasound may demonstrate substantial coronary atherosclerosis with remodeling and preserved luminal patency. (3) A nonischemic cardiomyopathy is present but coronary vasospasm or emboli may have led to an MI. Tests for abnormal coronary reactivity or the appropriate clinical scenario (e.g., the presence of intracardiac thrombus) may be helpful in this situation. (4) A nonischemic cardiomyopathy is present but the hyperenhancement pattern mimics that of myocardial infarction. Examples are shown in Fig. 24.10, and it is worthwhile to remember that certain nonischemic disorders (i.e., infiltrative CM) are more likely to present with CAD-type hyperenhancement than others.

Finally, when discerning the pattern of hyperenhancement, some caveats should be mentioned. Novices should be cautioned against a quick decision for non-CAD-type hyperenhancement. Here, it is important to distinguish between patterns that are clearly non-CAD-type (such as is often found in myocarditis, see Fig. 24.5), and one or two small, patchy lesions that vaguely appear to spare the subendocardium. For the latter (and when in doubt), one should opt for CAD-type hyperenhancement. It is more likely that CAD can present slightly atypically than for a more rare nonischemic disorder to be present. In nearly 70% of patients, the cause of heart failure is ischemic heart disease.[141] Moreover, the penalty for misdiagnosis is not symmetric. It is in those with ischemic heart disease that effective therapy including revascularization may substantially change patient outcome. Other common sources of error in interpreting hyperenhancement patterns are listed in Table 24.2, and shown in Figs. 24.11 and 24.12.

CLINICAL VALIDATION OF A DE-CMR-BASED APPROACH

CMR as Gatekeeper in New-Onset Heart Failure

CMR has been used as a noninvasive gatekeeper to left heart catheterization. Assomull et al.[142] studied a cohort of

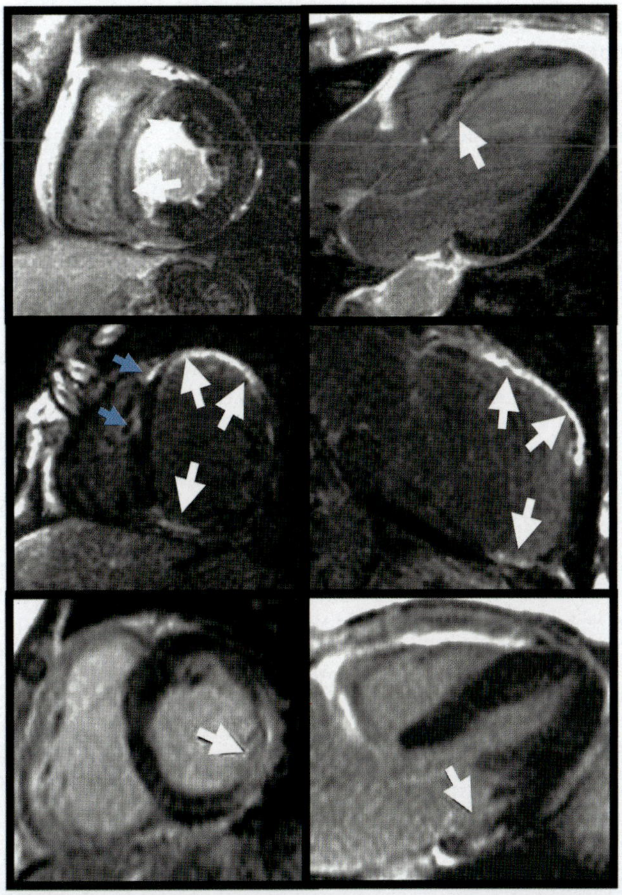

FIG. 24.10 Hyperenhancement (*white arrows*) in nonischemic cardiomyopathies mimicking that of coronary artery disease. (Upper row) Biopsy-proven HHV6 myocarditis and no coronary artery disease by angiography. (Middle row) Cardiac sarcoidosis with transmural scarring resulting in wall thinning similar to myocardial infarction. Note, the patient also has classic non-CAD type HE on the RV side of the septum (*blue arrows*). (Bottom row) Anderson–Fabry disease usually results in intramural HE, except for a few cases where the subendocardium can also be affected. (Modified with permission from. Moon J., Gadolinium enhanced cardiovascular magnetic resonance in Anderson-Fabry disease Evidence for a disease specific abnormality of the myocardial interstitium. *Eur Heart J.* 2003;24(23):2151–2155.)

120 patients with newly diagnosed HF who were scheduled to undergo coronary angiography as part of their clinical workup. Two expert consensus panels ascribed diagnoses based on either CMR results or coronary angiography results, which were then compared to the definitive diagnosis of a gold standard panel that reviewed all clinical data. The sensitivity of 100%, specificity of 96%, and diagnostic accuracy of 97% for DE-CMR were equivalent to coronary angiography (sensitivity, 93%; specificity, 96%; and diagnostic accuracy, 95%). Notably, using DE-CMR as an initial diagnostic step safely avoided catheterization in approximately 75% of DCM patients. Moreover, this strategy proved to be more cost-effective.

Mixed Cardiomyopathy

Bawaskar et al.[143] investigated the prevalence and prognostic significance of nonischemic CM in 3023 patients with documented obstructive CAD. Patients were divided into three categories of cardiomyopathy using a CMR-based interpretation algorithm: CAD and ischemic CM, CAD and nonischemic CM, or CAD and dual/mixed CM (both, nonischemic CM and ischemic CM). The authors identified nonischemic CM or mixed CM in one in six patients, although half of the cohort had no clinical suspicion of a nonischemic etiology prior to CMR. Furthermore, CAD patients with nonischemic CM or mixed CM had a higher risk of the primary outcome of all-cause death or hospitalization for heart failure than CAD patients with ischemic CM alone. The authors suggest that the limited prognostic benefit of coronary revascularization reported in previous studies may be partly attributable to concomitant, undiagnosed nonischemic CM. These findings indicate that CMR is superior to routine tests such as echocardiography in evaluating these patients, and raise the question of whether CMR should be used routinely prior to coronary revascularization, in order to improve patient selection and long-term outcomes.[143]

Use in Non-ST Elevation Myocardial Infarction (NSTEMI)

In contrast with the usual findings in STEMI patients, in whom the infarct-related artery is often identified, in many patients with NSTEMI the culprit artery is often not apparent from the x-ray angiogram. This challenge may occur if there has been intervening clot dissolution, or if the affected artery is a branch vessel that is flush occluded at its origin. In addition, NSTEMI patients

TABLE 24.2 Common sources of error in interpreting hyperenhancement patterns.

PITFALLS	COMMENTS/TEACHING POINTS
Patients with ischemic CM who appear to have non-CAD-type HE	
• Small and/or patchy HE which appears to spare the subendocardium	a. It is more likely that CAD can present slightly atypically than for a more rare nonischemic disorder to be present. When in doubt, one should opt for CAD-type hyperenhancement
• The most basal aspect of a myocardial infarction can spare the subendocardium (Fig. 24.10)	a. The coronary artery is epicardial and the most basal (proximal) aspect of its perfusion territory can involve only the epicardial portion of the LV wall b. When deciding that HE is of non-CAD type, i.e., "spares the subendocardium," note that this sparing refers to the entire extent of HE and not merely a part of the HE
• No-reflow zone can mimic normal myocardium (i.e., appear black), thus suggesting that HE does not involve the subendocardium (Fig. 24.11)	a. Use DE-CMR with a long inversion time (600 ms); with this technique, the no-reflow zone will appear black while normal myocardium will be gray b. Repeat imaging at a later time point; the no-reflow zone should at least partly fill in while normal myocardium would appear unchanged
Patients with nonischemic CM who appear to have CAD-type HE	
• In many nonischemic cardiomyopathies, in addition to non-CAD-type HE, it is common to have subendocardial or transmural HE (e.g., sarcoidosis)	a. Search for definite non-CAD type HE (i.e., epicardial HE). If definite non-CAD type HE coexists with other regions that have CAD-type HE, then the diagnosis is likely nonischemic CM rather than mixed CM
Miscellaneous	
• Midwall striae of HE at the base of the LV may be found in myocarditis, idiopathic dilated CM, and/or various genetic CMs, but may also be a nonspecific finding	a. Obtain DE-CMR images in orthogonal planes to adequately delineate the scar; nonspecific fibrosis tends to be contiguous with the fibrous skeleton of the heart
• In amyloidosis it might be difficult to find the null point of normal myocardium	a. Use phase-sensitive reconstructed DE and/or TI scout images; if myocardium has shorter T_1 relaxation time than blood (i.e., myocardium is brighter than cavity blood pool) then this is pathognomonic for cardiac amyloidosis. For TI scout images, the majority of myocardium nulls at a shorter time than blood in LV cavity (i.e., myocardium has shorter T_1 relaxation time).

CAD, coronary artery disease; *CM*, cardiomyopathy; *DE-CMR*, delayed enhancement cardiac magnetic resonance; *HE*, hyperenhancement; *LV*, left ventricle; *RV*, right ventricle; *TI*, inversion time.

more commonly manifest multivessel disease, which further complicates the assessment. The ability of CMR to distinguish even small MIs and to determine alternative diagnoses makes it an appealing technique for the evaluation of patients presenting with NSTEMI. A recent study of patients with NSTEMI undergoing x-ray coronary angiography and CMR found that in over half the patients the infarct-related artery (IRA) either could not be identified (37%) or was incorrectly assigned by coronary angiography (14%).[144] In addition, 15% of the patients had a noncoronary diagnosis made by CMR. Importantly, of the patients undergoing revascularization based on angiography, 27% had revascularization solely of nonculprit arteries, which presumably was not the operator's intent. From this and other studies of patients with NSTEMI, it is apparent that correct assignment of the IRA can be challenging, and that CMR can supply useful information aiding in this determination and in differentiation from noncoronary etiologies. In this regard it is important to note that the CARMENTA study comparing a CMR-first strategy to a standard evaluation with invasive coronary angiography showed that the CMR-first approach was safe, with no deleterious change in outcomes, while reducing the number of negative invasive coronary angiograms.[145] In this study, both CMR and coronary computed tomographic angiography (CTA) served as effective gatekeepers, with a greater reduction in invasive catheterizations in the CTA arm; nonetheless, those with negative anatomic imaging (coronary CT or invasive angiography) frequently proceeded to CMR (67% of cases) in order to establish a definitive diagnosis.

MINOCA

Similar to the spectrum of cardiomyopathies, patients with a working diagnosis of MINOCA represent a heterogeneous cohort. Society guidelines emphasize that the diagnosis of MINOCA is inherently descriptive and is just a "working" diagnosis that should prompt physicians to seek the underlying cause. Society guidelines also emphasize that the final diagnosis of MINOCA should be reserved solely for patients who are thought to have an ischemic cause, hence patients with nonischemic etiologies of myocardial injury (e.g., myocarditis) should be excluded.[146] A recent study confirms CMR as a key test in the contemporary diagnosis of MINOCA.[7] There were several important findings. First, CMR allowed ruling out a final diagnosis of true MINOCA in over half the patients (e.g., non-CAD-type hyperenhancement was detected on DE-CMR). Second, over a follow-up time of up to 10 years, CMR provided incremental prognostic value over conventional clinical factors. Third, the specific CMR diagnoses of acute MI, myocarditis, and nonischemic CM were independently associated with adverse outcome. Finally, a normal CMR exam portended a benign prognosis. Indeed, the 10-year event rate of a major adverse cardiac event (MACE) was 3.5%, and in line with age-matched, population-based cohorts completely free of clinical cardiovascular disease. These results underline the importance of performing CMR for both diagnostic and prognostic purposes in patients with the working diagnosis of MINOCA.[7]

SUMMARY

In conclusion, DE-CMR may be a valuable tool in evaluating the etiology of cardiomyopathy. As it provides direct

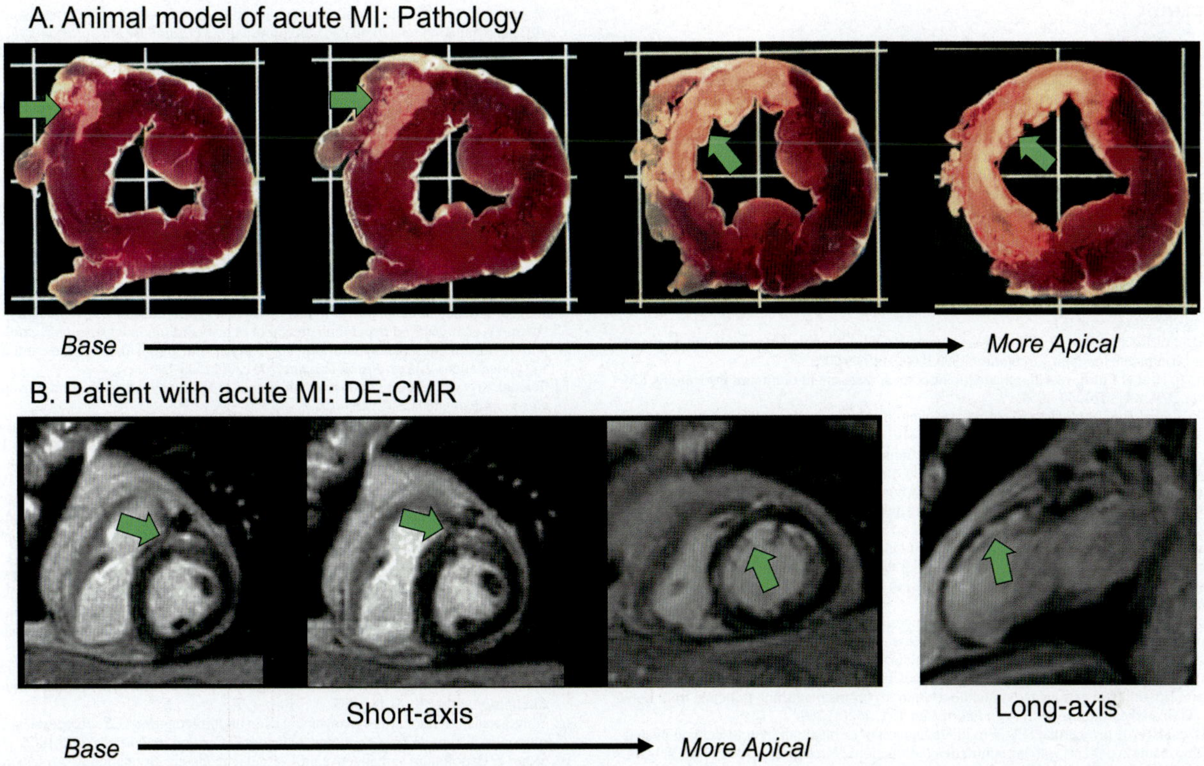

FIG. 24.11 The most basal aspect of a myocardial infarction can spare the subendocardium as illustrated by gross pathology in a canine heart with acute MI (A; modified with permission from Kim et al.[8]) and in vivo DE-CMR images from a patient with acute infarction (B); arrows point to infarcted myocardium. Examining the more distal contiguous slices and orthogonal views demonstrates the subendocardial involvement by the infarction. Thus, before deciding that HE is non-CAD-type, for example, "spares the subendocardium," note that subendocardial sparing refers to the entire extent of HE and not merely a small portion.

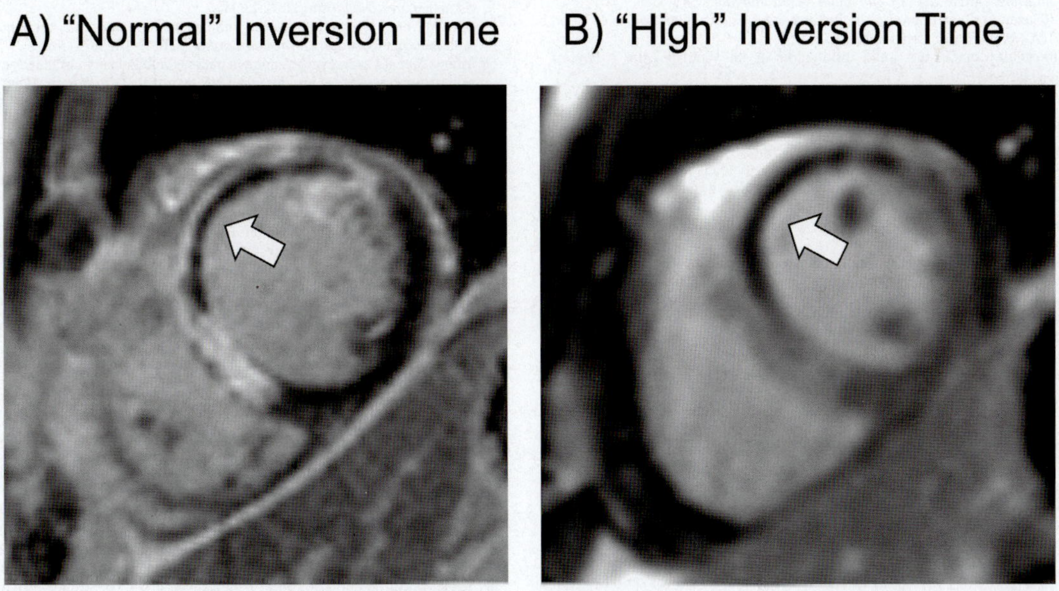

FIG. 24.12 It may be difficult to differentiate normal myocardium from no-reflow zones within the core of an acute MI (*arrow*, A) using inversion times to null the normal myocardium since both regions appear black. However, with higher inversion times (~600 ms), the no-reflow region that remains black may be reliably differentiated from normal myocardium, which is now gray in appearance (B).

assessment of myopathic processes, it represents a fundamentally different approach than traditionally undertaken, which consists of tests to determine the presence or absence of coronary artery disease. A stepwise algorithm for interpreting CMR images is presented, which accounts for differences in the presence, location, and pattern of myocardial hyperenhancement among cardiomyopathies. Additionally, a combination of DE-CMR with assessment of coronary anatomy and/or functional testing for ischemia may allow delineation of patients with nonischemic CM and incidental CAD and patients with mixed cardiomyopathy. In the future, this approach should be evaluated in larger populations for diagnostic accuracy, cost-effectiveness, and ultimately to determine if patient outcome can be improved.

REFERENCES

1. Alderman EL, et al. Results of coronary artery surgery in patients with poor left ventricular function (CASS). *Circulation*. 1983;68(4):785–795.
2. Lawton JS, et al. 2021 ACC/AHA/SCAI guideline for coronary artery revascularization: executive summary: a report of the American college of cardiology/American heart association joint committee on clinical practice guidelines. *Circulation*. 2022;145(3):e4–e17.
3. Felker GM, Shaw LK, O'Connor CM. A standardized definition of ischemic cardiomyopathy for use in clinical research. *J Am Coll Cardiol*. 2002;39(2):210–218.
4. Narins CR, et al. Arrhythmic and mortality outcomes among ischemic versus nonischemic cardiomyopathy patients receiving primary ICD therapy. *JACC Clin Electrophysiol*. 2022;8(1):1–11.
5. Packer M, et al. Effect of carvedilol on survival in severe chronic heart failure. *N Engl J Med*. 2001;344(22):1651–1658.
6. Felker GM, et al. Underlying causes and long-term survival in patients with initially unexplained cardiomyopathy. *N Engl J Med*. 2000;342(15):1077–1084.
7. Konst RE, et al. Prognostic value of cardiac magnetic resonance imaging in patients with a working diagnosis of MINOCA-an outcome study with up to 10 years of follow-up. *Circ Cardiovasc Imaging*. 2023;16(8):e014454.
8. Kim RJ, et al. Relationship of MRI delayed contrast enhancement to irreversible injury, infarct age, and contractile function. *Circulation*. 1999;100(19):1992–2002.
9. Mahrholdt H, et al. Cardiovascular magnetic resonance assessment of human myocarditis. *Circulation*. 2004;109(10):1250–1258.
10. Moon JCC, et al. The histologic basis of late gadolinium enhancement cardiovascular magnetic resonance in hypertrophic cardiomyopathy. *J Am Coll Cardiol*. 2004;43(12):2260–2264.
11. Wu E, et al. Visualisation of presence, location, and transmural extent of healed Q-wave and non-Q-wave myocardial infarction. *Lancet*. 2001;357(9249):21–28.
12. Wagner A, et al. Effects of time, dose, and inversion time for acute myocardial infarct size measurements based on magnetic resonance imaging-delayed contrast enhancement. *J Am Coll Cardiol*. 2006;47(10):2027–2033.
13. Ricciardi MJ, et al. Visualization of discrete microinfarction after percutaneous coronary intervention associated with mild creatine kinase-MB elevation. *Circulation*. 2001;103(23):2780–2783.
14. Uretsky BF, et al. Acute coronary findings at autopsy in heart failure patients with sudden death. *Circulation*. 2000;102(6):611–616.
15. Corya BC, et al. Echocardiographic features of congestive cardiomyopathy compared with normal subjects and patients with coronary artery disease. *Circulation*. 1974;49(6):1153–1159.
16. Wallis DE, et al. Segmental wall motion abnormalities in dilated cardiomyopathy: a common finding and good prognostic sign. *J Am Coll Cardiol*. 1984;4(4):674–679.
17. Glamann DB. Utility of various radionuclide techniques for distinguishing ischemic from nonischemic dilated cardiomyopathy. *Arch Intern Med*. 1992;152(4):769.
18. Wu YW, et al. Tl-201 myocardial SPECT in differentiation of ischemic from nonischemic dilated cardiomyopathy in patients with left ventricular dysfunction. *J Nucl Cardiol*. 2003;10(4):369–374.
19. Rahman JE, et al. Noninvasive diagnosis of biopsy-proven cardiac amyloidosis. *J Am Coll Cardiol*. 2004;43(3):410–415.
20. Kubo N, et al. Feasibility of diagnosing chronic myocarditis by endomyocardial biopsy. *Heart Vessel*. 1997;12(4):167–170.
21. Kronmal RA, et al. Risk factors for the progression of coronary artery calcification in asymptomatic subjects. *Circulation*. 2007;115(21):2722–2730.
22. Kim RJ, et al. The use of contrast-enhanced magnetic resonance imaging to identify reversible myocardial dysfunction. *N Engl J Med*. 2000;343(20):1445–1453.
23. Shah D, Judd R, Kim R. Myocardial viability. *Clin Magn Reson Imaging*. 2006;233.
24. Koenig SH, et al. Relaxation of water protons in the intra– and extracellular regions of blood containing Gd(DTPA). *Magn Reson Med*. 1986;3(5):791–795.
25. Polimeni PI. Extracellular space and ionic distribution in rat ventricle. *Am J Physiol*. 1974;227(3):676–683.
26. Rehwald WG, et al. Myocardial magnetic resonance imaging contrast agent concentrations after reversible and irreversible ischemic injury. *Circulation*. 2002;105(2):224–229.
27. Reimer KA, et al. The wavefront phenomenon of ischemic cell death. 1. Myocardial infarct size vs duration of coronary occlusion in dogs. *Circulation*. 1977;56(5):786–794.
28. Bello D, et al. Gadolinium cardiovascular magnetic resonance predicts reversible myocardial dysfunction and remodeling in patients with heart failure undergoing β-blocker therapy. *Circulation*. 2003;108(16):1945–1953.
29. Schuster EH, Bulkley BH. Ischemic cardiomyopathy: a clinicopathologic study of fourteen patients. *Am Heart J*. 1980;100(4):506–512.
30. Boucher CA, et al. Cardiomyopathic syndrome caused by coronary artery disease. III: Prospective clinicopathological study of its prevalence among patients with clinically unexplained chronic heart failure. *Heart*. 1979;41(5):613–620.
31. Roberts WC, Siegel RJ, McManus BM. Idiopathic dilated cardiomyopathy: analysis of 152 necropsy patients. *Am J Cardiol*. 1987;60(16):1340–1355.
32. McCrohon JA, et al. Differentiation of heart failure related to dilated cardiomyopathy and coronary artery disease using gadolinium-enhanced cardiovascular magnetic resonance. *Circulation*. 2003;108(1):54–59.
33. Topol EJ, Yadav JS. Recognition of the importance of embolization in atherosclerotic vascular disease. *Circulation*. 2000;101(5):570–580.
34. Arroyo L. Mechanisms of plaque rupture mechanical and biologic interactions. *Cardiovasc Res*. 1999;41(2):369–375.
35. Assomull RG, et al. Cardiovascular magnetic resonance, fibrosis, and prognosis in dilated cardiomyopathy. *J Am Coll Cardiol*. 2006;48(10):1977–1985.
36. Gulati A, et al. Association of fibrosis with mortality and sudden cardiac death in patients with nonischemic dilated cardiomyopathy. *JAMA*. 2013;309(9):896–908.
37. Soriano CJ, et al. Noninvasive diagnosis of coronary artery disease in patients with heart failure and systolic dysfunction of uncertain etiology, using late gadolinium-enhanced cardiovascular magnetic resonance. *J Am Coll Cardiol*. 2005;45(5):743–748.
38. Matoh F, et al. The usefulness of delayed enhancement magnetic resonance imaging for diagnosis and evaluation of cardiac function in patients with cardiac sarcoidosis. *J Cardiol*. 2008;51(3):179–188.
39. Halliday Brian P, et al. Outcome in dilated cardiomyopathy related to the extent, location, and pattern of late gadolinium enhancement. *JACC Cardiovasc Imaging*. 2019;12(8_Part_2):1645–1655.
40. Augusto JB, et al. Dilated cardiomyopathy and arrhythmogenic left ventricular cardiomyopathy: a comprehensive genotype-imaging phenotype study. *Eur Heart J Cardiovasc Imaging*. 2020;21(3):326–336.
41. Yang Y, et al. Ringlike late gadolinium enhancement provides incremental prognostic value in non-classical arrhythmogenic cardiomyopathy. *J Cardiovasc Magn Reson*. 2023;25(1):72.
42. Vaz A, et al. Ring-like late gadolinium enhancement: differential diagnosis and mimics. *Radiol Bras*. 2025;58:e20240111.
43. de Frutos F, et al. Late gadolinium enhancement distribution patterns in non-ischaemic dilated cardiomyopathy: genotype-phenotype correlation. *Eur Heart J Cardiovasc Imaging*. 2023;25(1):75–85.
44. Hasselberg NE, et al. Lamin A/C cardiomyopathy: young onset, high penetrance, and frequent need for heart transplantation. *Eur Heart J*. 2017;39(10):853–860.
45. Holmström M, et al. Late gadolinium enhanced cardiovascular magnetic resonance of lamin A/C gene mutation related dilated cardiomyopathy. *J Cardiovasc Magn Reson*. 2011;13(1):30.
46. Raman S, et al. Mid-myocardial fibrosis by cardiac magnetic resonance in patients with lamin A/C cardiomyopathy: possible substrate for diastolic dysfunction. *J Cardiovasc Magn Reson*. 2007;9(6):907–913.
47. Strach K, et al. Clinical, genetic, and cardiac magnetic resonance imaging findings in primary desminopathies. *Neuromuscul Disord*. 2008;18(6):475–482.
48. He Y, et al. Myocardial fibrosis in desmin-related hypertrophic cardiomyopathy. *J Cardiovasc Magn Reson*. 2010;12(1):68.
49. Chen Z, et al. Features of myocardial injury detected by cardiac magnetic resonance in a patient with desmin-related restrictive cardiomyopathy. *ESC Heart Fail*. 2021;8(6):5560–5564.
50. Choudhury L, et al. Myocardial scarring in asymptomatic or mildly symptomatic patients with hypertrophic cardiomyopathy. *J Am Coll Cardiol*. 2002;40(12):2156–2164.
51. Wilson JM, et al. Magnetic resonance imaging of myocardial fibrosis in hypertrophic cardiomyopathy. *Tex Heart Inst J*. 2002;29(3):176–180.
52. Moon JCC, et al. Toward clinical risk assessment inhypertrophic cardiomyopathy withgadolinium cardiovascular magnetic resonance. *J Am Coll Cardiol*. 2003;41(9):1561–1567.
53. Amano Y, et al. Delayed hyper–enhancement of myocardium in hypertrophic cardiomyopathy with asymmetrical septal hypertrophy: comparison with global and regional cardiac MR imaging appearances. *J Magn Reson Imaging*. 2004;20(4):595–600.
54. Teraoka K, et al. Delayed contrast enhancement of MRI in hypertrophic cardiomyopathy. *Magn Reson Imaging*. 2004;22(2):155–161.
55. Moon JC. Myocardial late gadolinium enhancement cardiovascular magnetic resonance in hypertrophic cardiomyopathy caused by mutations in troponin I. *Heart*. 2005;91(8):1036–1040.
56. Soler R, et al. Magnetic resonance imaging of delayed enhancement in hypertrophic cardiomyopathy. *J Comput Assist Tomogr*. 2006;30(3):412–420.
57. Dumont C, et al. Clinical significance of late gadolinium enhancement on cardiac magnetic resonance in patients with hypertrophic cardiomyopathy. *Rev Esp Cardiol*. 2007;60(1):15–23.
58. Melacini P, et al. Cardiovascular magnetic resonance signs of ischemia in hypertrophic cardiomyopathy. *Int J Cardiol*. 2008;128(3):364–373.
59. Payá E, et al. Variables associated with contrast-enhanced cardiovascular magnetic resonance in hypertrophic cardiomyopathy: clinical implications. *J Card Fail*. 2008;14(5):414–419.
60. Suk T, et al. Myocardial scar detected by contrast-enhanced cardiac magnetic resonance imaging is associated with ventricular tachycardia in hypertrophic cardiomyopathy patients. *Heart Lung Circ*. 2008;17(5):370–374.
61. Chan RH, et al. Prognostic value of quantitative contrast-enhanced cardiovascular magnetic resonance for the evaluation of sudden death risk in patients with hypertrophic cardiomyopathy. *Circulation*. 2014;130(6):484–495.
62. Yang S, et al. Subendocardial involvement as an underrecognized LGE subtype related to adverse outcomes in hypertrophic cardiomyopathy. *JACC Cardiovasc Imaging*. 2023;16(9):1163–1177.
63. Moon J. Gadolinium enhanced cardiovascular magnetic resonance in Anderson-Fabry disease evidence for a disease specific abnormality of the myocardial interstitium. *Eur Heart J*. 2003;24(23):2151–2155.
64. Weidemann F, et al. The variation of morphological and functional cardiac manifestation in fabry disease: potential implications for the time course of the disease. *Eur Heart J*. 2005;26(12):1221–1227.
65. Beer M, et al. Impact of enzyme replacement therapy on cardiac morphology and function and late enhancement in fabry's cardiomyopathy. *Am J Cardiol*. 2006;97(10):1515–1518.
66. Aquaro GD, et al. Cardiac magnetic resonance in fabry disease: morphological, functional, and tissue features. *Diagnostics*. 2022;12(11).
67. Silva MC, et al. Myocardial delayed enhancement by magnetic resonance imaging in patients with muscular dystrophy. *J Am Coll Cardiol*. 2007;49(18):1874–1879.
68. Yilmaz A, et al. Cardiac involvement in patients with Becker muscular dystrophy: new diagnostic and pathophysiological insights by a CMR approach. *J Cardiovasc Magn Reson*. 2008;10(1):50.
69. Puchalski MD, et al. Late gadolinium enhancement: precursor to cardiomyopathy in duchenne muscular dystrophy? *Int J Cardiovasc Imaging*. 2008;25(1):57–63.
70. Almogheer B, et al. Diagnostic and prognostic value of cardiovascular magnetic resonance in neuromuscular cardiomyopathies. *Pediatr Cardiol*. 2022;43(1):27–38.
71. Maceira AM, et al. Cardiovascular magnetic resonance in cardiac amyloidosis. *Circulation*. 2005;111(2):186–193.
72. Perugini E. Non-invasive evaluation of the myocardial substrate of cardiac amyloidosis by gadolinium cardiac magnetic resonance. *Heart*. 2005;92(3):343–349.
73. Hosch W, et al. Magnetresonanztomografie bei kardialer amyloidose–morphologie, funktion und late enhancement. *RöFo*. 2008;180(7):639–645.
74. Vogelsberg H, et al. Cardiovascular magnetic resonance in clinically suspected cardiac amyloidosis. *J Am Coll Cardiol*. 2008;51(10):1022–1030.
75. Fontana M, et al. Prognostic value of late gadolinium enhancement cardiovascular magnetic resonance in cardiac amyloidosis. *Circulation*. 2015;132(16):1570–1579.
76. Dungu J, et al. Patterns of late gadolinium enhancement in 94 patients with AL or transthyretin cardiac amyloidosis. *J Cardiovasc Magn Reson*. 2012;14(Suppl 1):O87.
77. Dungu JN, et al. CMR-based differentiation of AL and ATTR cardiac amyloidosis. *JACC Cardiovasc Imaging*. 2014;7(2):133–142.
78. Stevenson A, et al. Prognostic value of late gadolinium enhancement detected on cardiac magnetic resonance in cardiac sarcoidosis. *JACC Cardiovasc Imaging*. 2023;16(3):345–357.
79. Mahrholdt H, et al. Presentation, patterns of myocardial damage, and clinical course of viral myocarditis. *Circulation*. 2006;114(15):1581–1590.
80. Aquaro GD, et al. Cardiac MR with late gadolinium enhancement in acute myocarditis with preserved systolic function: ITAMY study. *J Am Coll Cardiol*. 2017;70(16):1977–1987.
81. Laissy J-P, et al. Differentiating acute myocardial infarction from myocarditis: diagnostic value of early- and delayed-perfusion cardiac MR imaging. *Radiology*. 2005;237(1):75–82.
82. Yelgec NS, et al. Value of MRI in patients with a clinical suspicion of acute myocarditis. *Eur Radiol*. 2007;17(9):2211–2217.
83. Gutberlet M, et al. Suspected chronic myocarditis at cardiac MR: diagnostic accuracy and association with immunohistologically detected inflammation and viral persistence. *Radiology*. 2008;246(2):401–409.
84. Cadour F, et al. Cardiac MRI features and prognostic value in immune checkpoint inhibitor-induced myocarditis. *Radiology*. 2022;303(3):512–521.
85. Lerchner T, et al. Cardiac magnetic resonance imaging in patients with suspected myocarditis from immune checkpoint inhibitor therapy–a real-world observational study. *Int J Cardiol Heart Vasc*. 2025;56:101581.
86. Zhang L, et al. Cardiovascular magnetic resonance in immune checkpoint inhibitor-associated myocarditis. *Eur Heart J*. 2020;41(18):1733–1743.
87. Rochitte CE, et al. Myocardial delayed enhancement by magnetic resonance imaging in patients with Chagas' disease. *J Am Coll Cardiol*. 2005;46(8):1553–1558.
88. Volpe Gustavo J, et al. Left ventricular scar and prognosis in chronic Chagas cardiomyopathy. *JACC J Am Coll Cardiol*. 2018;72(21):2567–2576.
89. Torreão JA, et al. Myocardial tissue characterization in Chagas' heart disease by cardiovascular magnetic resonance. *J Cardiovasc Magn Reson*. 2015;17(1):97.
90. Regueiro A, et al. Myocardial involvement in Chagas disease: insights from cardiac magnetic resonance. *Int J Cardiol*. 2013;165(1):107–112.

91. Senra T, et al. Long-term prognostic value of myocardial fibrosis in patients with Chagas cardiomyopathy. *J Am Coll Cardiol*. 2018;72(21):2577–2587.
92. Abdel-Aty H, et al. Myocardial tissue characterization in systemic lupus erythematosus: value of a comprehensive cardiovascular magnetic resonance approach. *Lupus*. 2008;17(6):561–567.
93. Feng X, et al. The presence, location, and degree of late gadolinium enhancement in relation to myocardial dysfunction and poor prognosis in patients with systemic lupus erythematosus. *J Cardiovasc Dev Dis*. 2023;10(11):451.
94. du Toit R, et al. Myocardial injury in systemic lupus erythematosus according to cardiac magnetic resonance tissue characterization: clinical and echocardiographic features. *Lupus*. 2020;29(11):1461–1468.
95. Seneviratne MG, et al. Prevalence, distribution and clinical correlates of myocardial fibrosis in systemic lupus erythematosus: a cardiac magnetic resonance study. *Lupus*. 2016;25(6):573–581.
96. Myhr KA, et al. Myocardial fibrosis associates with lupus anticoagulant in patients with systemic lupus erythematosus. *Int J Cardiovasc Imaging*. 2024;40(1):127–137.
97. Tzelepis GE, et al. Pattern and distribution of myocardial fibrosis in systemic sclerosis: a delayed enhanced magnetic resonance imaging study. *Arthritis Rheum*. 2007;56(11):3827–3836.
98. Kobayashi H, et al. Cardiac magnetic resonance imaging with pharmacological stress perfusion and delayed enhancement in asymptomatic patients with systemic sclerosis. *J Rheumatol*. 2009;36(1):106–112.
99. Naßenstein K, et al. Detection of myocardial fibrosis in systemic sclerosis by contrast-enhanced magnetic resonance imaging. *RöFo*. 2008;180(12):1054–1060.
100. Sano M, et al. Cardiac involvement in systemic sclerosis and the value of late gadolinium enhancement (LGE) in cardiac magnetic resonance (CMR). *Eur Heart J*. 2013;34(suppl_1):P2999.
101. Eitel I, et al. Differential diagnosis of suspected apical ballooning syndrome using contrast-enhanced magnetic resonance imaging. *Eur Heart J*. 2008;29(21):2651–2659.
102. Eitel I, et al. Clinical characteristics and cardiovascular magnetic resonance findings in stress (Takotsubo) cardiomyopathy. *JAMA*. 2011;306(3).
103. Schietinger BJ, et al. Patterns of late gadolinium enhancement in chronic hemodialysis patients. *JACC Cardiovasc Imaging*. 2008;1(4):450–456.
104. Mark PB, et al. Redefinition of uremic cardiomyopathy by contrast-enhanced cardiac magnetic resonance imaging. *Kidney Int*. 2006;69(10):1839–1845.
105. Debl K. Delayed hyperenhancement in magnetic resonance imaging of left ventricular hypertrophy caused by aortic stenosis and hypertrophic cardiomyopathy: visualisation of focal fibrosis. *Heart*. 2006;92(10):1447–1451.
106. Papanastasiou CA, et al. The prognostic role of late gadolinium enhancement in aortic stenosis: a systematic review and meta-analysis. *JACC Cardiovasc Imaging*. 2020;13(2, Part 1):385–392.
107. Musa TA, et al. Myocardial scar and mortality in severe aortic stenosis. *Circulation*. 2018;138(18):1935–1947.
108. Thornton GD, et al. Myocardial scar and remodelling predict long-term mortality in severe aortic stenosis beyond 10 years. *Eur Heart J*. 2024;45(22):2019–2022.
109. Maltês S, et al. LGE prevalence and patterns in severe aortic stenosis: when "junctional" means the same. *Int J Cardiol*. 2023;378:159–163.
110. Wassmuth R, et al. Cardiovascular magnetic resonance imaging detects cardiac involvement in churg-strauss syndrome. *J Card Fail*. 2008;14(10):856–860.
111. Karageorgiou I, et al. Cardiac magnetic resonance imaging findings in patients with antineutrophil cytoplasmic antibody-associated vasculitides: a systematic review. *ACR Open Rheumatol*. 2025;7(4):e70026.
112. Liori S, et al. Churg–strauss syndrome-associated heart failure and left ventricular thrombosis. *ESC Heart Failure*. 2023;10(3):2107–2112.
113. Baccouche H, et al. Images in cardiovascular medicine. Magnetic resonance assessment and therapy monitoring of cardiac involvement in Churg-strauss syndrome. *Circulation*. 2008;117(13):1745–1749.
114. Breuckmann F, et al. MR characterization of cardiac abnormalities in HIV+ individuals with increased BNP levels. *Eur J Med Res*. 2007;12(5):185–190.
115. Hudson JA, et al. Association of HIV infection with cardiovascular pathology based on advanced cardiovascular imaging: a systematic review. *JAMA*. 2022;328(10):951–962.
116. Luetkens JA, et al. Cardiac magnetic resonance reveals signs of subclinical myocardial inflammation in asymptomatic HIV-infected patients. *Circ Cardiovasc Imaging*. 2016;9(3):e004091.
117. Sanz J, et al. Prevalence and correlates of septal delayed contrast enhancement in patients with pulmonary hypertension. *Am J Cardiol*. 2007;100(4):731–735.
118. Swift AJ, et al. Diagnostic accuracy of cardiovascular magnetic resonance imaging of right ventricular morphology and function in the assessment of suspected pulmonary hypertension results from the ASPIRE registry. *J Cardiovasc Magn Reson*. 2012;14(1):40.
119. Swift AJ, et al. LGE patterns in pulmonary hypertension do not impact overall mortality. *JACC Cardiovasc Imaging*. 2014;7(12):1209–1217.
120. Freed BH, et al. Late gadolinium enhancement cardiovascular magnetic resonance predicts clinical worsening in patients with pulmonary hypertension. *J Cardiovasc Magn Reson*. 2012;14(1):11.
121. Mouquet F, et al. Characterisation of peripartum cardiomyopathy by cardiac magnetic resonance imaging. *Eur Radiol*. 2008;18(12):2765–2769.
122. Isaak A, et al. Peripartum cardiomyopathy: diagnostic and prognostic value of cardiac magnetic resonance in the acute stage. *Diagnostics*. 2022;12(2):378.
123. Liang Y-D, et al. Left ventricular function recovery in peripartum cardiomyopathy: a cardiovascular magnetic resonance study by myocardial T1 and T2 mapping. *J Cardiovasc Magn Reson*. 2020;22(1):2.
124. Schelbert EB, et al. Myocardial damage detected by late gadolinium enhancement cardiac magnetic resonance is uncommon in peripartum cardiomyopathy. *J Am Heart Assoc*. 2017;6(4):e005472.
125. Modi K, et al. Myocardial damage assessed by late gadolinium enhancement on cardiovascular magnetic resonance imaging in cancer patients treated with anthracyclines and/or trastuzumab. *Eur Heart J Cardiovasc Imaging*. 2020;22(4):427–434.
126. Carneiro AC, et al. A new typical finding in late gadolinium enhanced images for the diagnosis of endomyocardial fibrosis-the double V sign. *J Cardiovasc Magn Reson*. 2011;13(1):O40.
127. Salemi VM, et al. Late gadolinium enhancement magnetic resonance imaging in the diagnosis and prognosis of endomyocardial fibrosis patients. *Circ Cardiovasc Imaging*. 2011;4(3):304–311.
128. de Carvalho FP, Azevedo CF. Comprehensive assessment of endomyocardial fibrosis with cardiac mri: morphology, function, and tissue characterization. *Radiographics*. 2020;40(2):336–353.
129. Frederiksen CA, et al. Two different clinical presentations and stages of loeffler endocarditis diagnosed by multimodality investigations. *CASE*. 2023;7(12):496–501.
130. Polito MV, et al. Loeffler's endocarditis: an integrated multimodality approach. *J Am Soc Echocardiogr*. 2020;33(12):1427–1441.
131. Asadian S, Jahanshahi B, Rezaeian N. Follow-up CMR in a case of loeffler endocarditis. *Clin Case Rep*. 2021;9(1):599–600.
132. Arbelo E, et al. 2023 ESC guidelines for the management of cardiomyopathies. *Eur Heart J*. 2023;44(37):3503–3626.
133. Kim HW, et al. Patients with acute myocarditis following mRNA COVID-19 vaccination. *JAMA Cardiol*. 2021;6(10):1196–1201.
134. Muser D, et al. Prognostic value of nonischemic ringlike left ventricular scar in patients with apparently idiopathic nonsustained ventricular arrhythmias. *Circulation*. 2021;143(14):1359–1373.
135. Haugaa KH, et al. Comprehensive multi-modality imaging approach in arrhythmogenic cardiomyopathy—an expert consensus document of the European association of cardiovascular imaging. *Eur Heart J Cardiovasc Imaging*. 2017;18(3):237–253.
136. Kim RJ, Judd RM. Gadolinium-enhancedmagnetic resonance imagingin hypertrophic cardiomyopathy. *J Am Coll Cardiol*. 2003;41(9):1568–1572.
137. Iles LM, et al. Histological validation of cardiac magnetic resonance analysis of regional and diffuse interstitial myocardial fibrosis. *Eur Heart J Cardiovasc Imaging*. 2014;16(1):14–22.
138. Patel MR, et al. Detection of myocardial damage in patients with sarcoidosis. *Circulation*. 2009;120(20):1969–1977.
139. Mahrholdt H, et al. Delayed enhancement cardiovascular magnetic resonance assessment of non-ischaemic cardiomyopathies. *Eur Heart J*. 2005;26(15):1461–1474.
140. Kotani J-i, et al. Intravascular ultrasound analysis of infarct-related and non–infarct-related arteries in patients who presented with an acute myocardial infarction. *Circulation*. 2003;107(23):2889–2893.
141. Hunt SA, et al. ACC/AHA 2005 guideline update for the diagnosis and management of chronic heart failure in the adult. *Circulation*. 2005;112(12).
142. Assomull RG, et al. Role of cardiovascular magnetic resonance as a gatekeeper to invasive coronary angiography in patients presenting with heart failure of unknown etiology. *Circulation*. 2011;124(12):1351–1360.
143. Bawaskar P, et al. Nonischemic or dual cardiomyopathy in patients with coronary artery disease. *Circulation*. 2024;149(11):807–821.
144. Heitner JF, et al. Identifying the infarct-related artery in patients with non-ST-segment-elevation myocardial infarction. *Circ Cardiovasc Interv*. 2019;12(5):e007305.
145. Smulders MW, et al. The role of cardiovascular magnetic resonance imaging and computed tomography angiography in suspected non-ST-elevation myocardial infarction patients: design and rationale of the CARdiovascular magnetic rEsoNance imaging and computed tomography angiography (CARMENTA) trial. *Am Heart J*. 2013;166(6):968–975.
146. Tamis-Holland JE, et al. Contemporary diagnosis and management of patients with myocardial infarction in the absence of obstructive coronary artery disease: a scientific statement from the american heart association. *Circulation*. 2019;139(18):e891–e908.

25 Hypertrophic Cardiomyopathy

MICHAEL AYERS AND CHRISTOPHER M. KRAMER

INTRODUCTION

Hypertrophic cardiomyopathy (HCM) is a heterogenous disorder unified under the broad umbrella of significantly increased maximal left ventricular (LV) thickness without an underlying cause.[1] The disease involves the septum in 90% of cases, but numerous phenotypic configurations exist (Figs. 25.1A, B and 25.2). The estimated disease prevalence sits between 1:200 and 1:500. HCM inflicts a substantial cumulative burden with respect to morbidity and mortality.[2] Overall mortality rates are <1% per year, though patients diagnosed at younger ages (20–29 years) have fourfold increases in mortality compared to the general US population (Fig. 25.3).[2,3] Clinically, HCM is predominately characterized by heart failure and arrhythmias, though the symptoms and presentations are widely variable.[2] Between 20% and 40% of patients with HCM will suffer from atrial fibrillation, a rhythm which is often poorly tolerated due to the decreased LV compliance associated with HCM.[2] HCM remains one of the more common causes of sudden death in young adults, though associations between sudden death and exercise have become less clear.[4-7]

The earliest case reports date back to 1869 when Henri Liouville first described left ventricular outflow tract obstruction (LVOTO), a physiologic phenomenon seen in one third of HCM patients at rest and another third of HCM patients with provocation.[2,8] By the 1950s, Evans and Teare had both clearly documented the familial nature of HCM.[9,10] By the early 1990s, DNA sequencing revealed that an autosomal dominant mutation in myosin heavy chain 7 (*MHY7*) acted as a molecular genetic basis for the disease, with mutations in the myosin-binding protein C gene (*MYBPC3*) identified shortly thereafter.[11] Fast forward 30 plus years, the cardiology community has identified over 1400 mutations in at least eight causative genes, though *MHY7* and *MYBPC3* are still the most commonly identified. Despite these substantial gains in the understanding of the genetic underpinnings, only approximately 40% of patients with HCM have an identifiable genotype. Another 20–30% display an autosomal dominant pattern of disease inheritance within their family pedigree despite there being no clear causative gene identified.[12] The remainder are often seen with a sporadic or recessive inheritance pattern. Recently, evidence has increased that many sarcomere mutation-negative patients may possess a polygenic predisposition

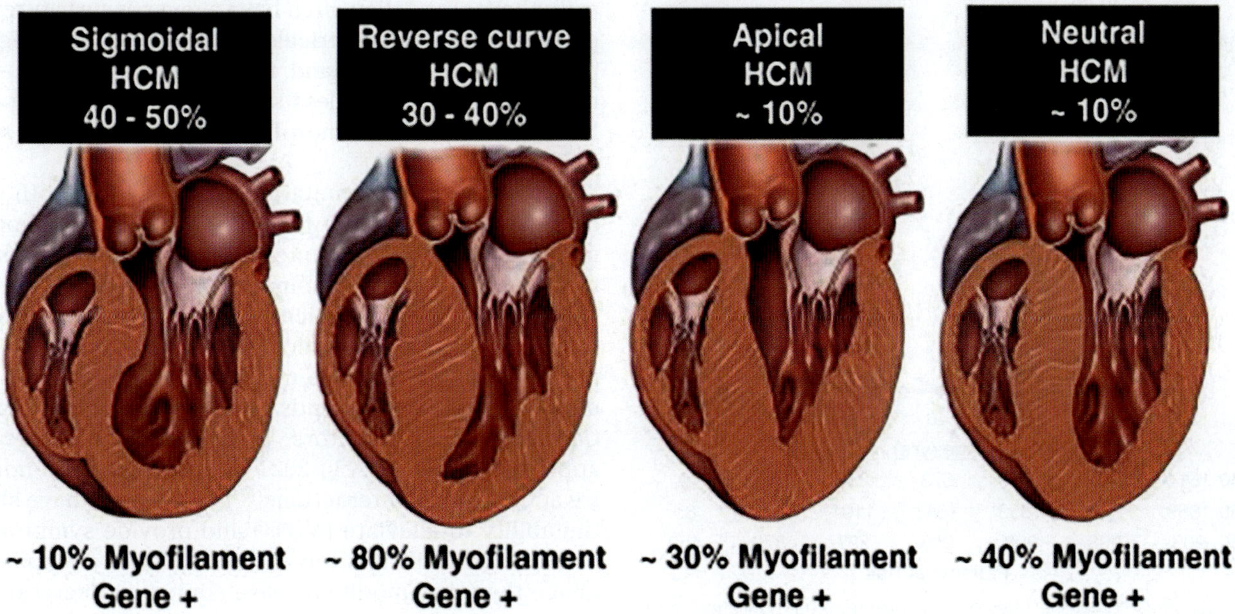

FIG. 25.1 The most common septal morphologies and the likelihood that each morphology has a detectable sarcomere mutation. (Bos J, Towbin J, Ackerman M. Diagnostic, prognostic, and therapeutic implications of genetic testing for hypertrophic cardiomyopathy. *JACC*. 2009;54[3]:201–211.)

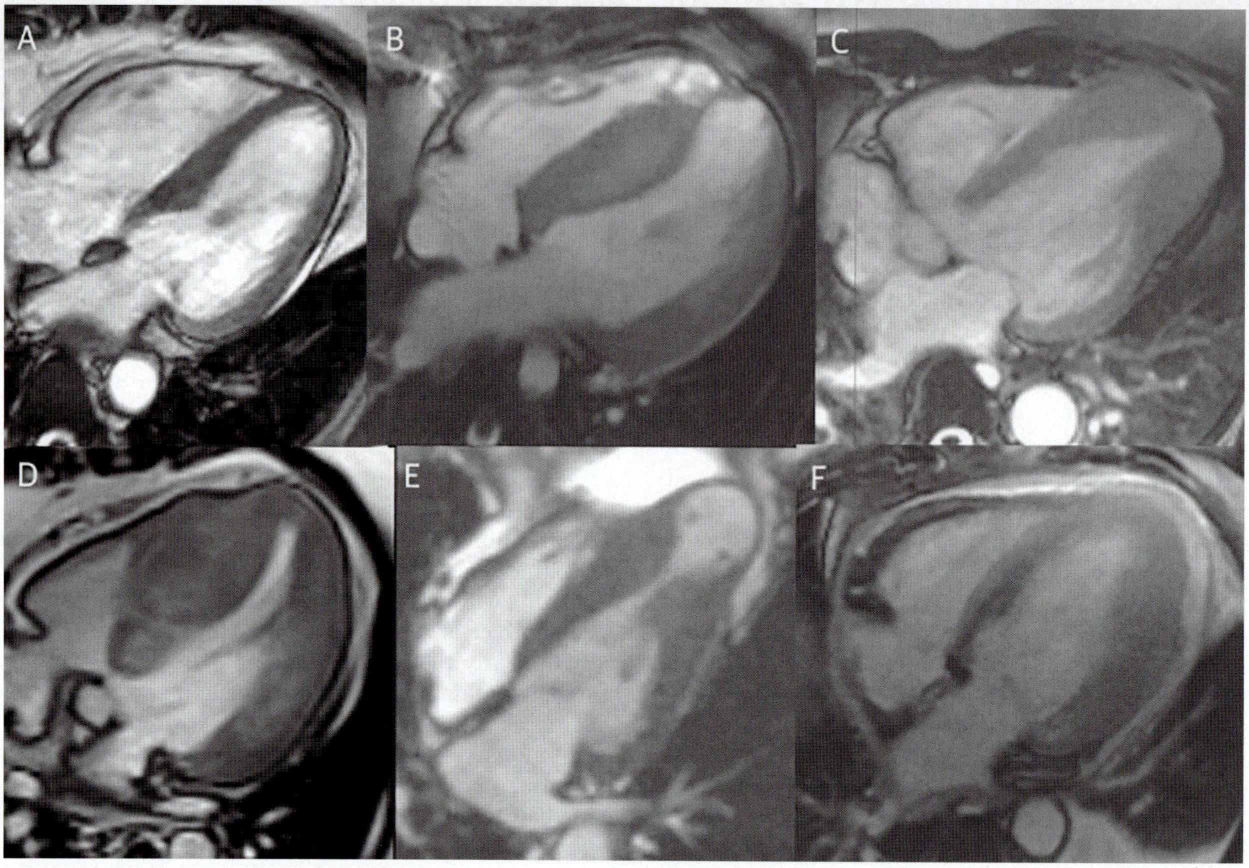

FIG. 25.2 CMR SSP four-chamber cine images from six morphological subtypes: (A) isolated basal septal, (B) reverse curvature, (C) apical, (D) concentric, (E) mid-cavitary obstruction with aneurysm, and (F) isolated lateral wall.

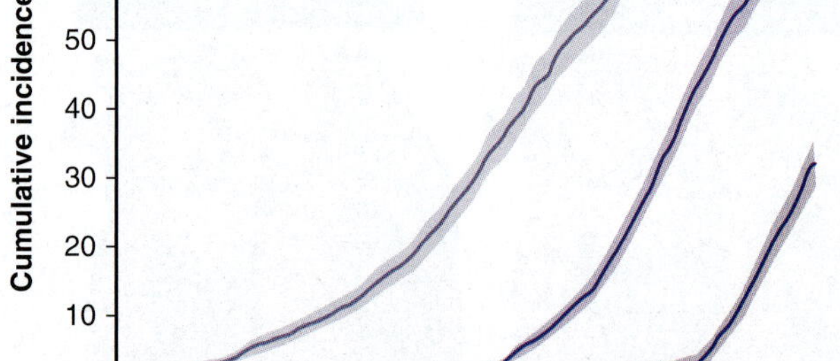

	10	20	30	40	50	60	70
<40	1614	1424	1068	573	238	55	9
40-60	1659	1658	1653	1643	1191	411	85
>60	909	908	908	905	897	879	452

FIG. 25.3 Overall composite rates of heart failure, atrial fibrillation, and sudden cardiac death based on age at time of diagnosis. (Ho et al Circulation 23 Aug 2018.)

to hypertrophy that is unveiled by environmental triggers such as hypertension and obesity.[13] The clinical relevance of the difference between the two groups—genotype-positive and genotype-negative patients—is significant. Genotype-positive patients on the whole experience earlier onset of disease, less LVOTO, more ventricular arrhythmias, and they often have a reverse curvature morphology to the interventricular septum. Genotype-negative patients, on the other hand, typically have a later onset of disease, more LVOTO, less sudden death, and they often have an isolated basal morphology of the increased septal thickness (Fig. 25.4).[14]

Known sarcomere mutations can result in both gains or losses of sarcomere function. While the pathogenic model is unlikely to be one-size-fits-all, almost all mutations result in some combination of altered contractility, reduced lusitropy, inefficient energy consumption, unmitigated myocyte proliferation, and fibrosis.[15] Increases in the understanding of the molecular pathogenesis of the disease have paid dividends with respect to management. Cardiac myosin inhibitors, a novel class of drugs first approved by the FDA in 2021, were designed to normalize actin–myosin interactions.[15] These agents have shown the ability to alleviate LVOTO and provide symptomatic benefit, and while it is too early to tell, there is some evidence they may modify disease course by decreasing LV thickness, left atrial size, left ventricular mass, and reducing progression of fibrosis.[16] It remains unclear whether

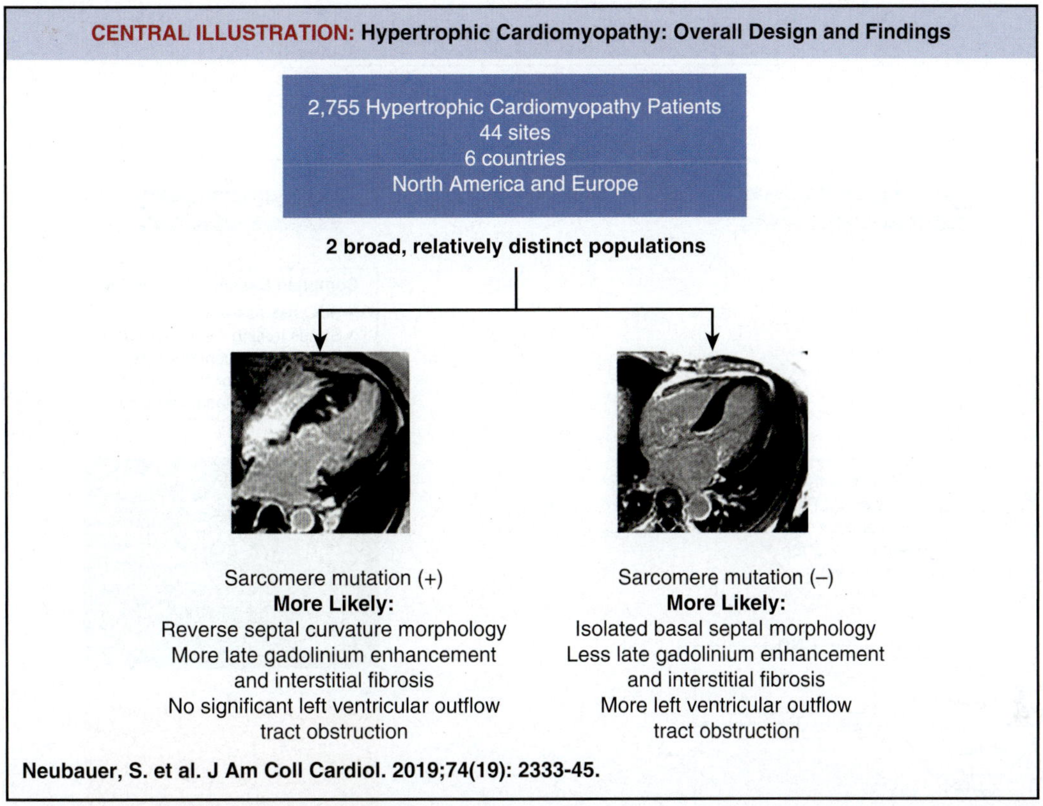

FIG. 25.4 Sarcomere-positive patients are more likely to have reverse curvature morphologies with more LGE, more interstitial fibrosis, a younger onset at age of diagnosis, and more sudden cardiac death, but are less likely to have significant LVOTO relative to the isolated basal phenotypes. (Neubauer et al. JACC 2019.)

the latter is simply due to the reduction in LVOTO or a primary effect of the drug.

Cardiovascular imaging plays a central role in HCM. Transthoracic echocardiography (TTE) serves as the work horse, with the benefit of widespread availability and expertise, lack of ionizing radiation, and the ability to assess hemodynamics via the Doppler principle. In the last 20 years, cardiac magnetic resonance imaging (CMR) has emerged as an irreplaceable tool in the diagnosis, management, and prognosis of HCM. In the 2020 AHA/ACC guidelines, CMR has a class I indication if the diagnosis of HCM is inconclusive after a TTE, to rule out alternative possible diagnoses, to risk stratify for sudden cardiac death (SCD), or to help elucidate the mechanism of obstruction (Fig. 25.5). CMR receives a class II recommendation for more accurate assessment of left ventricular ejection fraction (LVEF), wall thickness, to diagnose apical aneurysms, or to reassess late gadolinium enhancement (LGE) burden for patients at elevated risk of SCD.[17] This chapter will focus on the strengths of CMR with respect to diagnosing HCM, excluding phenocopies on the differential diagnosis, identifying specific HCM phenotypes, risk stratifying patients for sudden death, assessing the etiology of LVOTO, and identifying unique features such as mitral valve anomalies.

DIAGNOSIS

HCM is defined by an increase in LV wall thickness ≥15 mm in adults in the absence of another cause. While the extent of LV thickness does correlate with prognosis, 15 mm has as much statistical significance as it does prognostic: 15 mm of LV thickness is a value 6 standard deviations above population means.[17] When a known genotype or family history exists, the cutoff is decreased to ≥13–14 mm in LV thickness. It should be noted that maximal LV thickness, but not total LV mass, is required to make a diagnosis of HCM. LV mass can be normal in up to 20% of patients with HCM.[18] LV mass does demonstrate a modest relationship with maximal LV thickness, and increased LV mass is a sensitive but nonspecific marker for predicting adverse outcomes (100% sensitivity, 39% specificity). A maximal wall thickness >28–30 mm, however, is a more specific negative prognosticator (41% sensitivity, 90% specificity).[19] For this reason, massive LV thickness is included as a class IIA indication to consider primary prevention using an implantable cardiac defibrillator (ICD).

Echocardiography serves as the initial imaging modality to assess LV thickness, but has limitations. TTE can underestimate LV thickness if two-dimensional views do not transect the thickest segment of myocardium or if a patient has poor acoustic windows. Near-field artifact can hinder identification of apical hypertrophy when endomyocardial borders are not distinct. TTE can overestimate thickness if the two-dimensional views transect the myocardium at nonperpendicular angles or even more commonly if the septal measurements incorrectly include right ventricular structures such as trabeculations (Fig. 25.6). CMR creates three-dimensional images with high spatial resolution and signal- to-noise ratio. Cine steady-state free precession (SSFP) imaging allows sharp contrast between bright-blood and dark-myocardium allowing precise

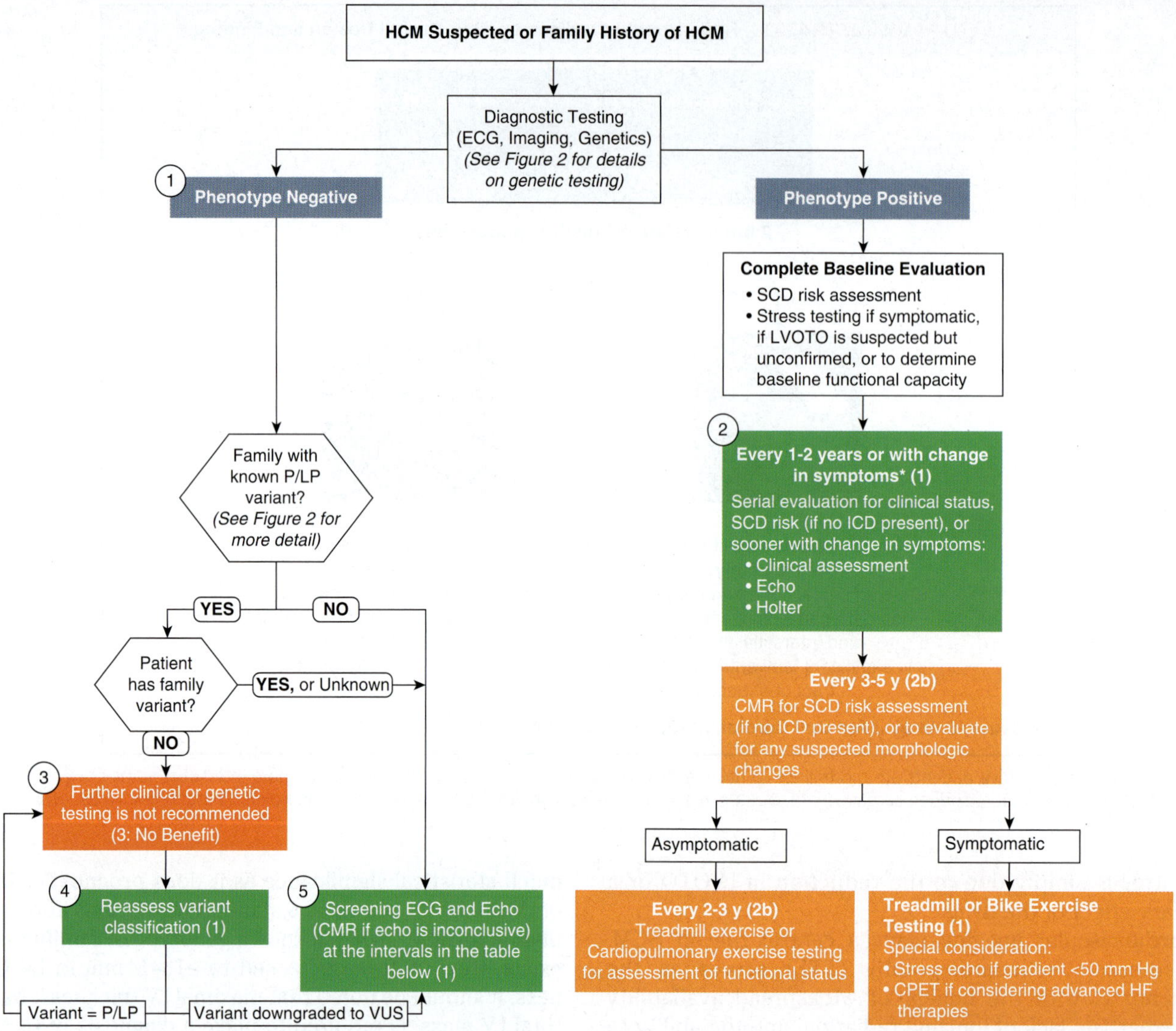

FIG. 25.5 The screening algorithm for HCM. (B, From Maron MS, Lesser JR, Maron BJ. Management implications of massive left ventricular hypertrophy in hypertrophic cardiomyopathy significantly underestimated by echocardiography but identified by cardiovascular magnetic resonance. *Am J Cardiol.* 2010;105:1842–1843. D, From Moon JC, Fisher NG, McKenna WJ, Pennell DJ. Detection of apical hypertrophic cardiomyopathy by cardiovascular magnetic resonance in patients with nondiagnostic echocardiography. *Heart.* 2004;90:645–649.)

measurements. When measuring LV thickness, the images should be first observed in motion in a short-axis series. This allows optimal visual differentiation of septum versus right ventricular (RV) moderator band or RV trabeculations. True septal cardiomyocytes should move with an inward radial motion toward the center of the LV cavity during systole, whereas RV components will move toward the center of the right ventricle or remain stationary. After observing the myocardium in motion, a static measurement should be made on end-diastolic images from epicardium to endocardium. In roughly half of cases, differences in echocardiographic and CMR measurements exceed 10%, with echocardiography both under- and overestimating LV thickness.[20] Discrepancies between TTE and CMR measurements can become dramatic in patients with massive LV thickness ≥28–30 mm.[21]

When a patient has an identifiable pathogenic genotype, his or her first-degree relatives are screened first with genetic testing. If a family member screens positive for the known pathogenic genetic mutation, TTE and EKG are recommended as the next steps to assess for a diagnostic phenotype. If a family member has a pathogenic genotype but the family member does not have an overt phenotype, surveillance screening should be performed every 1–2 years for adolescents and every 2–5 years for adults through the fourth or fifth decade of life.[17] When the probrand does not have an identifiable pathogenic genotype, TTE and EKG are recommended as the initial steps of screening for family members.[17] In instances where there is no identifiable genotype, family members should be screened with TTE and EKG at 1–5-year intervals.

In genotype-positive, phenotype-negative patients, CMR is helpful in confirming maximal LV thickness. Genotype-positive, phenotype-negative patients often have morphologic abnormalities even in the absence of increased LV thickness ≥13 mm. Common morphologic abnormalities include elongated anterior leaflets, myocardial clefts and crypts, or abnormal papillary muscles.[22] Such abnormalities can predate overt increases in LV thickness. In cases where the genotype is unknown, these findings can be clinical clues of an underlying sarcomere disorder (Fig. 25.7).

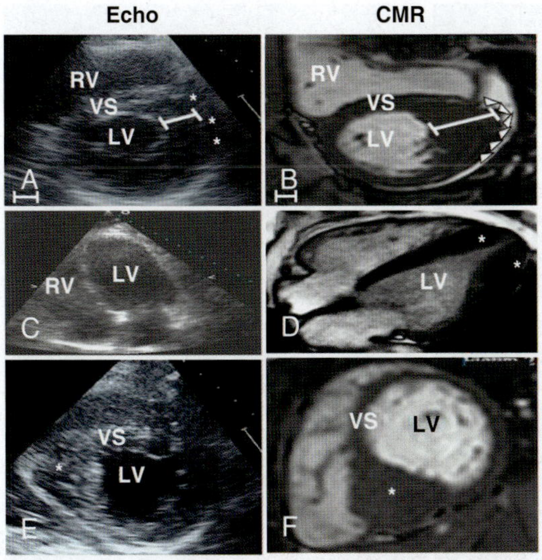

FIG. 25.6 Advantage of cardiovascular magnetic resonance (*CMR*) compared with two-dimensional (2D) transthoracic echocardiography. (A) 2D transthoracic echocardiography (TTE). Anterolateral left ventricular free wall is 18 mm; myocardial border and adjacent extracardiac structures are not well defined (*asterisks*). (B) CMR in the same patient shows well-delineated border of anterolateral wall (*arrowheads*), which is massively thickened (35 mm), creating a sudden cardiac death (SCD) risk factor. (C) 2D TTE. Nondiagnostic left ventricle (*LV*). (D) CMR in the same patient; segmental hypertrophy of left ventricular apex (*asterisks*), that is, apical hypertrophic cardiomyopathy. (E) 2D TTE. Inferior septal (*VS*) thickness is 21 mm (*asterisk*). (F) CMR in the same patient; massive hypertrophy (41 mm) (*asterisk*), creating an SCD risk marker. *RV*, Right ventricle. (B, From Maron MS, Lesser JR, Maron BJ. Management implications of massive left ventricular hypertrophy in hypertrophic cardiomyopathy significantly underestimated by echocardiography but identified by cardiovascular magnetic resonance. *Am J Cardiol.* 2010;105:1842–1843. D, From Moon JC, Fisher NG, McKenna WJ, Pennell DJ. Detection of apical hypertrophic cardiomyopathy by cardiovascular magnetic resonance in patients with nondiagnostic echocardiography. *Heart.* 2004;90:645–649.)

DIFFERENTIAL DIAGNOSIS

Physiologic Remodeling

When evaluating for HCM, the stipulation of increased thickness "in absence of another cause" can introduce diagnostic uncertainty. As many as one in four patients with hypertension have some degree of LVH.[23] Even with longstanding, severe, resistant hypertension, it is rare to exceed 18 mm in thickness. Measurements between 14–18 mm, however, can lie in a gray zone.[24] The majority of patients with severe hypertrophy from hypertension, however, will have concentric rather than an asymmetric remodeling pattern. Only 1% of HCM will present with a concentric pattern.[14] LVOTO should also lean the clinician toward a diagnosis of HCM rather than hypertensive cardiomyopathy, but LVOTO has been described in both entities.[25] Myocardial crypts, clefts, and mitral valve abnormalities are all more consistent with HCM.

Similar to hypertension, athletic remodeling can cause concentric LVH. With athletic remodeling, measurements rarely exceed 15 mm even in elite athletes.[26] In instances when hypertrophy is in the 13–15-mm range and athletic remodeling is on the differential, late gadolinium enhancement (LGE), T1 values, and extracellular volume (ECV) can aid in clarifying the diagnosis. Roughly one out of every three intensive endurance athletes will have some LGE, most typically at the RV insertion.[27] Nearly two out of three patients with HCM will have LGE, most commonly in the RV insertion and/or in the thickest areas of the septum.[28] Athletes typically have normal T1 values and normal to low ECV, unlike HCM where these values are typically elevated.[29] In rare cases of clinical uncertainty, detraining can be helpful to rule out HCM. A patient who regresses in wall thickness more than 2 mm after 2–3 months of detraining likely has athletic remodeling. Aortic stenosis, subaortic membrane, and supravalvular aortic stenosis typically elicit concentric patterns of hypertrophy, and the degree of increased thickness can exceed 15 mm. With these etiologies, hemodynamic assessment should reveal fixed rather than dynamic obstruction.

Infiltrative Processes

In pediatric populations, mitochondrial diseases, RASopathies such as Noonan syndrome, and storage disorders such as Pompe disease can all result in phenocopies of HCM, though each typically displays profound systemic involvement of the disease processes. In the adult population, wild-type transthyretin amyloidosis, hereditary transthyretin amyloidosis, and light-chain cardiac amyloidosis are increasingly identified during the workup for HCM.[30]

While classically thought of as a concentric process, many patients with amyloidosis can present with asymmetric remodeling.[31] Amyloidosis results in ECV elevations greater than with any other cardiomyopathy, and the LGE pattern tends to be diffuse subendocardial to transmural with concomitant right ventricular involvement. Other clinical clues or "red flags" such as bilateral carpal tunnel syndrome, bicep tendon rupture, neuropathy, lumbar stenosis, reduced voltage on surface electrocardiograms, or in the case of light-chain amyloidosis, an abnormal monoclonal immunoglobulin band in the serum or urine, further assist in the diagnosis. In earlier stages of disease with less significant hypertrophy, a technetium-99m pyrophosphate scan has excellent sensitivity and specificity for transthyretin amyloidosis.

Other infiltrative cardiomyopathies include Friedreich's ataxia, hemochromatosis, PRKAG2-assocaited cardiomyopathy, Danon disease, and Anderson–Fabry disease. The first two diseases tend to result in a more mild, concentric LVH and typically present with noncardiac symptoms.[32] Friedreich's ataxia is a relentless neurodegenerative disease, but rarely pediatric patients can present with cardiac symptoms.[33] Hemochromatosis has a prevalence of nearly one in 300 in the US population, and patients usually experience arthralgias, endocrinopathies, liver disease, and abdominal pain.[34] Hemochromatosis has a pathognomonic CMR finding on T2* sequences, resulting in values that can be less than 20 ms in the setting of LV dysfunction (normal 50 ms). This sequence is not routinely performed, and so some index of suspicion is required in order to correctly protocol image acquisition. Genetic testing for HFE mutations for hemochromatosis has excellent sensitivity.[35] PRKAG2 mutations cause abnormal function of the adenosine monophosphate kinase leading to accumulation of glycogen within the cardiac myocyte. The degree and pattern of hypertrophy in these patients is highly variable, from concentric, to isolated lateral wall, to asymmetric septal hypertrophy.[36] Patients may have multiple accessory atrioventricular pathways, and sudden arrhythmogenic death remains a major clinical concern.[37]

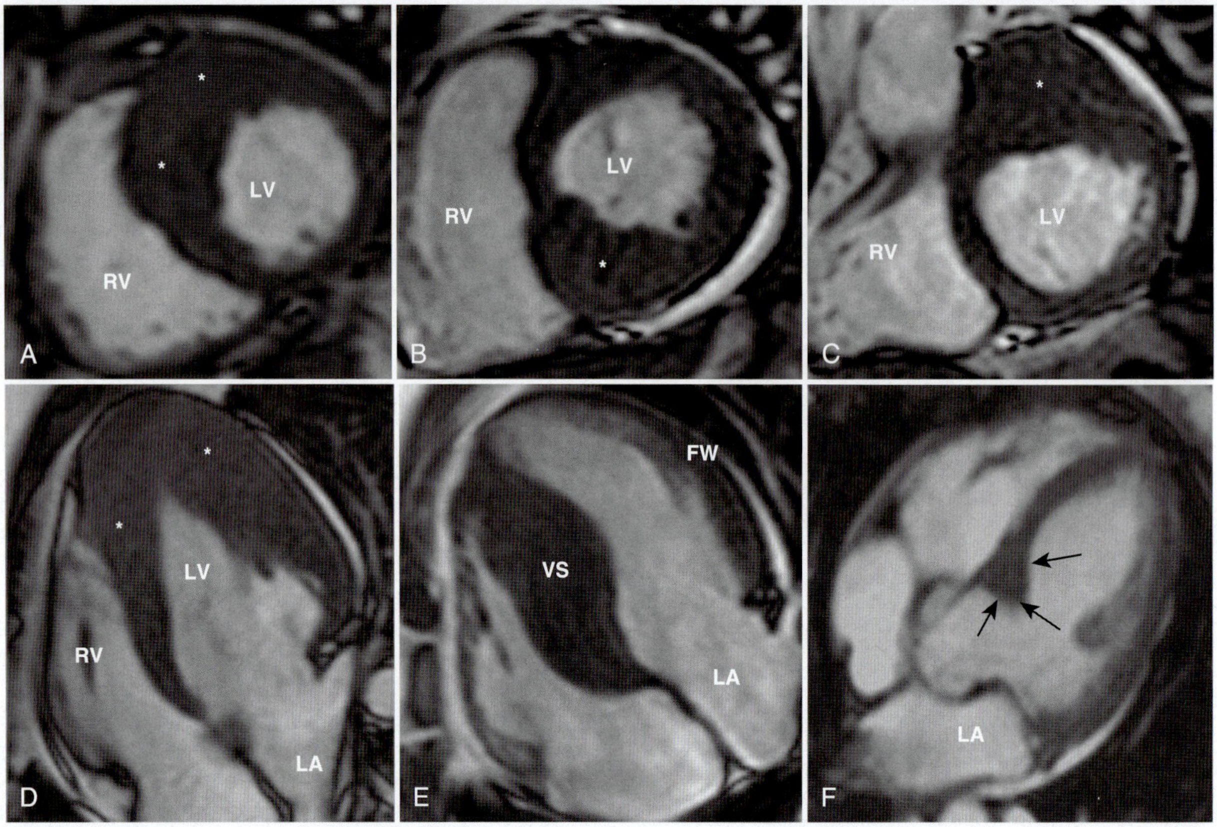

FIG. 25.7 Cardiovascular magnetic resonance (CMR) end-diastolic images demonstrating the diverse patterns of left ventricular (*LV*) hypertrophy in hypertrophic cardiomyopathy (*HCM*). (A–C) Short-axis CMR images demonstrating (A) hypertrophy of the basal anterior free wall and a portion of the continuous anterior septum (*asterisks*), representing the most common area of LV hypertrophy in HCM. (B) Prominent hypertrophy in the basal posterior ventricular septum (*asterisk*), (C) massive hypertrophy (wall thickness of 31 mm) confined to the basal anterior free wall (*asterisk*). (D–F) Long-axis four-chamber CMR images demonstrating (D) hypertrophy localized to the LV apex (*asterisks*), (E) hypertrophy throughout the ventricular septum (*VS*) but sparing the LV free wall (*FW*), (F) focal area of hypertrophy confined to the basal anterior septum (*arrows*). *LA*, left atrium; *LV*, left ventricle; *RV*, right ventricle.

The final two diseases, Anderson–Fabry disease and Danon disease, present in late adolescence to early adulthood. Anderson–Fabry is an X-linked multisystem glycogen storage disorder resulting from mutations in the α-galactosidase A gene, leading to toxic cellular accumulation of glycosphingolipids in tissues. This systemic illness is associated with neuropathy, autonomic disturbances, gastrointestinal pain, and renal disease. Electrocardiogram findings include preexcitation and prolonged QRS. In early to mid-stages, T1 parametric mapping will reveal profoundly reduced T1 values and concentric remodeling. Scarring typically initiates in the inferolateral segments and can progress to involve other segments in later stages of the disease. As replacement fibrosis progresses, T1 values can normalize or even become elevated.[38] Enzyme replacement therapy has drastically improved the outlook for patients with this disease, particularly when diagnosed earlier in the disease course.[39] Danon disease is a lysosomal storage disorder from a mutation in lysosomal associated membrane protein 2 (LAMP2), leading to an accumulation of intracellular vacuoles with resultant cardiac, skeletal, and cognitive abnormalities. Disease progression is typically accelerated, with significant LGE. Cardiac disease often causes death before age 25 (Fig. 25.8).[40]

PHENOTYPE

Ninety percent of cases of HCM will involve thickening of the septum, but the pattern is variable. The most common location of thickening involves the continuity of the basal anterior and basal anteroseptal segments.[14] When the basal septum is involved in isolation, the phenotype is referred to as an isolated basal subtype, occurring in 40–50% of HCM cases. If the thickness is greater in the mid-septal segments, it often creates a convex protrusion into the ventricular cavity. This configuration is referred to as a reverse curvature subtype. If the septum is uniformly thickened in the basal to mid segments, but lacks the convexity of the reverse curvature subtype, the configuration is referred to as a neutral subtype.

In 8–10% of cases, only apical segments are involved, often in a symmetric pattern. The apical subtype is more common in southeast Asian cohorts, representing around 25% of cases associated with this ancestry.[41] In general, apical HCM has a more favorable prognosis. An exception to this occurs when the increased thickness extends into the midventricular segments creating midventricular obstruction (about 3% of all HCM). Midventricular obstruction is a high-risk form of HCM due to the risk of the formation of apical aneurysms. Smaller aneurysms can be difficult to detect on TTE, particularly without the use of ultrasound-enhancing agents. Patients with apical aneurysms have poorer prognoses due to high rates of ventricular arrhythmias and sudden death arising from the arrhythmogenic, dense apical replacement fibrosis. Large aneurysms, as defined by those with >4 cm width, are nearly threefold more likely to result in heart failure, stroke, or sudden death.[42] The presence of an apical aneurysm is a class

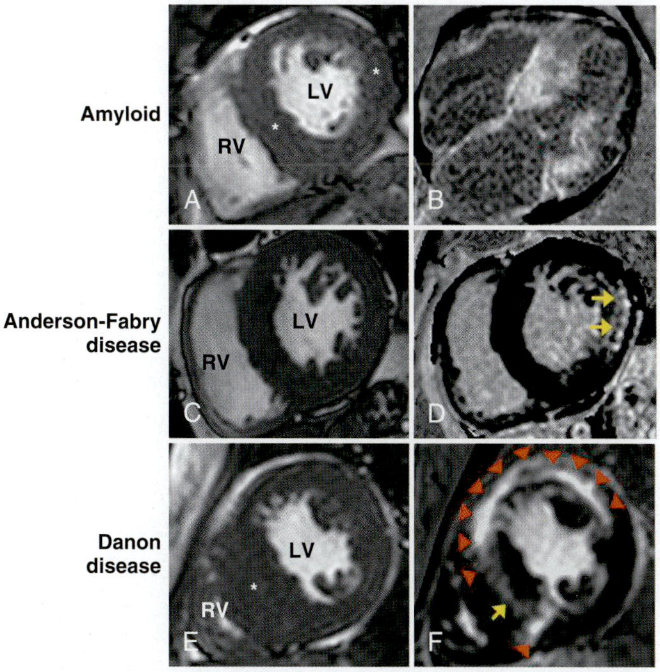

FIG. 25.8 Cardiovascular magnetic resonance (CMR) for differentiation of etiology of left ventricular (LV) hypertrophy. (A) A 64-year-old male with concentric LV hypertrophy (maximum LV wall thickness of 18 mm in septum and 14 mm in lateral wall). (B) Late gadolinium enhancement (LGE) image in the same patient demonstrates early contrast washout with transmural LGE in septum and lateral wall (*arrows*) features consistent with cardiac amyloid. The patient underwent cardiac biopsy confirming the diagnosis of amyloid. (C) A 44-year-old female with concentric LV hypertrophy (maximum wall thickness of 16 mm in septum and 13 mm in the lateral wall). (D) LGE image in the same patient demonstrates LGE confined to the basal inferolateral wall (*arrows*), a location of LGE typical for Anderson–Fabry disease. The patient underwent genetic testing, which demonstrated pathogenic mutation in the GLA gene, confirming the diagnosis of Anderson–Fabry disease. (E) A 21-year-old male demonstrated massive LV hypertrophy (wall thickness of 32 mm) confined to the ventricular septum (*asterisk*). (F) LGE images in the same patient demonstrated transmural LGE throughout the anterior and lateral walls (*arrowheads*) with mid-myocardial LGE throughout the septum (*arrow*) in a pattern atypical for HCM. Genetic testing was sent and revealed a pathogenic mutation in the *LAMP2* gene, consistent with Danon cardiomyopathy. *LV*, left ventricle; *RV*, right ventricle.

IIA indication for consideration of a primary prevention ICD (Fig. 25.9). Patients with apical aneurysm also suffer from high rates of cerebrovascular accidents due to clot forming in the area of dyskinesis, though empiric anticoagulation is not recommended in the absence of known LV thrombus (Fig. 25.10).[43] Isolated mid-cavitary, concentric, RV predominant, and isolated lateral wall variants have also been described, but represent less than 5% of cases.[14] Increased RV wall thickness is typically seen at the junction of the insertion sites but can also be diffuse. It is unclear if increased RV wall thickness is a sequela of pulmonary hypertension or a direct effect of the sarcomere mutation itself.[44]

LATE GADOLINIUM ENHANCEMENT

While gains in understanding have been made, the exact pathogenesis of HCM remains unknown. Early in the disease, there is architectural disruption of normal myocardial fiber orientation, a phenomenon known as myocyte disarray. Gradually, there is associated increased wall thickness on a gross anatomic level. Myocyte disarray and increased LV thickness diminish myocardial blood flow from the arterioles and capillaries, accelerating myofibrillar apoptosis via ischemia, upregulating the TGF-beta fibrotic pathways, and causing collage deposition and fibrosis.[45] The resultant scar is thought to be a nidus for ventricular arrhythmias and to contribute to reductions in systolic function (Figs. 25.11A, B and 25.12).

CMR serves as the gold standard to quantify scar burden in patients with HCM. Semiautomated programs quantify LGE pixels and calculate the degree to which the pixels deviate above the mean signal intensity of the reference normal myocardium. A threshold of 6 SD above the mean reference myocardium best represents macroscopic scar devoid of myocytes, known as replacement fibrosis.[46] This bright signal can similarly be readily identified on visual assessment. Lesser degrees of LGE represent varying degrees of collagen intermixed with cardiomyocytes and are known as interstitial fibrosis.[28] The ability to quantify LGE hinges upon the interpreter to correctly identify a segment of normal myocardium and to ensure areas included in the LGE calculation are a full 6 SDs above the reference segment. This method is preferred over the full-width half-maximum approach. While multiple thresholds have been published, a higher cutoff point increases the reproducibility of measurements.[47] Numerous obstacles to accurate quantification exist, including image quality, inversion times, surface coil intensity, and artifact.

The distinction between interstitial fibrosis and replacement fibrosis is an important one, as the quantification of LGE can drive decision-making regarding the placement of primary prevention ICD.[17] LGE is reported as a percentage of total left ventricular mass. In the international multicenter Hypertrophic Cardiomyopathy Registry (HCMR), roughly half of patients with HCM have some degree of LGE, though the majority of these have a burden of <5% of total myocardium.[47] While overall burden of LGE linearly correlates with incident nonsustained ventricular tachycardia, sudden death, heart failure, and all-cause mortality,[47] one-fourth of patients experiencing SCD will have <10% LGE. Thus, decreased or even complete absence of LGE decreases but does not obviate risk of SCD. The burden of LGE correlates with maximal LV thickness, younger age at time of diagnosis, and genotype positivity.[14] Extensive LGE is defined as >15–20% of myocardial mass. Extensive LGE confers a twofold increased risk of SCD and serves as a class IIB indication for primary prevention ICD in the 2020 ACC/AHA Guidelines.[17,48] More recent data have supported a lower cutoff of >10% LGE to improve prognostic power.[49] Many patterns of scar have been described, though the most typical pattern is one of patchy involvement of the area of greatest wall thickness and/or at the RV insertion sites. At present, no correlation between LGE pattern and prognosis exists, likely due to the enormous diversity of patterns observed.[14] When quantifying LGE in HCM, areas of ischemic scar should be distinguished from nonischemic scar, as it is unclear how ischemic scar contributes to adverse HCM-related outcomes. Discernment of ischemic versus nonischemic scar can be difficult, as transmural LGE in HCM is well described, though HCM scar should not necessarily follow coronary distributions.[50]

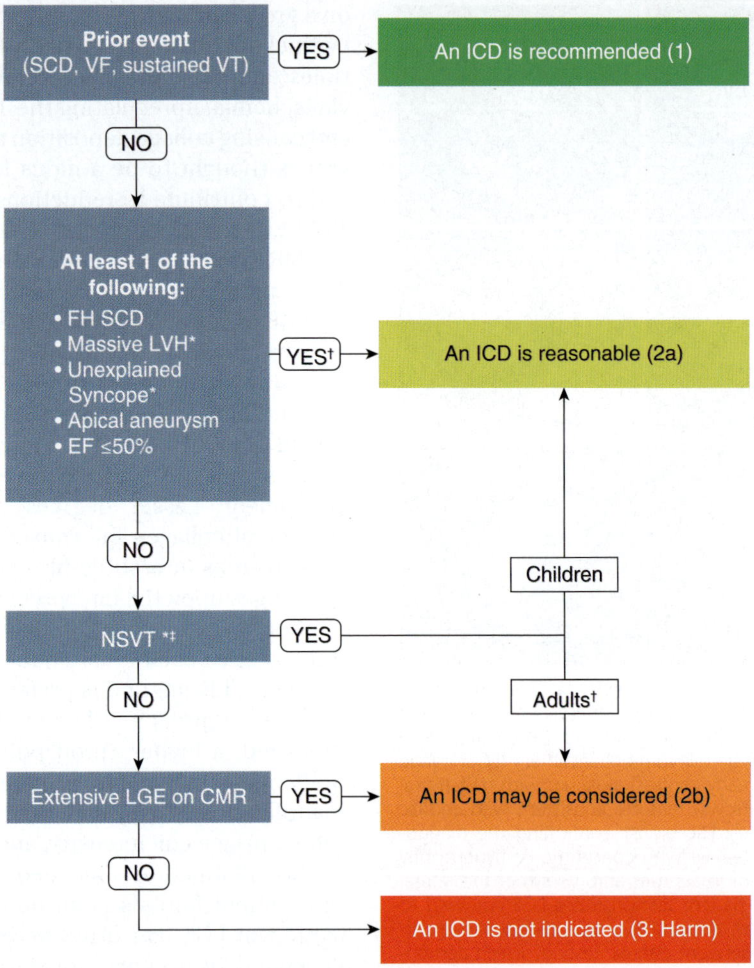

FIG. 25.9 ICD indications. ICD recommendations from 2020 AHA/ACC guidelines for management of HCM. In pediatric patients, more than one of the risk factors with an * should be present. ‡ For NSVT, frequent, longer, faster, and more recent runs of NSVT should carry more weight. Notably, CMR assists in diagnosing massive LVH >28–30 mm, apical aneurysms, reduced ejection fraction <50%, and extensive LGE. Also notable, LGE is not included in the HCM risk assessment tool endorsed by the ESC.

While much of the focus of LGE quantification centers around assessing the risk of SCD, to a lesser degree, LGE may also serve as a risk factor for progression to systolic dysfunction. Around one in 20 patients with HCM will progress to have a reduced ejection fraction <50%, and these patients experience very high rates of adverse outcomes including progression to heart transplant.[17,51] Progression of LGE between interval scans is associated with worsened outcomes.[49,50,52] The current guidelines offer a IIB recommendation to consider repeat CMR at 3–5-year intervals due to a lower level of evidence.[52]

One particular area of immense excitement is virtual native enhancement imaging. This is a deep-learning CMR technology that generates images resembling LGE without requiring gadolinium-based contrast agents[53] by superimposing T1 maps on SSFP cine images. In HCMR, VNE achieved excellent agreement with LGE with respect to quantification and distribution. Virtual native enhancement (VNE) shows promise to reduce both cost and scan times, potentially expanding CMR availability to more HCM patients. There are significantly more robust data correlating the degree of LGE with clinical outcomes, but VNE has the potential to be paradigm changing. As HCMR is completed, further insight into the relationship of LGE, SCD, advanced heart failure, VNE, and the value of repeated scans is to be expected.

LVOT OBSTRUCTION, SYSTOLIC FUNCTION, AND STRAIN

Over the last several decades, the physiologic understanding of the mechanisms of outflow tract obstruction has evolved. The initial hypothesis centered around the Venturi effect; increased velocity of fluid through a narrowed outflow tract pulled the mitral valve further into the outflow tract, worsening obstruction.[54] While Venturi forces are present, the magnitude of their influence is much smaller than initially presumed. Instead, outflow tract obstruction is primarily due to drag forces directly pushing on the mitral valve apparatus, further exaggerating systolic anterior motion (SAM) of the anterior leaflet. Significant obstruction is defined as > 30 mm Hg difference between the left ventricle and the aorta in systole under resting conditions, or >50 mmHg difference with provocation. Valsalva maneuver, when sustained for longer than 6–8 seconds, can decrease LV preload, LV end-diastolic volume, and in turn can worsen outflow tract obstruction. Exercise can worsen obstruction by increasing LV contractility and decreasing the time for diastolic filling.[17] Continuous-wave Doppler with TTE remains the preferred technique to quantify LVOT gradient, CMR provides visualization of SAM and

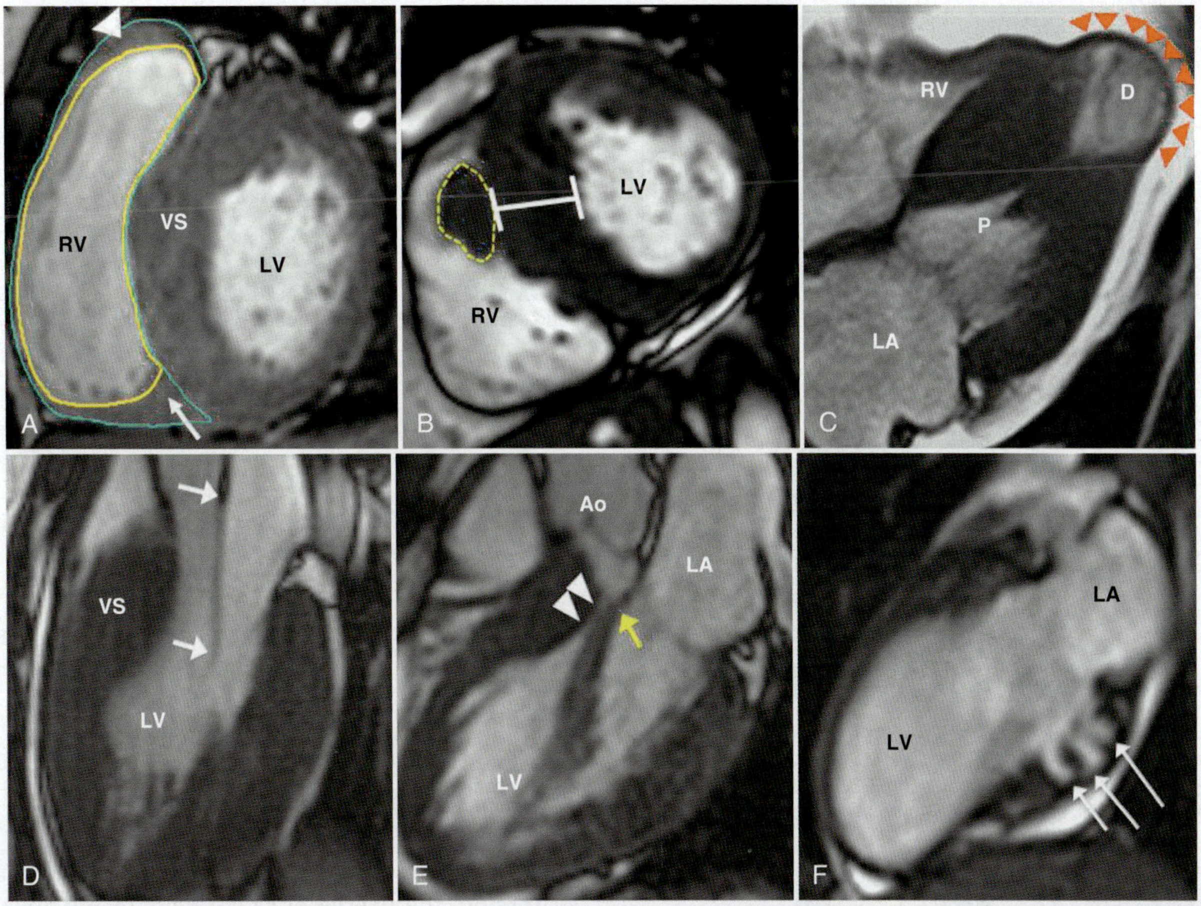

FIG. 25.10 Cardiovascular magnetic resonance (CMR) end-diastolic images demonstrating diversity of the phenotypic expression within hypertrophic cardiomyopathy (HCM). (A) Increased wall thickness in the superior segment (*arrowhead*) and inferior segment (*arrow*) of the right ventricular (*RV*) free wall. (B) Prominent and hypertrophied crista supraventricularis (*outlined structure*) and RV muscle structure. It is important not to include this muscle structure in the measurement of ventricular septum because this can lead to overestimation of maximal left ventricular (*LV*) wall thickness. (C) Medium-sized LV apical aneurysm (*arrowheads*) and maximum wall thickness at midventricular level with muscular apposition of the ventricular septum and LV free wall producing distinct proximal (*P*) and distal (*D*) chamber. (D) Elongation of the anterior mitral valve leaflet (*arrows*), contributing to LV outflow obstruction in this patient. (E) Muscular midcavitary obstruction attributable to the insertion of anomalous anterolateral papillary muscle directly into anterior leaflet (*arrow*), contacting the midventricular septum in systole (*arrowheads*). (F) Asymptomatic genotype-positive, phenotype-negative patient with three deep myocardial crypts in the basal inferior LV wall. *Ao*, Aorta; *LA*, left atrium; *LV*, left ventricle; *RV*, right ventricle; *VS*, ventricular septum. ((A) Modified from Maron MS, Hauser TH, Dubrow E, et al., Right ventricular involvement in hypertrophic cardiomyopathy. *Am J Cardiol.* 2007;100:1293–1298. D, Modified from Maron MS, Olivotto I, Harrigan C, et al., Mitral valve abnormalities identified by cardiovascular magnetic resonance represent a primary phenotypic expression of hypertrophic cardiomyopathy. *Circulation.* 2011;124:40–47. F, From Maron MS, Rowin EJ, Lin D, et al. Prevalence and clinical profile of myocardial crypts in hypertrophic cardiomyopathy. *Circ Cardiovasc Imaging.* 2012;5:441–447.)

septal contact to help differentiate the mechanism from subaortic stenosis or other obstructive lesions. Occasionally, hemodynamic assessment with cardiac catheterization is required to supplement these imaging modalities. Initial management of obstruction focuses on hydration, avoidance of vasodilating medications, and negative inotropic agents such as beta-blockers or calcium channel blockers. Refractory symptoms can be managed with cardiac myosin inhibitors, disopyramide, or with mechanical options such as alcohol septal ablation or surgical myectomy (Figs. 25.13A–C, 25.14, and 25.15).[17]

It is imperative to understand the mechanism of any mitral valve regurgitation prior to deciding on a management approach for residual symptoms of outflow tract obstruction. In obstructive HCM, the average length of the anterior mitral leaflet is 34 mm compared to 24 mm in normal hearts.[55] In classic, SAM-dependent regurgitation, the anterior leaflet is pulled into the LVOT via drag forces and the shorter posterior leaflet remains outside of the LVOT. This creates a funnel with fluid coursing along the atrial aspects of the anterior and posterior leaflets in an anteroseptal to posterolateral direction. One out of five HCM patients will have significant SAM-independent regurgitation.[56] HCM patients may have SAM-independent MR due to anomalous insertions of the papillary muscle directly into the mitral leaflet, apical or anterolateral displacement of the papillary muscle bundles, degeneration of the mitral apparatus, very severe elongation of the anterior mitral leaflet, or concomitant elongation of the posterior leaflet. A centrally or anteroseptally directed jet should provide a clinical clue of a SAM-independent etiology. In these instances, the MR and the patient's symptoms may persist despite medical therapies or alcohol septal reduction. In such cases, a surgical strategy may be preferred to address the mitral anomalies (Fig. 25.16). Anomalous mitral valves can necessitate extended resections, concomitant mitral repair, or even mitral valve replacement.

As is true with other disease states, CMR is considered the gold standard for assessment of ejection fraction in HCM. As mentioned previously, an ejection fraction <50% portends a particularly poor short-term risk in HCM, with median freedom to survival from advanced therapies

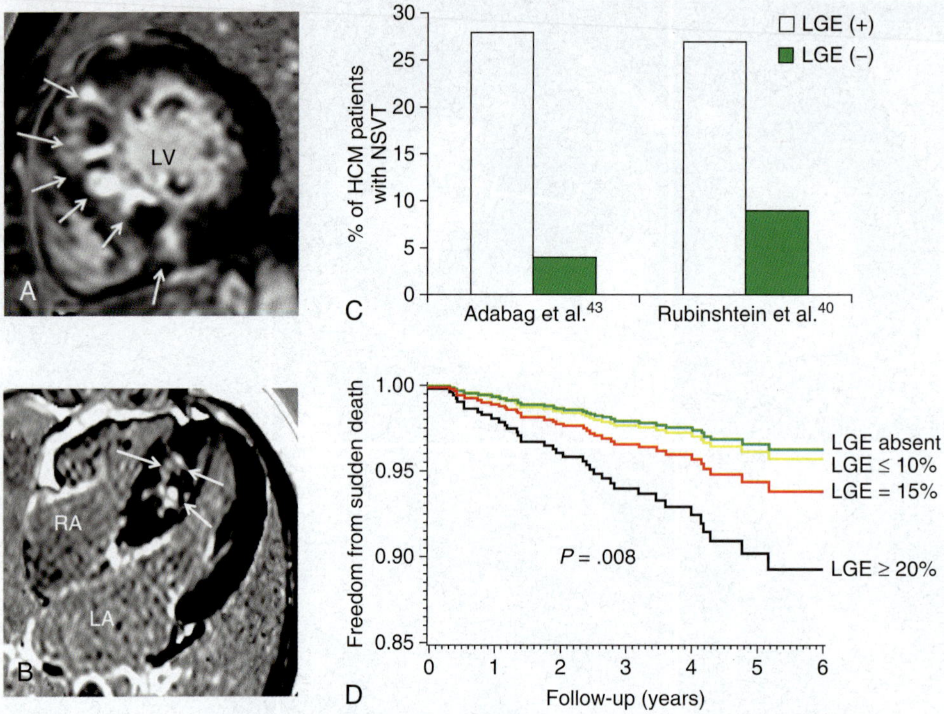

FIG. 25.11 Relationship between late gadolinium enhancement (*LGE*) and sudden death risk in hypertrophic cardiomyopathy (*HCM*). (A, B) LGE CMR images in two different HCM patients, each with extensive LGE (*arrows*) throughout the ventricular septum. (C) Nonsustained ventricular tachycardia (*NSVT*) on 24-hour Holter electrocardiogram (ECG) is sevenfold more common in HCM patients with LGE compared with those without LGE. (D) Relation between extent of LGE and sudden death events in 1293 patients with HCM. *LV*, Left ventricle; *RV*, right ventricle.

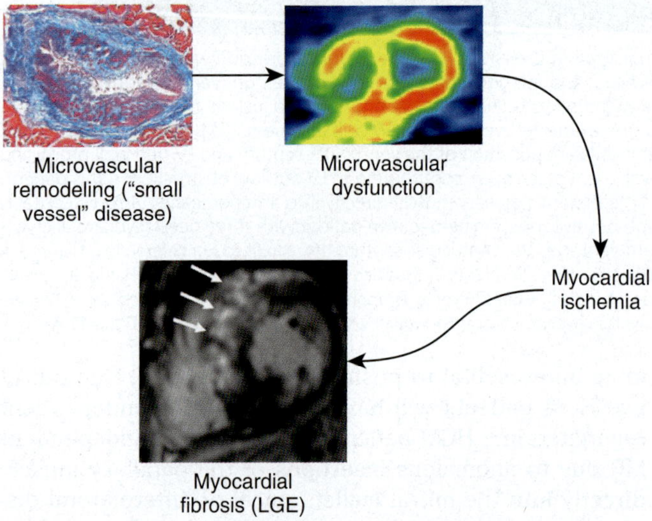

FIG. 25.12 Proposed mechanism for late gadolinium enhancement (*LGE*) in hypertrophic cardiomyopathy (HCM). Structurally abnormal intramural coronary arteries are responsible for microvascular ischemia. Over time, myocyte cell death and a process of repair with replacement fibrosis can be imaged as LGE in HCM. (Modified from Chan RH, Maron BJ, Olivotto I, et al. Prognostic value of quantitative contrast-enhanced cardiovascular magnetic resonance for the evaluation of sudden death risk in patients with hypertrophic cardiomyopathy. *Circulation* 2014;130:484–513.)

or death of 8.4 years.[57] Patients with borderline reduced ejection fractions in the 50–59% range are at heightened risk for progression. Given that patients with asymmetric ventricles or more significant hypertrophy have more challenging ejection fractions to interpret on TTE, CMR plays an important role in confirming ventricular function.

Early studies on HCM with CMR elucidated a potential roll for left ventricular strain both for the pathophysiologic understanding of the disease and for prognostication.[58] LV torsion, the degree of radial twist of the apex about the long axis relative to the base, is preserved in HCM. The rate of twisting, however, has been linked to myocardial fibrosis.[59] Untwisting rates are perturbed early in the disease course, oftentimes before overt phenotypes emerge. This may suggest a pathologic dissociation of actin and myosin in patients with sarcomere mutations due to abnormal calcium handling. A global longitudinal strain has been shown on both TTE and CMR to correlate with adverse outcomes, and also correlates with other demographic factors such as reverse curvature and apical morphologies, extent of LGE, abnormal biomarkers, female patients, and black patients. How and if these features will be early, independent predictors of the disease course remains to be seen.

FUTURE DIRECTIONS

As therapeutic options expand within HCM, there is renewed interest in identifying imaging and biochemical parameters that might predict disease progression or serve as markers of disease modification. Ideally, these novel markers could either indicate who may benefit from a therapy or to monitor the response to a therapy. Within HCMR, baseline T1 mapping using the Shortened Modified Look-Locker Inversion recovery technique was used to calculate extracellular volume as a percent of LV mass. Native mean T1 values recorded before administration of gadolinium contrasts agents and ECV calculations based on changes in the myocardium during gadolinium administration both correlate in

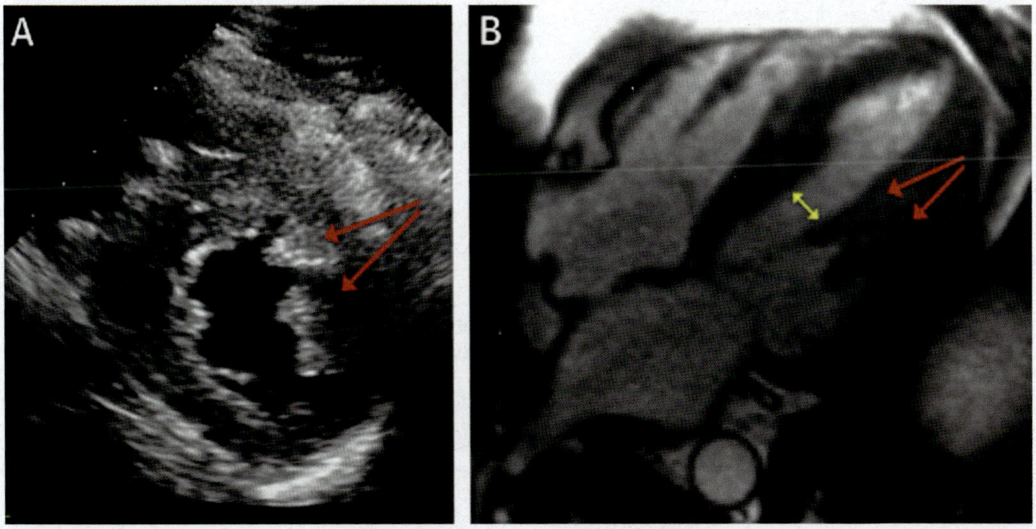

FIG. 25.13 Side-by-side comparison of a bifid papillary abnormality on short-axis with TTE (A) and four-chamber SSFP with CMR (B). (*Sherrid M. V., Balaram S., Kim B., Axel L., Swistel D. G. The mitral valve in obstructive hypertrophic cardiomyopathy: a test in context. J Am Coll Cardiol 2016;67(15):1846-1858.*)

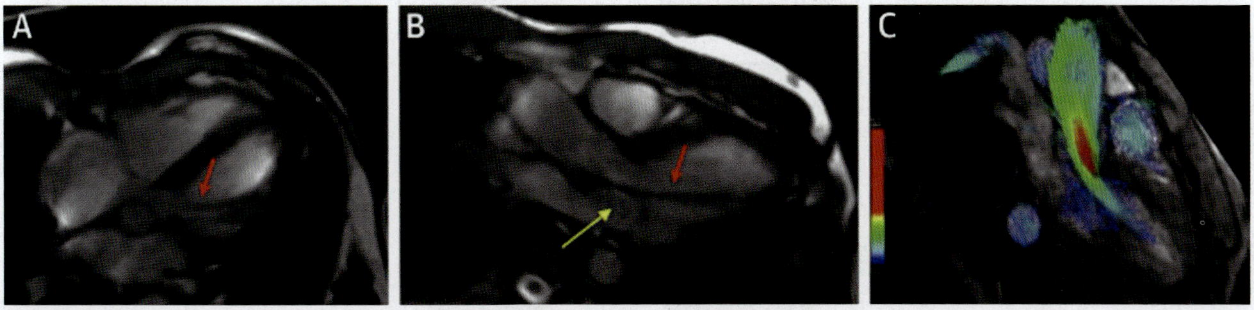

FIG. 25.14 In early systole, the four-chamber (A) and three-chamber views (B) demonstrate an anomalous papillary muscle with a narrow LVOT. Four-dimensional imaging demonstrates elevated flow velocities in the outflow tract consistent with obstruction (C).

a graded fashion with maximum wall thickness, LGE, elevations in cardiac biomarkers, genotype positivity, and arrhythmia burden.[14] ECV has been shown to correlate with outcomes even in the absence of overt replacement fibrosis.[60] T1 mapping and ECV show promise as earlier markers of disease, as histologic interstitial fibrosis predates replacement fibrosis seen with LGE. T1 and ECV are well established to differentiate HCM from other disease, as discussed previously. Stronger associations between T1, ECV, and outcomes may become apparent with the data from HCMR.[14]

While the compendium of evidence overwhelmingly supports the notion that scar is a negative prognosticator, the underlying drivers of fibrosis have been difficult to detect and quantify. One hypothesis is that myofibrillar disarray and microvascular dysfunction are the sine qua non of scar formation. In that vein, there has been exploration of imaging modes to measure microvascular health and myofibrillar structure. CMR perfusion sequences can assess myocardial blood flow (MBF) during rest and stress. Resting MBF correlates with LGE, burden of nonsustained ventricular tachycardia (NSVT), and New York Heart Association (NYHA) class.[60]

Another emerging technique is cardiac diffusion tensor imaging (cDTI). cDTI measures the diffusion of water within an imaging voxel in an attempt to quantify the degree of myofibrillar disorder. The technique is histologically validated and contrast free (Fig. 25.16). The absolute second eigenvector angel (E2A) is a component of cDTI thought to correspond with cardiomyocyte tension and lusitropy. Patients with overt increases in wall thickness have decreased cDTI and E2A relative to genotype-positive, phenotype-negative patients. Genotype-positive patients without overt hypertrophy have reduced cDTI and E2A values relative to normal controls. Cardiac diffusion tensor imaging also indirectly assesses myocyte integrity by measuring the freedom with which water diffuses, reporting mean diffusivity (MD) and fractional anisotropy (FA). Both values are abnormally reduced in HCM, but not to the same extent as some phenocopies such as amyloidosis. Supporting the hypothesis that cellular and histologic abnormalities predate overt increases in wall thickness, it has been demonstrated that for HCM patients even segments of normal myocardial thickness have decreased MD, FA, and increased E2A relative to normal controls. Within the same segment of myocardium, MD and FA are more significantly reduced in the subendocardial layers, which are known to have relative reductions of blood flow in HCM.[61] These data hint at the potential of MBF, cDTI, E2A, MD, and FA as early-phenotype biomarkers in HCM, as well as the potential to differentiate HCM from other diseases, though sufficient follow-up studies have not been completed.[61]

CENTRAL ILLUSTRATION: The Mitral Valve in Obstructive Hypertrophic Cardiomyopathy: Anomalies of the Mitral Valve and Papillary Muscle

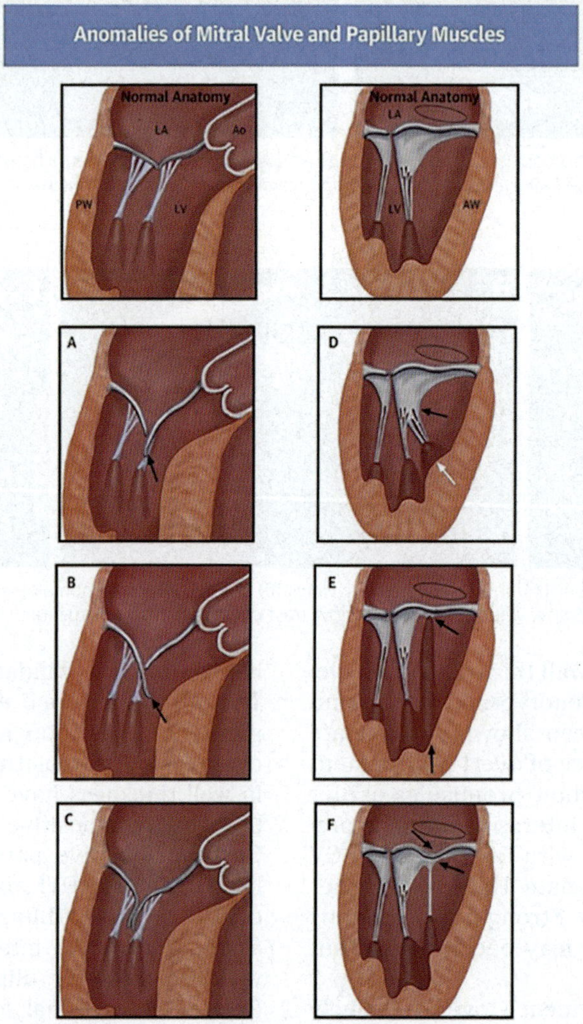

Sherrid, M.V. et al. J Am Coll Cardiol. 2016;67(15):1846-58.

FIG. 25.15 A myriad of mitral anomalies that have been described in HCM. The top images show normal mitral anatomy. (A) Elongated anterior leaflet; (B) elongated posterior leaflet. (C) Bileaflet elongation. (D) Anterior displacement of a bifid anterolateral papillary muscle. (E) Anomalous insertion of the papillary muscle head. (F) A chord inserting into the midportion of the anterior leaflet, causing tenting into the LVOT. *Ao*, aorta; *AW*, anterior wall; *LA*, left atrium; *LV*, left ventricle; *LVOT*, left ventricular outflow tract; *PW*, posterior wall. (Sherrid et al., *JACC*. 2016.)

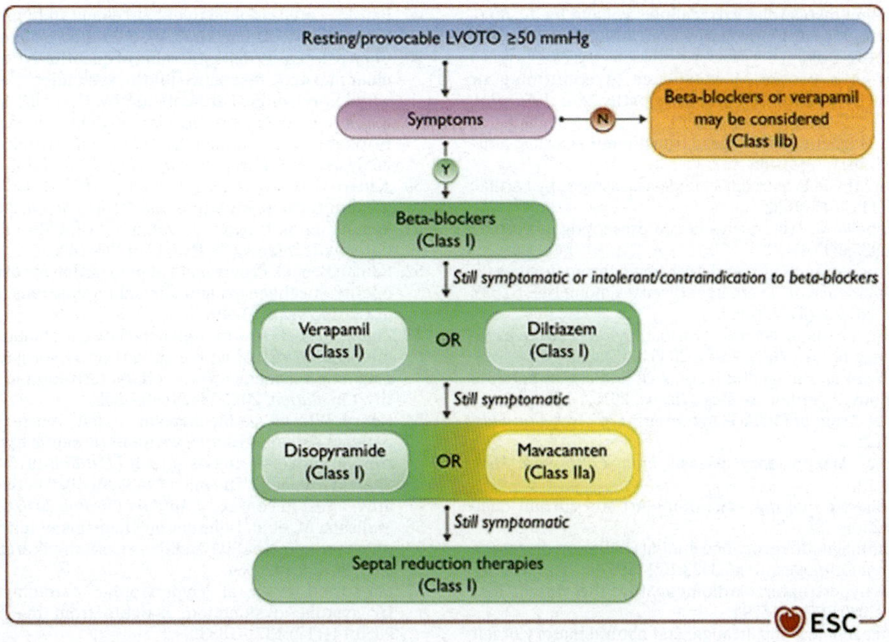

FIG. 25.16 ESC guidelines for the management of LVOTO. This flowchart suggests contemporary management of LVOTO. As more trial data regarding long-term safety of cardiac myosin inhibition and trials with head-to-head comparison of beta blockers to cardiac myosin inhibitors emerge, the order of suggested treatments may change. (Arbelo et al., *EHJ*. 2023.)

CONCLUSION

HCM is an incredibly heterogeneous and underdiagnosed disorder that can exact a heavy toll of comorbidities on patients. CMR is an irreplaceable tool in the world of HCM, confirming diagnoses, excluding phenocopies, characterizing phenotypes, aiding in decision-making around ICD placement, prognosticating, monitoring for disease progression, and assisting in the selection of gradient reduction therapies. As therapies for HCM continue to improve and expand, cardiac imaging will only continue to grow in importance. High-volume centers of expertise in HCM must have comprehensive CMR programs to deliver appropriate care.

REFERENCES

1. Elliott PM, et al. 2014 ESC Guidelines on diagnosis and management of hypertrophic cardiomyopathy: the task force for the diagnosis and management of hypertrophic cardiomyopathy of the European Society of Cardiology (ESC). *Eur Heart J*. 2014;35(39):2733–2779.
2. Ho CY, et al. Genotype and lifetime burden of disease in hypertrophic cardiomyopathy: insights from the sarcomeric human cardiomyopathy registry (SHaRe). *Circulation*. 2018;138(14):1387–1398.
3. Maron BJ. Hypertrophic cardiomyopathy: a systematic review. *JAMA*. 2002;287(10):1308–1320.
4. Stroumpoulis KI, Pantazopoulos IN, Xanthos TT. Hypertrophic cardiomyopathy and sudden cardiac death. *World J Cardiol*. 2010;2(9):289–298.
5. Weissler-Snir A, et al. Hypertrophic cardiomyopathy-related sudden cardiac death in young people in ontario. *Circulation*. 2019;140(21):1706–1716.
6. Lampert R, et al. Vigorous exercise in patients with hypertrophic cardiomyopathy. *JAMA Cardiol*. 2023;8(6):595–605.
7. Martinez KA, et al. Return-to-play for elite athletes with genetic heart diseases predisposing to sudden cardiac death. *J Am Coll Cardiol*. 2023;82(8):661–670.
8. Marian AJ, Roberts R. The molecular genetic basis for hypertrophic cardiomyopathy. *J Mol Cell Cardiol*. 2001;33(4):655–670.
9. Evans W. Familial cardiomegaly. *Br Heart J*. 1949;11(1):68–82.
10. Teare D. Asymmetrical hypertrophy of the heart in young adults. *Br Heart J*. 1958;20(1):1–8.
11. Burke MA, et al. Clinical and mechanistic insights into the genetics of cardiomyopathy. *J Am Coll Cardiol*. 2016;68(25):2871–2886.
12. Teekakirikul P, et al. Hypertrophic cardiomyopathy: an overview of genetics and management. *Biomolecules*. 2019;9(12).
13. Watkins H. Time to think differently about sarcomere-negative hypertrophic cardiomyopathy. *Circulation*. 2021;143(25):2415–2417.
14. Neubauer S, et al. Distinct subgroups in hypertrophic cardiomyopathy in the NHLBI HCM Registry. *J Am Coll Cardiol*. 2019;74(19):2333–2345.
15. Toepfer CN, et al. Myosin sequestration regulates sarcomere function, cardiomyocyte energetics, and metabolism, informing the pathogenesis of hypertrophic cardiomyopathy. *Circulation*. 2020;141(10):828–842.
16. Saberi S, et al. Mavacamten favorably impacts cardiac structure in obstructive hypertrophic cardiomyopathy: EXPLORER-HCM cardiac magnetic resonance substudy analysis. *Circulation*. 2021;143(6):606–608.
17. Ommen SR, et al. 2020 AHA/ACC guideline for the diagnosis and treatment of patients with hypertrophic cardiomyopathy: executive summary: a report of the american college of cardiology/american heart association joint committee on clinical practice guidelines. *Circulation*. 2020;142(25):e533–e557.
18. Maron MS, et al. Hypertrophic cardiomyopathy phenotype revisited after 50 years with cardiovascular magnetic resonance. *J Am Coll Cardiol*. 2009;54(3):220–228.
19. Olivotto I, et al. Assessment and significance of left ventricular mass by cardiovascular magnetic resonance in hypertrophic cardiomyopathy. *J Am Coll Cardiol*. 2008;52(7):559–566.
20. Hindieh W, et al. Discrepant measurements of maximal left ventricular wall thickness between cardiac magnetic resonance imaging and echocardiography in patients with hypertrophic cardiomyopathy. *Circ Cardiovasc Imaging*. 2017;10(8).
21. Bois JP, et al. Comparison of maximal wall thickness in hypertrophic cardiomyopathy differs between magnetic resonance imaging and transthoracic echocardiography. *Am J Cardiol*. 2017;119(4):643–650.
22. van Velzen HG, et al. Prognostic significance of anterior mitral valve leaflet length in individuals with a hypertrophic cardiomyopathy gene mutation without hypertrophic changes. *J Ultrasound*. 2018;21(3):217–224
23. Cuspidi C, et al. High normal blood pressure and left ventricular hypertrophy echocardiographic findings from the PAMELA population. *Hypertension*. 2019;73(3):612–619.
24. Geske JB, Ommen SR, Gersh BJ. Hypertrophic cardiomyopathy: clinical update. *JACC Heart Fail*. 2018;6(5):364–375.
25. Yoshida N, et al. Left ventricular outflow tract obstruction caused by massive mitral annular calcification in a patient with hypertensive heart disease. *J Cardiol Cases*. 2015;12(3):87–90.
26. Engel DJ, Schwartz A, Homma S. Athletic cardiac remodeling in US professional basketball players. *JAMA Cardiol*. 2016;1(1):80–87.
27. Domenech-Ximenos B, et al. Prevalence and pattern of cardiovascular magnetic resonance late gadolinium enhancement in highly trained endurance athletes. *J Cardiovasc Magn Reson*. 2020;22(1):62.
28. Green JJ, et al. Prognostic value of late gadolinium enhancement in clinical outcomes for hypertrophic cardiomyopathy. *JACC Cardiovasc Imaging*. 2012;5(4):370–377.

29. Swoboda PP, et al. Assessing myocardial extracellular volume by T1 mapping to distinguish hypertrophic cardiomyopathy from athlete's heart. *J Am Coll Cardiol.* 2016;67(18):2189–2190.
30. Farrar E, et al. Impact of a center of excellence in confirming or excluding a diagnosis of hypertrophic cardiomyopathy. *Am J Cardiol.* 2023;208:83–91.
31. Martinez-Naharro A, et al. Magnetic resonance in transthyretin cardiac amyloidosis. *J Am Coll Cardiol.* 2017;70(4):466–477.
32. Meyer C, et al. Cardiomyopathy in Friedreich's ataxia-assessment by cardiac MRI. *Mov Disord.* 2007;22(11):1615–1622.
33. Sharratt GP, Jacob JC, Hobeika C. Friedreich's ataxia presenting as cardiac disease. *Pediatr Cardiol.* 1985;6(1):41–42.
34. Grosse SD, et al. Clinical penetrance in hereditary hemochromatosis: estimates of the cumulative incidence of severe liver disease among HFE C282Y homozygotes. *Genet Med.* 2018;20(4):383–389.
35. Cheong B, et al. Evaluation of myocardial iron overload by T2* cardiovascular magnetic resonance imaging. *Tex Heart Inst J.* 2005;32(3):448–449.
36. Pöyhönen P, et al. Cardiovascular magnetic resonance findings in patients with PRKAG2 gene mutations. *J Cardiovasc Magn Reson.* 2015;17:89.
37. Porto AG, et al. Clinical spectrum of PRKAG2 syndrome. *Circ Arrhythm Electrophysiol.* 2016;9(1):e003121.
38. Umer M, Kalra DK. Cardiac MRI in fabry disease. *Front Cardiovasc Med.* 2022;9:1075639.
39. Azevedo O, et al. Fabry disease therapy: state-of-the-Art and current challenges. *Int J Mol Sci.* 2020;22(1).
40. Liu X, et al. Cardiovascular magnetic resonance findings in Danon disease: a case series of a family. *Front Cardiovasc Med.* 2023;10:1159576.
41. Hughes RK, et al. Apical hypertrophic cardiomyopathy: the variant less known. *J Am Heart Assoc.* 2020;9(5):e015294.
42. Maron MS, et al. Prevalence, clinical significance, and natural history of left ventricular apical aneurysms in hypertrophic cardiomyopathy. *Circulation.* 2008;118(15):1541–1549.
43. Perillo EF, et al. Diagnosis and clinical implication of left ventricular aneurysm in hypertrophic cardiomyopathy. *Diagnostics.* 2023;13(11).
44. Maron MS, et al. Right ventricular involvement in hypertrophic cardiomyopathy. *Am J Cardiol.* 2007;100(8):1293–1298.
45. Schlittler M, et al. Myocardial fibrosis in hypertrophic cardiomyopathy: a perspective from fibroblasts. *Int J Mol Sci.* 2023;24(19).
46. Moravsky G, et al. Myocardial fibrosis in hypertrophic cardiomyopathy: accurate reflection of histopathological findings by CMR. *JACC Cardiovasc Imaging.* 2013;6(5):587–596.
47. Pan JA. Late Gadolinium enhancement in hypertrophic cardiomyopathy: is there more to it than size? *JACC Cardiovasc Imaging.* 2023;17:498–500.
48. Chan RH, et al. Prognostic value of quantitative contrast-enhanced cardiovascular magnetic resonance for the evaluation of sudden death risk in patients with hypertrophic cardiomyopathy. *Circulation.* 2014;130(6):484–495.
49. Kiaos A, et al. Quantitative late gadolinium enhancement cardiac magnetic resonance and sudden death in hypertrophic cardiomyopathy: a meta-analysis. *JACC Cardiovasc Imaging.* 2023;17:489–497.
50. Aquaro GD, et al. Diagnostic and prognostic role of late gadolinium enhancement in cardiomyopathies. *Eur Heart J Suppl.* 2023;25(Suppl C):C130–C136.
51. Weng Z, et al. Prognostic value of LGE-CMR in HCM: a meta-analysis. *JACC Cardiovasc Imaging.* 2016;9(12):1392–1402.
52. Raman B, et al. Progression of myocardial fibrosis in hypertrophic cardiomyopathy: mechanisms and clinical implications. *Eur Heart J Cardiovasc Imaging.* 2019;20(2):157–167.
53. Zhang Q, et al. Toward replacing late gadolinium enhancement with artificial intelligence virtual native enhancement for gadolinium-free cardiovascular magnetic resonance tissue characterization in hypertrophic cardiomyopathy. *Circulation.* 2021;144(8):589–599.
54. Henry WL, et al. Mechanism of left ventricular outlfow obstruction in patients with obstructive asymmetric septal hypertrophy (idiopathic hypertrophic subaortic stenosis). *Am J Cardiol.* 1975;35(3):337–345.
55. Sherrid MV, et al. The mitral valve in obstructive hypertrophic cardiomyopathy: a test in context. *J Am Coll Cardiol.* 2016;67(15):1846–1858.
56. Molisana M, et al. Different mechanisms of mitral regurgitation in hypertrophic cardiomyopathy: A clinical case and literature review. *Front Cardiovasc Med.* 2022;9:1020054.
57. Marstrand P, et al. Hypertrophic cardiomyopathy with left ventricular systolic dysfunction: insights from the SHaRe registry. *Circulation.* 2020;141(17):1371–1383.
58. Young AA, et al. Three-dimensional left ventricular deformation in hypertrophic cardiomyopathy. *Circulation.* 1994;90(2):854–867.
59. Rigopoulos AG, et al. Speckle tracking imaging in hypertrophic cardiomyopathy. *Herz.* 2019;44(3):265.
60. Yang EY, et al. Myocardial extracellular volume fraction adds prognostic information beyond myocardial replacement fibrosis. *Circ Cardiovasc Imaging.* 2019;12(12):e009535.
61. Das A, et al. Phenotyping hypertrophic cardiomyopathy using cardiac diffusion magnetic resonance imaging: the relationship between microvascular dysfunction and microstructural changes. *Eur Heart J Cardiovasc Imaging.* 2022;23(3):352–362.

26 Role of Cardiovascular Magnetic Resonance in Dilated Cardiomyopathy

ROBERT S. ZHANG, PABLO VILLAR CALLE, JIWON KIM, AND JONATHAN W. WEINSAFT

BACKGROUND

Dilated cardiomyopathy (DCM) is a condition defined by left ventricular systolic dysfunction and dilatation not explained by abnormal loading conditions (hypertension, valvular disease) or coronary artery disease.[1] DCM is common, with an estimated prevalence as high as 1 in 250 individuals in the general population.[2] Genetic mutations, particularly those encoding structural proteins of the sarcomere and desmosome, have been implicated in DCM. Titin (TTN) truncating mutations are the most common cause of genetically mediated DCM, occurring in approximately 25% of familial cases and 18% of sporadic cases.[3,4] Nongenetic forms of DCM may arise from an array of etiologies, including myocarditis, exogenous exposures, and systemic conditions. Despite advances in heart failure (HF) treatment, morbidity and mortality associated with DCM remain substantial, making it a leading indication for cardiac transplantation.[5] Primary causes of death in DCM patients include HF and arrhythmia,[6] but patients with DCM may also demonstrate subtle structural cardiac abnormalities and arrhythmogenic features on CMR prior to developing—symptoms[7–9], highlighting the importance of early detection by CMR.

Key clinical challenges for patients with DCM include differentiation from other phenotypically similar conditions, identifying those at greatest risk for life-threatening arrhythmias, and defining groups most likely to experience poor responses to HF medications for whom advanced care (mechanical support, transplant) is most warranted. CMR provides a powerful tool to address these clinical challenges: It enables highly accurate assessment of myocardial function and geometry capable of detecting subtle abnormalities not discernible by conventional methods such as ultrasound and/or radionuclide imaging. In parallel, CMR enables myocardial tissue characterization, thus providing insight into the mechanistic basis of contractile dysfunction and enhancing diagnostic yield as well as prognostic risk stratification. This chapter provides an overview of CMR for the evaluation and management of DCM, including established and emerging CMR methods for diagnosis, prognostic risk assessment, and therapeutic decision-making that may enhance clinical outcomes for patients with this condition.

CARDIAC GEOMETRY AND CONTRACTILE FUNCTION

LV Morphology/Function

The diagnosis and therapeutic management of patients with DCM relies on detailed assessment of LV geometry and function. CMR provides an accurate assessment of LV chamber size, global and regional contractility, and is well-established as a noninvasive reference standard for LV chamber remodeling.[10]

LV structure and functional indices can be assessed by CMR using dynamic ECG-gated ("cine") imaging; steady-state free precession (SSFP) pulse sequences are the typically used approach for this purpose. Cine-CMR quantification of LV parameters is based on analysis of contiguous short-axis images. This enables 3D volumetric assessment based on planimetry of endocardial contours during systole and diastole; end-diastolic epicardial contours are typically attained to quantify myocardial mass (Fig. 26.1). Using this method, LV ejection fraction, myocardial mass, and stroke volume can be quantified using volumetric data without the need for geometric assumptions. In clinical practice, cine-CMR assessment of regional wall motion is primarily based on visual analysis. If quantitative assessment is necessary, myocardial tagging methods can be used for the assessment of regional contractility. Tagging can be performed using tailored pulse sequences (methods whereby saturation prepulses are applied to the myocardium, producing a grid-like pattern that is deformed as a function of regional contractility), or by postprocessing of conventional cine-CMR data (a method referred to as "feature tracking").[11] Tagging sequences have been used to assess precise changes in regional myocardial contractility, and have been shown to be capable of discerning alterations in myocardial energetics and regional contractility not discernible by conventional wall motion assessment.[12]

Cine-CMR provides an array of data particularly important for the assessment of DCM. LVEF as quantified on CMR has been shown to predict prognosis (including arrhythmic risk) and provides a rationale for prophylactic therapies (e.g., internal cardiac defibrillator implantation).[13] Regional wall motion can provide both prognostic and diagnostic value, including differentiation of DCM from other

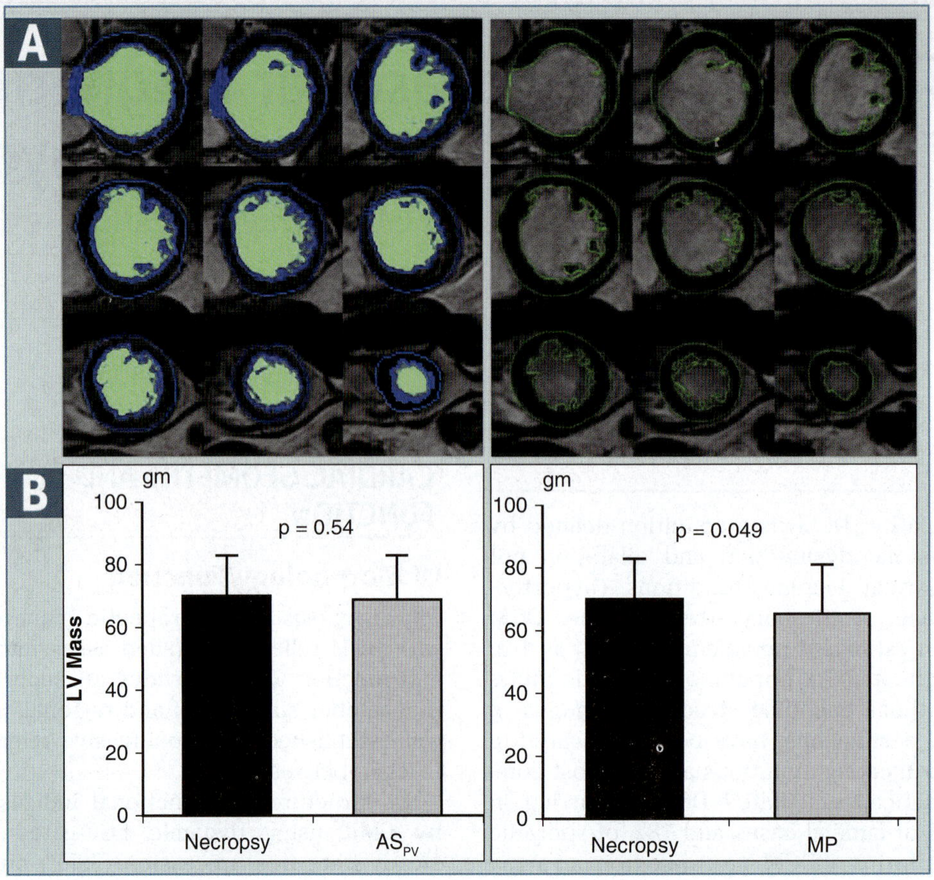

FIG. 26.1 Representative example of left ventricular volumes and mass quantification using manual planimetry (A, *top right*) and automated segmentation (A, *top left*). Note that, whereas both methods yield close agreement with phantom validated chamber volumes and necropsy quantified left ventricular mass (B, *bottom*), automated segmentation with partial voxel interpolation yields improved performance as evidenced by nonsignificant differences with necropsy data. (Adapted from Codella et al. Circ Cardiovasc Imaging. 2012 Jan;5(1):137–146. Elsevier editorial permission will be needed for use of this figure).

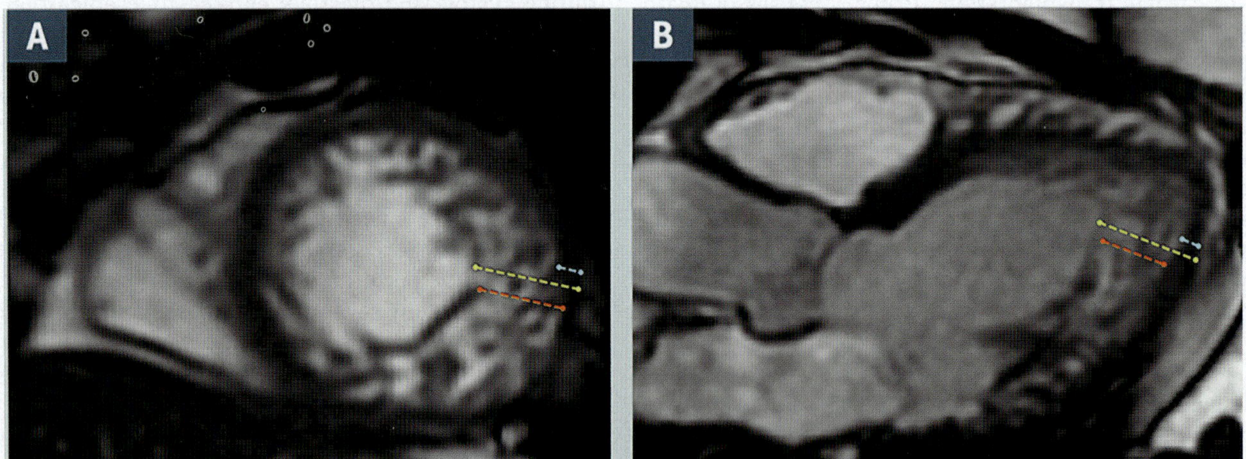

FIG. 26.2 Representative example of left ventricular noncompaction (LVNC) on cine-CMR at end-diastole. Apical short-axis (A) and three-chamber long-axis (B) orientations demonstrate prominent trabeculations and deep intertrabecular recesses involving the apical segments of the left ventricle. The dashed red lines represent the noncompacted myocardial layer, the light blue dashed line denotes the compacted myocardial layer, and the yellow dashed includes compacted and noncompacted myocardium. The maximum noncompacted to compacted (NC/C) myocardial thickness ratio, measured at end-diastole, is 3.7, meeting the diagnostic threshold for LVNC.

mimickers such as stress ("Takotsubo") and ischemic cardiomyopathy—each of which is characterized by regional contractile dysfunction patterns distinct from global dysfunction as a hallmark of DCM. Regarding strain, myocardial feature tracking is increasingly being recognized for its incremental utility. To this end, prognostic outcome studies in patients with DCM have shown cine-CMR-derived global longitudinal strain (GLS) to predict adverse outcomes independent of conventional clinical indices as well as imaging parameters such as LVEF.[11]

DCM can be accompanied by alterations in myocardial architecture that can be well discerned on CMR. Cine-CMR provides high-resolution endocardial definition—including delineation of trabeculations, intratrabecular recesses, as well as developmental phenotype as defined by compacted and noncompacted components (Fig. 26.2). These data provide potential value in the assessment of patients with suspected DCM, in that they can potentially differentiate this condition from other causes of nonischemic cardiomyopathy. For example, increased trabeculations have been described in the context of LV noncompaction cardiomyopathy (LVNC), for which an exaggerated noncompacted/compacted ratio is a diagnostic criterion.[14] With respect to prognosis, outcome studies among patients referred for CMR have yielded mixed results with respect to predictive utility of increased trabeculations. For example, among a cohort of 700 patients referred for CMR, Ivanov et al. reported that increased LV trabeculations (as assessed by four distinct criteria for LVNC) did not predict clinical outcomes during nearly 7 years of follow-up, thus raising the question of the utility of this area of focus among heart failure populations, including patients with DCM.[15]

RV Morphology/Function

DCM can be accompanied by functional and structural changes throughout the heart, which may be due to diffuse alterations in cardiac myocyte biology and/or secondary changes attributable to LV-induced alterations in loading conditions. While the mechanism remains uncertain, it is well known that adverse remodeling in structures other than the LV can modify the therapeutic response and impact prognosis, and is thus important to characterize in patients with DCM.

Adverse right ventricular (RV) remodeling has been shown to be common in DCM—having been reported to occur in up to 30%–60% of patients.[16] Paralleling LV assessment, RV quantification can be attained from cine-CMR via planimetry of short-axis datasets from which chamber size and function can be derived. CMR is particularly well suited for the RV, given its thin-walled structure and irregularly contoured shape. Consistent with this concept, cine-CMR has been shown to provide precise measurements of both RV chamber size and function, including high reproducibility in both normative controls as well as patients with heart failure.[17]

With respect to clinical application, it is well-known that adverse RV remodeling as discerned by cine-CMR is prognostically important in DCM. For example, among a cohort of 250 patients with DCM prospectively undergoing CMR, Gulati et al. reported that RV systolic dysfunction (RVSD; defined by RVEF ≤45%) was present in 34% and was strongly predictive of adverse outcomes. During a median follow-up of 6.8 years, a composite endpoint of all-cause mortality or cardiac transplantation was nearly fivefold more common among patients with RVSD (49% vs. 10%; hazard ratio [HR]; 5.90 [95% confidence interval (CI) 3.35–10.37]; $P<.001$): RVSD remained independently predictive of the primary endpoint of all-cause mortality/transplant (HR 3.90; [CI 2.16–7.04]; $P<.001$), and of secondary outcomes of cardiovascular mortality or transplantation (HR 3.35; 95% CI 1.76–6.39; $P<.001$) even after adjustment for left-sided indices.[16] These data are consistent with other studies in patients with ischemic[18] and nonischemic cardiomyopathy,[19] highlighting the importance of RV assessment in patients for whom the diagnosis of DCM is suspected but not yet established.

Atrial Remodeling and Valvular Regurgitation

Given that adverse ventricular dilation and dysfunction are hallmarks of DCM, it is reasonable to expect that altered loading forces would provide a nidus for both adverse atrial remodeling as well as impaired (mitral, tricuspid) valve integrity. While the prevalence of these findings has not been a particular area of study in patients with DCM, it is well accepted that CMR is well suited for their assessment.

Left (LA) and right atrial (RA) quantification are conventionally assessed via cine-CMR chamber planimetry using the biplane area–length method.[20] This compares favorably against other noninvasive imaging methods because of its excellent endocardial border definition and multiplanar imaging ability.[21] Emerging approaches include feature tracking-derived strain imaging, which has been shown to provide a marker of ventricular noncompliance and diastolic dysfunction.[22] Cine-CMR-derived LA chamber size and strain have been shown to predict prognosis among an array of clinical groups—including patients with DCM.[23,24] As evidence of this concept, Raafs et al. studied a cohort of 488 DCM patients, among whom 14% ($n=70$) reached the primary study endpoint (sudden or cardiac death, HF hospitalization, life-threatening arrhythmia) during a median follow-up interval of 6 (IQR 4–9) years: impaired LA conduit strain (<12%) on cine-CMR was strongly associated with adverse prognosis, and remained independently predictive (HR 3.65 [95% CI 2.01–6.64]; $P<.001$) after adjustment for clinical heart failure severity (NYHA class >2, HR 1.81 [95% CI 1.05–3.02]; $P=.033$) as well as the presence of LGE-evidenced myocardial fibrosis (HR 2.22 [95% CI 1.42–3.85]; $P<.001$). Right atrial strain has also been tested as a prognostic variable in patients with DCM, for whom it has been shown to predict clinical outcomes.[25] Taken together, these data support the concept that adverse atrial remodeling impacts clinical outcomes and provide further evidence of the utility of CMR as a powerful multiparametric tool for prognostic assessment of patients with DCM.

It is well-established that both mitral and tricuspid valve integrity are closely linked to ventricular performance, and that adverse ventricular remodeling (dilation and/or dysfunction) can provide a nidus for ("functional") valvular regurgitation. In this context, it is not unexpected that regurgitant valve disease is common in patients with DCM. For example, among a retrospective cohort of 1256 DCM patients, 73% had at least mild mitral regurgitation (MR), with 24% of patients having severe functional MR.[26] Regarding MR assessment, regurgitant volume (and fraction) can be calculated as the difference between aortic forward flow volume (via phase contrast CMR) and total LV stroke volume (via cine-CMR), as is illustrated in Fig. 26.3. An equivalent approach can be applied for TR, for which regurgitant volume and fraction can be quantified based on pulmonic and RV stroke volume indices. Alternative approaches include differential LV–RV stroke volume (in the absence of aortic or pulmonic valve pathology),

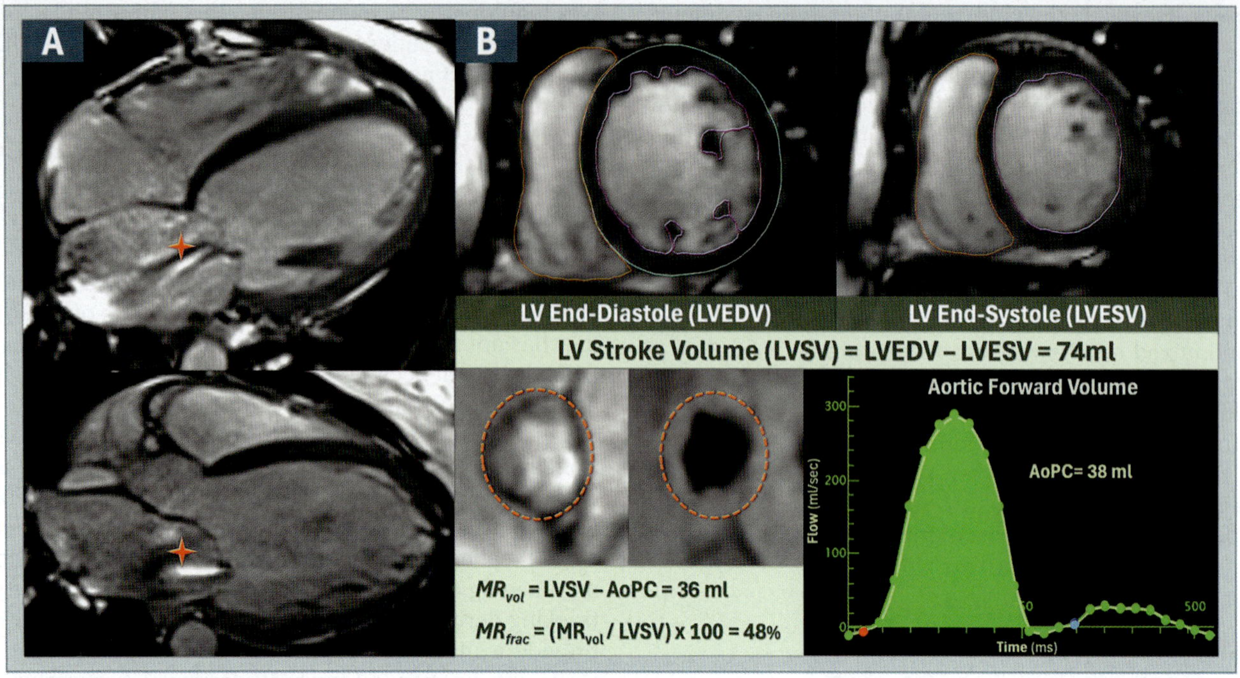

FIG. 26.3 Representative example of functional mitral regurgitation (MR) quantification based on differential stroke volumes derived from cine-CMR and phase-contrast imaging. Cine-CMR in four-chamber and three-chamber orientations demonstrates a central MR jet (*red stars*), consistent with leaflet tethering (A). Left ventricular stroke volume (LVSV) calculated by cine-CMR, based on the difference between end-diastolic and end-systolic volumes (LVSV = LVEDV − LVESV = 74 mL) (B). Phase-contrast velocity-encoded imaging acquired orthogonal to the ascending aorta (AoPC) demonstrates forward stroke volume of 38 mL. MR volume (MR_{vol}) is calculated as the difference between LVSV and AoPC flow (MR_{vol} = 36 mL), with corresponding MR fraction (MR_{frac}) derived as MR_{vol}/LVSV × 100 = 48% (D).

direct quantification of atrio-ventricular regurgitant flow on phase contrast CMR, and qualitative assessment of regurgitant jet size/depth based on cine-CMR dephasing.

Regarding prognosis, both MR and TR as assessed by CMR have been shown to impact outcomes in DCM. For example, in the above-referenced DCM cohort, Rossi et al. reported that severe MR was independently associated with the outcome of all-cause mortality and heart failure hospitalization (HR 2.0 [95% CI 1.4–2.7], $P < .0001$).[26] Other groups have reported on the prognostic impact of TR in heart failure cohorts, inclusive of patients with DCM. It is also important to recognize that accurate assessment of the presence and severity of valvular regurgitation impacts therapeutic decision-making: MR severity as quantified by CMR has been shown to provide incremental utility (vs. echocardiography) for the prediction of reverse remodeling after mitral valve surgery,[27] and to predict postprocedural outcomes among patients with DCM. Regarding therapeutic response, Li et al. studied 112 patients with DCM, among whom the primary study endpoint (all-cause death or unplanned hospitalization for HF) was less common among patients who underwent mitral valve repair compared to those treated medically (44.8% vs. 68.5%; HR 0.28 [CI 0.14–0.55]; $P < .001$).[28] Further studies are ongoing to test these concepts among patients undergoing percutaneous valve repair, including whether CMR-informed interventions impact quality of life and clinical outcomes.

CMR TISSUE CHARACTERIZATION

A key advantage of CMR in the assessment of DCM is its unique ability to provide insight into myocardial tissue characteristics, so as to inform underlying mechanisms responsible for alterations in chamber morphology and contractile function. This is particularly important in the assessment of patients with known or suspected DCM, for whom contractile dysfunction can occur due to an array of processes (including primary myocardial [nonischemic] pathology, systemic disorders, ischemic injury, and mixed pathology). Several CMR approaches have been shown to provide utility in DCM—the most common of which are LGE CMR (for focal replacement fibrosis) and parametric mapping methods (for diffuse fibrosis). Rationale and clinical utility of key CMR pulse sequences as applied to the assessment of DCM are further detailed below.

Late Gadolinium Enhancement

One of the histologic hallmarks of DCM, common to all causes of heart failure, is myocardial fibrosis.[29,30] There are two main forms of fibrosis detected histologically: interstitial and replacement fibrosis. Interstitial fibrosis describes an increase in the collagen volume fraction with expansion of the extracellular matrix, whereas replacement fibrosis describes discrete areas of myocardial scarring resulting from myocyte cell death.[31]

LGE CMR is well validated as a tool to detect focal myocardial fibrosis. Cross-sectional studies have reported focal LGE in approximately 30% of patients with DCM, typically in a linear distribution involving the septum (Fig. 26.4).[32] While mechanisms for mid-wall LGE in the context of DCM are uncertain, prior data from our group and others have suggested that fibrosis occurs in association with increased left ventricular wall stress, which may provide a substrate for myocyte cell death.[33]

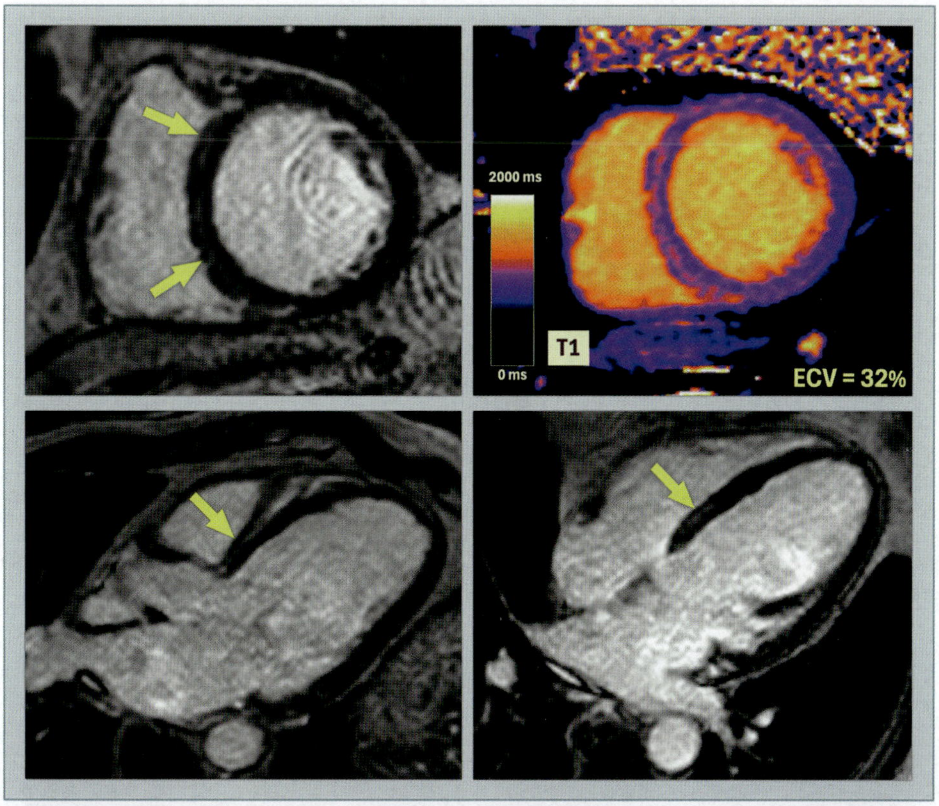

FIG. 26.4 Representative example of midwall myocardial fibrosis in dilated cardiomyopathy. LGE-CMR basal short-axis image (*top left*) with midwall hyperenhancement involving the interventricular septum (*yellow arrow*), consistent with nonischemic fibrosis. Corresponding T1 color map (*top right*) with native T1 values at the upper limit of normal and mildly elevated extracellular volume fraction (ECV = 32%). Long-axis imaging confirms the presence of midwall septal fibrosis (*bottom*).

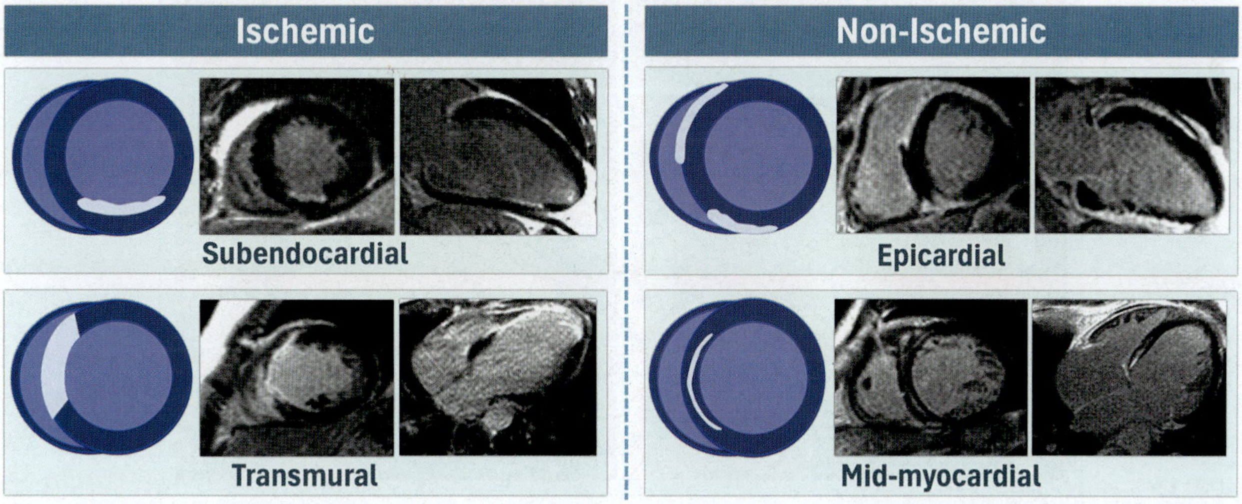

FIG. 26.5 Characteristic LGE patterns distinguishing ischemic from nonischemic cardiomyopathy. Left panel shows ischemic patterns with subendocardial and transmural enhancement corresponding to coronary artery territories. Right panel demonstrates nonischemic patterns including epicardial and mid-myocardial enhancement that does not follow coronary distributions. (Adapted from Mahrholdt et al, Eur Heart J. 2005 Aug;26(15):1461–1474. Elsevier editorial permission will be needed for use of this figure).

DIAGNOSTIC UTILITY OF LGE

The LGE pattern can be useful to differentiate DCM from other diagnostic mimickers. Among patients with DCM, LGE is typically absent or (when present) localized to the mid or epicardial aspect of the interventricular septum—possibly reflecting adverse geometric remodeling with associated increased wall stress. In contrast, LGE in the setting of ischemic cardiomyopathy is typically subendocardial or transmural (Fig. 26.5).[34] Prior studies have shown that relying solely on coronary angiography to diagnose DCM may misdiagnose up to 13% of patients.[32] As evidence of this, Bawaskar et al. used CMR to study a retrospective cohort of 3023 patients with obstructive CAD—8.2% had CAD and no cardiomyopathy (no LGE, preserved LVEF), 64.8% had CAD with ischemic cardiomyopathy, 9.3% had CAD with nonischemic cardiomyopathy, and 7.7% had CAD with dual (ischemic and nonischemic) cardiomyopathy (Fig. 26.6).[35] The presence

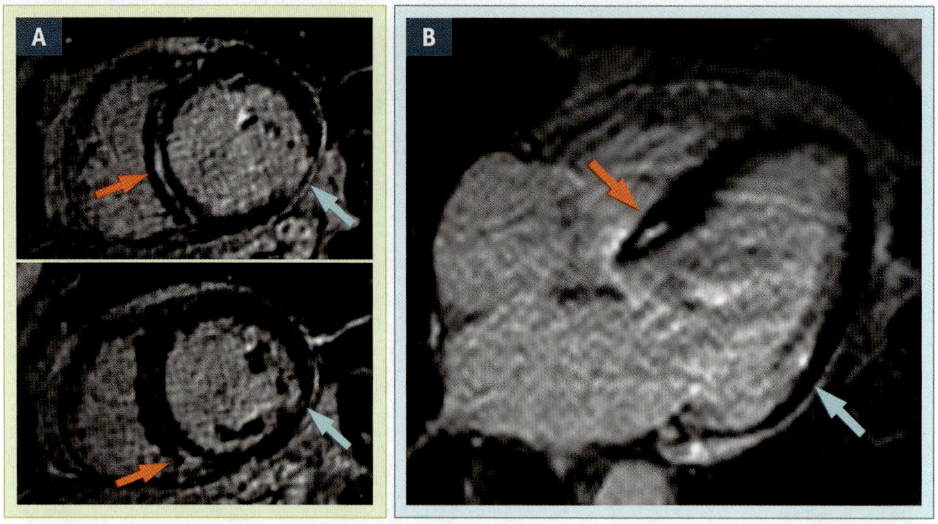

FIG. 26.6 Representative example of coexisting ischemic and nonischemic scar patterns in the same patient. LGE-CMR in short-axis (A) and four-chamber (B) orientations, demonstrating midwall fibrosis in the interventricular septum (*orange arrow*) consistent with nonischemic pattern, and near-transmural myocardial infarction in the basal-mid-inferolateral wall (*blue arrow*) consistent with ischemic pattern.

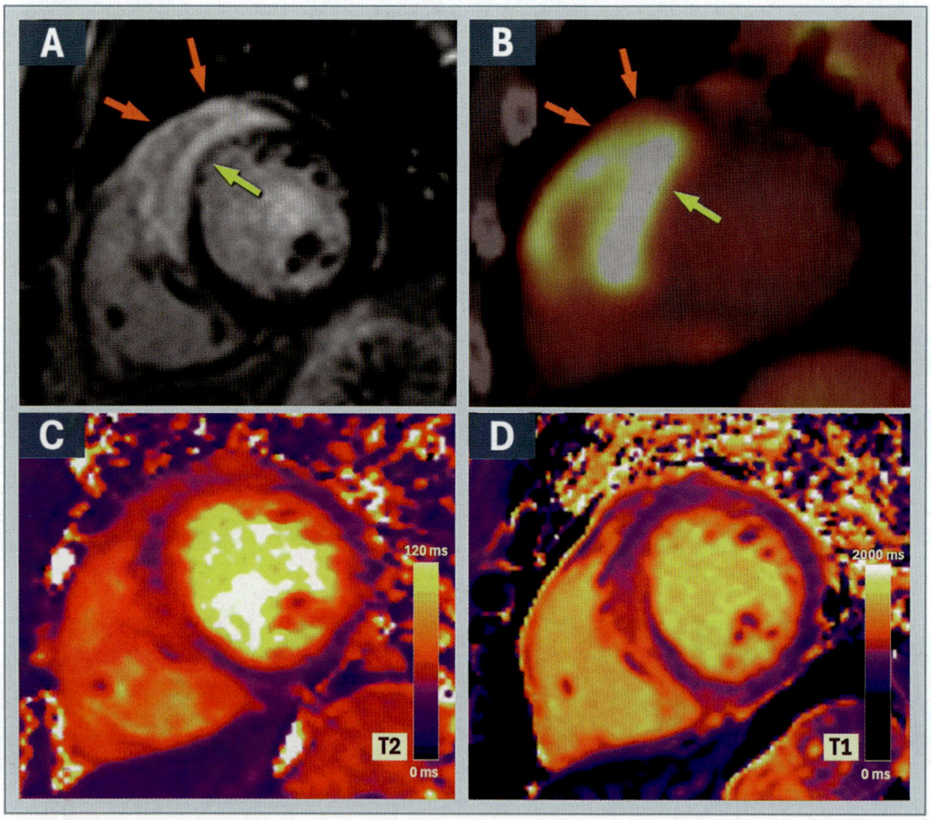

FIG. 26.7 Representative example of myocardial involvement in sarcoidosis. LGE-CMR in short-axis orientation with extensive epicardial scar involving the anteroseptum (*yellow arrow*) and extension into the right ventricular free wall (*orange arrows*), forming the characteristic "hook sign" (A). FDG PET/CT with radiotracer uptake in the same region, consistent with active myocardial inflammation (B). Parametric T2 mapping with elevated T2 relaxation time in the interventricular septum, consistent with associated inflammation (C). Corresponding parametric T1 mapping with increased native T1 and extracellular volume fraction (ECV = 43%) in the mid-anteroseptum (D).

of concomitant nonischemic cardiomyopathy in 17% of patients in the study highlights the potential utility of LGE-CMR in cardiomyopathy patients with obstructive CAD, and underscores a key role of CMR to distinguish ischemic cardiomyopathy from DCM.

LGE also provides value to differentiate DCM from other causes of nonischemic cardiomyopathy (NICM). For example, sarcoidosis is a common form of NICM that can be nonspecific in clinical presentation and imaging manifestations—including LV dilation or dysfunction that can be challenging to differentiate from other cardiomyopathies. With respect to tissue characteristics, certain LGE patterns have been described as "pathology-frequent" and "pathology-rare." Subepicardial LGE involvement of the septum with extension into the right ventricle suggests a very high likelihood of cardiac sarcoidosis (>90%) (Fig.

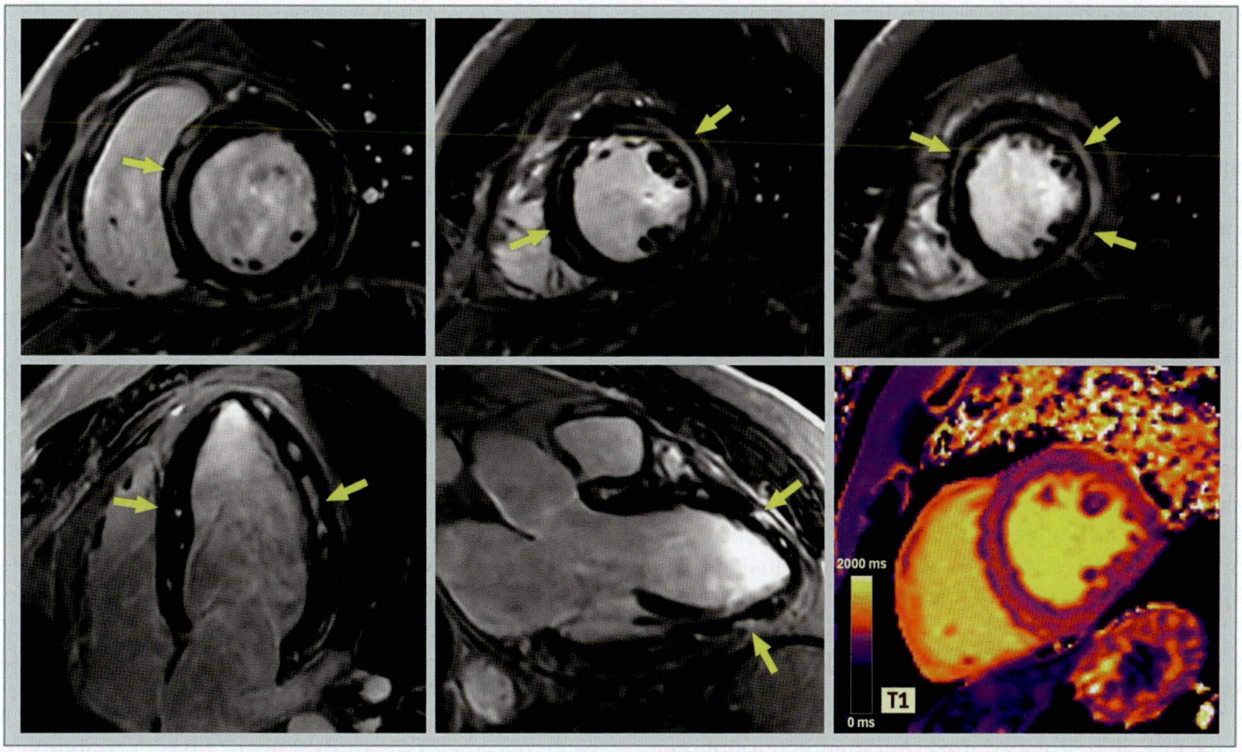

FIG. 26.8 Representative example of genetically mediated cardiomyopathy associated with desmoplakin mutation. LGE-CMR in short-axis (*top row*) and long-axis orientations (bottom left: four-chamber; bottom middle: three-chamber) demonstrates extensive mid-myocardial and epicardial scar (*yellow arrows*) involving all left ventricular walls, forming a ring-like pattern. Parametric T1 mapping (*bottom right*) demonstrates diffusely elevated native T1 relaxation times, consistent with myocardial fibrosis.

26.7).[36] Similarly, multifocal LGE has been associated with a high likelihood of cardiac sarcoidosis (50%–90%).[37] Conversely, in patients with no enhancement or focal subendocardial enhancement, cardiac sarcoidosis is highly unlikely (<10%).[36,37]

CMR also provides utility to differentiate between DCM subtypes. Emerging evidence highlights a strong phenotype–genotype correlation in forms of genetically mediated cardiomyopathy, with a "ring-like" scar pattern associated with the presence of pathogenic/likely pathogenic mutations of genes like filamin C (FLNC), desmoplakin (DSP), and phospholamban (PLN), among others, in up to 60% of patients (Fig. 26.8).[38]

PROGNOSTIC UTILITY OF LGE

LGE is well-established as a powerful predictor of poor prognosis—including adverse ventricular remodeling, HF hospitalization, and increased all-cause mortality.[19] This concept has been demonstrated in patients with DCM, and more broadly. In a prospective, longitudinal study of 472 DCM patients, those with LGE evidenced midwall fibrosis had higher all-cause mortality (26.8% vs. 10.6%) and sudden cardiac death (29.6% vs. 7.0%; both $P<.001$) during a median follow-up of 5.3 years.[39] In a meta-analysis by Becker et al. of 34 studies ($n=4554$), the presence of LGE was associated with increased cardiovascular mortality (OR 3.40 [95% CI 2.01–5.67]) and rehospitalization for HF (OR 2.66 [95% CI 1.67–4.24]).[19] Taken together, these data support the concept that myocardial injury detected by LGE is a key determinant of adverse outcomes and highlight the prognostic utility of CMR for evaluation of patients with DCM.

LGE is also important with respect to prediction of arrhythmic risk. From a pathophysiological standpoint, this association is unsurprising, as myocardial scar is a primary substrate for ventricular arrhythmias.[40,41] Prognostic utility of LGE for arrhythmic events has been well-demonstrated. A meta-analysis of 29 studies ($n=2948$) by Di Marco et al. demonstrated that patients with LGE were significantly associated with the arrhythmic endpoint (sustained VA, appropriate ICD therapy, or sudden cardiac death [SCD]) in the overall population (OR 4.3 [95% CI 3.3–5.8]; $P<.001$), when including only those studies that performed multivariate analysis (HR 6.7 [95% CI 3.6–12.5]; $P<.001$),[42] and in analysis restricted to studies with mean LVEF >35% (OR 5.2 [95% CI 3.4–7.9]; $P<.001$).[42]

Despite emerging data supporting the link between LGE and arrhythmic risk, LVEF remains the primary accepted criterion for primary prevention implantable cardioverter-defibrillators (ICDs). Despite this, only about 20% of DCM patients who receive primary prevention ICDs experience appropriate device therapies.[43] The DANISH trial (Danish ICD Study in Patients With Dilated Cardiomyopathy) randomized 1,116 patients with symptomatic systolic heart failure with LVEF ≤35% due to DCM to ICD placement vs. standard care. At a median follow-up of 68 months, there was no difference in the primary endpoint of all-cause mortality between the two groups (21.6% vs. 23.4% $P=.28$). Of the patients who received an ICD, 5.9% of the patients received inappropriate shocks. These results underscore the high rate of inappropriate ICD therapies in patients with DCM receiving ICDs and lack of clear survival benefit in DCM patients on guideline-directed medical therapy. These findings also highlight the imprecision of current risk stratification tools for ventricular arrhythmias, leading to a potential overtreatment of patients with markedly impaired LVEF (<35%) but low arrhythmic risk and the undertreatment of others in whom LVEF is minimally impaired, but risk for sudden death is markedly increased. Incorporating LGE status into selection criteria for primary prevention ICDs has the potential to inform treatment for patients at higher arrhythmic risk (LGE positive), while sparing patients without LGE the risk of potential complications from an intracardiac device that is unlikely to improve their prognosis.

Ongoing clinical trials, such as CMR GUIDE (Cardiovascular magnetic resonance-Guided management of mild to moderate left ventricular systolic dysfunction)[44] and the BRITISH (using cardiovascular magnetic resonance identified scar as the Benchmark Risk Indication Tool for Implantable cardioverter defibrillators in patients with Non-Ischemic Cardiomyopathy and Severe systolic Heart failure) trial[45] are testing LGE as a decision-making tool for ICD implantation. The studies are respectively enrolling NICM patients with LGE and moderate (EF 36%–50%) or severe (EF ≤35%) LV dysfunction to compare outcomes between ICD therapy and implantable loop recorder in these populations. Treatments targeted at preventing or reversing LGE also provide future therapeutic possibilities.

RESPONSE TO MEDICAL AND INTERVENTIONAL THERAPIES

Despite advances in medical therapies for heart failure, the individual patient response to treatment varies. LGE-CMR holds the potential to inform therapeutic response.[46,47] For instance, Leong et al. studied 68 patients with newly diagnosed DCM, among whom 24% ($n = 12$) had LGE, which was typically located in the septal midwall and/or RV insertion sites.[46] Follow-up CMR was performed 5 months after initiation of optimal medical therapy using an LVEF improvement of >5% as the threshold of therapeutic response, which revealed that 28% ($n = 19$) of patients were nonresponders. LGE burden was higher in nonresponders compared to responders (0.9 ± 0.9 g vs. 0.2 ± 0.6 g, $P < .001$), and LGE size was independently associated with change in LVEF over time ($P < .001$) even after controlling for contractile dysfunction (strain dyssynchrony index)—highlighting the potential role of LGE for prediction of response to medical therapies for patients with DCM.

Similar to medical therapy, response to electrophysiologic interventions is highly variable, and may be informed by LGE-CMR. This concept has been tested in the context of cardiac resynchronization therapy (CRT)—an established treatment for DCM patients with concomitant left bundle branch block conduction pattern and markedly impaired LVEF (≤35%).[13] At present, up to 30%–50% of patients receiving CRTs are nonresponders (lack of EF improvement).[48] Several studies have shown that the presence of posterolateral wall LGE is associated with an impaired CRT response[49–51]—a finding explained by the notion that LV lead placement in areas of nonviable myocardium results in poor mechanical capture and absence of contractile recovery. A study by Becker et al. involving 44 patients with end-stage heart failure (NYHA class III/IV, LVEF ≤35%) and left bundle branch block (QRS duration >120 ms) examined the impact of posterolateral myocardial scar on the efficacy of CRT. The findings revealed that patients with transmural posterolateral scar (>50% of LV wall thickness) had a significantly lower response rate to CRT (14%) compared to those without posterolateral scar tissue (81%; $P < .05$).[49] In a separate cohort of 98 DCM patients, LGE and degree of dyssynchrony (defined as time-to-peak strain) were independently associated with LVEF nonresponse and poor clinical outcomes.[52]

Left bundle branch area pacing (LBBAP) has emerged as an alternative strategy to improve CRT response, especially in patients with DCM.[53,54] Akin to conventional CRT, LBBAP response varies and is associated with the LGE pattern.[55] A retrospective observational study of 147 patients with NICM, wide QRS (≥130 ms), and reduced LVEF (≤35% despite optimal medical treatment or LVEF <50% with expected high ventricular pacing burden >40%) demonstrated that the extent of septal scar (based on a median of 5.7% of myocardial mass) stratified patients into those who did better with LBBAP vs. conventional biventricular pacing (BVP).[56] In the low septal scar group, LBBAP resulted in significantly increased LVEF and reduced LV end-diastolic dimension compared to BVP. In patients with high septal scar, there was a trend to significant improvement in the same parameters with BVP over LBBAP. Variability in CRT response among DCM patients highlights the need for improved patient selection strategies—LGE distribution, particularly septal and posterolateral wall scar, respectively, may identify nonresponders to LBBAP or BVP, and thus inform optimal electrophysiologic approaches prior to device implantation.

Lipomatous Metaplasia

As an adjunct to LGE, CMR can also discern tissue characterization indices that differentiate between acute and chronic myocardial injury. Whereas acute injury is typically characterized by edema and inflammation (as delineated on T2-weighted CMR), chronic infarct is often accompanied by lipomatous metaplasia (LM) (which appears bright on T1-weighted CMR). Regarding the clinical significance of the LM, it is well known that intramyocardial fat provides a pro-arrhythmic substrate.[57] LM can be present in the setting of both ischemic and nonischemic cardiomyopathy—including among patients with DCM. In cross-sectional studies, LM has been reported to be present in approximately 24%–57% of patients with DCM.[58,59] Xu et al. conducted a retrospective study of 113 patients with NICM (79% DCM) to evaluate the prevalence and prognosis of LM.[59] LM was identified using a combination of CMR and cardiac computed tomography. The study found that LM was present in 83% of patients with VT compared to 57% without VT, and in 100% of the patients with recurrent VT.

LM can be identified using several different CMR approaches. Conventional CMR approaches have employed (precontrast) T1-weighted spin echo pulse sequences for this purpose, on which fat appears bright (high-signal intensity). LGE data can also be leveraged to confirm the presence of LM based on differential inversion recovery between fat (short T1 recovery) and both viable and infarcted myocardium (Fig. 26.9). On steady-state free

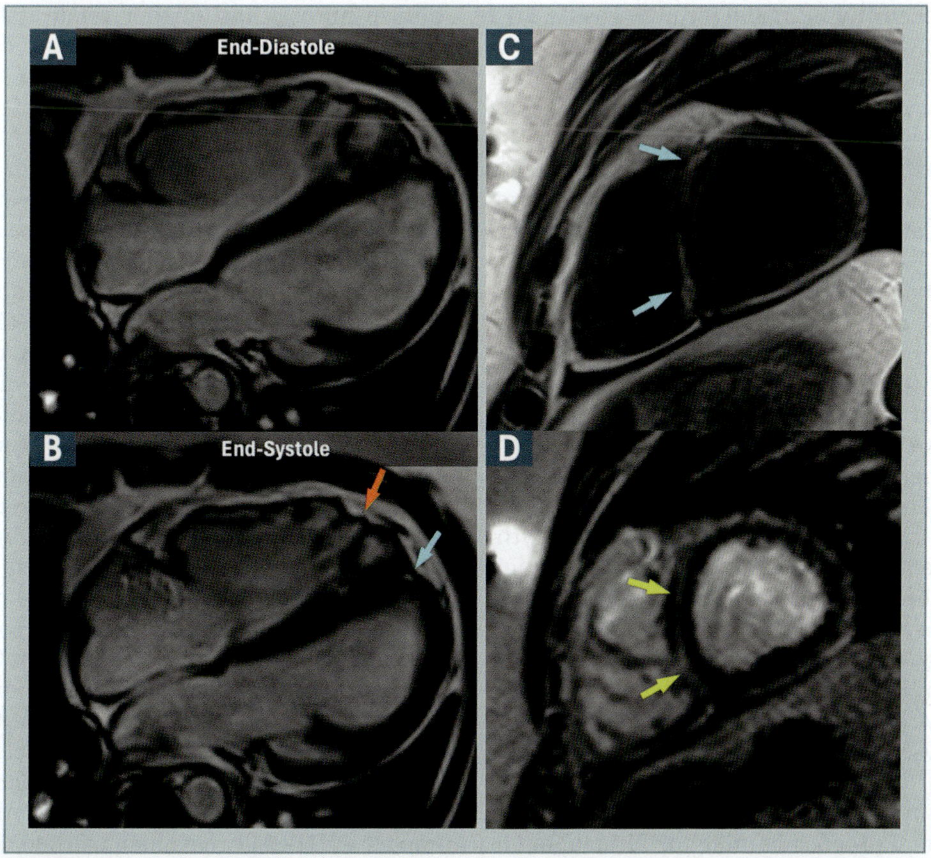

FIG. 26.9 Representative example of lipomatous metaplasia in arrhythmogenic cardiomyopathy (ACM) with biventricular involvement. Cine-CMR in four-chamber orientation (A: end-diastole; B: end-systole) with focal dyskinesia in the right ventricular free wall (*red arrow*) and chemical shift artifact in the distal interventricular septum (*blue arrow*), suggestive of lipomatous metaplasia. T1-weighted black blood imaging (C) with high signal intensity in the distal septum, consistent with lipomatous metaplasia. Corresponding short-axis LGE-CMR (D) with associated hyperenhancement in the epicardial aspect of the distal septum (*yellow arrow*).

precession pulse sequences—as is typically employed for cine-CMR (a key component of nearly all CMR exams)—LM can be identified based on the presence of a "chemical shift artifact" (Fig. 26.9), which is characterized by a region of central high-signal intensity surrounded by a low-signal intensity band due to intravoxel cancellation between admixed fat- and water-containing regions.[60] However, one key limitation of SSFP for the assessment of LM is that it is particularly sensitive to magnetic field inhomogeneity, especially in the presence of metallic implanted devices. Given its importance as a mechanism for arrhythmic events, direct comparisons of the diagnostic and prognostic yields of different CMR approaches for LM in patients with DCM is an important area for future research.

T1 Mapping

T1 mapping has emerged as a promising CMR approach capable of further refining tissue characterization and risk assessment for patients with DCM. Several different pulse sequences have been used for this purpose, which share a common theme of acquiring multiple co-registered datasets with different T1 weightings (acquired at different time points after an inversion or saturation prepulse), and then fitting measured signal intensities using an equation for T1 relaxation. "Native" T1 is measured on precontrast T1 images. Co-registered data from pre- and postcontrast T1 mapping data can be integrated to obtain the "extracellular volume fraction" (ECV). ECV is a measure of the extracellular space outside the myocytes, and an increased ECV provides a marker of diffuse myocardial fibrosis (distinct from focal fibrosis as reflected by LGE-CMR).[61] Pre- and postcontrast T1 mapping data can be readily acquired (typical acquisition time <30 seconds per pulse sequence), thus facilitating their integration into routine clinical CMR exams so as to further enhance multiparametric tissue characterization.

Given that diffuse interstitial fibrosis has been reported to be a histologic finding in patients with DCM and other nonischemic cardiomyopathies, substantial research has focused on use of T1 mapping indices for noninvasive tissue characterization of these cohorts. Elevation of ECV in even mild phenotypes of DCM, compared with controls, has been demonstrated.[62] It has also been shown that elevated T1 indices are common in patients with DCM, in whom elevated T1 and ECV reflect histological fibrosis.[24,63] Among 88 patients DCM patients who underwent CMR and endomyocardial biopsy (EMB) within a 3-month timespan, investigators from the Maastricht Cardiomyopathy Registry reported that 36% ($n = 32$) had increased T1 based on a center-specific cutoff (>1052 ms).[24] With respect to histological validation, data from this study demonstrated that diagnostic accuracy for moderate histologic fibrosis (defined as collagen volume fraction >10%) for T1 was 0.91 (CI 0.85–0.97; $P < .0001$) with an optimal cutoff of 1056 ms (sensitivity 96%, specificity 77%) and for ECV was 0.82 (CI 0.73–0.91; $P<.0001$) with an optimal cutoff of 28.9% (sensitivity 88%, specificity 64%). Integration of T1 and ECV data further improved diagnostic performance, as evidenced by an area under the curve of 0.95. These data support the notion that elevated T1 indices are common in patients with DCM—and that these noninvasive CMR indices provide a marker of histologically evidenced diffuse myocardial fibrosis.

Several studies have reported that T1 mapping-derived ECV provides prognostic value for patients with DCM. In a prospective study of 407 DCM patients, Zhou et al. reported that ECV (cutoff of 32.8%) was associated with an increased risk of the primary endpoint (composite of HF death, SCD, aborted SCD, and heart transplantation), even after adjusting for LGE (HR 5.92 [CI 2.56, 13.66], $P<.001$).[64] In another study that encompassed 99 DCM patients, Rubis et al. reported that ventricular arrhythmic burden (defined as presence of ventricular or a high burden of premature ventricular contractions) was associated with increased ECV as measured using T1 mapping: ECV was higher in patients with, as compared to those without, increased arrhythmic burden (global ECV: 27.9 ± 4.9 vs. 30.3 ± 4.2; $P<.02$), whereas neither qualitative nor quantitative LGE assessment differentiated between groups.[65]

Despite promising results in several studies, data regarding incremental prognostic utility of T1 mapping in patients with DCM is mixed. For example, a recent meta-analysis demonstrated that ECV (OR 1.09 [95% CI 0.91–1.30], per 1% increase) and T1 relaxation time (OR 1.03 [95% CI 0.93–1.13], per 10 ms increase) were not associated with HF events (defined as any combination of HF death, cardiac transplant, left ventricular assist device implantation, or HF hospitalization).[66] However, T1 relaxation time was associated with increased arrhythmic (OR 1.07 [CI 1.01–1.14]) events and major adverse cardiovascular events (OR 1.06 [CI 1.01–1.11]). Regarding prognosis, it is also uncertain whether CMR-derived T1 mapping indices are modifiable via targeted pharmacotherapies (e.g., ACE inhibitors or angiotensin receptor blockers, each of which have antifibrotic potential), and whether change in T1 is paralleled by differential clinical outcomes. Taken together, diffuse myocardial fibrosis as delineated by T1 mapping indices may be extremely valuable tools to stratify clinical prognosis and therapeutic response for patients with DCM, but further research is warranted to confirm these issues.

Despite conceptual strengths and prognostic potential, several challenges remain that impede widespread utilization of T1 mapping as a tool to inform routine clinical decision-making. These include a lack of standardization in acquisition methods (including pulse sequence type and measurement techniques), normative cutoffs, and potential confounders (e.g., co-existent tissue properties such as intramyocardial fat that can impact T1 and thus impede parametric mapping as a marker of fibrosis, heart rate variability). Technical advances in CMR are well suited to address these issues and facilitate broader application of robust T1 mapping methods to quantify diffuse fibrosis and further refine risk stratification for patients with DCM.

EMERGING TECHNIQUES

Diffuse Tensor CMR

Diffusion tensor CMR (DT-CMR) is an emerging CMR technique that provides insight into cardiac microstructure. DT-CMR can demonstrate cardiomyocyte helical architecture, which impacts cardiac systolic and diastolic function. Additionally, this approach can reveal dynamic reorientation of sheetlets, functional units of cardiomyocytes separated by shear layers, between diastole and systole so as to elucidate mechanisms by which microstructural changes impact cardiac function.[67] Further, DT-CMR can quantify tissue diffusion through parameters such as fractional anisotropy, reflecting cardiomyocyte organization, and mean diffusivity, indicative of cardiomyocyte packing.[67] Abnormalities in myocyte orientation and sheetlet dynamics have been identified in DCM patients.[68,69] Nielles-Vallespin et al. studied 19 normative controls and 19 DCM patients, among whom diffusion tensor CMR demonstrated differences between groups: Among controls, sheetlet orientation moved by 45 degrees from a tangential plane to a more radial direction during systole whereas in DCM patients, systolic redirection was blunted (20 degrees) whereas diastolic values were similar. Although the clinical impact of DT-CMR remains uncertain, its ability to detect preclinical myocardial microstructural changes holds promise for its utility in early diagnosis and improved risk stratification in DCM.

Quantitative Susceptibility Mapping (QSM)

Quantitative susceptibility mapping is an MRI technique that relies on the phase of the MR signal to directly estimate susceptibility, a measure of how tissue is magnetized when placed in an external magnetic field. QSM has been predominantly applied in neurological disorders associated with iron accumulation, such as Parkinson and Alzheimer diseases. However, QSM also holds significant potential for cardiovascular imaging, enabling the assessment of critical indicators of cardiac disease, including blood oxygenation levels, hemorrhage, myocardial iron content, and calcification.

QSM-derived blood oxygenation also has potential in patients with DCM, as it can measure mixed venous oxygen saturation (Fig. 26.10) and identify patients in low output states to optimize therapy. In an initial validation study, Wen et al. tested a 3D free-breathing QSM technique in healthy controls ($n=10$) and patients being considered for invasive cardiac catheterization.[70] Among cardiac patients, QSM was successful in 87% and yielded higher differential (LV–RV) oxygenation (ΔSaO_2) than in controls ($P<.001$). Regarding heart failure, QSM-calculated ΔSaO_2 was higher among patients with, as compared to those without, LV dysfunction ($29.4 \pm 5.9\%$ vs. $20.9 \pm 5.7\%$, $P<.001$). Invasive catheterization measurements ($n=15$) obtained within a mean interval of 4 ± 3 days from CMR demonstrated QSM to yield high correlation ($r=0.87$, $P<.001$), small bias (–0.1%),

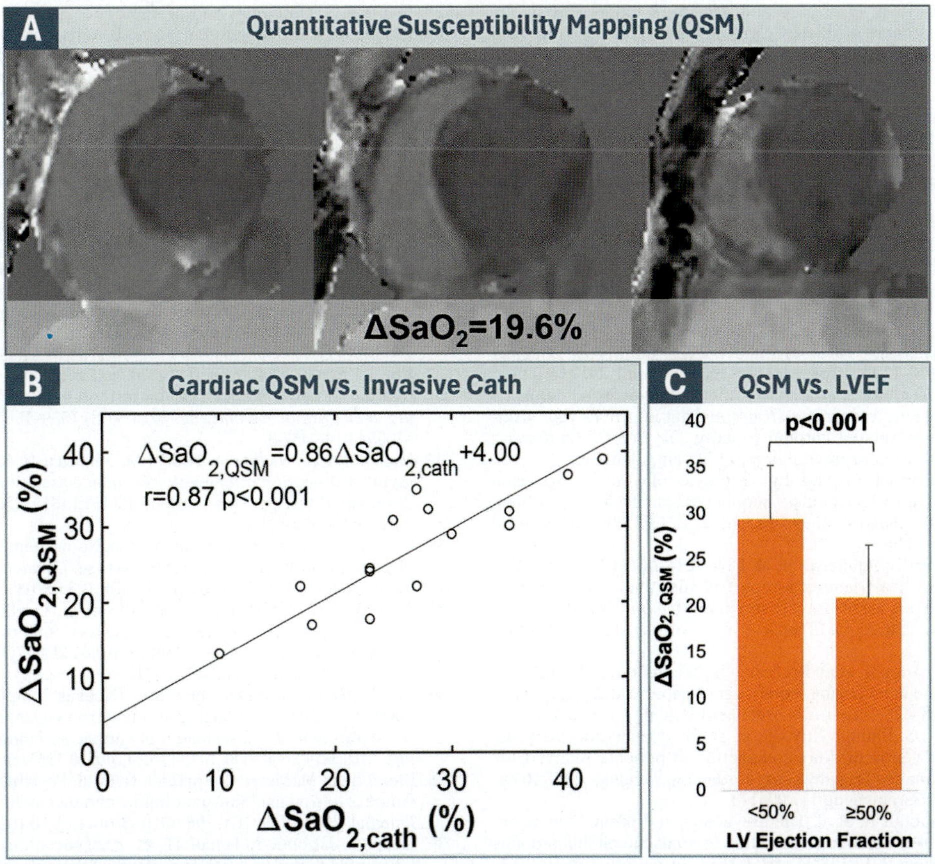

FIG. 26.10 Representative application of quantitative susceptibility mapping (QSM) for myocardial oxygenation in dilated cardiomyopathy. QSM parametric map (A) in a patient with dilated cardiomyopathy demonstrates differential blood oxygenation between cardiac chambers. QSM-derived differential blood pool oxygenation between the left and right ventricles (ΔSaO_2) correlates strongly with invasive catheter-based measurements (B). QSM-derived ΔSaO_2 values are significantly higher in patients with reduced left ventricular ejection fraction (LVEF <50%) compared to those with preserved LVEF, indicating impaired myocardial oxygen extraction (C). (Adapted from Wen et al J Cardiovasc Magn Reson. 2019 Nov 18;21(1):70. Elsevier editorial permission will be needed for use of this figure).

and good limits of agreement (±8.6%) with invasively measured ΔSaO_2. Nonetheless, numerous technical challenges remain, particularly related to cardiac motion, blood flow dynamics, and susceptibility-induced distortions. Current research is focused on addressing these challenges to enable widespread use of QSM in clinical practice and testing the prognostic value of QSM among patients with DCM and other cardiomyopathic processes.

CONCLUSION

In summary, CMR provides a powerful tool for multiparametric assessment of cardiac morphology, function, and tissue characteristics within a single noninvasive examination that offers unique diagnostic and prognostic insights for the assessment of DCM. CMR provides a highly precise tool to assess myocardial performance to inform the physiologic basis of patient symptoms and track response to therapy. In parallel, myocardial tissue characterization, as uniquely enabled by CMR, provides a powerful means of informing the mechanism of contractile dysfunction and enhancing prognostic prediction—including stratification of response to interventional treatments and risk for clinical outcomes such as heart failure hospitalization, arrhythmic events, and death. Emerging CMR techniques are well poised to augment the assessment of key aspects of cardiovascular physiology—including myocardial architecture and oxygen-based metabolism—and thus further enhance diagnostics and risk prediction. Ongoing research is focused on testing the incremental utility of CMR in relation to conventional assessment in large-scale epidemiologic cohorts toward the goal of improving clinical outcomes for patients with DCM.

REFERENCES

1. Pinto YM, Elliott PM, Arbustini E, et al. Proposal for a revised definition of dilated cardiomyopathy, hypokinetic non-dilated cardiomyopathy, and its implications for clinical practice: a position statement of the ESC working group on myocardial and pericardial diseases. *Eur Heart J.* 2016;37(23):1850–1858. https://doi.org/10.1093/eurheartj/ehv727.
2. Hershberger RE, Hedges DJ, Morales A. Dilated cardiomyopathy: the complexity of a diverse genetic architecture. *Nat Rev Cardiol.* 2013;10(9):531–547. https://doi.org/10.1038/nrcardio.2013.105.
3. Gerull B, Gramlich M, Atherton J, et al. Mutations of TTN, encoding the giant muscle filament titin, cause familial dilated cardiomyopathy. *Nat Genet.* 2002;30(2):201–204. https://doi.org/10.1038/ng815.
4. Herman DS, Lam L, Taylor MR, et al. Truncations of titin causing dilated cardiomyopathy. *N Engl J Med.* 2012;366(7):619–628. https://doi.org/10.1056/NEJMoa1110186.
5. Lund LH, Edwards LB, Dipchand AI, et al. The registry of the international society for heart and lung transplantation: thirty-third adult heart transplantation report-2016; focus theme: primary diagnostic indications for transplant. *J Heart Lung Transplant.* 2016;35(10):1158–1169. https://doi.org/10.1016/j.healun.2016.08.017.

6. Halliday BP, Gulati A, Ali A, et al. Sex- and age-based differences in the natural history and outcome of dilated cardiomyopathy. *Eur J Heart Fail.* 2018;20(10):1392–1400. https://doi.org/10.1002/ejhf.1216.
7. Donal E, Delgado V, Bucciarelli-Ducci C, et al. Multimodality imaging in the diagnosis, risk stratification, and management of patients with dilated cardiomyopathies: an expert consensus document from the European association of cardiovascular imaging. *Eur Heart J Cardiovasc Imaging.* 2019;20(10):1075–1093. https://doi.org/10.1093/ehjci/jez178.
8. Fatkin D, Yeoh T, Hayward CS, et al. Evaluation of left ventricular enlargement as a marker of early disease in familial dilated cardiomyopathy. *Circ Cardiovasc Genet.* 2011;4(4):342–348. https://doi.org/10.1161/circgenetics.110.958918.
9. Taylor MR, Fain PR, Sinagra G, et al. Natural history of dilated cardiomyopathy due to lamin A/C gene mutations. *J Am Coll Cardiol.* 2003;41(5):771–780. https://doi.org/10.1016/s0735-1097(02)02954-6.
10. Patel AR, Kramer CM. Role of cardiac magnetic resonance in the diagnosis and prognosis of nonischemic cardiomyopathy. *JACC, Cardiovasc Imaging.* 2017;10(10_Part_A):1180–1193. https://doi.org/10.1016/j.jcmg.2017.08.005.
11. Buss SJ, Breuninger K, Lehrke S, et al. Assessment of myocardial deformation with cardiac magnetic resonance strain imaging improves risk stratification in patients with dilated cardiomyopathy. *Eur Heart J Cardiovasc Imaging.* 2015;16(3):307–315. https://doi.org/10.1093/ehjci/jeu181.
12. Ibrahim el SH. Myocardial tagging by cardiovascular magnetic resonance: evolution of techniques-pulse sequences, analysis algorithms, and applications. *J Cardiovasc Magn Reson.* 2011;13(1):36. https://doi.org/10.1186/1532-429x-13-36.
13. Heidenreich PA, Bozkurt B, Aguilar D, et al. 2022 AHA/ACC/HFSA guideline for the management of heart failure: a report of the American college of cardiology/American heart association joint committee on clinical practice guidelines. *Circulation.* 2022;145(18):e895–e1032. https://doi.org/10.1161/cir.0000000000001063.
14. Petersen SE, Jensen B, Aung N, et al. Excessive trabeculation of the left ventricle: JACC: cardiovascular imaging expert panel paper. *JACC, Cardiovasc Imaging.* 2023;16(3):408–425. https://doi.org/10.1016/j.jcmg.2022.12.026.
15. Ivanov A, Dabiesingh DS, Bhumireddy GP, et al. Prevalence and prognostic significance of left ventricular noncompaction in patients referred for cardiac magnetic resonance imaging. *Circ Cardiovasc Imaging.* 2017;10(9). https://doi.org/10.1161/circimaging.117.006174.
16. Gulati A, Ismail TF, Jabbour A, et al. The prevalence and prognostic significance of right ventricular systolic dysfunction in nonischemic dilated cardiomyopathy. *Circulation.* 2013;128(15):1623–1633. https://doi.org/10.1161/circulationaha.113.002518.
17. Grothues F, Moon JC, Bellenger NG, Smith GS, Klein HU, Pennell DJ. Interstudy reproducibility of right ventricular volumes, function, and mass with cardiovascular magnetic resonance. *Am Heart J.* 2004;147(2):218–223. https://doi.org/10.1016/j.ahj.2003.10.005.
18. Pouleur AC, Rousseau MF, Ahn SA, et al. Right ventricular systolic dysfunction assessed by cardiac magnetic resonance is a strong predictor of cardiovascular death after coronary bypass grafting. *Ann Thorac Surg.* 2016;101(6):2176–2184. https://doi.org/10.1016/j.athoracsur.2015.11.035.
19. Becker MAJ, Cornel JH, van de Ven PM, van Rossum AC, Allaart CP, Germans T. The prognostic value of late gadolinium-enhanced cardiac magnetic resonance imaging in nonischemic dilated cardiomyopathy: a review and meta-analysis. *JACC, Cardiovasc Imaging.* 2018;11(9):1274–1284. https://doi.org/10.1016/j.jcmg.2018.03.006.
20. Peters DC, Lamy J, Sinusas AJ, Baldassarre LA. Left atrial evaluation by cardiovascular magnetic resonance: sensitive and unique biomarkers. *Eur Heart J Cardiovasc Imaging.* 2021;23(1):14–30. https://doi.org/10.1093/ehjci/jeab221.
21. Sade LE, Faletra FF, Pontone G, et al. The role of multi-modality imaging for the assessment of left atrium and left atrial appendage: a clinical consensus statement of the European association of cardiovascular imaging (EACVI), European heart rhythm association (EHRA) of the European society of cardiology (ESC). *Eur Heart J Cardiovasc Imaging.* 2025;26(3):385–413. https://doi.org/10.1093/ehjci/jeaf014.
22. Kim J, Yum B, Palumbo MC, et al. Left atrial strain impairment precedes geometric remodeling as a marker of post-myocardial infarction diastolic dysfunction. *JACC, Cardiovasc Imaging.* 2020;13(10):2099–2113. https://doi.org/10.1016/j.jcmg.2020.05.041.
23. Gulati A, Ismail TF, Jabbour A, et al. Clinical utility and prognostic value of left atrial volume assessment by cardiovascular magnetic resonance in non-ischaemic dilated cardiomyopathy. *Eur J Heart Fail.* 2013;15(6):660–670. https://doi.org/10.1093/eurjhf/hft019.
24. Raafs AG, Adriaans BP, Henkens MTHM, et al. Myocardial fibrosis assessment using T1 and ECV mapping with histologic validation in chronic dilated cardiomyopathy. *JACC, Cardiovasc Imaging.* 2022;15(10):1828–1830. https://doi.org/10.1016/j.jcmg.2022.05.002.
25. Li Y, Guo J, Li W, et al. Prognostic value of right atrial strain derived from cardiovascular magnetic resonance in non-ischemic dilated cardiomyopathy. *J Cardiovasc Magn Reson.* 2022;24(1):54. https://doi.org/10.1186/s12968-022-00894-w.
26. Rossi A, Dini FL, Faggiano P, et al. Independent prognostic value of functional mitral regurgitation in patients with heart failure. A quantitative analysis of 1256 patients with ischaemic and non-ischaemic dilated cardiomyopathy. *Heart.* 2011;97(20):1675–1680. https://doi.org/10.1136/hrt.2011.225789.
27. Uretsky S, Gillam L, Lang R, et al. Discordance between echocardiography and MRI in the assessment of mitral regurgitation severity: a prospective multicenter trial. *J Am Coll Cardiol.* 2015;65(11):1078–1088. https://doi.org/10.1016/j.jacc.2014.12.047.
28. Li J, Wei X. Outcomes and predictors of patients with moderate or severe functional mitral regurgitation and nonischemic dilated cardiomyopathy. *Clin Cardiol.* 2023;46(8):922–929. https://doi.org/10.1002/clc.24067.
29. Beltrami CA, Finato N, Rocco M, et al. The cellular basis of dilated cardiomyopathy in humans. *J Mol Cell Cardiol.* 1995;27(1):291–305. https://doi.org/10.1016/s0022-2828(08)80028-4.
30. Marijianowski MM, Teeling P, Mann J, Becker AE. Dilated cardiomyopathy is associated with an increase in the type I/type III collagen ratio: a quantitative assessment. *J Am Coll Cardiol.* 1995;25(6):1263–1272. https://doi.org/10.1016/0735-1097(94)00557-7.
31. López B, Ravassa S, Moreno MU, et al. Diffuse myocardial fibrosis: mechanisms, diagnosis and therapeutic approaches. *Nat Rev Cardiol.* 2021;18(7):479–498. https://doi.org/10.1038/s41569-020-00504-1.
32. McCrohon JA, Moon JC, Prasad SK, et al. Differentiation of heart failure related to dilated cardiomyopathy and coronary artery disease using gadolinium-enhanced cardiovascular magnetic resonance. *Circulation.* 2003;108(1):54–59. https://doi.org/10.1161/01.Cir.0000078641.19365.4c.
33. Kim J, Kochav JD, Gurevich S, et al. Left ventricular geometric remodeling in relation to non-ischemic scar pattern on cardiac magnetic resonance imaging. *Int J Cardiovasc Imaging.* 2014;30(8):1559–1567. https://doi.org/10.1007/s10554-014-0487-8.
34. Mahrholdt H, Wagner A, Judd RM, Sechtem U, Kim RJ. Delayed enhancement cardiovascular magnetic resonance assessment of non-ischaemic cardiomyopathies. *Eur Heart J.* 2005;26(15):1461–1474. https://doi.org/10.1093/eurheartj/ehi258.
35. Bawaskar P, Thomas N, Ismail K, et al. Nonischemic or dual cardiomyopathy in patients with coronary artery disease. *Circulation.* 2024;149(11):807–821. https://doi.org/10.1161/circulationaha.123.067032.
36. Athwal PSS, Chhikara S, Ismail MF, et al. Cardiovascular magnetic resonance imaging phenotypes and long-term outcomes in patients with suspected cardiac sarcoidosis. *JAMA Cardiol.* 2022;7(10):1057–1066. https://doi.org/10.1001/jamacardio.2022.2981.
37. Vita T, Okada DR, Veillet-Chowdhury M, et al. Complementary value of cardiac magnetic resonance imaging and positron emission tomography/computed tomography in the assessment of cardiac sarcoidosis. *Circ Cardiovasc Imaging.* 2018;11(1):e007030. https://doi.org/10.1161/circimaging.117.007030.
38. Bietenbeck M, Meier C, Korthals D, et al. Possible causes and clinical relevance of a "ring-like" late gadolinium enhancement pattern. *JACC, Cardiovasc Imaging.* 2024;17(1):104–106. https://doi.org/10.1016/j.jcmg.2023.08.004.
39. Gulati A, Jabbour A, Ismail TF, et al. Association of fibrosis with mortality and sudden cardiac death in patients with nonischemic dilated cardiomyopathy. *JAMA.* 2013;309(9):896–908. https://doi.org/10.1001/jama.2013.1363.
40. Hsia HH, Marchlinski FE. Electrophysiology studies in patients with dilated cardiomyopathies. *Card Electrophysiol Rev.* 2002;6(4):472–481. https://doi.org/10.1023/a:1021109130276.
41. Pogwizd SM, McKenzie JP, Cain ME. Mechanisms underlying spontaneous and induced ventricular arrhythmias in patients with idiopathic dilated cardiomyopathy. *Circulation.* 1998;98(22):2404–2414. https://doi.org/10.1161/01.cir.98.22.2404.
42. Marco AD, Anguera I, Schmitt M, et al. Late gadolinium enhancement and the risk for ventricular arrhythmias or sudden death in dilated cardiomyopathy. *JACC (J Am Coll Cardiol): Heart Fail.* 2017;5(1):28–38. https://doi.org/10.1016/j.jchf.2016.09.017.
43. Kadish A, Dyer A, Daubert JP, et al. Prophylactic defibrillator implantation in patients with nonischemic dilated cardiomyopathy. *N Engl J Med.* 2004;350(21):2151–2158. https://doi.org/10.1056/NEJMoa033088.
44. Selvanayagam JB, Hartshorne T, Billot L, et al. Cardiovascular magnetic resonance-GUIDEd management of mild to moderate left ventricular systolic dysfunction (CMR GUIDE): Study protocol for a randomized controlled trial. *Ann Noninvasive Electrocardiol.* 2017;22(4). https://doi.org/10.1111/anec.12420.
45. Flett A, Cebula A, Nicholas Z, et al. Rationale and study protocol for the BRITISH randomized trial (using cardiovascular magnetic resonance identified scar as the benchmark risk indication tool for implantable cardioverter defibrillators in patients with nonischemic cardiomyopathy and severe systolic heart failure). *Am Heart J.* 2023;266:149–158. https://doi.org/10.1016/j.ahj.2023.09.008.
46. Leong DP, Chakrabarty A, Shipp N, et al. Effects of myocardial fibrosis and ventricular dyssynchrony on response to therapy in new-presentation idiopathic dilated cardiomyopathy: insights from cardiovascular magnetic resonance and echocardiography. *Eur Heart J.* 2012;33(5):640–648. https://doi.org/10.1093/eurheartj/ehr391.
47. Bello D, Shah DJ, Farah GM, et al. Gadolinium cardiovascular magnetic resonance predicts reversible myocardial dysfunction and remodeling in patients with heart failure undergoing beta-blocker therapy. *Circulation.* 2003;108(16):1945–1953. https://doi.org/10.1161/01.Cir.0000095029.57483.60.
48. Birnie DH, Tang AS. The problem of non-response to cardiac resynchronization therapy. *Curr Opin Cardiol.* 2006;21(1):20–26. https://doi.org/10.1097/01.hco.0000198983.93755.99.
49. Bleeker GB, Kaandorp TA, Lamb HJ, et al. Effect of posterolateral scar tissue on clinical and echocardiographic improvement after cardiac resynchronization therapy. *Circulation.* 2006;113(7):969–976. https://doi.org/10.1161/circulationaha.105.543678.
50. White JA, Yee R, Yuan X, et al. Delayed enhancement magnetic resonance imaging predicts response to cardiac resynchronization therapy in patients with intraventricular dyssynchrony. *J Am Coll Cardiol.* 2006;48(10):1953–1960. https://doi.org/10.1016/j.jacc.2006.07.046.
51. Bilchick KC, Kuruvilla S, Hamirani YS, et al. Impact of mechanical activation, scar, and electrical timing on cardiac resynchronization therapy response

and clinical outcomes. *J Am Coll Cardiol*. 2014;63(16):1657–1666. https://doi.org/10.1016/j.jacc.2014.02.533.

52. Song Y, Chen X, Yang K, et al. Cardiac MRI-derived myocardial fibrosis and ventricular dyssynchrony predict response to cardiac resynchronization therapy in patients with nonischemic dilated cardiomyopathy. *Radiol Cardiothorac Imaging*. 2023;5(5):e220127. https://doi.org/10.1148/ryct.220127.
53. Wang Y, Zhu H, Hou X, et al. Randomized trial of left bundle branch vs biventricular pacing for cardiac resynchronization therapy. *J Am Coll Cardiol*. 2022;80(13):1205–1216.
54. Diaz JC, Sauer WH, Duque M, et al. Left bundle branch area pacing versus biventricular pacing as initial strategy for cardiac resynchronization. *Clin Electrophysiol*. 2023;9(8_Part_2):1568–1581.
55. Chen Z, Ma X, Gao Y, et al. Cardiac magnetic resonance–derived myocardial scar is associated with echocardiographic response and clinical prognosis of left bundle branch area pacing for cardiac resynchronization therapy. *EP Europace*. 2023;25(11). https://doi.org/10.1093/europace/euad326.
56. Chen Z, Ma X, Wu S, et al. A comparison of the association of septal scar burden on responses to LBBAP-CRT and BVP-CRT. *JACC (J Am Coll Cardiol): Clin Electrophysiol*. 2024;10(7, Part 1):1439–1451. https://doi.org/10.1016/j.jacep.2024.03.005.
57. Xu L, Khoshknab M, Berger RD, et al. Lipomatous metaplasia enables ventricular tachycardia by reducing current loss within the protected corridor. *JACC Clin Electrophysiol*. 2022;8(10):1274–1285. https://doi.org/10.1016/j.jacep.2022.07.005.
58. Baroldi G, Silver MD, De Maria R, Parodi O, Pellegrini A. Lipomatous metaplasia in left ventricular scar. *Can J Cardiol*. 1997;13(1):65–71.
59. Xu L, Khoshknab M, Moss J, et al. Lipomatous metaplasia is associated with ventricular tachycardia recurrence following ablation in patients with nonischemic cardiomyopathy. *JACC Clin Electrophysiol*. 2024;10(6):1135–1146. https://doi.org/10.1016/j.jacep.2024.02.024.
60. Shriki JE, Surti KS, Farvid AF, et al. Chemical shift artifact on steady-state free precession cardiac magnetic resonance sequences as a result of lipomatous metaplasia: a novel finding in chronic myocardial infarctions. *Can J Cardiol*. 2011;27(5):664.e17–664.e23. https://doi.org/10.1016/j.cjca.2010.12.074.
61. Flett AS, Hayward MP, Ashworth MT, et al. Equilibrium contrast cardiovascular magnetic resonance for the measurement of diffuse myocardial fibrosis: preliminary validation in humans. *Circulation*. 2010;122(2):138–144. https://doi.org/10.1161/circulationaha.109.930636.
62. aus dem Siepen F, Buss SJ, Messroghli D, et al. T1 mapping in dilated cardiomyopathy with cardiac magnetic resonance: quantification of diffuse myocardial fibrosis and comparison with endomyocardial biopsy. *Eur Heart J Cardiovasc Imaging*. 2015;16(2):210–216. https://doi.org/10.1093/ehjci/jeu183.
63. Nakamori S, Dohi K, Ishida M, et al. Native T1 mapping and extracellular volume mapping for the assessment of diffuse myocardial fibrosis in dilated cardiomyopathy. *JACC, Cardiovasc Imaging*. 2018;11(1):48–59. https://doi.org/10.1016/j.jcmg.2017.04.006.
64. Zhou D, Zhu L, Wu W, et al. A novel cardiac magnetic resonance-based personalized risk stratification model in dilated cardiomyopathy: a prospective study. *Eur Radiol*. 2024;34(6):4053–4064. https://doi.org/10.1007/s00330-023-10415-7.
65. Rubiś PP, Dziewięcka EM, Banyś P, et al. Extracellular volume is an independent predictor of arrhythmic burden in dilated cardiomyopathy. *Sci Rep*. 2021;11(1):24000. https://doi.org/10.1038/s41598-021-03452-z.
66. Eichhorn C, Koeckerling D, Reddy RK, et al. Risk stratification in nonischemic dilated cardiomyopathy using CMR imaging: a systematic review and meta-analysis. *JAMA*. 2024;332(18):1535–1550. https://doi.org/10.1001/jama.2024.13946.
67. Khalique Z, Ferreira PF, Scott AD, Nielles-Vallespin S, Firmin DN, Pennell DJ. Diffusion tensor cardiovascular magnetic resonance imaging: a clinical perspective. *JACC, Cardiovasc Imaging*. 2020;13(5):1235–1255. https://doi.org/10.1016/j.jcmg.2019.07.016.
68. Nielles-Vallespin S, Khalique Z, Ferreira PF, et al. Assessment of myocardial microstructural dynamics by in vivo diffusion tensor cardiac magnetic resonance. *J Am Coll Cardiol*. 2017;69(6):661–676.
69. Von Deuster C, Sammut E, Asner L, et al. Studying dynamic myofiber aggregate reorientation in dilated cardiomyopathy using in vivo magnetic resonance diffusion tensor imaging. *Circ: Cardiovasc Imaging*. 2016;9(10):e005018.
70. Wen Y, Weinsaft JW, Nguyen TD, et al. Free breathing three-dimensional cardiac quantitative susceptibility mapping for differential cardiac chamber blood oxygenation—initial validation in patients with cardiovascular disease inclusive of direct comparison to invasive catheterization. *J Cardiovasc Magn Reson*. 2019;21(1):70. https://doi.org/10.1186/s12968-019-0579-7.

27 Infiltrative Cardiomyopathies

CHETAN SHENOY

INTRODUCTION

Infiltrative cardiomyopathies represent a diverse group of disorders characterized by the abnormal deposition of substances within the myocardium, leading to progressive cardiac dysfunction and, in some cases, life-threatening complications. These conditions pose a significant diagnostic challenge due to their varied etiologies, clinical presentations, and subtle early findings. Cardiovascular magnetic resonance (CMR) imaging has emerged as a pivotal tool in the evaluation and management of infiltrative cardiomyopathies, providing unparalleled insights into cardiac structure, function, and tissue characteristics.

In this chapter, we will delve into the role of CMR in the assessment and understanding of infiltrative cardiomyopathies, highlighting its unique capabilities in diagnosing, differentiating, and monitoring these complex cardiac disorders. We will explore the key CMR findings, diagnostic algorithms, and the impact of CMR on clinical management, as well as discuss emerging techniques and future directions in this field.

PATHOPHYSIOLOGY OF INFILTRATIVE CARDIOMYOPATHIES

Infiltrative cardiomyopathies are characterized by the abnormal deposition of substances within the myocardium, leading to progressive cardiac dysfunction. The pathophysiology of these conditions can be diverse, with various etiologies and underlying mechanisms contributing to the disease process.

The common pathways in infiltrative cardiomyopathies include:

1. Protein misfolding and aggregation: Conditions such as cardiac amyloidosis involve the deposition of misfolded proteins, such as light chains (AL amyloidosis) or transthyretin (ATTR amyloidosis), within the myocardium.
2. Metabolic disturbances: Disorders like Fabry disease and glycogen storage diseases are characterized by the accumulation of specific metabolites or storage products within the myocardium, causing cellular dysfunction and structural changes.
3. Inflammatory processes: Although technically an inflammatory cardiomyopathy, cardiac sarcoidosis has traditionally been considered an infiltrative cardiomyopathy because it involves the formation of noncaseating granulomas within the myocardium, leading to tissue damage.
4. Excessive metal deposition: Iron overload cardiomyopathy is characterized by the deposition of excessive iron within the myocardium, often seen in hereditary hemochromatosis or secondary to multiple blood transfusions.

The progressive deposition of these substances within the myocardium can result in various pathological changes, including myocyte injury, interstitial fibrosis, and impaired cardiac function. These structural and functional alterations are the key targets for assessment and monitoring using CMR imaging.

ROLE OF CARDIOVASCULAR MAGNETIC RESONANCE

CMR has emerged as a pivotal tool in the evaluation and management of infiltrative cardiomyopathies, offering unparalleled insights into cardiac structure, function, and tissue characteristics.

The unique capabilities of CMR in the assessment of infiltrative cardiomyopathies include:

1. Tissue characterization: CMR provides a comprehensive assessment of myocardial tissue composition, allowing for the detection and distinction of various infiltrative processes based on signal intensities, relaxation times, and late gadolinium enhancement (LGE) patterns.
2. Functional assessment: CMR cine imaging enables the evaluation of ventricular volumes, ejection fraction, and regional wall motion abnormalities, which can be indicative of the severity and progression of infiltrative cardiomyopathies.
3. Quantitative analysis: Advanced CMR techniques, such as T1 and T2 mapping, allow for the quantification of specific tissue properties, providing objective markers of disease severity and response to treatment.
4. Multiparametric evaluation: The integration of various CMR sequences, including cine, T1/T2 mapping, LGE, and others, enables a comprehensive and tailored assessment of infiltrative cardiomyopathies.
5. Noninvasive nature: CMR is a noninvasive imaging modality free of radiation, which is particularly advantageous in the longitudinal monitoring of patients with infiltrative cardiomyopathies, as it avoids the risks associated with repeated invasive procedures and repeated radiation.

In the following sections, we will explore the key CMR findings (Table 27.1), diagnostic algorithms, and clinical applications in the most common infiltrative cardiomyopathies.

TABLE 27.1 Key Cardiovascular Magnetic Resonance findings in common infiltrative cardiomyopathies.

CONDITION	LATE GADOLINIUM ENHANCEMENT	MYOCARDIAL T1/T2	VENTRICULAR MORPHOLOGY	MYOCARDIAL STRAIN
Cardiac amyloidosis	Diffuse subendocardial or transmural	Increased native T1, increased extracellular volume (ECV)	Biatrial enlargement, ventricular wall thickening	Reduced global longitudinal strain
Cardiac sarcoidosis	Subepicardial, multifocal, septal, right ventricular free wall late gadolinium enhancement (LGE)	Increased T2 (active inflammation)	Regional or global ventricular dysfunction	Reduced regional/ global strain
Fabry disease	Patchy or diffuse midwall LGE	Increased native T1	Left ventricular hypertrophy	Reduced global longitudinal strain
Iron overload cardiomyopathy	Diffuse subtle LGE	Decreased T2*	Impaired systolic and diastolic function	Reduced global longitudinal strain

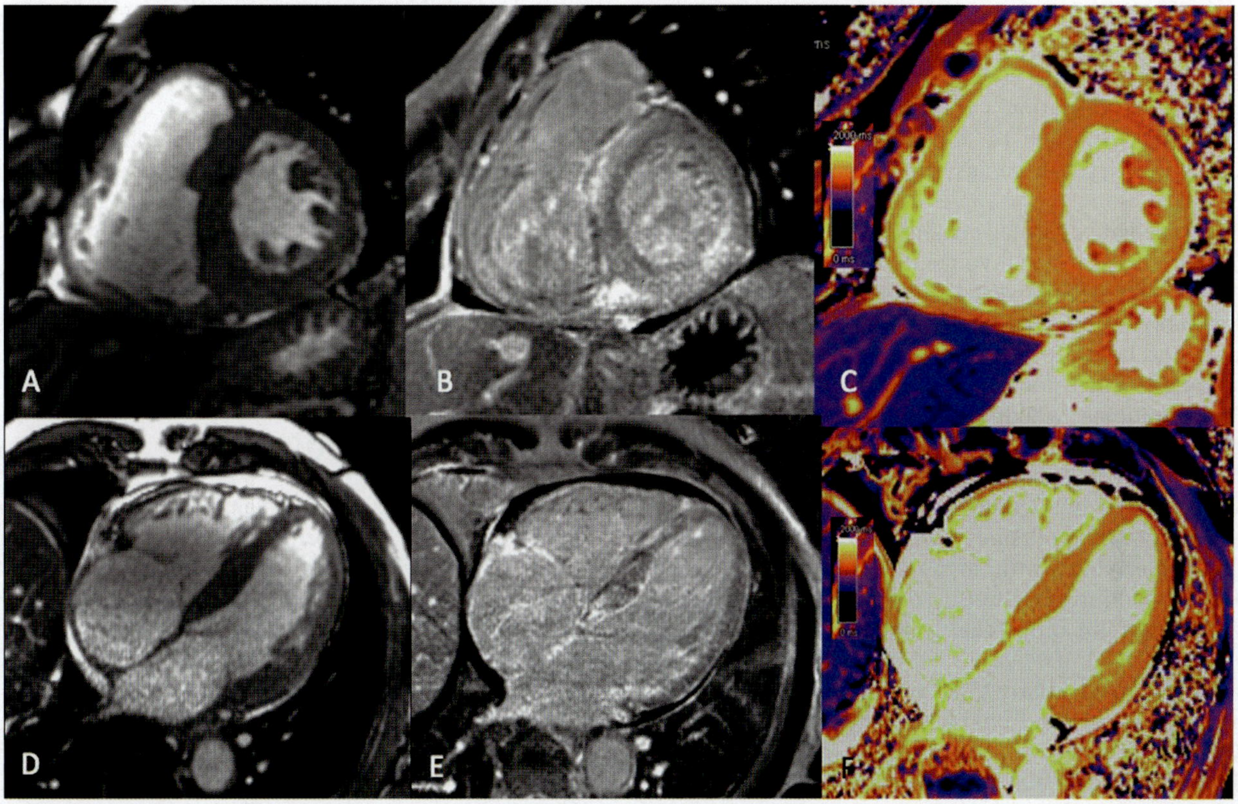

FIG. 27.1 Cardiac amyloidosis. Steady state free precession (SSFP) cine (A, D), late gadolinium enhancement (LGE) (B, E), and native T1 map (C, F) images in a patient with AL cardiac amyloidosis demonstrate concentric hypertrophy and diffuse, abnormal enhancement on LGE images (B, E). The native T1 maps (C, F) show elevated values at 1450 ms.

CARDIAC AMYLOIDOSIS

Cardiac amyloidosis is the exemplar infiltrative cardiomyopathy, characterized by the deposition of misfolded proteins within the myocardium. The two most common subtypes are transthyretin (ATTR) amyloidosis and immunoglobulin light chain (AL) amyloidosis, each with distinct etiologies, clinical features, and prognostic implications.

Cardiovascular Magnetic Resonance Findings in Cardiac Amyloidosis

CMR plays a crucial role in the evaluation of cardiac amyloidosis, as it can provide characteristic findings (Fig. 27.1) that aid in the diagnosis, and often the distinction of the various subtypes.

1. LGE:

- Diffuse subendocardial LGE: The characteristic pattern of LGE reflects the infiltrative process, with preferential involvement of the subendocardium. This pattern is often seen in both AL and ATTR amyloidosis.
- Transmural LGE: In advanced stages of cardiac amyloidosis, the LGE pattern may become transmural, with involvement of the entire myocardial wall.
- Since AL amyloid is more toxic, causing small-vessel involvement and ischemia, patients with AL amyloidosis tend to present earlier in the disease course with only subendocardial LGE. On the contrary, ATTR amyloid is not as toxic, and the fibrils deposit diffusely and extensively with transmural involvement before patients clinically present with heart failure. Thus, patients with AL amyloidosis are more likely to present with subendocardial LGE, while those with ATTR amyloidosis are more likely to present with transmural LGE.[1]

2. Increased myocardial native T1 and extracellular volume (ECV) fraction:
   - The infiltration of amyloid proteins within the myocardium leads to an increase in native T1 values and ECV fraction, which can be quantified using T1 mapping.
   - Elevated native T1 and ECV are sensitive markers of cardiac amyloid deposition, often preceding the development of overt cardiac dysfunction.
3. Biatrial enlargement and ventricular wall thickening:
   - Amyloid deposition can result in biventricular hypertrophy, with characteristic biatrial enlargement and ventricular wall thickening.
   - The degree of wall thickening, however, may be less pronounced in ATTR amyloidosis compared to AL amyloidosis.
4. Impaired myocardial strain:
   - Amyloid infiltration compromises myocardial contractility, leading to reduced global longitudinal strain, which can be assessed using feature-tracking CMR.
   - Impaired myocardial strain may serve as an early marker for cardiac involvement in amyloidosis, even in the absence of overt structural changes.

The combination of these CMR findings, along with clinical data and laboratory tests, enables accurate diagnosis and provides clues for the distinction between AL and ATTR amyloidosis, which is crucial for guiding targeted treatment strategies.

We recommend CMR as the first-line imaging technique in patients with suspected cardiac amyloidosis, rather than bone scintigraphy, since CMR helps identify the cause of the underlying cardiomyopathy—including cardiac amyloidosis and many other cardiomyopathies—whereas bone scintigraphy only reliably identifies ATTR cardiac amyloidosis.

Patients with very early ATTR amyloidosis can only have abnormalities in tissue characterization—mild elevation in ECV (<0.40) or very subtle subendocardial LGE—with no significant changes in structure and function, whereas those with more advanced disease have all the typical functional and structural changes typical of cardiac amyloidosis. Thus, patients with very early ATTR amyloidosis may be missed on CMR since mild elevation in ECV is clinically common and nonspecific. These patients may have low-grade (grade 1) cardiac uptake on bone scintigraphy.[2] Nevertheless, the absence of LGE in a patient who has CMR for increased ventricular wall thickening excludes the possibility of cardiac amyloidosis, since ventricular wall thickening is not seen with very early cardiac amyloidosis.

While bone scintigraphy has a high sensitivity for ATTR cardiac amyloidosis, the absence of cardiac uptake on bone scintigraphy does not exclude AL cardiac amyloidosis. There is also disproportionately low cardiac uptake in certain variants of ATTR cardiac amyloidosis such as the Ser77Tyr, Phe64Leu19, Y114C, and Val30Met *TTR* variants.[2]

AApoAI cardiac amyloidosis is a rare form of cardiac amyloidosis that produces distinctive features of disproportionate right-sided involvement comprising right ventricular (RV) free wall thickening, RV free wall LGE, right atrial (RA) wall thickening, tricuspid valve thickening, and septal leaflet tethering, resulting in restricted mobility and eccentric regurgitation. If seen, these novel findings should prompt genetic screening for underlying AApoAI.[3]

AApoAIV cardiac amyloidosis is another rare form of cardiac amyloidosis that presents most commonly with heart failure and always displays classical cardiac amyloidosis CMR features, mimicking the common forms of cardiac amyloidosis.[3]

Clinical Implications

The accurate diagnosis and distinction of cardiac amyloidosis subtypes using CMR are crucial, as they have distinct treatment approaches and prognoses. For example, targeted therapies for AL amyloidosis (e.g., chemotherapy, stem cell transplantation) differ from the management of ATTR amyloidosis (e.g., TTR stabilizers, gene-silencing therapies).

CMR data also carry prognostic implications. ECV is also an independent predictor of prognosis in systemic AL amyloidosis and can help define the hematological response associated with better long-term outcomes for each patient and potentially inform treatment strategies.[4] Changes in native T1 and ECV in response to chemotherapy in AL amyloidosis predict survival incremental to known predictors.[5,6]

CARDIAC SARCOIDOSIS

Cardiac sarcoidosis is an inflammatory cardiomyopathy characterized by the formation of noncaseating granulomas within the myocardium. Early detection and management of cardiac sarcoidosis are crucial, as it can lead to sudden death, life-threatening arrhythmias, and heart failure.

Cardiovascular Magnetic Resonance Findings in Cardiac Sarcoidosis

CMR plays a pivotal role in the diagnosis of cardiac sarcoidosis, demonstrating characteristic findings that aid in the assessment and management of this condition.

Cardiac sarcoidosis can lead to regional or global ventricular dysfunction, which can be assessed using cine CMR. The degree of functional impairment closely correlates with the extent of cardiac damage as seen by LGE.[7] This distinguishes it from some genetic dilated cardiomyopathies in which the LV dysfunction is worse out of proportion to the LGE.

Cardiac sarcoidosis is often labeled a "great masquerader," with features that overlap with many other cardiomyopathies, but this was proven not to be true in a systematic review of gross pathology images from patients with cardiac histology–proven cardiac sarcoidosis who had autopsy or cardiac transplantation.[8]

LGE features that are seen frequently in patients with cardiac sarcoidosis include: left ventricular (LV) subepicardial, LV multifocal, septal, and RV free wall involvement[8] (Fig. 27.2). LGE features that are rarely or never seen include isolated LV midmyocardial involvement, isolated

LV subendocardial involvement, isolated LV transmural involvement, and absence of septal involvement.[8] The absence of LGE excludes the diagnosis in patients presenting with clinical signs or symptoms suspicious for cardiac sarcoidosis.[8,9]

T2-weighted imaging and T2 mapping techniques can detect areas of myocardial edema and inflammation, reflecting the active inflammatory process in cardiac sarcoidosis. However, since inflammation is nonspecific and can be seen with a large variety of cardiomyopathies including inflammatory, genetic, ischemic, and infectious cardiomyopathies, the presence of inflammation on T2 mapping is not very helpful in making the diagnosis of cardiac sarcoidosis. This is also true of 18F-fluorodeoxyglucose uptake on positron emission tomography (FDG-PET).

The diagnosis of cardiac sarcoidosis should be made integrating CMR features of cardiac sarcoidosis with histological evidence of sarcoidosis, ideally from the heart or from outside the heart at the very minimum (Table 27.2). We do not recommend diagnosing cardiac sarcoidosis based solely on imaging.

Since cardiac sarcoidosis is a highly morbid cardiomyopathy with a high risk of ventricular arrhythmias and heart failure, a diagnosis of cardiac sarcoidosis has prognostic implications as well. The close ties between the implications of the diagnosis on prognosis are highlighted in Fig. 27.3.

Among patients with histologically proven sarcoidosis, CMR features suggestive of cardiac sarcoidosis are associated with a high risk of ventricular arrhythmias, sudden cardiac death, and heart failure.[7,10]

The CMR findings in cardiac sarcoidosis are also helpful for guiding endomyocardial biopsy, as the LGE patterns can help identify the most appropriate targets for biopsy. The yield of endomyocardial biopsy is proportional to the extent of LGE on the right ventricular aspect of the septum—the targeted location for biopsy.

While CMR can be used to longitudinally track changes in ventricular function and the extent of LGE, FDG-PET is the standard imaging technique for this purpose. T2 mapping has not been studied for monitoring the response to immunosuppressive therapy in cardiac sarcoidosis. T2 mapping in its current form is unlikely to replace FDG-PET for treatment monitoring, since the quantitative data are affected by off-resonance errors in the presence of cardiac devices, which are common in patients with cardiac sarcoidosis.

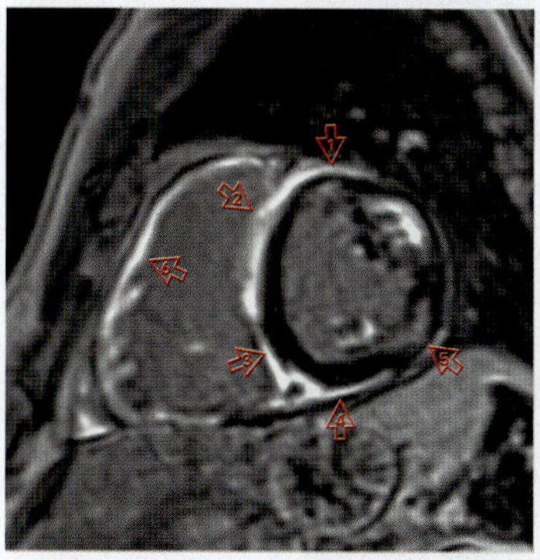

FIG. 27.2 Cardiac sarcoidosis. Late gadolinium enhancement (*LGE*) image shows the characteristic LGE features of cardiac sarcoidosis.

FABRY CARDIOMYOPATHY

Fabry disease is a rare, inherited lysosomal storage disorder characterized by the accumulation of globotriaosylceramide (Gb3) within various tissues, including the myocardium. Early recognition and management of cardiac involvement are essential, as it can lead to significant morbidity and mortality.

Cardiovascular Magnetic Resonance Findings in Fabry Cardiomyopathy

CMR plays a pivotal role in the evaluation of Fabry cardiomyopathy, providing characteristic findings (Fig. 27.4) that aid in the diagnosis and monitoring of this condition.

1. Ventricular hypertrophy:
   - Fabry disease can lead to LV hypertrophy, which can be assessed using CMR.
   - The degree of hypertrophy may correlate with the severity of cardiac involvement and disease progression.
2. Impaired myocardial strain:
   - Gb3 deposition can compromise myocardial contractility, resulting in reduced global longitudinal strain, which can be evaluated using feature-tracking CMR.

TABLE 27.2 Interpreting Cardiovascular Magnetic Resonance features of cardiac sarcoidosis with histological data.

CMR FEATURES OF CARDIAC SARCOIDOSIS	SARCOIDOSIS IN EXTRACARDIAC TISSUE	SARCOIDOSIS IN CARDIAC TISSUE	INTERPRETATION	COMMENTS
Present	Present	Present	Cardiac sarcoidosis	Ideal
Present	Absent	Present	Cardiac sarcoidosis	Ideal
Present	Present	Absent	Cardiac sarcoidosis	Acceptable
Present	Absent	Absent	Needs tissue diagnosis	Incomplete
Absent	Present	Present	Not clinically relevant cardiac sarcoidosis	Very rare
Absent	Absent	Present	Not clinically relevant cardiac sarcoidosis	Very rare
Absent	Present	Absent	Not cardiac sarcoidosis	
Absent	Present	Absent	Not cardiac sarcoidosis	
Absent	Absent	Absent	Not cardiac sarcoidosis	

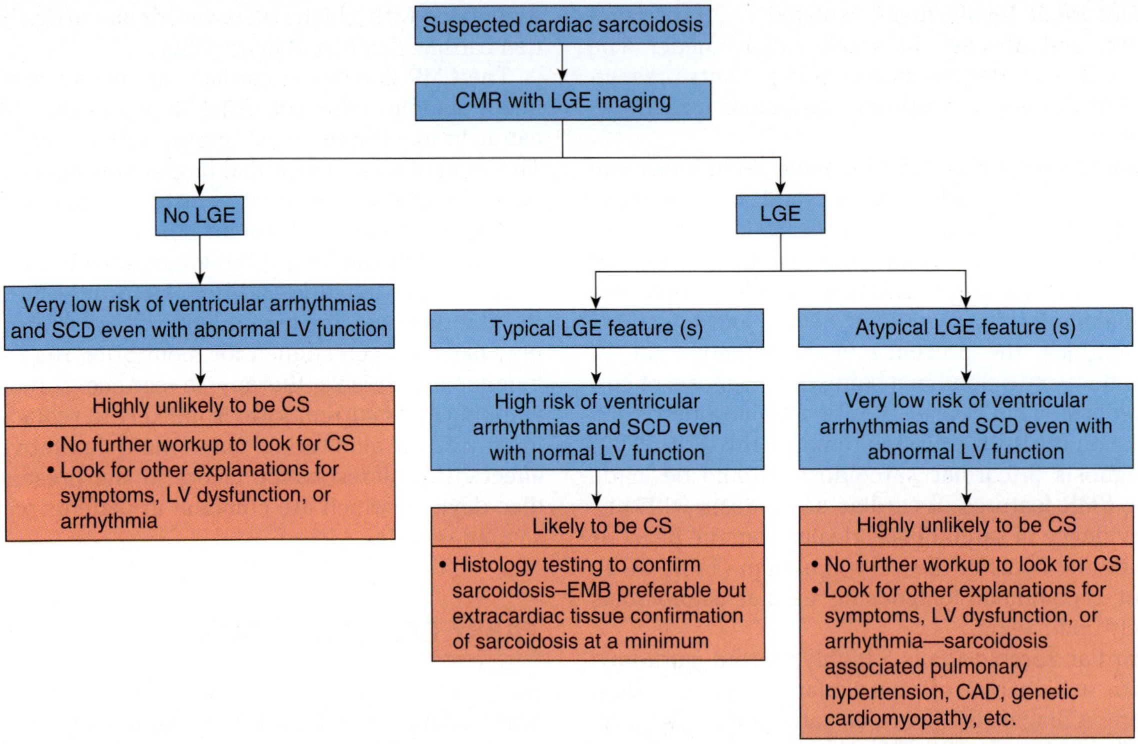

FIG. 27.3 Algorithm for the diagnosis and prognostication of cardiac sarcoidosis using cardiac magnetic resonance (*CMR*). The text in the blue boxes is supported by data. The text in the salmon boxes are our interferences and recommendations. *CS*, cardiac sarcoidosis; *LGE*, late gadolinium enhancement; *SCD*, sudden cardiac death; *LV*, left ventricle; *CAD*, coronary artery disease; *EMB*, endomyocardial biopsycad.

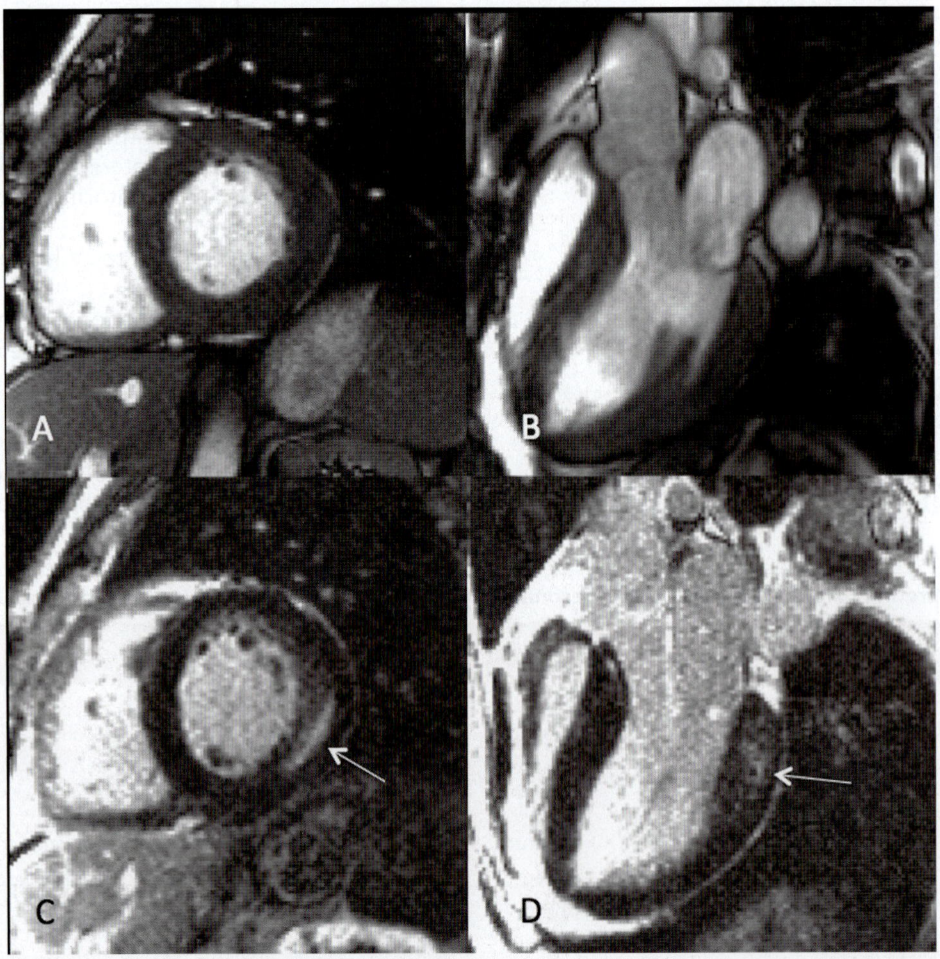

FIG. 27.4 Fabry cardiomyopathy. Steady state free precession (SSFP) cine images (A, B) in a patient with Fabry cardiomyopathy show concentric left ventricular hypertrophy. Late gadolinium enhancement (LGE) images (C, D) show midmyocardial patchy LGE in the basal inferolateral segment, which is characteristic of this cardiomyopathy.

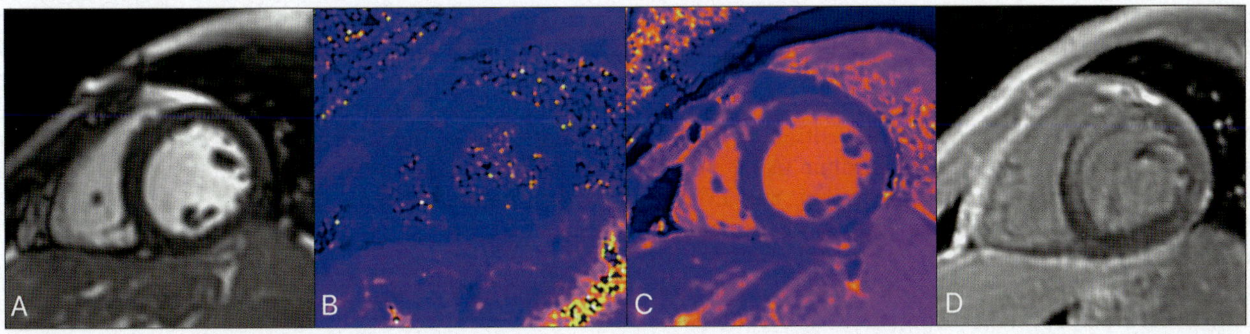

FIG. 27.5 Iron overload cardiomyopathy. Steady state free precession (SSFP) cine (A), T2* mapping (B), native T1 (C), and late gadolinium enhancement (LGE) (D) images in a patient with iron overload cardiomyopathy show characteristic findings including a dark appearance of the left ventricular myocardium on cine imaging (A), low T2* at 4.8 ms (B), low native T1 at 670 ms (C), and diffuse mild patchy enhancement of the myocardium on LGE imaging (D).

3. Increased myocardial native T1 values:
   - The accumulation of Gb3 within the myocardium leads to an increase in native T1 values, which can be quantified using CMR.
   - Elevated native T1 values are a sensitive marker of early cardiac involvement in Fabry disease, even in the absence of overt structural changes.
4. Patchy LGE:
   - Myocardial fibrosis and scarring, a consequence of Gb3 deposition, can be visualized as areas of LGE, often in a midwall or subepicardial distribution.
   - The pattern and extent of LGE can provide insights into the severity and progression of cardiac involvement.
   - Impaired myocardial strain may serve as an early marker of cardiac involvement, even before the development of overt structural changes.

CMR is invaluable in the early detection of cardiac involvement, monitoring disease progression and evaluating the response to enzyme replacement therapy in patients with Fabry cardiomyopathy. CMR-derived parameters, such as native T1 and LGE, can serve as sensitive markers of disease progression and response to therapy, allowing for personalized management strategies and improved patient outcomes.

IRON OVERLOAD CARDIOMYOPATHY

Iron overload cardiomyopathy is a rare condition characterized by the deposition of excessive iron within the myocardium, often seen in hereditary hemochromatosis or secondary to multiple blood transfusions.

Cardiovascular Magnetic Resonance Findings in Iron Overload Cardiomyopathy

CMR plays a crucial role in the assessment and management of iron overload cardiomyopathy, providing characteristic findings (Fig. 27.5) that aid in the evaluation and monitoring of this condition.

1. Reduced myocardial T2* values:
   - The presence of excess myocardial iron deposition leads to a reduction in T2* relaxation time, which can be quantified using specialized CMR techniques.
   - Decreased myocardial T2* values are a hallmark feature of iron overload cardiomyopathy and can serve as a sensitive marker of cardiac iron deposition.
2. Impaired ventricular function:
   - Iron overload can compromise cardiac contractility, resulting in systolic and diastolic dysfunction, which can be evaluated using cine CMR.
   - The degree of ventricular dysfunction correlates with the severity of myocardial iron deposition.
3. Myocardial fibrosis:
   - Chronic iron deposition may lead to the development of myocardial fibrosis, which can be detected using LGE imaging.
   - The presence and extent of myocardial fibrosis can provide insights into the long-term consequences of iron overload and guide management strategies.

Quantification of myocardial T2* is particularly valuable in the early detection of cardiac iron overload, allowing for timely initiation of iron chelation therapy and monitoring of treatment response.

Native T1 mapping has a complementary use with T2* mapping for the detection of mild iron overload by increasing the sensitivity. However, it is less specific than T2* mapping for iron overload since myocardial fat and fibrosis can both influence T1 values.

Other Infiltrative Cardiomyopathies

In addition to the conditions mentioned above, CMR has also proven invaluable in the assessment of other infiltrative cardiomyopathies, such as Anderson-Fabry disease, glycogen storage diseases, and endomyocardial fibrosis.

ANDERSON-FABRY DISEASE

- CMR findings: increased myocardial native T1 values and characteristic patterns of LGE, aiding in the diagnosis and distinction from other hypertrophic cardiomyopathies.

GLYCOGEN STORAGE DISEASES

- CMR findings: evaluation of myocardial involvement in conditions like Pompe disease and Danon (LAMP2) disease, using a combination of cine, T1/T2 mapping, and LGE imaging to characterize the pattern and extent of myocardial infiltration and its impact on cardiac structure and function. Danon cardiomyopathy typically manifests with LVH and LGE in various, often extensive, patterns, but always sparing the midseptum.

ENDOMYOCARDIAL FIBROSIS

- CMR findings: assessment of the deposition of fibrous tissue within the ventricular endocardium using a combination of cine imaging, T1/T2 mapping, and LGE to characterize the extent and distribution of the infiltrative process.

The comprehensive assessment of these less common infiltrative cardiomyopathies using CMR is essential for accurate diagnosis, risk stratification, and guiding targeted therapeutic interventions.

CONCLUSIONS

CMR has revolutionized the evaluation and management of infiltrative cardiomyopathies, significantly enhancing patient outcomes through earlier diagnosis and tailored treatment strategies. By offering detailed insights into cardiac structure, function, and tissue characteristics, CMR facilitates accurate distinction among various subtypes of infiltrative cardiomyopathy. Its characteristic findings, including LGE and quantitative tissue parameters, are pivotal for guiding targeted therapies and monitoring disease progression. Ultimately, the integration of CMR into clinical practice is essential for improving patient care and advancing our understanding of infiltrative cardiomyopathies.

SUMMARY

CMR has transformed how infiltrative cardiomyopathies are assessed and managed, leading to improved patient outcomes through earlier detection and customized treatment approaches. By providing comprehensive details about cardiac structure, function, and tissue properties, CMR allows for precise distinction between the various subtypes of infiltrative cardiomyopathy. Key findings such as LGE and quantitative tissue metrics play a crucial role in directing targeted therapies and tracking disease progression. Incorporating CMR into clinical practice is vital for enhancing patient care and deepening our understanding of infiltrative cardiomyopathies.

REFERENCES

1. Dungu JN, Valencia O, Pinney JH, et al. CMR-Based differentiation of AL and ATTR cardiac amyloidosis. *JACC Cardiovasc Imaging*. 2014;7:133–142.
2. Ioannou A, Patel RK, Razvi Y, et al. Multi-imaging characterization of cardiac phenotype in different types of amyloidosis. *JACC Cardiovasc Imaging*. 2023;16:464–477.
3. Ioannou A, Porcari A, Patel RK, et al. Rare forms of cardiac amyloidosis: diagnostic clues and phenotype in apo AI and AIV amyloidosis. *Circ Cardiovasc Imaging*. 2023;16:523–535.
4. Porcari A, Masi A, Martinez-Naharro A, et al. Redefining cardiac involvement and targets of treatment in systemic immunoglobulin AL amyloidosis. *JAMA Cardiol*. 2024;9:e242555.
5. Martinez-Naharro A, Patel R, Kotecha T, et al. Cardiovascular magnetic resonance in light-chain amyloidosis to guide treatment. *Eur Heart J*. 2022;43:4722–4735.
6. Ioannou A, Patel RK, Martinez-Naharro A, et al. Tracking treatment response in cardiac light-chain amyloidosis with native T1 mapping. *JAMA Cardiol*. 2023;8:848–852.
7. Athwal PSS, Chhikara S, Ismail MF, et al. Cardiovascular magnetic resonance imaging phenotypes and long-term outcomes in patients with suspected cardiac sarcoidosis. *JAMA Cardiol*. 2022;7:1057–1066.
8. Okasha O, Kazmirczak F, Chen KA, Farzaneh–Far A, Shenoy C. Myocardial involvement in patients with histologically diagnosed cardiac sarcoidosis: a systematic review and meta–analysis of gross pathological images from autopsy or cardiac transplantation cases. *J Am Heart Assoc*. 2019;8:e011253.
9. Shenoy C, Bawaskar PH. Late gadolinium enhancement on cardiac magnetic resonance in suspected cardiac sarcoidosis. *JACC Cardiovasc Imaging*. 2023;16:358–360.
10. Mathijssen H, Bawaskar PH, Rochlani Y, et al. Prediction of ventricular arrhythmic outcomes in suspected cardiac sarcoidosis: a comparison of cardiovascular magnetic resonance phenotyping vs. societal recommendations for implantable cardioverter-defibrillator placement. *Eur Heart J*. 2025;46(36):3583–3896. https://doi.org/10.1093/eurheartj/ehaf338.

28 Cardiac Iron Loading and Cardiovascular Magnetic Resonance

AMNA ABDEL-GADIR AND MARK A. WESTWOOD

IRON OVERLOAD

Iron is an essential element for many metabolic processes including oxygen transport, mitochondrial respiration, nucleic acid replication, and signaling, but excess iron in its free form can be toxic. A healthy male human body contains approximately 35 to 45 mg of iron per kilogram of body weight, with lower amounts found in premenopausal females as a result of menstruation.[1] More than two-thirds of iron is incorporated into hemoglobin in developing erythroid precursors and mature red cells, and 10%–15% is present in myoglobin, enzymes, and cytochromes. The remaining body iron serves as storage depots in hepatocytes, in the form of ferritin, and in reticuloendothelial macrophages.[1]

Circulating iron is mainly bound to transferrin, the major iron transport protein. In healthy adults, approximately one-third of transferrin is saturated with iron, and virtually all circulating iron is bound to transferrin.[2]

Iron storage is an important component of iron hemostasis, providing a reservoir of nontoxic iron that can be used for future needs. Ferritin, the major intracellular iron storage protein, is found in all cells of the body with high concentrations in bone marrow macrophages, the spleen, and the liver.

The regulation of iron metabolism is complex, as the human body does not have an active regulatory mechanism for its excretion.[1] Control is based on a finely balanced system of iron absorption from the gastrointestinal tract and loss via sloughing of the intestinal mucosa, desquamation of skin, and menstrual blood loss. The circulating peptide hormone hepcidin plays a key role in the regulation of systemic iron homeostasis. Produced mainly by hepatocytes, hepcidin modulates serum iron levels by inhibiting iron release from duodenal enterocytes, macrophages, and hepatocytes.[1] Hepcidin reduces iron release into the plasma by binding to the iron exporter ferroportin.

Under normal physiological conditions, total body iron is approximately 3 to 5 g. In conditions of iron excess, iron exceeds the carrying capacity of transferrin and a toxic nontransferrin-bound iron (NTBI) is measurable in the plasma. Labile plasma iron, a component of NTBI, can be taken up by organs including the liver, pancreas, and heart.

CARDIAC IRON LOADING AND CONDITIONS ASSOCIATED WITH CARDIAC IRON LOADING

Cardiac iron loading can occur via two distinct mechanisms: first, primary disruption of iron regulation (genetic hemochromatosis syndromes), in which excess gastrointestinal absorption is slow and symptoms often present in middle age; and, second, via transfusional iron overload, in which the iron accumulation rate is much faster—children can develop cardiac iron accumulation within a few years of initiating regular transfusion therapy. The degree of iron loading is affected by the underlying diagnosis and the intensity and duration of transfusions. Iron accumulation from transfusion is on average 40-fold faster than from gastrointestinal iron absorption in nontransfused anemic patients. Excess iron cannot be naturally excreted in humans because of the lack of such a regulatory excretory pathway.

There are several conditions that can potentially lead to cardiac iron loading, which encompass a wide range of inherited and acquired conditions. Table 28.1 shows the most common pathology leading to iron accumulation, beta-thalassemia. This is a genetic condition with severe reduction or absent production of the beta-globin chain constituent of hemoglobin A. Excess alpha-chains result from ineffective erythropoiesis, and there is a life-threatening anemia by 2 years of age. Clinically, β-thalassemia is subdivided into transfusion-dependent thalassemia, also known as thalassemia major (TM), and nontransfusion-dependent thalassemia (NTDT). Patients with TM require treatment with regular, lifelong, repeated blood transfusions, which is compounded by a mild increase in gastrointestinal iron uptake related to hepcidin suppression.[3] TM predominantly occurs where malaria is endemic because heterozygous genetic hemoglobin mutations confer resistance. In other parts of the world, it occurs primarily through.

The detail of the hemoglobinopathy plays a role in the pattern and pathology of iron loading. In patients with NTDT, pulmonary hypertension and thrombosis play a greater clinical role and iron loading occurs at a later age.[4,5] In sickle cell disease (SCD), the defining clinical features include sickle cell crises (intermittent attacks of severe pain), pulmonary hypertension, thrombosis, and stroke.[6] Even when SCD patients are transfused to prevent cardiovascular complications, extrahepatic iron deposition is lower compared with other transfusional anemias. Manual and automated exchange transfusions result in mild degrees of iron overload, and in some cases, iron deficiency. Conversely, in Diamond-Blackfan anemia, in which the intrinsic bone marrow activity is low, patients are very prone to nonhepatic tissue iron accumulation.

PREVALENCE OF CARDIAC IRON OVERLOAD AND CARDIOMYOPATHY

The introduction of chelation therapy in the 1960s with desferrioxamine changed the natural progression of TM patients receiving regular transfusions, for whom the most common cause of death was heart failure at a very young age. Despite therapeutic developments and the availability of chelating agents, cardiac iron overload remains a major cause of morbidity and mortality, accounting for 70% of deaths. In the current millennium, data using T2* from TM patients across the world show that cardiac iron overload continues to be common, based on definitions of T2* values from cardiovascular magnetic resonance (CMR) for severe cardiac iron loading of <10 ms, and for mild to moderate cardiac iron loading of 10 to 20 ms (Table 28.2). The worldwide variability of myocardial involvement may be explained by differences in thalassemia genotypes, the availability of chelation therapies, and techniques for iron quantification guiding treatment.

The prevalence of iron-related cardiomyopathy is more difficult to measure. It can be estimated from either the prevalence of clinical heart failure or the presence of detectable left ventricular (LV) dysfunction, with the latter being higher in any given population. The prevalence of cardiomyopathy increases with age and decreases with more recent year of birth. For example, in a cohort of patients born before 1976, 37% had heart disease, defined as need for inotropic or antiarrhythmic medications, but in a survey in 2004, the number of TM patients of all ages receiving cardiac medication was only 10%. In a more recent long-term follow-up study of 24.9 years, patients with thalassemia born after 1980 had a lower risk of cardiac complications and death compared to those born before 1980.

TABLE 28.1 Iron overload syndromes. Syndromes broadly divided into two groups: inherited and acquired (also commonly referred to as secondary).

INHERITED IRON OVERLOAD SYNDROMES	ACQUIRED IRON OVERLOAD SYNDROMES
HFE-related hemochromatosis (type 1) C282Y/C282Y C282Y/H63D Other HFE mutations	**Iron-loading anemias** Thalassemias Sideroblastic anemia Aplastic anemia Pyruvate kinase deficiency
Juvenile hemochromatosis (type 2) Subtype A—Hemojuvelin mutations Subtype B—Hepcidin mutations	**Acquired anemias** Myelodysplasia Myelofibrosis Leukemia Long term dialysis
Transferrin receptor 2 hemochromatosis (type 3)	**Chronic liver disease** Hepatitis C infections NAFLD Alcoholic liver disease
Ferroportin diseases (type 4) Classical Nonclassical	**Miscellaneous** Friedreich ataxia Aceruloplasminemia Increased dietary intake

HFE, Human factors engineering; *NAFLD*, non-alcoholic liver disease.
Adapted from Siddique A., et al. Review article: the iron overload syndromes. Aliment Pharmacol Ther. 2012;35(8):876–93 and Kremastinos D.T., et al. Iron overload cardiomyopathy in clinical practice. Circulation. 2011;124(20):2253–63.

MECHANISMS OF CARDIAC IRON ENTRY AND TOXICITY

The mechanism of human cardiac iron loading is incompletely understood. In vitro and animal studies suggest that iron, in its ferrous form, enters myocytes via DMT1

TABLE 28.2 Incidence of cardiac iron overload from published data around the world.

COUNTRY	SAMPLE SIZE	SEVERE	MILD TO MODERATE	NORMAL
		T2* <10 ms	T2* 10–20 ms	T2* >20 ms
Australia[7]	30	37%	27%	37%
Brazil[8]	136	12.6%	23.4%	64%
Egypt[9]	89	25% <20 ms		75%
Greece[10]	201	7% <20 ms		90.5%
Hong Kong[11]	180	26%	24%	50%
Italy[8]	167	13% (<8 ms)	52% (8–20 ms)	35%
Italy[12]	220	30% <20 ms		66%
India	103	29% <20 ms		71%
Indonesia[13]	162	5%	10%	85%
Oman[14]	81	24%	22%	54%
Pakistan[15]	83	47%	16%	37%
Thailand	405	2.5%	2.7%	94.8%
Thailand	97	10.3%	5.2%	84.5%
Turkey[16]	28	46%	39%	14%
United Kingdom[17]	109	20%	43%	37%
United States of America[18]	141	13%	21%	66%
Worldwide survey[19]	3445	20%	22%	58%

Modified from Pennell DJ, Udelson JE, Arai AE, et al. American Heart Association committee on heart failure and transplantation of the council on clinical cardiology and council on cardiovascular radiology and imaging. Cardiovascular function and treatment in β-thalassemia major: a consensus statement from the American heart association. *Circulation*. 2013;128:281–308.

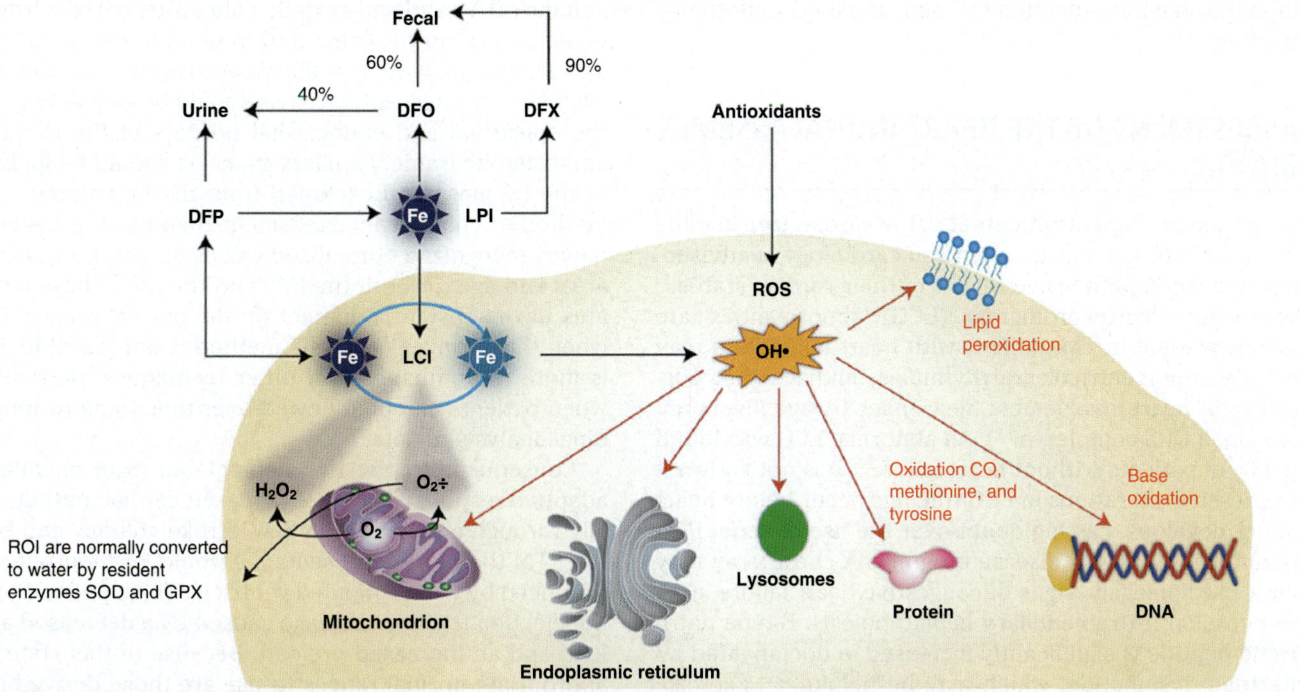

FIG. 28.1 Amelioration of free iron species (labile plasma iron *[LPI]* and labile cell iron *[LCI]*) by iron chelators and antioxidants. LPI penetrates through the cell membrane with a consequent accumulation of LCI. Both LPI and LCI react with reactive oxygen intermediate *(ROI)* producing noxious reactive oxygen species *(ROS)*, for example, *OH'* radicals, which are highly reactive and oxidize DNA, proteins, and lipid components of the cell. Deferiprone *(DFP)* chelates LCI alone or in combination with LPI by deferoxamine *(DFO)*. Deferasirox *(DFX)* mainly removes LPI. (From Rachmilewitz EA, Giardina PJ. How I treat thalassemia. *Blood*. 2011;118:3479–3488.)

and L-type and T-type calcium channels.[20–23] The addition of amlodipine, an L-type calcium channel blocker, to standard chelation therapy has been shown to improve cardiac iron in small-sample pediatric and adult patient studies, but further work is required in this domain.[24–26]

Accumulation of myocardial iron eventually leads to increased levels of intracellular free iron. The toxicity of free iron is mediated via several mechanisms (Fig. 28.1)[27,28]: (1) membrane damage caused by lipid peroxidation; (2) mitochondrial damage and perturbation of the respiratory enzyme chain[29,30]; (3) altered electrical function, including ryanodine release channel interference[31,32]; (4) cardiac fibrosis, which was reported as prominent in early autopsy studies; and (5) changes in gene expression.[33] Iron that is safely stored in ferritin or hemosiderin is nontoxic, yielding hearts with low T2* and normal function. However, high iron stores predispose patients to the development of cardiac dysfunction in the future. The result is that the natural history and clinical course in untreated patients is one of a long asymptomatic phase of progressive myocardial iron accumulation with sudden onset of either malignant arrhythmias or acutely impaired myocardial function in early adulthood. There is significant mortality once symptomatic,[34,35] and 5-year survival for patients presenting with heart failure is only 48%.[36] One factor behind this is that although evidence suggests that intensive iron chelation therapy can completely restore cardiac function in most patients with asymptomatic cardiac dysfunction and even in some with clinical heart failure,[37–39] there is a risk of relapse caused by a lag between the clearance of cardiac iron and improvements in systolic function. Even in asymptomatic patients, treatment of severe cardiac siderosis by aggressive chelation therapy is associated with improvements in ventricular function.[40] Improved life expectancy for TM patients in the United Kingdom has resulted from the increasing availability of T2* CMR and earlier escalation of therapy. Even with modern-day chelation regimens, it is important to avoid New York Heart Association stage IV heart failure in thalassemia as in-hospital mortality remains in excess of 50%.

Of significant clinical interest is that cardiac iron loading is commonly associated with complications including hypothyroidism, diabetes, hypoadrenalism, growth hormone deficiency, and hypoparathyroidism. This suggests a common or similar iron uptake mechanism. In untreated cardiac iron accumulation, historical series also showed more cardiac complications, such as pericarditis and myocarditis, which occurred in addition to heart failure and arrhythmias.[34,41] Chelation seems to have altered this, with myocarditis and pericarditis now being unusual. Chelation has also led to a significant reduction in the historical occurrence of dense replacement fibrosis of myocytes, even in those who die from heart failure, although occasional small patches of fibrosis may be present.[34,41–44] In the modern era of chelation therapy, dilated cardiomyopathy (with restrictive features) and arrhythmia (predominantly atrial fibrillation) persist. Ventricular arrhythmias are more common in severe cardiac iron loading. Iron deposition throughout the myocardium in TM patients is nonuniform, being preferentially deposited in the subepicardium, but no systematic variation occurs between myocardial regions such that iron deposition in the interventricular septum is highly representative of total cardiac iron. There are other cardiac changes such as decreased left atrial (LA) function,[45] impaired right ventricular (RV) function,[46] impaired diastolic function,[47–49] and impaired endothelial function.[50–52]

ASSESSMENT OF THE HEART IN THALASSEMIA MAJOR

Annual assessment of patients at risk of cardiac iron loading by cardiology specialists in red cell cardiology is advised, allowing a comprehensive review of their cardiac status.[53] New-onset electrocardiogram (ECG) abnormalities are usually evident in TM patients with heart failure and may include supraventricular arrhythmias, findings that suggest right heart involvement, new-onset T-wave inversion, and small QRS complexes.[54,55] An abnormal ECG was found in 46% of patients without heart failure.[56] It is not known if progressive alterations in ECG tracings occur before heart failure develops, casting doubt over the use of serial ECG monitoring to assess disease progress. A chest x-ray may show cardiomegaly, signs of congestive heart failure, and, on occasion, extramedullary hematopoiesis. B-type natriuretic peptide is significantly increased in documented LV diastolic dysfunction, which may be helpful.[57,58] Exercise stress testing may be able to unmask subclinical LV dysfunction in TM, but results are influenced by many other factors, and it seems to have questionable value.

Before the development of CMR-derived T2*, cardiac function was the key marker of disease progression despite a number of factors limiting its use.[59] The limitations and reproducibility of echocardiography around operator experience and acoustic windows are well documented[17] but should be tempered against the widespread, safe, economical, and routinely available nature of this test. Before the advent of three-dimensional techniques, the need to make geometric assumptions for the quantification of volumes and mass, which often break down in abnormal remodeled ventricles, led to significant interobserver variability.[60] Despite this, impaired resting LV function based on echocardiography correlated with increased cardiac mortality over 12 years.[61] Echocardiography provides less accurate quantification than CMR, and accuracy decreases with worsening LV function as geometric assumptions become an ever-greater approximation. Echocardiography is the preferred second-line technique after CMR. It is important that echo is done in experienced centers used to scanning large numbers of TM patients.[62,63]

CMR is noninvasive, reliable, and free of ionizing radiation. Although increasingly seen as a mainstream cardiology investigation, the widespread use of CMR is limited by its cost and claustrophobia, although the latter is less of an issue with new-generation, wide-bore scanners. The limitation with implanted cardiac devices is progressively being overcome.[64] For the assessment of LV and RV function, the lack of geometric assumptions optimizes accuracy and reproducibility. Indeed, CMR is widely accepted as the gold standard for all biventricular measurements and indices. Routine use of steady-state free precession-based acquisitions for cine imaging with end-expiratory breath-hold are acquired in the four-chamber and two-chamber long-axis views along with contiguous short-axis cines from the atrioventricular ring to the apex. The optimal end-diastolic volume (EDV) and end-systolic volume are derived from LV volume/time curves generated from all frames of all cines and should include systolic valve tracking to adjust for systolic valve descent. LV mass should be calculated using the epicardial and endocardial borders of the LV in the end-diastolic frame. Papillary muscles should be included in the LV mass and excluded from the LV volumes. This method of volumetric assessment then has the benefit of having recognized normalized values for sex, body surface area, and age for both the LV[65] and the RV.[66] These covariates have substantial impact on the normal ranges. Even when this stringent analysis method is not possible, CMR is more reproducible than other techniques, particularly when patients can be followed over time to allow longitudinal analysis of data.[67,68]

Consequent to the low hemoglobin from anemia, an adaptive response leads to increased cardiac output, usually through an increase in EDV, stroke volume, and heart rate. TM therefore represents a chronic, high-output state produced by volume-loaded ventricles (high preload), with the ejection fraction increase caused by a decreased afterload and an increased preload. Because of this state, the appropriate normal ranges to use are those derived from nonanemic TM patients, because for both the LV[69] and RV[70] there are differences compared with standard normal cohorts. Pediatric normal ranges are also available.[71,72] The hyperdynamic circulation also leads to an increased LV mass. The same pattern is true for the RV indices, but the differences are not as marked.[70] Using these adjusted "normal for TM" ranges may enhance diagnostic accuracy for detection of cardiomyopathy.

Whereas CMR offers several other techniques such as late gadolinium enhancement for the detection of myocardial fibrosis and myocarditis, and myocardial perfusion imaging for coronary artery disease, these are uncommon findings in this group of patients and routine cardiac assessment with these techniques is not advocated.[73] Although possible, diastolic function assessed using CMR is time consuming and more operator dependent and in clinical practice is more readily assessed using echocardiography.[74,75]

CARDIOVASCULAR MAGNETIC RESONANCE OF CARDIAC IRON USING T2*

In simple terms, radiofrequency (RF) pulses cause spinning protons to be deflected from their equilibrium state. Immediately after this RF pulse, protons begin to return to equilibrium by two separate processes: T1 recovery and T2 relaxation. Magnetic field inhomogeneity accelerates these processes whereby the protons return to equilibrium. As myocardial iron stores increase in the heart, ferritin breakdown increases into particulate hemosiderin, which is a form of ferrihydrite (hydrated iron oxide). The hemosiderin to ferritin ratio is significantly higher in cardiac siderosis than in normal hearts.[76] It is this particulate intracellular iron that markedly increases magnetic field inhomogeneity and thereby accelerates both T1 and T2 relaxation. Because the influence on these parameters as a result of particulate iron is much greater than normal

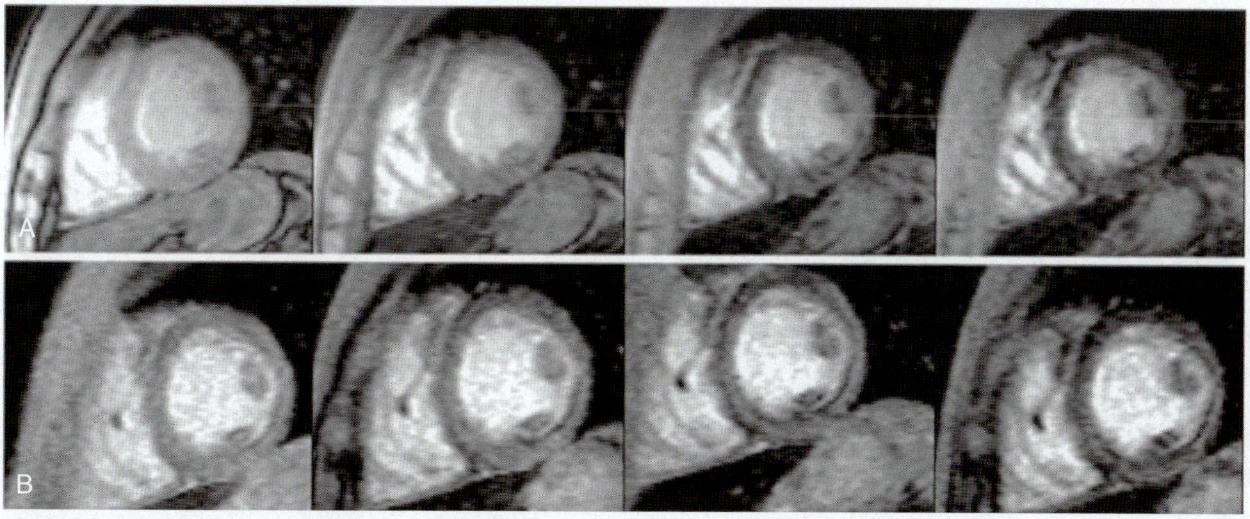

FIG. 28.2 T2* multiecho images. (A) A single breath-hold was used and (B) multiple breath-holds were used to acquire images of the myocardium with increasing echo time (TE). Note the better registration of the position of the diaphragm with the breath-hold technique. The signal intensity of the myocardium falls as the TE increases according to the myocardial T2*. (From Westwood M, Anderson LJ, Firmin DN, et al. A single breath-hold multiecho T2* cardiovascular magnetic resonance technique for diagnosis of myocardial iron overload. *J Magn Reson Imaging*. 2003;18:33–39.)

field inhomogeneity, changes in these parameters become a biomarker for myocardial iron deposition. Magnetic resonance (MR) relaxometry is the use of specific MR sequences that repeatedly sample image data every few milliseconds, from which relaxation or recovery curves can be derived. These techniques do not require contrast media.

Given that increased field inhomogeneity is affected by increased iron deposition, it follows that the sequence most sensitive to this parameter should be chosen. Gradient echo sequences are much more susceptible to field inhomogeneity than spin-echo sequences and are particularly affected by particles of hemosiderin iron. Gradient echo sequences measure T2*, whereas spin-echo sequences measure T1 and T2.

In addition, a T2* multiecho gradient echo can repeatedly sample image data at different echo times (TEs) in a single 10- to 15-second breath-hold from which T2* can be derived, and such sequences are T1 independent (Fig. 28.2). Bright-blood and dark-blood sequences are validated and widely used clinically. Bright-blood images are acquired immediately after the R wave to reduce artifact generated by blood flow and myocardial wall motion. Dark-blood sequences use a double inversion recovery pulse to null the signal from the blood.[43,69,77,78]

T2* and T2 are related by the formula $1/T2^* = 1/T2 + 1/T2'$, where T2′ represents magnetic inhomogeneity. There is no particular advantage to a multislice method, which has been reported,[79] because iron concentration in the septum is representative of mean total iron concentration.[80–82]

The method of calculating T2* values from raw datasets may be prone to error if care is not taken. Susceptibility artifacts at tissue borders, such as the lung myocardial interface and near the great cardiac veins in the anterior and posterior interventricular grooves, need to be minimized. For this reason, for routine analysis of T2*, a full-thickness region of interest (ROI) in the interventricular septum should be chosen to measure mean signal intensity for each echo time, thereby avoiding the above areas. Care is needed to ensure that the blood-pool signal and other artifacts are excluded from the ROI, which can be easier with a black-blood image. Signal intensity is plotted against TE, and a monoexponential decay curve is fitted to derive T2*, which represents the time taken for the signal intensity to decay to 37% of its initial value (Fig. 28.3). The signal intensity (SI) at each echo time is given by the following equation (where SI_0 represents the signal intensity at time zero and TE represents the echo time):

$$\text{Signal intensity (SI)} = SI_0.e^{-TE/T2*} \qquad \text{Eq. 28.1}$$

In severe myocardial iron loading, the myocardial signal obtained from the images with longer echo times becomes predominantly background noise, motion, and blood-pool artifacts. Because the true decay at these low signal values is masked by these effects, this will affect T2* calculations and may lead to spuriously high values. The simplest way to deal with these points at long TEs, which are in effect just noise, is to delete them from the analysis and curve fitting, which is known as truncation (Figs. 28.4 and 28.5).[83] To ensure the most robust analysis, dedicated and validated analysis software is preferable.

T2* is highly robust and has a high interobserver and intraobserver reproducibility, as well as high reproducibility between different studies performed a few hours or days apart and across different sites and scanner platforms.[84–86] Critically, this means that T2* measurements at 1.5 T are independent of the scanner, site, or country where they were obtained. Although it is also possible to derive T2* using a 3 T scanner, clinical experience is much more limited in TM, and there are potentially more artifacts.[87,88] The current recommendation is to perform clinical T2* MR at 1.5 T.[89] Finally, in very simple terms, increasing cardiac iron will lead to a decrease in the measured cardiac T2* value.

Although T2* has become the established technique for the assessment of myocardial iron loading, previous work used the ratio of signal intensity between the myocardium and skeletal muscle on a T2-weighted spin-echo image. Because T2-weighted images are less susceptible to field

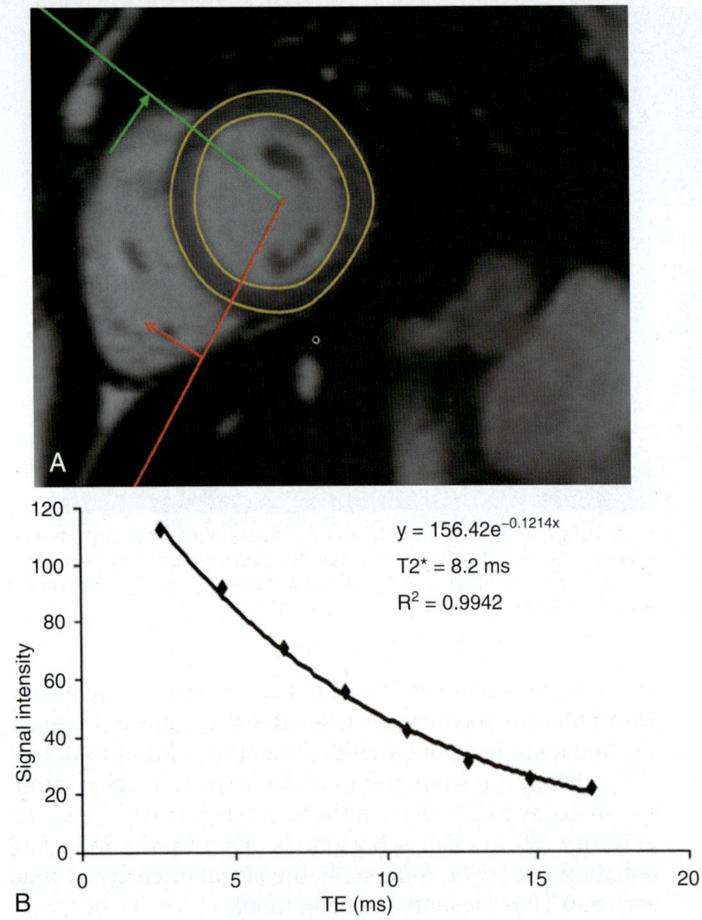

FIG. 28.3 (A) Image analysis software is used to measure the signal intensity of the interventricular septum. The endocardial and epicardial contours are drawn, and the full thickness septal region of interest is shown as the arc between the *red* and *green* radial lines, which is a region of interest that is not perturbed by susceptibility effects from deoxygenated hemoglobin in the anterior and inferior cardiac veins, nor the lung interface. (B) Decay curve and T2* calculation. The plot of septal signal intensity against echo time *(TE)* can be fitted with an exponential curve, yielding the decay constant T2*. (A, From He T, Zhang J, Carpenter JP, et al. Automated truncation method for myocardial T2* measurement in thalassemia. *J Magn Reson Imaging*. 2013;37:479–483. B, From He T, Gatehouse PD, Kirk P, et al. Black-blood T2* technique for myocardial iron measurement in thalassemia. *J Magn Reson Imaging*. 2007;25:1205–1209.)

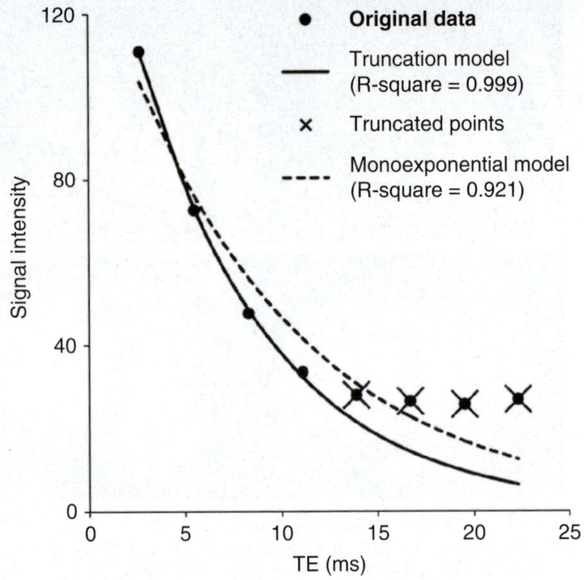

FIG. 28.4 Truncation curve analysis. When myocardial T2* is very short, the myocardial signal may decay to near the level of noise by the third or fourth echo time *(TE)*. The later points in the graph simply measure noise, but this has the unwanted effect of not allowing the exponential line-fit to drop to zero, which artificially increases the calculated T2* value, making it incorrect. This can easily be determined because the curve does not fit the first time points properly. Software tools are therefore used to truncate the signal values at long TEs, so that the exponential curve fits the first points correctly. This gives a significantly lower T2* value, which is more accurate, and in this example increases the *R-square* of fit from 0.921 to 0.999. (From He T, Zhang J, Carpenter JP, et al. Automated truncation method for myocardial T2* measurement in thalassemia. *J Magn Reson Imaging*. 2013;37:479–483.)

inhomogeneity (indeed, part of the refocusing of the RF pulse in a spin-echo image is designed to mitigate effects attributed to field inhomogeneity), small changes in imaging parameters had a significant effect on these results, and reproducibility was poor. It is, however, possible to construct multiecho spin-echo sequences from which T2 can be derived in a similar way to T2*. Although T2 does shorten with increasing myocardial iron load, T2 assessment has not been validated to the same extent as T2*, and is not routinely used.

CARDIOVASCULAR MAGNETIC RESONANCE OF CARDIAC IRON USING T1 MAPPING

As with T2*, T1 sequences can be used to produce a map of T1 values for the heart. T1 is an intrinsic magnetic property that represents the longitudinal relaxation time after excitation of hydrogen atoms. At selected magnetic field strengths, each tissue has a characteristic range of values, and deviation from these values implies disease. T1 values, measured in milliseconds, are increased with the expansion of the extracellular compartment by fibrosis, edema, and amyloid, and reduced with iron accumulation, lipid accumulation, and hemorrhage.[90–94] These changes may be detectable in early disease, and prognostic in some diseases.[89,95,96]

T1 measurements were first introduced in the 1970s using the Look-Locker sequence.[97] This original sequence required multiple breath-holds to obtain a series of images along the T1 recovery curve following an initial inversion pulse. This method, however, had recognized limitations, including significant in-plane and through-plane motion artifacts, leading to inaccurate T1 values. Several improved approaches have since been described using: 1) inversion recovery–based methods including modified Look-Locker inversion (MOLLI) recovery and shortened MOLLI (ShMOLLI), and 2) saturation recovery–based methods such as saturation recovery single-shot acquisition (Fig. 28.6).[98–101]

Improvements in the original method to make the MOLLI sequence have overcome some of the challenges associated with cardiac and respiratory motion, enabling the acquisition of T1 measurements over a single breath-hold to generate a color map. The MOLLI 5(3)3 variant is most commonly used for T1 mapping, whereby images are acquired over 11 heartbeats in diastole. A 180-degree inversion pulse over five heartbeats is followed by a rest period of three heartbeats, with a further inversion pulse

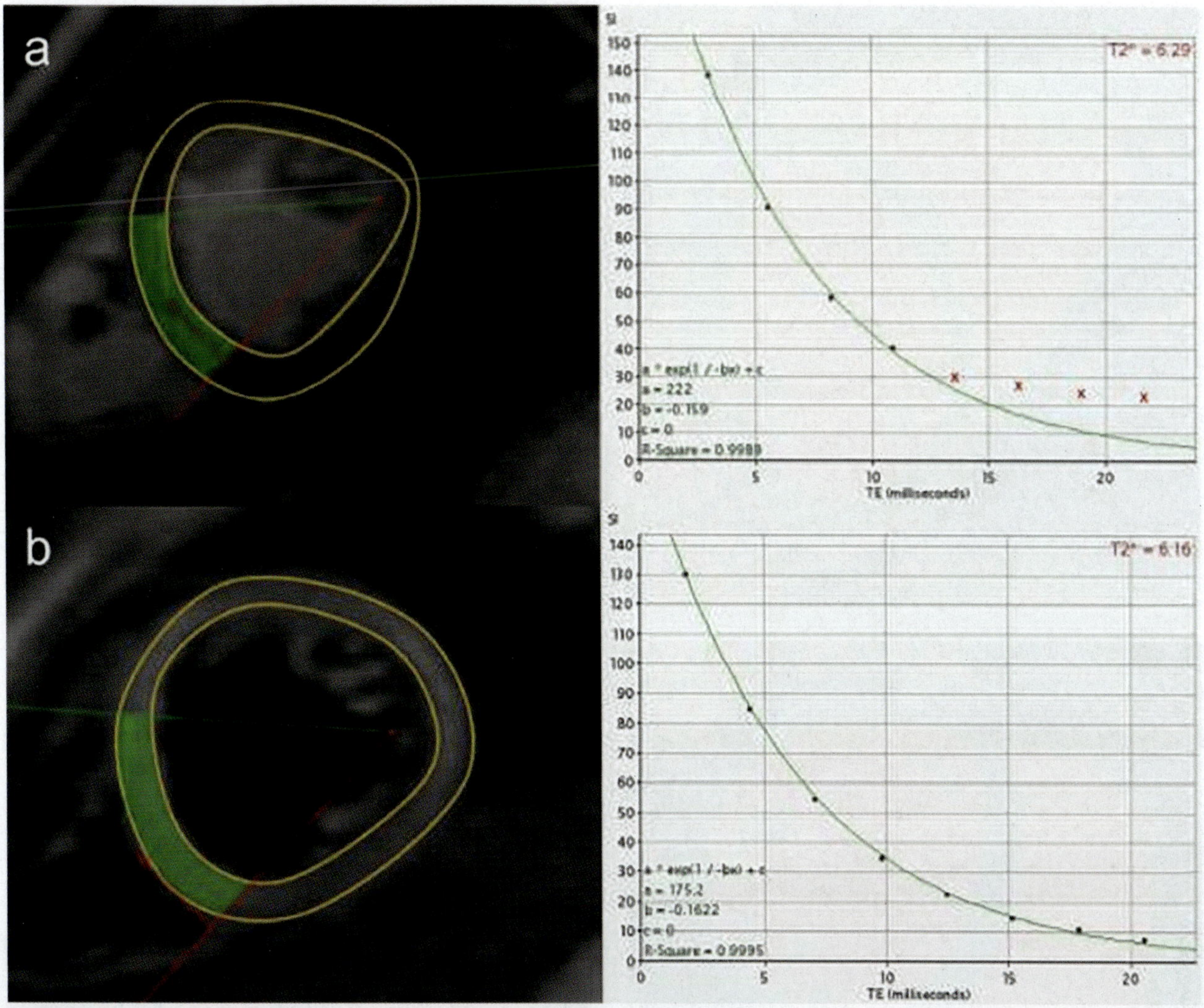

FIG. 28.5 (A) Cardiovascular magnetic resonance bright-blood T2* demonstrating the region of interest in the interventricular septum in a patient with severe myocardial iron loading secondary to transfusion-dependent thalassemia. The last four points are background noise and removed to improve the curve fit using the truncating method ($R^2=0.9989$, T2* 6.29 ms). (B) The same patient's dark-blood T2* sequence ($R^2=0.9995$, T2* 6.16 ms). *TE*, echo time. (Adapted from Menacho et al. T2* mapping techniques: iron ovelroad assessment and other potential clnical application. Magn Reson Imaging Clin N Am. 2019 August;27(3):439–451.)

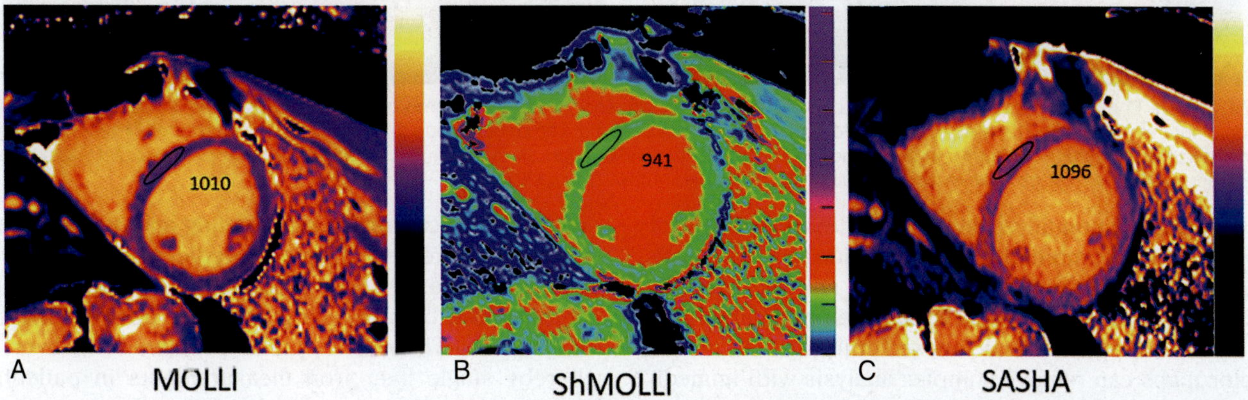

FIG. 28.6 Examples of native T1 maps from a healthy volunteer. Three different T1 sequences are shown, each demonstrating regions of interest and their values. (A) Modified Look-Locker inversion (*MOLLI*). (B) Shortened MOLLI (*ShMOLLI*). (C) Saturation recovery single-shot acquisition (*SASHA*). Note the difference in T1 values with each sequence and the difference in look-up tables on the right of each image. (Adapted from Abdel-Gadir A., et al. Myocardial T1 mapping: where are we now and where are we going? Res Rep Clin Cardiol. 2014;5:339–347.)

and three image acquisitions. The ShMOLLI technique allows further shortening of the acquisition time, requires a short breath-hold, and has been shown to have very little heart rate dependence.[100]

To date, T1 in the detection of iron has been promising at both 1.5 and 3 T, and has been shown to correlate with cardiac iron in vitro.[102,103] T1 mapping for iron has increasingly shown excellent reproducibility and correlation with

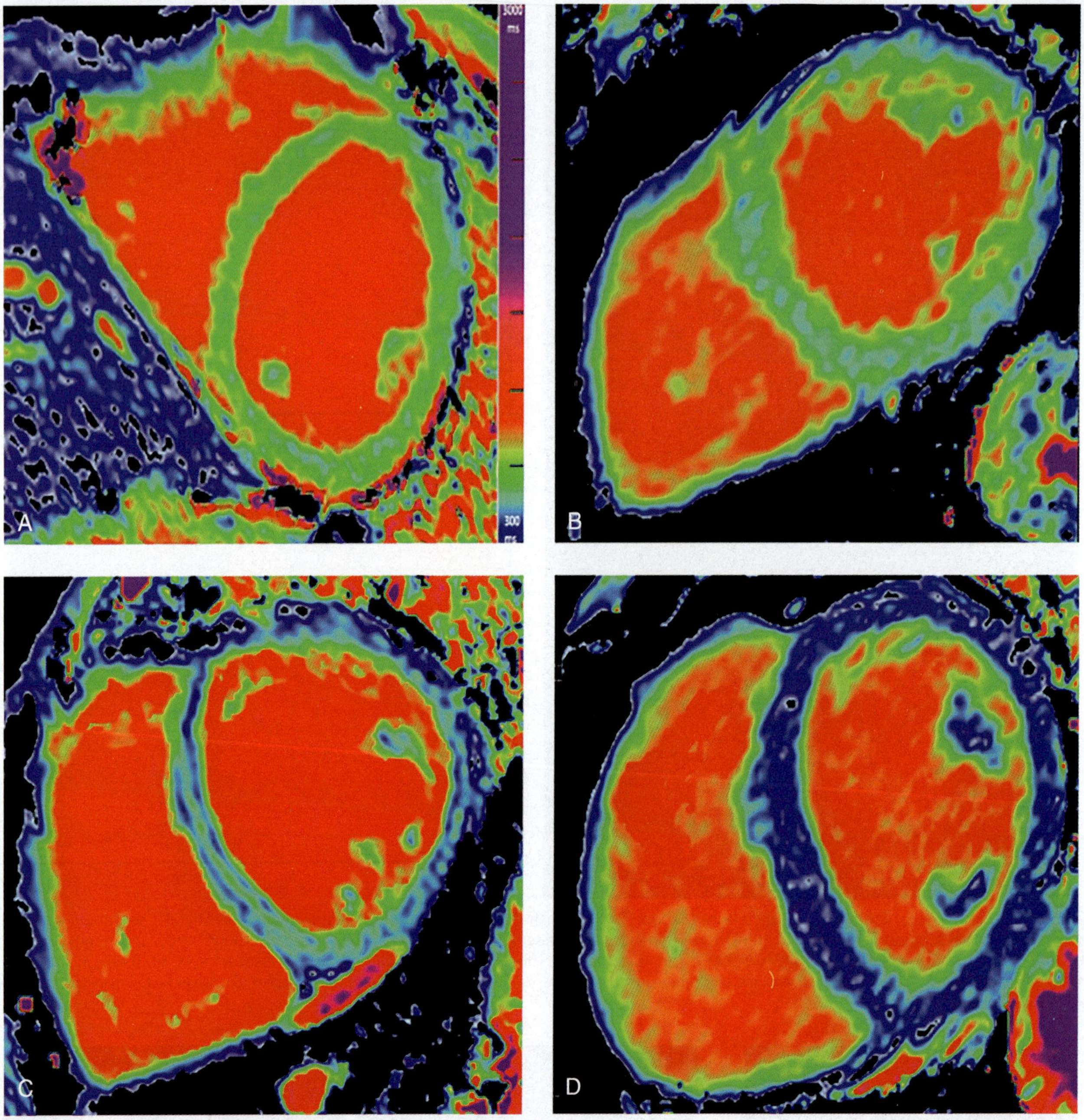

FIG. 28.7 Native T1 mapping (shortened modified Look-Locker inversion sequence) in myocardial iron overload demonstrating (A) healthy volunteer (with a region of interest drawn) and (B) mild, (C) moderate, and (D) severe iron overload. The color look-up table means that with shorter T1 times, the presence of iron allows the myocardium to appear blue. (Adapted from Sado DM, Maestrini V, Piechnik SK, et al., Noncontrast myocardial T1 mapping using cardiovascular magnetic resonance for iron overload. *J Magn Reson Imaging*. 2015 Jun;41(6):1505-11. doi: 10.1002/jmri.24727.)

T2* and cardiac complications.[94,104–108] The assessment of T2* and T1, in combination, may provide a more sensitive measure of early cardiac siderosis, and the addition of both values in clinical reports has been recommended, with T1 values reported as decreased or normal.[109] The use of color maps can remove complex analysis with immediate identification of iron loading (Fig. 28.7).

T2*, PREDICTION OF HEART FAILURE, AND PROGNOSIS

Serum ferritin measurements are simple to undertake and are widely available. Although trends in ferritin are useful for monitoring the direction of body iron loading, they do not fully predict cardiac iron loading and, critically, a low ferritin measurement does not predict the future absence of heart failure.[61,110,111] In particular, a single ferritin measurement can be misleading and does not reflect cardiac iron burden. There is a similar problem with liver iron, whereby single liver iron measurements in patients on long-term iron chelation may be misleading because they do not correlate with cardiac iron levels.[37] Over time, poor liver iron control may increase the risk of cardiac iron loading.[111,112] Similarly, noncompliance with chelation therapy leading to elevated serum ferritin levels (and thereby elevated liver iron) is a major predictive factor for cardiac iron loading in patients.[113] Therefore, high liver iron levels per se may not be the best way to view the cardiac risk associated with liver iron loading, and although control of

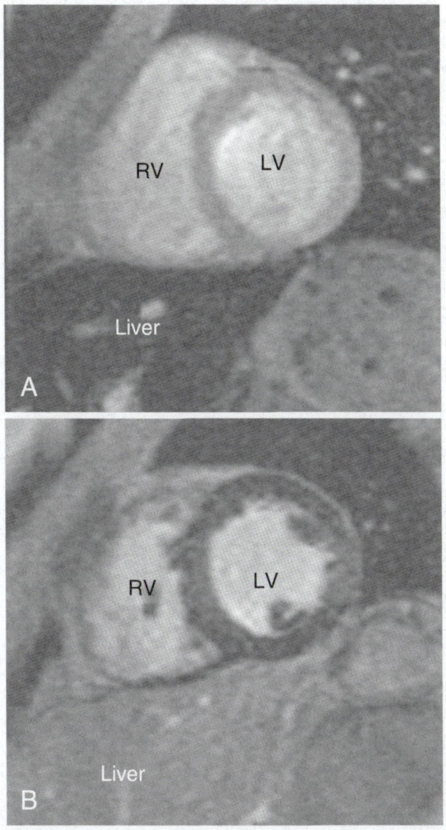

FIG. 28.8 Disparate heart and liver loading. (A) A dark liver signal but normal myocardium, indicating iron loading in the liver but not the heart. (B) The reverse is shown, with normal liver signal but dark myocardium indicating cardiac iron loading in the absence of liver iron loading. The latter patient is at risk from heart failure, but in previous decades before T2* cardiovascular magnetic resonance (CMR), it was the former patient who would have received intensified iron chelation treatment. This disparate iron loading between organs helps explain the high mortality burden from heart disease that occurred before T2* CMR was available to directly identify patients at risk of heart failure. *LV*, Left ventricle; *RV*, right ventricle. (From Anderson LJ, Holden S, Davis B, et al. Cardiovascular T2-star [T2*] magnetic resonance for the early diagnosis of myocardial iron overload. *Eur Heart J.* 2001;22:2171–2179.)

liver iron over time is likely to be important in the prevention of cardiac iron accumulation, low liver iron does not guarantee absence of cardiac iron loading.[112] Early on in the development of myocardial T2*, differential organ iron loading became apparent and disparate loading between the liver and heart was revealed as the reason for the limitations of these biomarkers (Fig. 28.8).

An increased risk of clinical heart failure has been demonstrated for patients with a falling left ventricular ejection fraction (LVEF) or absolute values below the lower limit of the normal range.[61] Limitations of the use of LVEF are that it requires meticulous attention to detail and that, more importantly, changes in LVEF are a late event compared with falling T2* levels <20 ms, and with low to moderate levels of cardiac iron, the change in LVEF is modest if at all present. Although absolute LVEF measurements vary between centers, volumetric analysis by CMR is superior to echocardiography.[67,68] There is a tipping point at which a marked deterioration in LVEF will occur with only a slight additional increase in cardiac iron loading. Because it is free iron that is toxic (T2* measures storage iron in the form of hemosiderin), the LVEF will improve rapidly with intensive chelation treatment. However, the storage iron loading of the heart will have only decreased marginally in this time period. Prolonged periods of chelation are therefore required to remove all the stored iron in the heart. Although most focus has been on deteriorating LV function, myocardial iron deposition is also strongly associated with RV dysfunction.[114,115]

Cardiac T2* has been directly calibrated to human cardiac iron concentration (Fig. 28.9).[81,82,116] The practical and commonly used lower limit of normal is 20 ms, although it is not appropriate to consider cardiac iron as a dichotomous variable. Historical data suggest that the upper limit of normal for cardiac iron is approximately 0.5 mg/g dry weight.[117] The probability of a reduced ejection fraction (EF) increases as cardiac iron increases,[59] and a cardiac T2* <10 ms predicts heart failure.[118] In one study, 98% of patients who developed heart failure had a myocardial T2* <10 ms and patients with a cardiac T2* <6 ms had a 50% likelihood of developing heart failure within 12 months (Fig. 28.10).[118] A normal cardiac T2* has a very high negative predictive value for exclusion of heart failure for at least 12 months. T2* is the most significant predictor of the development of heart failure compared with liver iron or serum ferritin.[118]

The high basal cardiac output in TM masks subtle but significant alterations in systolic function and a significant deterioration in LVEF occurs at a late stage of the iron overload; hence, myocardial T2* is the most appropriate biomarker to use to assess risk. In a cohort of 652 TM patients followed up for 1 year in whom 80 episodes of heart failure occurred, the mean LVEF assessed by CMR within a median time of 158 days from the heart failure event was 43.1%.[118] In nearly all patients, the myocardial T2* was <10 ms and the mean T2* was 6.7 ms. Furthermore, the risk of developing heart failure within 1 year without intensifying chelation therapy rises rapidly as the myocardial T2* progressively falls below 10 ms. For severe myocardial iron loading, a myocardial T2* value <6 ms conferred a relative risk of 270 compared with T2* values >10 ms for heart failure within 1 year. No additional prognostic information was provided from other biomarkers of cardiac iron (serum ferritin or liver iron). Receiver operating characteristic curve analysis shows that T2* is significantly superior in predicting heart failure compared with serum ferritin and liver iron, and should therefore always be used.[118] From this, the currently accepted T2* "risk ranges" for cardiac complications are T2* <10 ms representing high risk, 10 to 20 ms intermediate risk, and >20 ms low risk.

Although myocardial T2* assesses the risk of heart failure, the key next step is to change therapy to reduce that risk. Once a low T2* has been identified, it is necessary to intervene with intensive chelation treatment to lower cardiac iron quickly. This greatly reduces the risk of developing heart failure, which is important because once heart failure is established, it can precipitate an irreversible spiral of progressive deterioration in cardiac function, leading to death. Randomized controlled trials indicate that combining deferiprone with deferoxamine has the highest cardiac iron clearance rate and improves ventricular function. Intervention with intensified chelation appears to be very effective, as evidenced by a 71% reduction in cardiac

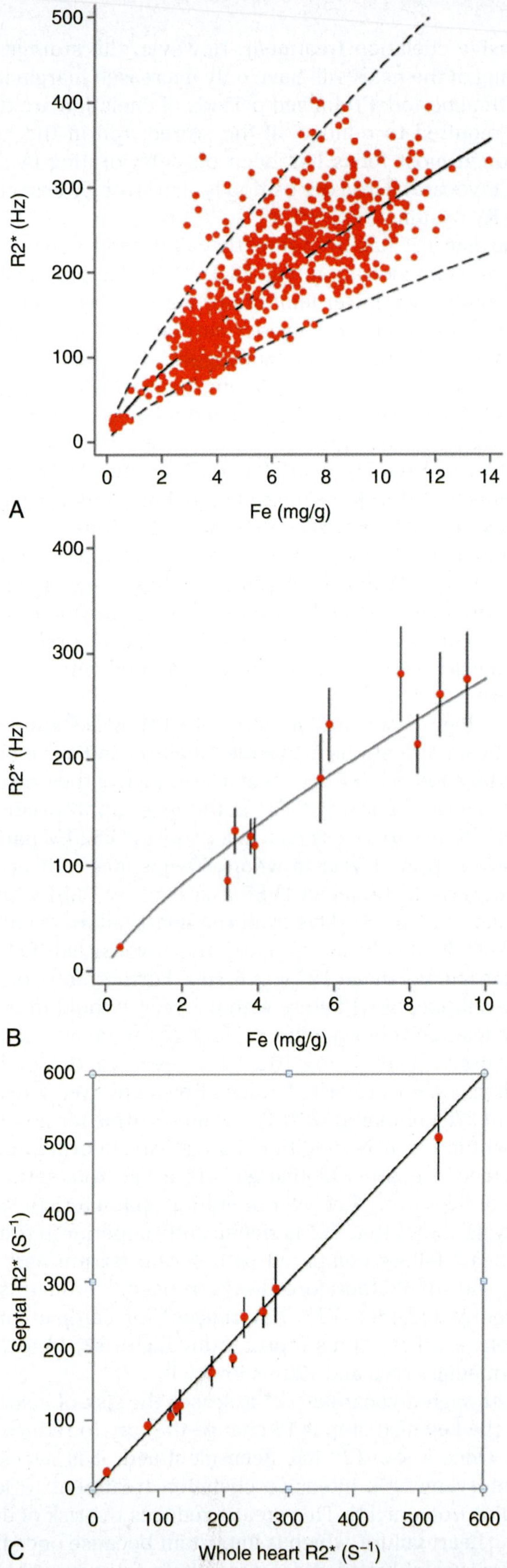

FIG. 28.9 Calibration of T2* to human iron. (A) The calibration of human R2* (equal to the reciprocal of T2*) for >500 myocardial samples against iron concentration measured by emission spectroscopy. The relationship is $[Fe] = 45 \bullet T2^{*-1.22}$. (B) A similar graph but using the mean whole-heart iron R2* (N=11) vs. iron concentration. (C) The relationship between whole-heart R2* and the septal R2* for each heart, confirming that using a septal region of interest alone was highly representative of average whole-heart iron concentration. (From Carpenter JP, He T, Kirk P, et al. On T2* magnetic resonance and cardiac iron. *Circulation*. 2011;123:1519–1528.)

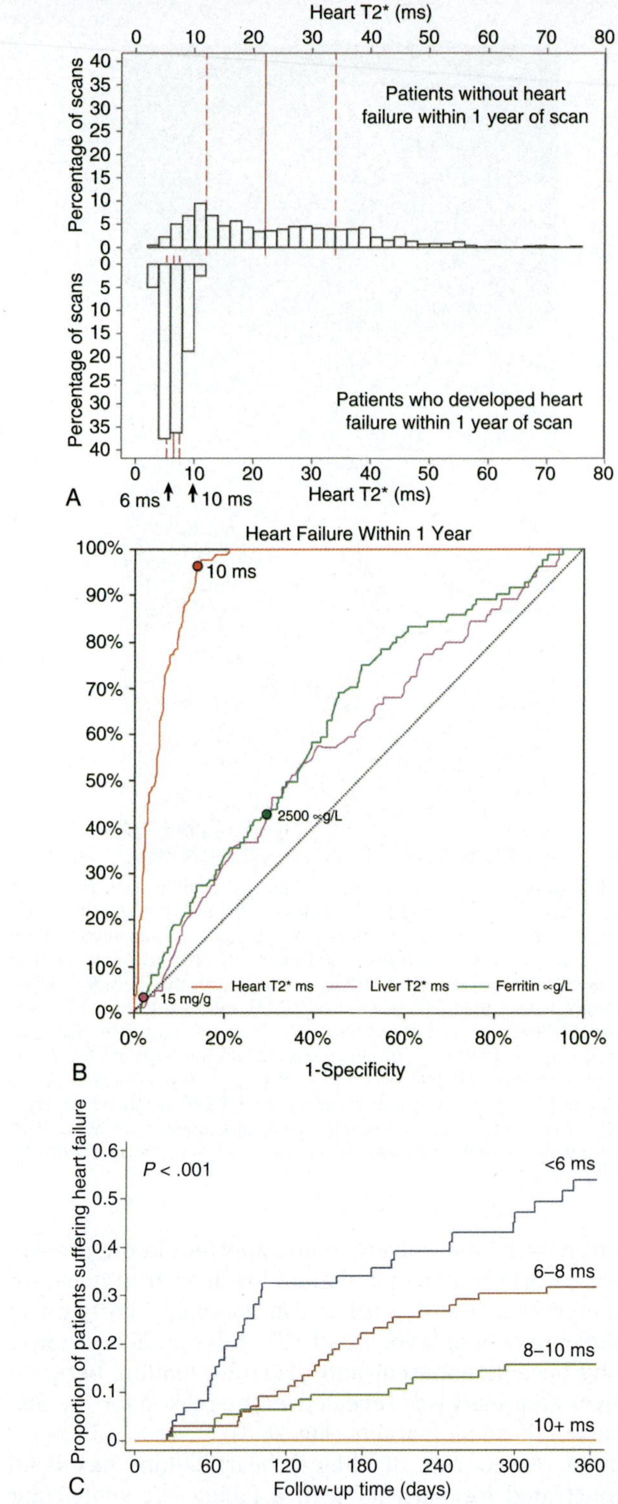

FIG. 28.10 T2* predicts heart failure and arrhythmia. (A) The top portion of the graph shows the distribution of myocardial T2* in patients who had a baseline cardiovascular magnetic resonance (CMR) scan and did not develop heart failure within 1 year. Note that the mean T2* was ~22 ms and there was a broad range of values. The lower portion of the graph shows the distribution of patients who did develop heart failure within 1 year of the baseline T2* CMR scan. Note the strong leftward shift of values, with a mean of ~7 ms. Nearly all patients had a T2* value <10 ms, and therefore this threshold is used clinically to indicate "high risk" of cardiac events. (B) Receiver operating curve analysis of the relative power of cardiac T2*, serum ferritin, and liver iron to predict future heart failure. Cardiac T2* greatly outperformed the conventional measures. Note the relative strength of performance of conventional thresholds of serum ferritin of 2500 µg/L, liver iron of 15 mg/g dry weight, and cardiac T2* of 10 ms. (C) Kaplan-Meier curves of the incremental likelihood of developing heart failure according to the cardiac T2* value. Patients with a T2* <6 ms had an approximately 50% likelihood of developing heart failure over 1 year. (From Kirk P, Roughton M, Porter JB, et al. Cardiac T2* magnetic resonance for prediction of cardiac complications in thalassemia major. *Circulation*. 2009;120:1961–1968.)

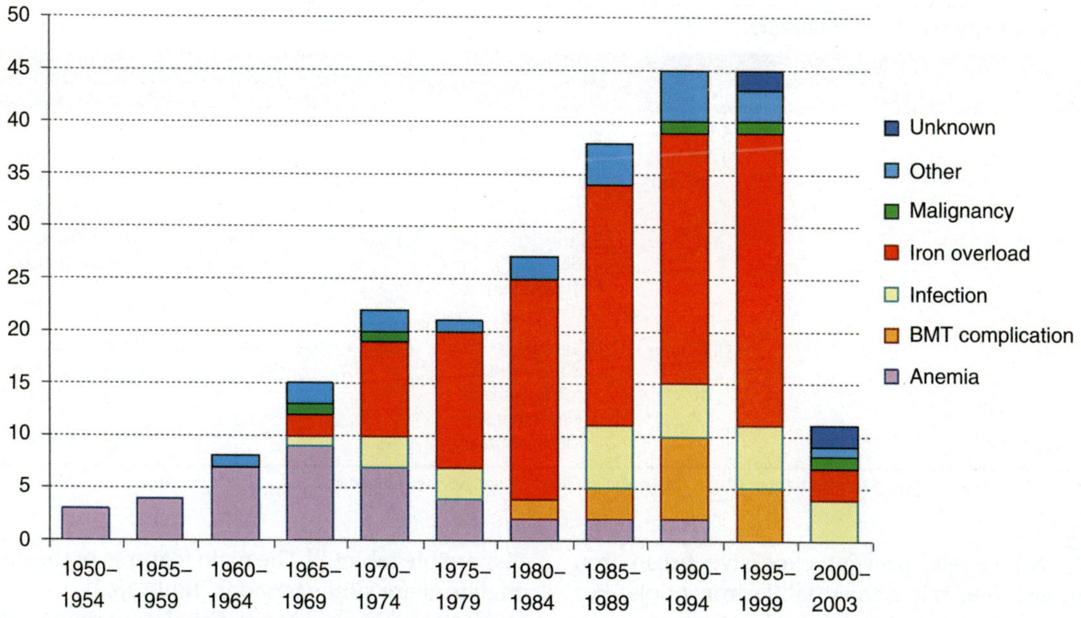

FIG. 28.11 UK mortality graph in thalassemia major (TM). The vertical axis shows the number of deaths in the United Kingdom in TM patients for each 5-year period from 1950 to after 2000. The portion of each column in *red* is the deaths from cardiac iron overload. After the introduction of cardiac T2* cardiovascular magnetic resonance in 1999, the mortality rate from cardiac iron overload fell by 71%. *BMT,* bone marrow transplantation. (From Modell B, Khan M, Darlison M, et al. Improved survival of thalassemia major in the UK and relation to T2* cardiovascular magnetic resonance. *J Cardiovasc Magn Reson*. 2008;10:42.)

deaths in the 5 years after the introduction of myocardial T2* in the United Kingdom in 1999 (Fig. 28.11).[119]

HEART FAILURE CAUSED BY CARDIAC IRON LOADING

Because the historic death rate from heart failure was 50% within 1 year, the current emphasis is to intervene early to prevent heart failure.[34,35] In 52 patients with mean LVEF 36%, there was 48% survival after 5 years with no change in iron chelator or use of cardiac medications.[36] Data to guide optimal management of iron chelator treatment are sparse, as there are few trials in acute heart failure. One follow-up study showed a mortality of only 1 in 7 patients in acute heart failure treated with continuous uninterrupted intravenous deferoxamine for 12 months.[37,120] The only randomized controlled trial in acute heart failure in TM was terminated early after only 23% recruitment.[120] It is therefore very underpowered and the results are difficult to interpret. It showed that the EF after 1 year on combination treatment of deferoxamine with deferiprone (EF + 8.4%) was higher (but not significantly higher) than the standard of care of monotherapy with deferoxamine (EF + 4.1%). It is critical to remember that even with a preserved LVEF, without escalation in therapy, the prospective risk for developing heart failure in 1 year is 47% if cardiac T2* is <6 ms, with a relative risk of 270 compared with patients with a T2* >10 ms (only 1 out of 80 episodes of heart failure in a trial over 7 years occurred in patients with a myocardial T2* >10 ms).[118] Because the relative risk of overt heart failure is so great and coupled with a poor prognosis,[38] many centers treat patients with a myocardial T2* <6 ms and those with overt heart failure with the same intensified chelation regimens. Many symptoms that are common in anemia are also typically present in heart failure, which makes the diagnosis of heart failure difficult on clinical grounds, which further cements the rationale for this approach.[121] Traditional signs of heart failure may appear late and may further delay treatment.[40,121] Sepsis may precipitate sudden, acute heart failure, possibly by disrupting iron stores, and is the second leading cause of death in TM patients with severe cardiac iron loading.[122,123]

Patients with severe cardiac iron loading (T2* less than 10 ms) require intensified chelation therapy.[62] Patients with mild to moderate cardiac iron loading (T2* between 10 and 20 ms) can be managed more conservatively by modifying chelator dose, improving patient compliance, or using alternative chelating agents. Any reduction in cardiac function with the presence of any myocardial iron loading warrants escalation in chelation therapy, even in asymptomatic cases.[124] Patients with myocardial iron loading in whom ventricular function measurements show a trend of deterioration (even though the absolute values may remain in the normal range) require intensification of chelation. If this fails to stabilize the situation, then a change in iron chelator regimen is required. In general, assessment of myocardial T2* every 2 years is sufficient in the absence of cardiac iron. In the presence of significant iron loading, more frequent assessment is required (every year with midiron loading, and every 6 months in patients with severe cardiac iron). More frequent assessment is also required if there is an impaired LVEF.

TREATMENT OF THALASSEMIA MAJOR AND IRON CHELATORS

Iron chelating agents have two functions: first, to tightly bind iron and prevent it from acting as a catalyst for redox reactions, and second, to allow iron to be transported and then excreted from the body. Hence, iron chelators should

TABLE 28.3 Main features of iron chelators.

DRUG	FDA-APPROVED	EU-APPROVED	ROUTE	TYPICAL CHRONIC DOSING	FREQUENCY	EXCRETION	MAIN ADVERSE EFFECTS
Deferoxamine	Yes	Yes	SC (IV in heart failure)	20–50 mg/kg/day	8–14 h infusion for 5–7 days/week	60% urine 40% feces	Sensorineural deafness, visual disturbance, skeletal abnormality, growth retardation
Deferiprone	Yes	Yes	Oral	25 mg/kg × 3 per day, maximum 100 mg/kg per day	×3/day	75%–90% urine	Agranulocytosis, GI disturbance, arthropathy
Deferasirox	Yes	Yes	Oral	Dosing depends on the specific formula used. Please consult local formulary.	usually ×1/day	~90% feces	Rash, GI disturbance, rise in creatinine

EU, European Union; *FDA*, US Food and Drug Administration; *GI*, gastrointestinal; *IV*, intravenous; *SC*, subcutaneous.

reduce tissue iron levels, prevent excessive organ iron accumulation, and neutralize toxic labile iron pools. For a chelating agent, diffusion through biologic membranes, and hence absorption from the gastrointestinal tract, and cellular penetration are governed not only by molecular size but also by lipophilicity and net molecular charge.[125] There are three commercially available iron chelators, each with very different properties.

The oldest iron chelator is deferoxamine, which was the first approved for use in the 1960s. It is not absorbed effectively by the gastrointestinal tract. This property, coupled with a short plasma half-life,[126] necessitates parenteral administration (usually subcutaneous) as a prolonged infusion or a continuous infusion for severe iron loading. Compliance is markedly adversely affected by the need for long parenteral administration. Other side effects include local infusion site reactions (induration, erythema, swelling, and itching), ophthalmologic and audiologic complications, renal toxicity, and, in high doses, even adult respiratory distress syndrome.[127]

The next chelator to be marketed was deferiprone. This is rapidly absorbed from the upper gastrointestinal tract and is administered orally three times daily because of its short half-life.[128] The iron chelator complex is renally excreted.[128] Minor side effects include gastrointestinal symptoms (nausea, vomiting, and abdominal pain) and a transient increase of liver enzymes. Agranulocytosis and neutropenia are more serious side effects that can necessitate either temporary or permanent cessation of therapy.

The most recent chelating agent, deferasirox, obtained FDA approval in 2005. Deferasirox is rapidly absorbed from the gastrointestinal tract and, because of its longer half-life, once daily administration is possible.[129] There are two preparations of deferasirox available: the original dispersible tablet formulation and the new formulation approved in 2015. The main route of excretion is fecal. Minor side effects include transient gastrointestinal disturbances (nausea, vomiting, diarrhea, and abdominal pain), diffuse maculopapular skin rash, and increased alanine aminotransferase and serum creatinine.[113] More severe side effects include Fanconi syndrome and auditory and ocular toxicities. The newer film-coated preparation has fewer gastrointestinal side effects compared to the original dispersible tablet.[127] The main features of the common iron chelators are summarized in Table 28.3.

All three commonly used chelators remove cardiac iron if given in adequate doses, and there is good patient compliance. However, each medication has advantages and disadvantages, and optimal therapy must be tailored to each patient. There are many reviews on this subject.[127,130,131] The following recommendations are specific to patients with detectable, asymptomatic cardiac iron overload. There are several randomized trials of cardiac iron treatment using chelating agents. The introduction of deferoxamine in the 1970s had a profound effect on reducing mortality in TM,[132] and deferiprone, which followed, has been associated with reduced cardiac mortality in many countries including the United Kingdom, Italy, Cyprus, and Taiwan.[119,133–135] The drastic improvement in cardiac mortality is probably multifactorial, including early identification of patients at cardiac risk from cardiac T2*, improved compliance with chelation therapy, and the use of specific agents alone or in combination.[119]

From a cardiac perspective, deferoxamine is only able to slowly remove cardiac iron, with rates varying from 1.1% to 2.2% per month, up to nearly 5% for constant 24/7 intravenous infusions.[37,136] Long-term infusions are inconvenient and uncomfortable, leading to reduced patient compliance. Although deferoxamine is the conventional chelating agent for TM, a change in therapy is probably warranted if compliance is poor. Deferiprone monotherapy offers superior cardiac protection[137–139] and improves survival compared with deferoxamine monotherapy.[140] In the only prospective randomized study comparing deferoxamine and deferiprone monotherapy, deferiprone reduced cardiac iron at nearly double the rate of deferoxamine.[136] Deferiprone is therefore suitable for patients with cardiac siderosis, either as monotherapy or in combination with deferoxamine.[141] It is noteworthy that the use of either deferoxamine or deferasirox alone in mild to moderate cardiac iron loading does not improve LVEF,[136,142–144] which is in contrast to deferiprone, which does improve LVEF.[133,136,137,139] Deferasirox monotherapy can be used in patients with cardiac iron loading and preserved systolic function with clearance rates similar to deferoxamine. Currently, there are few data on the use of deferasirox in patients with severe cardiac iron loading or a reduced LVEF.

There is evidence of a synergistic effect between deferiprone and deferoxamine,[30,145] and these agents have been successfully combined to improve cardiac and hepatic iron clearance.[146,147] Combination therapy can rapidly improve myocardial iron loading with an associated improvement in LVEF and has been shown to lead to a near doubling in the rate of increase of myocardial T2* when compared with deferoxamine monotherapy.[141,148–151] This accelerated cardiac iron clearance is associated with improved outcomes in severe cardiac iron loading.[134] Combination therapy is used for moderate to severe cardiac iron loading or where there is LV impairment. The beneficial effects of combination treatment have also been shown in mild to moderate cardiac iron loading with impaired RV function.[152] Although it is possible to combine deferiprone and deferasirox, there are currently limited data on the utility of this combination.[153,154] Combination deferoxamine and deferasirox has also been tested.[155] American Heart Association guidelines on the heart in TM, the use of T2*, and the treatment of cardiac iron loading have been published,[156] and expert opinion[11,53] and numerous national guidelines are in accord with these.[7,14,16,18,62]

EMERGING CHALLENGES AND TREATMENTS

As we now enter an age of much improved survival, and patients with TM enter their sixth decade of life and greater, new challenges to cardiac health are emerging. Diabetes caused by iron infiltration of the pancreas is a common finding in TM and is a risk factor for coronary artery disease. There is endothelial dysfunction even in the absence of iron loading. The prevalence of coronary artery disease in this population, which will occur as they age, is unknown. Additionally, the risk of arrhythmias such as atrial fibrillation attributed to altered hemodynamics in the left and right atrium is unknown, but may also be higher than that in the general population. T1 mapping is able to assess myocardial iron and characterize diffuse fibrosis, which does still occur with severe iron loading. However, these two processes have the opposite effect on T1 values, which may lead to challenges in interpretation of T1 values. The prognostic value of iron loading as assessed by T1 mapping is yet to be determined. Although recent trials on the use of calcium channel blockers to block cardiac iron uptake in TM are of great interest, much more work is needed to understand the prevention of heart failure. Finally, the ultimate goal would be to eradicate the defect in hemoglobin synthesis using advances in gene therapy such as *CRISPR-Cas9* gene editing, which has so far been demonstrated in stem cells from patients with sickle cell anemia and thalassemia. Clinical trials are ongoing, with recent authorization led by the United Kingdom's Medicines and Healthcare products Regulatory Agency.

REFERENCES

1. Andrews NC. Disorders of iron metabolism. *N Engl J Med.* 1999;341(26):1986–1995.
2. Chifman J, Laubenbacher R, Torti SV. A systems biology approach to iron metabolism. *Adv Exp Med Biol.* 2014;844:201–225.
3. Origa R, et al. Liver iron concentrations and urinary hepcidin in beta-thalassemia. *Haematologica.* 2007;92(5):583–588.
4. Aessopos A, et al. Heart disease in thalassemia intermedia. *Hemoglobin.* 2009;33(suppl 1):S170–S176.
5. Musallam KM, et al. Iron overload in non-transfusion-dependent thalassemia: a clinical perspective. *Blood Rev.* 2012;26(suppl 1):S16–S19.
6. Voskaridou E, Christoulas D, Terpos E. Sickle-cell disease and the heart: review of the current literature. *Br J Haematol.* 2012;157(6):664–673.
7. Angelucci E, et al. Italian society of hematology practice guidelines for the management of iron overload in thalassemia major and related disorders. *Haematologica.* 2008;93(5):741–752.
8. Chapchap EC, et al. Cardiac iron overload evaluation in thalassaemic patients using T2* magnetic resonance imaging following chelation therapy: a multicentre cross-sectional study. *Hematol Transfus Cell Ther.* 2023;45(1):7–15.
9. El Beshlawy A, El Tagui M, Hamdy M, et al. Low prevalence of cardiac siderosis in heavily iron loaded Egyptian thalassemia major patients. *Ann Hematol.* 2014;93:375–379.
10. Aessopos A, Fragodimitri C, Karabatsos F, et al. Cardiac magnetic resonance imaging R2* assessments and analysis of historical parameters in patients with transfusion-dependent thalassemia. *Haematologica.* 2007;92:131–132.
11. Rachmilewitz EA, Giardina PJ. How I treat thalassemia. *Blood.* 2011;118(13):3479–3488.
12. Positano V, Pepe A, Santarelli MF, et al. Multislice multiecho T2* cardiac magnetic resonance for the detection of heterogeneous myocardial iron distribution in thalassaemia patients. *NMR Biomed.* 2009;22:707–715.
13. Wahidiyat PA, Liauw F, Sekarsari D, Putriasih SA, Berdoukas V, Pennell DJ. Evaluation of cardiac and hepatic iron overload in thalassemia major patients with T2* magnetic resonance imaging. *Hematology.* 2017;22:501–507.
14. Ho PJ, et al. Australian guidelines for the assessment of iron overload and iron chelation in transfusion-dependent thalassaemia major, sickle cell disease and other congenital anaemias. *Intern Med J.* 2011;41(7):516–524.
15. Alvi N, Tipoo FA, Imran A, et al. Burden of cardiac siderosis in a thalassemia-major endemic population: a preliminary report from Pakistan. *J Pediatr Hematol Oncol.* 2016;38:378–383.
16. UKTS. Standards for the clinical care of children and adults living with thalassaemia in the UK. 2023.
17. Bellenger NG, et al. Comparison of left ventricular ejection fraction and volumes in heart failure by echocardiography, radionuclide ventriculography and cardiovascular magnetic resonance; are they interchangeable? *Eur Heart J.* 2000;21(16):1387–1396.
18. Sayani F, Warner M, Wu J, Wong-Rieger D, Humphreys K, Odame I. *Guidelines for the Clinical Care of Patients With Thalassaemia in Canada.* Thalassemia Foundation of Canada; 2009. https://www.thalassemia.ca/wp-content/uploads/Thalassemia-Guidelines_LR.pdf.
19. Carpenter JP, Roughton M, Pennell DJ. Myocardial Iron in Thalassemia (MINT) Investigators. International survey of T2* cardiovascular magnetic resonance in β-thalassemia major. *Haematologica.* 2013;98:1368–1374.
20. Ludwiczek S, et al. Ca2+ channel blockers reverse iron overload by a new mechanism via divalent metal transporter-1. *Nat Med.* 2007;13(4):448–454.
21. Oudit GY, et al. Role of L-type Ca2+ channels in iron transport and iron-overload cardiomyopathy. *J Mol Med (Berl).* 2006;84(5):349–364.
22. Kumfu S, et al. T-type calcium channel as a portal of iron uptake into cardiomyocytes of beta-thalassemic mice. *Eur J Haematol.* 2011;86(2):156–166.
23. Zhabyeyev P, et al. Amlodipine rescues advanced iron overload cardiomyopathy in hemojuvelin knockout murine model: Clinical implications. *Front Cardiovasc Med.* 2023;10:1129349.
24. Fernandes JL, et al. Amlodipine reduces cardiac iron overload in patients with thalassemia major: a pilot trial. *Am J Med.* 2013;126(9):834–837.
25. Khaled A, et al. A randomized controlled trial evaluating the effects of amlodipine on myocardial iron deposition in pediatric patients with thalassemia major. *Drug Des Dev Ther.* 2019;13:2427–2436.
26. Gupta V, et al. Comparison of the effects of calcium channel blockers plus iron chelation therapy versus chelation therapy only on iron overload in children and young adults with transfusion-dependent thalassemia: a randomized double-blind placebo-controlled trial. *Pediatr Blood Cancer.* 2022;69(6):e29564.
27. Murphy CJ, Oudit GY. Iron-overload cardiomyopathy: pathophysiology, diagnosis, and treatment. *J Card Fail.* 2010;16(11):888–900.
28. Hershko C. Pathogenesis and management of iron toxicity in thalassemia. *Ann N Y Acad Sci.* 2010;1202:1–9.
29. Link G, Pinson A, Hershko C. Ability of the orally effective iron chelators dimethyl- and diethyl-hydroxypyrid-4-one and of deferoxamine to restore sarcolemmal thiolic enzyme activity in iron-loaded heart cells. *Blood.* 1994;83(9):2692–2697.
30. Link G, et al. Exploring the "iron shuttle" hypothesis in chelation therapy: effects of combined deferoxamine and deferiprone treatment in hypertransfused rats with labeled iron stores and in iron-loaded rat heart cells in culture. *J Lab Clin Med.* 2001;138(2):130–138.
31. Wood JC, et al. Physiology and pathophysiology of iron cardiomyopathy in thalassemia. *Ann N Y Acad Sci.* 2005;1054:386–395.
32. Kim E, Giri SN, Pessah IN. Iron(II) is a modulator of ryanodine-sensitive calcium channels of cardiac muscle sarcoplasmic reticulum. *Toxicol Appl Pharmacol.* 1995;130(1):57–66.
33. Eaton JW, Qian M. Molecular bases of cellular iron toxicity. *Free Radic Biol Med.* 2002;32(9):833–840.
34. Engle MA, Erlandson M, Smith CH. Late cardiac complications of chronic, severe, refractory anemia with hemochromatosis. *Circulation.* 1964;30:698–705.
35. Engle MA. Cardiac involvement in Cooley's anemia. *Ann N Y Acad Sci.* 1964;119:694–702.
36. Kremastinos DT, et al. Heart failure in beta thalassemia: a 5-year follow-up study. *Am J Med.* 2001;111(5):349–354.
37. Anderson LJ, et al. Myocardial iron clearance during reversal of siderotic cardiomyopathy with intravenous desferrioxamine: a prospective study using T2* cardiovascular magnetic resonance. *Br J Haematol.* 2004;127(3):348–355.
38. Davis BA, Porter JB. Long-term outcome of continuous 24-hour deferoxamine infusion via indwelling intravenous catheters in high-risk beta-thalassemia. *Blood.* 2000;95(4):1229–1236.
39. Miskin H, et al. Reversal of cardiac complications in thalassemia major by long-term intermittent daily intensive iron chelation. *Eur J Haematol.* 2003;70(6):398–403.
40. Tanner MA, et al. Combined chelation therapy in thalassemia major for the treatment of severe myocardial siderosis with left ventricular dysfunction. *J Cardiovasc Magn Reson.* 2008;10(1):12.
41. Buja LM, Roberts WC. Iron in the heart. Etiology and clinical significance. *Am J Med.* 1971;51(2):209–221.
42. Kirk P, et al. Post-mortem study of the association between cardiac iron and fibrosis in transfusion dependent anaemia. *J Cardiovasc Magn Reson.* 2017;19(1):36.
43. Pepe A, et al. Myocardial scarring by delayed enhancement cardiovascular magnetic resonance in thalassaemia major. *Heart.* 2009;95(20):1688–1693.

44. Kirk P, et al. Low prevalence of fibrosis in thalassemia major assessed by late gadolinium enhancement cardiovascular magnetic resonance. *J Cardiovasc Magn Reson.* 2011;13(1):8.
45. Trikas A, et al. Exercise capacity in patients with beta-thalassemia major: relation to left ventricular and atrial size and function. *Am Heart J.* 1998;136(6):988–990.
46. Hamdy AM, Zein El-Abdin MY, Abdel-Hafez MA. Right ventricular function in patients with beta thalassemia: relation to serum ferritin level. *Echocardiography.* 2007;24(8):795–801.
47. Vogel M, et al. Tissue Doppler echocardiography in patients with thalassaemia detects early myocardial dysfunction related to myocardial iron overload. *Eur Heart J.* 2003;24(1):113–119.
48. Marci M, et al. Detection of early cardiac dysfunction in patients with Beta thalassemia by tissue Doppler echocardiography. *Echocardiography.* 2011;28(2):175–180.
49. Westwood MA, et al. Left ventricular diastolic function compared with T2* cardiovascular magnetic resonance for early detection of myocardial iron overload in thalassemia major. *J Magn Reson Imaging.* 2005;22(2):229–233.
50. Cheung YF, Chan GC, Ha SY. Arterial stiffness and endothelial function in patients with beta-thalassemia major. *Circulation.* 2002;106(20):2561–2566.
51. Cheung YF, Chan GC, Ha SY. Effect of deferasirox (ICL670) on arterial function in patients with beta-thalassaemia major. *Br J Haematol.* 2008;141(5):728–733.
52. Kukongviriyapan V, et al. Endothelial dysfunction and oxidant status in pediatric patients with hemoglobin E-beta thalassemia. *Pediatr Cardiol.* 2008;29(1):130–135.
53. Shah FT, et al. Guidelines for the monitoring and management of iron overload in patients with haemoglobinopathies and rare anaemias. *Br J Haematol.* 2022;196(2):336–350.
54. Mancuso L, et al. Electrocardiographic abnormalities in thalassemia patients with heart failure. *Cardiovasc Hematol Disord: Drug Targets.* 2009;9(1):29–35.
55. Russo V, et al. Electrocardiographic Presentation, Cardiac arrhythmias, and their management in beta-thalassemia major patients. *Ann Noninvasive Electrocardiol.* 2016;21(4):335–342.
56. Ramazzotti A, et al. Standardized T2* map of a normal human heart to correct T2* segmental artefacts; myocardial iron overload and fibrosis in thalassemia intermedia versus thalassemia major patients and electrocardiogram changes in thalassemia major patients. *Hemoglobin.* 2008;32(1-2):97–107.
57. Kremastinos DT, et al. Predictive value of B-type natriuretic peptides in detecting latent left ventricular diastolic dysfunction in beta-thalassemia major. *Am Heart J.* 2010;159(1):68–74.
58. Delaporta P, et al. Correlation of NT-proBNP levels and cardiac iron concentration in patients with transfusion-dependent thalassemia major. *Blood Cells Mol Dis.* 2013;50(1):20–24.
59. Anderson LJ, et al. Cardiovascular T2-star (T2*) magnetic resonance for the early diagnosis of myocardial iron overload. *Eur Heart J.* 2001;22(23):2171–2179.
60. Giakoumis A, et al. Comparison of echocardiographic (US) volumetry with cardiac magnetic resonance (CMR) imaging in transfusion dependent thalassemia major (TM). *Cardiovasc Ultrasound.* 2007;5:24.
61. Hahalis G, et al. Cardiac mortality in beta-thalassemia major: resting but not dobutamine stress echocardiography predicts mortality among initially cardiac disease-free patients in a prospective 12-year study. *Eur J Heart Fail.* 2009;11(12):1178–1181.
62. Farmakis D, et al. 2021 Thalassaemia international federation guidelines for the management of transfusion-dependent thalassemia. *HemaSphere.* 2022;6(8):e732.
63. Nagueh SF, et al. Recommendations for the evaluation of left ventricular diastolic function by echocardiography. *Eur J Echocardiogr.* 2009;10(2):165–193.
64. Bhuva A, et al. Joint British society consensus recommendations for magnetic resonance imaging for patients with cardiac implantable electronic devices. *Heart.* 2024;110(4):e3.
65. Maceira AM, et al. Normalized left ventricular systolic and diastolic function by steady state free precession cardiovascular magnetic resonance. *J Cardiovasc Magn Reson.* 2006;8(3):417–426.
66. Maceira AM, et al. Reference right ventricular systolic and diastolic function normalized to age, gender and body surface area from steady-state free precession cardiovascular magnetic resonance. *Eur Heart J.* 2006;27(23):2879–2888.
67. Grothues F, et al. Comparison of interstudy reproducibility of cardiovascular magnetic resonance with two-dimensional echocardiography in normal subjects and in patients with heart failure or left ventricular hypertrophy. *Am J Cardiol.* 2002;90(1):29–34.
68. Grothues F, et al. Interstudy reproducibility of right ventricular volumes, function, and mass with cardiovascular magnetic resonance. *Am Heart J.* 2004;147(2):218–223.
69. Westwood MA, et al. Normalized left ventricular volumes and function in thalassemia major patients with normal myocardial iron. *J Magn Reson Imaging.* 2007;25(6):1147–1151.
70. Carpenter JP, et al. Right ventricular volumes and function in thalassemia major patients in the absence of myocardial iron overload. *J Cardiovasc Magn Reson.* 2010;12(1):24.
71. Fernandes JL, et al. Left and right ventricular function and volume assessment in young thalassemia major patients with no related myocardial iron overload. *Ann Hematol.* 2012;91(12):1839–1844.
72. Meloni A, et al. Comparison of biventricular dimensions and function between pediatric sickle-cell disease and thalassemia major patients without cardiac iron. *Am J Hematol.* 2013;88(3):213–218.
73. Roghi A, et al. Unexpected myocarditis in thalassaemia major patient screened for iron load cardiomyopathy. *BMJ Case Rep.* 2009;2009.
74. Plein S, et al. Training and accreditation in cardiovascular magnetic resonance in Europe: a position statement of the working group on cardiovascular magnetic resonance of the European Society of Cardiology. *Eur Heart J.* 2011;32(7):793–798.
75. Kramer CM, et al. Standardized cardiovascular magnetic resonance imaging (CMR) protocols, society for cardiovascular magnetic resonance: board of trustees task force on standardized protocols. *J Cardiovasc Magn Reson.* 2008;10(1):35.
76. Fitchett DH, et al. Cardiac involvement in secondary haemochromatosis: a catheter biopsy study and analysis of myocardium. *Cardiovasc Res.* 1980;14(12):719–724.
77. He T, et al. Black-blood T2* technique for myocardial iron measurement in thalassemia. *J Magn Reson Imaging.* 2007;25(6):1205–1209.
78. Smith GC, et al. Value of black blood T2* cardiovascular magnetic resonance. *J Cardiovasc Magn Reson.* 2011;13(1):21.
79. Pepe A, et al. Multislice multiecho T2* cardiovascular magnetic resonance for detection of the heterogeneous distribution of myocardial iron overload. *J Magn Reson Imaging.* 2006;23(5):662–668.
80. Ghugre NR, et al. Improved R2* measurements in myocardial iron overload. *J Magn Reson Imaging.* 2006;23(1):9–16.
81. Ghugre NR, et al. MRI detects myocardial iron in the human heart. *Magn Reson Med.* 2006;56(3):681–686.
82. Carpenter JP, et al. On T2* magnetic resonance and cardiac iron. *Circulation.* 2011;123(14):1519–1528.
83. He T, et al. Automated truncation method for myocardial T2* measurement in thalassemia. *J Magn Reson Imaging.* 2013;37(2):479–483.
84. Westwood MA, et al. Interscanner reproducibility of cardiovascular magnetic resonance T2* measurements of tissue iron in thalassemia. *J Magn Reson Imaging.* 2003;18(5):616–620.
85. Westwood MA, et al. Intercentre reproducibility of magnetic resonance T2* measurements of myocardial iron in thalassaemia. *Int J Cardiovasc Imaging.* 2005;21(5):531–538.
86. Kirk P, et al. International reproducibility of single breathhold T2* MR for cardiac and liver iron assessment among five thalassemia centers. *J Magn Reson Imaging.* 2010;32(2):315–319.
87. Storey P, et al. R2* imaging of transfusional iron burden at 3T and comparison with 1.5T. *J Magn Reson Imaging.* 2007;25(3):540–547.
88. Meloni A, et al. Feasibility, reproducibility, and reliability for the T*2 iron evaluation at 3 T in comparison with 1.5 T. *Magn Reson Med.* 2012;68(2):543–551.
89. Puntmann VO, et al. Native T1 and ECV of noninfarcted myocardium and outcome in patients with coronary artery disease. *J Am Coll Cardiol.* 2018;71(7):766–778.
90. Bull S, et al. Human non-contrast T1 values and correlation with histology in diffuse fibrosis. *Heart.* 2013;99(13):932–937.
91. Ferreira VM, et al. Non-contrast T1-mapping detects acute myocardial edema with high diagnostic accuracy: a comparison to T2-weighted cardiovascular magnetic resonance. *J Cardiovasc Magn Reson.* 2012;14(1):42.
92. Karamitsos TD, et al. Noncontrast T1 mapping for the diagnosis of cardiac amyloidosis. *JACC, Cardiovasc Imaging.* 2013;6(4):488–497.
93. Sado DM, et al. Identification and assessment of Anderson-Fabry disease by cardiovascular magnetic resonance noncontrast myocardial T1 mapping. *Circ Cardiovasc Imaging.* 2013;6(3):392–398.
94. Sado DM, et al. Noncontrast myocardial T1 mapping using cardiovascular magnetic resonance for iron overload. *J Magn Reson Imaging.* 2015;41(6):1505–1511.
95. Banypersad SM, et al. T1 mapping and survival in systemic light-chain amyloidosis. *Eur Heart J.* 2015;36(4):244–251.
96. Martinez-Naharro A, et al. Magnetic resonance in transthyretin cardiac amyloidosis. *J Am Coll Cardiol.* 2017;70(4):466–477.
97. Look DC, Locker DR. Time saving in measurement of NMR and EPR relaxation times. *Rev Sci Instrum.* 2003;41(2):250–251.
98. Messroghli DR, et al. Modified look-locker inversion recovery (MOLLI) for high-resolution T1 mapping of the heart. *Magn Reson Med.* 2004;52(1):141–146.
99. Messroghli DR, et al. Optimization and validation of a fully-integrated pulse sequence for modified look-locker inversion-recovery (MOLLI) T1 mapping of the heart. *J Magn Reson Imaging.* 2007;26(4):1081–1086.
100. Piechnik SK, et al. Shortened modified look-locker inversion recovery (ShMOLLI) for clinical myocardial T1-mapping at 1.5 and 3 T within a 9 heartbeat breathhold. *J Cardiovasc Magn Reson.* 2010;12(1):69.
101. Chow K, et al. Saturation recovery single-shot acquisition (SASHA) for myocardial T(1) mapping. *Magn Reson Med.* 2014;71(6):2082–2095.
102. Wood JC, et al. Cardiac iron determines cardiac T2*, T2, and T1 in the gerbil model of iron cardiomyopathy. *Circulation.* 2005;112(4):535–543.
103. Krittayaphong R, et al. Assessment of cardiac iron overload in thalassemia with MRI on 3.0-T: high-field T1, T2, and T2* quantitative parametric mapping in comparison to T2* on 1.5-T. *JACC, Cardiovasc Imaging.* 2019;12(4):752–754.
104. Torlasco C, et al. Role of T1 mapping as a complementary tool to T2* for non-invasive cardiac iron overload assessment. *PLoS One.* 2018;13(2):e0192890.
105. Abdel-Gadir A, et al. Ultrafast magnetic resonance imaging for iron quantification in thalassemia participants in the developing world: the TIC-TOC study (Thailand and UK international collaboration in thalassaemia optimising ultrafast CMR). *Circulation.* 2016;134(5):432–434.
106. Medina KM, et al. Use of rapid cardiac magnetic resonance imaging to guide chelation therapy in patients with transfusion-dependent thalassaemia in India: UMIMI study. *Eur Heart J Qual Care Clin Outcomes.* 2022;8(3):289–297.
107. Singh SP, et al. Diagnostic value of T1 mapping in detecting iron overload in Indian patients with thalassemia major: a comparison with T2* mapping. *Indian J Radiol Imaging.* 2024;34(1):54–59.
108. Krittayaphong R, et al. Detection of cardiac iron overload with native magnetic resonance T1 and T2 mapping in patients with thalassemia. *Int J Cardiol.* 2017;248:421–426.
109. Hundley WG, et al. Society for cardiovascular magnetic resonance (SCMR) guidelines for reporting cardiovascular magnetic resonance examinations. *J Cardiovasc Magn Reson.* 2022;24(1):29.
110. Olivieri NF, et al. Survival in medically treated patients with homozygous beta-thalassemia. *N Engl J Med.* 1994;331(9):574–578.
111. Telfer PT, et al. Hepatic iron concentration combined with long-term monitoring of serum ferritin to predict complications of iron overload in thalassaemia major. *Br J Haematol.* 2000;110(4):971–977.
112. Noetzli LJ, et al. Longitudinal analysis of heart and liver iron in thalassemia major. *Blood.* 2008;112(7):2973–2978.
113. Delea TE, et al. Consequences and costs of noncompliance with iron chelation therapy in patients with transfusion-dependent thalassemia: a literature review. *Transfusion.* 2007;47(10):1919–1929.
114. Mancuso L, et al. Left ventricular diastolic dysfunction in beta-thalassemia major with heart failure. *Hemoglobin.* 2018;42(1):68–71.
115. Alpendurada F, et al. Relation of myocardial T2* to right ventricular function in thalassaemia major. *Eur Heart J.* 2010;31(13):1648–1654.
116. Jensen PD, et al. In vivo calibration of the T2* cardiovascular magnetic resonance method at 1.5 T for estimation of cardiac iron in a minipig model of transfusional iron overload. *J Cardiovasc Magn Reson.* 2021;23(1):27.
117. Collins W, Taylor WH. Determination of iron in cardiac and liver tissues by plasma emission spectroscopy. *Ann Clin Biochem.* 1987;24(Pt 5):483–487.
118. Kirk P, et al. Cardiac T2* magnetic resonance for prediction of cardiac complications in thalassemia major. *Circulation.* 2009;120(20):1961–1968.
119. Modell B, et al. Improved survival of thalassaemia major in the UK and relation to T2* cardiovascular magnetic resonance. *J Cardiovasc Magn Reson.* 2008;10(1):42.
120. Porter JB, et al. Treatment of heart failure in adults with thalassemia major: response in patients randomised to deferoxamine with or without deferiprone. *J Cardiovasc Magn Reson.* 2013;15(1):38.
121. Forni GL, Derchi G. Typical manifestation of acute congestive heart failure in patients with Thalassaemia major causing diagnostic delay in the emergency room. *Eur J Heart Fail.* 2003;5(5):607–608.
122. Rahav G, et al. Severe infections in thalassaemic patients: prevalence and predisposing factors. *Br J Haematol.* 2006;133(6):667–674.
123. Adamkiewicz TV, et al. Infection due to Yersinia enterocolitica in a series of patients with beta-thalassemia: incidence and predisposing factors. *Clin Infect Dis.* 1998;27(6):1362–1366.
124. Davis BA, et al. Value of sequential monitoring of left ventricular ejection fraction in the management of thalassemia major. *Blood.* 2004;104(1):263–269.

125. Hider RC, Liu ZD. Emerging understanding of the advantage of small molecules such as hydroxypyridinones in the treatment of iron overload. *Curr Med Chem.* 2003;10(12):1051–1064.
126. Lee P, et al. Intravenous infusion pharmacokinetics of desferrioxamine in thalassaemic patients. *Drug Metab Dispos.* 1993;21(4):640–644.
127. Entezari S, et al. Iron chelators in treatment of iron overload. *J Toxicol.* 2022;2022:4911205.
128. al-Refaie FN, et al. Pharmacokinetics of the oral iron chelator deferiprone (L1) in patients with iron overload. *Br J Haematol.* 1995;89(2):403–408.
129. Galanello R, Campus S, Origa R. Deferasirox: pharmacokinetics and clinical experience. *Expert Opin Drug Metab Toxicol.* 2012;8(1):123–134.
130. Porter JB. Optimizing iron chelation strategies in beta-thalassaemia major. *Blood Rev.* 2009;23(suppl 1):S3–S7.
131. Brittenham GM. Iron-chelating therapy for transfusional iron overload. *N Engl J Med.* 2011;364(2):146–156.
132. Modell B, et al. Survival and desferrioxamine in thalassaemia major. *Br Med J (Clin Res Ed).* 1982;284(6322):1081–1084.
133. Maggio A, et al. Improving survival with deferiprone treatment in patients with thalassemia major: a prospective multicenter randomised clinical trial under the auspices of the Italian society for thalassemia and hemoglobinopathies. *Blood Cells Mol Dis.* 2009;42(3):247–251.
134. Telfer PT, et al. Improved survival in thalassemia major patients on switching from desferrioxamine to combined chelation therapy with desferrioxamine and deferiprone. *Haematologica.* 2009;94(12):1777–1778.
135. Chuang TY, et al. Combined chelation with high-dose deferiprone and deferoxamine to improve survival and restore cardiac function effectively in patients with transfusion-dependent thalassemia presenting severe cardiac complications. *Ann Hematol.* 2020;99(10):2289–2294.
136. Pennell DJ, et al. Randomized controlled trial of deferiprone or deferoxamine in beta-thalassemia major patients with asymptomatic myocardial siderosis. *Blood.* 2006;107(9):3738–3744.
137. Anderson LJ, et al. Comparison of effects of oral deferiprone and subcutaneous desferrioxamine on myocardial iron concentrations and ventricular function in beta-thalassaemia. *Lancet.* 2002;360(9332):516–520.
138. Pepe A, et al. Evaluation of the efficacy of oral deferiprone in beta-thalassemia major by multislice multiecho T2. *Eur J Haematol.* 2006;76(3):183–192.
139. Pepe A, et al. Deferasirox, deferiprone and desferrioxamine treatment in thalassemia major patients: cardiac iron and function comparison determined by quantitative magnetic resonance imaging. *Haematologica.* 2011;96(1):41–47.
140. Borgna-Pignatti C, et al. Cardiac morbidity and mortality in deferoxamine- or deferiprone-treated patients with thalassemia major. *Blood.* 2006;107(9):3733–3737.
141. Tanner MA, et al. A randomized, placebo-controlled, double-blind trial of the effect of combined therapy with deferoxamine and deferiprone on myocardial iron in thalassemia major using cardiovascular magnetic resonance. *Circulation.* 2007;115(14):1876–1884.
142. Pennell DJ, et al. Continued improvement in myocardial T2* over two years of deferasirox therapy in beta-thalassemia major patients with cardiac iron overload. *Haematologica.* 2011;96(1):48–54.
143. Pennell DJ, et al. Deferasirox for up to 3 years leads to continued improvement of myocardial T2* in patients with beta-thalassemia major. *Haematologica.* 2012;97(6):842–848.
144. Pennell DJ, et al. Efficacy of deferasirox in reducing and preventing cardiac iron overload in beta-thalassemia. *Blood.* 2010;115(12):2364–2371.
145. Evans P, et al. Mechanisms for the shuttling of plasma non-transferrin-bound iron (NTBI) onto deferoxamine by deferiprone. *Transl Res.* 2010;156(2):55–67.
146. Wonke B, Wright C, Hoffbrand AV. Combined therapy with deferiprone and desferrioxamine. *Br J Haematol.* 1998;103(2):361–364.
147. Kattamis A, et al. Combined therapy with desferrioxamine and deferiprone in thalassemic patients: effect on urinary iron excretion. *Haematologica.* 2003;88(12):1423–1425.
148. Farmaki K, et al. Normalisation of total body iron load with very intensive combined chelation reverses cardiac and endocrine complications of thalassaemia major. *Br J Haematol.* 2010;148(3):466–475.
149. Jetsrisuparb A, et al. Retrospective study on the combination of desferrioxamine and deferasirox for treatment of iron-overloaded thalassemic patients: first evidence of more than 2 years. *J Pediatr Hematol Oncol.* 2010;32(5):400–403.
150. Farmaki K, Tzoumari I, Pappa C. Oral chelators in transfusion-dependent thalassemia major patients may prevent or reverse iron overload complications. *Blood Cells Mol Dis.* 2011;47(1):33–40.
151. Mourad FH, et al. Comparison between desferrioxamine and combined therapy with desferrioxamine and deferiprone in iron overloaded thalassaemia patients. *Br J Haematol.* 2003;121(1):187–189.
152. Alpendurada F, et al. Effects of combined deferiprone with deferoxamine on right ventricular function in thalassaemia major. *J Cardiovasc Magn Reson.* 2012;14(1):8.
153. Song TS, et al. Combined versus monotherapy or concurrent therapy for treatment of thalassaemia. *In Vivo (Athens).* 2014;28(4):645–649.
154. Elalfy MS, et al. Efficacy and safety of a novel combination of two oral chelators deferasirox/deferiprone over deferoxamine/deferiprone in severely iron overloaded young beta thalassemia major patients. *Eur J Haematol.* 2015;95(5):411–420.
155. Aydinok Y, et al. Effects of deferasirox-deferoxamine on myocardial and liver iron in patients with severe transfusional iron overload. *Blood.* 2015;125(25):3868–3877.
156. Pennell DJ, et al. Cardiovascular function and treatment in beta-thalassemia major: a consensus statement from the American heart association. *Circulation.* 2013;128(3):281–308.

29 Arrhythmogenic Cardiomyopathies

AIDEN ABIDOV

CARDIAC MAGNETIC RESONANCE IN DIAGNOSING ARRHYTHMOGENIC CARDIOMYOPATHY: GENERAL CONCEPTS AND CLINICAL CONSIDERATIONS

In their 1982 article, Frank Marcus from the University of Arizona and Guy Fontaine with a group of investigators from the *Hôpital de La Salpêtrière* provided a detailed description of a disease they called "arrhythmogenic right ventricular dysplasia," or ARVD.[1] They defined ARVD as a disorder of the heart muscle that leads to arrhythmias and predominantly involves the right ventricular (RV) myocardium, causing progressive fibrofatty replacement of the RV free wall and subsequent RV enlargement and focal regional wall motion abnormalities (Fig. 29.1). In the original 1982 paper, Marcus et al. described the following clinical picture of the disease: "The typical patient is a young or middle-aged male who presents with palpitations, tachycardia, or syncope. Ventricular tachycardia is of left bundle branch block configuration. Physical examination is surprisingly normal, but a fourth heart sound may be present. During sinus rhythm, the ECG may show incomplete or complete right bundle branch block, T wave inversion in V1 to V4 is usually present. The heart is moderately enlarged, and the pulmonary vasculature is normal." This description is still applicable to the typical appearance of the main clinical form of this disorder. Subsequent research defined important genetic features of this heritable pathology[2] and also described arrhythmogenic left ventricular cardiomyopathy (ALVC)[3,4] and biventricular arrhythmogenic cardiomyopathies (BiV-ACMs).[5] Importantly, the principle of combined diagnostic criteria for arrhythmogenic right ventricular cardiomyopathy (ARVC) emerged in 1994 as Task Force criteria (TFC) based on the major and minor criteria composed of anatomic, histologic, electrocardiographic, arrhythmic, and historical data.[6] A subsequent 2010 modification of the TFC[2] defined anatomic information based predominantly on noninvasive imaging modalities: echocardiography and cardiac magnetic resonance (CMR).

Arrhythmogenic cardiomyopathy (ACM) is now more frequently diagnosed as it is becoming better known to cardiac imagers and general clinical professionals. It is estimated to occur in 1:1000–1:5000 individuals[7] but have a higher incidence since one may have a pathological gene for this disease yet have little or no clinical manifestations during the "concealed phase" of the disease. This is known as a lack of association of genotype and phenotype. In addition, since ACM is one of the leading causes of sudden cardiac death (SCD) in the young,[8] it is important to be able to recognize the disease in a very early phase to prevent this catastrophic outcome.

One may ask, why should we focus our attention predominantly on one imaging modality, CMR, particularly when it is more expensive and less readily available than echocardiography? In contrast to echocardiography, magnetic resonance imaging (MRI) can provide a more accurate quantitative evaluation of left ventricular (LV) and RV function and structure. Specifically, it can accurately access LV and RV volumes and ejection fraction as well as segmental wall motion abnormalities.

Based on hundreds of published papers, cardiac MRI is a crucial diagnostic imaging modality in patients with suspected or known ACM, and is particularly valuable since important limitations of MRI (e.g., the need for prolonged breath-holding, inability to scan patients with permanent pacemakers or implantable cardioverters-defibrillators [ICDs]) have largely been overcome. For years now, the standard clinical practice has been to confirm the finding of abnormal RV function or structure suspected on two-dimensional echocardiogram in a patient with a possible ACM/ARVC on CMR since the latter is more reliable for diagnosis. It is also important that the cardiac imager who interprets the CMR must be aware of normal variants of the RV contractility patterns, particularly that of an apparent bulging of the RV free wall at the insertion of the RV papillary muscle (moderator band).

Other questions include the age at which ACM manifests. Should an MRI be done in children who have genetic abnormality but no clinical manifestation of the disease? How rapidly do morphological RV and/or LV features change in this disease? This would determine how frequently the CMR should be reassessed in first-degree relatives who may have no or minimal symptoms.

The excellent spatial resolution and safety of CMR make it an ideal methodology for follow-up and sequential imaging of patients with known or suspected ACM. CMR is useful in a differential diagnosis that includes several conditions mimicking ACM/ARVC, such as cardiac sarcoidosis, left-to-right supraventricular shunts, and myocarditis. The use of a gadolinium-based contrast agent (GBCA) to detect and localize scar/fibrosis in the LV or RV myocardium with a very high degree of diagnostic accuracy is unique to CMR, as is the its ability to provide effective tissue characterization and phenotyping of cardiomyopathies based on the disease-specific pattern of the late gadolinium enhancement (LGE) distribution.

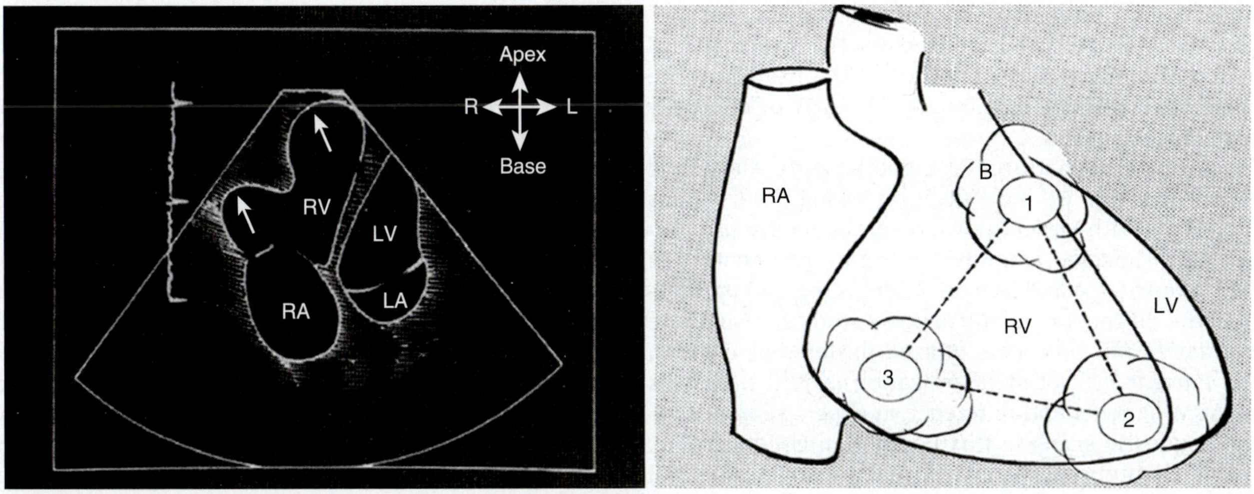

FIG. 29.1 Illustrations from the 1982 F. Marcus et al. paper "Right ventricular dysplasia: A report of 24 adult cases." (A) Two-dimensional echocardiogram shows two areas of dyskinesia (*arrows* in the right ventricle [*RV*]). They are at the apex and junction of the anterior, lateral, and inferior borders of the RV. (B) The most frequent sites of dysplasia: (1) the anterior infundibulum, (2) the right ventricular apex, and (3) the inferior or diaphragmatic aspect of the RV. These constitute the "triangle of dysplasia." *LV*, Left ventricle; *RA*, right atrium. (Reproduced, with permission from Marcus FI, Fontaine GH, Guiraudon G et al. Right ventricular dysplasia: a report of 24 adult cases. *Circulation*. 1982;65:384–398.)

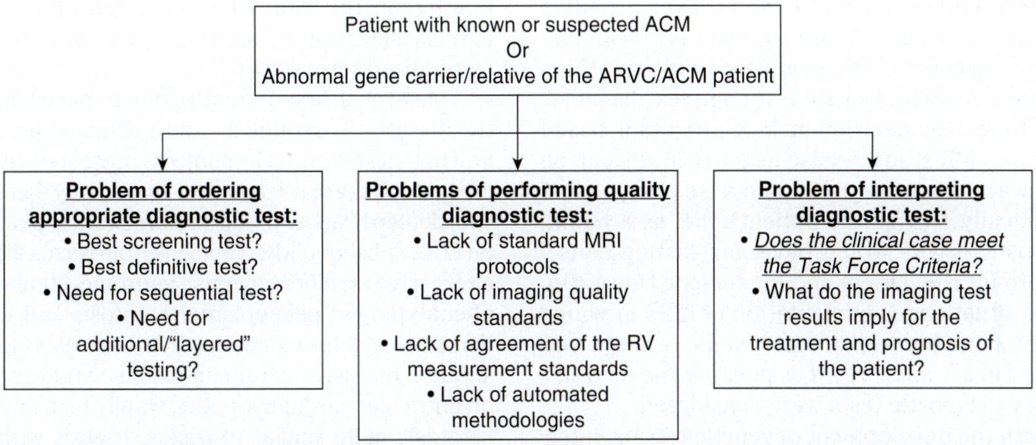

FIG. 29.2 Problems encountered in evaluation and management of patients with known or suspected arrhythmogenic cardiomyopathy. *ACM*, arrhythmogenic cardiomyopathy; *ARVC*, arrhythmogenic right ventricular cardiomyopathy; *MRI*, Magnetic resonance imaging. (Modified, with permission from Abidov A, Oliva IB, Marcus FI. Cardiac MRI in the Diagnosis, Clinical Management and Prognosis of Arrhyhtmogenic Right Ventricular Cardiomyopathy/Dysplasia. Academic Press/Elsevier, 2016.)

An important consideration is the increased safety of CMR, especially the absence of exposure to ionizing radiation and nephrotoxic iodine contrast. This allows sequential CMR studies in young patients without an increased associated risk.

Finally, CMR is useful in a differential diagnosis that includes several conditions mimicking ACM, such as cardiac sarcoidosis, left-to-right supraventricular shunts, and myocarditis, as well as some cases of "athlete's heart" and pericardial disease.

Based on the exceptional diagnostic capabilities listed above, CMR became a very important part of the original 1994 and modified 2010 TFC for ARVC and is truly an imaging foundation of the most recently published criteria for ACM.[9]

Advances in the field of echocardiography, cardiac computed tomography angiography (CTA), and nuclear cardiology have brought about many interesting applications that could significantly enhance the armamentarium of clinicians in the diagnosis and management of ACM, especially when combined with the results of CMR as part of the multimodality imaging assessment of this population. Increased utilization of artificial intelligence (AI) in cardiovascular imaging in the last few years has added significantly to the diagnostic power of imaging applications, including CMR.

In summary, there are many important clinical areas of interest reflecting the role of CMR and other rapidly developing cardiac imaging methodologies in patients with ACM/ARVC. In this chapter, we provide readers with a convenient overview of these areas. However, there are three types of problems with cardiac imaging in general, and cardiac MRI in particular, for the evaluation of ACM (Fig. 29.2):

1. The problem of ordering the right test for the patient's age and clinical presentation. Patients with known or suspected ACM are a highly heterogeneous group and include patients with confirmed ACM, asymptomatic gene carriers, and relatives of patients with ACM, as well as patients with suspected or possible ACM.

There is significant disagreement about which test should be utilized in these populations, which one is the most effective for screening, and whether the layered testing concept should be considered for "borderline" cases. The Modified TFC focused on the specificity of echo and MRI measurements of ARVC/D, possibly at the expense of sensitivity, particularly for early or clinically "silent" disease cases.

2. The problem of performing a good-quality diagnostic CMR. For years, we have been reviewing CMR studies of patients with either known or probable disease performed in imaging laboratories from many centers in the United States and abroad. There is marked variability in the diagnostic quality of these studies. Also, there are many CMR protocols utilized in different centers. The current lack of standardization of MRI protocols for ACM patients and difference in expertise in obtaining diagnostic scans in this population is concerning. In this chapter, we share with readers some potential solutions and algorithms allowing more uniformity in this field.
3. The problem of interpreting the results of the CMR study. There is a significant difference in clinical expertise in the interpretation of scans in patients with suspected ACM among different imaging centers. Even negative results in particular clinical populations may mean just one negative diagnostic criterion among many others that must be considered in such a complex diagnosis as ACM. At times, the decision-making process is based completely on CMR study. A false-negative study can be associated with increased risk, and a false-positive test may dramatically change the patient's life; as a result, both diagnostic errors would have long-lasting consequences both for the patient and for society. One example of these situations is implantation of ICDs in young patients who have borderline test results, or tests that are negative but are interpreted as positive and no other confirmatory diagnostic tests were considered.

Recently, with the development of genetic testing, interpretation of imaging test results in association with genetic defects in asymptomatic individuals has raised important clinical dilemmas. Genotype-positive patients may be subjected to changes in their occupation and limitations in their athletic activities (such as college sports) and lifestyle even though their actual clinical data do not suggest an increased risk.

In our chapter, we address these concerns and provide quick access to evidence-based algorithms and methods currently utilized in state-of-the-art imaging laboratories. Easy access to these data may save time and effort in reaching important clinical decisions and utilize an important principle of modern precision medicine: "the right test for the right patient."

THE HISTORY OF ARRHYTHMOGENIC CARDIOMYOPATHY

ACM represents one of the "ancient diseases," with knowledge of the clinical presentation and course of the disease dating back centuries.[10]

Based on the available evidence, the early description of the disease probably belongs to the pathologist Giovanni Maria Lancisi, who first reported the history of a family with disease recurrence in four generations, featuring cardiac palpitations and sudden death.[11] Dilatation and aneurysm of the right ventricle, which filled the right chest, were observed at autopsy of fatal cases.

Doctor René Laennec, in 1819, first drew attention to the relationship between fatty tissue in the right ventricle and sudden death.[12] In 1905, William Osler, in his famous treatise "The Principles and Practice of Medicine," described a case of a 40-year-old man who died suddenly while climbing up a hill. The heart showed biventricular massive myocardial atrophy with very thin walls, and was named "parchment heart."[13]

In 1982, Marcus and Fontaine[1] defined ARVD and reported a series of adult patients with this disorder presenting with ventricular arrhythmias with left bundle branch block morphology. Microscopic examination of myocardial samples, removed at surgical disconnection of the right from the left ventricle, disclosed fibrofatty replacement that the authors interpreted as a maldevelopmental defect, and so called the disease "right ventricular dysplasia." Subsequently, the term "dysplasia" was replaced by "cardiomyopathy" in the World Health Organization nomenclature and classification of heart muscle disease to create a more generalized term (ARVC).[14]

Thiene et al. first drew attention to the malignant aspect of the disease, presenting in youth with sudden death, even at first manifestation.[15] The subjects presented inverted T waves in right precordial leads and apparently benign premature ventricular beats with left bundle branch block morphology on ECG. Subsequently, clinicians from Naxos island described a recessive cardiocutaneous syndrome, combining the ARVC phenotype and palmoplantar keratosis and woolly hair.[16] A dermatologist from Ecuador, Luis Carvajal-Huerta, described another recessive cardiocutaneous syndrome consisting of biventricular cardiomyopathy, woolly hair, and palmoplantar keratosis quite similar to Naxos disease, with pump failure and rare polymorphic ventricular arrhythmias.[17]

Even very early in the development of ACM research, CMR demonstrated extraordinary diagnostic capability for detecting both morphofunctional (e.g., abnormal global and regional contractility, ventricular dilatation, aneurysms) and tissue characterization, with visualization of both fatty tissue on T2 sequences and myocardial fibrosis by LGE methodology. The use of LGE sequences was proven to be extremely effective in detecting LV involvement.[18]

Meanwhile, great steps forward have been achieved in the prevention of premature death in ARVC. As with the initial diagnosis of ACM, CMR is effectively utilized in defining prognosis and developing management plans for patients with established disease.[19]

DEFINITION, CLASSIFICATION, AND TASK FORCE CRITERIA FOR ARRHYTHMOGENIC RIGHT VENTRICULAR DYSPLASIA/ ARRHYTHMOGENIC CARDIOMYOPATHY

Frank Marcus and Guy Fontaine defined ARVD as a disorder of the heart muscle that leads to arrhythmias and predominantly involves the RV myocardium, causing

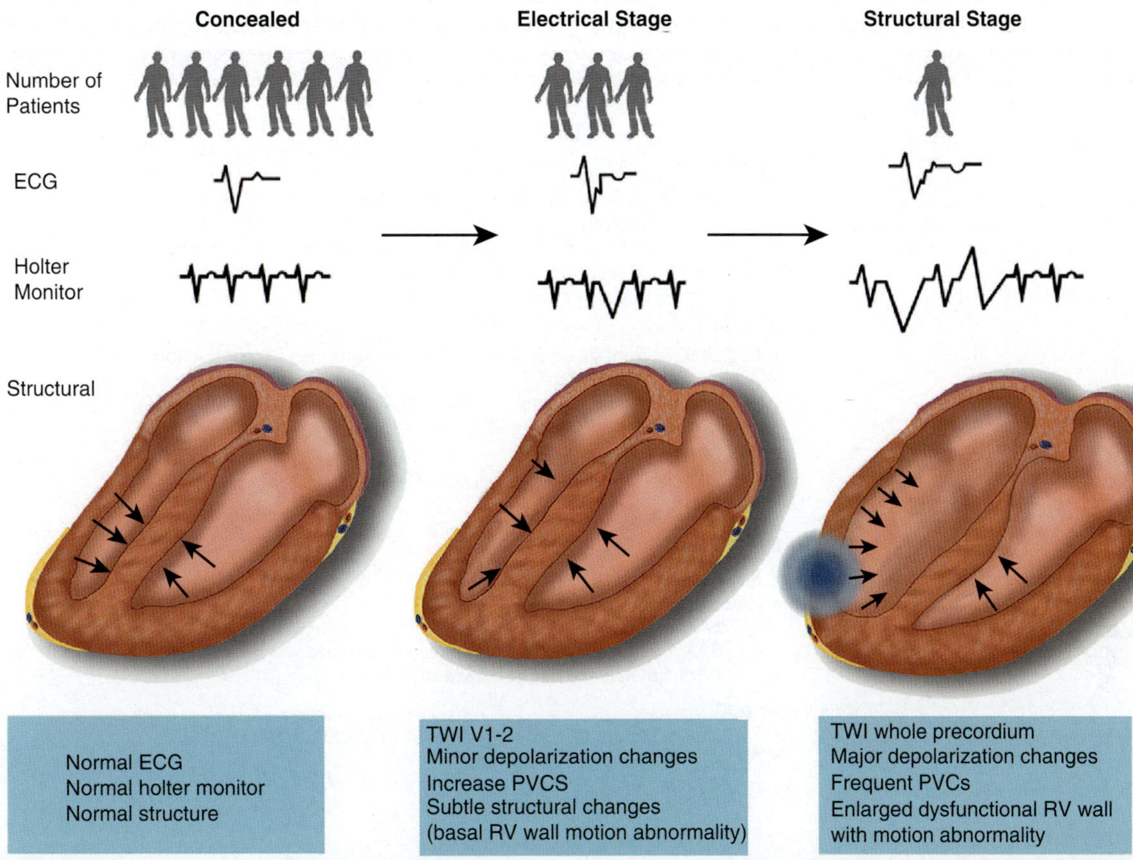

FIG. 29.3 Disease progression in ARVC. Family members of a proband with ARVC have a long latent stage without signs or symptoms of disease (*concealed stage*). Electrical changes on electrocardiogram or Holter monitoring are usually the first sign of disease, and structural abnormalities may be observed later. Disease progression is typically slow. *ECG*, electrocardiogram; *PVC*, premature ventricular complex; *RV*, right ventricular; *TWI*, T-wave inversion. (Reproduced, with permission from te Riele AS, James CA, Rastegar N et al. Yield of serial evaluation in at-risk family members of patients with ARVD/C. *J Am Coll Cardiol*. 2014;64:293–301.)

progressive fibrofatty replacement of the RV free wall and subsequent RV enlargement and focal regional wall motion abnormalities.

These authors described in detail imaging-based features of ARVD. Utilizing RV angiography and echocardiography, they revealed involvement of specific regions of the right ventricle (RV inflow tract and outflow tract and RV apex) defining it as "the triangle of dysplasia" (Fig. 29.1).

However, the clinical spectrum of the arrhythmogenic RV pathology is not limited by a single "typical" dysplastic structural phenotype, and thus, the term "arrhythmogenic right ventricular cardiomyopathy" or ARVC could combine all the disorders with RV anatomic and functional abnormalities and arrhythmogenic potential. Importantly, all these clinical types of ARVC/D follow some "general rules," including slow progression of the disease (Fig. 29.3).[20]

Several forms of ACM, including Carvajal syndrome and Naxos disease, are subtypes of cardiocutaneous syndromes.[21–23] Clinical features in these patients consist of a triad of RV cardiomyopathy, woolly hair, and plantar keratoderma. Both clinical disorders are autosomal recessive; while patients with Naxos disease have predominantly RV involvement and nonepidermolytic keratoderma, patients with Carvajal syndrome more frequently have biventricular involvement and epidermolytic cutaneous lesions.[23]

Another distinctive form of ARVC is Uhl disease, described predominantly in the pediatric population. This anomaly is characterized by the absence of myocardium in the RV free wall that gives the appearance of a "paper-thin" RV wall, or "parchment heart."

Due to a lack of specific symptoms and signs, TFC for the clinical diagnosis of ARVC were proposed in 1994.[6] There was agreement that there is no single diagnostic modality to confirm the disease. The multitude of criteria included structural, histological, ECG, arrhythmic, and familial features of the disease. The abnormalities were categorized into major and minor criteria.

The diagnosis of ARVC is fulfilled by the presence of two major or one major plus two minor criteria or four minor criteria from different groups.[6]

Diagnostic terminology based on the 2010 modified ARVC/D TFC[2] requires more definitive imaging-based thresholds of the RV structural and functional abnormalities (Table 29.1) and is summarized as follows:

1. Definitive diagnosis: two major or one major plus two minor criteria or four minor criteria from different categories.
2. Borderline diagnosis: one major and one minor or three minor criteria from different categories.
3. Possible diagnosis: one major or two minor criteria from different categories.

Establishing the diagnosis of ACM remains a clinical challenge, as there is no single test to establish the

TABLE 29.1 Comparison of 1994 Original and 2010 Revised Arrhythmogenic Right Ventricular Cardiomyopathy Task Force Criteria.

ORIGINAL TASK FORCE CRITERIA	REVISED TASK FORCE CRITERIA
I. Global or regional dysfunction and structural alterations[a] Major	
	By 2D echo:
• Severe dilatation and reduction of RV ejection fraction with no (or only mild) LV impairment • Localized RV aneurysms (akinetic or dyskinetic areas with diastolic bulging) • Severe segmental dilatation of the RV	• Regional RV akinesia, dyskinesia or **aneurysm** • And one of the fallowing (end diastole): — PLAXCRVOT ≥32 mm (corrected for body size [PLAX/BSA] ≥19 mm/m^2) — PSAX RVOT ≥36 mm (corrected for body size [PSAX/BSA] ≥21 mm/m^2) — Or fractional area change ≤33%
	By MRI • Regional RV akinesia or dyskinesia or dyssynchronous RV contraction • And one of the following: — Ratio of RV end-diastolic volume to BSA ≥110 mL/m^2 (male) or ≥100 mL/m^2 (female) — Or RV ejection fraction ≤40% **By RV angiography:** • Regional RV akinesia, dyskinesia, or aneurysm
Minor	
	By 2D echo:
• Mild global RV dilatation and/or ejection fraction reduction with normal LV • Mild segmental dilatation of the RV • Regional RV hypokinesis	• Regional RV akinesia or dyskinesia • And one of the following (end diastole): — PLAX RVOT ≥29 to <32 mm (corrected for body size[PLAX/BSA]≥ 16 to <19 mm/m^2) — PSAX RVOT ≥32 to <36 mm (corrected for body size [PSAX/BSA] ≥18 to <21 mm/m^2) — Or fractional area change >33% to ≤40%
	By MRI: • Regional RV akinesia or dyskinesia or dyssynchronous RV contraction • And one of the following: — Ratio of RV end diastolic volume to BSA ≥100 to <110 mL/m^2 (male) or — ≥90 to <100 mL/m^2 (female) — *or* RV ejection fraction >40% ta ≤45%
II. Tissue characterization of wall	
Major	
• Fibrofatty replacement of myocardium on endomyocardial biopsy	• Residual myocytes <60% by morphometric analysis (or <50% if estimated), with fibrous replacement of the RV free wall myocardium ≥1 sample, with or without fatty replacement of tissue on endomyocardial biopsy
Minor	• Residual myocytes 60%–75% by morphometric analysis (or 50%–65% if estimated), with fibrous replacement of the RV free wall myocardium in ≥1 sample, with or without fatty replacement of tissue on endomyocardial biopsy
III. Repolarization abnormalities	
Major	• Inverted T waves in right precordial leads (V_1, V_2, and V_3) or beyond in individuals >14 years of age (in the absence of complete right bundle-branch block QRS ≥120 ms)
Minor	
• Inverted T waves in right precordial leads (V_2 and V_3) (people age >12 years, in absence of right bundle-branch block)	• Inverted T waves in leads V_1 and V_2 in individuals >14 years of age (in the absence of complete right bundle-branch block) or in V_4, V_5, or V_6
	• Inverted T waves in leads V_1, V_2, V_3. and V_4 in individuals >14 years of age in the presence of complete right bundle-branch block
IV. Depolarization/conduction abnormalities Major	
• Epsilon waves or localized prolongation (>110 ms) of the QRS complex in right precordial leads (V_1 to V_3.)	• Epsilon wave (reproducible low-amplitude signals between end of QRS complex to onset of the T wave) in the right precordial leads (V_1 to V_3)
Minor	
• Late potentials (SAECG)	• Late potentials by SAECG in ≥1 of 3 parameters in the absence of a QRS duration of ≥110 ms on the standard ECG
	• Filtered QRS duration (fQRS)≥ 114 ms
	• Duration of terminal QRS <40 µV (low-amplitude signal duration) µ 38 ms
	• Root-mean-square voltage of terminal 40 ms ≤ 20 µV
	• Terminal activation duration of QRS ≥55 ms measured from the nadir of the S wave to the end of the QRS, including R′, in V_1, V_2, or V_3 in the absence of complete right bundle-branch block
V. Arrhythmias Major	• Nonsustained or sustained ventricular tachycardia of left bundle-branch morphology with superior axis (negative or indeterminate QRS in leads II, III, and aVF and positive in lead aVL)

Continued

TABLE 29.1 Comparison of 1994 Original and 2010 Revised Arrhythmogenic Right Ventricular Cardiomyopathy Task Force Criteria.—cont'd

ORIGINAL TASK FORCE CRITERIA	REVISED TASK FORCE CRITERIA
Minor	
• Left bundle-branch block-type ventricular tachycardia (sustained and nonsustained) (ECG, Holter, exercise)	• Nonsustained or sustained ventricular tachycardia of RV outflow configuration, left bundle-branch block morphology with inferior axis (positive QRS in leads II, III and aVF and negative in lead aVL) or of unknown axis
• Frequent ventricular extrasystoles (>1000 per 24 hours) (Holter)	• > 500 ventricular extrasystoles per 24 hours (Holter)
VI. Family history Major	
• Familial disease confirmed at necropsy or surgery	• ARVC/D confirmed in a first-degree relative who meets current task force criteria
	• ARVC/D confirmed pathologically at autopsy or surgery in a first-degree relative
Minor	• Identification of a pathogenic mutation[b] categorized as associated or probably associated with ARVC/D in the patient under evaluation
• Family history of premature sudden death (<35 years of age) due to suspected ARVC/D	• History of ARVC/D in a first-degree relative in whom it is not possible or practical to determine whether the family member meets current task force criteria
• Familial history (clinical diagnosis based on present criteria)	• Premature sudden death (<35 years of age) due to suspected ARVC/D in a first-degree relative
	• ARVC/D confirmed pathologically or by current task force criteria m second degree relative

[a]Hypokinesis is not included in this or subsequent definitions of RV regional wall motion abnormalities for the proposed modified criteria.

A pathogenic mutation is a DNA alteration associated with ARVC/D that alters or is expected to alter the encoded protein, is unobserved or rare in a large non-ARVC/D control population, and either alters or is predicted to alter the structure or function of the protein or has demonstrated linkage to the disease phenotype in a conclusive pedigree. *PLAX*, parasternal long-axis view; *RVOT*, RV outflow tract; *BSA*, body surface area; *PSAX*, parasternal short-axis view; *aVF*, augmented voltage unipolar left foot lead; *aVL*, augmented voltage unipolar left arm lead. Diagnostic terminology for original 1994 criteria: This diagnosis is fulfilled by the presence of two major, or one major plus two minor criteria or four minor criteria from different groups. Diagnostic terminology for revised 2010 criteria: Definite diagnosis: two major or one major and two minor criteria or four minor from different categories; borderline: one major and one minor or three minor criteria from different categories; possible: one major or two minor criteria from different categories.

Adopted with permission from Marcus FI, McKenna WJ, Sherrill D et al. Diagnosis of arrhythmogenic right ventricular cardiomyopathy/dysplasia: proposed modification of the task force criteria. *Circulation*. 2010;121:1533–1541.

identity of the disease due to its varied genotypic and phenotypic presentation. It should be noted that the cutoff values for RV volumetrics are different according to age, raising the concern of universality of the criteria in diagnosing ARVC.

In the last 2 decades, extensive cardiac imaging and clinical genetics-based research led to a much better understanding of the ARVC/D phenotype-genotype correlation. Based on this research, experts clearly recognized that the disease may actually frequently involve the left ventricle, resulting in biventricular or left-dominant phenotypic variants.[24] Accordingly, the term "ARVC/D" now defines a "traditional" subtype of the disease; to better describe the broader phenotypic spectrum of this disorder, a new term ("arrhythmogenic cardiomyopathy") has been introduced and is widely used by the clinical community.[24,25]

In order to further improve the diagnostic performance of the 2010 TFC, the following key points were proposed by an international panel of experts, which identify specific areas of the 2010 document requiring update to incorporate the research and clinical data on ACM gathered since the modified TFC were published[24]:

- The absence of specific criteria for diagnosing left-sided variants
- The crucial role of CMR imaging, not only in evaluating volumes, systolic function, and wall motion abnormalities, but particularly in the assessment of myocardial fibrosis based on LGE methodology[26]
- The inclusion of genetic testing as a major diagnostic criterion, even in probands. This approach potentially enables a diagnosis in cases lacking morphofunctional ventricular abnormalities or tissue changes. Of note, other cardiovascular diseases recommend genetic testing only in probands who meet clinical diagnostic criteria.

In 2020, based on the above considerations, updated diagnostic ACM criteria were proposed (Table 29.2 "Padua criteria").[9] More recently, based on the Padua criteria, the Task Force of the European Reference Network for rare, low prevalence, and complex diseases of the heart (ERN-GUARD-Heart) proposed a new set of criteria (Table 29.3 "European Task Force criteria").[27] These newest European TFC define ACM as primarily a "scarring" myocardial disease stemming from myocyte death and fibrofatty repair processes and leading to an increased risk of ventricular arrhythmias/sudden death and progressive systolic dysfunction.

The genetics of ACM are complex and represent an area of active ongoing research. For the typical ARVC patient, there is incomplete penetrance and highly variable expressivity. Typically, ARVD is a disease of the cell-to-cell junctions with many cases showing a predilection for mutations directly affecting desmosomal proteins.[28] It is associated with desmosomal gene mutations, and a total of five desmosomal genes may be found in these patients (plakophilin-2, desmoglein-2, desmocollin-2, desmoplakin, and junctional plakoglobin). Notably, nondesmosomal gene mutations (phospholamban, transforming growth factor beta-3, cardiac ryanodine receptor-2, tumor protein p63, desmin, lamin A/C, alpha T-catenin, and titin) are not uncommon in patients with ARVC and are more frequently associated with left dominant ACM (Fig. 29.4)[29] or biventricular involvement and with specific ECG findings (of low voltage in the standard leads and T wave inversion in V3–5).

The phenotypes of ACM are characterized as having three general clinical patterns: classic right, present in

TABLE 29.2 "Padua Criteria" for Diagnosis of Arrhythmogenic Cardiomyopathy.

CATEGORY	RIGHT VENTRICLE (UPGRADED 2010 ITF DIAGNOSTIC CRITERIA)	LEFT VENTRICLE (NEW DIAGNOSTIC CRITERIA)
I. Morphofunctional ventricular abnormalities II. Structural myocardial abnormalities III. Repolarization abnormalities IV. Depolarization abnormalities V. Ventricular arrhythmias VI. Family history/genetics	By echocardiography, CMR or angiography: Major • Regional RV akinesia, dyskinesia, or bulging plus one of the following: - Global RV dilatation (increase of RV EDV according to the imaging test specific nomograms) - Global RV systolic dysfunction (reduction of RV EF according to the imaging test specific diagrams) Minor • Regional RV akinesia, dyskinesia or aneurysm of RV free wall By CE-CMR: Major • Transmural LGE (stria pattern) of ≥1 RV region(s) (inlet, outlet, and apex in 2 orthogonal views) By EMB (limited indications): Major • Fibrous replacement of the myocardium in ≥1 sample, with or without fatty tissue Major • Inverted T waves in right precordial leads (V1,V2, and V3) or beyond in individuals with complete pubertal development (in the absence of complete RBBB) Minor • Inverted T waves in leads V1 and V2 in individuals with completed pubertal development (in the absence of complete RBBB) • Inverted T waves in V1, V2, V3, and V4 in individuals with completed pubertal development in the presence of complete RBBB Minor • Epsilon wave (reproducible low-amplitude signals between end of QRS complex to onset of the T wave) in the right precordial leads (V1 to V3) • Terminal activation duration of QRS ≥55 ms measured from the nadir of the S wave to the end of the QRS, including R′, in V1, V2, or V3 (in the absence of complete RBBB) Major • Frequent ventricular extrasystoles (N500 per 24 h), nonsustained or sustained ventricular tachycardia of LBBB morphology Minor • Frequent ventricular extrasystoles (N500 per 24 h), nonsustained or sustained ventricular tachycardia of LBBB morphology with inferior axis ("RVOT pattern") Major • ACM confirmed in a first-degree relative who meets diagnostic criteria • ACM confirmed pathologically at autopsy or surgery in a first degree relative • Identification of a pathogenic or likely pathogenetic ACM mutation in the patient under evaluation Minor • History of ACM in a first-degree relative in whom it is not possible or practical to determine whether the family member meets diagnostic criteria • Premature sudden death (<35 years of age) due to suspected ACM in a first-degree relative • ACM confirmed pathologically or by diagnostic criteria in a second-degree relative	By echocardiography, CMR or angiography: Minor • Global LV systolic dysfunction (depression of LV EF or reduction of echo- cardiographic global longitudinal strain), with or without LV dilatation (increase of LV EDV according to the imaging test specific nomograms for age, sex, and BSA) Minor • Regional LV hypokinesia or akinesia of LV free wall, septum, or both By CE-CMR: Major • LV LGE (stria pattern) of ≥1 Bull's eye segment(s) (in 2 orthogonal views) of the free wall (subepicardial or midmyocardial), septum, or both (excluding septal junctional LGE) Minor • Inverted T waves in left precordial leads (V4–V6) (in the absence of complete LBBB) Minor • Low QRS voltages (b0.5 mV peak to peak) in limb leads (in the absence of obesity, emphysema, or pericardial effusion) Minor • Frequent ventricular extrasystoles (N500 per 24 h), nonsustained or sustained ventricular tachycardia with an RBBB morphology (excluding the "fascicular pattern")

ACM, arrhythmogenic cardiomyopathy; *BSA*, body surface area; *EDV*, end diastolic volume; *EF*, ejection fraction; *EMB*, endomyocardial biopsy, *ITF*, international task force; *LBBB*, left bundle-branch block; *LGE*, late gadolinium enhancement; *LV*, left ventricle; *RBBB*, right bundle-branch block; *RV*, right ventricle; *RVOT*, right ventricular outflow tract.
Adopted with permission from Corrado D, Perazzolo Marra M, Zorzi A et al. Diagnosis of arrhythmogenic cardiomyopathy: the Padua criteria. *Int J Cardiol*. 2020;319:106–114.

39% of cases; left dominant, present in 5% of cases; and biventricular, present in 56% of cases.[30] The average age of onset is often generally in the early 30s, with a median age of onset of 26.[30,31] It is rare to demonstrate clinical signs or symptoms prior to the age of 12 or develop onset of symptoms after the age of 60. Palpitations and syncope are the most common presenting symptoms.[30,31]

Classic ARVC is a right heart–dominant disease characterized by four distinct phases.[32] In the early "concealed phase," the patients are often asymptomatic with little or no RV abnormality, but still have a risk of SCD.[15] In the "overt electrical phase," symptomatic ventricular arrhythmias are present, including premature ventricular complexes, nonsustained ventricular tachycardia (VT), sustained VT, or ventricular fibrillation. At this stage, RV morphological abnormalities are revealed on CMR. Disease progression leads to a third phase of RV failure, in which fibrofatty replacement of normal RV myocardium leads to impaired RV dynamics and varying degrees of RV failure. Finally, the disease can progress to biventricular failure, an advanced stage in which fibrofatty replacement of myocardium involves the septum and left ventricle, leading to left-sided heart failure. This stage can resemble dilated cardiomyopathy.[28]

The left-dominant pattern can be distinguished from classic ARVC/D in that it has mild right heart involvement with early and prominent LV involvement (Fig. 29.5).[32] The biventricular pattern differs from the classic pattern in that it demonstrates parallel RV and LV involvement rather than sequential RV and LV involvement (Fig. 29.6).[28] The prevalence of these subtypes may be underrepresented due to the clinical syndrome being attributed to other diseases and the lack of specific diagnostic guidelines for these entities.

According to the 2020 Padua criteria for ACM, while in patients with biventricular ACM the concomitant fulfillment of RV diagnostic criteria guarantees the disease specificity of the left-sided abnormalities, in patients with left-dominant ACM and no clinically detectable RV involvement, demonstration of a pathogenic mutation in ACM-related genes (major criterion) is necessary for diagnosis, because it is the most specific finding linking the LV phenotypic features to ACM.[9]

Extensive research demonstrates that the diagnosis of ALVC relies heavily on CMR data. However, considering the wide spectrum of LV disorders presenting with myocardial

TABLE 29.3 2023 European Task Force Criteria for Diagnosis of Arrhythmogenic Cardiomyopathy.

CATEGORY	RV PHENOTYPE	LV PHENOTYPE
I. Morphofunctional ventricular abnormalities	***Major*** • Regional RV akinesia, dyskinesia, or aneurysm *plus* one of the following: • Global RV dilatation (increase of RV EDV according to the imaging test specific nomograms for age, sex, and BSA)[a] or • Global RV systolic dysfunction I reduction of RV EF according to the imaging test specific nomograms for age and sex)[a] ***Minor*** • Regional RV akinesia, dyskinesia or aneurysm of RV free wall	***Minor*** • Global LV systolic dysfunction, with or without LV dilatation (increase of LV EDV according to the imaging test specific nomograms for age, sex, and BSA)[a]
II. Structural alterations	***Major*** • Fibrous replacement of the myocardium in ≥1 sample, with or without fatty tissue, at histology ***Minor*** • Unequivocal RV LGE (confirmed in 2 orthogonal views in ≥1 RV region(o) (excluding tricuspid valve)	***Major*** • "Ringlike" LV LGE (subepicardial or midmyocardial stria pattern) of ≥3 segments (confirmed in 2 orthogonal views) ***Minor*** • LV LGE (subepicardial or midmyocardial stria pattern) of 1 or 2 Bull's eye segment(o) (in 2 orthogonal views) of the free wall, septum, or both (excluding patchy, focal or septal junctional LGE[b])
III. Repolarization abnormalities	***Major*** • Negative T waves in right precordial leads 1 V_1, V_2, and V_3) or beyond in individuals ≥14 year-old (in the absence of complete RBBB and not preceded by J-point/ST-segment elevation) ***Minor*** • Negative T waves in leads VI and V2 in males ≥14-year-old (in the absence of RBBB and not preceded by J-point/ST segment elevation) • Negative T waves beyond V3 in the presence of complete RBBB • Negative T waves beyond V3 in individuals <14 years old	***Minor*** • Negative T waves in left precordial leads (V_4–V_6) (in the absence of complete LBBB)
IV. Depolarization and conduction abnormalities	***Minor*** • Epsilon wave (reproducible low-amplitude signals between end of QRS complex to onset of the T wave) in the right precordial leads (V1 to V3) • Terminal activation duration of QRS ≥55 ms measured from the nadir of the S wave to the end of the QRS, including R'. in VI, V2, or VS (in the absence of complete RBBB)	***Major*** • Low QRS voltage: (0.5 mV peak to peak) in all limb leads in the absence of other causes (e.g., cardiac amyloidosis, obesity, emphysema, or pericardial effusion)
V. Arrhythmias	***Major*** • Frequent ventricular extrasystoles (>500 per 24 h). Nonsustained or sustained ventricular tachycardia of LBBB morphology with noninferior axis ***Minor*** • Frequent ventricular extrasystoles (>500 per 24 h). nonsustained or sustained ventricular tachycardia of LBBB morphology with inferior axis ("RVOT pattern"!) • History of cardiac arrest due to ventricular fibrillation er sustained ventricular tachycardia of unknown morphology	***Minor*** • Frequent (>500 per 24 h) or exercise-induced ventricular extrasystoles with an RBBB morphology or multiple RBBB morphologies (excluding the "fascicular pattern") • Nonsustained or sustained ventricular tachycardia with an RBBB morphology (excluding the "fascicular pattern") • History of cardiac arrest due to ventricular fibrillation or sustained ventricular tachycardia of unknown morphology
VI. Family history/genetics	***Major*** • Identification of a pathogenic ACM-gene variant in the patient under evaluation • ACM confirmed in a first-degree relative who meets diagnostic criteria • ACM confirmed pathologically at autopsy or surgery in a first-degree relative ***Minor*** • Identification of a likely pathogenic ACM gene variant in patient under evaluation • History of ACM in a first-degree relative in whom it is not possible or practical to determine whether the family member meets diagnostic criteria • Premature sudden death (<35 years of age) due to suspected ACM in a first-degree relative • ACM confirmed pathologically or by diagnostic criteria in second-degree relative	

[a]Cut-off values of EDV and EF of the European TF criteria for, respectively, RV dilatation and systolic dysfunction are reported in Table 29.2.
[b]Septal junctional LGE at the RV insertion points.
ACM, arrhythmogenic cardiomyopathy; *BSA*, body surface area; *EDV*, end diastolic volume; *EF*, ejection fraction; *ITF*, international task force; *LBBB*, left bundle branch block; *LGE*, late gadolinium enhancement; *LV*, left ventricle; *RBBB*, right bundle-branch block; *RV*, right ventricle; *RVOT*, right ventricular outflow tract.
Adopted, with permission from Corrado D, Anastasakis A, Basso C et al. Proposed diagnostic criteria for arrhythmogenic cardiomyopathy: European task force consensus report. *Int J Cardiol*. 2024;395:131447.

fibrosis/scar and global or regional LV dysfunction, many experts in the field consider it to be difficult to reliably establish an isolated/predominant ALVC diagnosis based only on imaging without genetic or tissue-based confirmation.

Based on 2008 data from Sen-Chowdhry et al.,[33] which included the first detailed description of an LV-dominant ACM population, defined by the authors as desmoplakin disease, the CMR features of ALVC included LV LGE in 100% of the patients, with subepicardial and midwall LGE in 57.5%, and the majority of patients demonstrating LGE in the inferior and inferolateral wall. LV wall motion abnormalities (WMAs) were found in 61% of these patients, while mean LV ejection fraction (LVEF) and RV ejection fraction (RVEF) were preserved (54 ± 11% and 53 ± 7%). T-wave inversions in left precordial leads in the absence of complete left bundle branch block (LBBB) were noted in 40% of the patients.

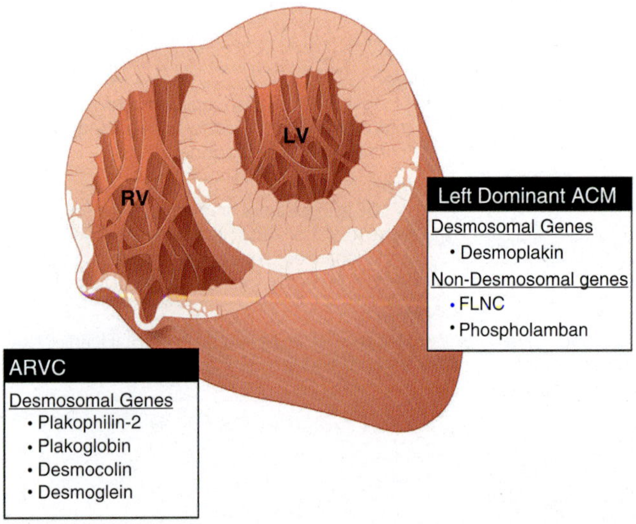

FIG. 29.4 Arrhythmogenic cardiomyopathy (*ACM*) phenotypes associated with different gene variants. Arrhythmogenic right ventricular cardiomyopathy (*ARVC*) is usually associated with variants in genes that encode desmosomal proteins, while both desmosomal and nondesmosomal genetic variants are seen in arrhythmogenic left ventricular cardiomyopathy. (Modified, with permission from Galizia MS, Attili AK, Truesdell WR et al. Imaging features of arrhythmogenic cardiomyopathies. *Radiographics*. 2024;44:e230154.)

Other very important data describing features in ALVC were provided by Casella et al.[4] In this important paper, the authors presented their carefully selected cohort of patients with ALVC based on the following strict diagnostic criteria:

1. Presence of a subepicardial LGE pattern with nonischemic distribution and fatty infiltration on CMR affecting exclusively the LV
   PLUS one of the following diagnostic features:
2. Positive genetic testing for pathogenic (class V)/likely pathogenic (class IV) variants associated with ARVC with LV involvement (namely desmoplakin, desmoglein-2 [DSG2], desmocollin-2, and plakoglobin [JUP])
3. Presence of fibrous AND fatty infiltration on an endomyocardial biopsy sample obtained from the left ventricle in one of the areas presenting LGE on CMR

The authors excluded patients without genetic testing or with known myocardial disease from their analysis. On CMR, subepicardial LGE and fibrofatty replacement in the left ventricle was detected in 100% patients.

According to the 2020 ACM "Padua criteria"[9], genetic testing is a crucial initial step for the diagnosis of ALVC, but LV enlargement was not required as a diagnostic criterion for ALVC (Table 29.2). A combination of LV structural criteria and ACM gene mutation and absence of the RV structural criteria defined the AVLC. Importantly, in this patient population, no transthoracic echocardiography or CMR study yielded a major criterion for ARVC diagnosis according to the 2010 TFC criteria.

Most recent 2023 European TFC[27] take into consideration a combination of genetic, historical/familial, histological (based on the endomyocardial biopsy results), ECG, and morphofunctional factors, similar to the diagnosis of ARVC based on the 2010 TFC. In contrast to the 2010 TFC, this new set of ACM criteria separately defines the RV and LV ACM phenotypes (Table 29.3). This new comprehensive set of TFC, in our understanding, brings a significant improvement in diagnostic accuracy, allowing the identification of many patients who may clearly present with a typical ALVC phenotype but would otherwise be missed by the 2010 TFC.

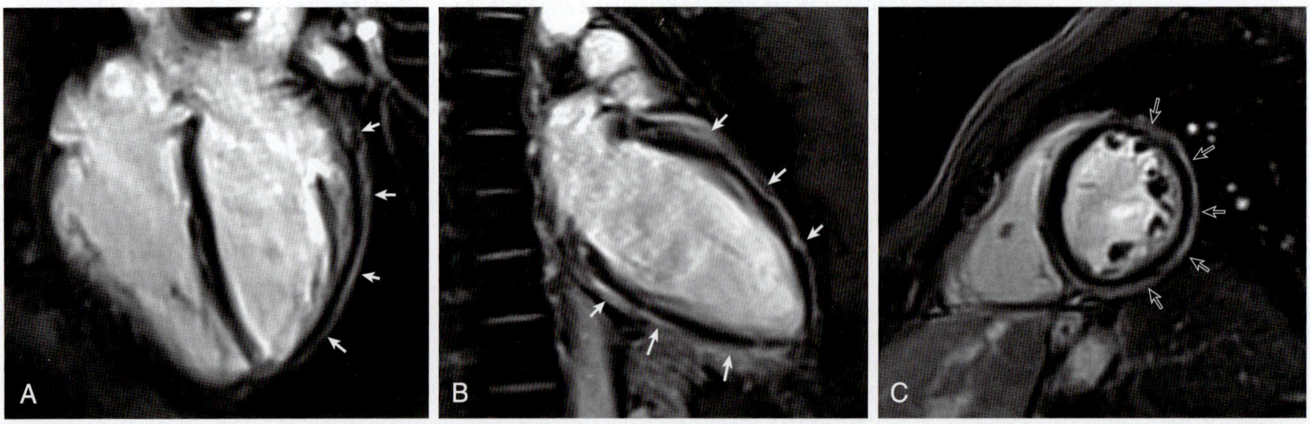

FIG. 29.5 LGE/myocardial fibrosis in arrhythmogenic left ventricular cardiomyopathy (ALVC or left-dominant ACM) phenotype. CMR images of a 24-year-old patient with a pathogenic desmoplakin gene variant. Postcontrast images: long-axis 4-chamber view (A) and long-axis 2-chamber view (B) showing a large amount of LV subepicardial LGE (*solid arrows*) extending from basal-to-apical segments. The involvement of the LV free wall and septum with a "ringlike" pattern in the short-axis view is noted (C, *open arrows*). *ACM*, Arrhythmogenic cardiomyopathy; *ALVC*, arrhythmogenic left ventricular cardiomyopathy; *CMR*, cardiac magnetic resonance; *LGE*, late gadolinium enhancement; *LV*, left ventricular. (Reproduced, with permission from Corrado D, Anastasakis A, Basso C, et al. Proposed diagnostic criteria for arrhythmogenic cardiomyopathy: European task force consensus report. *Int J Cardiol*. 2024;395:131447.)

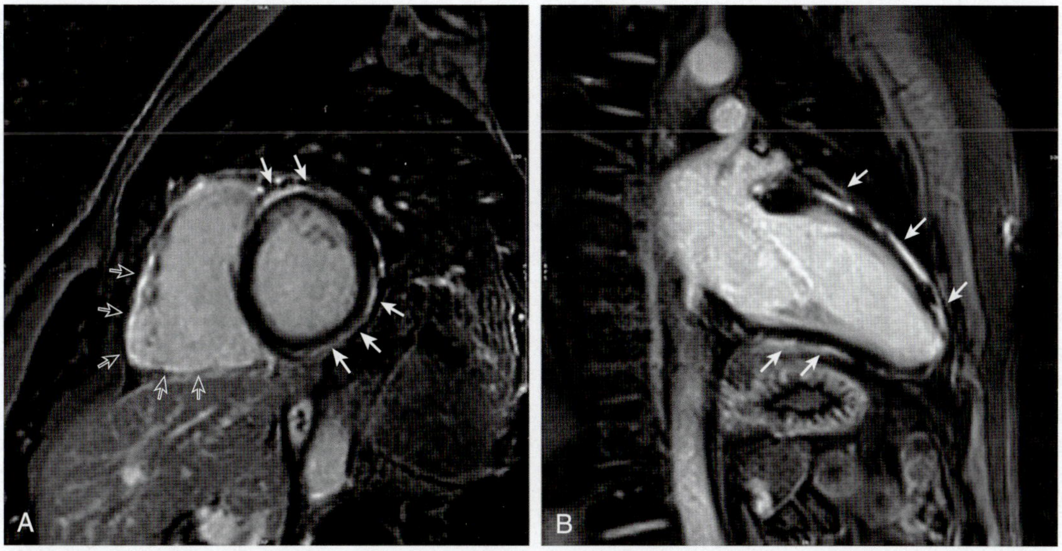

FIG. 29.6 **LGE/myocardial fibrosis in biventricular arrhythmogenic cardiomyopathy phenotype.** CMR images of a 40-year-old patient with a pathogenic DSG-2 gene variant. Postcontrast images: short-axis view (A) and long-axis 2-chamber view (B) showing LGE/myocardial fibrosis in the basal anterolateral RV wall (*open arrows*) and anterior and inferior/inferolateral LV wall (*solid arrows*). *ACM*, arrhythmogenic cardiomyopathy; *CMR*, cardiac magnetic resonance; *DSG-2*, desmoglein-2 gene; *LGE*, late gadolinium enhancement; *LV*, left ventricle; *RV*, right ventricle. (Reproduced, with permission from Sen-Chowdhry S, Morgan RD, Chambers JC, McKenna WJ. Arrhythmogenic cardiomyopathy: etiology, diagnosis, and treatment. *Annu Rev Med.* 2010;61:233–253.)

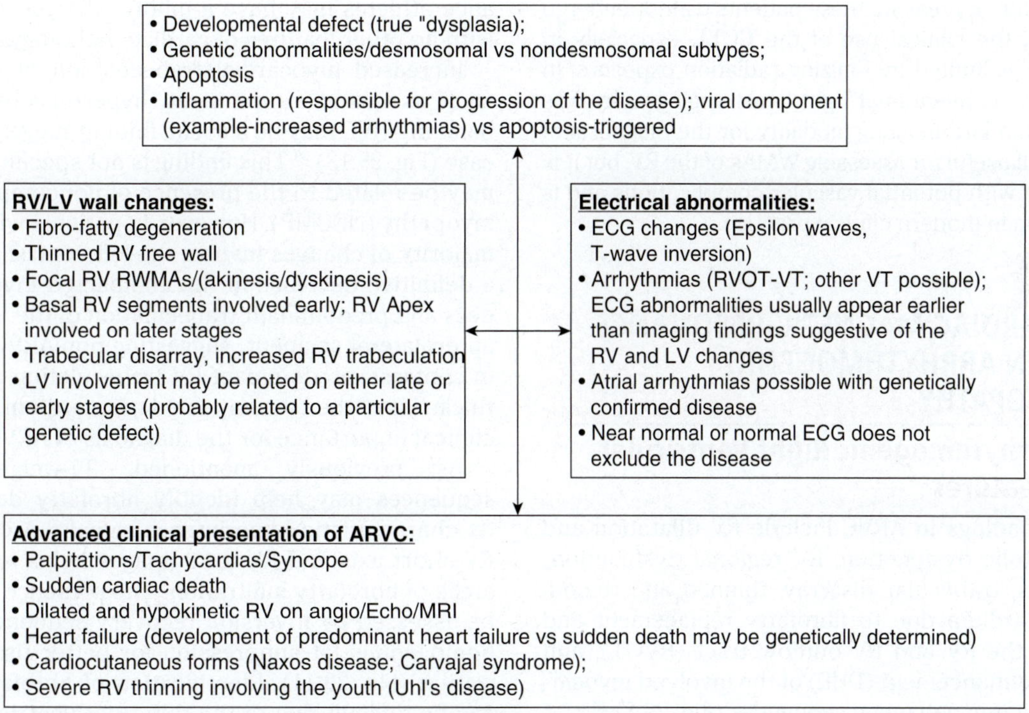

FIG. 29.7 Etiopathological considerations in arrhythmogenic cardiomyopathies. *ECG*, electrocardiogram; *LV*, left ventricle; *MRI*, magnetic resonance imaging; *RV*, right ventricle; *RVOT*, right ventricular outflow tract; *RWMA*, regional wall motion abnormality; *VT*, ventricular tachycardia. (Reproduced, with permission from Abidov A, Oliva IB, Marcus FI. Cardiac MRI in the Diagnosis, Clinical Management and Prognosis of Arrhyhtmogenic Right Ventricular Cardiomyopathy/Dysplasia. Academic Press/Elsevier, 2016.)

The complexity of clinical and diagnostic findings in patients with known and suspected ACM is presented in Fig. 29.7.[34] Regardless of the ACM subtype, careful evaluation of the patient's clinical history as well as the results of any relevant testing prior to the index CMR, is needed. This is one of the mandatory rules for cardiac imagers supervising the scan for patients with known or suspected ACM. When the patient has a history of palpitations and syncope, family history of sudden death, abnormal ECG with inverted T waves in right precordial leads (in case of suspected ARVC) or left precordial leads in the absence of complete LBBB (with suspected ALVC), frequent premature ventricular contractions (PVCs) on Holter monitor, and evidence of RV or LV global and/or regional dysfunction or enlargement on a recent echocardiogram, the level of pretest likelihood of this patient having ACM is high. Accordingly, the significance of any CMR abnormality in the patient is weighed differently from a patient with a low pretest likelihood of ACM. If the pretest likelihood of ACM is high, but the CMR appears normal, the cardiologist should consider additional testing and close follow-up to make sure that the patient is safe. During the follow-up, the focus may switch to identification of electrical abnormalities such as ECG or Holter monitoring.

It is important to note that the diagnosis of ACM does not always require an abnormal CMR. Various imaging techniques are available for evaluating the morphological changes of ACM and include two-dimensional transthoracic echocardiography, CMR radionuclide angiography, multidetector cardiac computed tomography (CT), and RV angiography. The conventional two-dimensional transthoracic echocardiogram (TTE) and three-dimensional TTE are readily available with no radiation exposure. The echocardiogram is useful to assess regional LV and RV akinesia, dyskinesia, or focal aneurysms and assess RV dimensions, which are an important part of the TFC.[2] However, the diagnostic accuracy may decrease when there is a poor acoustic window, especially with a dilated right ventricle. Cardiac CTA (CCTA) can also aid in assessing the myocardial changes in ACM such as RV and LV dilatation, prominent trabeculation, and scalloped surface of the RV free wall by providing three-dimensional assessment and even revealing fatty infiltration of the LV or RV myocardium; CCTA may be useful in patients with ICDs or pacemakers if, for any reason, these patients cannot undergo CMR. However, the clinical use of the CCTA, especially in young patients, is limited by ionizing radiation exposure. In the original TFC, conventional right heart angiography was considered a standard imaging modality for the diagnosis of ARVC and is still useful for assessing WMAs of the RV, but it is an invasive test with potential vascular complications and is very uncommon in modern clinical practice.

TYPICAL CARDIAC MAGNETIC RESONANCE FINDINGS IN ARRHYTHMOGENIC CARDIOMYOPATHY

"Classic" Arrhythmogenic Right Ventricular Dysplasia Features

Typical CMR findings in ARVC include RV dilatation and global RV systolic dysfunction, RV regional dysfunction/regional WMAs, trabecular disarray, thinned and remodeled RV myocardium due to fibrofatty replacement and aneurysms of the RV and RV outflow tract (RVOT), and delayed hyperenhancement (DHE) of the involved myocardium on gadolinium-enhanced sequences (Fig. 29.8).[35]

The 2010 ARVC TFC require the presence of qualitative WMAs and increased indexed end diastolic volume (EDV) or reduced ejection fraction (Fig. 29.9). If either RV size or RVEF abnormality fit the TFC and there is RV WMA, the patient would be classified as having a major criterion. The sensitivity of RV size or dysfunction alone is reported to range from 41% to 50% for major criteria and 31%–41% for minor criteria. The sensitivity increases from 79% to 89% for major criteria and from 68% to 78% for minor criteria when using indexed RVEDV (area) or RVEF (function).[2] The role of CMR in the diagnosis of ACM includes demonstrating and identifying intramyocardial fat deposits, pathological myocardial wall inflammation, and fibrosis leading to thinning and aneurysmal changes in the myocardium.

Fatty infiltration of the RV appears bright on T1-weighted sequences in an otherwise normal myocardium that has intermediate intense signal (Fig. 29.10).[36–38] A similar process was shown to involve the left ventricle (Fig. 29.11).

The ventricular anatomical and functional assessment is usually done with T1-weighted, bright-blood, steady-state free precession (SSFP) sequences. These sequences help assess the presence of aneurysms or dilatation of the right ventricle. Cine sequences of the ventricle permit an assessment of the WMAs and volumetric quantification of RV function. It also helps to assess involvement of the RVOT and left ventricle. This is particularly valuable in evaluating patients with different phenotypes who may have a BiV-ACM or LV dominant disease, such as those with desmoplakin gene mutations in whom there is marked involvement of the left ventricle with relative sparing of the right ventricle.[33]

The most important CMR finding to determine the presence of ARVC is assessment of RV size (one of the major TFC). However, the size of the RV is not a specific sign of ARVC (Fig. 29.12): RV enlargement may be present in many other pathological conditions, such as pulmonary embolus, congenital diseases causing RV volume/pressure overload, RV infarction, and cor pulmonale. Some endurance athletes may have a mildly enlarged RV cavity size, with no other features of cardiac pathology.

Increased myocardial trabeculation of the right ventricle as well as a prominent (hyperreflective) moderator band in ARVC may be a useful finding suggestive of the disease (Fig. 29.13).[39] This finding is not specific for ARVC and may be related to the presence of noncompaction cardiomyopathy (NCCMP). However, in patients with NCCMP, the majority of changes involve the left ventricle, and there is a definitive decrease in the compacted myocardial thickness and predominant trabeculation of the apex and distal anterolateral segment, suggesting non-ARVC/D pathology. In contrast, predominant RV trabeculation and preserved thickness of the LV compacted myocardium are findings of clinical importance for the diagnosis of ARVC.

As previously mentioned, T1-weighted imaging sequences may help identify fibrofatty deposition with its characteristic hyperintense signal.[40] A combination of RV short axis and RV axial images helps analyze smaller areas of fibrofatty infiltration. The presence of fat can also be assessed by inversion recovery sequences that cause homogenous fat suppression for better tissue characterization (Fig. 29.11). Identification of fibrofatty infiltration can be difficult due to the thin right ventricle and motion artifacts of the RV free wall. Arrhythmias may decrease the sensitivity of this identification. The presence of intramyocardial fat deposition is not pathognomonic for ARVC as it may be found in normal hearts.[41]

Assessment of Global and Regional Myocardial Function

ACM (and especially, ARVC) is characterized by infiltrative and subsequent inflammatory changes of the involved ventricle that lead to regional as well as global myocardial dysfunction. The morphological changes may not be readily apparent in the early subclinical phase. The MRI cine sequences with SSFP methodology can assist in assessing

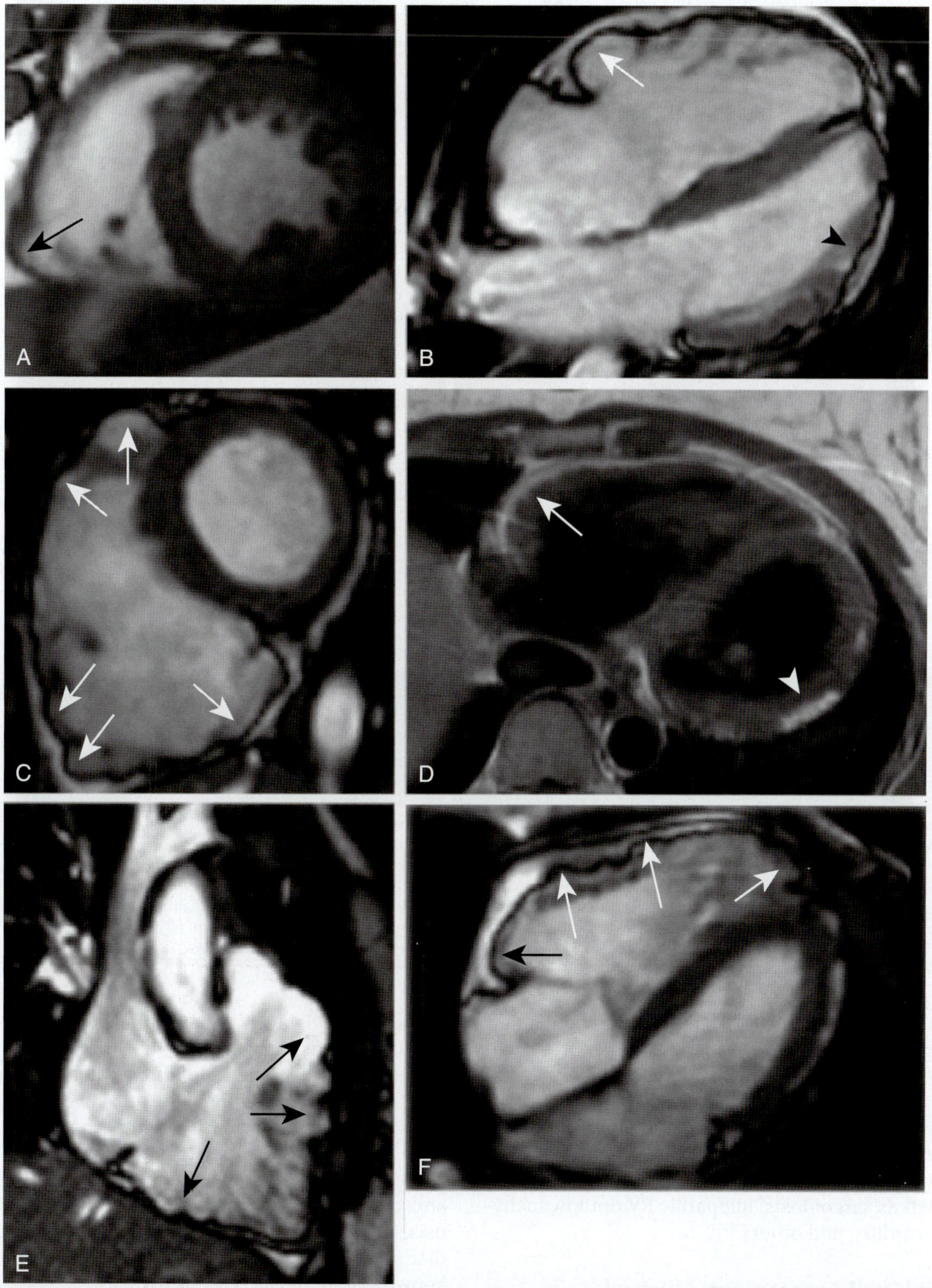

FIG. 29.8 CMR evidence of focal and regional RV systolic dysfunction and abnormal RV structure in ARVC. (A) Short-axis bright-blood image showing dyskinesis of the acute angle (*arrow*). (B) Horizontal long-axis bright-blood image showing subtricuspid bulging (*arrow*). Subepicardial fatty infiltration and wall thinning of the LV apicolateral region (*arrowhead*) is present. (C) Short-axis bright-blood image showing a dilated RV with microaneurysms and dyskinesis of the inferior wall, acute angle, and anterior wall of the RV (*arrows*). (D) T1-weighted image reveals moderate subepicardial fat infiltration of the RV anterior wall, extending as "fingers" into the myocardium (*arrow*). Note fatty infiltration in the LV lateral wall (*arrowhead*). (E) RVOT bright-blood image showing dyskinesis of the RVOT and RV inferior wall (*arrows*). (F) Horizontal long-axis bright-blood image showing dyskinesis of the subtricuspid region, RV anterior wall, and RV apex (*arrows*). *ARVD/C*, arrhythmogenic right ventricular dysplasia/cardiomyopathy; *CMR*, cardiac magnetic resonance; *RV*, right ventricular; *RVOT*, right ventricular outflow tract. (Reproduced with permission from Te Riele AS, James CA, Philips B, et al. Mutation-positive arrhythmogenic right ventricular dysplasia/cardiomyopathy: the triangle of dysplasia displaced. *J Cardiovasc Electrophysiol*. 2013;24:1311–1320.)

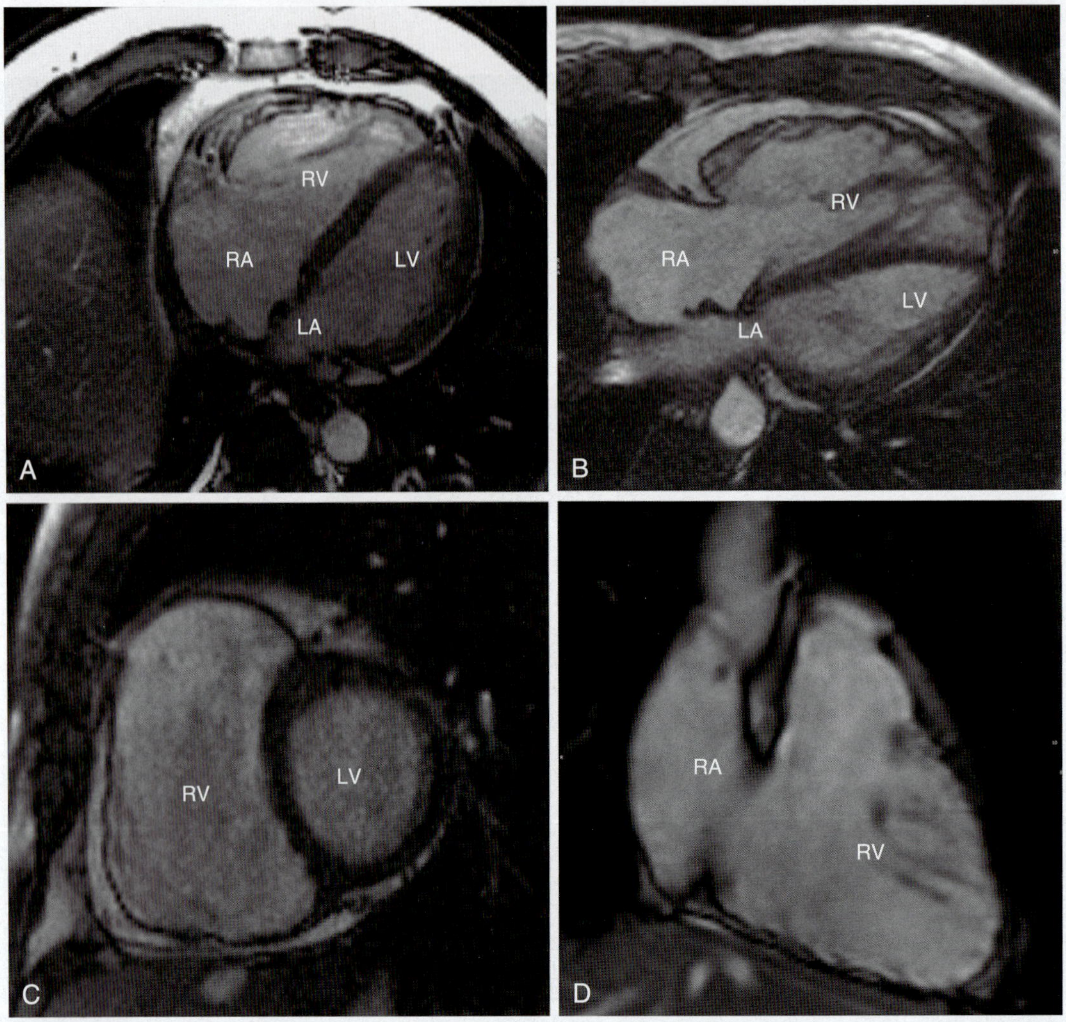

FIG. 29.9 Arrhythmogenic right ventricular cardiomyopathy appearance on cardiac magnetic resonance images. The images represent a balanced steady-state free precession sequences of patients with confirmed arrhythmogenic right ventricular cardiomyopathy/dysplasia. On all images, the right ventricle (*RV*) is dilated; cine images confirmed the presence of RV systolic dysfunction, with right ventricular ejection fraction (RVEF) <40%. (A) Axial view of predominantly basal/subtricuspid enlargement of the RV with relatively spared RV apex. (B and C) Axial and short-axis views showing diffuse RV enlargement with multiple small focal RV free wall outpouchings. (D) Dedicated RV inflow/outflow view, showing multiple small focal RV posterior wall outpouchings and focal RV outflow aneurysm. *LA*, left atrium; *LV*, left ventricle; *RA*, right atrium. (Reproduced with permission from Abidov A, Oliva IB, Marcus FI. Cardiac MRI in the Diagnosis, Clinical Management and Prognosis of Arrhyhtmogenic Right Ventricular Cardiomyopathy/Dysplasia. Academic Press/Elsevier, 2016.)

regional and global LV and RV function. For right-sided disease, regional WMAs can be seen in the RV free wall, outflow tract, and apex and can be homogenous or heterogeneous in distribution. As the disease progresses, CMR can definitively identify increased RV volume (increased RVEDV) and lower RV output (RVEF).[42]

CMR also helps to differentiate ARVC/D from mimicking diseases such as sarcoidosis, idiopathic RV outflow tachycardia, myocarditis, and others.[43–49]

Myocardial Wall Assessment: "Virtual Histology" Assessment Using Cardiac Magnetic Resonance

One of the hallmarks of ARVC is the development of myocardial fibrofatty infiltration and fibrosis. The resulting scarring can be readily identified with LGE images (Fig. 29.14).

In the fibrotic or scarred myocardium, there is an increase in the volume of distribution of gadolinium due to interstitial space expansion. This results in a hyperintense signal in the delayed enhancement images in those myocardial regions.[50] Ever since LGE sequences were introduced, it has become helpful to evaluate the presence of scar in the myocardium. The presence of LGE has been shown to correlate well with histopathology and to predict future occurrence of ventricular tachycardia.[51,52]

Delayed hyperenhancement is not specific for ARVC/D and can be seen in mimics of ARVC/D including sarcoidosis, myocarditis, and even in RV infarction. Overall, cardiac imagers should consider their findings following known LGE patterns (Fig. 29.15).[53]

Cardiac Magnetic Resonance Features of Arrhythmogenic Right Ventricular Dysplasia and Biventricular Arrhythmogenic Cardiomyopathy

By definition, the diagnosis of BiV-ACM requires the presence of disease features in both ventricles. As ARVC is a more common type of ACM, the presence of fibrofatty or

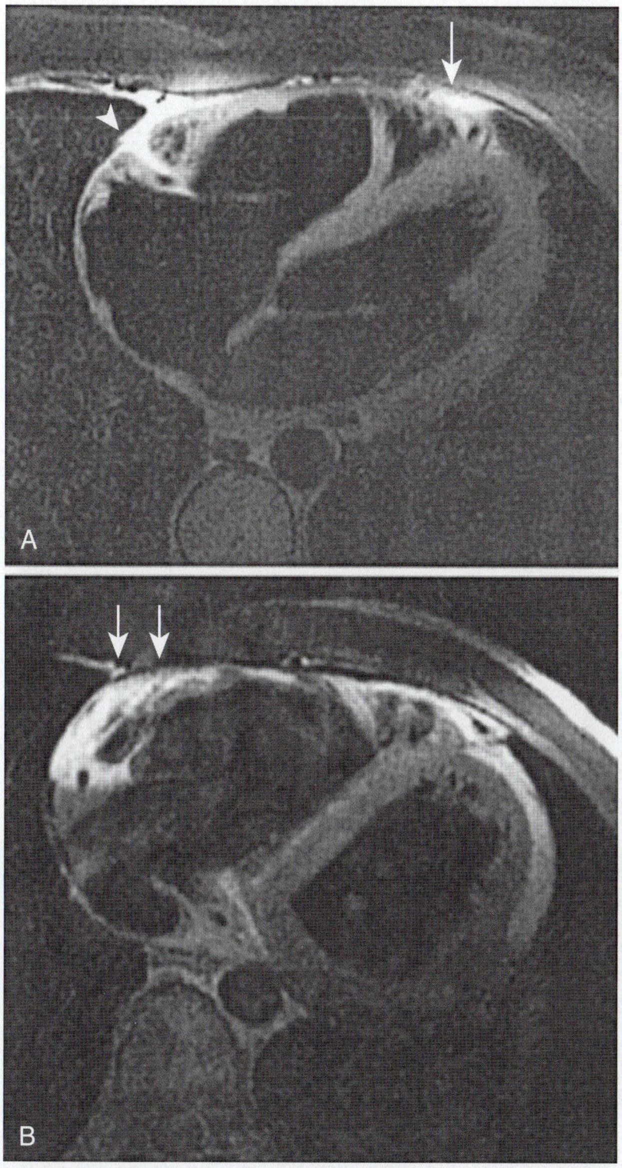

FIG. 29.10 Differences in epicardial fat appearance in normal volunteer versus patient with arrhythmogenic right ventricular cardiomyopathy. (A) Axial black-blood image from a normal volunteer showing a clear line of demarcation between the epicardial fat and underlying myocardium. Also note the abundance of epicardial fat in the atrioventricular groove (*arrowhead*) and at the apex (*arrow*). (B) Axial black-blood image from a patient with right ventricular dysplasia showing lack of demarcation between epicardial fat and myocardium (*arrows*). (Reproduced with permission from Tandri H, Bomma C, Calkins H, Bluemke DA. Magnetic resonance and computed tomography imaging of arrhythmogenic right ventricular dysplasia. *J Magn Reson Imaging*. 2004;19:848–858.)

fibrotic LV changes, especially LGE, with or without global LV dysfunction or dilatation and/or regional LV WMAs, that is unexplained by any other condition in patients with an otherwise established diagnosis of ARVC, leads to a diagnosis of BiV-ACM. In a less frequent scenario, a patient with established/dominant ALVC may also have CMR features suggestive of RV involvement.

Both possible clinical scenarios above require a cardiac imager to perform an exhaustive image analysis for both ventricles, even in cases with a well-defined right-sided disease.

According to Sen-Chowdhry et al.,[33] CMR features of ALVC include LV LGE in 100% of patients, subepicardial and midwall LGE in 57.5%, and LGE in the inferior and inferolateral wall in the majority of patients (Fig. 29.16). In the LV-dominant subtype of ACM, 55% of patients had septal involvement, while the LGE in "classic" ARVC typically spares septum.

According to M. Casella et al.,[4] subepicardial LGE and fibrofatty replacement in the left ventricle on CMR was detected in 100% of patients. Disease distribution showed a marked preference for the lateral (76%) and posterior basal (72%) LV segments, with only 2 (8%) patients presenting with nonisolated LV septal involvement.

Based on "Padua criteria,"[9] genetic testing is a crucial initial step for the diagnosis of ALVC, but LV enlargement is not required as a diagnostic criterion. Importantly, in this patient population, no transthoracic echocardiography or CMR study yielded a major criterion for ARVC diagnosis according to the 2010 TFC criteria. RV parameters in these patients were within normal limits.

Most recent 2023 European TFC[27] provided separate sets of major and minor diagnostic criteria for the RV and LV ACM phenotypes (Table 29.3). Based on these criteria, specific LV LGE predicting myocardial scar shows a distinct appearance, typically in the subepicardial or occasionally in the midmyocardial layers of the LV free wall, mainly in the inferolateral region. The 2023 TFC document further states that due to its high specificity, LV LGE involving ≥3 segments on the short-axis (SAX) myocardial fibrosis polar map, either contiguous in the same slice with a "ringlike" pattern or is continuous, is considered a major criterion. Segmental LV LGE affecting 1 or 2 LV polar map segments is classified as a minor criterion. Patchy or focal LV LGE is considered nondiagnostic and lacks clinical relevance in the absence of other abnormal findings. The document further notes that "septal junctional" LGE at RV insertion points is not indicative of ACM due to its nonpathological significance. Also, while the finding of fatty tissue alone is not considered a diagnostic criterion, its identification using CMR or multidetector computed tomography (MDCT)–dedicated sequences in regions of LGE/scar strengthen diagnostic specificity.[54]

Contrary to the RV phenotype criteria (in which RV dilatation and/or RV global systolic dysfunction in addition to RV focal regional wall motion abnormalities [RWMAs] are major diagnostic criteria for RV-ACM), the new 2023 TFC consider LV LGE in a specific, extensive (≥3 segments), ringlike subepicardial or midmyocardial pattern a major ALVC criterion, while global LV dysfunction with or without LV dilatation (increase in the LVEDV indexed to BSA; Table 29.4) is only a minor LV-ACM criterion.

Limitations of Cardiac Magnetic Resonance

CMR has several limitations in evaluating ACM. The protocols are operator dependent. Experienced CMR technicians are likely to obtain a diagnostic study compared to those with a weak knowledge of the diagnostic targets. The presence of an expert physician during acquisition may significantly improve the diagnostic yield of the test. The ability of the patient to cooperate with the study protocol, breath-holds, and

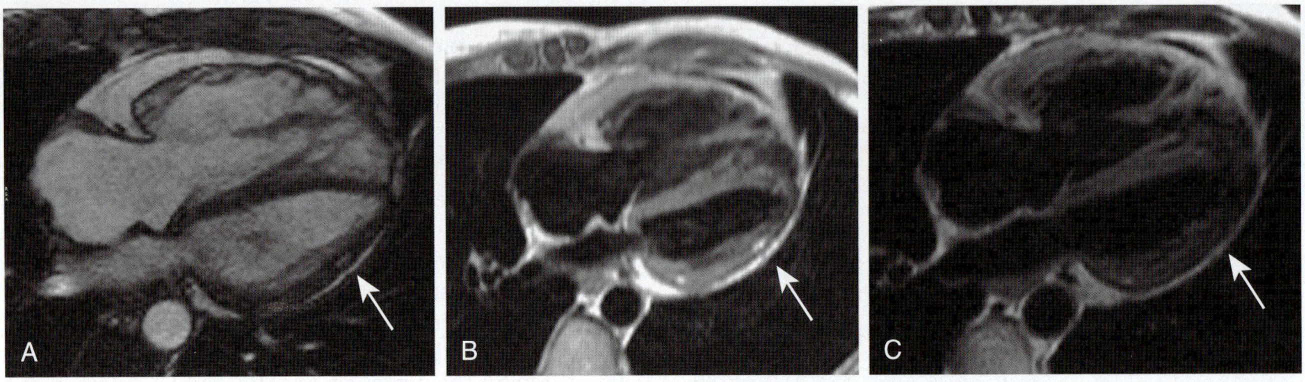

FIG. 29.11 Tissue characterization of cardiac magnetic resonance allows differentiation of left ventricular (LV) fatty infiltration in a patient with arrhythmogenic right ventricular cardiomyopathy (ARVC). All images were obtained on the same slice position for consistency. (A) Steady-state free precession (*bright-blood*) axial image revealing a pathological right ventricle with ARVC/dysplasia features as well as a small focal subepicardial signal in the distal anterolateral left ventricular (LV) wall. (B) Turbo-spin echo (TSE) (*black-blood*, T2-weighted) images show a hyperintense signal (comparable in brightness with the subcutaneous fat) in the same area of the LV. (C) Triple inversion recovery sequence (STIR) suppressing fat signal and demonstrating a hypointense signal in the distal anterolateral LV wall, thus confirming the lipid-rich composition of the LV wall lesion. (Reproduced with permission from Abidov A, Oliva IB, Marcus FI. Cardiac MRI in the Diagnosis, Clinical Management and Prognosis of Arrhyhtmogenic Right Ventricular Cardiomyopathy/Dysplasia. Academic Press/Elsevier, 2016.)

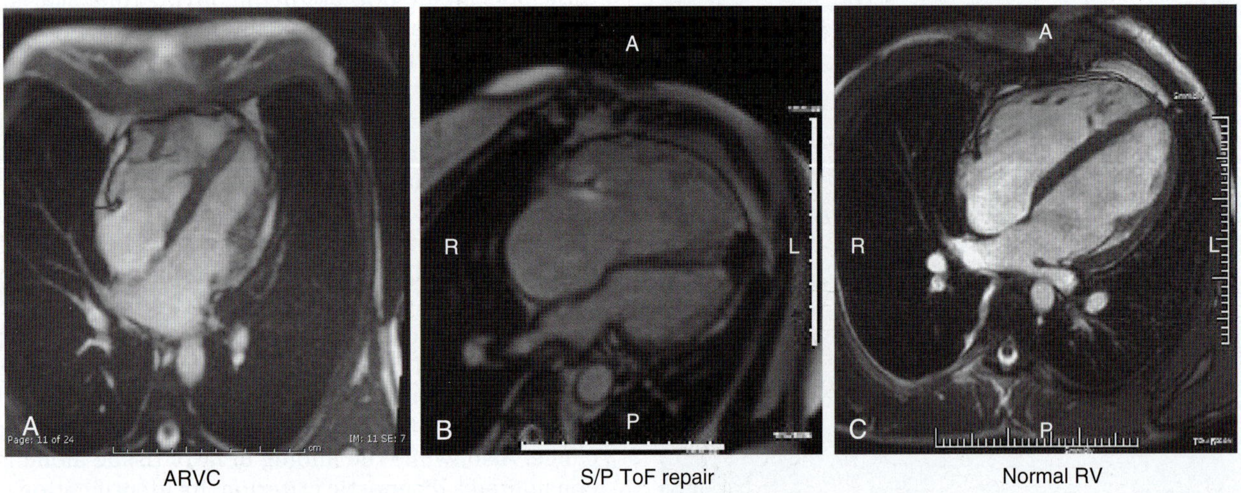

FIG. 29.12 Examples of the right ventricular enlargement on cardiac magnetic resonance. (A) A patient with advanced arrhythmogenic right ventricular cardiomyopathy. (B) A patient with severe pulmonary regurgitation and s/p tetralogy of Fallot repair. (C) Endurance athlete with no cardiac pathology. (Reproduced with permission from Abidov A, Oliva IB, Marcus FI. Cardiac MRI in the Diagnosis, Clinical Management and Prognosis of Arrhyhtmogenic Right Ventricular Cardiomyopathy/Dysplasia. Academic Press/Elsevier, 2016.)

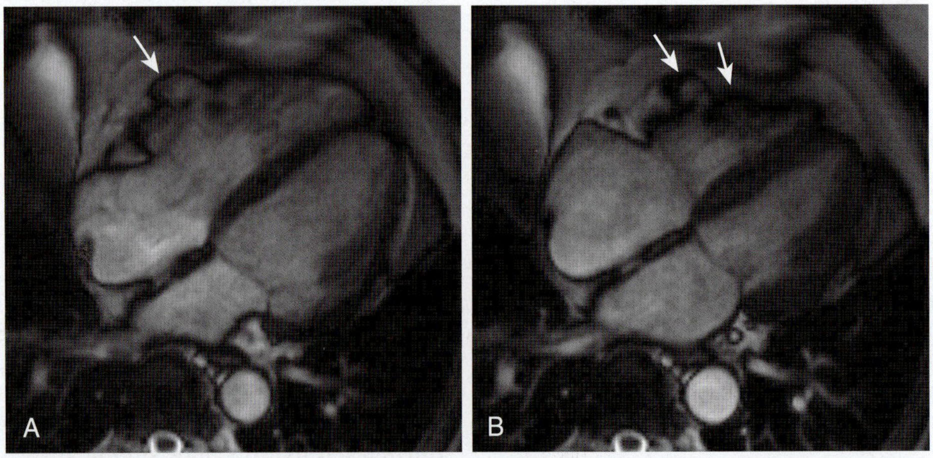

FIG. 29.13 Typical cardiac magnetic resonance features of a patient with arrhythmogenic right ventricular cardiomyopathy; dilated right ventricle, global right ventricular (RV) systolic dysfunction; trabecular disarray, focal aneurysms of the RV free wall. (A) Diastole. (B) Systole. (Reproduced with permission from Karamitsos TD, Francis JM, Myerson S, Selvanayagam JB, Neubauer S. The role of cardiovascular magnetic resonance imaging in heart failure. *J Am Coll Cardiol*. 2009;54:1407–1424.)

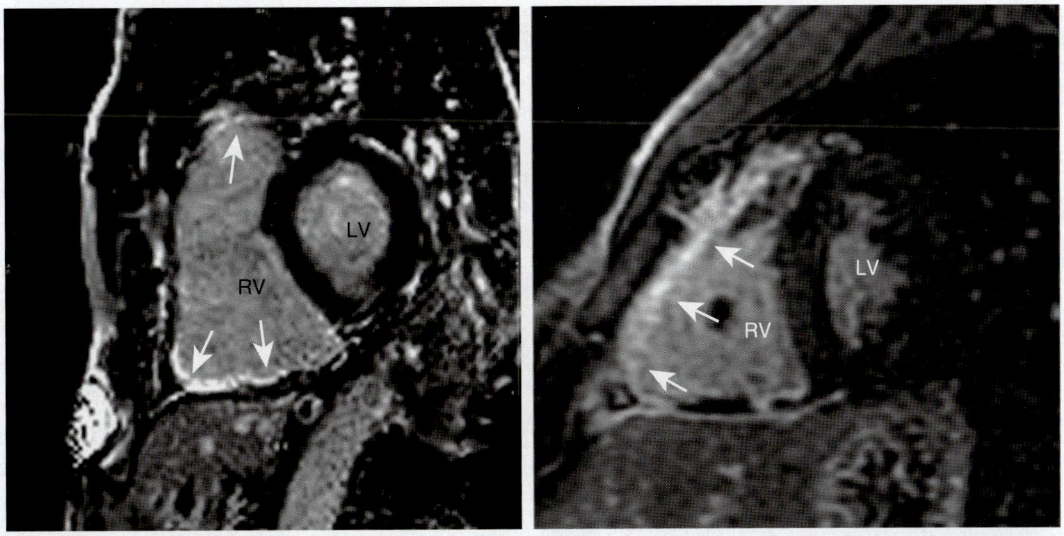

FIG. 29.14 Evidence of extensive right ventricular fibrotic changes (*white arrows*) **in patients** with advanced arrhythmogenic right ventricular cardiomyopathy on delayed-enhancement cardiac magnetic resonance imaging. *LV*, left ventricle; *RV*, right ventricle. (Reproduced with permission from Abidov A, Oliva IB, Marcus FI. Cardiac MRI in the Diagnosis, Clinical Management and Prognosis of Arrhyhtmogenic Right Ventricular Cardiomyopathy/Dysplasia. London, UK: Academic Press/ Elsevier, 2016.)

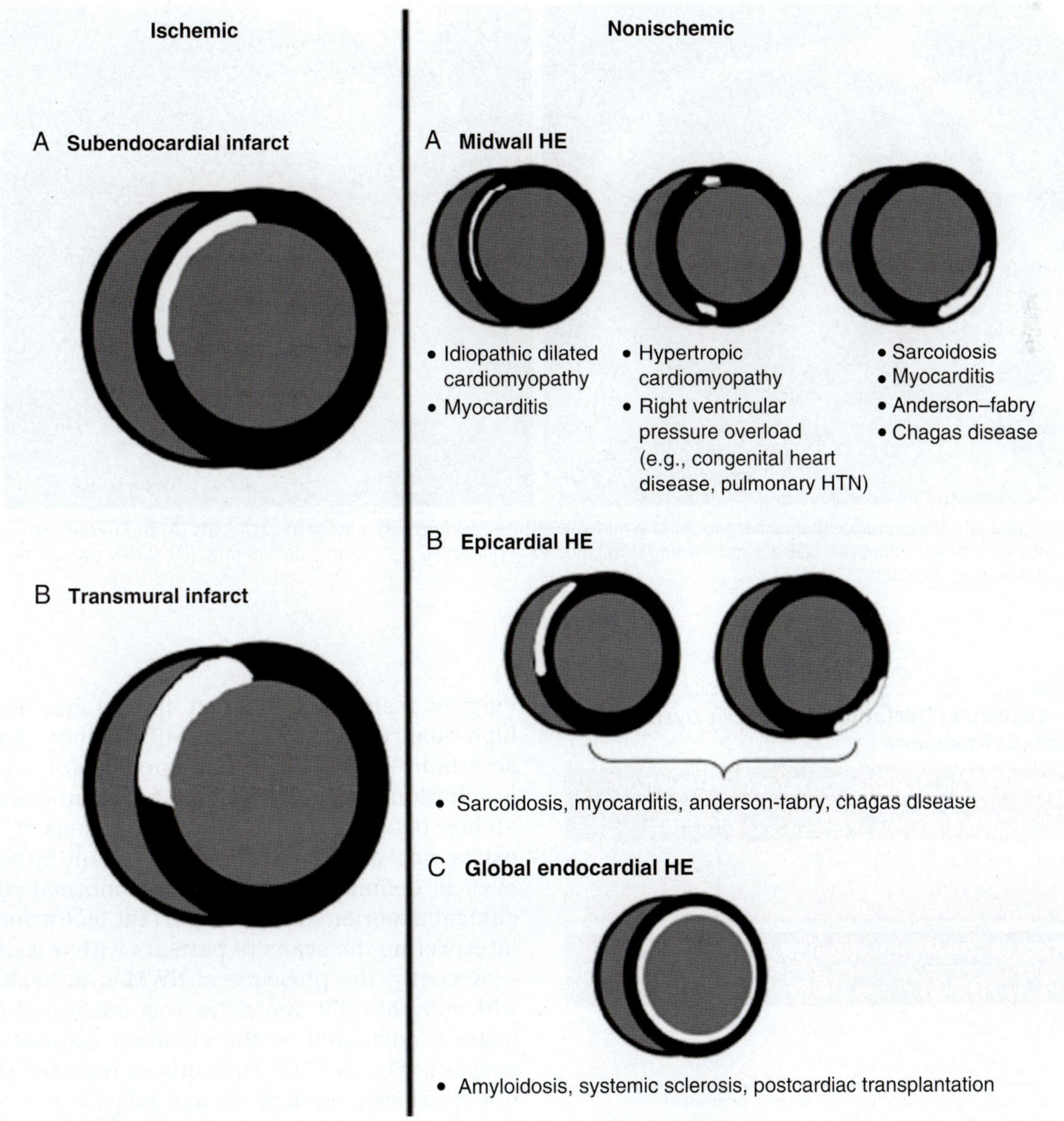

FIG. 29.15 Patterns of delayed gadolinium hyperenhancement on cardiac magnetic resonance. *HE, h*yperenhacement; *HTN*, hypertension. (From Edelman RR, et al., eds. Clinical Magnetic Resonance Imaging, 3rd ed. Elsevier Press; 2005.)

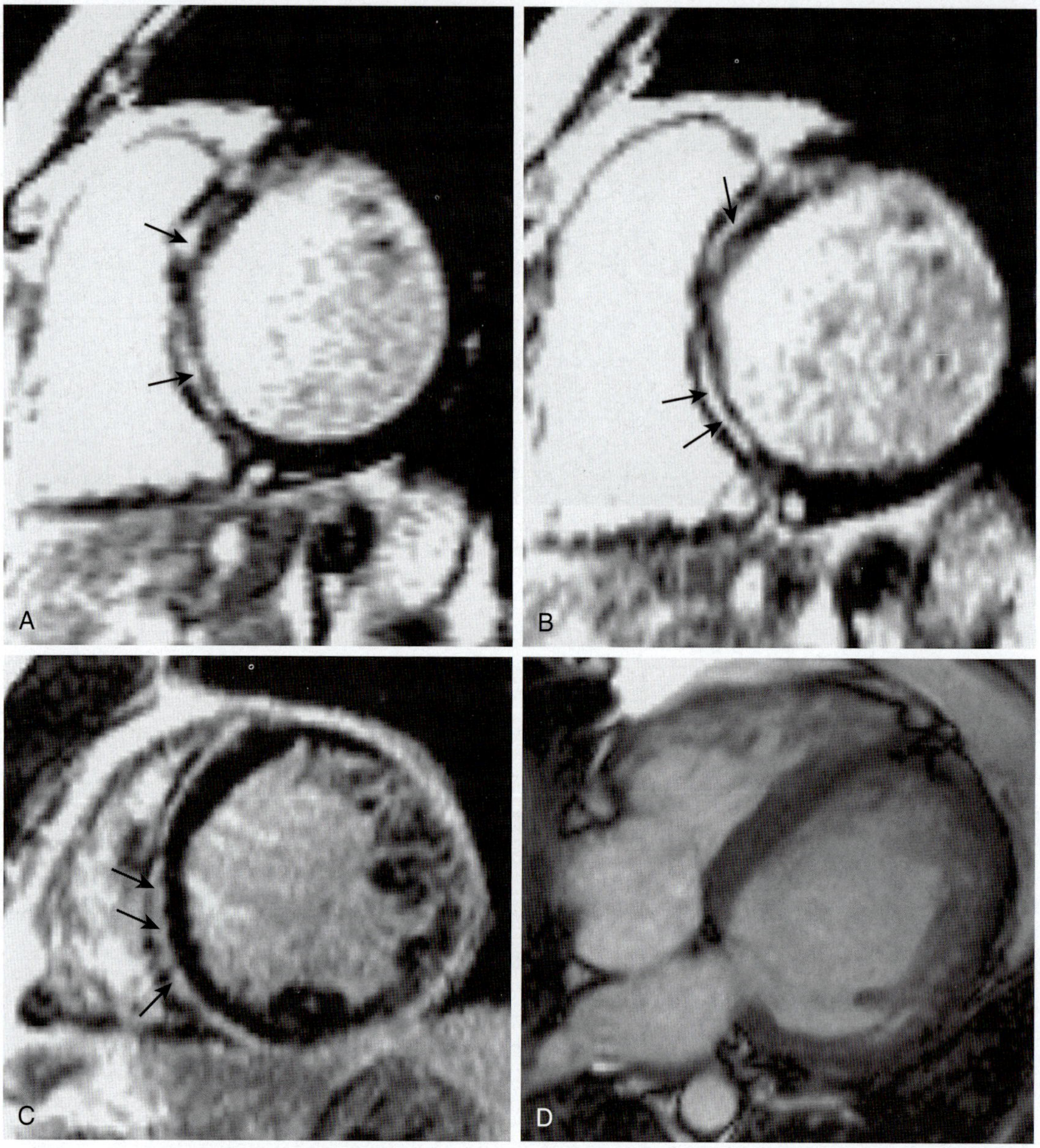

FIG. 29.16 The first had late gadolinium enhancement (LGE) in a midwall distribution (*arrows*), patchy in basal cuts (A) but becoming more confluent at midlevel (B). The second had circumferential LGE (C) and marked LV dilation with preserved right ventricular volumes (D), far exceeding the LV enlargement observed in the remainder of the cohort.

TABLE 29.4 Ventricular Dilatation and Systolic Dysfunction By Cardiac Magnetic Resonance.

RIGHT VENTRICULAR DILATATION AND SYSTOLIC DYSFUNCTION			
	FEMALES	MALES	ATHLETES
EDV/BSA (mL/m²)	>112	>121	>130
EF (%)	<51	<52	<52

LEFT VENTRICULAR DILATATION AND SYSTOLIC DYSFUNCTION			
	FEMALES	MALES	ATHLETES
EDV/BSA (mL/m²)	>96	>105	>122
EF (%)	<57	<57	<58

BSA, body surface area; *EDV*, end-diastolic volume; *EF*, ejection fraction.
Adopted, with permission from Corrado D, Anastasakis A, Basso C et al. Proposed diagnostic criteria for arrhythmogenic cardiomyopathy: European task force consensus report. *Int J Cardiol*. 2024;395:131447.

lengthy testing, is of great importance for obtaining high-quality CMR images. CMR findings that are characteristic of ACM are not specific for the disease.[51] In addition, there can be significant intraobserver variability between interpreting physicians.[40,55] Variability exists not only in defining the quantitative data, but even in defining normal versus abnormal scans. Again, clinical experience is an important factor for accurately interpreting the scans of patients with possible ACM.

Recently, the presence of RWMAs in healthy subjects with normal right ventricles was confirmed by 3-T CMR imaging compared to the standard acquisition on 1.5-T magnets (Fig. 29.17).[56] The authors reported the presence of hypokinesis, dyskinesis, and bulging in 92% of healthy patients and involvement of two or more segments in 60% of cases.

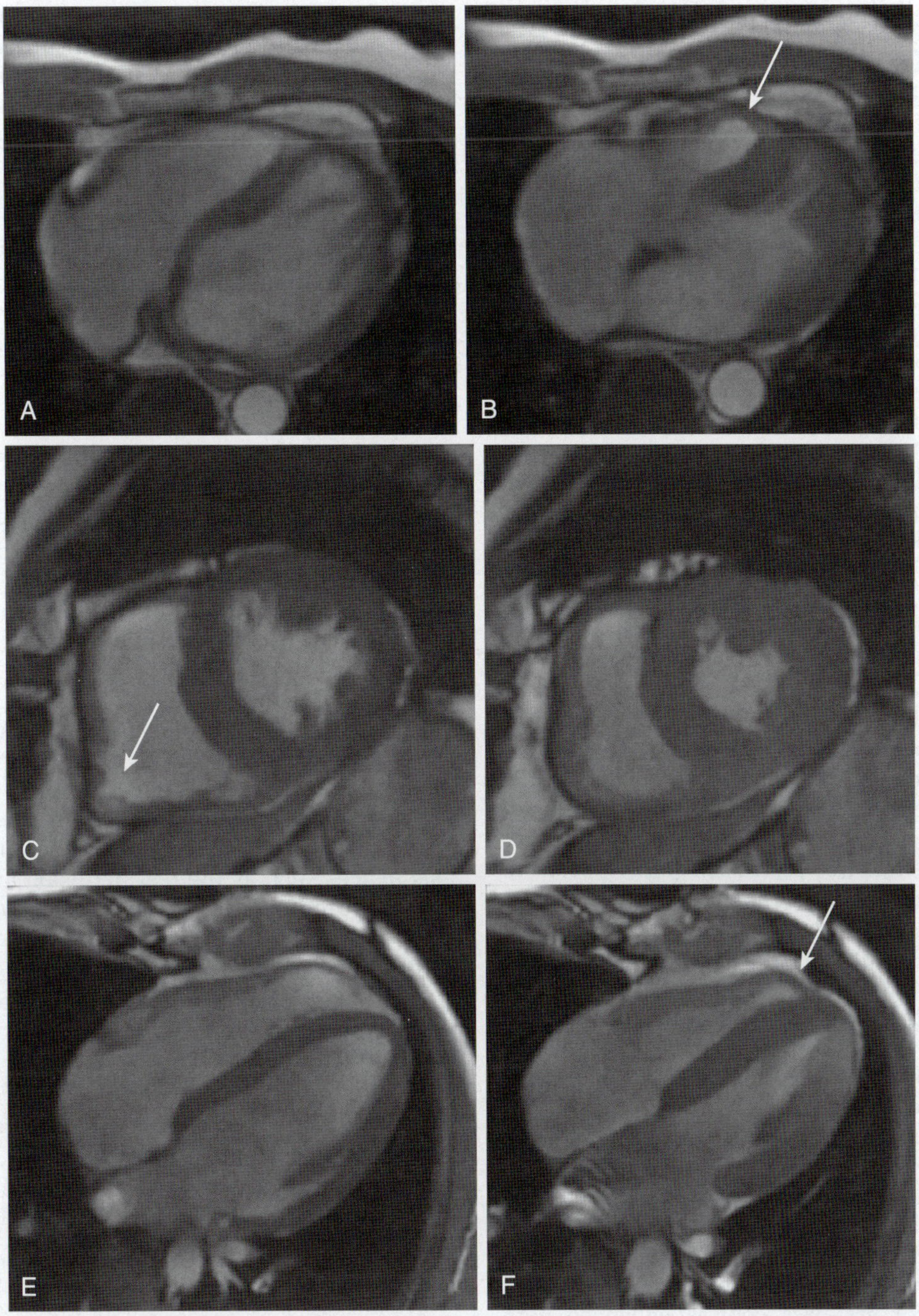

FIG. 29.17 Right ventricular (RV) global and regional function in healthy subjects scanned by 3-T cardiac magnetic resonance. Images of the RV wall motion in diastole (A, C, E) and systole (B, D, F) acquired in different planes. (A and B) Transverse view showing dyskinesia in the mediolateral segment in systole (A, *white arrow*). (C and D) Short-axis view with prominent bulging in the inferolateral segment in diastole (C, *white arrow*). (E and F) Horizontal long-axis view demonstrating dyskinesia in systole in apicolateral segment (F, *white arrow*). (Reproduced with permission from Quick S, Speiser U, Kury K, Schoen S, Ibrahim K, Strasser R. Evaluation and classification of right ventricular wall motion abnormalities in healthy subjects by 3-tesla cardiovascular magnetic resonance imaging. *Neth Heart J.* 2015;23:64–69.)

Importantly, the size of the focal WMA was small, and no WMAs were found in the basal region of the right ventricle. In this study, normal patients had regional WMAs predominantly in the apical-lateral and mediolateral segments with a close spatial relation to the moderator band (79.3%) and trabecular muscle (19.3%).[56] This observation may help to distinguish a "typical" pattern of a basal location of the abnormal focal RV geometry in "classic" ARVC.

Despite its limitations, CMR has an exceptionally important role in the evaluation of patients with known or suspected ACM and is a true "one-stop-shop" diagnostic test.

CARDIAC MAGNETIC RESONANCE IMAGING PROTOCOLS FOR KNOWN AND SUSPECTED ARRHYTHMOGENIC CARDIOMYOPATHY

CMR is a versatile imaging methodology capable of successfully resolving diagnostic challenges encountered by clinicians working with known or suspected ARVC/D patients.

While CMR is an excellent diagnostic tool, it requires skill and expertise, and it appears to have a "learning curve" for both the physician and technician. It requires close collaboration and communication with the entire clinical team, starting with the referring physicians and their understanding of the appropriateness of the test they have ordered for their patient.

A dedicated CMR protocol for image acquisition is probably the most important part of the diagnostic triangle ("appropriate order-right image-correct interpretation") that we described earlier. Different CMR scanner vendors provide sequence terminologies and methodologies specific for their software and hardware, which adds additional complexity in the image acquisition process.

In general, all MRI manufactures provide a robust and well-balanced methodology for CMR acquisition and thus, our protocol can be used in any scanner.

We will use general terminology to describe the CMR sequences. Our predominant sequence on a 1.5-T magnet for the assessment of global and regional RV and LV function is a balanced steady-state free precession (bSSFP) sequence. Rarely, we may need to utilize the gradient echo (GRE)–based cine images, mostly when significant valvular regurgitation is suggested or when the patient has a pacemaker/ICD.

Different centers may utilize magnets with different field strengths. Currently, 1.5-T scanners are most frequently utilized for ACM studies. However, there is a definitive trend showing an increase in CMR studies obtained on 3-T systems. Kramer et al.[57] summarized differences in CMR acquisition on 3- vs. 1.5-T scanners as follows:

1. ECG gating may be more problematic at 3 T than at 1.5 T. In cases where the ECG signal is unreliable, peripheral pulse gating may succeed for acquisitions that are amenable to retrospective gating, such as cine imaging.
2. As a result of improved signal-to-noise ratio, 3 T may be advantageous for first-pass contrast-enhanced perfusion imaging and LGE. Furthermore, tagging sequences and 4D flow techniques may benefit from imaging at 3 T.
3. bSSFP is well established as the default method of choice for cine imaging at 1.5 T. At 3 T, however, the increased sensitivity of bSSFP to off-resonance effects tends to worsen dark banding and flow artifacts. To mitigate these artifacts, it may be necessary to perform careful shimming. In rare cases, patient-specific frequency adjustment may be required.
4. Of note, devices that have been tested and determined to be safe at 1.5 T may not be safe at 3 T. The authors recommend checking specific information relating to CMR safety of devices at higher magnetic field strengths.

Clinically utilized ACM protocols among all experienced cardiac imaging centers are fairly standardized and provide structural and functional data for both ventricles since LV involvement is an important clinical and prognostic factor in this disorder. We recommend implementation of the standardized CMR protocols provided by C. Kramer et al. in the 2020 update of the Society for Cardiovascular Magnetic Resonance (SCMR) Board of Trustees Task Force.[57] This excellent document summarizes both a general CMR protocol and disease-specific acquisition protocols. For ACM, the document defines the CMR goal as "measuring RV and LV volumes and global and regional function (by cine imaging) and assessing RV and LV scar (LGE)."

In this regard, Kramer et al. recommend the following acquisition protocol in patients with suspected ACM:

1. LV structure and function—consider 5–6 mm slice thickness
2. Transaxial or oblique transaxial bSSFP cine images (slice thickness 5–6 mm) covering the right ventricle including RVOT. An RV vertical long-axis view aligned with tricuspid inflow is recommended
3. Optional sequences:
   a. Selected transaxial or oblique transaxial black-blood images (double inversion recovery T1-weighted fast spin-echo [FSE])
   b. Repeat same geometry with fat suppression
4. LGE. Consider T1 nulling for right ventricle

In addition, there are many clinical conditions that may mimic ARVC/ACM and, thus, the CMR data should have enough information to successfully differentiate these disorders. For these reasons, our protocol includes additional sequences such as the rest perfusion and phase-contrast data. The protocol may be further adjusted and customized

TABLE 29.5 Diagnostic Criteria for Cardiac Sarcoidosis.

Histologic diagnosis group	
Cardiac sarcoidosis is confirmed when endomyocardial biopsy specimens demonstrate noncaseating epithelioid cell granulomas with histologic or clinical diagnosis of extracardiac sarcoidosis.	
Clinical diagnosis group	
Although endomyocardial biopsy specimens do not demonstrate noncaseating epithelioid cell granulomas, extracardiac sarcoidosis is diagnosed histologically or clinically and satisfies the following conditions and more than one in six basic diagnostic criteria. 1. Two or more of the four major criteria are satisfied. 2. One of four of the major criteria and two or more of the five minor criteria are satisfied.	
Major criteria	Minor criteria
1. Advanced atrioventricular block. 2. Basal thinning of the interventricular septum. 3. Positive ^{67}gallium uptake in the heart. 4. Depressed ejection fraction of the LV (<50%).	1. Abnormal ECG findings: ventricular arrhythmias (ventricular tachycardia, multifocal or frequent PVCs). CRBBB, axis deviation or abnormal Q wave. 2. Abnormal echocardiography: regional abnormal wall motion or morphologic abnormality (ventricular aneurysm, wall thickening). 3. Nuclear medicine: perfusion defect detected by ^{201}Thallium or ^{99m}Technetium myocardial scintigraphy. 4. Gadolinium-enhanced CMR imaging: delayed enhancement of myocardium. 5. Endomyocardial biopsy: interstitial fibrosis or monocyte infiltration over moderate grade.

CMR, cardiac magnetic resonance; *CRBBB*, complete right bundle branch block; *ECG*, electrocardiogram; *LV*, left ventricle; *PVC*, premature ventricular contraction.
Reproduced with permission from no a. [Diagnostic guideline and criteria for sarcoidosis --2006]. Nippon Ganka Gakkai zasshi. 2007;111:117–121.

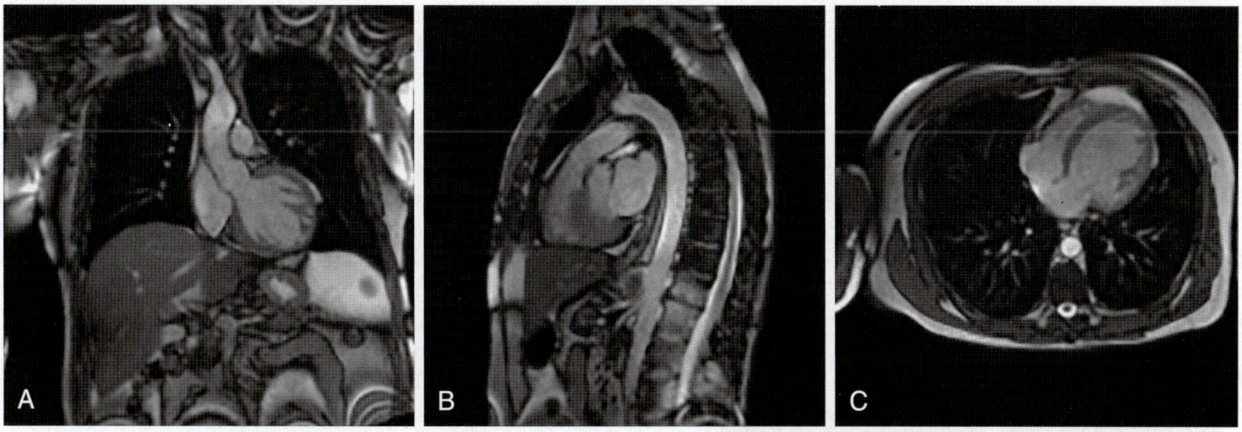

FIG. 29.18 Standard cardiac localizers: (A) Coronal. (B) Sagittal. (C) Transaxial.

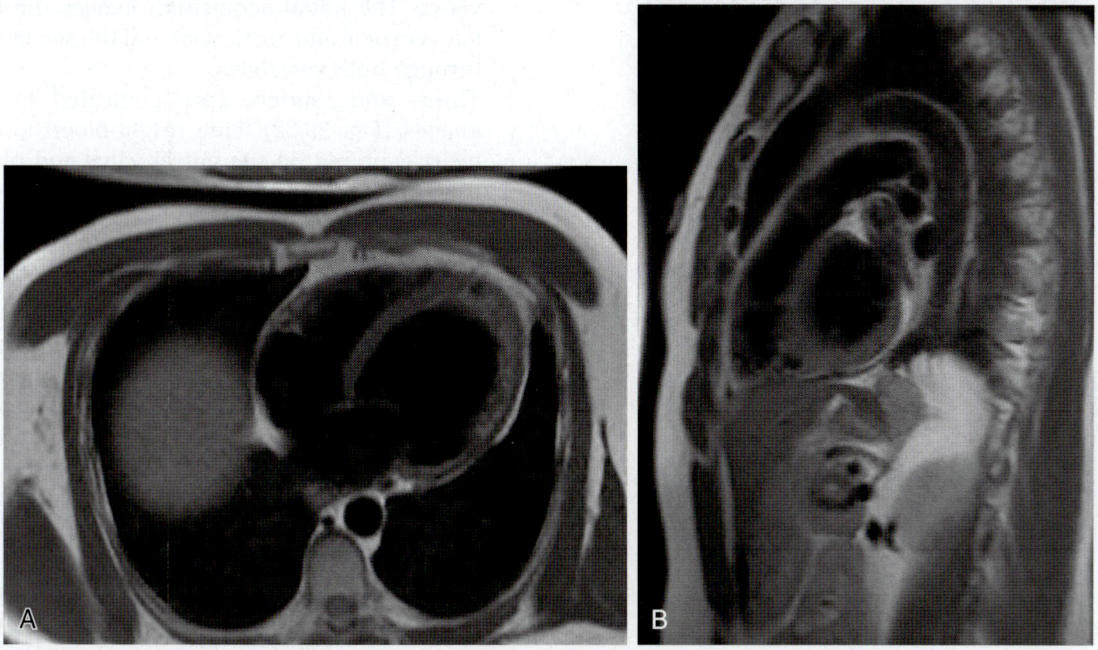

FIG. 29.19 Dark-blood imaging. Half-Fourier acquisition single-shot turbo spin-echo (HASTE) sagittal view centered on the right ventricular outflow tract (RVOT), planned from the axial black-blood images with the line of planning positioned parallel to the main pulmonary artery and passing through the RVOT. These images can be used to plan dedicated right ventricular (RV) views in the axial plane to assess RV free wall motion and characterize tissue (*fat deposition*). (A) HASTE axial view. (B) HASTE sagittal views.

by the physician after reviewing initial images on the scanner. We strongly recommend physician review while the patient is still on the scanner, since we frequently see findings requiring change or the addition of new sequences and views. Every possible effort should be made to obtain the most informative and effective CMR study to aid in establishing the right diagnosis for every patient referred to the imaging lab.

The CMR protocol we recommend for patients with known or suspected ACM is shown in Table 29.5.

It is important to note that axial imaging is considered the most informative methodology for RV-dedicated views (compared to the standard cardiac double oblique views for LV-dedicated imaging). Any dedicated axial stacks should include the entire right ventricle. We recommend including 6 to 8 slices in the stack with 1-cm intervals.

1. Cardiac localizers (Fig. 29.18): A few images are acquired through the chest in the axial, sagittal, and coronal planes using the single-shot fast spin echo technique. These images provide a general assessment of the intrathoracic anatomy and location of the heart. They are essential for the planning of dedicated cardiac views.
2. Dark-blood imaging (Fig. 29.19): half-Fourier acquisition single-shot turbo spin-echo (HASTE) axial views of the chest to assess anatomy and aid in the planning of follow-up images. This acquisition is planned from the three-plane localizer images. The blood is nulled by double inversion recovery (DIR) technique. Stagnant blood within the LV trabeculations will demonstrate high signal and should not be confused with subendocardial edema.

The single-shot technique allows the acquisition of multiple images in a single breath-hold. DIR images are always gated to the ECG to remove cardiac motion. In some ARVC/ACM imaging centers, breath-hold DIR Fast SE (DIR T1-weighted fast spin-echo [FSE]) sequences are preferred and the HASTE technique is not recommended due to the potential for cardiac motion artifact [4]. However, in our center we have consistently adequate clinical performance of the HASTE sequences; in case of suspected positive findings on HASTE, we may switch to breath-hold acquisition for clarity. In this regard, it is important that the CMR physicians review the initial images prior to contrast injection to establish the need for additional sequences before GBCA exposure.

3. Vertical long-axis (two-chamber) SSFP cine (Fig. 29.20): bright-blood technique that can be acquired using either a balanced steady-state free precession (bSSFP) technique or the conventional GRE sequence. The use of SSFP is preferable due to its higher contrast resolution and signal-to-noise ratio. GRE has lower contrast-to-noise ratio but should be used in patients with pacemaker/ICDs.

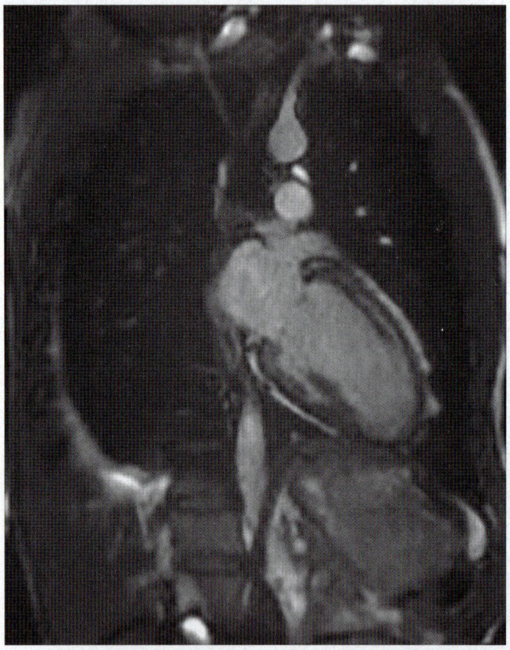

FIG. 29.20 Bright-blood technique can be acquired using either a balanced steady-state free precession technique or conventional gradient echo sequence.

Images are ECG gated and relatively long; therefore, usually one slice is acquired per breath-hold. The line of planning should pass through the center of the mitral valve, including the left atrium (LA) and LV apex. SSFP is a GRE sequence that acquires images by repeatedly applying a gradient with low flip angle and short TR, which leads to a steady state of longitudinal magnetization. The SSFP images are strongly susceptible to metal artifact and are heavily dependent on homogeneity of the magnetic field.

4. SAX scout (Fig. 29.21): cine bSSFP technique acquired through the base of the heart and midventricle and prescribed from the two-chamber view. These images are vital for the planning of three- and four-chamber views. The initial acquisition images the base of the left ventricle and aortic root and the second plane goes through both ventricles.
5. Three- and four-chamber dedicated LV SSFP cine images (Fig. 29.22): cine bright-blood images of the heart centered on the mitral valve and planned from the combination of the SAX scout and two-chamber views. The three-chamber view is acquired when positioning the line of planning through the center of the mitral valve and middle of the LA and left ventricle on the two-chamber view, and through the left ventricular outflow tract (LVOT) and aortic root on the first image of the SAX scout acquisition. The four-chamber view is acquired when positioning the line of planning through the mitral valve and middle of the LA and left ventricle on the two-chamber view, and through the mid-LV cavity on the second image of the SAX scout acquisition. It is important to rotate the line toward the largest position of the right ventricle.
6. Dedicated RV cine views (Fig. 29.23): We recommend obtaining dedicated RV inflow and outflow cine images

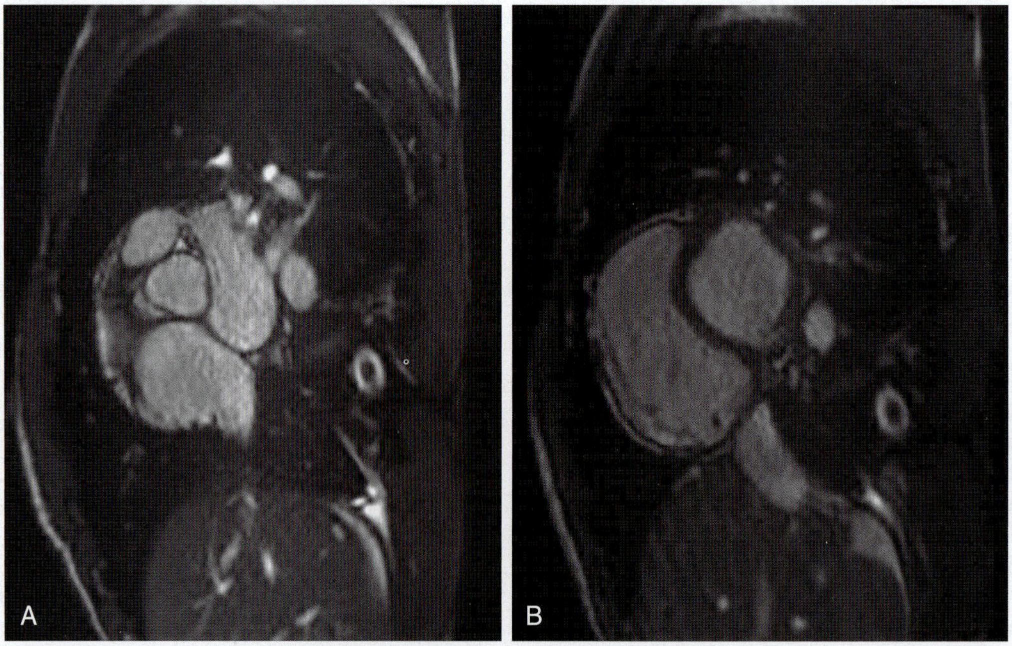

FIG. 29.21 (A) Basal short axis; (B) mid short axis.

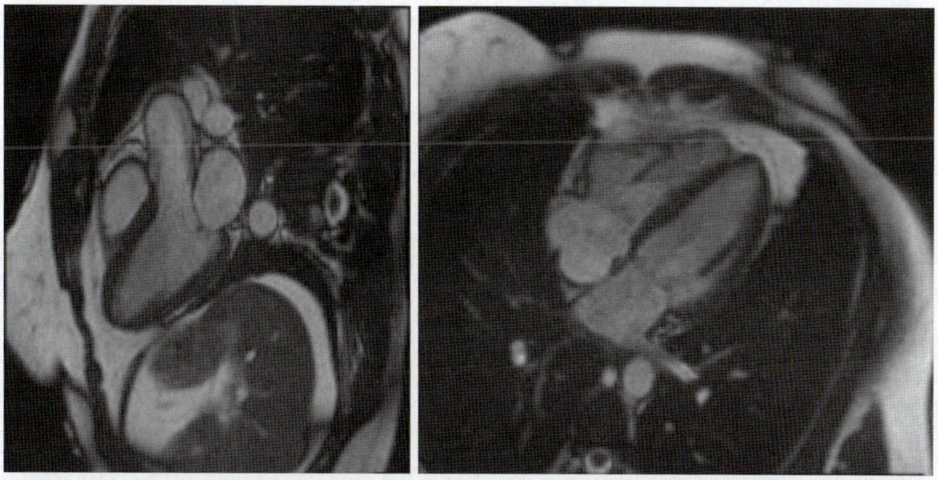

FIG. 29.22 Three- and four-chamber steady-state free precession images.

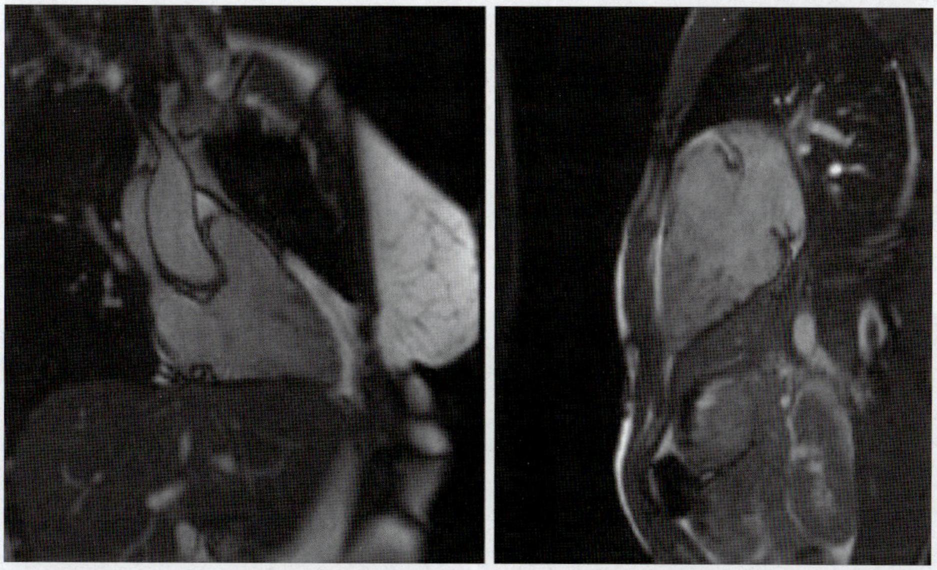

FIG. 29.23 Dedicated right ventricular cine views.

since these provide optimal visualization of the triangle of dysplasia, tricuspid valve, and pulmonic valve. These are planned from the sagittal black-blood images and are intended to evaluate wall motion of the RV free wall. Motion of the RVOT can also be assessed in this plane.

7. Axial cine view through the RV (Fig. 29.24): cine bSSFP images through the right ventricle on the axial plane.
8. T1-weighted images of the RV (Fig. 29.25): black-blood T1-weighted spin echo images acquired through the RV to assess for fat deposition in the anterior and free walls. We recommend two separate acquisitions: the initial acquisition is made through the right ventricle on the axial plane to assess the anterior RV wall. The slices should be exactly the same as the axial cine RV images so one can correlate the areas of fat deposition with abnormal wall motion. The second acquisition is done in the coronal or sagittal plane to analyze the inferior RV wall. If a hyperintense focus is seen within the RV myocardium, this sequence is repeated with the addition of chemical fat saturation to confirm fat deposition.

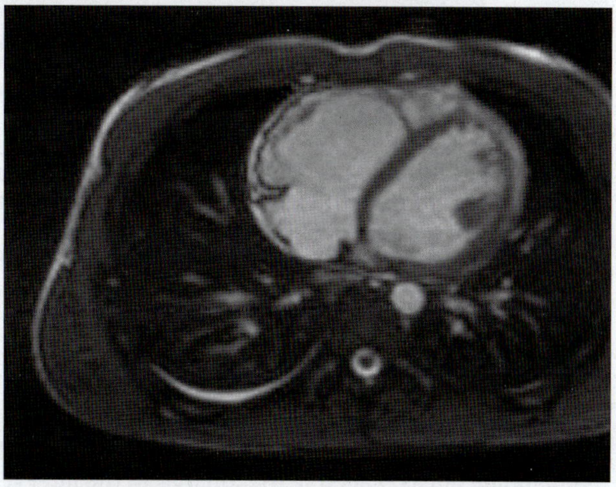

FIG. 29.24 Axial right ventricle–centered cine images.

9. Rest perfusion (Fig. 29.26): First-pass rest perfusion images are acquired in the SAX (three slices: basal-mid-apical SAX) and four-chamber (one slice) planes as part of the routine examination. This is a T1-weighted

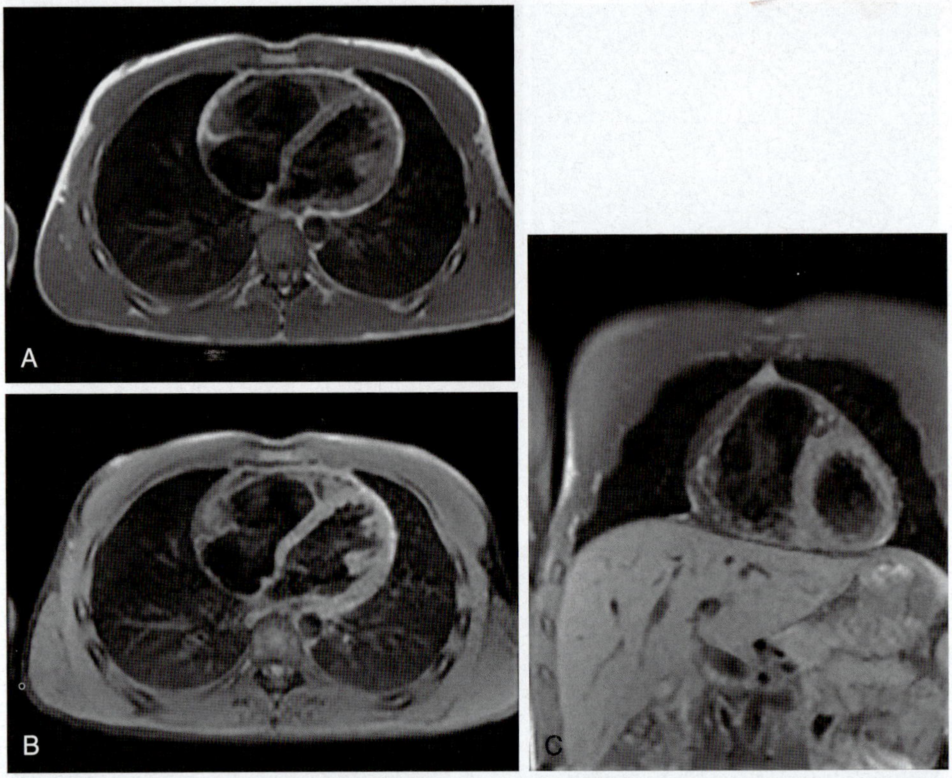

FIG. 29.25 Axial black-blood T1W SE (T1 Weighted Spin Echo) without (A) and with (B) fat supression. SE without fat saturation (C).

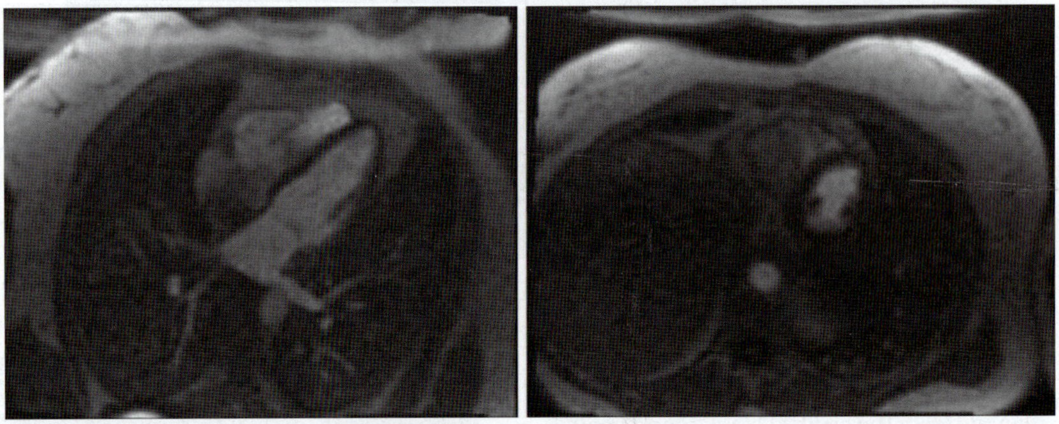

FIG. 29.26 Rest perfusion images.

sequence with images acquired immediately after intravenous administration of the gadolinium-based contrast. We use a 0.05 mmol/kg dose injected at 3 cm^3/s. After image acquisition is completed, the patient receives an additional half dose of contrast to allow appropriate delayed-enhancement imaging.

10. SAX SSFP cine stack (Fig. 29.27): cine bright-blood images through the ventricles. This sequence is planned from the four- and two-chamber views to insure that both ventricles are included in their entirety. A planning line is placed perpendicular to the interventricular septum in the four-chamber view and parallel to the mitral valve in the two-chamber view. These images are required to calculate ventricular volume and ejection fraction, both of which are included in the revised TFC for ARVC. They are also used to assess both LV and RV wall motion as well as the function of the mitral and tricuspid valves.
11. LVOT SSFP cine images (Fig. 29.28): cine bright-blood image through the ascending thoracic aorta planned from the three-chamber view. This sequence is used in conjunction with the three-chamber view to evaluate the aortic root and aortic valves. Both these planes are also used to plan the cine images of the aortic valve and phase-contrast imaging through the ascending aorta.
12. Aortic valve SSFP cine (Fig. 29.29): cine bright-blood image through the aortic valve planned from the LVOT and three-chamber cine images. Three slices are usually acquired (at, below, and above the valve). These images are used to accurately measure the dimensions of the aortic sinuses, give an

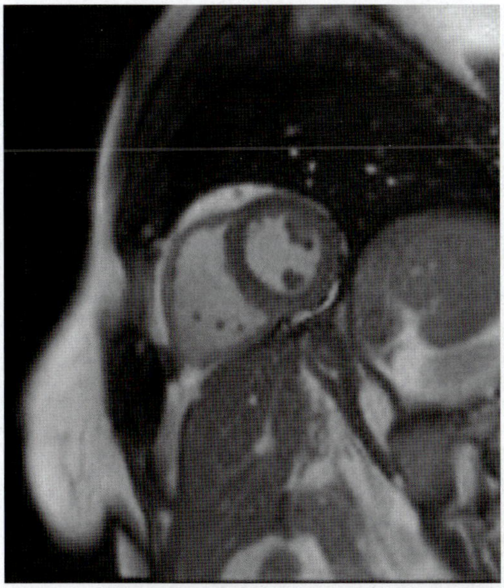

FIG. 29.27 Short-axis steady-state free procession cine stack images.

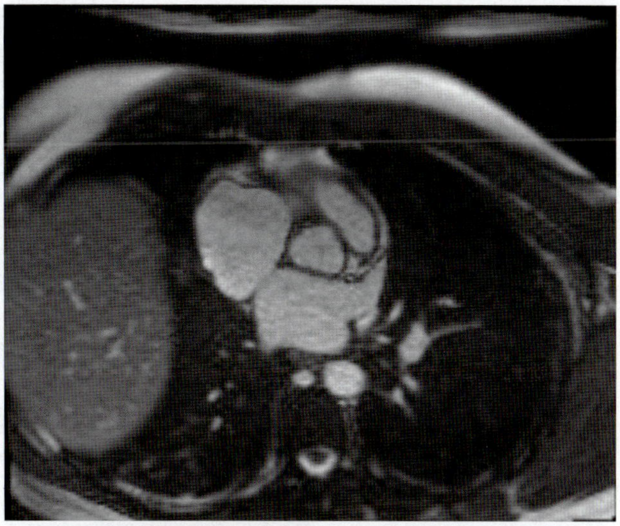

FIG. 29.29 Aortic valve cine images.

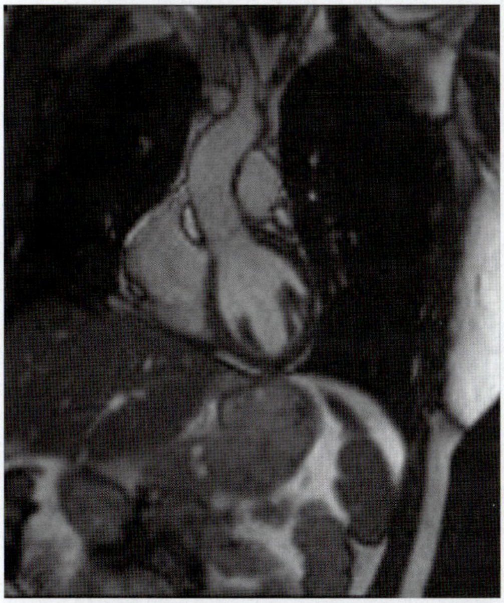

FIG. 29.28 Left ventricular outflow tract cine images.

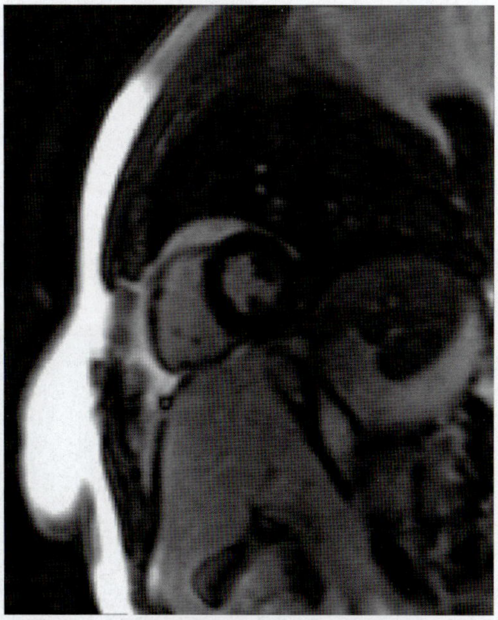

FIG. 29.30 Inversion time scout.

appropriate view of the aortic valve leaflets, and assess for dissection flaps.

13. Inversion time (TI) scout (Fig. 29.30): Single ECG-gated slice through the middle of the left ventricle acquired 9–10 min after intravenous administration of contrast. This image is planned from the four-chamber view and is used to determine the appropriate time of inversion for the delayed enhancement images.
14. Myocardial delayed enhancement (MDE) (Fig. 29.31): ECG-gated image through the heart obtained by copying the position of the previously acquired SAX stack as well as two-, three-, and four-chamber planes. The MDE is a T1-weighted GRE sequence that uses an inversion recovery pulse to null the normal myocardium. The appropriate time of inversion is copied from the TI scout. When evaluating patients with known/suspected ARVC/D we also include stack images of the right ventricle to evaluate the anterior and inferior walls of the RV. The TI for the RV myocardium is generally 50 ms shorter than that for the LV myocardium, but an RV-dedicated TI scout can be performed if needed. We use a single-shot technique for acquisition of seven to eight slices in one breath-hold. This technique can also be performed with free breathing due to its inherent fast time of acquisition. The segmented technique can be used if indeterminate areas of delayed enhancement are seen within the myocardium. This technique has a longer acquisition time (one slice per breath-hold) but provides images that have higher contrast-to-noise ratio and spatial resolution. Both single-shot and segmented MDE sequences provide magnitude and phase sensitivity images for each slice.
15. Phase-contrast imaging (Fig. 29.32): The GRE sequence is used to measure blood flow, direction, and velocity by measuring the phase shift of the protons in the blood when moving through a magnetic

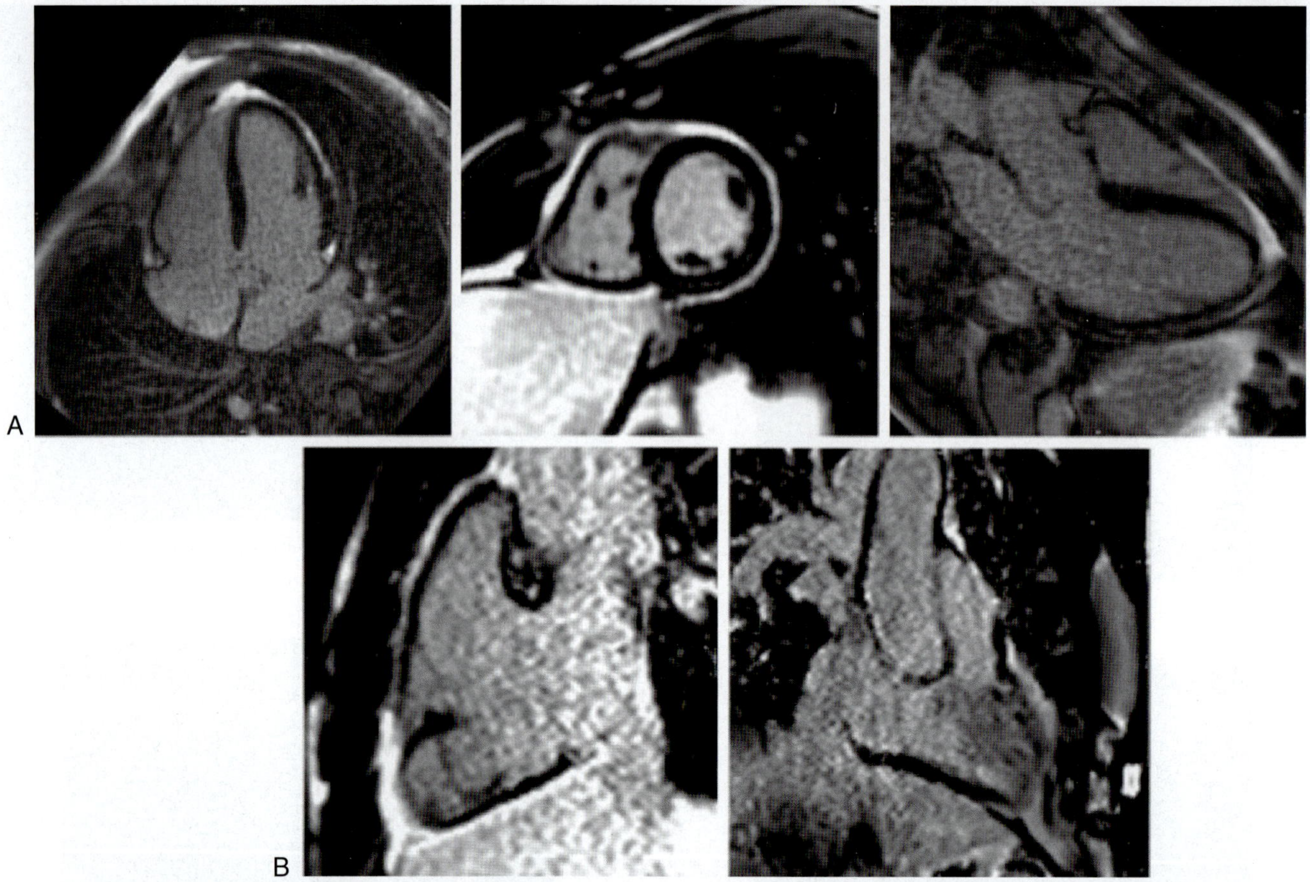

FIG. 29.31 Myocardial delayed enhancement (MDE) images: (A) Left ventricle–dedicated MDE images. (B) Right ventricle–dedicated MDE images.

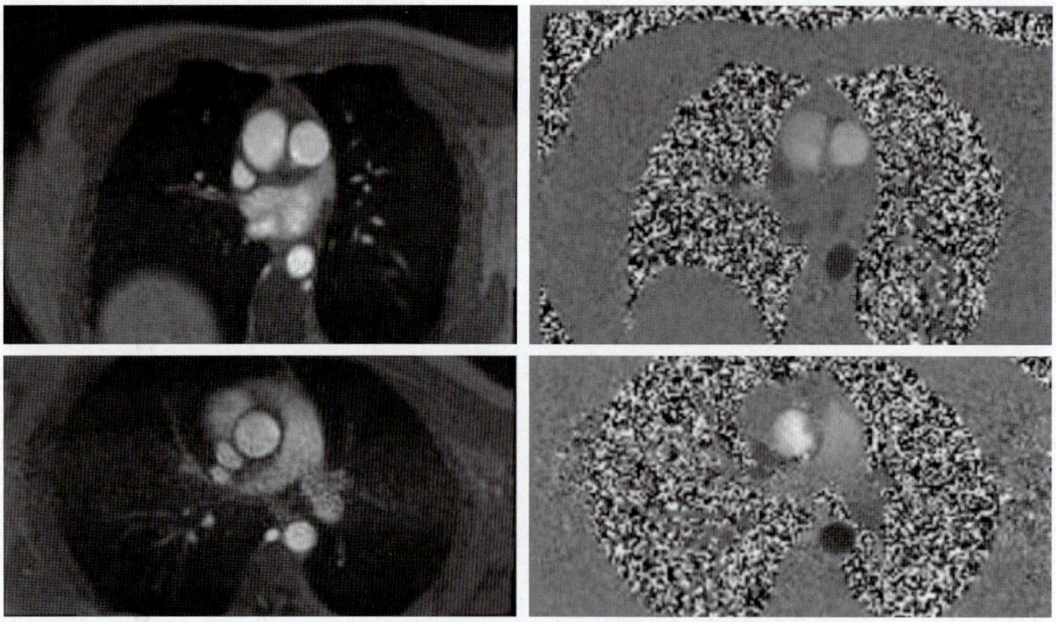

FIG. 29.32 Phase-contrast images of the pulmonary artery (*top row*) and aorta (*bottom row*).

field. Quantitated peak systolic velocity is used to calculate pressure gradient, which is essential when evaluating patients with suspected/known valvular stenosis. This sequence is planned through the midascending aorta and main pulmonary artery. The three-chamber and LVOT images are used to plane the phase contrast through the aorta, and the dedicated RVOT images are used to plane the phase contrast through the main pulmonary artery. Forward volumes are compared to the stroke volumes derived from the cine SAX stack sequence. Blood volumes and direction are also used to estimate shunt fraction (Qp:Qs) and assess the severity of valvular insufficiency.

16. Optional: If anomalous coronaries are suspected, the navigator sequence for visualization of the coronary arteries should be considered.

Other imaging centers utilize similar protocols. The main difference is the use of high-resolution dark-blood sequences in our practice instead of HASTE, used in their protocols.

For patients with suspected ARVC, we recommend acquiring axial cine SSFP images to evaluate wall motion of the RV anterior wall; the slices could be modified/customized to further investigate any abnormality if visualization of these findings is suboptimal on standard views. We usually obtain 10 slices with a 20% gap. Especially important is a clear visualization of the subtricuspid area, not easily visible in other cardiac-dedicated views.

We recommend obtaining the same axial images using T1-weighted black-blood HASTE to look for fatty deposition in the RV anterior wall and in the left ventricle. In addition to the axial black-blood imaging (HASTE), we also obtain a coronal black-blood HASTE to evaluate the RV inferior wall.

The perfusion images have a magnetization preparation pulse that is nonselective with a TI of 100 ms. Delayed contrast enhancement (DCE) images also require a nonselective magnetization preparation pulse.

The TI for the RV myocardium is about 50 ms less than the TI for the left ventricle. Therefore, we can either scan the SAX DCE twice after adjusting the TI for the RV (subtracting 50 ms from that for the left ventricle) or obtain another TI scout specifically for the right ventricle. We use the first approach when we are not able to obtain adequate nulling of the RV myocardium on the initial SAX MDE that was aimed for the LV myocardium.

All sequences use generalized autocalibrating partially parallel acquisitions with an acceleration factor of 2.[58] All sequences are performed during breath-hold and the number of concatenations depends on the patient's heart rate (HR). A faster HR allows acquisition of more images during the same breath-hold. Images are acquired by the RR interval. Therefore, a faster HR means more RR intervals in a given time compared to slower HRs, so the number of concatenations can be decreased. Exceptions to this rule are black-blood images, since they need a preparation pulse. We can only acquire one slice per breath-hold, regardless of the patient's HR.

General CMR image analysis and interpretation principles have been nicely summarized in the 2020 SCMR Task Force Standardized CMR interpretation and postprocessing update.[59]

We would like to emphasize that LV morphofunctional assessment is relatively well established and uniform, while a significant variability is noted in the RV assessment from different laboratories. Current RV volumetric assessment is similar for all commercially available software and is based (with some variations) on Simpson's rule. It has all the flaws due to multiple geometric assumptions and simplification of the complex RV geometry. The major problem with RV volume assessment is that the same principles used for the left ventricle are "forcefully" applied to the right ventricle, despite the fact that the right ventricle has a distinctly different geometry. A challenging part of the measurement methodology for the right ventricle is the infundibular segment. Future CMR developments will undoubtedly include a significant level of standardization and computer assessment of RV function and morphology. There are a few relatively simple rules to maintain good repeatability and reproducibility of the results. These rules were recently summarized by Tavano et al.[60] as follows (Fig. 29.33):

1. When Simpson's disk method is utilized, it is important to include the RV infundibulum in the measurement of RV volumes, as it can account for 25%–30% of RV volume.
2. The most basal level of the right ventricle should be carefully identified using the short axis (SAX) and long axis (LAX) views. The atrioventricular (AV) groove should be used to separate the right ventricle from the right atrium.
3. Endocardial contouring of the ventricle should be performed with inclusion of the RV trabeculae in the RV cavity.

Cardiac Magnetic Resonance Imaging in Pediatric Patients with Known or Suspected Arrhythmogenic Cardiomyopathy

Modern clinical practice considers either a phenotype-first or genotype-first approach in the diagnosis and management of ACM (Fig. 29.34A and B).[61] The ACM phenotype is identified mostly in young to middle-age adulthood. Accordingly, performing CMR in a pediatric population may not be clinically effective. This situation becomes even more complex in asymptomatic children with a positive ACM genotype, which is a frequent clinical finding in families of ACM patients. Children of an individual with the diagnosis of ARVC and associated genetic abnormality have a 50% chance of having the genetic abnormality. Therefore, at what age should the child of an affected parent be evaluated for the clinical manifestations of the disease? What methods should be used to test if the child is clinically affected? Is sudden arrhythmic death a problem in young children with the genetic abnormality? Is it possible to prevent the disease from developing in the offspring or at least slow its development? There are answers for some but not all of these important questions.

Let us first address the problem of ACM inheritability. Genetic testing is advised in a child when a parent has one of the five desmosomal genetic abnormalities of ACM. If the child has the same genetic defect as the parent, then the child has inherited the risk of becoming clinically affected with ACM. There is the unlikely possibility of the parent having two abnormal desmosomal genes, which occurs in 4%–17% of patients with ACM.[62–64] If the child also has more than one abnormal gene, then the likelihood of the child developing the disease, as well as an increased possibility of having severe clinical symptoms, is substantial. Conversely, if the parent has an abnormal desmosomal gene but the child does not, then the child's risk is minimal.

What if the parent has the clinical disease but does not have any of the desmosomal abnormalities? If so, there is probably no reason to check the child for the

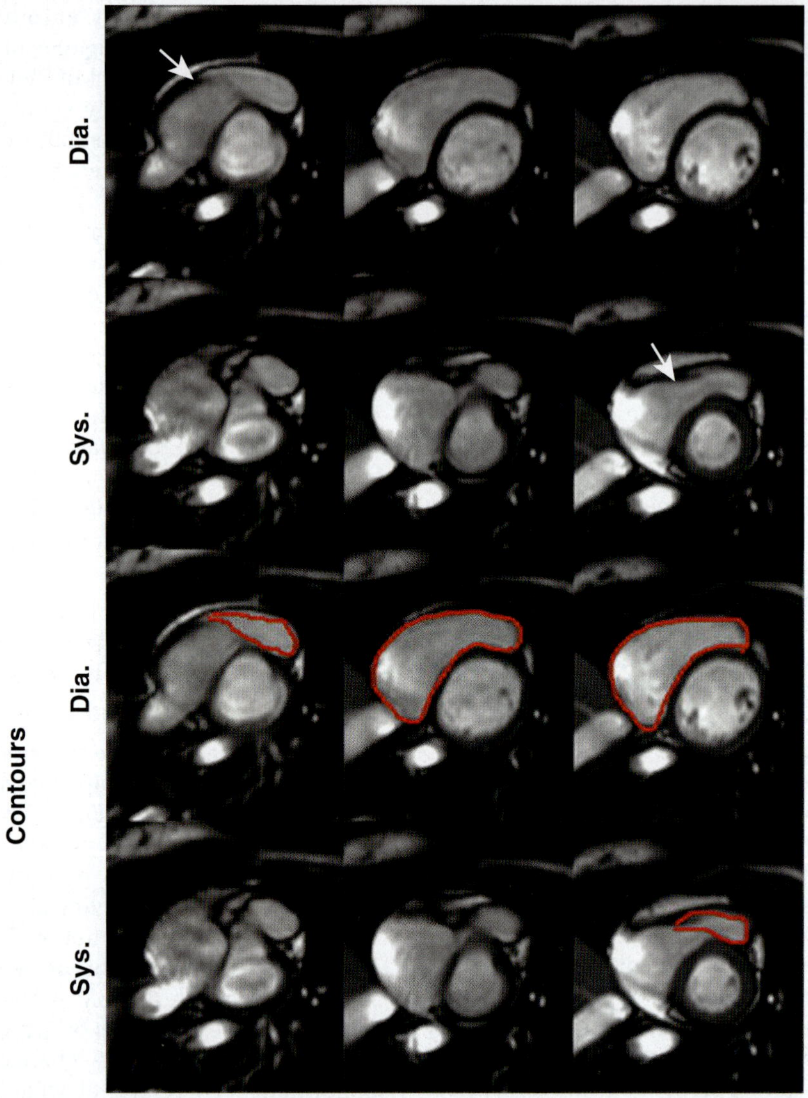

FIG. 29.33 Technique to measure the ejection fraction of the right ventricle (RV): The systole (*Sys.*) and diastole (*Dia.*) frames are selected. The most basal slice of the RV is different in systole and diastole. It is important to include the infundibulum in the measurement; the border between the infundibulum and right atrium is visualized on the short-axis plane by the atrioventricular groove (*arrow*). (Reproduced, with perrmission from Tavano A, Maurel B, Gaubert JY et al. MR imaging of arrhythmogenic right ventricular dysplasia: what the radiologist needs to know. *Diagnos Interv Imaging*. 2015;96:449–460.)

desmosomal abnormality, since it is extremely unlikely that a known desmosomal gene will be found in the child. However, the child of a patient with ACM who does not have a mutation still has a risk of developing symptomatic disease.[64]

Under these circumstances, the child of the affected parent should also be advised not to engage in endurance athletics since there is an increased risk of developing the disease.[65] These observations are probably due to the presence of yet unknown genetic abnormalities.

The earliest manifestation of the disease appears to be electrical, including ventricular arrhythmias such as PVCs and nonsustained or sustained VT. Therefore, obtaining an ECG, Holter monitoring, or exercise testing is a reasonable approach to see if the child has developed clinical evidence of ACM/ARVC. Structural abnormalities, such as RV enlargement or focal akinesia or dyskinesia, appear later than the electrical findings, although this is controversial.

The appearance of electrical findings prior to the detection of structural abnormalities by MRI is regarded as the usual sequence of events and has been demonstrated in a mouse model of ARVC.[66] This is an important concept, since it impacts the decision of how to screen children for the clinical presence of the disease. Based on the above assumptions, it would appear reasonable to perform serial ECGs, Holter monitoring, and possibly exercise testing to determine whether there is electrical instability during childhood in genetically affected children.

A baseline CMR may also be obtained as the study does not carry a risk of radiation exposure. This testing should probably be initiated at ages 9 to 10, especially if any electrical abnormalities are present. Positive CMR findings shift the probability of ACM in a young patient from probable to definite (Fig. 29.35).[67] Tests for electrical abnormalities should be repeated at yearly intervals or sooner if there are symptoms such as palpitations or evidence of VT. The question of how often to repeat these tests is unknown, but it is suggested that they be performed at yearly intervals until age 25. If negative, then ECGs and Holter studies may be repeated every 3 years thereafter until ages 40–50; after

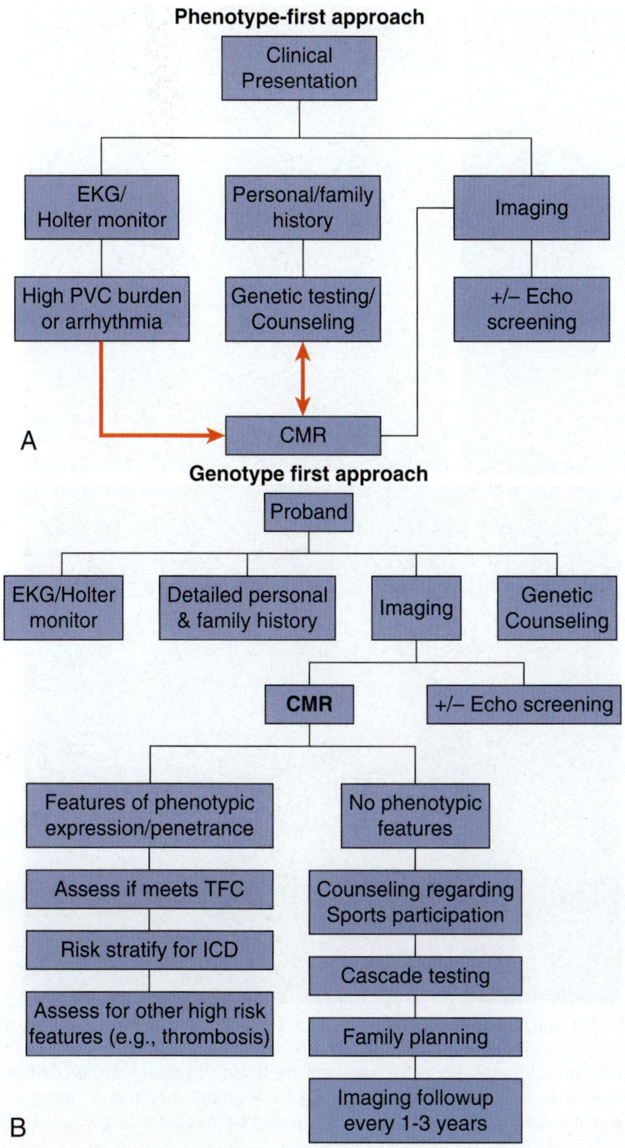

FIG. 29.34 (A) Phenotype-first approach for comprehensive assessment of arrhythmogenic cardiomyopathy (ACM) and the role of cardiac magnetic resonance (*CMR*) in such evaluation. (B) Genotype-first approach for comprehensive assessment of ACM. *ICD*, implantable cardioverter-defibrilator; *PVC*, Premature ventricular contraction; *TFC*, Task Force criteria. (Reproduced with permission from Basharat SA, Hsiung I, Garg J, Alsaid A. Arrhythmogenic cardiomyopathy: evolving diagnostic criteria and insight from cardiac magnetic resonance imaging. *Heart Fail Clin*. 2023;19:429–444.)

this age, and if the patient demonstrates consistently normal results, the tests may be obtained at 5-year intervals (Fig. 29.36).

In conclusion, it is reasonable to suggest that ECGs and Holter monitoring be performed at yearly intervals after the age of 8 or 10 years, supplemented by MRI studies if electrical abnormalities are present. Evidence has accumulated both experimentally and clinically that frequent, prolonged, and vigorous athletic activity is a risk factor for SCD and can exacerbate the rate of progression of the disease (Fig. 29.37).[65,69] Therefore, these types of activity should be avoided by probands or family members who are prone to develop the disease. Therapy by antiarrhythmic drugs or insertion of an ICD alone or in combination in asymptomatic children of probands with ACM will require further evaluation.

Utilization of Cardiac Magnetic Resonance in a Differential Diagnosis of Arrhythmogenic Cardiomyopathy

RIGHT VENTRICULAR SIZE AND FUNCTION-BASED ARRHYTHMOGENIC RIGHT VENTRICULAR CARDIOMYOPATHY CRITERIA: NORMAL VARIANTS AND ARTIFACTS

Morphofunctional changes in the ventricles are categorized as either major or minor diagnostic ACM markers. Accordingly, focal RV functional abnormalities (focal akinesia, dyskinesia, or dyssynchronous RV contractility) and either RV enlargement with a sex-specific RV end diastolic volume index (REDVI) or RV systolic dysfunction are the CMR-based parameters defining the disease. Tissue abnormalities suggestive of inflammation, fibrosis, or fibrofatty degeneration on standard CMR examination were not included in the 2010 TFC due to potential variability in the interpretation of these abnormalities.[2] However, LV LGE is an important part of the major and minor ACM criteria based on the 2023 European TFC.[27]

It is particularly important to follow CMR criteria in endurance athletes, who may present with borderline ECG changes.[70–76] Correct diagnosis of athletes with ACM requires utilization of the entirety of ECG, hemodynamic, and imaging findings, which can distinguish between ACM (mostly ARVC) and athlete's hearts.

In borderline cases, sequential CMR imaging may provide important information including progressive worsening of RV focal and global systolic function and RV enlargement. The latter findings suggest significant RV pathology, whereas decreased RV dimensions and/or improved function following a decrease in the amount of endurance training may be consistent with the "physiologic adaptation phenomenon" observed in the athlete's heart.[77]

Luijkx et al.[78] demonstrated that compared to the RVEDVI, RVEF is more likely to distinguish ACM from physiologic cardiac adaptation in athletes by CMR. They also noted that a good diagnostic alternative in athletes is the LV/RV EDV ratio, representing a normal proportionate adaptation of both ventricles in athletes.

CMR is a useful diagnostic modality to distinguish "traditional" ARVC and other RV cardiomyopathies as well as RV-specific disorders (Fig. 29.38).[79] The combination of a negative family history, absence of significant conduction abnormalities and arrhythmias by ECG and Holter, and absence of tissue abnormalities (such as delayed hyperenhancement or fibrofatty changes) on CMR suggests a low likelihood of ACM.

Compared to echocardiography, LV or RV RWMAs diagnosed by CMR are more precise due to a higher spatial resolution of CMR. However, there are several pitfalls. First, the possibility of an artifact of the observed WMA on cine images should be considered (Fig. 29.39).[60] The sequence should be repeated with a change in the image settings if

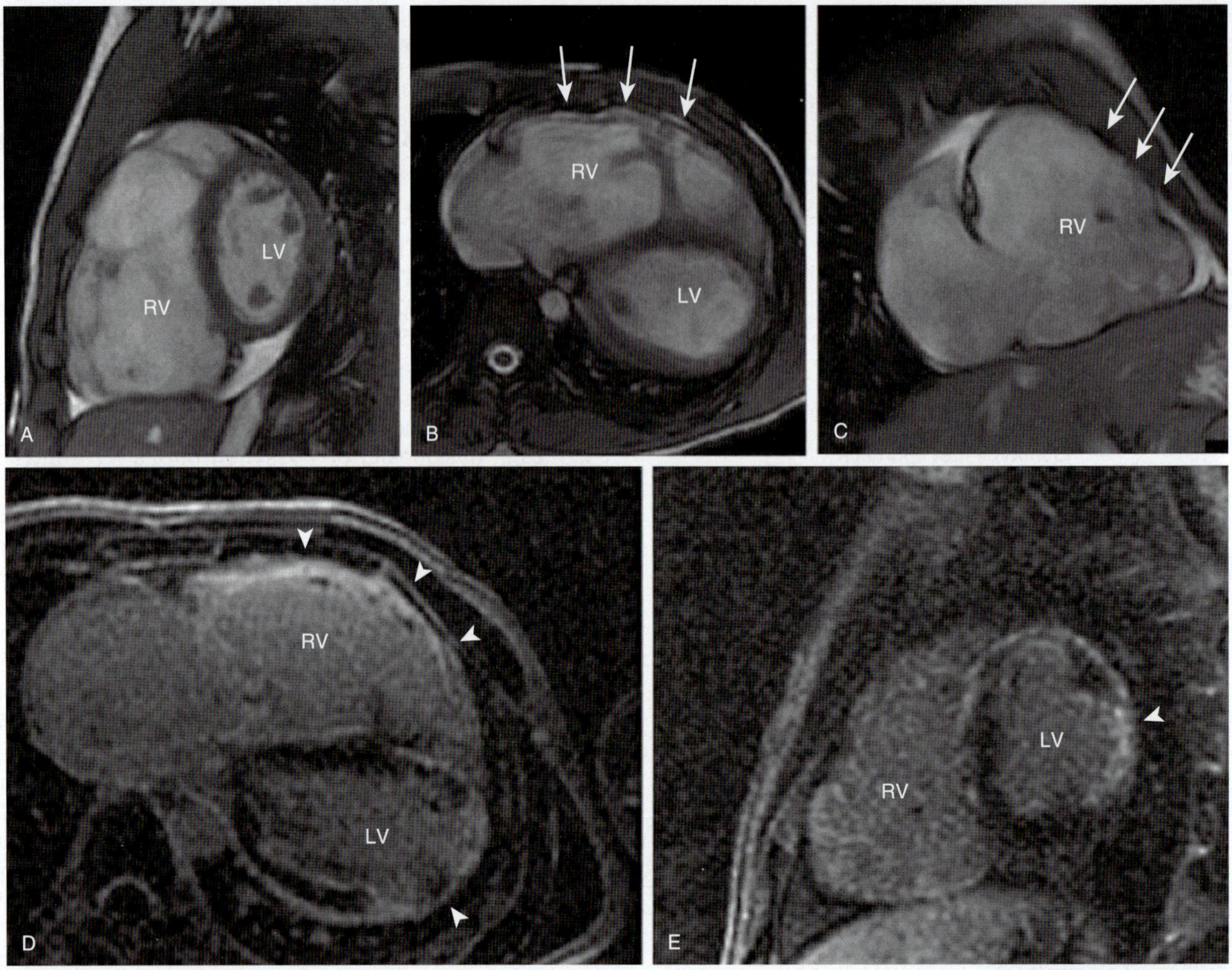

FIG. 29.35 Cardiac magnetic resonance evidence of arrhythmogenic right ventricular cardiomyopathy/dysplasia in a 13-year-old boy with palpitations, sustained ventricular tachycardia requiring cardioversion, and epsilon waves on his ECG. Short-axis (A), axial (B), and dedicated right ventricle (*RV*) (C) steady-state free precession images. Axial (D) and short-axis (E) delayed hyperenhancement images. Focal RV free wall aneurysms (*arrows*); areas of RV and the left ventricle (*LV*) delayed hyperenhancement (*arrowheads*). (Reproduced with permission from Saprungruang A, Tumkosit M, Kongphatthanayothin A. The presence of epsilon waves in all precordial leads (V1–V6) in a 13-year-old boy with arrhythmogenic right ventricular dysplasia (ARVD). *Ann Noninvasive Electrocardiol.* 2013;18:484–486.)

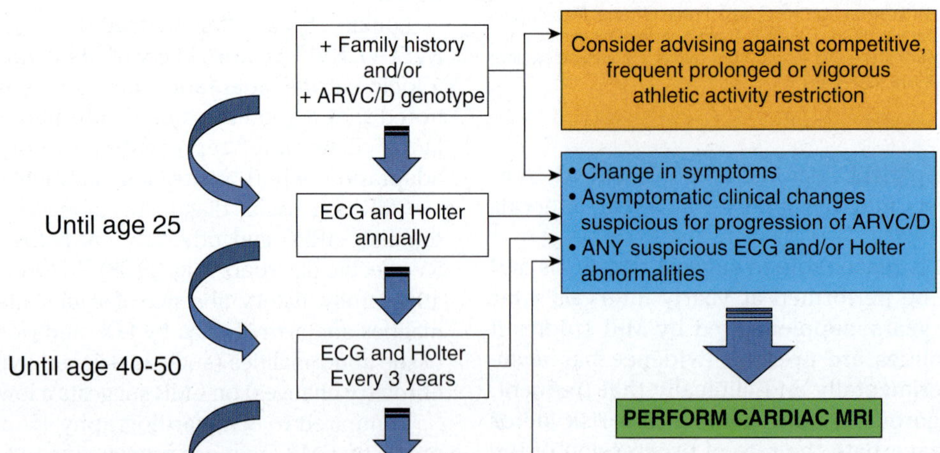

FIG. 29.36 Possible clinical algorithm for follow-up of children with positive arrhythmogenic right ventricular cardiomyopathy/dysplasia (*ARVC/D*) or arrhythmogenic cardiomyopathy genotype. *MRI*, Magnetic resonance imaging. (Reproduced with permission from Abidov A, Oliva IB, Marcus FI. Cardiac MRI in the Diagnosis, Clinical Management and Prognosis of Arrhyhtmogenic Right Ventricular Cardiomyopathy/Dysplasia. Academic Press/Elsevier, 2016.)

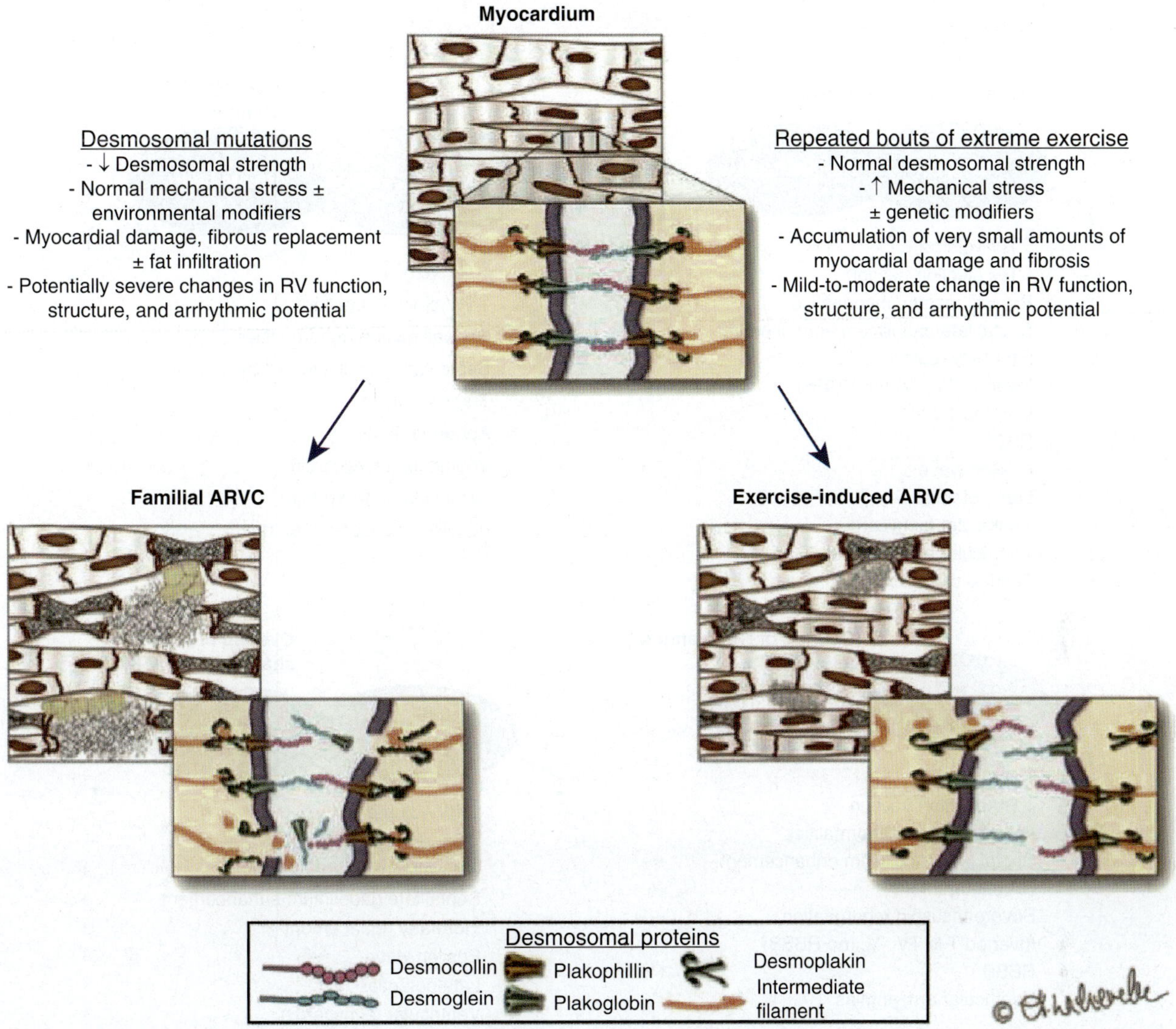

FIG. 29.37 Recommendations for participation in leisure-time physical activity and competitive sports of patients with arrhythmias and potentially arrhythmogenic conditions. (Reproduced with permission from Heidbuchel H, Corrado D, Biffi A et al. Recommendations for participation in leisure-time physical activity and competitive sports of patients with arrhythmias and potentially arrhythmogenic conditions. Part II: ventricular arrhythmias, channelopathies and implantable defibrillators. *Eur J Cardiovasc Prev Rehabil*. 2006;13:676–686.[68])

there is any concern of the validity of the recordings. Suspicion of regional wall motion changes may represent normal variants and are especially prominent at the RV apex, even on 3-T magnets.[56]

It is important to note that, in the majority of ARVC cases, regional RV WMAs predominantly involve basal (especially subtricuspid) segments, RV outflow tract, and midfree (lateral) and inferior RV wall. Involvement of the RV apex is rare in ARVC and is seen mostly in the advanced stages of the disease when the imaging features of ARVC resemble those in dilated cardiomyopathy. In ALVC, "ringlike" subepicardial or midwall LGE involving the inferolateral wall, septum, or both, is a characteristic lesion not seen in normal hearts or other nonischemic cardiomyopathies.

CARDIAC SARCOIDOSIS—AN ARRHYTHMOGENIC CARDIOMYOPATHY MIMIC

Cardiac sarcoidosis (CS) can be a difficult diagnosis by imaging methods. It may require a multidisciplinary approach similar to that for ACM. Diagnostic criteria for CS are based on minor and major criteria[80] and include a combination of imaging and nonimaging findings (Table 29.5).

Some structural abnormalities in CS on CMR may resemble those mentioned in the TFC for the diagnostic criteria of ACM. Among the findings mimicking ACM/ARVC, there may be RV enlargement and RV dysfunction as well as regional wall motion abnormalities. Fig. 29.40 demonstrates an example of a patient with sarcoid who had a positive biopsy and RV enlargement and dysfunction (both global and regional), fulfilling a major TFC for ARVC.[81] In these cases, a high level of clinical suspicion and understanding of the disease pathophysiology may encourage further evaluation by cardiac positron emission tomography (PET). PET appears to provide a high diagnostic yield in CS for the confirmation of myocardial inflammation and matching of lesions on T2-weighted CMR imaging with areas of increased fludeoxyglucose (18F) (F18-FDG) uptake in patients with CS (Fig. 29.41).[82–84] PET-CT is a powerful diagnostic tool for revealing extracardiac sarcoidosis, especially in the mediastinum/pulmonary hila (Fig. 29.42).[84] In addition to pulmonary involvement in CS, significant LV involvement is frequently present in CS patients. Although LGE is not specific or pathognomonic in either disorder, evidence

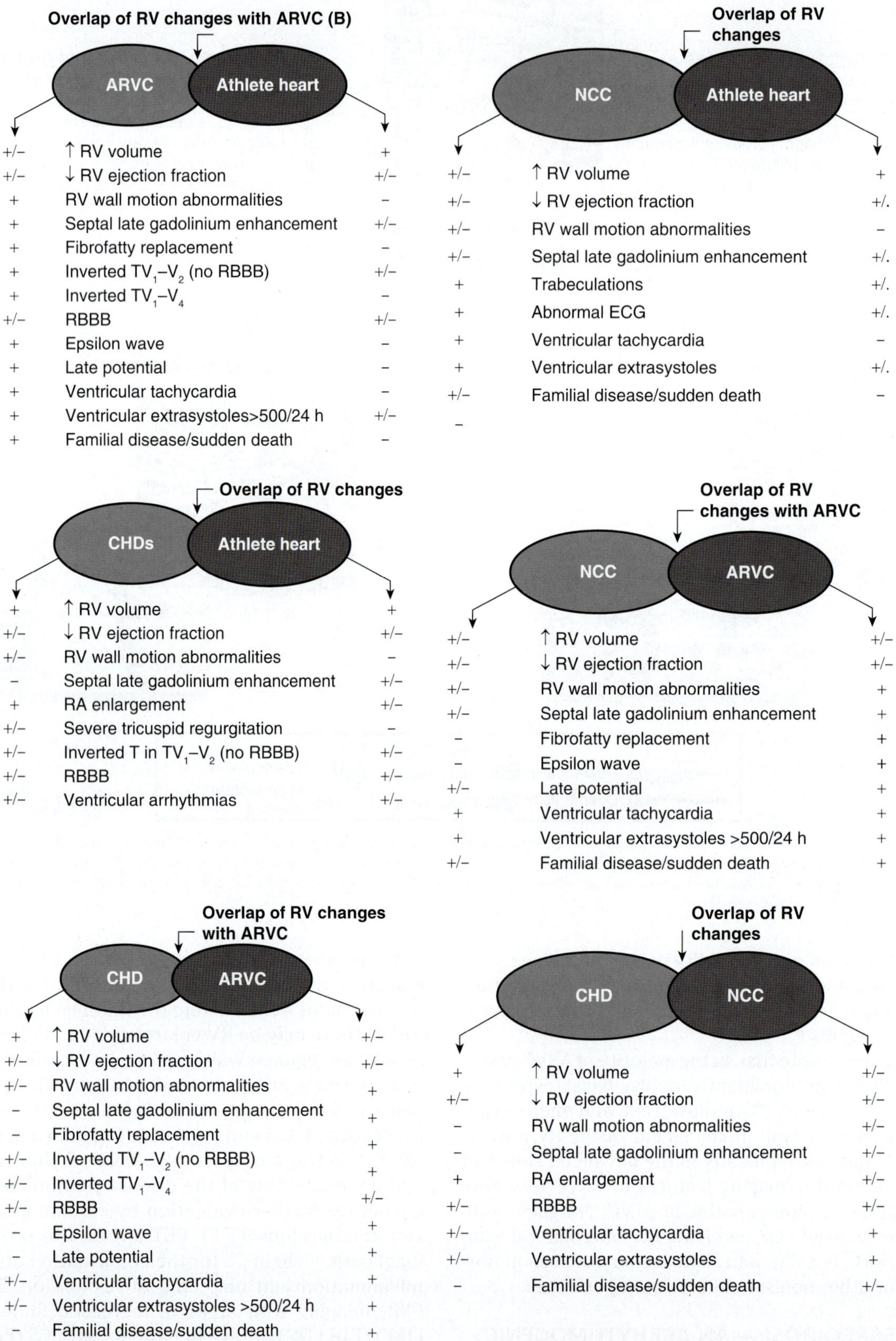

FIG. 29.38 Differential diagnosis of some right ventricular (*RV*) cardiomyopathies. *ARVC*, arrhythmogenic right ventricular cardiomyopathy; *CHD*, congenital heart disease; *NCC*, noncompaction cardiomyopathy; *RBBB*, right bundle branch block. (Reproduced with permission from Limongelli G, Rea A, Masarone D et al. Right ventricular cardiomyopathies: a multidisciplinary approach to diagnosis. *Echocardiography*. 2014;32:S75–S94.)

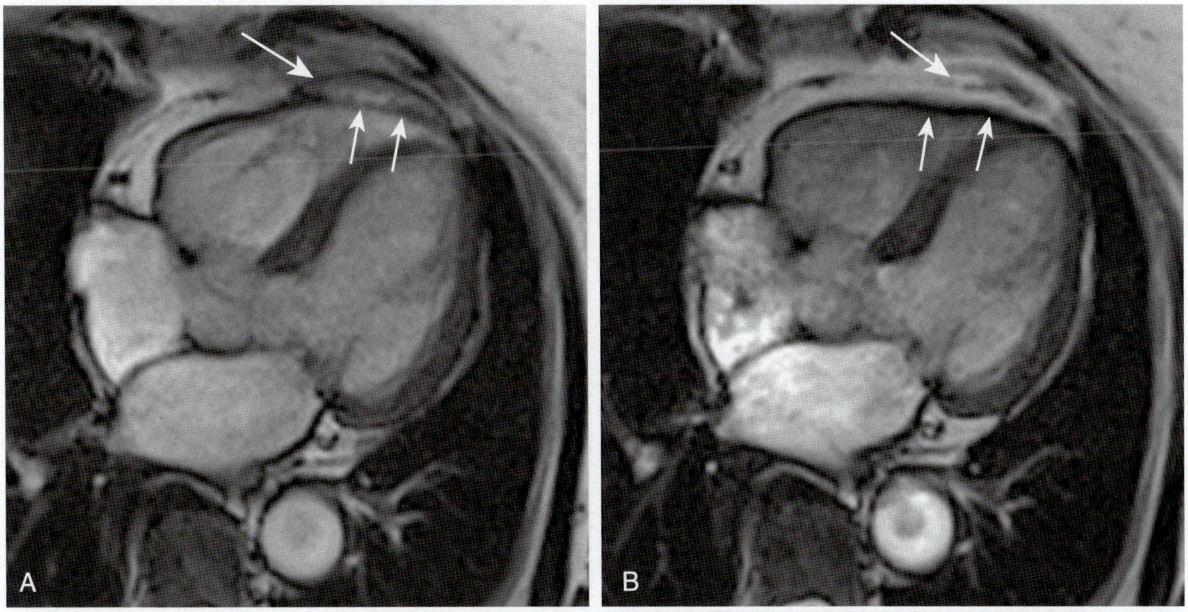

FIG. 29.39 Artifact mimicking a focal right ventricular (RV) wall motion abnormality on cine cardiac magnetic resonance images. (A) Cine steady-state free precession four-chamber view showing an artifact at the apex of the right ventricle (*broad arrow*) in front of the RV wall (*small white arrows*). (B) Absence of the artifact in the same four-chamber view, but with a slightly different radiofrequency (*open arrow*). (Reproduced with permission from Tavano A, Maurel B, Gaubert JY et al. MR imaging of arrhythmogenic right ventricular dysplasia: what the radiologist needs to know. *Diagnos Interv Imaging*. 2015;96:449–460.)

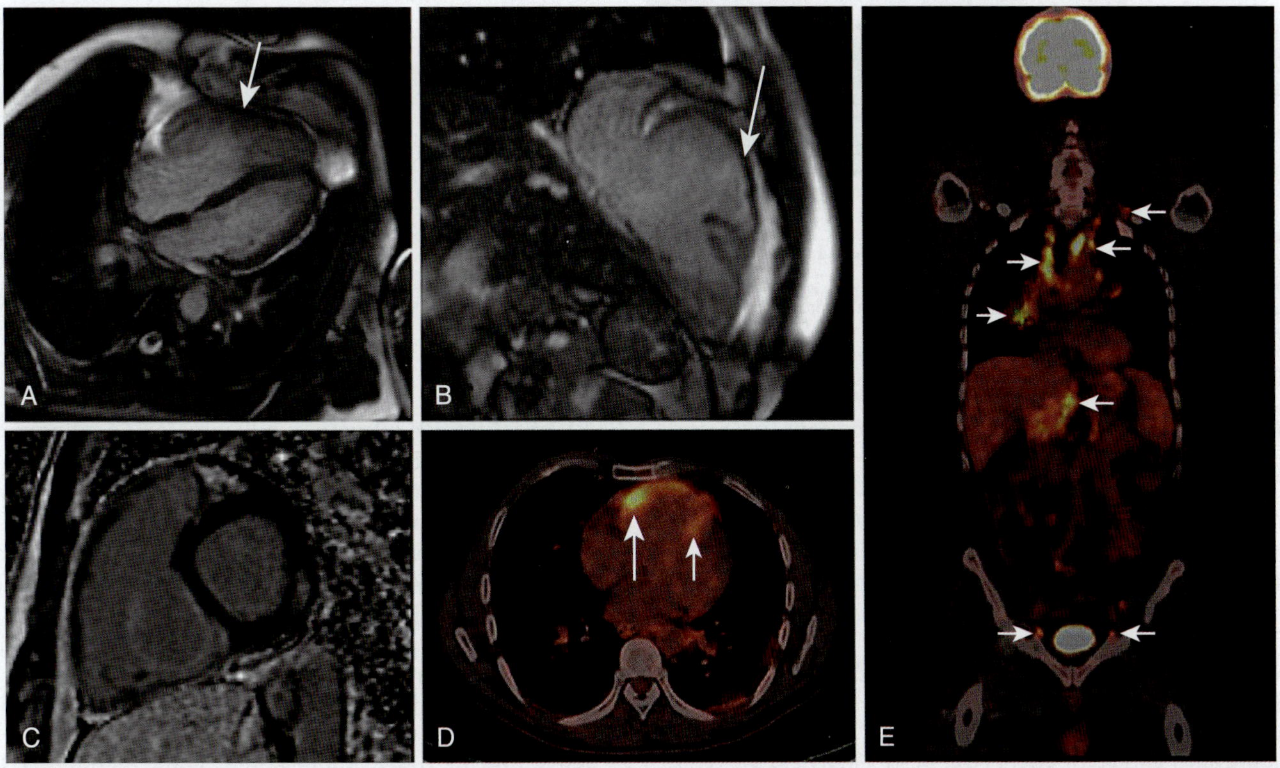

FIG. 29.40 Role of cardiac positron emission tomography (PET) in diagnosing cardiac sarcoidosis "mimicking" arrhythmogenic right ventricular cardiomyopathy. (A) Cardiac magnetic resonance imaging (MRI) showing dilated right ventricle (*arrow*) with indexed right ventricular (RV) end diastolic volume of 113 mL/m^2 and indexed RV end systolic volume of 71 mL/m^2. (B) Cardiac magnetic resonance demonstrates aneurysm in the inflow region (*arrow*) and apical hypokinesia with RV ejection fraction (RVEF) of 37%. (C) Cardiac MRI showing midwall-delayed gadolinium enhancement in the basal inferolateral segment of the left ventricle. (D) Axial-fused PET/CT image demonstrates intense focal fludeoxyglucose (FDG) uptake in the right ventricular free wall (*thick arrow*) and lesser uptake in the right ventricular septum (*thin arrow*). (E) Coronal-fused PET/CT demonstrates intense FDG uptake in enlarged neck, mediastinal, retroperitoneal, and groin nodes (*arrows*). Sites of bone uptake are not shown. (Reproduced with permission from Choo WK, Denison AR, Miller DR, Dempsey OJ, Dawson DK, Broadhurst PA. Cardiac sarcoid or arrhythmogenic right ventricular cardiomyopathy: a role for positron emission tomography (PET)? *J Nucl Cardiol*. 2013;20:479–480.)

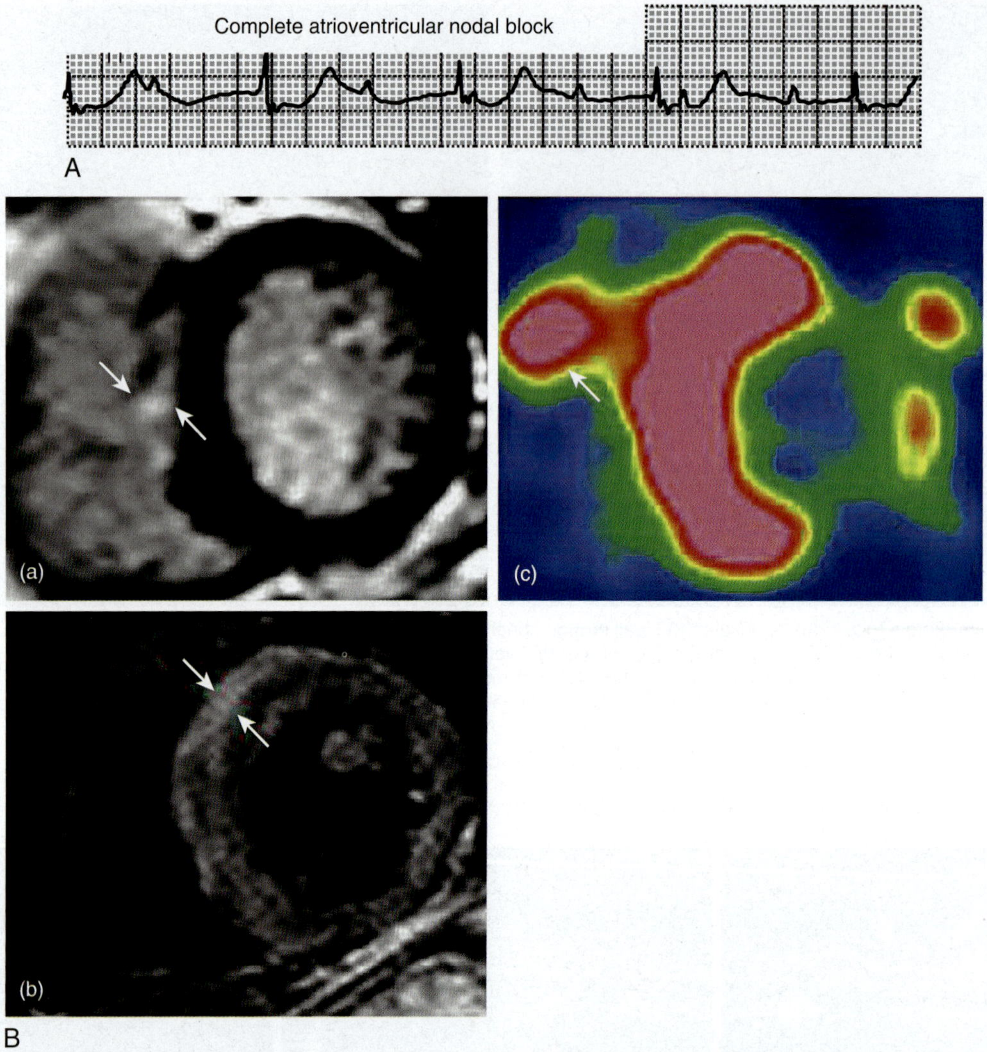

FIG. 29.41 Representative images from cardiac magnetic resonance (CMR) and cardiac positron emission tomography (PET) in a patient with pathologically proven cardiac sarcoid. Legend from the original publication: (A and B) CMR shows areas of delayed enhancement (DE) (A) and increased T2-weighted signal (B) in the anteroseptal wall of the left ventricle (LV) (*white and red arrows*). (C) 18F fludeoxyglucose (18F-FDG) PET shows focal 18F-FDG uptake in the anteroseptal LV and right ventricle (*black arrow*). (Reproduced with permission from Orii M, Imanishi T, Akasaka T. Assessment of cardiac sarcoidosis with advanced imaging modalities. *BioMed Res Int*. 2014;2014:897956.)

suggests that septal scarring is more frequent in CS and is rarely found in typical ARVC.[85]

Other useful clinical features suggestive of CS are older age of the patient at onset, mediastinal lymphadenopathy, presentation with conduction abnormalities rather than with ventricular arrhythmias, predominant LV dysfunction, and septal wall motion abnormalities.

OTHER ARRHYTHMOGENIC CARDIOMYOPATHY MIMICS: DIAGNOSTIC DILEMMAS

Based on an analysis of a series of 657 CMR studies in patients with known or suspected ACM, Quarta et al.[86] suggested the following classification of ARVC mimics:

1. Cardiac displacement (pectus excavatum, scoliosis, or other severe musculoskeletal problems involving the thoracic spine or rib cage; congenital absence of the pericardium) (Fig. 29.43)[29]
2. RV overload (pulmonary hypertension; severe tricuspid regurgitation, atrial septal defect [ASD], etc.)
3. RV scarring (RV infarction; inflammatory cardiomyopathies or sarcoidosis; myocarditis)

Based on our clinical experience, we propose adding to this classification RV functional abnormalities related to the pericardium and postthoracotomy changes as another ARVC mimic.

For ALVC/BiV-ACM, one must consider a much longer list of potential disease mimics; based on the 2023 TFC, the clinical pretest probability of the disease and genetic testing in addition to the imaging modalities become a very important diagnostic step in the assessment of these patients.

Each one of these mimics may have distinctive features. Clinical presentation, history, and careful evaluation of all imaging data may help to define the disorder. For suspected ARVC mimics, musculoskeletal abnormalities are relatively easily seen on CMR images. An additional comparison of the x-ray and CT scan may assist in reaching the correct diagnosis. RV overload mimics include congenital heart disorders (both simple and complex congenital heart disease). It is important to review all the data available on the images. CMR is a versatile methodology and evidence of the anomalies in the great vessels or cardiac structures (patent ductus arteriosus, partial anomalous venous return, Ebstein's anomaly, unroofed coronary sinus, and sinus venosus ASD) are among the disorders that CMR may assist in diagnosing in patients with enlarged and dysfunctional right ventricles. It is helpful to perform the phase-contrast analysis with calculation of the Qp/QS and estimates of cardiac shunting in these cases (Fig. 29.44).[87] For patients with evidence of delayed hyperenhancement (LGE), it is important to analyze for the presence of biventricular involvement, as well as for scar in the interventricular septum and the pattern of DHE in the left ventricle (midwall [in dilated cardiomyopathies] vs. epicardial [in some inflammatory cardiomyopathies] or subendocardial to transmural [specific for myocardial infarction]) (Fig. 29.15).[53] Basal involvement, especially in the subtricuspid area, is frequent in patients with "classic" ARVC. Inflammatory changes are frequently seen in patients with myocarditis and CS (see previous section) and are rarely observed in ARVC. Cardiac PET may

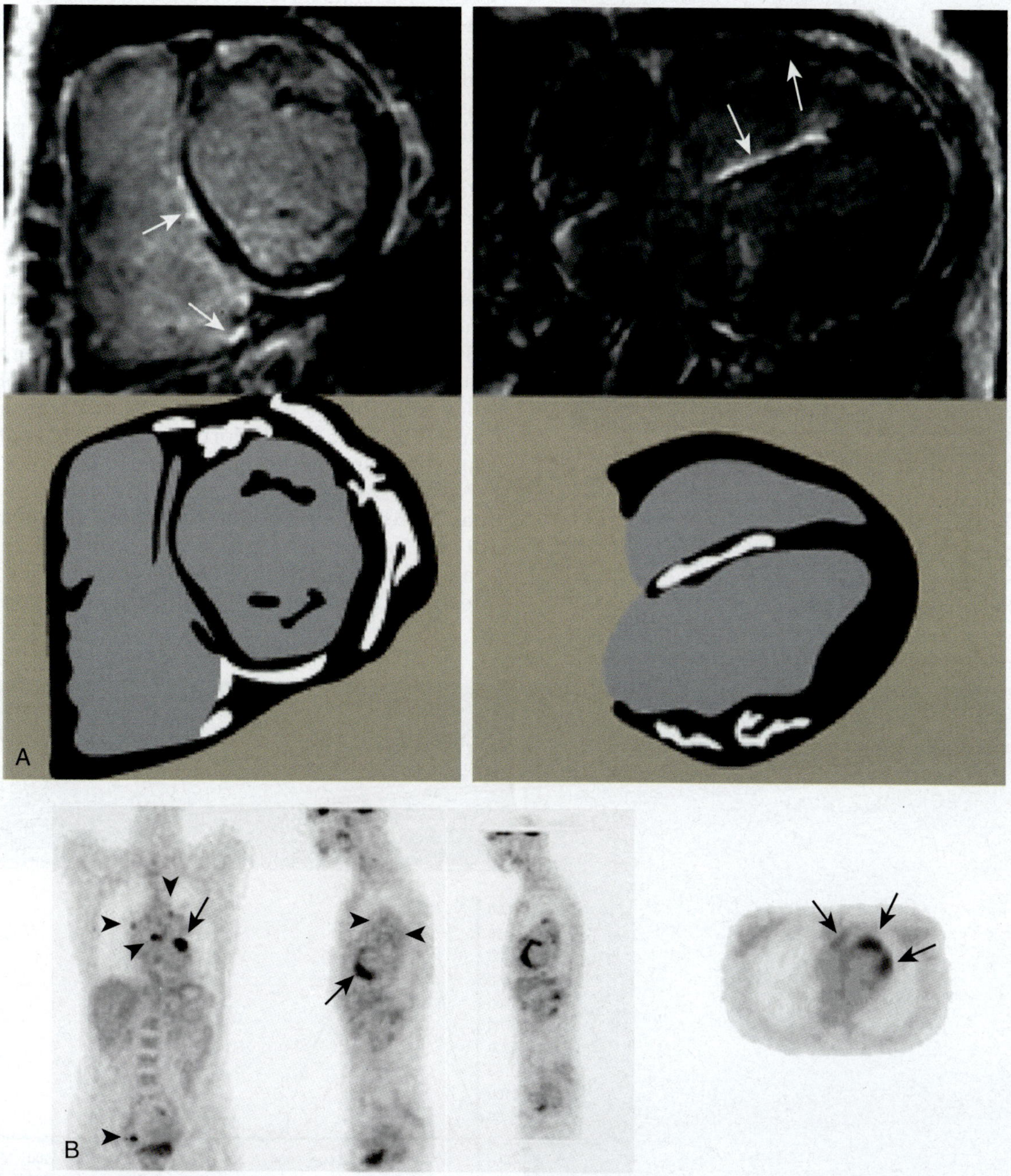

FIG. 29.42 Contrast-enhanced cardiac magnetic resonance (A) and fludeoxyglucose positron emission tomography (FDG PET) (B) study in a patient with biventricular congestive heart failure. Left-sided panel: inversion recovery gradient echo sequence, short-axis view demonstrates enhancement of the right-sided interventricular septum and inferior right ventricular insertion point. The horizontal long-axis view of the patient demonstrates enhancement of the right ventricular (RV) free wall and right-sided interventricular septum (right-sided panel, inversion-recovery gradient echo sequence). (B) FDG PET of this patient demonstrates sarcoid lymphadenopathy (*triangles*) and active inflammation of the anteroapical left ventricular segments and RV free wall (*arrows*). (Reproduced with permission from Smedema JP, Ainslie G, Crijns HJGM. Contrast-enhanced magnetic resonance in the diagnosis and management of cardiac sarcoidosis. Progress in Cardiovascular Diseases 2020; 63(3):271–307.)

increase the diagnostic accuracy of the images, confirming the location and pattern of inflammation seen on CMR, by an increased F18-FDG. Advanced CMR applications such as T1 and T2 mapping of the myocardium[88] can prove to be a useful addition to the standard ACM protocols when myocarditis is suspected.

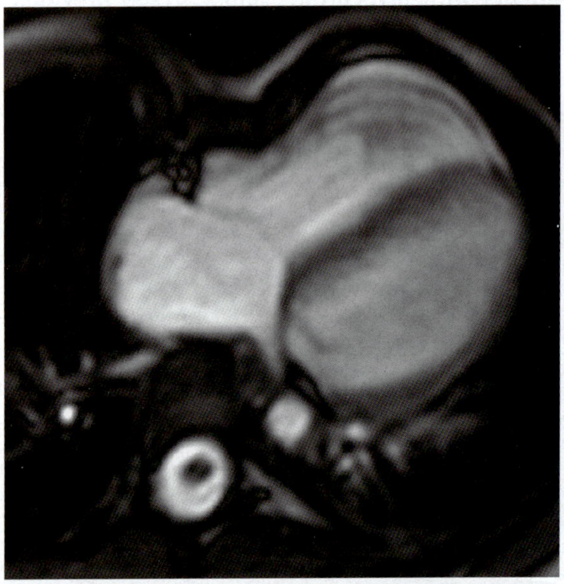

FIG. 29.43 Arrhythmogenic cardiomyopathy mimics: Chest deformities. Pectus excavatum in a 47-year-old male. Axial magnetic resonance image in a patient shows distortion of the right ventricle, with compression of the right ventricular (RV) base and a consequent relative enlargement of the RV apex. This can make assessment of wall motion abnormalities as well as contouring RV volumes challenging. (Reproduced, with permission from Galizia MS, Attili AK, Truesdell WR et al. Imaging features of arrhythmogenic cardiomyopathies. *Radiographics*. 2024;44:e230154.)

Finally, in our practice, we frequently observe RV focal abnormalities in patients who have had a sternotomy. This is probably due to pericardial adhesion to the posterior sternal surface. Paradoxical postoperative septal motion may also be seen in these patients. This adds to the difficulty in calculating RV volumes and RVEF, since the interventricular septum has dyssynchronous motion and may interact with the Simpson's disk method assumptions.

Prognostic Value of Cardiac Magnetic Resonance in Arrhythmogenic Cardiomyopathy

ACM is a clinically heterogeneous disease due to its incomplete penetrance and variable expression. Symptoms related to ACM range from palpitations, fatigue, and chest pain to more severe presentations such as lightheadedness and near syncope due to rapid monomorphic VT, as well as heart failure and SCD. However, many patients are asymptomatic, especially in the early stages of disease. Fibrofatty replacement of the RV or the LV myocardium interferes with normal electrical impulse conduction in the cardiac tissue and may precipitate SCD. Progressive myocardial cell loss also results in ventricular dysfunction and heart failure. Both these factors influence the natural history of ACM.[31,89–91] Areas of myocardial fibrosis may lead to reentry, which can cause hemodynamically stable or unstable ventricular arrhythmias in patients with relatively stable disease (Fig. 29.45).[92–95] Unfortunately, in ACM patients, the very first clinical presentation may be SCD.

What is the magnitude of the problem? Typical ARVC has a prevalence estimated between 1:2000 and 1:5000 of the general population and is one of the leading causes of SCD in youth.[15] ARVC accounts for 3%–4% of deaths in sports and 5% of SCD in people younger than

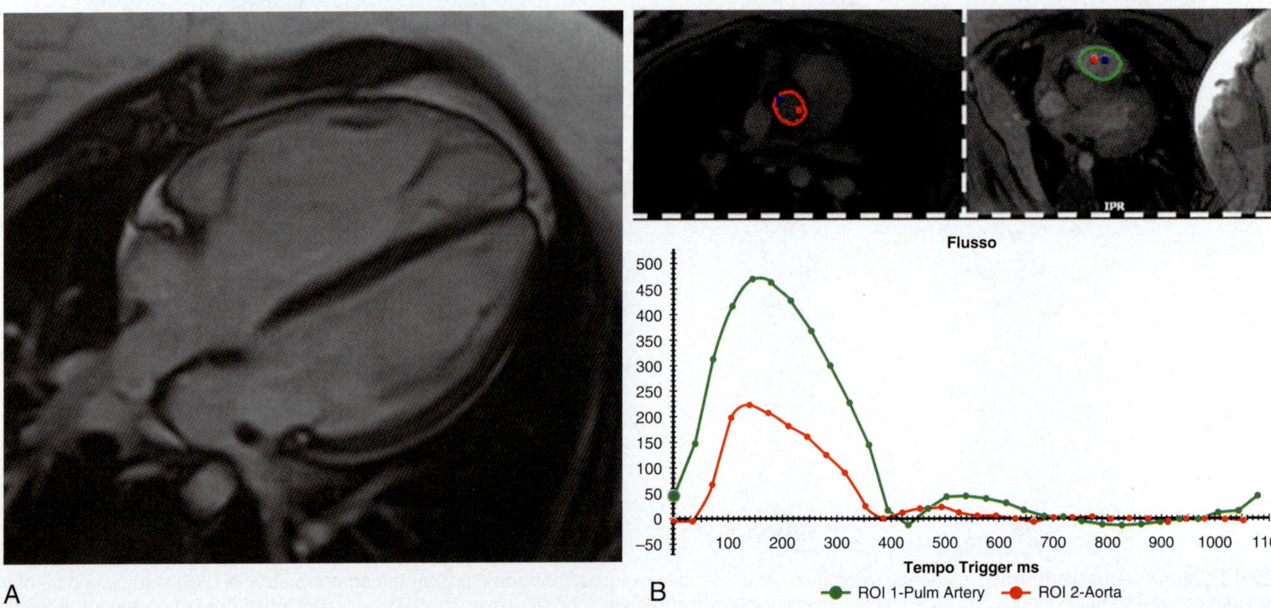

FIG. 29.44 Arrhythmogenic cardiomyopathy mimics: Adult congenital heart disease. Cardiac magnetic resonance (CMR) images in a 21-year-old admitted for effort-related syncope. (A) Severe right ventricular dilatation. (B) Flow CMR demonstrated the differences in cardiac output between aorta and pulmonary artery, suggestive of left-to-right shunt (Qp/Qs 2.5). The patient was diagnosed with atrial septal defect (*upper sinus venosus type*) and partial anomalous pulmonary venous return. *ROI*, region of interest. (Reproduced, with permission from Cipriani A, Mattesi G, Bariani R et al. Cardiac magnetic resonance imaging of arrhythmogenic cardiomyopathy: evolving diagnostic perspectives. *Eur Radiol*. 2023;33:270–282.)

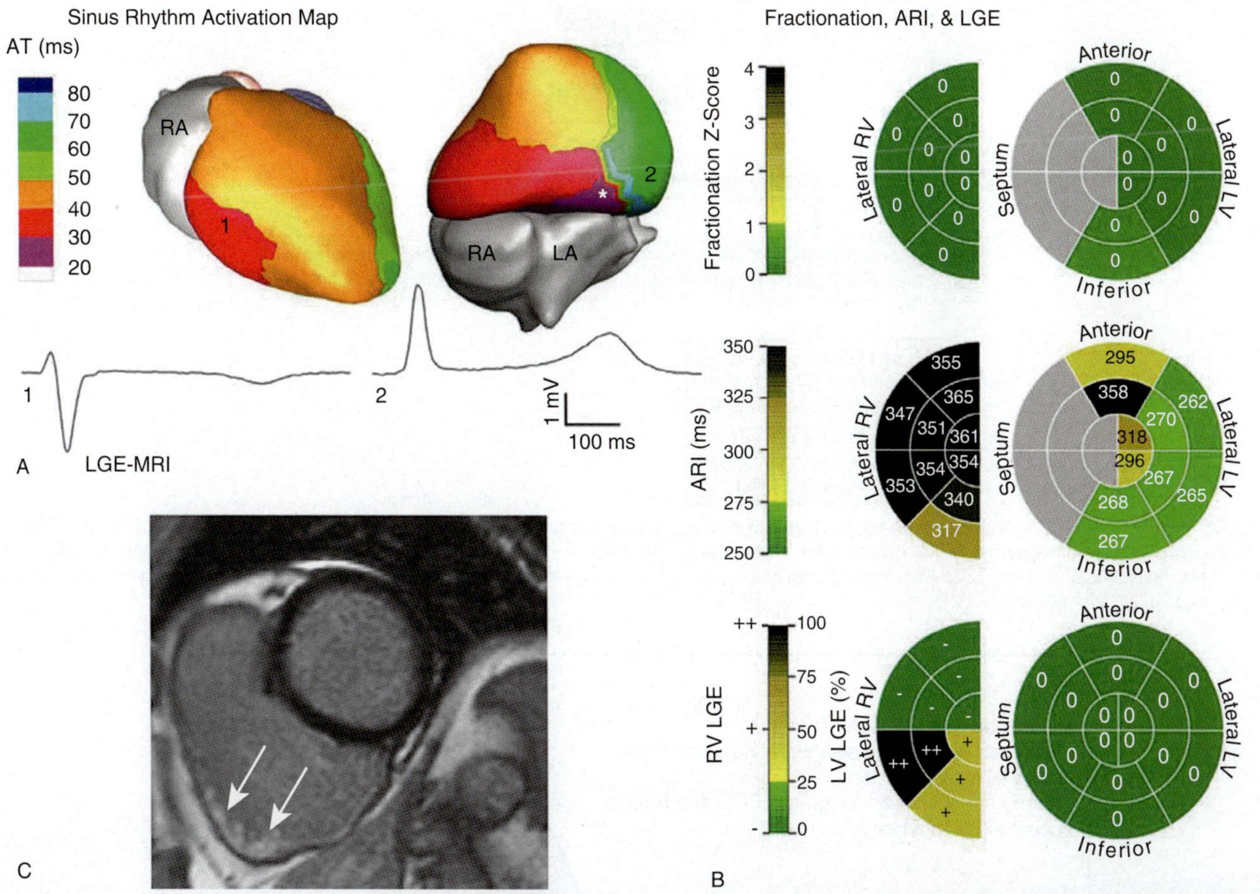

FIG. 29.45 Electric substrate of a patient with advanced arrhythmogenic right ventricular cardiomyopathy and a high premature ventricular contraction rate. (A) Ventricular epicardial breakthrough during sinus rhythm was abnormal, with earliest activation originating from the basal inferior left ventricle (*LV*; asterisk). Right ventricle (*RV*; 1) and LV (2) unipolar electrograms (EGMs) had normal QRS morphology. (B) EGM fractionation was not abnormal compared with controls (*top*). Fridericia-corrected activation-recovery intervals (*ARIs*) were prolonged compared with control values (*middle*). Concentrated late gadolinium enhancement (*LGE*) was visible in the inferior RV (*bottom*). (C) Cardiac magnetic resonance shows extensive LGE, which was confined to the subepicardial RV (indicated by *yellow arrows*). AT indicates activation time; *LA*, left atrium; and *RA*, right atrium. (Reproduced, with permission from Andrews CM, Srinivasan NT, Rosmini S et al. Electrical and structural substrate of arrhythmogenic right ventricular cardiomyopathy determined using noninvasive electrocardiographic imaging and late gadolinium magnetic resonance imaging. *Circ Arrhythm Electrophysiol*. 2017;10:e005105.)

65 years of age.[15,96] SCD can occur at any time during the course of the disease, with an incidence varying from 0.1% to 3% per year.[11] Evidence suggests that SCD is caused by hemodynamically unstable VT or ventricular fibrillation (VF). SCD in young asymptomatic patients is usually due to VF that occurs during the active phase of acute myocyte death and reactive inflammation.[92–94] Thus, appropriate screening and risk stratification is pivotal in patients with ACM due to the associated risk of SCD.

CMR findings and evidence of electrical instability allow initial screening and selection of patients at expected high risk among those patients with known or suspected ACM (Figs. 29.46 and 29.47).[97,98]

In this regard, the presence of the unique LGE is associated with incremental diagnostic and prognostic value in ACM. It allows the identification of patients at higher risk among survivors of aborted cardiac arrest and reveals an arrhythmic substrate in 76% of cases.[98] Risk stratification of patients at a high risk of major adverse cardiac events (MACEs) based on the amount of LGE is effective not only in ACM but also in other cardiac disorders leading to arrhythmias; the threshold of LGE >8% is clearly associated with increased MACE risk (Fig. 29.48).[98]

The role of CMR is not limited by the baseline, initial diagnosis of ACM. Regardless of the severity and clinical phase of the disease (early vs. advanced), an important question is what is the best approach to follow these patients? How soon after the initial diagnosis of ARVC/D should we rescan the patient? Current guidelines recommend serial screening of genetically predisposed patients using a combination of ECG, Holter monitoring, and imaging.[99] Several studies have focused on identifying parameters that can be used to determine the risk of SCD. The role of ECG is well established when stratifying patients with ARVC.

The presence of both electrical and CMR abnormalities identify patients at high risk who might benefit from prophylactic ICD placement, since sustained ventricular arrhythmias occur exclusively in patients with abnormal CMR results.[35]

Deac et al. analyzed the prognostic value of CMR in 369 patients with at least one criterion for ARVC and found that an abnormal CMR study was a significant

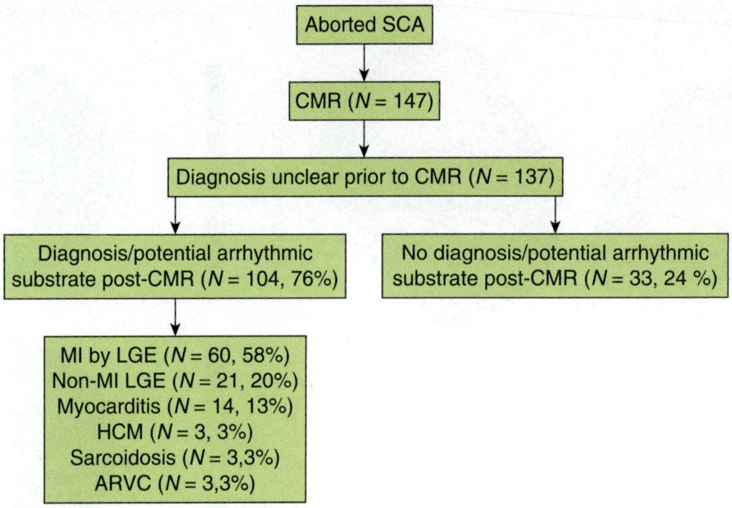

FIG. 29.46 Cardiac magnetic resonance (*CMR*)-based diagnosis of the potential arrhythmic source among survivors of sudden cardiac death (*SCD*). *ARVC*, arrhythmogenic RV cardiomyopathy; *HCM*, hypertrophic cardiomyopathy; *LGE*, late Gadolinium enhancement; *MI*, myocardial infarcton; *SCA*, sudden cardiac arrest. (Reproduced with permission from Neilan TG, Farhad H, Mayrhofer T et al. Late gadolinium enhancement among survivors of sudden cardiac arrest. *JACC Cardiovasc Imaging*. 2015;8:414–423.)

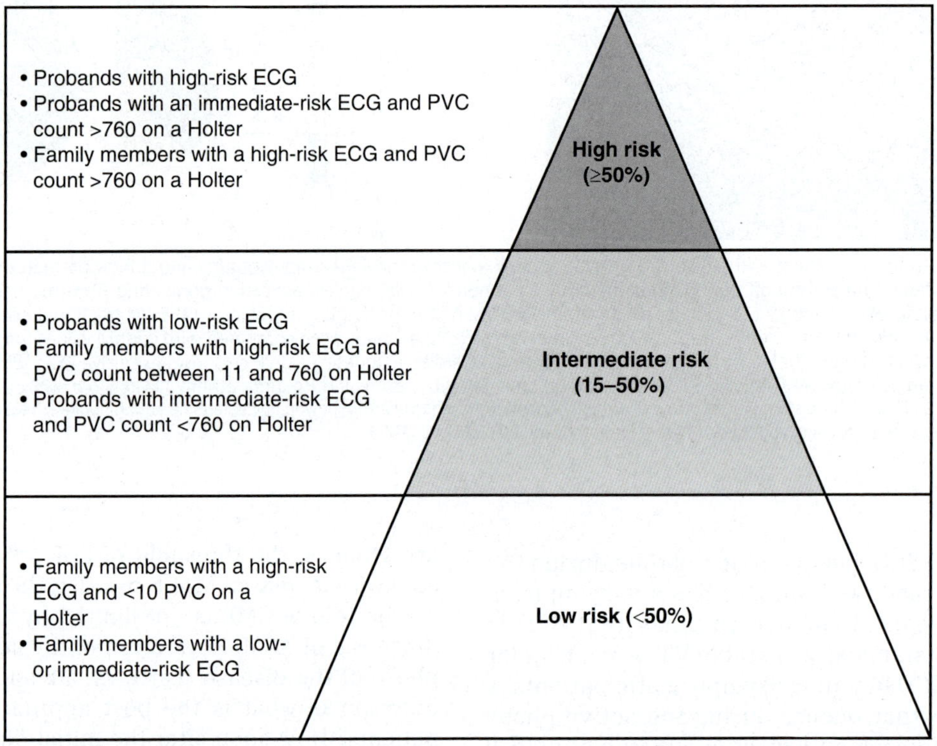

FIG. 29.47 Arrhythmic risk stratification among patients with ARVC-associated desmosomal mutations based on presentation, electrocardiogram (*ECG*), and Holter monitoring. *PVC*, Premature ventricular contractions. (Reproduced with permission from Bhonsale A, James CA, Tichnell C et al. Risk stratification in arrhythmogenic right ventricular dysplasia/cardiomyopathy-associated desmosomal mutation carriers. *Circ Arrhythm Electrophysiol*. 2013;6:569–578.)

predictor of an endpoint composite that included cardiac death, sustained VT, VF, and appropriate ICD discharge. The risk of an abnormal CMR was compared to traditional clinical parameters. After multivariable analysis, only abnormal CMR and VT remained significant predictors of outcomes.[100] This recent study corroborates the findings of the previous work of Aquaro et al. who found similar results. According to their analysis, the patients with an abnormal CMR were at increased risk of cardiac events.[54]

Future Perspectives of Cardiac Magnetic Resonance Utilization and Role of Artificial Intelligence for Diagnostic and Prognostic Assessment of Arrhythmogenic Cardiomyopathy

ACM is a variable disease with a wide spectrum of genetic abnormalities leading to the structural cardiac pathology. In many cases, we encounter discrepant phenotype-genotype findings.

In addition, even in the advanced disease phase, there are clinical findings not well aligned with the typical diagnostic criteria of the disease.

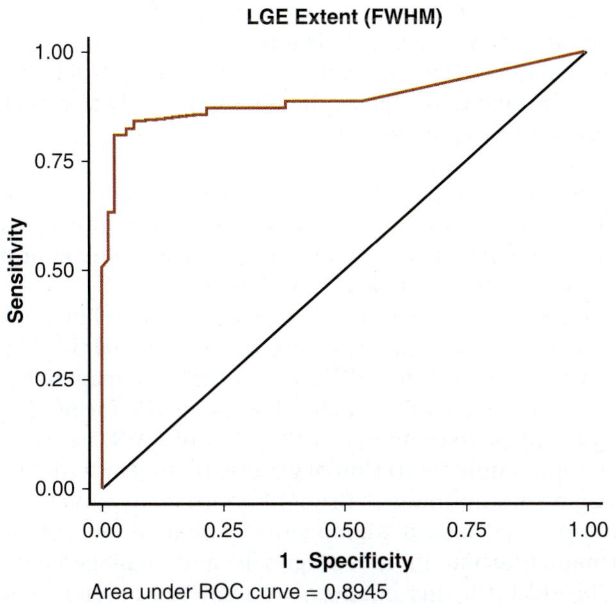

FIG. 29.48 ROC curve for prediction of major adverse cardiac events among survivors of sudden cardiac death. The cutoff of delayed hyperenhancement with the highest sensitivity and specificity (8.1%) was utilized. *FWHM,* full-width at half-maximum analysis; *LGE,* late Gadolinium enhancement; *ROC,* receiver operating characteristic. (Reproduced with permission from Neilan TG, Farhad H, Mayrhofer T et al. Late gadolinium enhancement among survivors of sudden cardiac arrest. *JACC Cardiovasc Imaging.* 2015;8:414–423.)

CMR is a crucial imaging methodology in establishing an accurate general ACM diagnosis as well as in defining a specific subtype of the disease ("classic" ARVC, ALVC, or BiV-ACM) (Fig. 29.49).[24]

In this regard, the measurement of global and regional LV and RV function and reliability of the measurements obtained by imagers with different level of clinical expertise, as well as the reproducibility and repeatability of sequential volumetric measurements, even within the same laboratory and for the same imaging expert, often become an area of concern.

The ability to effectively implement standardized segmentation of the LV and the RV and have an automated or semiautomated (physician-assisted) assessment of regional wall motion abnormalities and LV and RV global and regional systolic function, is, in our understanding, a "low-hanging fruit" in terms of utilizing artificial intelligence (AI) applications in cardiac imaging and, specifically, in the field of ACM imaging.

Considering the importance of calculating scar/fibrosis (both regional and total scar burden), AI may become a very important tool in developing reproducible LGE polar maps and highlighting any disease-specific LGE patterns for further diagnostic decision-making by the CMR reader, in addition to the scar burden calculation (often presented as a percent of the myocardium involved). The latter is closely associated with overall arrhythmic risk and a threshold of 15% scar burden is often used as a threshold

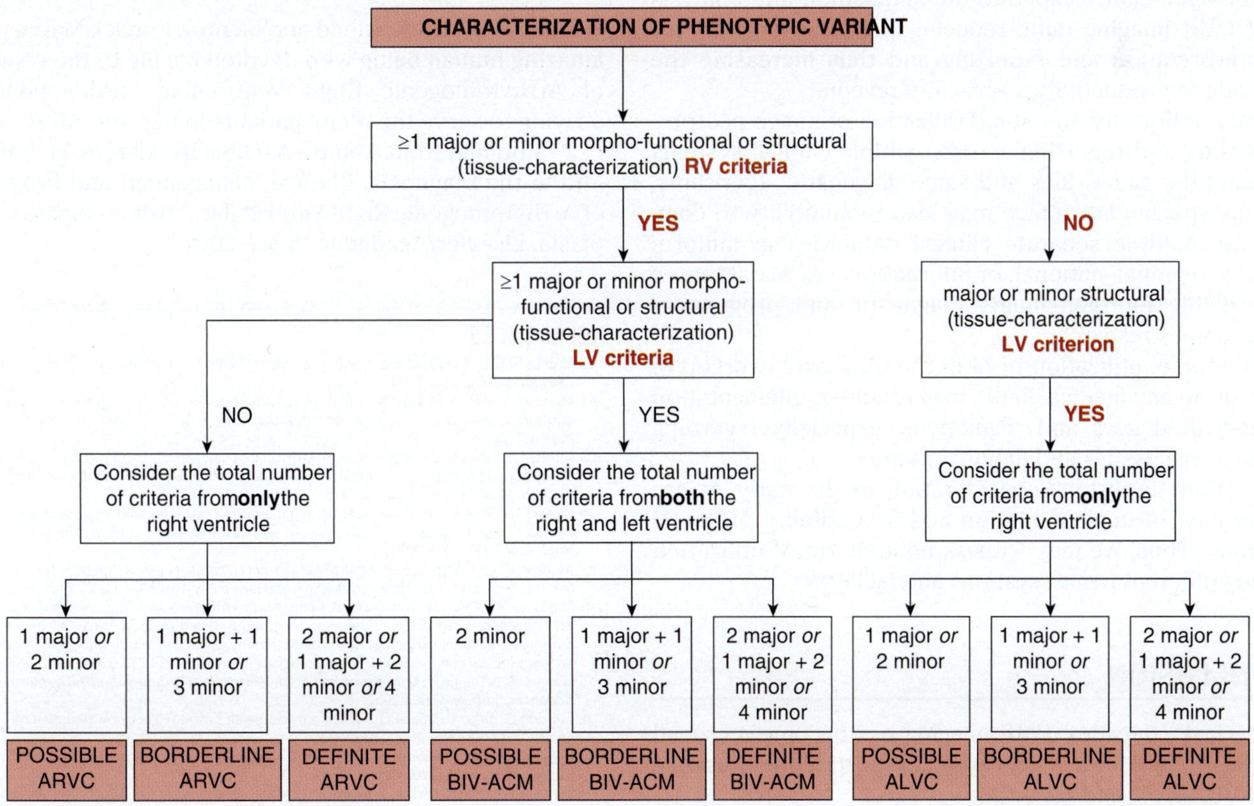

FIG. 29.49 Flowchart for phenotypic characterization of Arrhythmogenic cardiomyopathy based on 2023 European task force criteria.[27] *ALVC,* arrhythmogenic left ventricular cardiomyopathy; *ARVC,* arrhythmogenic right ventricular cardiomyopathy; *BIV-ACM,* biventricular arrhythmogenic cardiomyopathy; *LV,* left ventricle; *RV,* right ventricle. (From Corrado D, Anastasakis A, Basso C, et al. Proposed diagnostic criteria for arrhythmogenic cardiomyopathy: European task force consensus report. *Int J Cardiol.* 2024;395:131447.)

defining the need for ICD implantation for primary prophylaxis of sudden death.

Finally, the overall diagnosis of ACM is a very complicated process, with multiple criteria that need to be considered as a combined set in order to proceed with the probable, possible, or definitive disease statement. We believe that we may soon have AI-guided, clinically validated, and effective ACM probability calculators as well as ACM prognostic models, which, combined with CMR software, will allow customized patient-centered reporting. Moreover, the presence of large ACM databases allows to provide better input into the machine-learning algorithms defining these prognostic models and thus significantly improving their predictive power.

Among the expected advantages of utilizing AI to assist in the diagnostic workup of ACM, we can list the following:

1. Enhanced comprehensive assessment: AI can analyze complex clinical, historical, genetic, and imaging data to provide the most precise probability of ACM based on any of the TFC.
2. Improved diagnostic accuracy: AI-based algorithms can detect subtle changes in morphology, function, and tissue composition, leading to earlier detection of the disease and allowing a more accurate comparison of any sequential studies done to identify cases with ACM progression.
3. Personalized risk assessment: AI may provide patient-specific management recommendations based on an individual patient's clinical profile, and potentially improve outcomes.
4. Improved efficiency and productivity: Utilization of AI will significantly expedite the acquisition and analysis of CMR imaging data, reducing the time required for interpretation and reporting and thus increasing the reader's productivity and facility revenue.
5. Data uniformity and standardization of image postprocessing and reporting across multiple clinical systems using the same rules and same diagnostic algorithms. This specific advantage may lead to an ability to combine multiple separate clinical databases in uniform large regional, national, or international ACM databases available for high-quality diagnostic and prognostic/outcomes research.

Of course, utilization of AI in the diagnostic workup of ACM (as in any medical field), may require implementation of dedicated laws and regulations, especially regarding medico-legal issues and liability matters.

Another important consideration in the early AI era is the cost of implementation and accessibility of the AI systems. Thus, we may witness nonuniform AI utilization among different health systems and facilities.

CONCLUSION

In the last 2 decades, CMR imaging has become a crucial diagnostic tool for discovering and reporting the presence of ARVC, ALVC, and BiV-ACM.

Right-sided ACM is so-called "desmosomal" disease with predominantly autosomal dominant inheritance and a spectrum of clinical presentations in young individuals including characteristic morphofunctional changes of the right and left ventricle such as myocardial fibrosis secondary to fibrofatty degeneration, global and regional systolic dysfunction, and potentially fatal ventricular arrhythmias. Nondesmosomal genotypes are more common in ALVC and BiV-ACM, with differences in phenotype and specific imaging findings.

Importantly, since ACM is a proven risk factor for SCD, particularly in the young, it is important for cardiac imagers to be able to recognize the disease as early as possible to prevent this catastrophic event.

CMR is a unique versatile diagnostic tool that combines cardiac anatomy, function, perfusion, flow, and tissue characterization including the presence of scar/fibrosis and myocardial inflammation all in one concise clinical protocol that is obtained in less than 1 hour.

Based on its exceptional diagnostic capabilities, CMR became a very important part of the original 1994 and modified 2010 TFC for ARVC and is truly an imaging foundation of the most recent 2023 European TFC for ACM.

Recent developments in the field of CMR, as well as the rapid implementation of genetic testing and AI-based imaging methodologies brought about many novel applications that could significantly enhance our clinical armamentarium in the diagnosis and management of ACM/ARVC. In this chapter, we included a brief review of CMR-based diagnostic methodologies that are useful in the assessment and management of this complex pathology.

ACKNOWLEDGMENTS

*In memory of dear friend and mentor, Frank I. Marcus—an amazing human being who devoted his life to the research of Arrhythmogenic Right Ventricular Cardiomyopathy, striving to serve the many patients living with ARVC.

**Modified from Abidov A, Oliva IB, Marcus FI. Cardiac MRI in the Diagnosis, Clinical Management and Prognosis of Arrhythmogenic Right Ventricular Cardiomyopathy/Dysplasia. Elsevier/Academic Press; 2016.

REFERENCES

1. Marcus FI, Fontaine GH, Guiraudon G, et al. Right ventricular dysplasia: a report of 24 adult cases. *Circulation*. 1982;65:384–398.
2. Marcus FI, McKenna WJ, Sherrill D, et al. Diagnosis of arrhythmogenic right ventricular cardiomyopathy/dysplasia: proposed modification of the task force criteria. *Circulation*. 2010;121:1533–1541.
3. Cipriani A, Bauce B, De Lazzari M, et al. Arrhythmogenic right ventricular cardiomyopathy: characterization of left ventricular phenotype and differential diagnosis with dilated cardiomyopathy. *J Am Heart Assoc*. 2020;9:e014628.
4. Casella M, Gasperetti A, Sicuso R, et al. Characteristics of patients with arrhythmogenic left ventricular cardiomyopathy: combining genetic and histopathologic findings. *Circ Arrhythm Electrophysiol*. 2020;13:e009005.
5. Akdis D, Chen L, Saguner AM, et al. Novel plasma biomarkers predicting biventricular involvement in arrhythmogenic right ventricular cardiomyopathy. *Am Heart J*. 2022;244:66–76.
6. McKenna WJ, Thiene G, Nava A, et al. Diagnosis of arrhythmogenic right ventricular dysplasia/cardiomyopathy. Task force of the working group myocardial and pericardial disease of the European society of cardiology and of the scientific council on cardiomyopathies of the international society and federation of cardiology. *Br Heart J*. 1994;71:215–218.
7. Marcus FN A, Thiene G. *Arrhythmogenic Right Ventricular Cardiomyopathy/Dysplasia: Recent Advances*. Springer Verlag; 2007.
8. Corrado D, Basso C, Thiene G. Sudden cardiac death in young people with apparently normal heart. *Cardiovasc Res*. 2001;50:399–408.
9. Corrado D, Perazzolo Marra M, Zorzi A, et al. Diagnosis of arrhythmogenic cardiomyopathy: the Padua criteria. *Int J Cardiol*. 2020;319:106–114.
10. Thiene GR, Rizzo S, Pillichou K, Basso C. Arrhythmogenic cardiomyopathy: history and pathology. In: Abidov AO, Oliva IB, Marcus FI, eds. *Cardiac MRI in the Diagnosis, Clinical Management and Prognosis of Arrhythmogenic Right Ventricular Cardiomyopahy/dysplasia*. Elsevier; 2016:5–35.
11. Lancisi G. *De Motu Cordis et Aneurysmatibus*. Excudebat Felix-Carolus Musca; 1736.

12. Laennec RTH. *A Treatise on the Diseases of the Chest and on Mediate Auscultation*. Paris Brosson & Chaudé; 1819.
13. Osler W. *The Principles and Practice of Medicine*. D. Appleton & Co; 1905.
14. Richardson P, McKenna W, Bristow M, et al. Report of the 1995 world health organization/international society and federation of cardiology task force on the definition and classification of cardiomyopathies. *Circulation*. 1996;93:841–842.
15. Thiene G, Nava A, Corrado D, Rossi L, Pennelli N. Right ventricular cardiomyopathy and sudden death in young people. *N Engl J Med*. 1988;318:129–133.
16. Protonotarios N, Tsatsopoulou A, Scampardonis G. Arrhythmogenic cardiomyopathy with ectodermal dysplasia. *Am Heart J*. 1988;116:1651–1652.
17. Carvajal-Huerta L. Epidermolytic palmoplantar keratoderma with woolly hair and dilated cardiomyopathy. *J Am Acad Dermatol*. 1998;39:418–421.
18. Marra MP, Leoni L, Bauce B, et al. Imaging study of ventricular scar in arrhythmogenic right ventricular cardiomyopathy: comparison of 3D standard electroanatomical voltage mapping and contrast-enhanced cardiac magnetic resonance. *Circ Arrhythm Electrophysiol*. 2012;5:91–100.
19. Marcus FI, Abidov A. Arrhythmogenic right ventricular cardiomyopathy 2012: diagnostic challenges and treatment. *J Cardiovasc Electrophysiol*. 2012;23:1149–1153.
20. te Riele AS, James CA, Rastegar N, et al. Yield of serial evaluation in at-risk family members of patients with ARVD/C. *J Am Coll Cardiol*. 2014;64:293–301.
21. Protonotarios N, Tsatsopoulou A, Fontaine G. Naxos disease: keratoderma, scalp modifications, and cardiomyopathy. *J Am Acad Dermatol*. 2001;44:309–311.
22. Baykan A, Olgar S, Argun M, et al. Different clinical presentations of Naxos disease and Carvajal syndrome: case series from a single tertiary center and review of the literature. *Anatol J Cardiol*. 2015;15:404–408.
23. Protonotarios N, Tsatsopoulou A. Naxos disease and Carvajal syndrome: cardiocutaneous disorders that highlight the pathogenesis and broaden the spectrum of arrhythmogenic right ventricular cardiomyopathy. *Cardiovasc Pathol*. 2004;13:185–194.
24. Graziano F, Zorzi A, Cipriani A, et al. Contemporary diagnostic approach to arrhythmogenic cardiomyopathy: the three-step work-up. *Trends Cardiovasc Med*. 2024;35(2):107–113.
25. Graziano F, Zorzi A, Ungaro S, et al. The 2023 European task force criteria for diagnosis of arrhythmogenic cardiomyopathy: historical background and review of main changes. *Rev Cardiovasc Med*. 2024;25:348.
26. Perazzolo Marra M, Rizzo S, Bauce B, et al. Arrhythmogenic right ventricular cardiomyopathy. Contribution of cardiac magnetic resonance imaging to the diagnosis. *Herz*. 2015;40:600–606.
27. Corrado D, Anastasakis A, Basso C, et al. Proposed diagnostic criteria for arrhythmogenic cardiomyopathy: European task force consensus report. *Int J Cardiol*. 2024;395:131447.
28. Patel AML, Marcus FI. Association of phenotype and genotype in the diagnosis and prognosis of ARVC/D in the adult population. In: Abidov AO, Oliva IB, Marcus FI, eds. *Cardiac MRI in the Diagnosis, Clinical Management and Prognosis of Arrhythmogenic Right Ventricular Cardiomyopathy/Dysplasia*. Academic Press/Elsevier; 2016:89–103.
29. Galizia MS, Attili AK, Truesdell WR, et al. Imaging features of arrhythmogenic cardiomyopathies. *Radiographics*. 2024;44:e230154.
30. Sen-Chowdhry S, Syrris P, Ward D, Asimaki A, Sevdalis E, McKenna WJ. Clinical and genetic characterization of families with arrhythmogenic right ventricular dysplasia/cardiomyopathy provides novel insights into patterns of disease expression. *Circulation*. 2007;115:1710–1720.
31. Dalal D, Nasir K, Bomma C, et al. Arrhythmogenic right ventricular dysplasia: a United States experience. *Circulation*. 2005;112:3823–3832.
32. Sen-Chowdhry S, Morgan RD, Chambers JC, McKenna WJ. Arrhythmogenic cardiomyopathy: etiology, diagnosis, and treatment. *Annu Rev Med*. 2010;61:233–253.
33. Sen-Chowdhry S, Syrris P, Prasad SK, et al. Left-dominant arrhythmogenic cardiomyopathy: an under-recognized clinical entity. *J Am Coll Cardiol*. 2008;52:2175–2187.
34. Abidov A, Oliva IB, Marcus FI. *Cardiac MRI in the Diagnosis, Clinical Management and Prognosis of Arrhyhtmogenic Right Ventricular Cardiomyopathy/Dysplasia*. Academic Press/Elsevier; 2016.
35. te Riele AS, Bhonsale A, James CA, et al. Incremental value of cardiac magnetic resonance imaging in arrhythmic risk stratification of arrhythmogenic right ventricular dysplasia/cardiomyopathy-associated desmosomal mutation carriers. *J Am Coll Cardiol*. 2013;62:1761–1769.
36. Auffermann W, Wichter T, Breithardt G, Joachimsen K, Peters PE. Arrhythmogenic right ventricular disease: MR imaging vs angiography. *AJR Am J Roentgenol*. 1993;161:549–555.
37. White RD, Trohman RG, Flamm SD, et al. Right ventricular arrhythmia in the absence of arrhythmogenic dysplasia: MR imaging of myocardial abnormalities. *Radiology*. 1998;207:743–751.
38. Tandri H, Bomma C, Calkins H, Bluemke DA. Magnetic resonance and computed tomography imaging of arrhythmogenic right ventricular dysplasia. *J Magn Reson Imaging*. 2004;19:848–858.
39. Karamitsos TD, Francis JM, Myerson S, Selvanayagam JB, Neubauer S. The role of cardiovascular magnetic resonance imaging in heart failure. *J Am Coll Cardiol*. 2009;54:1407–1424.
40. Bluemke DA, Krupinski EA, Ovitt T, et al. MR Imaging of arrhythmogenic right ventricular cardiomyopathy: morphologic findings and interobserver reliability. *Cardiology*. 2003;99:153–162.
41. Burke AP, Farb A, Tashko G, Virmani R. Arrhythmogenic right ventricular cardiomyopathy and fatty replacement of the right ventricular myocardium: are they different diseases? *Circulation*. 1998;97:1571–1580.
42. Ferrari VA, Scott CH. Arrhythmogenic right ventricular cardiomyopathy: time for a new look. *J Cardiovasc Electrophysiol*. 2003;14:483–484.
43. Barbou F, Lahutte M, Gontier E. Cardiac sarcoidosis presenting as an arrhythmogenic right ventricular cardiomyopathy. *Heart*. 2012;98:1753–1754.
44. Chia PL, Subbiah RN, Kuchar D, Walker B. Cardiac sarcoidosis masquerading as arrhythmogenic right ventricular cardiomyopathy. *Heart Lung Circ*. 2012;21:42–45.
45. Corrado D, Thiene G. Cardiac sarcoidosis mimicking arrhythmogenic right ventricular cardiomyopathy/dysplasia: the renaissance of endomyocardial biopsy? *J Cardiovasc Electrophysiol*. 2009;20:477–479.
46. Tandri H, Bluemke DA, Ferrari VA, et al. Findings on magnetic resonance imaging of idiopathic right ventricular outflow tachycardia. *Am J Cardiol*. 2004;94:1441–1445.
47. Chimenti C, Calabrese F, Thiene G, Pieroni M, Maseri A, Frustaci A. Inflammatory left ventricular microaneurysms as a cause of apparently idiopathic ventricular tachyarrhythmias. *Circulation*. 2001;104:168–173.
48. Christensen AH, Svendsen JH. Myocarditis mimicking arrhythmogenic right ventricular cardiomyopathy. *J Am Coll Cardiol*. 2009;54:663–664; author reply 665-666.
49. Divakara Menon SM, Ganame J, Lira Lea Plaza G, et al. Right ventricular tachycardia: common presentation versus common disease. *Circulation*. 2013;128:e85–e87.
50. Tandri H, Saranathan M, Rodriguez ER, et al. Noninvasive detection of myocardial fibrosis in arrhythmogenic right ventricular cardiomyopathy using delayed-enhancement magnetic resonance imaging. *J Am Coll Cardiol*. 2005;45:98–103.
51. Sen-Chowdhry S, Prasad SK, Syrris P, et al. Cardiovascular magnetic resonance in arrhythmogenic right ventricular cardiomyopathy revisited: comparison with task force criteria and genotype. *J Am Coll Cardiol*. 2006;48:2132–2140.
52. Tandri H, Calkins H, Nasir K, et al. Magnetic resonance imaging findings in patients meeting task force criteria for arrhythmogenic right ventricular dysplasia. *J Cardiovasc Electrophysiol*. 2003;14:476–482.
53. Mahrholdt H, Wagner A, Judd RM, Sechtem U, Kim RJ. Delayed enhancement cardiovascular magnetic resonance assessment of non-ischaemic cardiomyopathies. *Eur Heart J*. 2005;26:1461–1474.
54. Aquaro GD, Barison A, Todiere G, et al. Usefulness of combined functional assessment by cardiac magnetic resonance and tissue characterization versus task force criteria for diagnosis of arrhythmogenic right ventricular cardiomyopathy. *Am J Cardiol*. 2016;118:1730–1736.
55. Tandri H, Calkins H, Marcus FI. Controversial role of magnetic resonance imaging in the diagnosis of arrhythmogenic right ventricular dysplasia. *Am J Cardiol*. 2003;92:649.
56. Quick S, Speiser U, Kury K, Schoen S, Ibrahim K, Strasser R. Evaluation and classification of right ventricular wall motion abnormalities in healthy subjects by 3-tesla cardiovascular magnetic resonance imaging. *Neth Heart J*. 2015;23:64–69.
57. Kramer CM, Barkhausen J, Bucciarelli-Ducci C, Flamm SD, Kim RJ, Nagel E. Standardized cardiovascular magnetic resonance imaging (CMR) protocols: 2020 update. *J Cardiovasc Magn Reson*. 2020;22:17.
58. Blaimer M, Breuer F, Mueller M, Heidemann RM, Griswold MA, Jakob PM. SMASH, SENSE, PILS, GRAPPA: how to choose the optimal method. *Top Magn Reson Imaging*. 2004;15:223–236.
59. Schulz-Menger J, Bluemke DA, Bremerich J, et al. Standardized image interpretation and post-processing in cardiovascular magnetic resonance—2020 update: society for cardiovascular magnetic resonance (SCMR): board of trustees task force on standardized post-processing. *J Cardiovasc Magn Reson*. 2020;22:19.
60. Tavano A, Maurel B, Gaubert JY, et al. MR imaging of arrhythmogenic right ventricular dysplasia: what the radiologist needs to know. *Diagnos Interv Imaging*. 2015;96:449–460.
61. Basharat SA, Hsiung I, Garg J, Alsaid A. Arrhythmogenic cardiomyopathy: evolving diagnostic criteria and insight from cardiac magnetic resonance imaging. *Heart Fail Clin*. 2023;19:429–444.
62. Bauce B, Rampazzo A, Basso C, et al. Clinical phenotype and diagnosis of arrhythmogenic right ventricular cardiomyopathy in pediatric patients carrying desmosomal gene mutations. *Heart Rhythm*. 2011;8:1686–1695.
63. Xu T, Yang Z, Vatta M, et al. Compound and digenic heterozygosity contributes to arrhythmogenic right ventricular cardiomyopathy. *J Am Coll Cardiol*. 2010;55:587–597.
64. Groeneweg JA, Bhonsale A, James CA, et al. Clinical presentation, long-term follow-up, and outcomes of 1001 arrhythmogenic right ventricular dysplasia/cardiomyopathy patients and family members. *Circ Cardiovasc Genet*. 2015;8(3):437–446.
65. Sawant AC, Bhonsale A, Te Riele AS, et al. Exercise has a disproportionate role in the pathogenesis of arrhythmogenic right ventricular dysplasia/cardiomyopathy in patients without desmosomal mutations. *J Am Heart Assoc*. 2014;3(6):e001471.
66. Gomes J, Finlay M, Ahmed AK, et al. Electrophysiological abnormalities precede overt structural changes in arrhythmogenic right ventricular cardiomyopathy due to mutations in desmoplakin-A combined murine and human study. *Eur Heart J*. 2012;33:1942–1953.
67. Saprungruang A, Tumkosit M, Kongphatthanayothin A. The presence of epsilon waves in all precordial leads (V1-V6) in a 13-year-old boy with arrhythmogenic right ventricular dysplasia (ARVD). *Ann Noninvasive Electrocardiol*. 2013;18:484–486.
68. Heidbuchel H, Corrado D, Biffi A, et al. Recommendations for participation in leisure-time physical activity and competitive sports of patients with arrhythmias and potentially arrhythmogenic conditions. Part II: ventricular arrhythmias, channelopathies and implantable defibrillators. *Eur J Cardiovasc Prev Rehabil*. 2006;13:676–686.
69. Heidbuchel H, Prior DL, La Gerche A. Ventricular arrhythmias associated with long-term endurance sports: what is the evidence? *Br J Sports Med*. 2012;46(suppl 1):i44–i50.
70. Zaidi A, Sheikh N, Jongman JK, et al. Clinical differentiation between physiological remodeling and arrhythmogenic right ventricular cardiomyopathy in athletes with marked electrocardiographic repolarization anomalies. *J Am Coll Cardiol*. 2015;65:2702–2711.
71. Major Z, Csajagi E, Kneffel Z, et al. Comparison of left and right ventricular adaptation in endurance-trained male athletes. *Acta Physiol Hung*. 2015;102:23–33.
72. Zaidi A, Ghani S, Sharma R, et al. Physiological right ventricular adaptation in elite athletes of African and Afro-Caribbean origin. *Circulation*. 2013;127:1783–1792.
73. Mangold S, Kramer U, Franzen E, et al. Detection of cardiovascular disease in elite athletes using cardiac magnetic resonance imaging. *Rofo*. 2013;185:1167–1174.
74. D'Andrea A, Riegler L, Golia E, et al. Range of right heart measurements in top-level athletes: the training impact. *Int J Cardiol*. 2013;164:48–57.
75. Heidbuchel H, La Gerche A. The right heart in athletes. Evidence for exercise-induced arrhythmogenic right ventricular cardiomyopathy. *Herzschrittmacherther Elektrophysiol*. 2012;23:82–86.
76. Scharf M, Brem MH, Wilhelm M, Schoepf UJ, Uder M, Lell MM. Cardiac magnetic resonance assessment of left and right ventricular morphologic and functional adaptations in professional soccer players. *Am Heart J*. 2010;159:911–918.
77. Knackstedt C, Schmidt K, Syrocki L, et al. Long-term follow-up of former world-class swimmers: evaluation of cardiovascular function. *Heart Vessels*. 2015;30:369–378.
78. Luijkx T, Velthuis BK, Prakken NH, et al. Impact of revised task force criteria: distinguishing the athlete's heart from ARVC/D using cardiac magnetic resonance imaging. *Eur J Prev Cardiol*. 2012;19:885–891.
79. Limongelli G, Rea A, Masarone D, et al. Right ventricular cardiomyopathies: a multidisciplinary approach to diagnosis. *Echocardiography*. 2014;32:S75–S94.
80. Choo WK, Denison AR, Miller DR, Dempsey OJ, Dawson DK, Broadhurst PA. Cardiac sarcoid or arrhythmogenic right ventricular cardiomyopathy: a role for positron emission tomography (PET)? *J Nucl Cardiol*. 2013;20:479–480.
81. Choo WK, Denison AR, Miller DR, Dempsey OJ, Dawson DK, Broadhurst PA. Cardiac sarcoid or arrhythmogenic right ventricular cardiomyopathy: a role for positron emission tomography (PET)? *J Nucl Cardiol*. 2013;20:479–480.
82. Orii M, Imanishi T, Akasaka T. Assessment of cardiac sarcoidosis with advanced imaging modalities. *BioMed Research International*. 2014;2014:897956.
83. Gazitt T, Kharouf F, Feld J, et al. Real-life utilization of criteria guidelines for diagnosis of cardiac sarcoidosis (CS). *J Clin Med*. 2023;12.
84. Smedema JP, Snoep G, van Kroonenburgh MP, et al. Evaluation of the accuracy of gadolinium-enhanced cardiovascular magnetic resonance in the diagnosis of cardiac sarcoidosis. *J Am Coll Cardiol*. 2005;45:1683–1690.
85. Philips B, Madhavan S, James CA, et al. Arrhythmogenic right ventricular dysplasia/cardiomyopathy and cardiac sarcoidosis: distinguishing features when the diagnosis is unclear. *Circ Arrhythm Electrophysiol*. 2014;7:230–236.
86. Quarta G, Husain SI, Flett AS, et al. Arrhythmogenic right ventricular cardiomyopathy mimics: role of cardiovascular magnetic resonance. *J Cardiovasc Magn Reson*. 2013;15:16.
87. Cipriani A, Mattesi G, Bariani R, et al. Cardiac magnetic resonance imaging of arrhythmogenic cardiomyopathy: evolving diagnostic perspectives. *Eur Radiol*. 2023;33:270–282.
88. Hagio T, Huang C, Abidov A, et al. T2 mapping of the heart with a double-inversion radial fast spin-echo method with indirect echo compensation. *J Cardiovasc Magn Reson*. 2015;17:24.
89. Corrado D, Basso C, Thiene G. Arrhythmogenic right ventricular cardiomyopathy: an update. *Heart*. 2009;95:766–773.
90. Basso C, Thiene G, Corrado D, Angelini A, Nava A, Valente M. Arrhythmogenic right ventricular cardiomyopathy. Dysplasia, dystrophy, or myocarditis? *Circulation*. 1996;94:983–991.
91. Corrado D, Basso C, Thiene G, et al. Spectrum of clinicopathologic manifestations of arrhythmogenic right ventricular cardiomyopathy/dysplasia: a multicenter study. *J Am Coll Cardiol*. 1997;30:1512–1520.
92. Basso C, Corrado D, Marcus FI, Nava A, Thiene G. Arrhythmogenic right ventricular cardiomyopathy. *Lancet*. 2009;373:1289–1300.

93. Corrado D, Basso C, Pilichou K, Thiene G. Molecular biology and clinical management of arrhythmogenic right ventricular cardiomyopathy/dysplasia. *Heart*. 2011;97:530–539.
94. Corrado D, Leoni L, Link MS, et al. Implantable cardioverter-defibrillator therapy for prevention of sudden death in patients with arrhythmogenic right ventricular cardiomyopathy/dysplasia. *Circulation*. 2003;108:3084–3091.
95. Andrews CM, Srinivasan NT, Rosmini S, et al. Electrical and structural substrate of arrhythmogenic right ventricular cardiomyopathy determined using noninvasive electrocardiographic imaging and late gadolinium magnetic resonance imaging. *Circ Arrhythm Electrophysiol*. 2017;10:e005105.
96. Peters S, Peters H, Thierfelder L. Risk stratification of sudden cardiac death and malignant ventricular arrhythmias in right ventricular dysplasia-cardiomyopathy. *Int J Cardiol*. 1999;71:243–250.
97. Bhonsale A, James CA, Tichnell C, et al. Risk stratification in arrhythmogenic right ventricular dysplasia/cardiomyopathy-associated desmosomal mutation carriers. *Circ Arrhythm Electrophysiol*. 2013;6:569–578.
98. Neilan TG, Farhad H, Mayrhofer T, et al. Late gadolinium enhancement among survivors of sudden cardiac arrest. *JACC Cardiovasc Imaging*. 2015;8:414–423.
99. Ackerman MJ, Priori SG, Willems S, et al. HRS/EHRA expert consensus statement on the state of genetic testing for the channelopathies and cardiomyopathies this document was developed as a partnership between the Heart Rhythm Society (HRS) and the European Heart Rhythm Association (EHRA). *Heart Rhythm*. 2011;8:1308–1339.
100. Deac M, Alpendurada F, Fanaie F, et al. Prognostic value of cardiovascular magnetic resonance in patients with suspected arrhythmogenic right ventricular cardiomyopathy. *Int J Cardiol*. 2013;168:3514–3521.

30 Myocarditis

CARLOS EDUARDO ROCHITTE AND ADRIANO CAMARGO DE CASTRO CARNEIRO

INTRODUCTION

The 1995 World Health Organization/International Society and Federation of Cardiology Task Force on the Definition and Classification of Cardiomyopathies defined myocarditis as an inflammatory disease of the myocardium diagnosed by established histological, immunological, and immunohistochemical criteria, and defined inflammatory cardiomyopathy as myocarditis in association with cardiac dysfunction.[1]

Regarding its etiologies, a broad range of infectious and noninfectious causes can lead to myocarditis, including viruses and other nonviral pathogens (e.g., *Trypanosoma cruzi* in Chagas cardiomyopathy), autoimmune diseases (immune-mediated myocarditis), vaccines (e.g., COVID-19 messenger RNA vaccine-related myocarditis), immune checkpoint inhibitor cancer therapies (immune checkpoint–associated myocarditis), drugs (hypersensitivity myocarditis), and exposure to toxins (toxic myocarditis).[2–4]

Although endomyocardial biopsy (EMB) remains the gold standard tool for the diagnosis of myocarditis, sampling errors and the potential risks of this invasive procedure limit its clinical use, particularly in patients with favorable prognosis and low likelihood that the biopsy results will modify their clinical management. Therefore, EMB is mainly reserved for clinical scenarios with a higher likelihood of finding specific treatable disorders.[2–5]

The introduction and development of cardiovascular magnetic resonance (CMR) as a valuable imaging tool in clinical practice in the past decades, especially by providing noninvasive myocardial tissue characterization with the detection of myocardial edema and fibrosis, have changed the workflow for the management of inflammatory heart diseases, supporting their diagnosis and adding prognostic information.[2–4,6–9]

The most recent consensus/statements on myocarditis strongly recommend the use of CMR in patients with clinically suspected myocarditis; its diagnosis is established when the CMR findings are consistent with nonischemic myocardial injury.[2,3,10,11] In the United States, the reported incidence of myocarditis per 100,000 persons gradually increased from 9.5 cases in 2005 to 14.4 cases in 2014, with no change in the trend of EMB, suggesting an important role for CMR in the diagnostic workup of these patients.[12]

This chapter reviews the current use of CMR in patients with suspected acute myocarditis and in those with suspected chronic inflammatory cardiomyopathy and discusses the techniques that should be applied to these specific diagnoses, included novel quantitative T1 and T2 mapping.

ACUTE MYOCARDITIS

Myocarditis may manifest with a wide spectrum of symptoms and signs, ranging from chest pain, dyspnea, palpitations, or syncope to more severe presentations like heart failure, arrhythmia, or conduction disturbances to life-threatening cardiogenic shock with hemodynamic compromise (fulminant myocarditis) or even death.[2,3] Acute myocarditis is suspected when a short time (usually <1 month) passed from the onset of the symptoms, and is also a common differential diagnosis (infarct-like myocarditis) in patients with acute chest pain, elevated troponin, and nonobstructive coronary arteries.[2,10,13]

The CMR examination has a class I recommendation in patients with suspected myocarditis in several cardiology guidelines, with an exceptional diagnostic accuracy in patients with acute myocarditis.[2,3,10,11] As myocardial edema decreases with time in the evolution of acute myocarditis, CMR should be performed early after the suspicion, preferably within 2 weeks after the initial presentation to achieve the highest sensitivity, except in patients with fulminant myocarditis, in whom CMR should be postponed until after clinical stabilization.[4,14]

Cardiovascular Magnetic Resonance in Acute Myocarditis

CMR is the most useful noninvasive examination for suspected acute myocarditis, since it can evaluate the morphology and function of both ventricles, as well as pericardial-associated involvement if present. In fact, CMR is the gold standard modality for these assessments and can remarkably detect myocardial inflammation using tissue characterization techniques, which allow greater accuracy compared with other imaging examinations.[1,2,10,11]

The late gadolinium enhancement (LGE) technique assesses the pattern of myocardial necrosis/fibrosis, which can differentiate ischemic from nonischemic injury and help to diagnose other etiologies beyond myocarditis.[6,11] Techniques like T2-weighted imaging, early gadolinium enhancement (EGE), and more recent techniques like T1 and T2 mapping allow for additional evidence of myocardial injury, improving the sensitivity and specificity of CMR for acute myocarditis (Fig. 30.1).[8,9,14,15]

Due to those important advantages, CMR can be considered the first-line diagnostic tool in this scenario.[2,3,10] A careful exception is patients with a significant pretest probability of acute coronary syndromes, in whom a

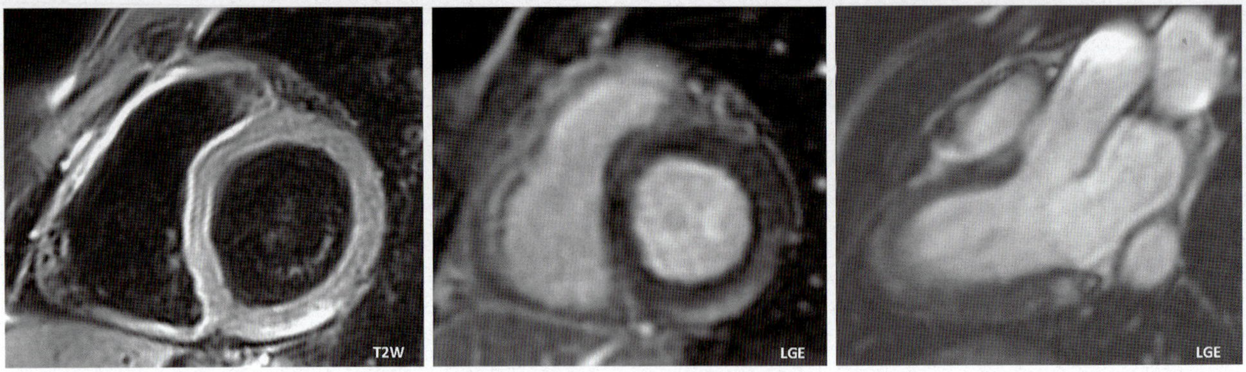

FIG. 30.1 Cardiovascular magnetic resonance in a 36-year-old male patient with acute chest pain, elevated troponin, and normal left ventricular systolic function showing the typical appearance of acute myocarditis. The T2-weighted image shows subepicardial edema in the basal inferior/inferolateral segment, with corresponding subepicardial necrosis in the late gadolinium enhancement images.

strategy with invasive coronary angiography or coronary computed tomography angiography might be chosen prior to CMR to avoid a possible delay if an urgent revascularization is required.[10,13]

Next is a detailed description of CMR techniques and their role in the diagnosis of acute myocarditis, followed by a discussion on the diagnostic criteria, prognosis, risk stratification, and CMR follow-up.

Morphological and Functional Abnormalities

For morphological and function abnormalities of the heart, cine imaging, preferably with a balanced steady-state free precession (bSSFP) sequence, must cover the entire myocardium using a short-axis stack covering both ventricles from base to apex and standard multiplanar long-axis views, which provide images for the calculation of the ventricles' volumes and systolic function. The presence and severity of any associated pericardial effusion can also be evaluated in the cine images.[7]

In acute myocarditis, a transient increase of the wall thickness of the left ventricle (LV), regional or global, can sometimes be seen and is associated with acute myocardial edema.[7] With respect to systolic function, it can be entirely normal in cases of uncomplicated acute myocarditis, even in the presence of myocardial edema and necrosis, or it can be regionally (e.g., hypokinesia of the basal inferolateral segment) or globally affected; however, systolic dysfunction could also have other ischemic and nonischemic causes.[7–9]

Although the recognition of regional or global left ventricle systolic dysfunction may be a supportive criterion for myocarditis, these functional abnormalities are neither sensitive nor specific findings for myocardial inflammation.[7,8] Therefore, further techniques to analyze tissue characterization are necessary (Fig. 30.2).

Myocardial Strain Analysis

Another technique that can be used to assess biventricular function is myocardial strain analysis. CMR feature-tracking is a quantitative software that uses cine images acquired in the CMR examination and quantifies myocardial deformation in different orientations. The global longitudinal, circumferential, and radial peak strains of both ventricles are calculated by the software after the epicardial and endocardial contours of the myocardium are automatically traced and manually corrected if necessary. The global peak longitudinal strain (GLS) is generated from long-axis views, and the global peak circumferential strain (GCS) and global peak radial strain (GRS) are generated from short-axis views.[16]

Myocardial strain analysis (GLS, GCS, and GRS) using CMR feature-tracking has proved to be more sensitive in detecting LV dysfunction in patients with acute myocarditis, especially when global left ventricle ejection fraction (LVEF) is preserved, creating more clinical scenarios of myocarditis cases compared with standard cine imaging.[16–18] Another advantage of this technique is its prognostic value, as myocardial strain was independently associated with all-cause mortality, major adverse cardiovascular events (MACE), and incomplete LV functional recovery in acute myocarditis.[16,19,20]

Despite these advantages, myocardial strain does not allow for direct visualization of myocardial inflammation, and like standard cine imaging, depends on other techniques to diagnose myocarditis.

Pericardial Involvement

Small and not circumferential pericardial effusion is physiological and generally seen in CMR examinations due to the high spatial resolution and independence of the acoustic window of the method, and therefore must be interpreted with caution to prevent overdiagnosis. In patients with acute myocarditis, pericardial effusion is commonly reported, and it is considered a supportive criterion for myocarditis, although its presence alone is not specific for pericardial or myocardial inflammation.[7,8]

CMR signs of pericardial inflammation such as pericardial thickness in fast spin echo T1 images, hyperintensity of the pericardium in T2-weighted or LGE images, and newer findings like low signal of the pericardial effusion in native T1 mapping (values ≤3015 ms are suggestive of exudate) can confirm a diagnosis of pericarditis.[21,22] Active pericardial inflammation is also a supportive criterion for myocarditis, and makes the diagnosis of associated myocarditis (myopericarditis) more likely, especially in patients with elevated troponin.[8]

T2-Weighted Imaging

T2-weighted images reveal increased water content in a tissue as a signal hyperintensity, and are used to detect

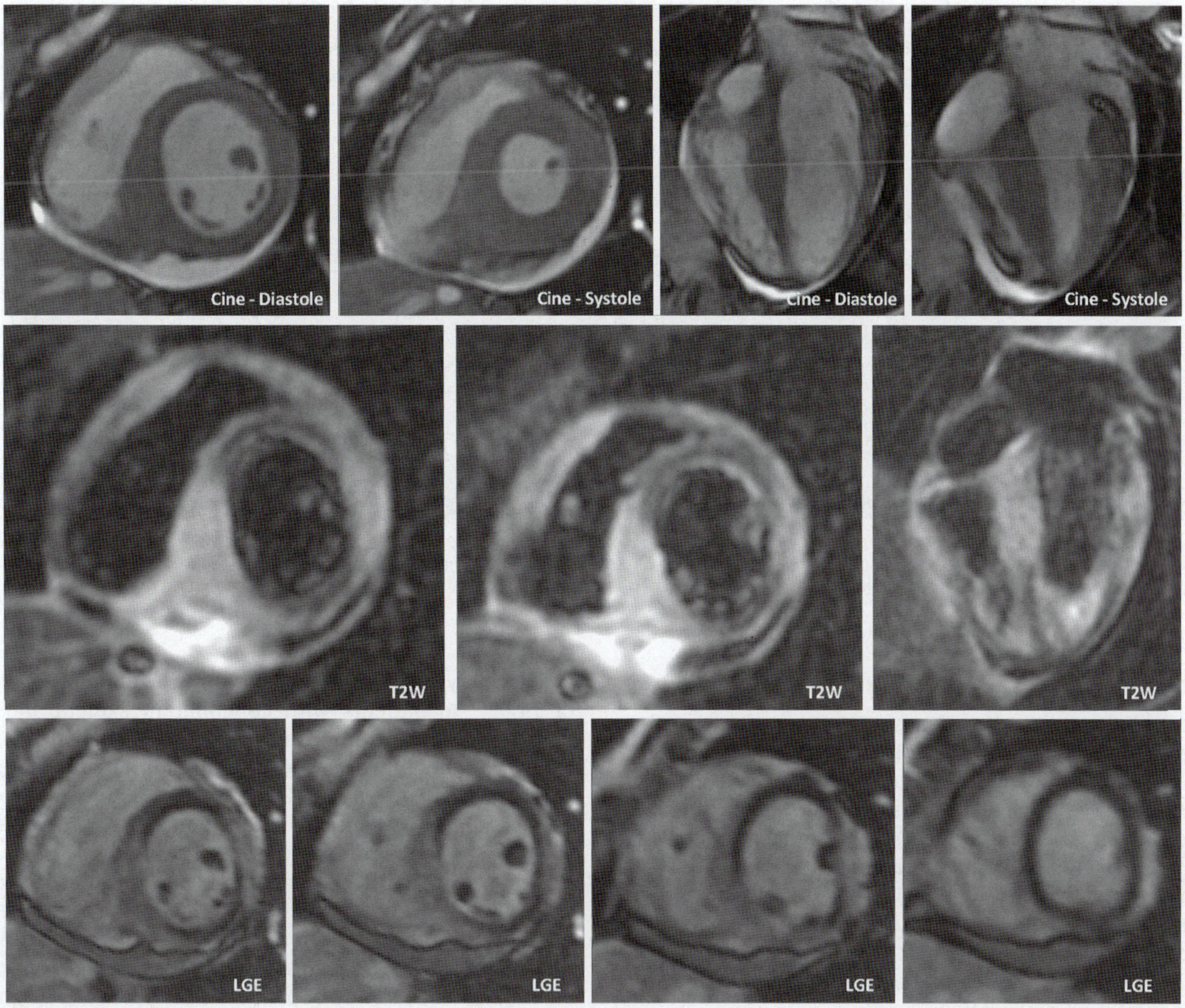

FIG. 30.2 Cardiovascular magnetic resonance in a 26-year-old male patient with acute chest pain and elevated troponin. Cine images show preserved left ventricular systolic function, pericardial effusion, and an increased wall thickness of the basal and midinferoseptal segments (*first row*). T2-weighted (*T2W*) images show transmural edema in the inferoseptal segment, subepicardial edema in the lateral segment, and pericardial edema adjacent to the left ventricle (*second row*). Late gadolinium enhancement (*LGE*) images show transmural necrosis in the inferoseptal segment, and subepicardial necrosis in the lateral segment (*third row*).

regional or global myocardial edema. Triple inversion recovery black-blood spin echo sequences with inversion pulses for blood flow and fat suppression are usually applied for this purpose; however, they can be susceptible to arrhythmia and motion-related artifacts and have an inherently low signal-to-noise ratio (SNR).[7] To improve image quality, the use of body or surface coils with signal intensity correction algorithms and thicker slices can reduce variation in signal homogeneity and increase SNR.[7–9]

T2-weighted images are generally acquired in short-axis views covering the left ventricle from base to apex, and can also be acquired in long-axis views in selected patients with abnormal cine images.

In myocarditis, myocardial edema is noticed as regional or global signal hyperintensity. Regional edema can be identified visually as a focal high signal compared with apparently normal myocardium, which mainly appears in a subepicardial or transmural pattern, or in a semiquantitative manner with appropriated software, where the signal intensity (SI) of the focal edema is more than 2 standard deviations above the mean signal intensity of the apparently normal myocardium within the same image.[7–9]

Myocardial edema can also be global in myocarditis and may not be detected by the previous exposed means. In this case, a ratio of the signal intensity of the myocardium relative to the signal intensity of the skeletal muscle (preferred measure in the serratus anterior muscle) greater than or equal to 1.9 (T2 signal intensity ratio ≥1.9), within the same image, has a good diagnostic accuracy to semiquantitatively detect global myocardial edema (sensitivity of 84%, specificity of 74%, and accuracy of 79%).[23] Nevertheless, this technique could have limitations in patients with concomitant myositis in a systemic inflammatory process, in whom a higher signal intensity of the skeletal muscle may lead to a false-negative result (Fig. 30.3).[7–9]

$$\text{T2 SIGNAL INTENSITY RATIO} = \frac{\text{MYOCARDIUM SI}}{\text{SKELETAL MUSCLE SI}}$$

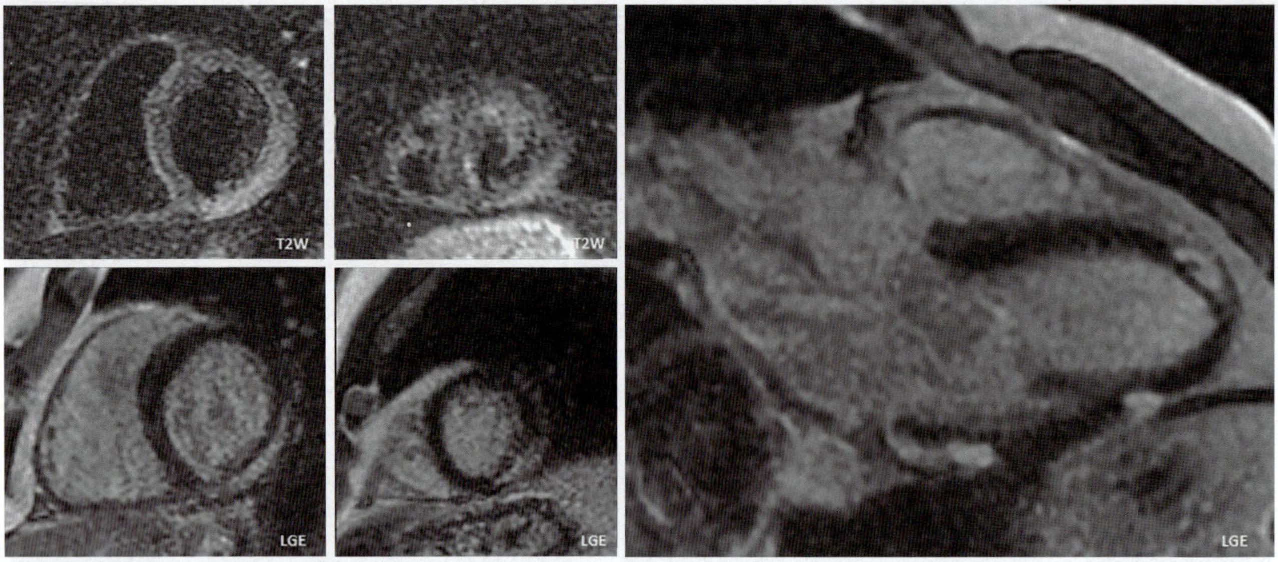

FIG. 30.3 Cardiovascular magnetic resonance in a 40-year-old male patient with acute chest pain, elevated troponin, and normal left ventricular ejection fraction. T2-weighted (*T2W*) images show subepicardial edema in the basal and apical inferior/inferolateral segments. Late gadolinium enhancement (*LGE*) images show corresponding subepicardial necrosis in these segments. The three-chamber view shows the patchy LGE distribution.

Early Gadolinium Enhancement

Myocardial inflammation leads to increased blood flow (hyperemia), increased vascular permeability (capillary leakage), and expansion of the extracellular space, which can be assessed through increased uptake of gadolinium-based contrast agent (GBCA) early after the contrast bolus.[23–26] The EGE technique attempts to estimate these changes and employ T1-weighted spin echo images in axial and short-axis views (usually three images) acquired before and within the first 3 minutes after intravenous GBCA injection, with identical parameters before and after the contrast administration.[24]

To analyze these changes, myocardial enhancement is defined as the percent increase of the myocardial signal intensity from precontrast to postcontrast images, and can be normalized to the skeletal muscle enhancement, defined as the percentage of the skeletal muscle intensity increase from precontrast to postcontrast images, through a variable-call early gadolinium enhancement ratio (EGEr), calculated by dividing the myocardial enhancement by the skeletal muscle enhancement.[23,24]

$$\text{MYOCARDIAL ENHANCEMENT}\,(\%) = \frac{(\text{POST-CONTRAST SI} - \text{PRE-CONTRAST SI}) \times 100}{\text{PRE-CONTRAST SI}}$$

$$\text{SKELETAL MUSCLE ENHANCEMENT}\,(\%) = \frac{(\text{POST-CONTRAST SI} - \text{PRE-CONTRAST SI}) \times 100}{\text{PRE-CONTRAST SI}}$$

$$\text{EGEr} = \frac{\text{MYOCARDIAL ENHANCEMENT}}{\text{SKELETAL MUSCLE ENHANCEMENT}}$$

According to the first proposed CMR diagnostic criteria for myocarditis, an EGE ratio greater than or equal to 4.0 (EGEr ≥4.0) is a good cutoff for this diagnosis, and achieved a sensitivity of 80%, a specificity of 68%, and an accuracy of 74%.[7,23] In patients with concomitant skeletal muscle involvement, the EGEr could have false-negative results, so for patients in whom the skeletal muscle enhancement is greater than or equal to 20% (≥20%), it is recommended to apply an absolute myocardial enhancement greater than 45% (>45%) as the threshold for myocarditis.[7,26]

Nowadays, the EGE technique is not routinely used in most centers; a comparative study that evaluated the diagnostic performance of shortened CMR protocols showed that the removal of EGE imaging does not change the overall diagnostic accuracy of protocols based on T2-weighted and LGE imaging, though this was associated with a significantly lower positive likelihood ratio for myocarditis.[24] Adding to that, the newest CMR diagnostic criteria for myocarditis, with the use of techniques like T1 and T2 mapping, exclude EGE from the required protocol, yet it still can be used in experienced centers and in those without access to parametric mapping techniques.[8]

Late Gadolinium Enhancement

The LGE technique has become the gold standard noninvasive method for evaluating irreversible myocardial injury, in either the acute (necrosis) or chronic stage (fibrosis), and the pattern of the myocardial injury visualized by LGE can accurately differentiate ischemic (the hyperenhancement should always involve the subendocardium and be located in an epicardial coronary artery territory) from nonischemic injury (the hyperenhancement generally spares the subendocardial layer or is located in a territory not consistent with the perfusion of an epicardial coronary artery).[6,11]

The LGE image is acquired using inversion recovery–based T1-weighted imaging, most commonly gradient-echo sequences, after intravenous GBCA injection (habitually after 10 minutes), with a proper inversion time to null the signal of the reference normal myocardium and to enhance

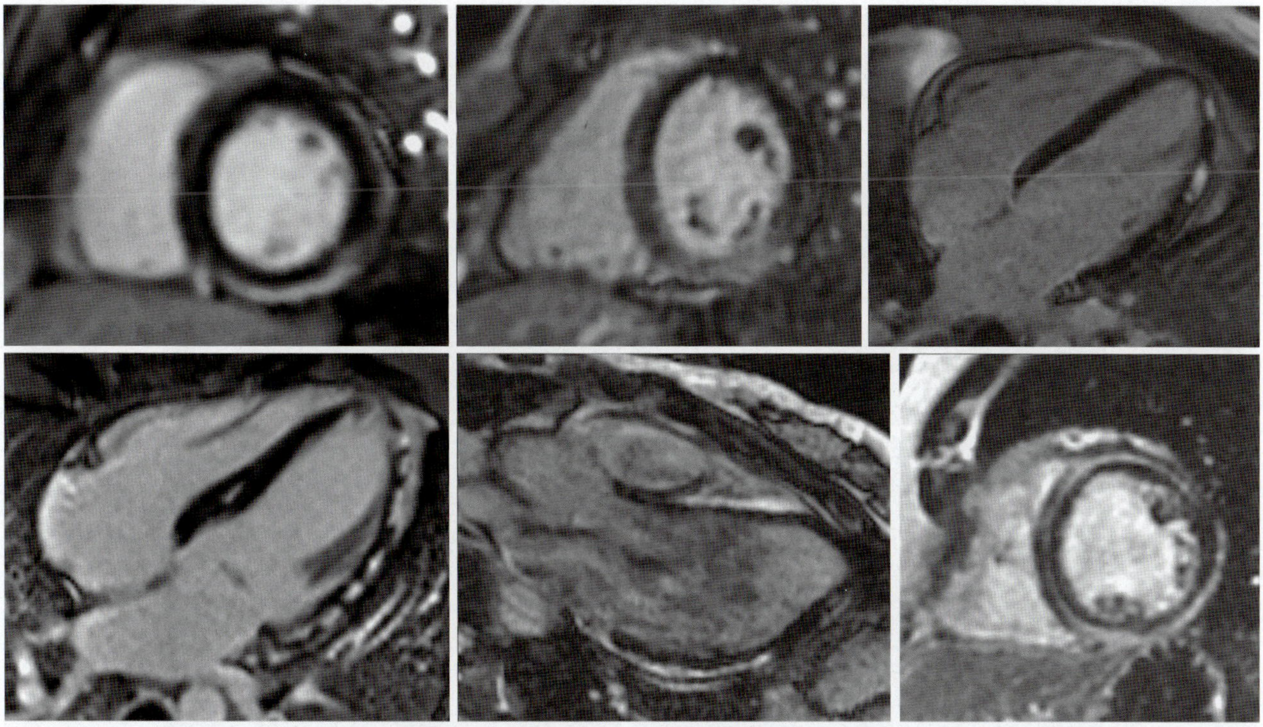

FIG. 30.4 Late gadolinium enhancement (*LGE*) patterns and distribution in myocarditis. (A) Subepicardial LGE in the basal inferior segment. (B) Transmural and heterogeneous LGE in the basal inferior segment. (C) Subepicardial LGE in the lateral wall in a patchy distribution. (D) Midwall LGE in the basal septal segment and subepicardial LGE in the lateral wall in a multifocal distribution. (E) Subepicardial LGE in the septal and lateral wall in a diffuse distribution. (F) Diffuse midwall and subepicardial LGE in a ringlike pattern.

the myocardium with an abnormal increase of GBCA concentration as bright areas.[6] The LGE image needs to fully cover both ventricles using a short-axis stack from base to apex, and standard multiplanar long-axis views must also be acquired in order for the areas of abnormal LGE to be confirmed in at least two orthogonal planes.

In myocarditis, LGE patterns are typically subepicardial and midwall, but transmural lesions can also occur in few cases with a more severe inflammation.[6–11] Regarding its distribution, LGE is usually focal or patchy in the basal to midinferolateral segment, and occasionally in the septal wall; however, LGE may sometimes be multifocal or diffuse (Fig. 30.4).[6–11]

It is important to note that although LGE can specifically detect nonischemic myocardial injury and has a high sensitivity in acute infarct-like myocarditis, it is not specific for active myocardial inflammation and could have a lower sensitivity in mild myocarditis cases; therefore, LGE is better used in combination with other techniques to achieve a higher diagnostic accuracy for acute myocarditis (Figs. 30.5 and 30.6).[7–9,23,24,27]

T1 Mapping

Mapping of T1 and T2 myocardial relaxation times allows a noninvasive spatial visualization and quantification of changes in myocardial composition, producing secondary images that correspond to pixel-by-pixel maps of the specific magnetic property.[28,29] In acute myocarditis, the edema increases myocardial water content, which prolongs the myocardial T1 and T2 relaxation times, making these parametric techniques helpful in this diagnosis. Also, the parametric mapping overcomes some limitations of the previous semiquantitative techniques by directly quantifying alterations in the myocardial structure, even if they are diffuse or associated with skeletal muscle inflammation.[8,9,28,29]

The T1 map is acquired before the administration of GBCA (native T1), using inversion recovery– or saturation recovery–based sequences (or hybrid methods), in at least one short-axis view (midventricular), but preferably three (basal, mid, and apical) or more (base to apex), and associated with long-axis views (four-chamber, two chamber, and/or three-chamber) depending on the center's protocol, the suspected diagnosis, and the findings in the previously acquired cine images.[28,30]

Since the measured native T1 relaxation time is highly affected by differences in acquisition schemes and postprocessing methods, its normal values must be locally validated and the site-specific normal range reported.[28,30] The native T1 relaxation time should be measured in areas of abnormal visual appearance for focal disease, and in the septum or entire left ventricle myocardium (global) for diffuse disease. In acute myocarditis, the global native T1 relaxation time may be more sensitive than the one measured within the midseptal segment.[28,30,31]

In myocarditis, native T1 is prolonged due to intracellular and extracellular increases in free water content, and can detect myocardial edema, vasodilatation, hyperemia, and expansion of the interstitial space, even areas of chronic regional and diffuse fibrosis. Thus, T1 mapping is highly sensitive for detecting diseased myocardium in acute myocarditis and an excellent way to rule out this diagnosis, but is not specific for the activity of myocarditis.[8,9,15,28] In

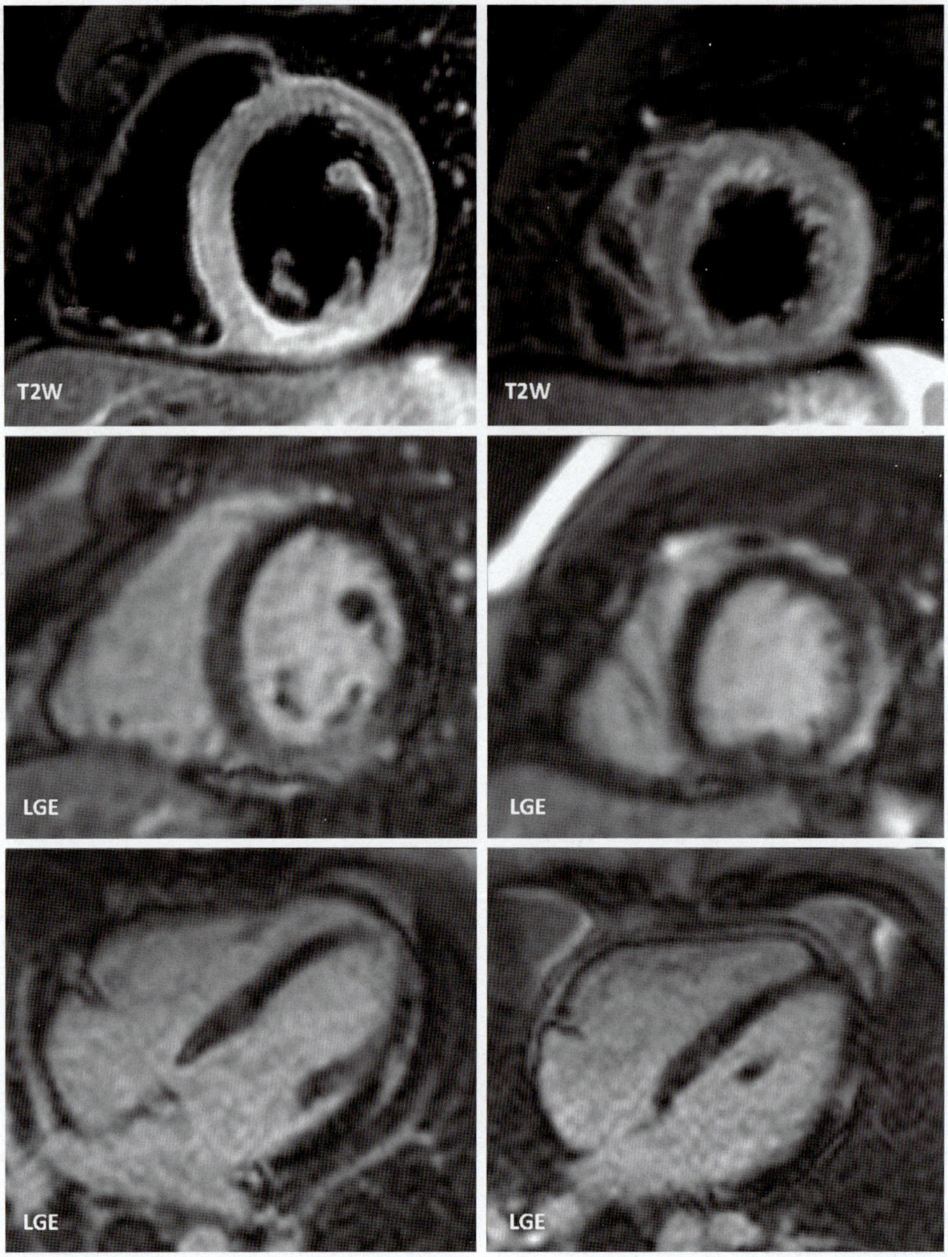

FIG. 30.5 Cardiovascular magnetic resonance (*CMR*) in a 34-year-old male patient who presented with acute chest pain, electrocardiogram with ST-segment elevation in the inferior wall, elevated troponin, echocardiography with hypokinesia of the basal inferior segment, and normal coronary arteries in invasive coronary angiography. T2-weighted (*T2W*) images show transmural edema in the basal inferior segment, and subepicardial edema in the mid and apical lateral segments. Late gadolinium enhancement (*LGE*) images show corresponding necrosis with the same patterns in these segments. This patient had a definitive diagnosis of acute myocarditis after the CMR examination.

a study published in 2019, the isolated T1 mapping technique achieved a sensitivity of 90%, a specificity of 77%, and an accuracy of 85% for acute myocarditis.[15]

Extracellular Volume Mapping

Extracellular volume (ECV) estimates the extracellular space (interstitial and extracellular matrix), and can detect an increase in this volume in myocarditis caused by myocardial edema and fibrosis. To assess the ECV, postcontrast T1 mapping should be performed 10 to 30 minutes after GBCA administration using the same scan parameters of native T1, and the patient's hematocrit should be collected immediately before the CMR examination, if possible, or within 24 hours of scanning.[25] To calculate the myocardial ECV fraction, measures of the myocardial and blood T1 relaxation times before and after GBCA injection are necessary, in addition to hematocrit, which represents the cellular fraction of blood, according to the formula below. Inline ECV maps can also be used as an alternative to manual ECV calculation.[28,30]

$$\mathrm{ECV}\,(\%) = (100 - \mathrm{HEMATOCRIT}) \times \frac{(1/\text{POST-CONTRAST Myo T1} - 1/\text{NATIVE Myo T1})}{(1/\text{POST-CONTRAST Blood T1} - 1/\text{NATIVE Blood T1})}$$

The ECV had an area under the curve of 0.81 for the diagnosis of acute myocarditis in a meta-analysis published in 2018.[32] As with native T1, the ECV can also detect areas of chronic fibrosis, and their use together with specific techniques for myocardial inflammation, like T2 mapping,

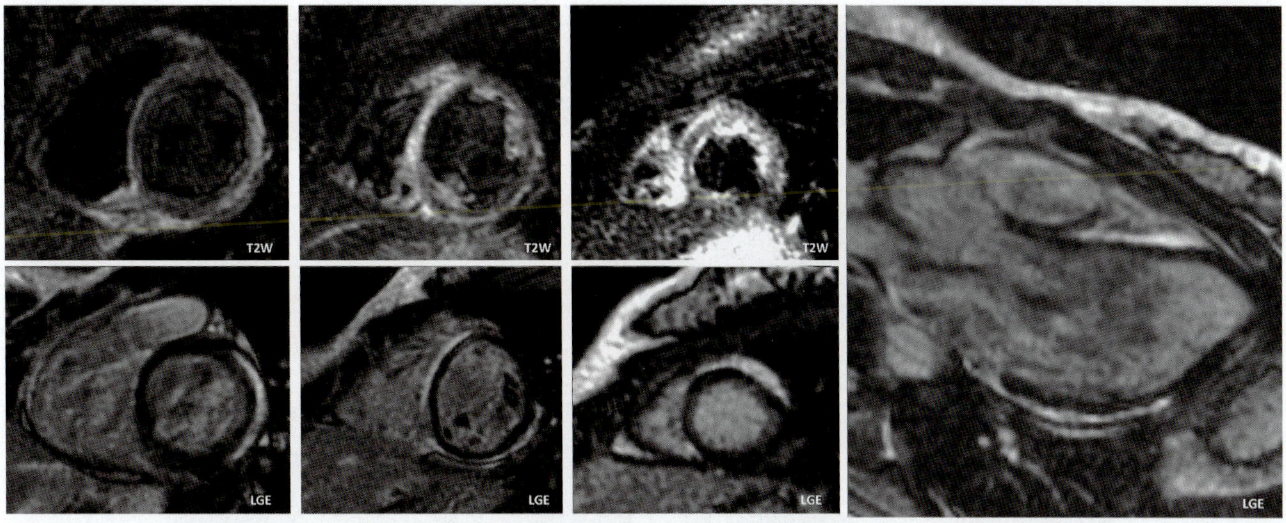

FIG. 30.6 Cardiovascular magnetic resonance in a 16-year-old female patient with acute chest pain, highly elevated troponin, and normal left ventricular ejection fraction. T2-weighted (*T2W*) and late gadolinium enhancement (*LGE*) images show diffuse subepicardial edema and necrosis in the lateral, septal, and inferior walls, and in the apical anterior segment.

may provide a more interesting evaluation of the activity of myocarditis.[8,9,15]

T2 Mapping

T2 mapping is highly sensitive and specific for myocardial edema, and can detect the activity of myocarditis since it is insensitive to identifying areas of chronic fibrosis. T2 mapping is acquired without GBCA administration, but with a T2 preparation module followed by multiecho readouts with bSSFP, gradient, or spin echo sequences, and at least three source images are recommended.[29,30] T2 maps can be acquired in any imaging plane, usually the same planes as T1 mapping, and the T2 relaxation times are measured in the same manner as T1 mapping (see above). Also, the range of its normal values must be locally validated and reported.[29,30]

In a study published in 2019, the isolated T2 mapping technique achieved a sensitivity of 85%, a specificity of 88%, and an accuracy of 86% for acute myocarditis.[15] Further, the T2 mapping generally normalized after the resolution of myocarditis, and the persistence of a prolonged T2 relaxation time after the acute phase can distinguish cases of healed from active myocarditis, and correlates with adverse cardiac events (Fig. 30.7).[33–36]

Lake Louise Criteria

CMR techniques to assess myocardial tissue characterization can identify different features of myocardial injury, like edema, hyperemia, capillary leak, necrosis, and fibrosis, and some are more sensitive to myocarditis, while others are more specific. In 2005, Abdel-Aty et al. published a study using the available techniques at that time to diagnose patients with suspected acute myocarditis, and the T2-weighted images and EGEr had higher sensitivities (84% and 80%), lower specificities (74% and 68%), and diagnostic accuracies of 79% and 74% respectively, while LGE had a sensitivity of just 44%, but a specificity of 100%, and a diagnostic accuracy of 71%. The best diagnostic performance was achieved when diagnostic criteria of any two of the three techniques were positive, with a 76% sensitivity, 95% specificity, and 85% diagnostic accuracy.[15]

In 2009, the first International Consensus on CMR in Myocarditis was published and proposed diagnostic criteria called the Lake Louise Criteria (2009 LLC), which state that in patients with clinically suspected myocarditis, if at least two of the following three techniques are positive, the CMR examination is consistent with myocarditis[7]:

- **T2-weighted imaging:** regional or global myocardial signal intensity increase (global: T2 signal intensity ratio ≥1.9)
- **EGE:** increased global myocardial EGE (EGEr ≥4.0 or myocardial enhancement >45% in patient with skeletal muscle enhancement ≥20%)
- **LGE:** one or more myocardial areas with high signal intensity in a nonischemic pattern

The 2009 LLC has two supportive findings that provide additional evidence for myocarditis[7]:

- Left ventricle dysfunction
- Pericardial effusion (Fig. 30.8)

The development of the T1 and T2 mapping, robust techniques for pixelwise quantitative characterization of myocardial tissue abnormalities, showed an excellent diagnostic performance in patients with acute myocarditis.[15,32] In 2018, a novel Expert Consensus Recommendations for renew the CMR diagnostic criteria for myocardial inflammation was published to include these parametric mapping techniques, and try to improve the diagnostic accuracy of the CMR exams.[8] Updated Lake Louise Criteria (2018 LLC) were proposed, which state that in patients with a significant clinical pretest probability of myocarditis, a CMR examination provides strong evidence for the diagnosis of acute myocardial inflammation if at least one criterion in each of the following two categories is positive:

- **T2-based marker for myocardial edema:**
  - ➢ **T2-weighted imaging:** regional or global myocardial signal intensity increase (global: T2 signal intensity ratio ≥1.9)
  - ➢ **T2 mapping:** regional or global increase of myocardial T2 relaxation time
- **T1-based marker for associated myocardial injury:**
  - ➢ **LGE:** one or more myocardial areas with high signal intensity in a nonischemic pattern

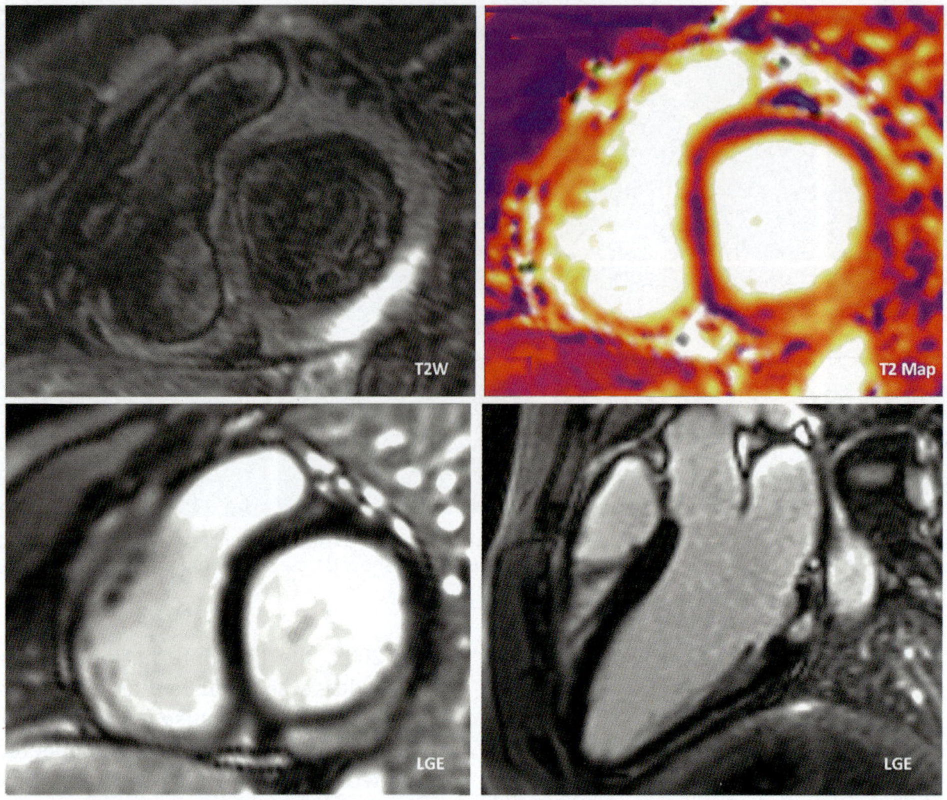

FIG. 30.7 Cardiovascular magnetic resonance in a 22-year-old male patient with acute chest pain, elevated troponin, and normal left ventricular ejection fraction showing a focal subepicardial injury in the basal inferior/inferolateral segments detected by T2-weighted (*T2W*), T2 mapping, and late gadolinium enhancement (*LGE*) images, compatible with acute myocarditis.

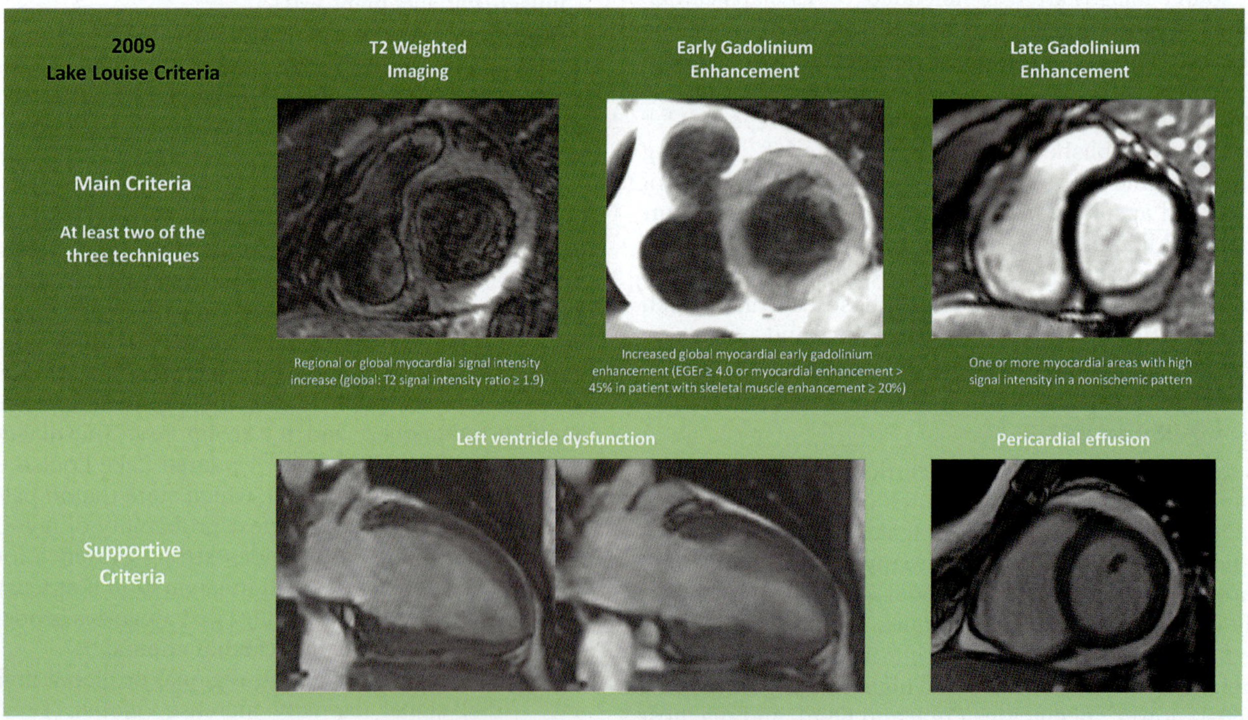

FIG. 30.8 Overview of the 2009 Lake Louise Criteria.

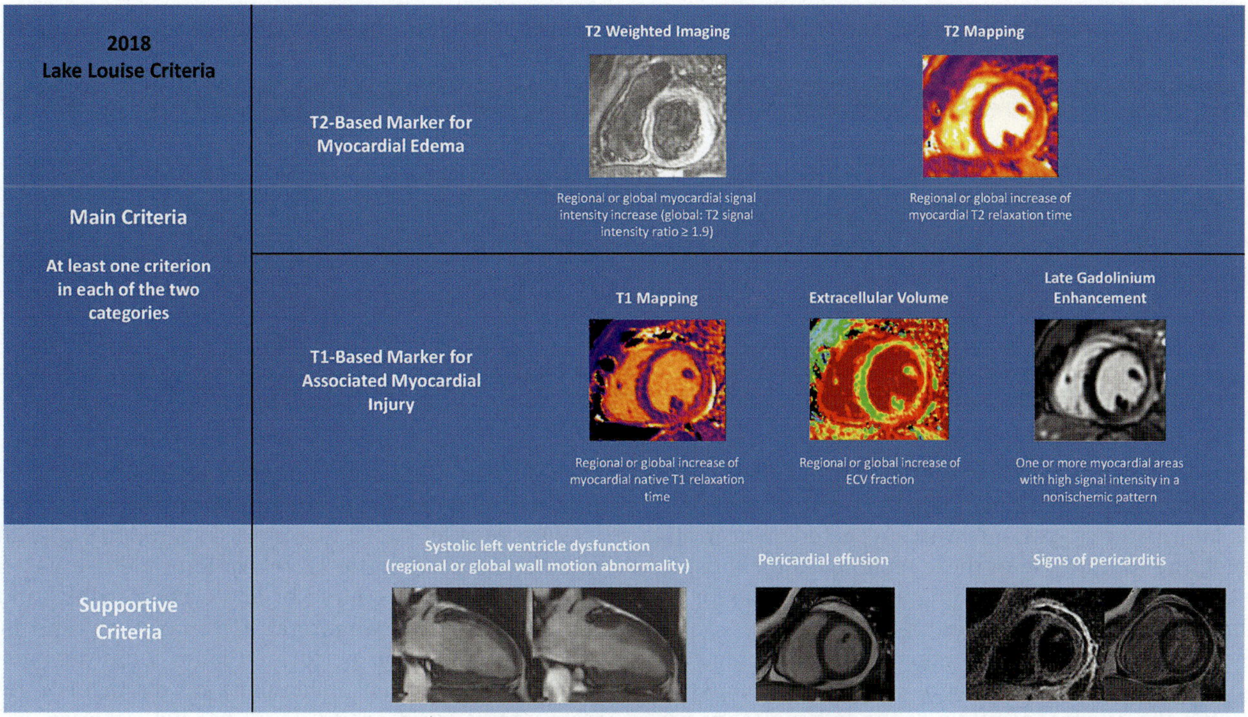

FIG. 30.9 Overview of the 2018 Lake Louise Criteria.

- ➢ **T1 mapping:** regional or global increase of myocardial native T1 relaxation time
- ➢ **ECV:** regional or global increase of ECV fraction

The 2018 LLC also has two supportive findings that provide additional evidence for myocarditis[8]:

- Systolic left ventricle dysfunction (regional or global wall motion abnormality)
- Pericardial effusion and/or signs of pericarditis (Fig. 30.9)

In a study that compared use of the 2009 LLC and 2018 LLC for diagnosis of patients with acute myocarditis, the updated criteria had a higher diagnostic accuracy (2018 LLC: 91% vs. 2009 LLC: 82%) due to a higher sensitivity (2018 LLC: 87% vs. 2009 LLC: 72%), with a similar specificity (both: 96%), which was mainly driven by the use of myocardial T1 and T2 mapping.[15]

It is pertinent to mention that although the use of combined criteria like the proposed Lake Louise Criteria is recommended, in patients with a high suspicion of acute myocarditis, the presence of only one abnormal criterion could still suggest this diagnosis, although with less specificity. This is often the case when only LGE is positive, which might be related to the higher spatial resolution and contrast-to-noise ratio of this robust technique. This may be even more relevant in CMR scans not yet equipped with the T1 and T2 mapping techniques, which is still a frequent situation around the world.

Prognostic Information

Beyond the diagnostic value in patients with suspected myocarditis, the CMR examination can add prognostic information in this scenario. In a study of 670 patients with suspected myocarditis with a median follow-up of 4.7 years, a normal CMR corresponded to low annual MACE and death rates.[37] In another study of 203 patients with acute myocarditis and an initial CMR-based diagnosis, in which all patients showed nonischemic LGE patterns (82% located in the subepicardial layer and 60% limited in the posterolateral LV wall), a lower LVEF detected by CMR was an independent predictor of adverse clinical outcome.[38]

As LGE represents irreversible myocardial injury, its presence in patients with myocarditis has been demonstrated to be the best independent predictor of all-cause and cardiac mortality. In a study of 222 patients with biopsy-proven myocarditis with a median follow-up of 4.7 years, a relevant long-term mortality rate was found (19.2% all cause, 15% cardiac, and 9.9% sudden cardiac death). The presence of LGE was associated with a hazard ratio (HR) of 8.4 for all-cause mortality and 12.8 for cardiac mortality, and no patient without LGE experienced sudden cardiac death, even those with left ventricle enlargement and dysfunction.[39]

The location, pattern, and extent of LGE are also significantly associated with MACE. In a study of patients with suspected myocarditis, when LGE was located in the septum (HR: 2.55), in the midwall (HR: 2.39), or in a patchy distribution (HR: 2.93), an increased MACE rate was found. Further, each 10% increase in the LGE extension corresponded to a 79% increase in the risk of MACEs (HR: 1.79 per 10% LGE increase).[37]

After the acute phase of myocarditis, the resolution of myocardial edema and the contraction of scar tissue could cause LGE lesions to shrink or even disappear (no longer be visible by CMR spatial resolution) in a subsequent CMR examination. In a study of a subgroup of 187 patients from the ITAMY registry (ITAlian study in MYocarditis), CMR was performed within the first week after symptom onset and after 6 months. Patients with an increased extent of LGE at the repeat CMR examination had worse prognosis than those with unchanged/decreased LGE.[40]

TABLE 30.1 Risk stratification and likelihood of indication for endomyocardial biopsy based on cardiac magnetic resonance parameters.

PROGNOSTIC RISK	CMR PARAMETER	SUGGESTED APPROACH	INDICATION FOR BIOPSY
Low	No changes in T1 and T2 No ventricular dysfunction	Clinical follow-up	No indication
Intermediate	Positive T1 or T2 No extensive LGE (<17 g and <13% of LV mass) Normal function or mild LV dysfunction	Clinical follow-up Repeat CMR at 1, 3, and 6 months	Stable: No indication Progressive dysfunction: Possible indication
High	Positive T1 or T2 Extensive LGE (>17 g or >13% of LV mass), or septal involvement Moderate or severe LV dysfunction	Clinical follow-up Repeat CMR at 1, 3, and 6 months	Possible indication

CMR, cardiovascular magnetic resonance; *LGE*, late gadolinium enhancement; *LV*, left ventricular.

Other techniques like T2-weighted imaging, EGE, native T1 mapping, ECV, and T2 mapping have also shown prognostic information in patients with suspected myocarditis, although the routine use of these techniques for this purpose still needs more study, with more enthusiasm for the parametric mapping techniques.[36,37,41–44]

One important clinical dilemma in the acute phase of myocarditis is the indication of myocardial biopsy to determine the etiopathogenesis of the inflammatory process. Myocardial biopsy is an invasive procedure not free from complications and with a low sensitivity in the scenario of a regional myocardial injury. For the first time, a recent guideline from the Brazilian Society of Cardiology proposed a risk stratification algorithm using CMR-only data to provide a probability of benefit from myocardial biopsy. The risk stratification CMR parameters included the T1 and T2 mapping techniques, the LV function, and the LGE presence, extent, and septal location (Table 30.1).[10] This cardiology society considered this risk stratification scheme useful for the management of patients with myocarditis, even though this algorithm has not yet been tested in a randomized clinical trial.

Follow-Up

Patients with a previous diagnosis of acute myocarditis should be followed up with clinical assessment and echocardiography to monitor symptoms and LVEF, as some patients may not achieve a full clinical recovery and some could experience complication such as dilated cardiomyopathy, ventricular arrhythmias, or high-degree atrioventricular block.[2,3] The use of serial CMR scans in the routine follow-up of asymptomatic patients with previous acute myocarditis is debatable, although its use in patients with persistent symptoms or in athletes is more acceptable, particularly in a minimum interval of 3 to 6 months after the initial illness.[2,3,45–47]

The follow-up CMR examination can accurately calculate the LVEF, an important measure that may change the clinical management, but mainly, the CMR can assess signs of ongoing myocardial inflammation, which in some cases may indicate an EMB.[3] The two parameters used for this purpose are extension of the LGE and T2 mapping. As seen above, after the acute phase of myocarditis, LGE lesions are expected to shrink or disappear, and in patients in whom an increased extent of the LGE was observed at the follow-up CMR scan 6 months after symptom onset, a higher rate of cardiac death was observed.[40]

With respect to T2 mapping, a technique specific for myocardial edema, the T2 relaxation time decreases and normalizes in the course of acute myocarditis, and the persistence of an abnormal T2 relaxation time in the follow-up CMR scan performed later could demonstrate ongoing myocardial inflammation, distinguish healed from active myocarditis, and predict adverse cardiac outcomes.[33–36]

According to the recent European Society of Cardiology Guidelines for the management of cardiomyopathies, which include evaluation of myocarditis, CMR has a class I-B indication at initial evaluation and a class IIa-C indication during follow-up to monitor disease progression and aid risk stratification and management. In the case of inflammatory cardiomyopathies, a class IIa-C indication is also considered for serial follow-up and assessment of therapeutic response.[11]

Recent European clinical practice guidelines have further framed myocarditis and pericarditis within a broader spectrum of inflammatory myopericardial syndromes, emphasizing the role of initial clinical presentation in guiding diagnostic pathways, intensity of evaluation, and follow-up. In this context, cardiovascular magnetic resonance remains the cornerstone noninvasive diagnostic modality, while endomyocardial biopsy is increasingly considered earlier in selected high-risk phenotypes when results are expected to influence management, ideally within multidisciplinary teams. Contemporary guidance also places stronger emphasis on structured follow-up after acute myocarditis, particularly in patients with arrhythmic presentations or residual myocardial injury, incorporating serial clinical assessment, rhythm monitoring, and repeat imaging to support risk stratification, guide return-to-activity decisions, and identify patients at risk for adverse outcomes or progression to inflammatory cardiomyopathy.[47a,47b,47c]

Specific Etiology: Myocarditis Associated with COVID-19

The coronavirus disease 2019 (COVID-19) is an infectious disease caused by the severe acute respiratory syndrome coronavirus 2 (SARS-CoV-2) that was first detected in December 2019 and has had an important impact worldwide. The World Health Organization characterized this virus outbreak as an ongoing pandemic in March 2020 and declared a Public Health Emergency of International Concern in January 2020, a status that was withdrawn more than 3 years later, in May 2023, when a drastic drop in the world mortality rate was observed.

This primarily respiratory virus was usually associated with a systemic inflammatory process and pneumonia in the first years of the pandemic, and cardiac involvement was also often described. The published prevalence of myocardial abnormalities identified by CMR in patients with COVID-19 ranges from 0% to 78%.[48–54] This wide range may be explained by differences in study participants (e.g., inpatient vs. outpatient, acute infection vs. convalescent patients, symptomatic vs. asymptomatic, athlete vs. non-athlete), the lack of control groups in some studies driven by the epidemiologic phase of the pandemic, and the change to a less severe disease after vaccines and newer variants of SARS-CoV-2.

In autopsy studies of the heart, SARS-CoV-2 was predominantly located within the pericytes and in the subendothelium, and macrophage infiltration, interstitial inflammation, and micro or macrovascular thrombi were also common histopathological findings.[55,56] In clinical practice, heterogeneous cardiac manifestations of non-ischemic and ischemic injuries were reported.[57–59]

Regarding systolic dysfunction, patients with COVID-19 could have both ventricles affected. In the context of severe lung parenchyma injury and hypoxia, right ventricle dilatation and dysfunction could occur due to increased afterload.[59] Left ventricle involvement is more frequently compromised in COVID-19, with dysfunction being regional or global depending on the etiology of the cardiac injury.

Nonischemic injury is more prevalent in patients with COVID-19 than ischemic injury, and can manifest as myocardial edema without fulfilling the Lake Louise Criteria for myocarditis, myocarditis, pericarditis, myopericarditis, stress cardiomyopathy (takotsubo syndrome), or as part of the multisystem inflammatory syndrome in children (MIS-C). Ischemic injury, such as infarction, microinfarction, or myocardial ischemia, can also occur and is not unusual in patients with COVID-19; it is a differential diagnosis in patients with SARS-CoV-2 infection and evidence of myocardial injury.[57–59] In an international retrospective study of 1047 patients with COVID-19 and suspected cardiac involvement referred for CMR, 20.9% had nonischemic injury patterns (7.9% with acute myocarditis) and 6.7% had ischemic injury patterns (1.9% with acute myocardial infarction).[57]

Myocardial edema could be identified by CMR in patients with active COVID-19, as increased T2 mapping is a prevalent abnormality in these patients, even in asymptomatic or mildly symptomatic patients recently recovered and without suspected cardiac involvement.[47,52] Myocarditis defined by the 2018 LLC is a well-described complication of this viral infection, and in a multicenter study of 342 patients with COVID-19 and an elevated troponin level who had a CMR scan, the prevalence of recent myocarditis was 6.7% compared with 1.7% in controls without COVID-19, and the presence of LGE was an independent predictor of MACE (Figs. 30.10 and 30.11).[54]

In MIS-C, a severe inflammatory response with multisystem involvement that typically begins 2 to 6 weeks after SARS-CoV-2 infection and requires hospitalization, cardiovascular manifestation could occur as systolic dysfunction, arrhythmias, myocarditis, pericarditis, or coronary ectasia/aneurysms. When CMR was performed in patients with MIS-C and cardiac involvement, abnormal T2-weighted images, and increased global T1 and T2 mapping were identified and generally related to mild or no myocardial LGE (Fig. 30.12).[58–64]

Specific Etiology: Myocarditis Associated with COVID-19 Vaccines

Myocarditis associated with COVID-19 vaccines is a rare complication following the COVID-19 mRNA vaccines BNT162b2 (Pfizer-BioNTech) and mRNA-1273 (Moderna), with the highest risk in male individuals aged 12–29 years after the second dose of the COVID-19 mRNA vaccine.[59,65–70] Most patients had acute chest pain and elevated troponin within a week after the vaccine, generally with a mild clinical presentation and a quick resolution of symptoms, although deaths were also reported.[66–68]

When CMR scans were performed in patients with suspected mRNA vaccine-related myocarditis, the majority of patients had LGE and fulfilled the LLC for myocarditis, and some had left ventricle dysfunction.[59,60,66,67,71] The most frequent location of LGE was subepicardial at the basal inferolateral segment, and compared with other causes of myocarditis, patients had a higher LVEF, less extensive LGE, and less involvement of the septal wall (Fig. 30.13).[71]

CHRONIC INFLAMMATORY CARDIOMYOPATHY

Chronic inflammatory cardiomyopathy represents the evolution of acute myocarditis, diagnosed or not in the acute phase, that caused morphological or functional abnormalities of the myocardium, generally with a clinical phenotype of dilated cardiomyopathy (presence of left ventricle dilatation and global or regional systolic dysfunction) or nondilated left ventricular cardiomyopathy (normal-sized left ventricle with systolic dysfunction or normal-sized left ventricle with nonischemic scarring despite the presence of wall motion abnormalities).[2,11] Chronic myocarditis could be defined as an intermediate stage between acute myocarditis and chronic inflammatory cardiomyopathy in patients with ongoing myocardial inflammation.[2]

In patients being evaluated for heart failure or ventricular arrhythmias of unknown etiology, inflammatory cardiomyopathy should be a suspected diagnosis, and a CMR examination is proposed at the initial evaluation of these patients as a class I recommendation.[2,3,10,11] The ability of CMR to provide noninvasive myocardial tissue characterization, particularly with the LGE technique for the detection of myocardial fibrosis, and to differentiate ischemic from nonischemic injury could help diagnose the possible etiologies of cardiomyopathy (Fig. 30.14).

When a nonischemic LGE pattern is identified by CMR in these clinical scenarios, a nonischemic etiology must

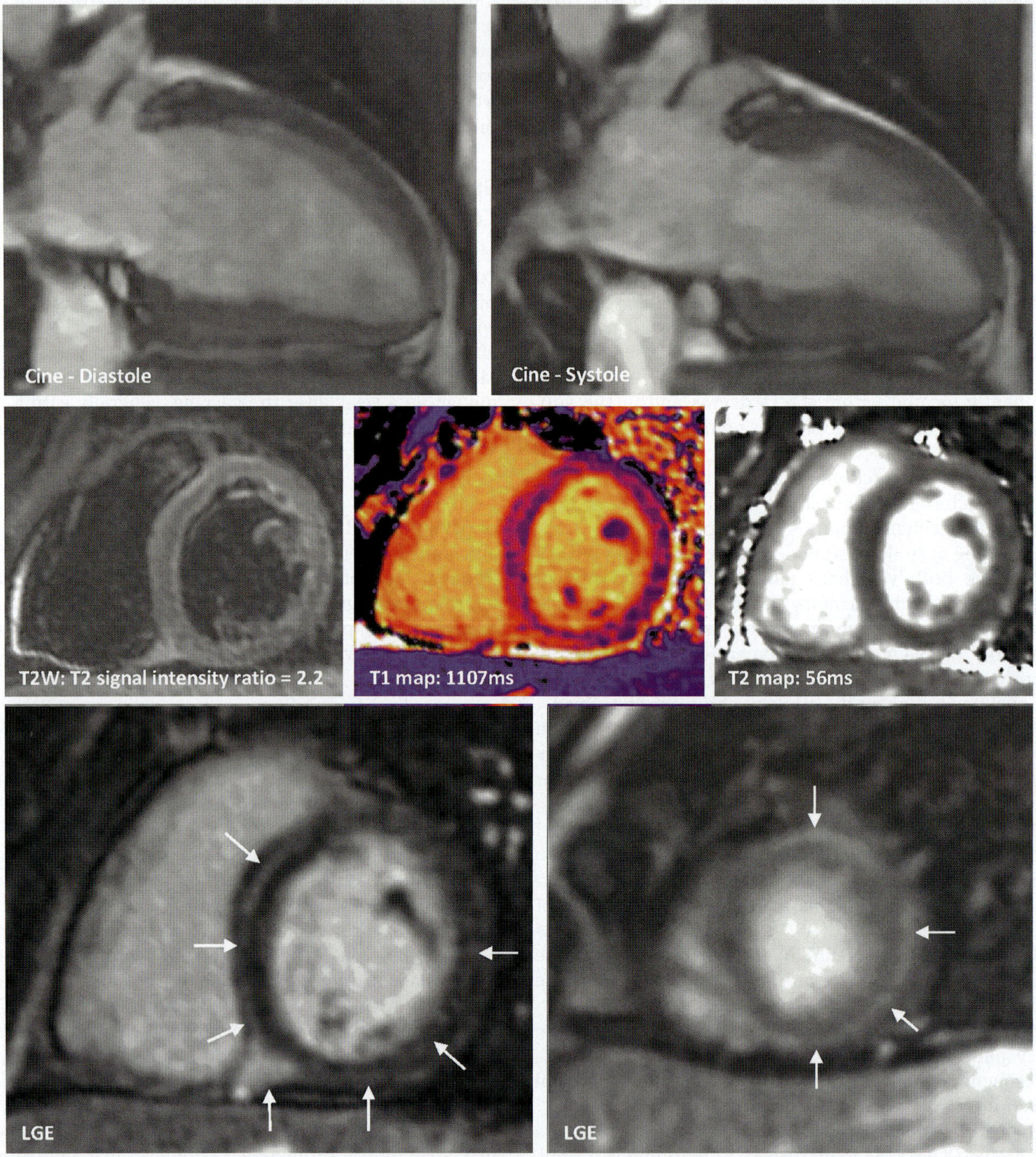

FIG. 30.10 Cardiovascular magnetic resonance in a 32-year-old male patient with acute COVID-19 infection who developed acute chest pain and elevated troponin within the first week of the initial symptoms. Cine images show global left ventricular systolic dysfunction (left ventricular ejection fraction = 42%), T2-weighted (*T2W*) image shows global myocardial signal increase with T2 signal intensity ratio of 2.2, T1 mapping shows global increase of myocardial native T1 relaxation time (1107 ms), and T2 mapping shows global increase of myocardial T2 relaxation time (56 ms). Late gadolinium enhancement (*LGE*) images show a diffuse midwall (*basal segments*) and subepicardial (*apical segments*) hyperintensity areas, including the right ventricular insertion point (*arrows*).

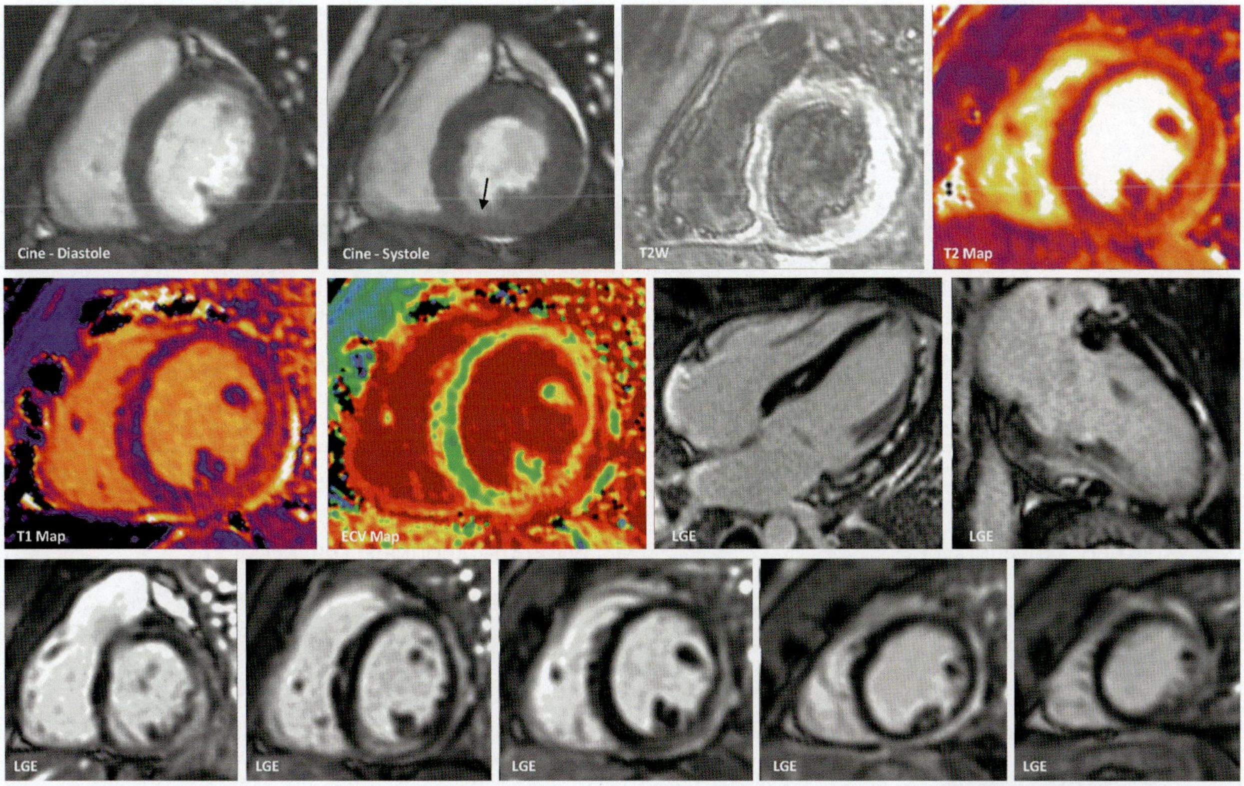

FIG. 30.11 Cardiovascular magnetic resonance in a 24-year-old male patient with acute COVID-19 infection who developed acute chest pain and elevated troponin within the first week of the initial symptoms. Cine images show a regional hypokinesia of the basal inferior segment (left ventricle ejection fraction = 51%). T2-weighted image (*T2W*), T2 mapping (61 ms), and extracellular volume (*ECV*) mapping (50%) show regional subepicardial abnormalities in the lateral and inferior walls. Native T1 mapping shows regional increase (1210 ms) in the basal septum and in the lateral and inferior walls. Late gadolinium enhancement (*LGE*) images show a multifocal distribution involving the basal septum (midwall) and the lateral and inferior walls (subepicardial and midwall).

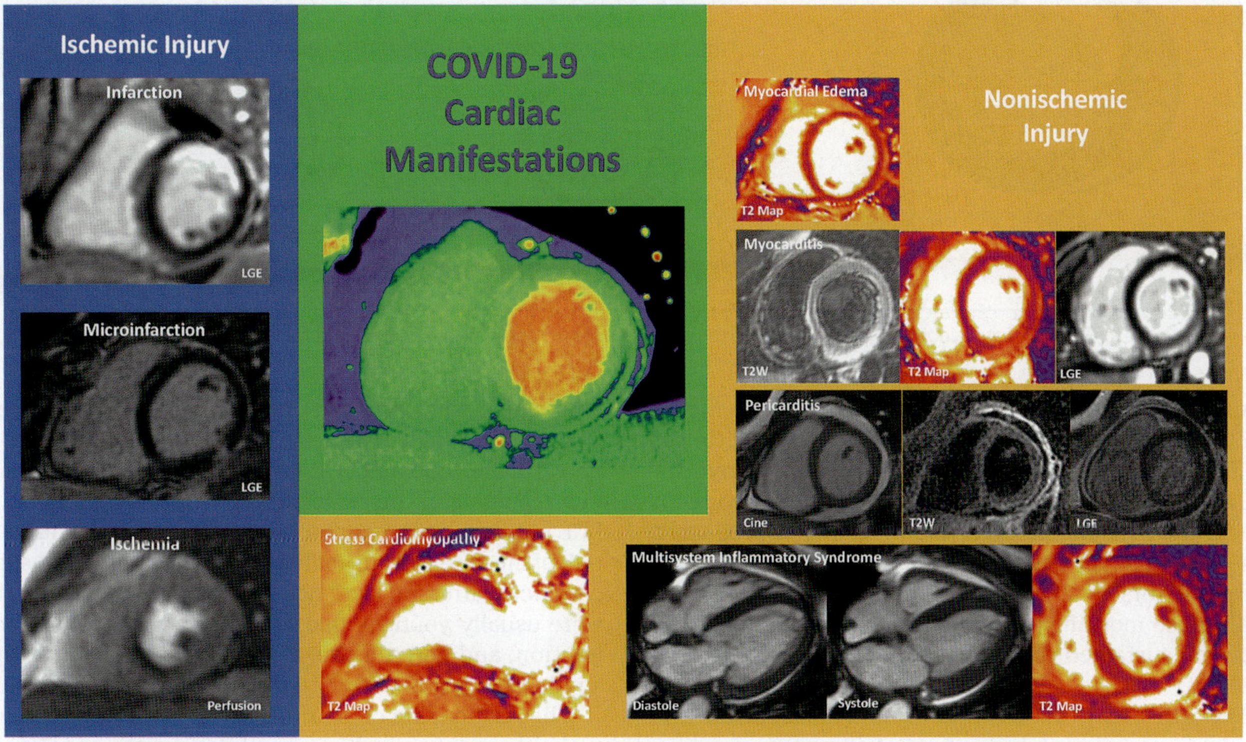

FIG. 30.12 Overview of the COVID-19 cardiac manifestations. *LGE*, Late gadolinium enhancement; *T2W*, T2 weighted.

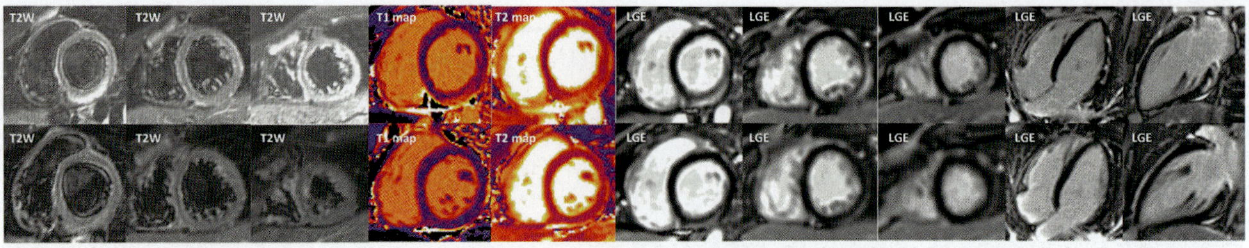

FIG. 30.13 Cardiovascular magnetic resonance (*CMR*) in a 15-year-old male patient who presented with acute chest pain, elevated troponin, and normal LVEF 3 days after the second dose of a COVID-19 mRNA vaccine (BNT162b2). The first row shows the admission CMR with subepicardial abnormalities involving the basal inferior/inferolateral segment, and the mid and apical lateral segments in T2-weighted (*T2W*) images, T1 mapping (1277 ms), T2 mapping (69 ms), and late gadolinium enhancement (*LGE*) images. The second row shows the follow-up CMR 45 days after admission with resolution of abnormalities in T2-weighted images, T1 mapping, and T2 mapping, and an important decrease of the LGE extension.

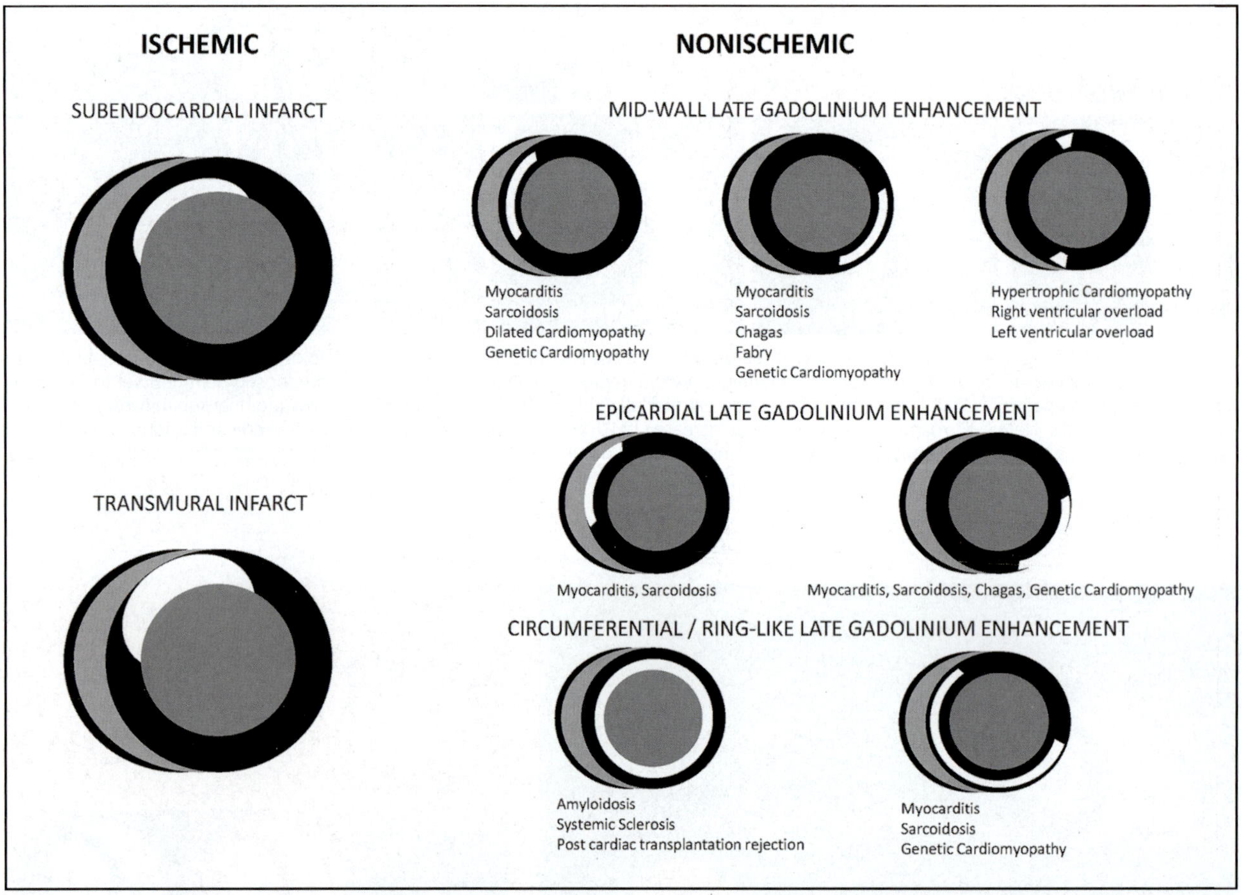

FIG. 30.14 Late gadolinium enhancement patterns, distributions, and possible etiologies (*differential diagnosis*).

be suspected, and inflammatory cardiomyopathy should be considered as a possible diagnosis, although with less specificity than in patients with suspected acute myocarditis. Another important detail that LGE could provide for patients with inflammatory cardiomyopathy is prognosis, as the presence, location, and extent of LGE are independent predictors of major adverse cardiovascular events like all-cause mortality, cardiac mortality, sudden cardiac death, and sustained ventricular arrhythmia, as described above.[37,39]

It is worth noting that some patterns of nonischemic LGE should raise suspicion for specific etiologies of myocarditis, as in cardiac sarcoidosis and Chagas cardiomyopathy, as described below.[11] A relevant pattern of nonischemic LGE found in some patients with suspected cardiomyopathy and which has received increasing attention in recent years is the ringlike pattern, defined as left ventricle subepicardial or midwall LGE involving at least three contiguous segments in the same short axis slice.[68,69] This ringlike LGE pattern is independently associated with an increased risk of life-threatening ventricular arrhythmias and sudden cardiac death, and patients that had the ringlike pattern were usually younger, had higher left ventricular ejection fraction, and had a higher prevalence of family history of sudden cardiac death or cardiomyopathy.[72,73]

The relationship of the ringlike LGE pattern with younger patients and family history make genetic cardiomyopathies an essential differential diagnosis when this pattern is detected, and genetic testing must be considered.[11] When genetic testing was performed in these patients, mutations

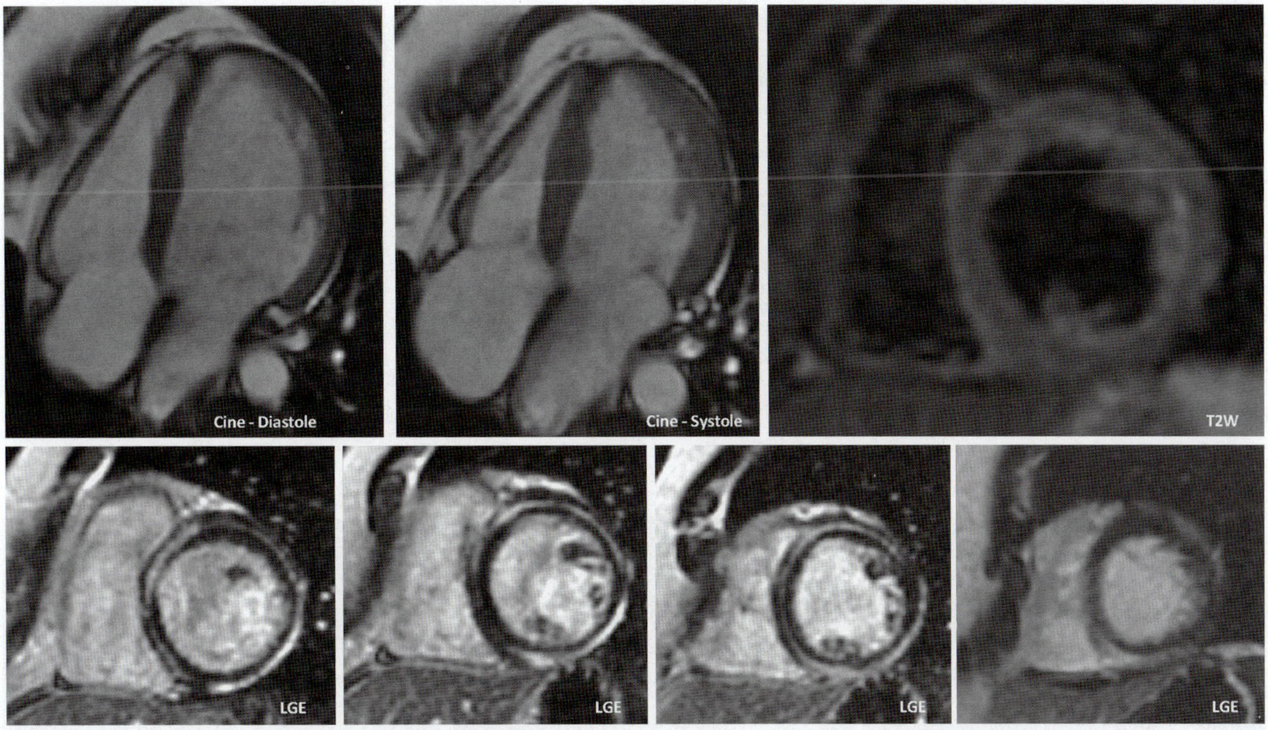

FIG. 30.15 Cardiovascular magnetic resonance (*CMR*) in a 38-year-old female patient who developed exertion dyspnea 5 months after admission in another center with acute chest pain, elevated troponin, normal echocardiography, and normal coronary arteries in coronary computed tomography angiography. CMR shows global left ventricular systolic dysfunction (left ventricle ejection fraction = 44%) in cine images, no edema in T2-weighted (*T2W*) image, and diffuse midwall and subepicardial fibrosis in a ringlike pattern in late gadolinium enhancement (*LGE*) images, consistent with previous myocarditis.

in genes encoding cardiac desmosomal proteins such as desmoplakin (DSP), and nondesmosomal genes such as desmin (DES), filamin C (FLNC), and lamin A/C (LMNA) were identified.[11,74–76] Although not specific, some subtle differences could suggest some etiologies. In myocarditis, despite a contiguous appearance in short-axis views, a patchy pattern could be recognized in long-axis views.[74] In filaminopathy (FLNC), a more contiguous midwall LGE pattern is common, more prevalent in the inferolateral segment, and in laminopathy (LMNA), a midwall LGE pattern in the basal septal segment is predominant.[11,74–76] In arrhythmogenic cardiomyopathy, a subepicardial LGE pattern more extensive in the inferolateral wall is observed, with a circumferential left ventricle involvement in DES mutation and biventricular involvement in DSP mutation (Fig. 30.15).[11,74–76]

Specific Etiology: Cardiac Sarcoidosis

Sarcoidosis is an inflammatory disease characterized by the presence of noncaseating granulomas, usually with multisystem involvement, with the lungs affected in more than 90% of patients. Although about 5% of patients with sarcoidosis develop clinical cardiac symptoms, the estimated prevalence of cardiac involvement is at least 25% in autopsy findings and in studies using CMR.[77–79]

The principal manifestations of cardiac sarcoidosis are heart failure, ventricular arrhythmias, and conduction disturbances, and patients with chronic heart failure and dilated cardiomyopathy who present with new ventricular arrhythmias or second-degree or third-degree heart block should have this etiology of myocarditis suspected.[2,80] Cardiac sarcoidosis can be diagnosed when there is histological evidence of sarcoidosis in myocardial tissue, or more commonly when there is a histological diagnosis of extracardiac sarcoidosis and a demonstration of cardiac involvement, often made by LGE on CMR examination or a patchy uptake on dedicated cardiac fluorodeoxyglucose-positron emission tomography (FDG-PET).[77]

LGE in cardiac sarcoidosis could occur in different patterns and locations.[77,79] In a study of 321 patients with biopsy-proven extracardiac sarcoidosis who underwent CMR for cardiac involvement screening, 29.9% of patients had diagnosed cardiac sarcoidosis. The left ventricle was involved in 93.5% of the cases, 68.8% with at least two different LV walls affected (multifocal), 71% in the septum, 51.6% in the lateral wall, 21.5% in the anterior wall, and 17.2% in the inferior wall. A nonischemic LGE pattern (subepicardial or midwall) was identified in the majority of cases and in all locations, though a potentially ischemic LGE pattern (subendocardial or transmural) involving mainly the lateral wall and the septum was found in 21.5% of patients with LGE (Fig. 30.16).[79]

In another retrospective study of 107 patients referred for evaluation of known or suspected cardiac sarcoidosis by both CMR and FDG-PET, the likelihood of cardiac sarcoidosis was estimated by the examinations' findings. By CMR, a multifocal LGE, defined as at least two noncontiguous areas of nonischemic LGE, had a probable likelihood (50%–90%) of cardiac sarcoidosis in these patients. And when there was LGE in the basal/mid anteroseptal or inferoseptal segments with contiguous extension into the right ventricle's anterior or inferior walls across the insertion points ("hook sign"), a high likelihood (>90%) was assigned (Fig. 30.17).[81]

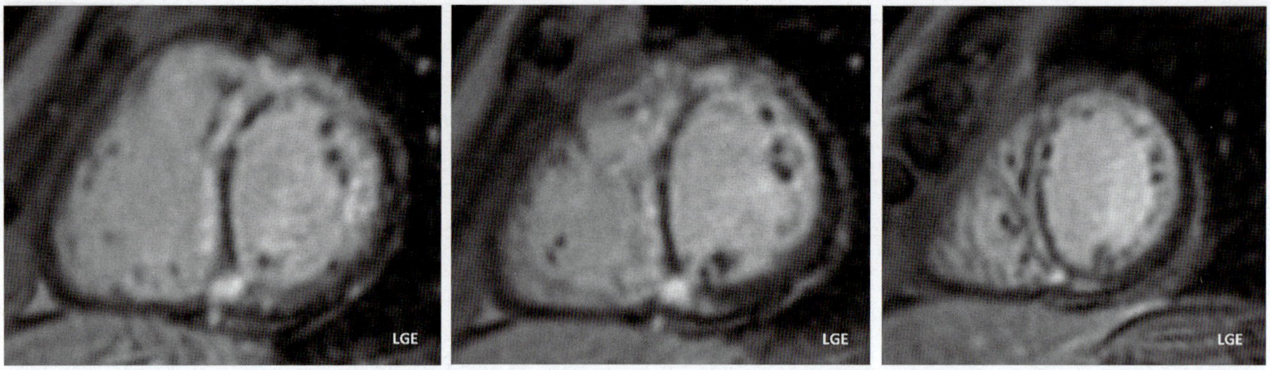

FIG. 30.16 Cardiovascular magnetic resonance in a 58-year-old male patient with extracardiac sarcoidosis who developed sustained ventricular tachycardia. Late gadolinium enhancement (*LGE*) images show predominant subepicardial fibrosis in the septal wall and in the right ventricle insertion points.

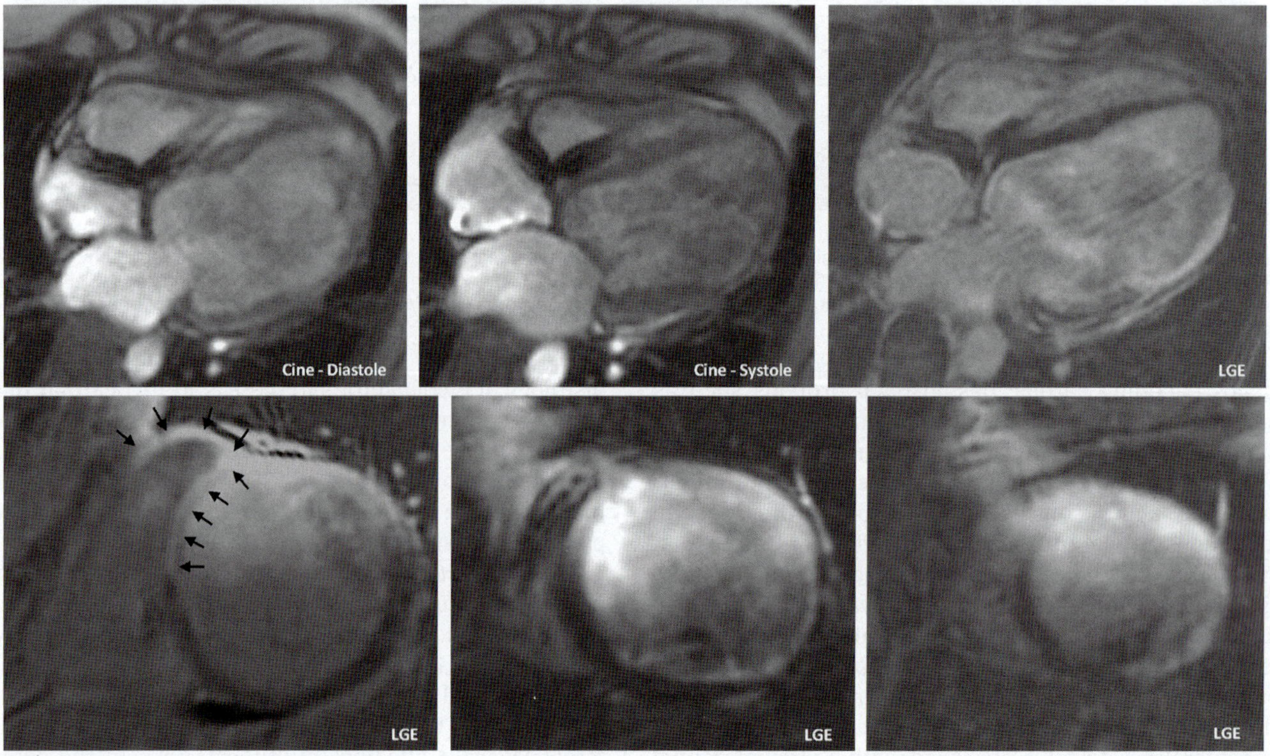

FIG. 30.17 Cardiovascular magnetic resonance in a 31-year-old female patient with dilated cardiomyopathy and sustained ventricular tachycardia submitted to an implantable cardioverter-defibrillator. Cine images show left ventricular dilatation and global systolic dysfunction (left ventricular ejection fraction = 24%), with akinesia of the basal anterior and anteroseptal segments, and of the mid and apical lateral segment. Late gadolinium enhancement (*LGE*) images show transmural fibrosis in the basal anterior and anteroseptal segments with extension into the right ventricular anterior wall (*"hook sign"/arrows*), and subendocardial fibrosis in the mid and apical lateral segment. A subsequent endomyocardial biopsy was consistent with cardiac sarcoidosis.

Regarding prognosis, the presence of LGE is an independent predictor of all-cause mortality and cardiac events.[79,82] In a meta-analysis of 10 studies that included 760 patients with known or suspected cardiac sarcoidosis and used CMR, patients with LGE had higher odds for all-cause mortality (odds ratio: 3.06) and higher odds for the composite outcome of arrhythmogenic events (ventricular arrhythmia, implantable cardioverter-defibrillator shock, and sudden cardiac death) plus all-cause mortality (odds ratio: 10.74) than those without LGE. The annualized event rate of the composite outcome was also increased in patients with LGE (11.9% vs. 1.1%).[82]

Specific Etiology: Chagas Cardiomyopathy

Chagas disease is an infectious disease caused by the protozoan parasite *Trypanosoma cruzi* and generally transmitted by a triatomine bug (vector-borne), although it can also be transmitted through consumption of *T. cruzi*–contaminated food, through blood transfusion, congenitally (maternal-fetal transmission), solid organ transplantation, and laboratory accidents. It is estimated that about 6 to 7 million people worldwide are infected with *T. cruzi*, mainly in endemic areas of Latin American countries, although the prevalence of Chagas disease is increasing in nonendemic regions like the United States, Canada, European countries

(Spain, Italy, and France), Japan, and Australia due to population migration over the previous decades.[83]

Chagas disease presents in two phases, an acute phase in which most patients are asymptomatic or have mild nonspecific symptoms of an infectious disease, and a chronic phase that could last 10 to 30 years before a manifestation related to organ involvement appears. This asymptomatic period of the chronic phase, when patients have evidence of Chagas disease (serology or parasitological test) and no evidence of cardiac involvement by electrocardiogram and chest radiography, is called the indeterminate form. About 30% of patients chronically infected with the indeterminate form develop a cardiac form, in which patients could be asymptomatic with abnormal electrocardiogram (e.g., right bundle branch block and left anterior fascicular block) or abnormal echocardiography without systolic dysfunction, or could develop a chronic Chagas cardiomyopathy with a dilated cardiomyopathy phenotype, and could have manifestations such as heart failure, ventricular arrhythmias, conduction disturbances, or thromboembolic events.[83]

The pathogenesis of chronic Chagas cardiomyopathy is a progressive and incessant myocarditis leading to myocardial fibrosis and dilated cardiomyopathy. The cardiac form of Chagas disease is associated with a higher mortality, and sudden cardiac death accounts for 55% to 65% of the deaths in Chagas disease, often by ventricular arrhythmias.[83,84]

When CMR was performed on 51 seropositive patients in the chronic phase of Chagas disease in a study, LGE was detected in 20% of patients with the indeterminate form and no previous evidence of cardiac involvement, in 84.6% of patients with the cardiac form and no evidence of ventricular arrhythmias, and in 100% of patients with Chagas cardiomyopathy and previously documented ventricular tachycardia. The quantified LGE extension was correlated with the severity of the disease, with higher New York Heart Association functional classes and lower LVEF. The LGE in Chagas cardiomyopathy was predominantly localized in the LV apex and the inferolateral wall, and could be found either in a nonischemic pattern (12.3% subepicardial and 34.6% midwall) or in a subendocardial or transmural pattern (53.1%) (Fig. 30.18).[85]

In another study, 54 patients in the chronic phase of Chagas disease were submitted to CMR using T2-weighted imaging, EGE, and LGE. LGE was present in 72.2% of all patients, in 12.5% of patients with the indeterminate form, in 94.1% of patients with the cardiac form and no LV systolic dysfunction, and in 100% of patients with the cardiac form and LV systolic dysfunction. Abnormal T2-weighted images and EGE were found in 77.8% and 73.8% of all patients, in 31.3% and 25% of patients with the indeterminate form, in 94.1% and 92.3% of patients with the cardiac form and no LV systolic dysfunction, and in 100% and 94.1% of patients with the cardiac form and LV systolic dysfunction, respectively. These findings supported ongoing myocardial inflammation in Chagas disease, and showed that all three techniques correlated with the severity of this condition.[86]

The prognostic information related to myocardial fibrosis detected by the LGE technique in Chagas disease was also reported in previous studies.[87–89] In a study of 130 patients with Chagas cardiomyopathy who had a previous CMR

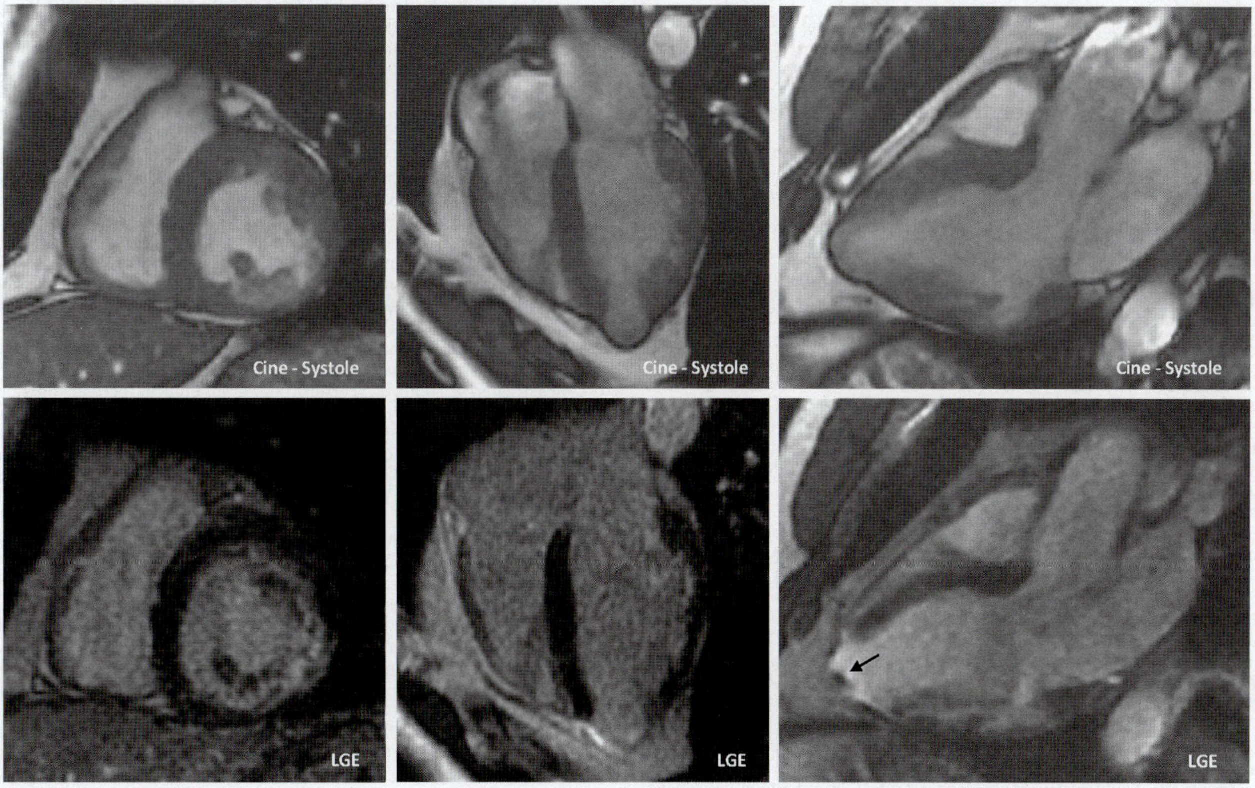

FIG. 30.18 Cardiovascular magnetic resonance in a 56-year-old male patient with Chagas cardiomyopathy. Cine images show systolic dysfunction (left ventricular ejection fraction = 49%) with myocardial thinning of the inferolateral wall and the LV apex (*aneurysm*). Late gadolinium enhancement (*LGE*) images show transmural fibrosis of the inferolateral wall and the LV apex, and a small thrombus in the left ventricular apex (*arrow*).

examination, clinical follow-up was retrospectively obtained concerning the primary outcome of all-cause mortality, heart transplantation, antitachycardia pacing or appropriate shock from an implantable cardioverter-defibrillator, and aborted sudden cardiac death. After a median follow-up of 5.05 years, 44.6% had a primary outcome, and 34.6% died. LGE was an independent predictor of adverse outcome and all-cause mortality, and each 1-gram increase in myocardial fibrosis was associated with a 3.1% increase in the primary outcome and with a 2.8% increase in mortality.[89]

SUMMARY AND FUTURE DIRECTIONS

The ability of CMR to provide noninvasive myocardial tissue characterization with the detection of myocardial edema and fibrosis have changed the workflow for the management of myocarditis, with a class I recommendation in patients with suspected inflammatory heart disease in several cardiology guidelines, excellent diagnostic accuracy in patients with acute myocarditis, and the ability to add relevant prognostic information.

The recent techniques of T1 and T2 mapping allowed for additional evidence of myocardial injury, improved the CMR sensitivity and specificity for acute myocarditis, and led updated CMR diagnostic criteria for myocarditis in 2018, including parametric techniques to achieve a higher diagnostic accuracy. Further studies with the use of T1 and T2 mapping in the follow-up of patients with myocarditis to guide EMB indication and immunosuppressive therapy will be expected in the near future.

The use of novel molecular contrast agents sensitive to immune cells may permit a more specific assessment of myocardial inflammation to guide novel therapies.[9] And the development of artificial intelligence with multiparametric CMR and clinical data should produce better outcome prediction and guide treatment strategies.[45]

REFERENCES

1. Richardson P, McKenna W, Bristow M, et al. Report of the 1995 world health organization/international society and federation of cardiology task force on the definition and classification of cardiomyopathies. *Circulation.* 1996;93(5):841–842.
2. Ammirati E, Frigerio M, Adler ED, et al. Management of acute myocarditis and chronic inflammatory cardiomyopathy: an expert consensus document. *Circ Heart Fail.* 2020;13(11):e007405.
3. Caforio AL, Pankuweit S, Arbustini E, European Society of Cardiology Working Group on Myocardial and Pericardial Diseases, et al. Current state of knowledge on aetiology, diagnosis, management, and therapy of myocarditis: a position statement of the European society of cardiology working group on myocardial and pericardial diseases. *Eur Heart J.* 2013;34(33):2636–2648. 2648a-2648d.
4. Basso C. Myocarditis. *N Engl J Med.* 2022;387(16):1488–1500.
5. Cooper LT, Baughman KL, Feldman AM, American Heart Association; American College of Cardiology; European Society of Cardiology; Heart Failure Society of America; Heart Failure Association of the European Society of Cardiology, et al. The role of endomyocardial biopsy in the management of cardiovascular disease: a scientific statement from the American heart association, the American college of cardiology, and the European society of cardiology. Endorsed by the heart failure society of America and the heart failure association of the European society of cardiology. *J Am Coll Cardiol.* 2007;50(19):1914–1931.
6. Mahrholdt H, Wagner A, Judd RM, et al. Delayed enhancement cardiovascular magnetic resonance assessment of non-ischaemic cardiomyopathies. *Eur Heart J.* 2005;26(15):1461–1474.
7. Friedrich MG, Sechtem U, Schulz-Menger J, et al. International consensus group on cardiovascular magnetic resonance in myocarditis. cardiovascular magnetic resonance in myocarditis: a JACC white paper. *J Am Coll Cardiol.* 2009;53(17):1475–1487.
8. Ferreira VM, Schulz-Menger J, Holmvang G, et al. Cardiovascular magnetic resonance in nonischemic myocardial inflammation: expert recommendations. *J Am Coll Cardiol.* 2018;72(24):3158–3176.
9. Lewis AJM, Burrage MK, Ferreira VM. Cardiovascular magnetic resonance imaging for inflammatory heart diseases. *Cardiovasc Diagn Ther.* 2020;10(3):598–609.
10. Montera MW, Marcondes-Braga FG, Simões MV, et al. Brazilian society of cardiology guideline on myocarditis - 2022. *Arq Bras Cardiol.* 2022;119(1):143–211.
11. Arbelo E, Protonotarios A, Gimeno JR, ESC Scientific Document Group, et al. 2023 ESC guidelines for the management of cardiomyopathies. *Eur Heart J.* 2023;44(37):3503–3626.
12. Pahuja M, Adegbala O, Mishra T, et al. Trends in the incidence of in-hospital mortality, cardiogenic shock, and utilization of mechanical circulatory support devices in myocarditis (analysis of national inpatient sample data, 2005-2014). *J Card Fail.* 2019;25(6):457–467.
13. Byrne RA, Rossello X, Coughlan JJ, ESC Scientific Document Group, et al. 2023 ESC guidelines for the management of acute coronary syndromes. *Eur Heart J.* 2023;44(38):3720–3826.
14. Isaak A, Bischoff LM, Faron A, et al. Multiparametric cardiac magnetic resonance imaging in pediatric and adolescent patients with acute myocarditis. *Pediatr Radiol.* 2021;51(13):2470–2480.
15. Luetkens JA, Faron A, Isaak A, et al. Comparison of original and 2018 Lake Louise Criteria for diagnosis of acute myocarditis: results of a validation cohort. *Radiol Cardiothorac Imaging.* 2019;1(3):e190010.
16. Fischer K, Obrist SJ, Erne SA, et al. Feature tracking myocardial strain incrementally improves prognostication in myocarditis beyond traditional CMR imaging features. *JACC Cardiovasc Imaging.* 2020;13(9):1891–1901.
17. Baeßler B, Schaarschmidt F, Dick A, et al. Diagnostic implications of magnetic resonance feature tracking derived myocardial strain parameters in acute myocarditis. *Eur J Radiol.* 2016;85(1):218–227.
18. Weigand J, Nielsen JC, Sengupta PP, et al. Feature tracking-derived peak systolic strain compared to late gadolinium enhancement in troponin-positive myocarditis: a case-control study. *Pediatr Cardiol.* 2016;37(4):696–703.
19. Lee JW, Jeong YJ, Lee G, et al. Predictive value of cardiac magnetic resonance imaging-derived myocardial strain for poor outcomes in patients with acute myocarditis. *Korean J Radiol.* 2017;18(4):643–654.
20. Soeiro AM, Bossa AS, César MC, et al. The association of myocardial strain with cardiac magnetic resonance and clinical outcomes in patients with acute myocarditis. *Front Cardiovasc Med.* 2023;10:1121083.
21. Bogaert J, Francone M. Cardiovascular magnetic resonance in pericardial diseases. *J Cardiovasc Magn Reson.* 2009;11(1):14.
22. Rosmini S, Seraphim A, Knott K, et al. Non-invasive characterization of pleural and pericardial effusions using T1 mapping by magnetic resonance imaging. *Eur Heart J Cardiovasc Imaging.* 2022;23(8):1117–1126.
23. Abdel-Aty H, Boyé P, Zagrosek A, et al. Diagnostic performance of cardiovascular magnetic resonance in patients with suspected acute myocarditis: comparison of different approaches. *J Am Coll Cardiol.* 2005;45(11):1815–1822.
24. Chu GC, Flewitt JA, Mikami Y, et al. Assessment of acute myocarditis by cardiovascular MR: diagnostic performance of shortened protocols. *Int J Cardiovasc Imaging.* 2013;29(5):1077–1083.
25. Friedrich MG, Strohm O, Schulz-Menger J, et al. Contrast media-enhanced magnetic resonance imaging visualizes myocardial changes in the course of viral myocarditis. *Circulation.* 1998;97(18):1802–1809.
26. Laissy JP, Messin B, Varenne O, et al. MRI of acute myocarditis: a comprehensive approach based on various imaging sequences. *Chest.* 2002;122(5):1638–1648.
27. Schwab J, Rogg HJ, Pauschinger M, et al. Functional and morphological parameters with tissue characterization of cardiovascular magnetic imaging in clinically verified "infarct-like myocarditis". *Rofo.* 2016;188(4):365–373.
28. Haaf P, Garg P, Messroghli DR, et al. Cardiac T1 mapping and extracellular volume (ECV) in clinical practice: a comprehensive review. *J Cardiovasc Magn Reson.* 2016;18(1):89.
29. O'Brien AT, Gil KE, Varghese J, et al. T2 mapping in myocardial disease: a comprehensive review. *J Cardiovasc Magn Reson.* 2022;24(1):33.
30. Messroghli DR, Moon JC, Ferreira VM, et al. Clinical recommendations for cardiovascular magnetic resonance mapping of T1, T2, T2* and extracellular volume: a consensus statement by the society for cardiovascular magnetic resonance (SCMR) endorsed by the European association for cardiovascular imaging (EACVI). *J Cardiovasc Magn Reson.* 2017;19(1):75. https://doi.org/10.1186/s12968-017-0389-8. Erratum in: J Cardiovasc Magn Reson. 2018 Feb 7;20(1):9.
31. Dabir D, Vollbrecht TM, Luetkens JA, et al. Multiparametric cardiovascular magnetic resonance imaging in acute myocarditis: a comparison of different measurement approaches. *J Cardiovasc Magn Reson.* 2019;21(1):54.
32. Kotanidis CP, Bazmpani MA, Haidich AB, et al. Diagnostic accuracy of cardiovascular magnetic resonance in acute myocarditis: a systematic review and meta-analysis. *JACC Cardiovasc Imaging.* 2018;11(11):1583–1590.
33. von Knobelsdorff-Brenkenhoff F, Schüler J, Dogangüzel S, et al. Detection and monitoring of acute myocarditis applying quantitative cardiovascular magnetic resonance. *Circ Cardiovasc Imaging.* 2017;10(2):e005242.
34. Bohnen S, Radunski UK, Lund GK, et al. Performance of t1 and t2 mapping cardiovascular magnetic resonance to detect active myocarditis in patients with recent-onset heart failure. *Circ Cardiovasc Imaging.* 2015;8(6):e003073.
35. Lurz P, Luecke C, Eitel I, et al. Comprehensive cardiac magnetic resonance imaging in patients with suspected myocarditis: the MyoRacer-trial. *J Am Coll Cardiol.* 2016;67(15):1800–1811.

36. Spieker M, Haberkorn S, Gastl M, et al. Abnormal T2 mapping cardiovascular magnetic resonance correlates with adverse clinical outcome in patients with suspected acute myocarditis. *J Cardiovasc Magn Reson.* 2017;19(1):38.
37. Gräni C, Eichhorn C, Bière L, et al. Prognostic value of cardiac magnetic resonance tissue characterization in risk stratifying patients with suspected myocarditis. *J Am Coll Cardiol.* 2017;70(16):1964–1976.
38. Sanguineti F, Garot P, Mana M, et al. Cardiovascular magnetic resonance predictors of clinical outcome in patients with suspected acute myocarditis. *J Cardiovasc Magn Reson.* 2015;17(1):78.
39. Grün S, Schumm J, Greulich S, et al. Long-term follow-up of biopsy-proven viral myocarditis: predictors of mortality and incomplete recovery. *J Am Coll Cardiol.* 2012;59(18):1604–1615.
40. Aquaro GD, Ghebru Habtemicael Y, et al. "Cardiac magnetic resonance" working group of the Italian society of cardiology. Prognostic value of repeating cardiac magnetic resonance in patients with acute myocarditis. *J Am Coll Cardiol.* 2019;74(20):2439–2448.
41. Vermes E, Childs H, Faris P, et al. Predictive value of CMR criteria for LV functional improvement in patients with acute myocarditis. *Eur Heart J Cardiovasc Imaging.* 2014;15(10):1140–1144.
42. Wagner A, Schulz-Menger J, Dietz R, et al. Long-term follow-up of patients paragraph sign with acute myocarditis by magnetic paragraph sign resonance imaging. *MAGMA.* 2003;16(1):17–20.
43. Thavendiranathan P, Zhang L, Zafar A, et al. Myocardial T1 and T2 mapping by magnetic resonance in patients with immune checkpoint inhibitor-associated myocarditis. *J Am Coll Cardiol.* 2021;77(12):1503–1516.
44. Gräni C, Bière L, Eichhorn C, et al. Incremental value of extracellular volume assessment by cardiovascular magnetic resonance imaging in risk stratifying patients with suspected myocarditis. *Int J Cardiovasc Imaging.* 2019;35(6):1067–1078.
45. Eichhorn C, Greulich S, Bucciarelli-Ducci C, et al. Multiparametric cardiovascular magnetic resonance approach in diagnosing, monitoring, and prognostication of myocarditis. *JACC Cardiovasc Imaging.* 2022;15(7):1325–1338.
46. Maron BJ, Udelson JE, Bonow RO, et al. Eligibility and disqualification recommendations for competitive athletes with cardiovascular abnormalities: task force 3: hypertrophic cardiomyopathy, arrhythmogenic right ventricular cardiomyopathy and other cardiomyopathies, and myocarditis: a scientific statement from the American heart association and American college of cardiology. *J Am Coll Cardiol.* 2015;66(21):2362–2371.
47. Pelliccia A, Solberg EE, Papadakis M, et al. Recommendations for participation in competitive and leisure time sport in athletes with cardiomyopathies, myocarditis, and pericarditis: position statement of the sport cardiology section of the European association of preventive cardiology (EAPC). *Eur Heart J.* 2019;40(1):19–33.
47a Schulz-Menger J, et al. 2025 ESC Guidelines for the management of myocarditis and pericarditis. *Eur Heart J.* 2025;46(40):3952–4041.
47b Drazner MH, et al. 2024 ACC expert consensus decision pathway on strategies and criteria for the diagnosis and management of myocarditis. *J Am Coll Cardiol.* 2025;85:391–431.
47c Ammiratti E, et al. Diagnosis and treatment of acute myocarditis: a review. *JAMA.* 2023;329(13):1098–1113.
48. Puntmann VO, Carerj ML, Wieters I, et al. Outcomes of cardiovascular magnetic resonance imaging in patients recently recovered from coronavirus disease 2019 (COVID-19). *JAMA Cardiol.* 2020;5(11):1265–1273.
49. Galea N, Marchitelli L, Pambianchi G, et al. T2-mapping increase is the prevalent imaging biomarker of myocardial involvement in active COVID-19: a cardiovascular magnetic resonance study. *J Cardiovasc Magn Reson.* 2021;23(1):68.
50. Joy G, Artico J, Kurdi H, COVID. Investigators, et al. Prospective case-control study of cardiovascular abnormalities 6 months following mild COVID-19 in healthcare workers. *JACC Cardiovasc Imaging.* 2021;14(11):2155–2166.
51. Rajpal S, Tong MS, Borchers J, et al. Cardiovascular magnetic resonance findings in competitive athletes recovering from COVID-19 infection. *JAMA Cardiol.* 2021;6(1):116–118.
52. Clark DE, Parikh A, Dendy JM, et al. COVID-19 myocardial pathology evaluation in athletes with cardiac magnetic resonance (COMPETE CMR). *Circulation.* 2021;143(6):e238.
53. Vago H, Szabo L, Dohy Z, et al. Cardiac magnetic resonance findings in patients recovered from COVID-19: initial experiences in elite athletes. *JACC Cardiovasc Imaging.* 2021;14(6):1279–1281.
54. Artico J, Shiwani H, Moon JC, , OxAMI (Oxford Acute Myocardial Infarction Study) Investigators; COVID-HEART Investigators†, Greenwood JP, et al. Myocardial involvement after hospitalization for COVID-19 complicated by troponin elevation: a prospective, multicenter, observational study. *Circulation.* 2023;147(5):364–374.
55. Basso C, Leone O, Rizzo S, et al. Pathological features of COVID-19-associated myocardial injury: a multicentre cardiovascular pathology study. *Eur Heart J.* 2020;41(39):3827–3835.
56. Pellegrini D, Kawakami R, Guagliumi G, et al. Microthrombi as a major cause of cardiac injury in COVID-19: a pathologic study. *Circulation.* 2021;143(10):1031–1042.
57. Vidula MK, Rajewska-Tabor J, Cao JJ, et al. Myocardial injury on CMR in patients with COVID-19 and suspected cardiac involvement. *JACC Cardiovasc Imaging.* 2023;16(5):609–624.
58. Petersen SE, Friedrich MG, Leiner T, et al. Cardiovascular magnetic resonance for patients with COVID-19. *JACC Cardiovasc Imaging.* 2022;15(4):685–699.
59. Ferreira VM, Plein S, Wong TC, et al. Cardiovascular magnetic resonance for evaluation of cardiac involvement in COVID-19: recommendations by the society for cardiovascular magnetic resonance. *J Cardiovasc Magn Reson.* 2023;25(1):21.
60. Clark DE, Aggarwal SK, Phillips NJ, et al. Cardiac magnetic resonance in the evaluation of COVID-19. *Card Fail Rev.* 2022;8:e09.
61. Blondiaux E, Parisot P, Redheuil A, et al. Cardiac MRI in children with multisystem inflammatory syndrome associated with COVID-19. *Radiology.* 2020;297(3):E283–E288.
62. Theocharis P, Wong J, Pushparajah K, et al. Multimodality cardiac evaluation in children and young adults with multisystem inflammation associated with COVID-19. *Eur Heart J Cardiovasc Imaging.* 2021;22(8):896–903.
63. Caro-Domínguez P, Navallas M, Riaza-Martin L, et al. Imaging findings of multisystem inflammatory syndrome in children associated with COVID-19. *Pediatr Radiol.* 2021;51(9):1608–1620.
64. Li DL, Davogustto G, Soslow JH, et al. Characteristics of COVID-19 myocarditis with and without multisystem inflammatory syndrome. *Am J Cardiol.* 2022;168:135–141.
65. Writing Committee, Gluckman TJ, Bhave NM, Allen LA, et al. 2022 ACC expert consensus decision pathway on cardiovascular sequelae of COVID-19 in adults: myocarditis and other myocardial involvement, post-acute sequelae of SARS-CoV-2 infection, and return to play: a report of the American college of cardiology solution set oversight committee. *J Am Coll Cardiol.* 2022;79(17):1717–1756.
66. Witberg G, Barda N, Hoss S, et al. Myocarditis after Covid-19 vaccination in a large health care organization. *N Engl J Med.* 2021;385(23):2132–2139.
67. Mevorach D, Anis E, Cedar N, et al. Myocarditis after BNT162b2 mRNA vaccine against covid-19 in Israel. *N Engl J Med.* 2021;385(23):2140–2149.
68. Oster ME, Shay DK, Su JR, et al. Myocarditis cases reported after mRNA-based COVID-19 vaccination in the US from December 2020 to August 2021. *JAMA.* 2022;327(4):331–340.
69. Patone M, Mei XW, Handunnetthi L, et al. Risk of myocarditis after sequential doses of COVID-19 vaccine and SARS-CoV-2 infection by age and sex. *Circulation.* 2022;146(10):743–754.
70. Naveed Z, Li J, Wilton J, Canadian Immunization Research Network (CIRN) Provincial Collaborative Network (PCN) Investigators, et al. Comparative risk of myocarditis/pericarditis following second doses of BNT162b2 and mRNA-1273 coronavirus vaccines. *J Am Coll Cardiol.* 2022;80(20):1900–1908.
71. Fronza M, Thavendiranathan P, Chan V, et al. Myocardial injury pattern at MRI in COVID-19 vaccine-associated myocarditis. *Radiology.* 2022;304(3):553–562.
72. Muser D, Nucifora G, Pieroni M, et al. Prognostic value of nonischemic ring-like left ventricular scar in patients with apparently idiopathic nonsustained ventricular arrhythmias. *Circulation.* 2021;143(14):1359–1373.
73. Chen W, Qian W, Zhang X, et al. Ring-like late gadolinium enhancement for predicting ventricular tachyarrhythmias in non-ischaemic dilated cardiomyopathy. *Eur Heart J Cardiovasc Imaging.* 2021;22(10):1130–1138.
74. Bietenbeck M, Meier C, Korthals D, et al. Possible causes and clinical relevance of a "ring-like" late gadolinium enhancement pattern. *JACC Cardiovasc Imaging.* 2024;17(1):104–106.
75. Segura-Rodríguez D, Bermúdez-Jiménez FJ, Carriel V, et al. Myocardial fibrosis in arrhythmogenic cardiomyopathy: a genotype-phenotype correlation study. *Eur Heart J Cardiovasc Imaging.* 2020;21(4):378–386.
76. Corrado D, Basso C. Arrhythmogenic left ventricular cardiomyopathy. *Heart.* 2022;108(9):733–743.
77. Birnie DH, Nery PB, Ha AC, et al. Cardiac sarcoidosis. *J Am Coll Cardiol.* 2016;68(4):411–421.
78. wai K, Tachibana T, Takemura T, et al. Pathological studies on sarcoidosis autopsy. I. Epidemiological features of 320 cases in Japan. *Acta Pathol Jpn.* 1993;43(7–8):372–376.
79. Kouranos V, Tzelepis GE, Rapti A, et al. Complementary role of CMR to conventional screening in the diagnosis and prognosis of cardiac sarcoidosis. *JACC Cardiovasc Imaging.* 2017;10(12):1437–1447.
80. Cooper Jr LT. Myocarditis. *N Engl J Med.* 2009;360(15):1526–1538.
81. Vita T, Okada DR, Veillet-Chowdhury M, et al. Complementary value of cardiac magnetic resonance imaging and positron emission tomography/computed tomography in the assessment of cardiac sarcoidosis. *Circ Cardiovasc Imaging.* 2018;11(1):e007030.
82. Coleman GC, Shaw PW, Balfour Jr PC, et al. Prognostic value of myocardial scarring on CMR in patients with cardiac sarcoidosis. *JACC Cardiovasc Imaging.* 2017;10(4):411–420.
83. Marin-Neto JA, Rassi Jr A, Oliveira GMM, et al. SBC guideline on the diagnosis and treatment of patients with cardiomyopathy of Chagas disease - 2023. *Arq Bras Cardiol.* 2023;120(6):e20230269.
84. Rassi Jr A, Rassi SG, Rassi A. Sudden death in Chagas' disease. *Arq Bras Cardiol.* 2001;76(1):75–96.
85. Rochitte CE, Oliveira PF, Andrade JM, et al. Myocardial delayed enhancement by magnetic resonance imaging in patients with Chagas' disease: a marker of disease severity. *J Am Coll Cardiol.* 2005;46(8):1553–1558.
86. Torreão JA, Ianni BM, Mady C, et al. Myocardial tissue characterization in Chagas' heart disease by cardiovascular magnetic resonance. *J Cardiovasc Magn Reson.* 2015;17:97.
87. Mello RP, Szarf G, Schvartzman PR, et al. Delayed enhancement cardiac magnetic resonance imaging can identify the risk for ventricular tachycardia in chronic Chagas' heart disease. *Arq Bras Cardiol.* 2012;98(5):421–430.
88. Uellendahl M, Siqueira ME, Calado EB, et al. Cardiac magnetic resonance-verified myocardial fibrosis in Chagas disease: clinical correlates and risk stratification. *Arq Bras Cardiol.* 2016;107(5):460–466.
89. Senra T, Ianni BM, Costa ACP, et al. Long-term prognostic value of myocardial fibrosis in patients with Chagas cardiomyopathy. *J Am Coll Cardiol.* 2018;72(21):2577–2587.

31 Cardio-Oncology

CORY R. TRANKLE, WENDY BOTTINOR, JENNIFER H. JORDAN, AND W. GREGORY HUNDLEY

ABBREVIATIONS

CMR cardiovascular magnetic resonance
CTRCD cancer therapy–related cardiac dysfunction
ECVF extracellular volume fraction
EF ejection fraction
HER2 human epidermal growth factor receptor two
LV left ventricular
TTE transthoracic echocardiography

INTRODUCTION

Although therapeutic advances have reduced cancer-related mortality for several malignancies, these improved oncologic outcomes have been partially offset by untoward adverse cardiovascular-related morbidity and mortality. Today, it has become acceptable to identify cancer survivors at the time of cancer diagnosis. In the care of cancer survivors, cardiovascular magnetic resonance (CMR) can serve as a useful diagnostic tool to diagnose adverse cancer therapy–related cardiovascular disease and thus enable the administration of targeted therapy to prevent a future cardiac event. In this chapter, the various mechanisms of cancer and cancer therapy–related cardiovascular disease (CTRCD) are described with accompanying CMR images along with descriptions regarding the use of CMR to diagnose subclinical cardiovascular disease and thereby inform therapeutic decisions to avoid cardiovascular events.

MECHANISMS OF CARDIOVASCULAR ABNORMALITIES

Several cancer therapies have the potential to contribute to cardiovascular dysfunction through a variety of often overlapping mechanisms. These include endothelial and myocellular injury and inflammation; activation of fibrotic and cellular senescent processes that promote accelerated aging; promotion of vascular thrombosis and disruption of microcirculatory function; fostering of atherosclerosis; initiation of inappropriate activation of the renin, angiotensin, and aldosterone axis; and facilitation of adverse atrial and biventricular arrhythmias.[1] These mechanisms—alone or in combination—and their adverse effects on cardiovascular morphology or function may in turn reduce exercise capacity, contribute to fatigue, reduce overall quality of life, and in some cases, promote an increased risk of cardiovascular-related mortality. The presentation of the utility of CMR in patients with cancer across assessments of left ventricular (LV) contractile function, LV myocardial volume and mass, cardiac masses, valvular heart disease, right ventricular (RV) function, and pericardial disease is shown in Fig. 31.1. Although several of the disease processes are discussed in greater depth in other dedicated chapters, they are also mentioned in this chapter as these adverse consequences may occur in those receiving treatment for cancer.[2]

Left Ventricular Contractile Dysfunction

Historically, measures of left ventricular ejection fraction (LVEF) have been utilized to identify suitability for the administration of many forms of cancer treatment.[3] Consequently, reductions in LVEF have formed a basis for diagnosing CTRCD. Today, transthoracic echocardiography (TTE) is used widely to assess LVEF and therefore CTRCD definitions have focused on readily obtainable TTE measures. Commonly, absolute reductions in LVEF by 10 percentage points to values < 53% identify CTRCD. Additionally, other investigators have incorporated echocardiographic measures of LV global longitudinal strain and/or cardiac blood serum–based biomarkers to identify clinical or subclinical LV dysfunction related to the administration of cancer treatments.[4]

While CMR may provide similar assessments of these previously developed TTE-based measures of CTRCD, CMR may also be used to identify information that subclinical cardiac injury and provides the mechanistic basis for the etiology of this injury. This latter aspect of CMR-based assessments can be highly advantageous to provider teams seeking to avoid subclinical and clinical cardiovascular events related to the administration of cancer therapy and maximize the administration of therapies associated with the successful treatment, remission, and cure of cancer.

DECREASED LEFT VENTRICULAR END DIASTOLIC VOLUME

Since reductions in LVEF are frequently used as criteria for CTRCD, it is important to note that the formula used for measuring LVEF ([LV end diastolic volume − LV end systolic volume]/LV end diastolic volume) may be influenced by changes in LV end diastolic volume. Indeed, patients receiving cancer treatment are often vulnerable to reductions in LV end diastolic volume precipitated by intravascular volume depletion due to decreased appetite, nausea, vomiting, and/or diarrhea. This decrease in LV preload

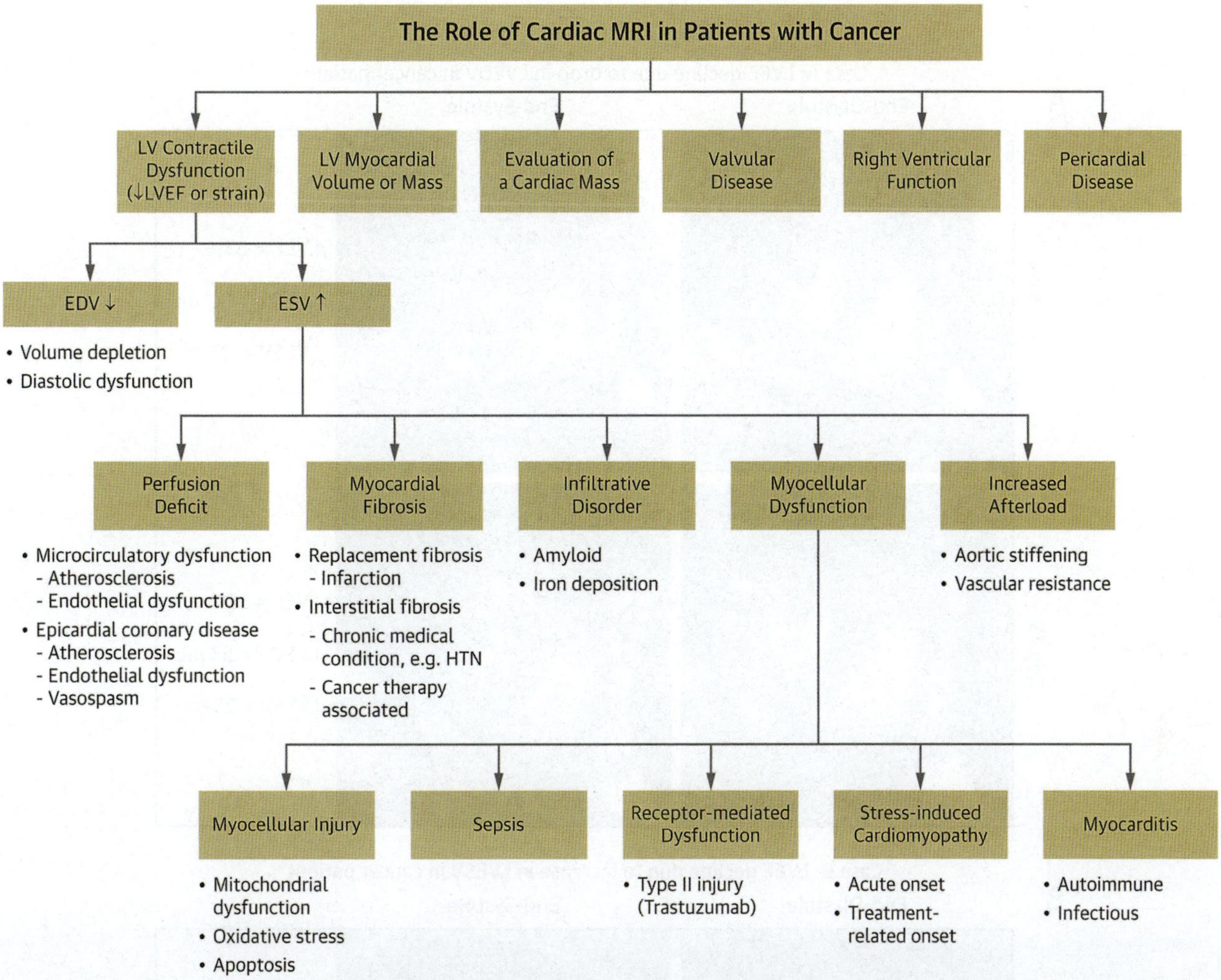

FIG. 31.1 Mechanisms of cardiovascular dysfunction in patients with cancer. Several pathways may lead to cardiovascular dysfunction in patients with cancer or cancer-related treatments. Cardiovascular magnetic resonance can be instrumental in characterizing the pathophysiology and potentially directing therapies toward the mechanism of dysfunction. *EDV,* end diastolic volume; *ESV,* end systolic volume; *HTN,* hypertension; *LV,* left ventricular; *LVEF,* left ventricular ejection fraction. (Permission obtained to reproduce from Jordan JH, Todd RM, Vasu S, Hundley WG. Cardiovascular magnetic resonance in the oncology patient. *JACC Cardiovasc Imaging*. 2018;11(8):1150–1172. doi:10.1016/j.jcmg.2018.06.004 Fig. 1.)

related to intravascular volume depletion (Fig. 31.2) can affect LV volumetric or strain measurements and may account for up to 20% of instances of declines in LVEF in those receiving potentially cardiotoxic chemotherapy. Relative to factors that impact LV contractility, reductions in LV end diastolic volume alone may reflect a lower risk of long-term reductions in LVEF.[5]

INCREASED LEFT VENTRICULAR END SYSTOLIC VOLUME

Increases in LV end systolic volume in those receiving potentially cardiotoxic chemotherapy may reflect intrinsic LV myocardial injury or increases in LV afterload that impede LV ejection. Potential mechanisms of LV end systolic volume rises that are pertinent to patients receiving cancer therapy are summarized in the following sections.

Left Ventricular Myocardial Perfusion Defects

As with the general population, patients with cancer are vulnerable to comorbid coronary atherosclerosis, which is influenced by age, sex, race, comorbid risk factors, socioeconomic status, cancer stage, and cancer subtype.[6] Whether resulting in flow-limiting stenosis of the large epicardial coronary vessels or disruption of microvascular vasodilatory function, this disease may manifest as abnormalities on vasodilator stress perfusion CMR studies. Furthermore, certain cancer therapies may accelerate coronary atherosclerosis (e.g., hormone antagonism, radiation therapy), precipitate vascular events such as myocardial infarction (e.g., immune checkpoint inhibitors, interleukin-2), or promote coronary vasospastic events (e.g., 5-fluorouracil).[1] In patients with cancer, CMR—particularly after intravenous administration of endothelial-independent vasodilators (e.g., adenosine)—may be of particular utility to identify coronary arterial epicardial or microcirculatory abnormalities that impair LV myocardial perfusion due to (1) its high diagnostic accuracy and prognostic capacity in general populations of patients with known or suspected coronary artery disease, (2) its ability to evaluate for mimics of ischemic disease that may be present in patients receiving cancer therapy (e.g., stress cardiomyopathy, myocarditis), and (3) increasingly available techniques designed to quantify myocardial blood flow, which are gaining more widespread use in recent years.[7] Case examples of the use of vasodilator stress CMR to help identify LV myocardial perfusion defects in those receiving cancer treatment are shown in Figs. 31.3 and 31.4.

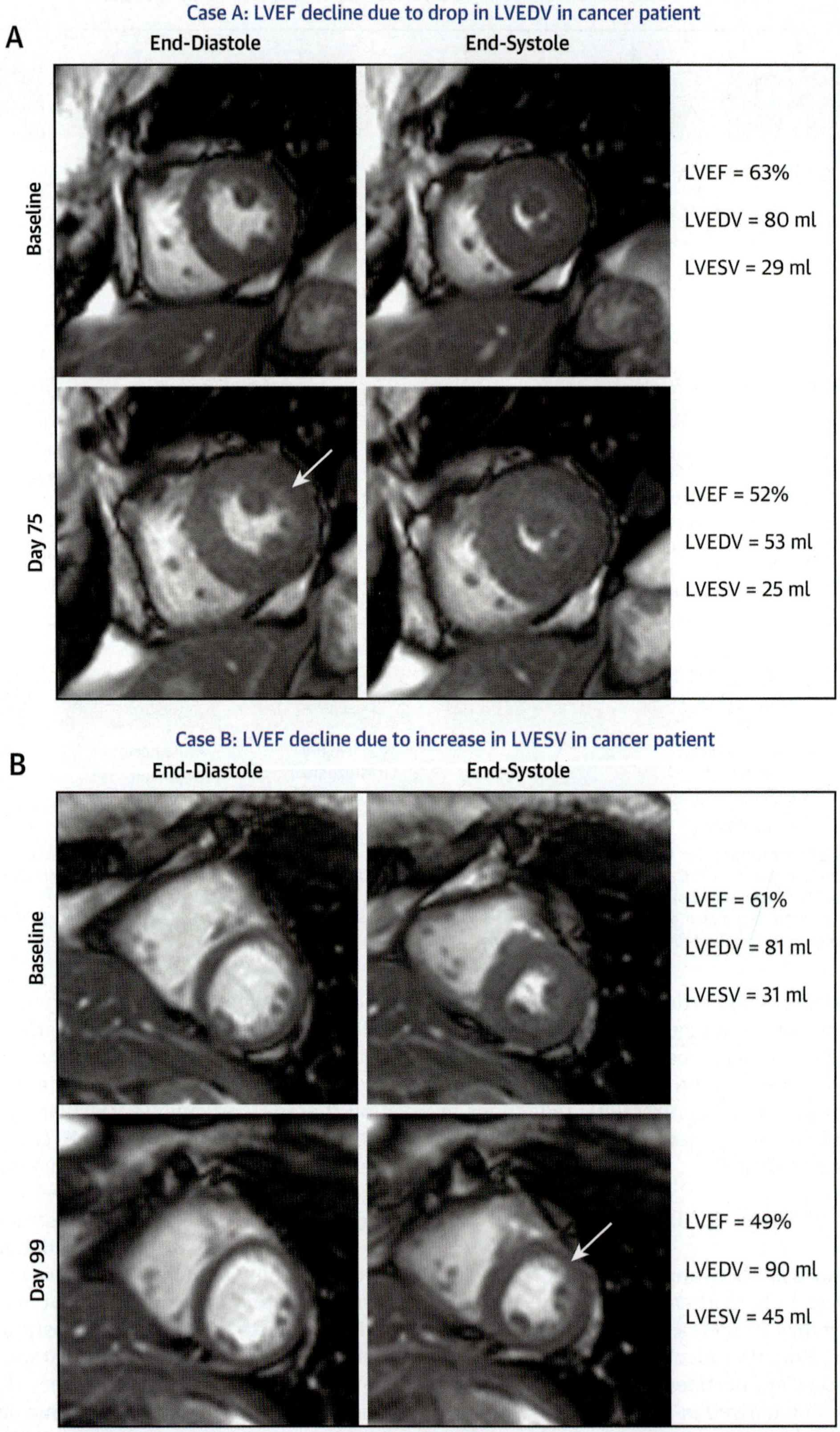

FIG. 31.2 Decline in left ventricular ejection fraction due to changes in end diastolic or end systolic volumes. Reductions in left ventricular ejection fraction during the course of cancer treatment may be due to decreased left ventricular end diastolic volume (panel A) or increased left ventricular end systolic volume (panel B)—or a combination of the two. Cardiovascular magnetic resonance allows for precise volumetric assessments to make this distinction across serial scans. *LVEDV*, left ventricular end diastolic volume; *LVESV*, left ventricular end systolic volume; *LVEF*, left ventricular ejection fraction. (Permission obtained to reproduce from Jordan JH, Todd RM, Vasu S, Hundley WG. Cardiovascular magnetic resonance in the oncology patient. *JACC Cardiovasc Imaging*. 2018;11(8):1150–1172. doi:10.1016/j.jcmg.2018.06.004 Fig. 3.)

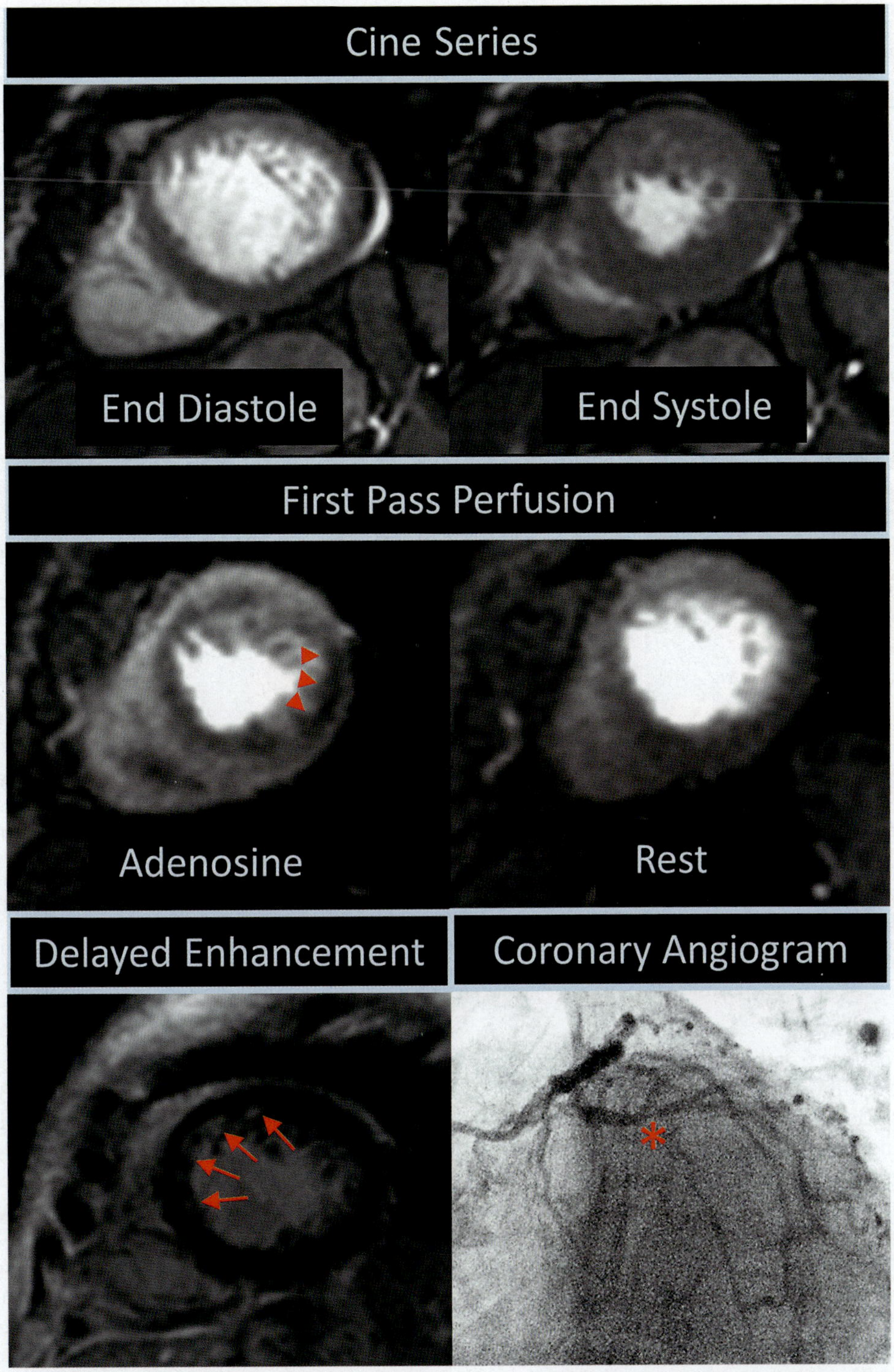

FIG. 31.3 Example of vasodilator stress perfusion study. A 77-year-old female with B-cell acute lymphoblastic leukemia experienced elevated blood pressure and chest discomfort with outpatient asciminib therapy. She was known to have a history of coronary artery disease with prior stenting in the left anterior descending artery and was referred for cardiovascular magnetic resonance to exclude progression of coronary perfusion deficits. Cine series (*top panels*) revealed low normal systolic function. Vasodilator stress perfusion demonstrated a reversible perfusion defect (*arrowheads*) compared to rest involving the inferolateral wall (*middle panels*), in addition to a perfusion defect involving the left anterior descending artery territory (anterior, septal walls). Late gadolinium-enhanced imaging (*lower left panel*) showed focal scar involving the left anterior descending artery territory (*arrows*) but not at the site of the inferolateral reversible perfusion defect. Coronary angiography (*lower right panel*) confirmed flow-limiting stenosis of the circumflex artery (*asterisk*) for which a drug-eluting stent was placed. Chest pain symptoms resolved, and the patient was able to continue asciminib therapy for her malignancy.

Myocardial Fibrosis

Patients with cancer may experience focal reactive fibrosis before or after therapy arising from localized cardiac injuries such as myocardial infarction or myocarditis. Such injuries can either be provoked by cancer treatment or related to underlying comorbidities. Standard late gadolinium-enhanced imaging techniques are instrumental in identifying those patterns of regional injury through pattern recognition, aiding in diagnosis and risk stratification. An example of this is shown in Fig. 31.5, in which standard late gadolinium-enhanced techniques allowed for determination of the mechanism of cardiomyocyte injury among a relatively broad differential.

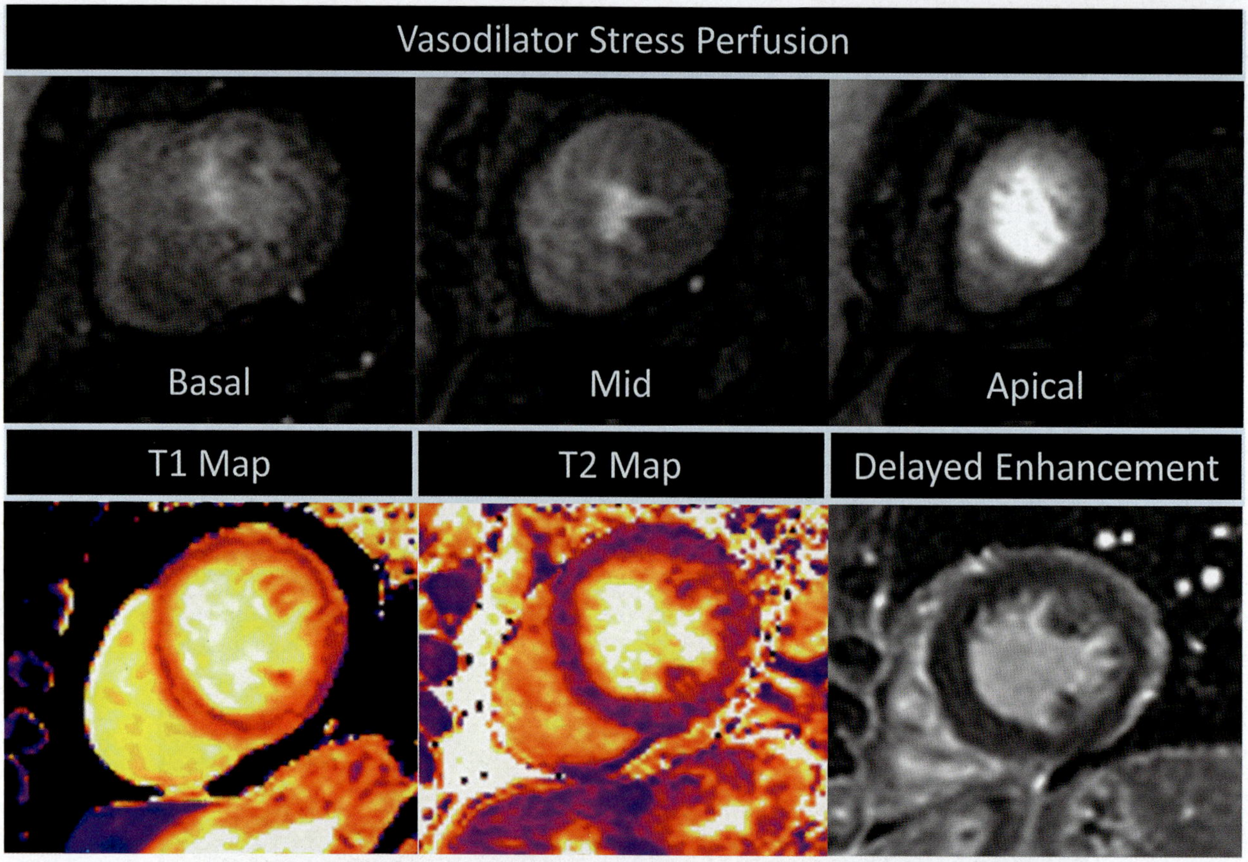

FIGURE 31.4 Example of acute chest pain presentation mimicking ST-elevation myocardial infarction during fluoropyrimidine therapy. A 60-year-old female with stage III adenocarcinoma of the colon developed sudden onset chest pain during her first infusion of folinic acid, fluorouracil, and oxaliplatin. She was referred to the emergency department with ST-segment elevation on electrocardiogram and elevated troponin levels. She underwent emergent coronary angiography showing no significant focal stenosis. She was referred for vasodilator stress cardiovascular magnetic resonance to evaluate for ischemic versus nonischemic injury pattern and help exclude flow-limiting lesions in the macrovascular or microvascular coronary arterial system. First-pass perfusion images during vasodilator (adenosine) stress (*top row*) demonstrated no perfusion defects. Tissue characterization with parametric mapping and late gadolinium-enhanced images (*bottom row*) showed no residual myocardial injury. The patient was thus restarted on fluorouracil as bolus dosing instead of infusions along with antispastic (diltiazem and nitroglycerin) pretreatment, with no further cardiovascular events on therapy.

However, some cancer treatments (e.g., anthracyclines) may promote a more diffuse myocardial injury, provoking fibroblast differentiation into myofibroblasts and secretion of collagen, resulting in a widespread LV myocardial interstitial fibrosis.[8] Due to the uniform distribution throughout the LV myocardium, this interstitial pattern of fibrosis does not produce the focal increases in signal intensity that are observed with late gadolinium-enhanced imaging methods. To this end, parametric mapping techniques can be a useful aid to identifying abnormal myocardial tissue characteristics in this population.

LV myocardial interstitial fibrosis raises CMR-based LV myocardial measures of T1 relaxation and extracellular volume fraction (ECVF).[9] For example, in survivors of pediatric malignancies with a preserved LVEF by TTE, elevations of LV myocardial ECVF have been correlated with exposure to anthracyclines, higher cumulative doses of anthracyclines, and reduced exercise capacity.[10] An example of suspected chronic elevation of ECVF in a patient with anthracycline exposure and LV systolic dysfunction is shown in Fig. 31.6.

Infiltrative Disorders

Infiltrative cardiomyopathies are discussed in depth separately (Chapter 28), but two such disorders are of particular relevance to the cardio-oncology population. One is cardiac amyloidosis, specifically light chain amyloidosis in the setting of multiple myeloma. In these cases, extracellular deposits of monoclonal immunoglobulin light chains produced in bone marrow plasma cell dyscrasias accumulate to cause myocardial wall thickening and functional compromise. In conjunction with other diagnostic modalities (e.g., cardiac scintigraphy, laboratory assessment of monoclonal gammopathy), expert consensus pathways highlight the potential for CMR to provide detailed tissue analysis in cases of suspected cardiac amyloidosis.[11] Cardiac amyloidosis has been associated with a constellation of abnormal findings on CMR including elevated LV myocardial ECVF, abnormal gadolinium contrast kinetics (manifested on postcontrast inversion time scout sequences displaying an abnormal nulling sequence, where the myocardium reaches the null point prior to the blood pool), atrial enlargement/stasis, pericardial effusion, and a diffuse pattern of late gadolinium enhancement with a subendocardial distribution. An example of light chain cardiac amyloidosis is shown in Fig. 31.7. In addition to diagnosing cases of suspected cardiac amyloidosis, CMR is well positioned to (1) evaluate for alternative thick heart cardiomyopathies that might mimic amyloidosis (e.g., hypertrophic cardiomyopathy,

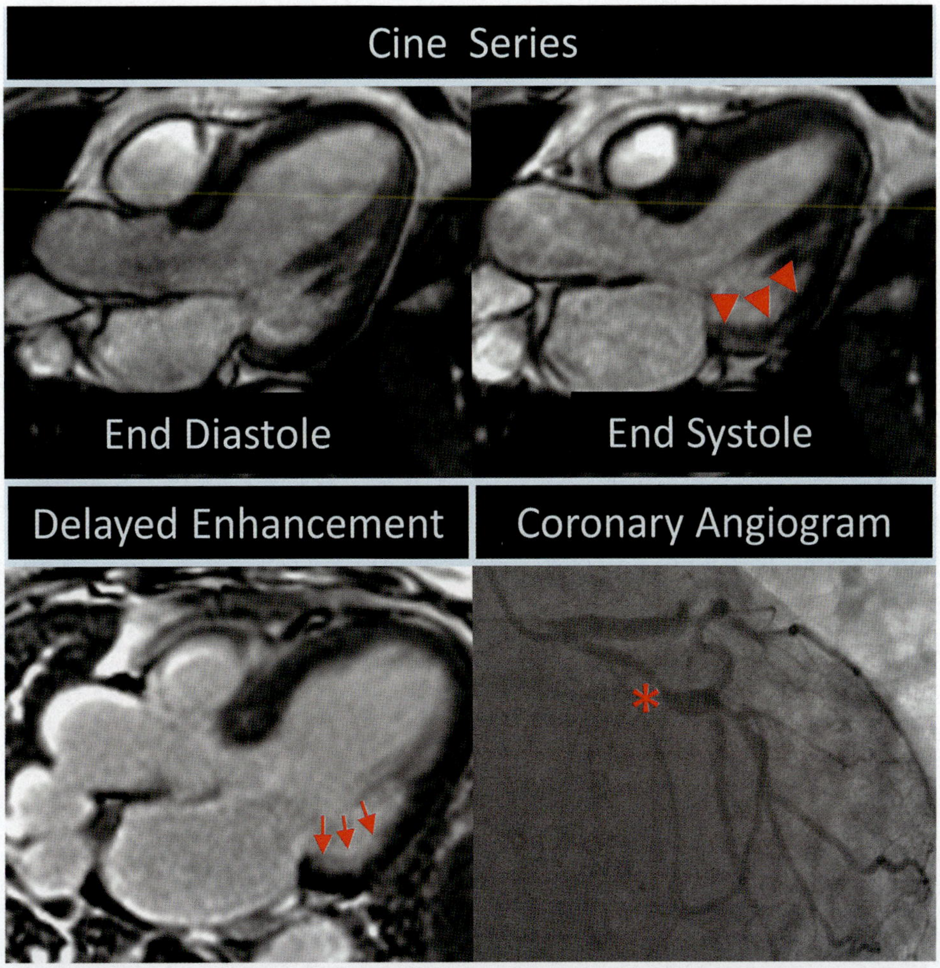

FIG. 31.5 Example of acute coronary syndrome experienced during immune checkpoint inhibitor therapy. A 71-year-old female with metastatic xanthogranuloma disseminatum presented after two cycles of the immune checkpoint inhibitor pembrolizumab with headache, photophobia, chest pain, and elevated troponin I levels. Initial differential diagnosis included acute coronary syndrome, myocarditis, and stress cardiomyopathy. The patient was referred for cardiovascular magnetic resonance, where cine sequences (*top row*) demonstrated new regional hypokinesis along the basal inferolateral wall (*arrowheads*). Late gadolinium-enhanced imaging (*bottom left*) demonstrated focal enhancement in the corresponding territory (*arrows*), with a subendocardial distribution suggestive of ischemic etiology. Subsequent coronary angiography (*bottom right*) demonstrated a midvessel 80% stenosis of the left circumflex artery (*asterisk*). (Case vignette and angiogram images reproduced from Menachery SM et al. CJC Open 2022;5:170–172. Open access publication which permits reproducing as long as work is properly cited. Does not require permission from the publisher.)

Fabry disease, hypertensive heart disease) and (2) evaluate complications of cardiac amyloidosis such as intracardiac thrombus.

Secondly, iron overload cardiomyopathy may also be a concern in patients who have forms of anemia requiring repeated transfusions (e.g., aplastic anemia, myelodysplasia) or conditions affecting iron absorption (e.g., hemochromatosis, which can overlap with the oncology field if patients develop hepatocellular carcinoma). Contrary to amyloidosis, ventricular wall thickness is not necessarily increased in early iron overload cardiomyopathy. There is typically early preservation of LVEF due to epicardial distribution of iron deposits, with late findings of a dilated or restrictive cardiomyopathy phenotype. In suspected cases, CMR is the only noninvasive diagnostic tool to quantify iron deposition through the use of T2* relaxation imaging sequences on 1.5 T imaging systems (T2* values < 20 ms indicating iron overload cardiomyopathy, <10 ms indicating severe overload). In addition to helping determine thresholds for chelation therapy, serial myocardial T2* imaging can assist with monitoring response to iron removal strategies.[12]

Myocellular Dysfunction

Direct myocellular injury is a potential complication of cancer treatment, with perhaps the best-known example of this being anthracycline-induced cardiomyocyte injury. A number of pathways likely contribute to this damage including oxidative stress, damage to deoxyribonucleic acid, and cardiomyocyte apoptosis, among others. Such changes may be uniquely reflected in CMR-derived tissue characterizations (e.g., elevated native T1 and T2 values representing acute myocardial inflammation and edema) even before the deterioration of LV function or onset of clinical symptoms.[9]

Patients receiving cancer therapies often become immunocompromised, increasing risk for infections with particular vulnerability during periods of neutropenia. Indeed, about half of patients who experience neutropenic fever develop sepsis—a condition that is itself known to promote septic cardiomyopathy through a variety of proposed mechanisms including high levels of circulating proinflammatory cytokines, nitric oxide handling, mitochondrial dysfunction, coronary microcirculatory hypoperfusion, and endothelial dysfunction resulting in depressed myocardial function. There are limited publications of CMR

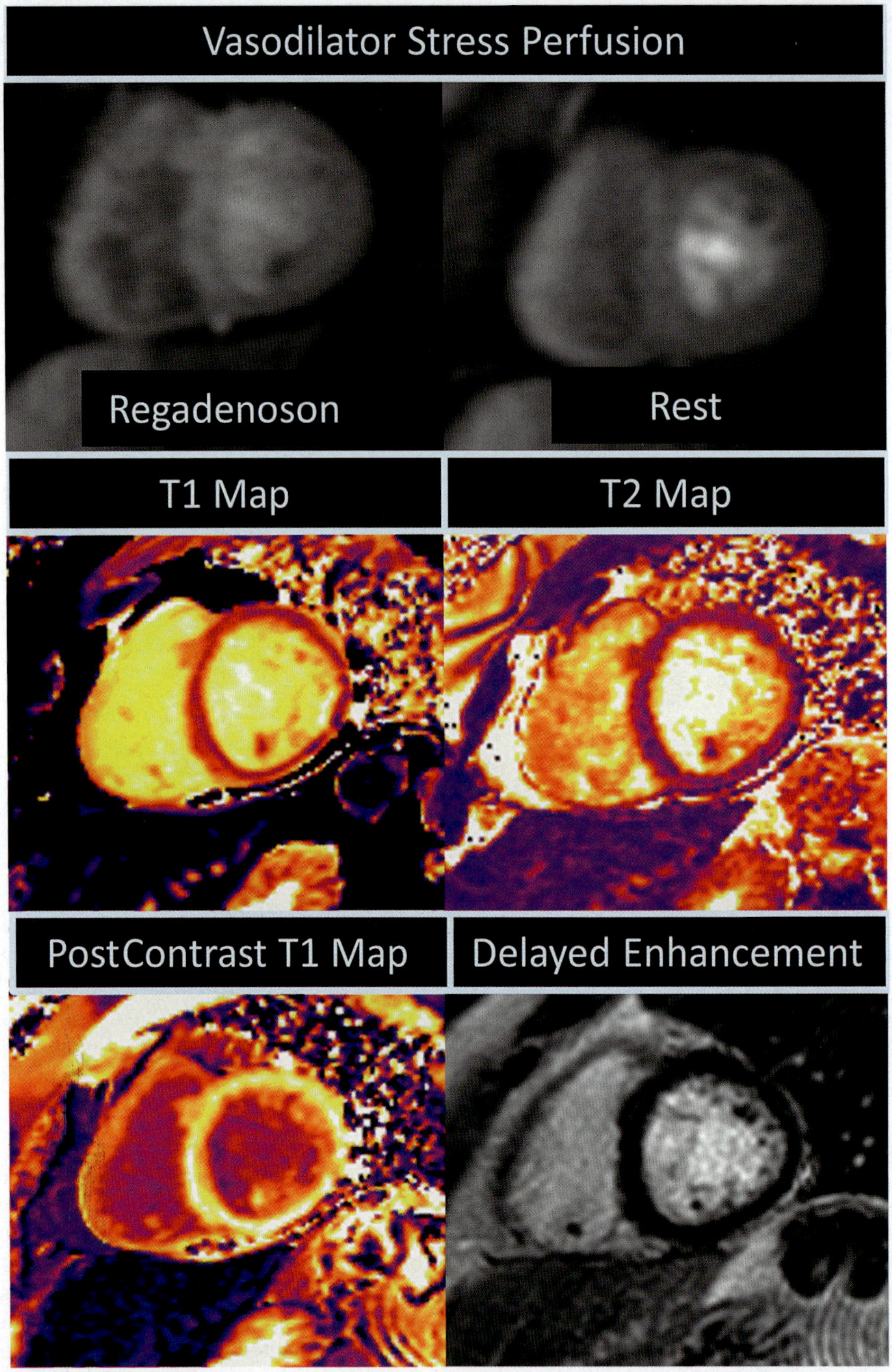

FIG. 31.6 Example of chronic systolic dysfunction after anthracycline exposure. A 31-year old-female with a history of myelodysplastic syndrome was the recipient of multiple lines of chemotherapy including the anthracycline daunorubicin and total body irradiation for allogeneic stem cell transplant. Echocardiography revealed mildly reduced left ventricular systolic function. The patient was referred for vasodilator stress cardiovascular magnetic resonance (CMR), where first-pass perfusion imaging (*top row*) demonstrated no reversible perfusion defects, precontrast parametric mapping (*middle row*) displayed upper normal myocardial T1 values and normal T2 values, and postcontrast imaging (*bottom row*) included late gadolinium enhancement showing no signs of focal scar with postcontrast T1 mapping (in conjunction with precontrast T1 maps and recent hematocrit) suggestive of increased extracellular volume fraction of 31%–34%. While there are no pathognomonic features for anthracycline toxicity without the aid of myocardial biopsy, the lack of other etiologies discovered on CMR along with strong clinical suspicion allowed for this presumptive diagnosis.

evaluations during septic cardiomyopathy, particularly those associated with cancer treatment. However, existing reports describe elevated native T2 values in those with reduced LVEF suggestive of myocardial edema, as well as a subset of individuals with wall motion patterns suggestive of stress cardiomyopathy (classic takotsubo variant).[13]

Similar to septic cardiomyopathy, patients with cancer or those receiving cancer-related therapy are at risk for stress cardiomyopathy. While this condition remains poorly understood, in general cohorts the described baseline risk factors include female sex, comorbid psychiatric conditions (including anxiety or depression), pulmonary

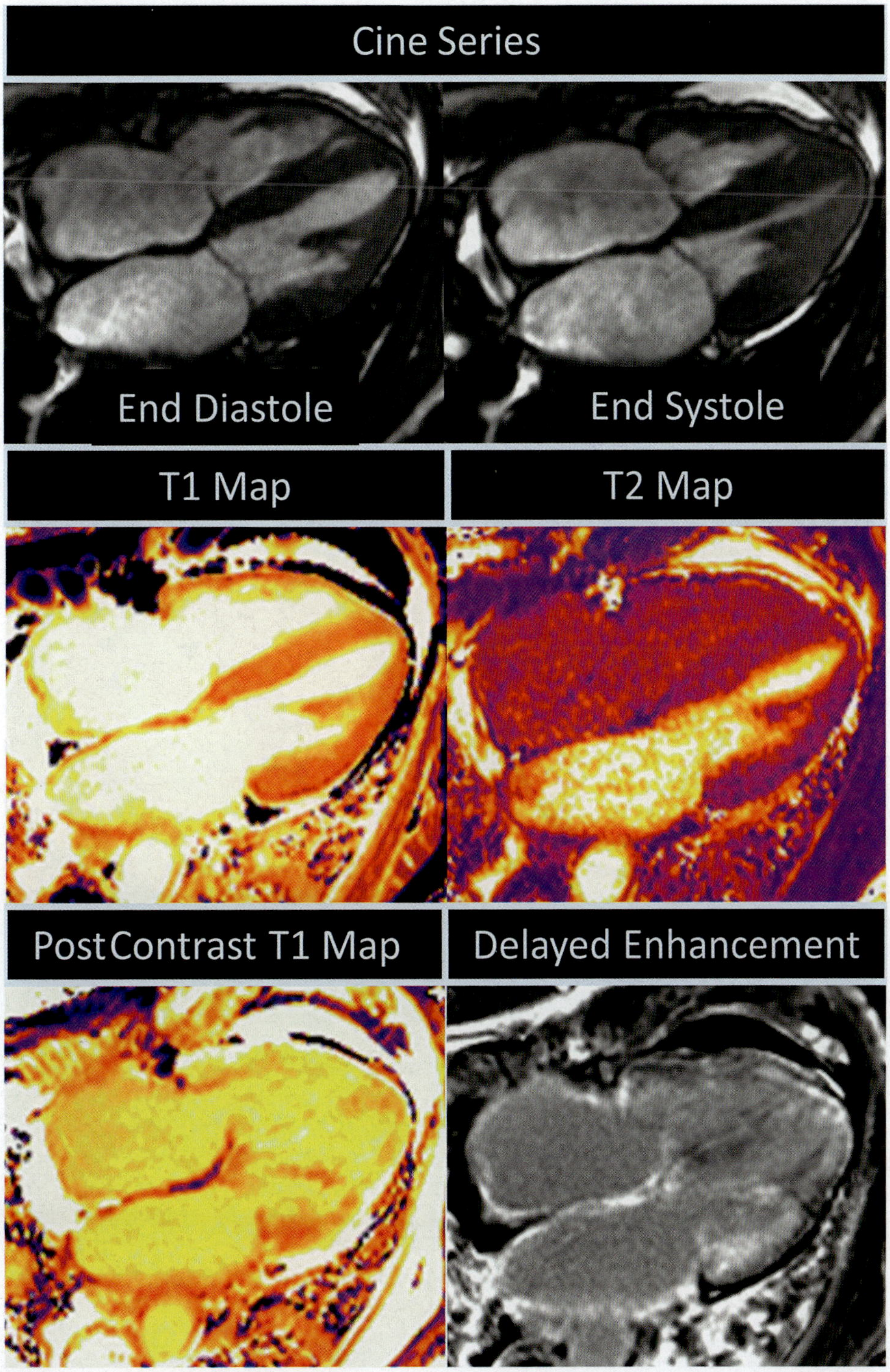

FIG. 31.7 **Example of light chain cardiac amyloidosis.** A 64-year-old female with a history of IgA lambda multiple myeloma that was diagnosed after surgical intervention of recurrent pleural effusion. She was referred for cardiovascular magnetic resonance to screen for cardiac amyloidosis. Cine images (*top row*) displayed several features concerning for cardiac involvement: thickened left ventricular (LV) walls to 1.5 cm, reduced LV end diastolic volume with mildly reduced ejection fraction (including relative apical preservation of contraction), atrial stasis, and pericardial effusion. Parametric mapping (*middle row*) demonstrated markedly elevated native T1 values (1400–1450 msec on a 3 T system, local normal ranges 1086–1292 msec) and normal T2 values. Postcontrast images revealed abnormal gadolinium kinetics (myocardium reached the null point before the blood pool on inversion recovery scout sequences) with widespread subendocardial late gadolinium enhancement (*bottom left*) and postcontrast T1 values that allowed for extracellular volume calculation—found to be markedly elevated in the range of 51%–57%.

disease, diabetes mellitus, and substance abuse disorders.[14] If coupled with a significant emotional or physical stressor, a series of proposed pathways can contribute to an abrupt and dramatic but temporary decline in LV systolic function that may closely mimic acute myocardial infarction on clinical and electrocardiographic assessment. Emotional stress and anxiety are common reactions to cancer diagnosis and treatment, and further physiologic burden from cancer therapies or associated complications may serve as acute triggers for stress cardiomyopathy events. Indeed, patients with a diagnosis of malignancy appear to have disproportionately high representation

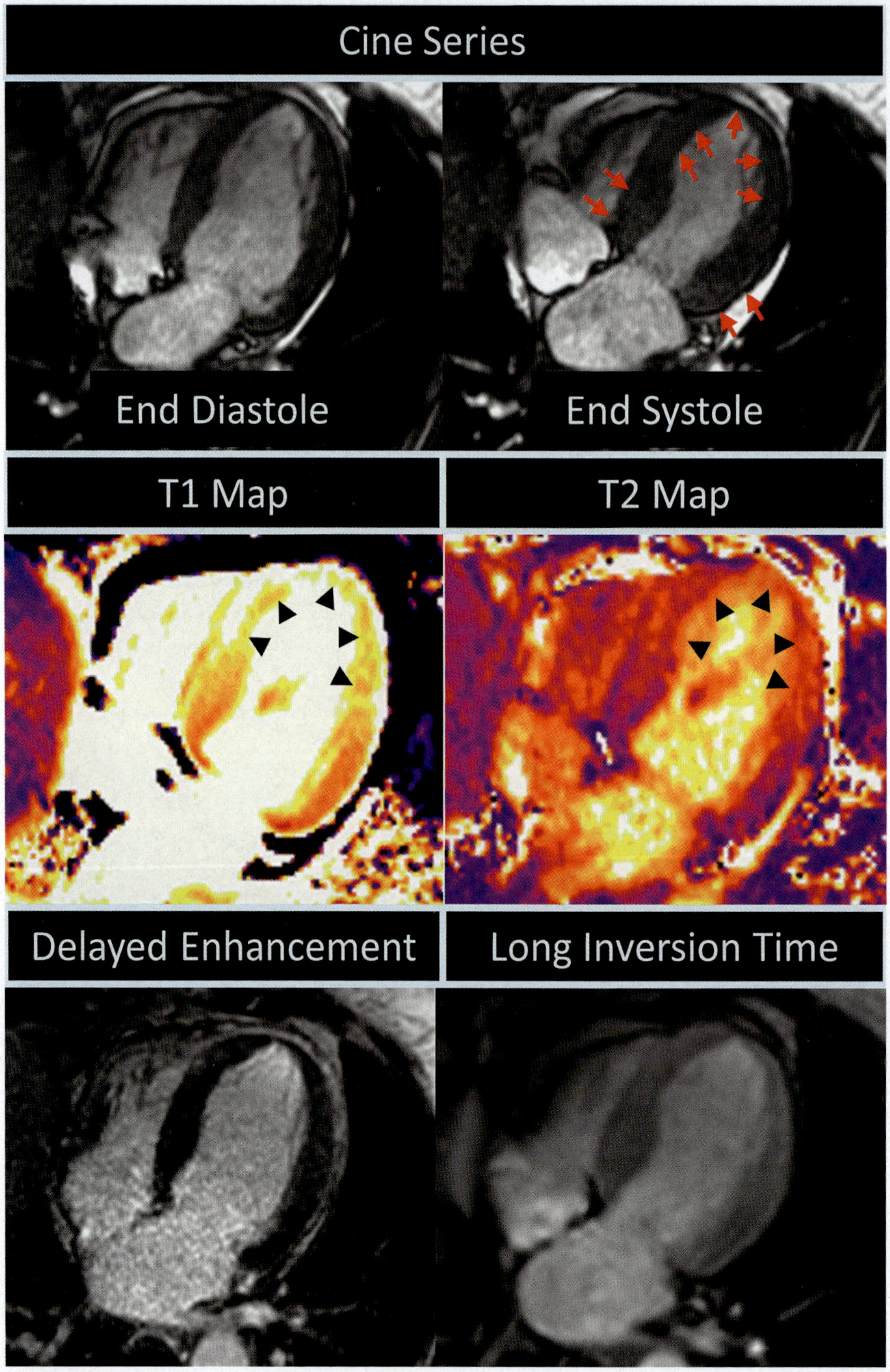

FIG. 31.8 Example of stress cardiomyopathy. A 55-year-old female with a history of extrahepatic cholangiocarcinoma status post Whipple surgery who declined adjuvant therapy due to recurrent nausea and vomiting. During an episode of vomiting she experienced sudden chest discomfort, associated with elevated troponin levels on presentation to the emergency department. Coronary angiogram was without obstructive findings, so she was referred for cardiovascular magnetic resonance. Cine sequences (*top row*) demonstrated basal hyperdynamic function with apical ballooning (wall motion indicated by *arrows*). Parametric mapping (*middle row*) demonstrated markedly elevated native T1 and T2 values in the affected territories (*arrowheads*). Postcontrast imaging (*bottom row*) was without late gadolinium enhancement or apical thrombus. Medical therapy was initiated for her systolic dysfunction, which normalized over the next several months.

in published cohorts of stress cardiomyopathy.[15] In this regard, CMR may be helpful in establishing the diagnosis in cases of abrupt LV systolic dysfunction. Cine sequences can reveal a classic "apical ballooning" appearance of takotsubo cardiomyopathy (the predominant phenotype) or one of the alternatively described wall motion patterns.[14] Parametric mapping tends to display elevations in native T1 and T2 values in the affected territories, with a lack of focal late gadolinium enhancement. Further, CMR has a high sensitivity for detecting complications of stress cardiomyopathy such as intracardiac thrombus, LV outflow tract obstruction, or structural complications including ventricular septal or free wall rupture. An example of stress cardiomyopathy is shown in Fig. 31.8.

A similar clinical entity is myocarditis, an inflammatory disorder affecting cardiomyocytes that typically manifests as chest pain, exhibits elevated cardiac biomarker levels, and is sometimes associated with compromised cardiac function, heart failure, arrhythmias, and even death. Triggers include infection and autoimmune conditions, the latter of particular importance in cardio-oncology with the introduction and increasingly expanded use of immune checkpoint inhibitors. While rare, myocarditis associated with immune checkpoint inhibitors is associated with high mortality. CMR has a well-established role in the diagnosis and prognosis of myocarditis from a general perspective, in which a combination of T2-based abnormalities (by T2 mapping or T2-weighted images) and T1-based abnormalities (by T1 mapping, late gadolinium enhancement, or extracellular volume fraction) is necessary to diagnose myocardial inflammation. However, it is important to note that in the case of immune checkpoint inhibitor–associated myocarditis, late gadolinium-enhanced and T2-weighted imaging may lack abnormalities if performed early (within 4 days) within the myoinflammatory course.[16] An example of immune checkpoint inhibitor–associated myocarditis is shown in Fig. 31.9.

A relatively unique mechanism of myocellular dysfunction may arise from treatment with trastuzumab, which targets human epidermal growth factor receptor 2 (HER2), which is overexpressed in approximately one in four breast cancers. It is thought that an off-target effect of HER2 blockade may involve modulation of cell survival pathways in cardiomyocytes, with increased risk of myocardial depression in those simultaneously receiving anthracyclines. However, LV dysfunction associated with HER2 inhibitors may not always involve cellular destruction and appears at least partially reversible upon interruption of therapy. Thus, early identification of this complication may be of paramount importance to allow for introduction of cardiac-supportive medications (e.g., beta blockers, angiotensin-converting enzyme inhibitors), and possible withdrawal of therapy in severe cases. To this end, CMR may be particularly helpful, especially in cases with challenging acoustic windows that limit the sensitivity of echocardiology to detect subtle changes in function. An example of HER2 antagonism–related cardiomyopathy is shown in Fig. 31.10.

Increased Afterload

Classes of anticancer treatments that have been implicated in direct vascular damage include anthracyclines, alkylating agents, tyrosine kinase inhibitors, and vascular endothelial growth factor inhibitors. Among other effects, such damage may increase aortic stiffness, thereby blunting LV systolic unloading and contributing to a reduction in LVEF by increasing LV end systolic volume.[17] Cine and phase-contrast CMR of the aorta may be helpful in examining this effect through measurement of aortic distensibility and pulse-wave velocity. Patients who receive cancer therapies that increase aortic stiffness can develop blunted aortic distensibility (represented by a decreased difference between maximum and minimum aortic cross-sectional luminal areas on cine imaging), leading to a more rapid transit time of blood flow through the aorta, which can be captured in a single axial plane using phase-contrast techniques.[17]

Left Ventricular Myocardial Volume and Mass

In addition to being the gold standard of chamber size measurements, CMR offers precise and reproducible assessments of LV myocardial mass. Loss of muscle mass, with or without replacement fibrosis, has been proposed as a mechanism by which some patients may experience decline in cardiac function following cancer therapy. Indeed, anthracycline exposure has been shown to be associated with about a 5% decline in LV mass as assessed by serial CMR, and is independently associated with increased heart failure symptoms (Fig. 31.11).[18] A cross-sectional analysis of patients who survived pediatric malignancies treated with anthracyclines similarly demonstrated low LV myocardial mass. Coined the "Grinch syndrome," this phenomenon has been associated with reductions in exercise capacity on cardiopulmonary exercise testing and hemodynamic measures consistent with restrictive cardiomyopathy.[19] How frequently this form of myocardial wasting is encountered and which therapeutic strategies may prevent its occurrence are important areas for future CMR investigation.

Cardiac Masses

The use of CMR in cardiac masses is described in depth elsewhere (Chapters 34, 35). In general, primary cardiac tumors are infrequent, particularly when compared to cardiac metastases, which are thought to be 20–40 times more common. It has been estimated that up to 12% of patients with malignancy have metastatic lesions to the cardiac/pericardial structures, most of which are clinically silent and only discovered on autopsy. The highest-risk malignancies for cardiac metastasis include melanomas, breast cancer, lung cancer, and esophageal cancer.[20] Additionally, hypercoagulability with malignancy (particularly upper gastrointestinal and hematological malignancies) may promote formation of intracardiac thrombus in patients with other predisposing conditions such as indwelling central venous catheter, atrial fibrillation, or left ventricular dysfunction. To that end, in patients with suspected cardiac tumors, CMR has shown a high level of diagnostic accuracy to distinguish among pseudomasses, thrombi, benign tumors, and malignant tumors, as well as to offer prognostic information.[21] A case example is shown in Fig. 31.12. Image sequences used to identify the etiology of abnormal LV myocardial masses include LV myocardial cine, perfusion, late enhancement, and mapping methods (before and after the administration of gadolinium contrast).

Valvular Disease

In addition to comorbid valvular disease unrelated to cancer diagnosis or treatment, patients who receive thoracic radiation are at elevated risk of valvular heart disease. While TTE is often the first-line modality for assessment

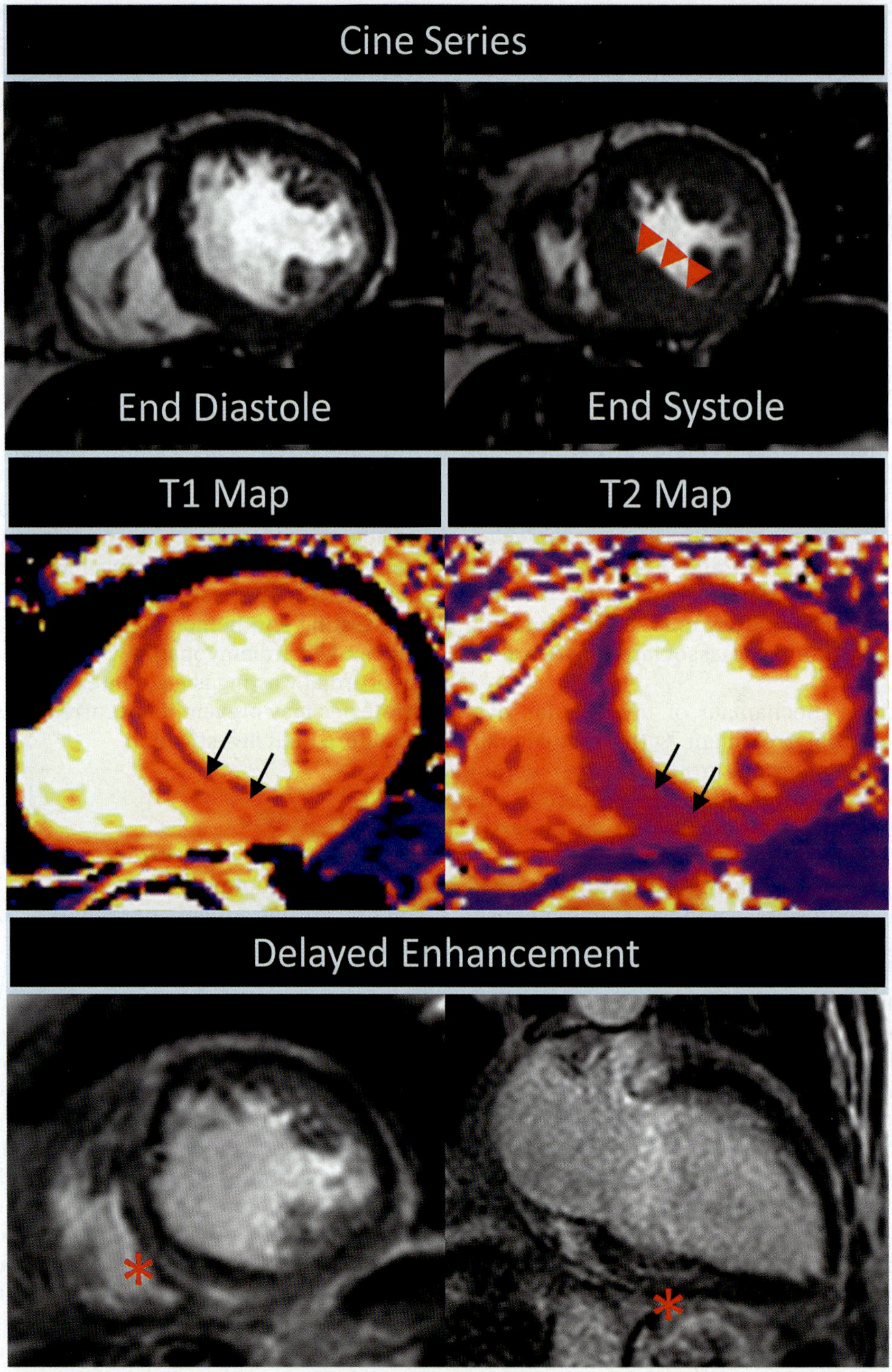

FIG. 31.9 Example of immune checkpoint inhibitor-associated myocarditis. A 71-year-old female with heart failure with recovered ejection fraction, metastatic renal cell carcinoma and end-stage renal disease presented after receiving her third infusion of two immune checkpoint inhibitors (ipilimumab and nivolumab) with symptomatic monomorphic ventricular tachycardia requiring cardioversion. Initial echocardiogram suggested left ventricular hypertrophy with inferior hypokinesis. Cardiovascular magnetic resonance was utilized to assess for potential etiologies of arrhythmia, with a differential including ischemic injury, hypertrophic cardiomyopathy, and myocarditis. Cine sequences (*top rows*) demonstrated focally thickened inferior/inferoseptal walls most evident during systole (*arrowheads*). Parametric mapping (*middle row*) displayed elevations in native T1 and T2 values in the corresponding regions (*arrows*), suggestive of active inflammation or edema. Late gadolinium-enhanced imaging (*bottom row*) demonstrated focal enhancement of the septum and inferior wall (*asterisk*), in a midmyocardial distribution. These findings were not consistent with hypertrophic or ischemic injury, and a diagnosis of immune checkpoint inhibitor-related myocarditis was made.

of known or suspected valvular heart disease, guidelines recommend consideration of alternative modalities such as CMR when further diagnostic testing is needed, including if there are discrepancies between clinical presentation and echocardiographic assessment of valvular function.[22]

While interrogation of valvular function is discussed extensively elsewhere, standard CMR sequences include cinematic assessment of valve morphology and function coupled with phase-contrast imaging to quantify stenotic pressure gradients or regurgitant flow.

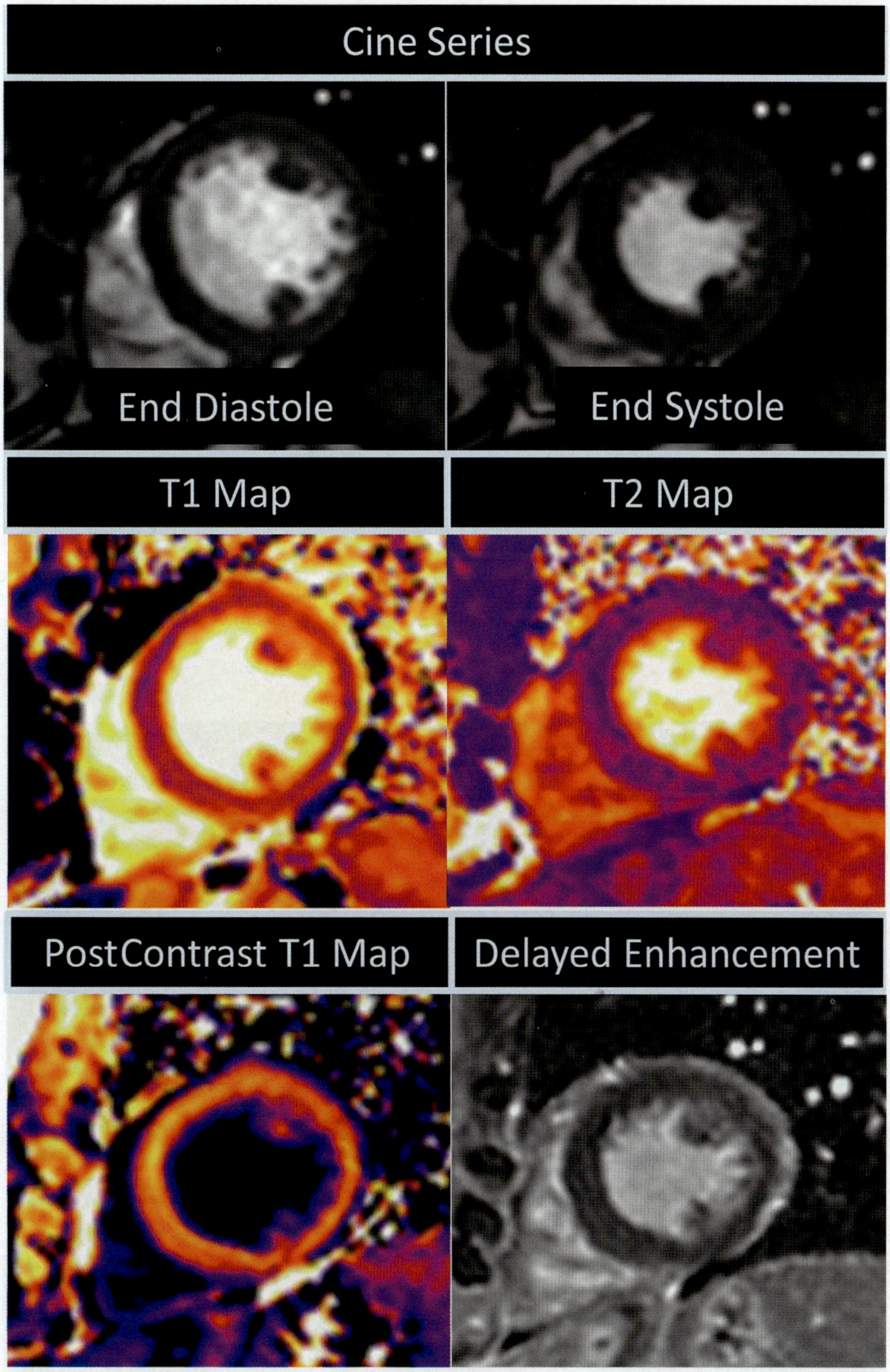

FIG. 31.10 Example of decline in left ventricular systolic function during HER2-targeted therapy. A 58-year-old female with a prior diagnosis of non-Hodgkin lymphoma treated with cyclophosphamide, doxorubicin, vincristine, and mantle radiation, as well as a family history of premature cardiovascular disease, presented after new diagnosis of breast cancer for which she was undergoing treatment with trastuzumab and paclitaxel. Routine echocardiogram demonstrated an acute decline in left ventricular ejection fraction (LVEF) from 56% to 20% over a 4-month span. Differential diagnosis included ischemic disease (e.g., from radiation-induced accelerated atherosclerosis), diffuse interstitial fibrosis from prior anthracycline exposure, stress cardiomyopathy, and HER2 antagonism–related cardiomyopathy. She was referred for cardiovascular magnetic resonance to help distinguish among these potential etiologies. Cine images (now after introduction of guideline-directed medical therapy for systolic dysfunction) demonstrated mildly reduced LVEF of 43% (*top row*). Parametric mapping revealed normal native T1 and T2 values (*middle row*), with postcontrast T1 maps incorporated for extracellular volume calculation, which was also normal. Late gadolinium-enhanced imaging was without localized enhancement, arguing against focal injury. Thus, after exclusion of several of the potential etiologies, the patient was diagnosed with HER2 antagonism related cardiomyopathy; after withdrawal of trastuzumab she experienced normalization of left ventricular systolic function.

Right Ventricular Dysfunction

In patients receiving cancer treatment who undergo serial imaging surveillance with transthoracic echocardiography, assessment of the right ventricle can be challenging due to its position immediately behind the sternum and unique geometry. In this regard, CMR can provide superior volumetric and functional assessment of the right ventricle despite its thin walls limiting options for tissue

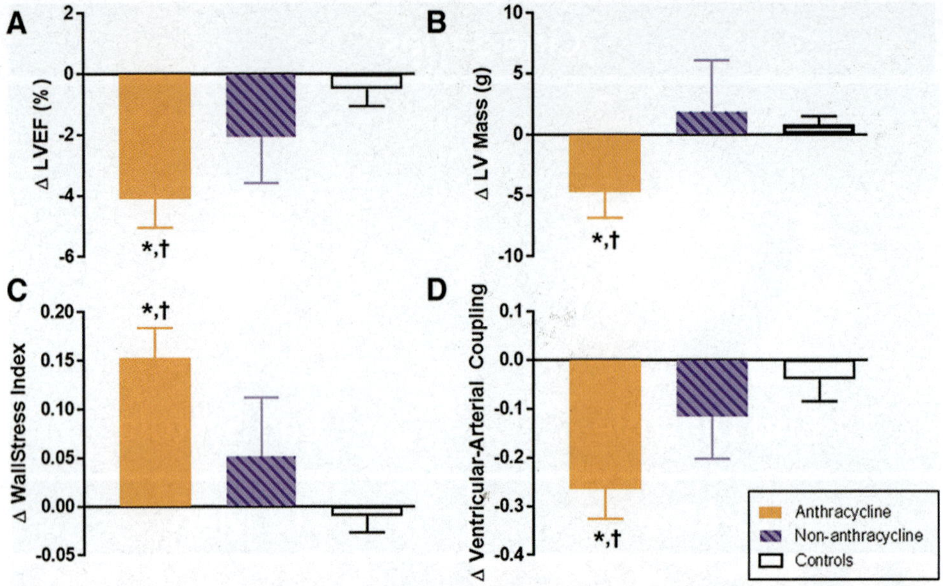

FIG. 31.11 Changes in left ventricular (*LV*) function, mass, and arterial interactions following anthracycline exposure. Patients treated with anthracyclines have been shown to have multiple adverse cardiovascular changes including more pronounced decreases in LV ejection fraction (*LVEF,* panel A), reductions in LV mass (panel B), increased wall stress indices (panel C), and worsened measures of ventricular-arterial coupling (panel D) compared to patients who received nonanthracycline treatment regimens. (Reproduced image from Jordan JH, Castellino SM, Meléndez GC et al. Left ventricular mass change after anthracycline chemotherapy. *Circ Heart Fail*. 2018;11(7):e004560. doi:10.1161/CIRCHEARTFAILURE.117.004560 Fig. 1.)

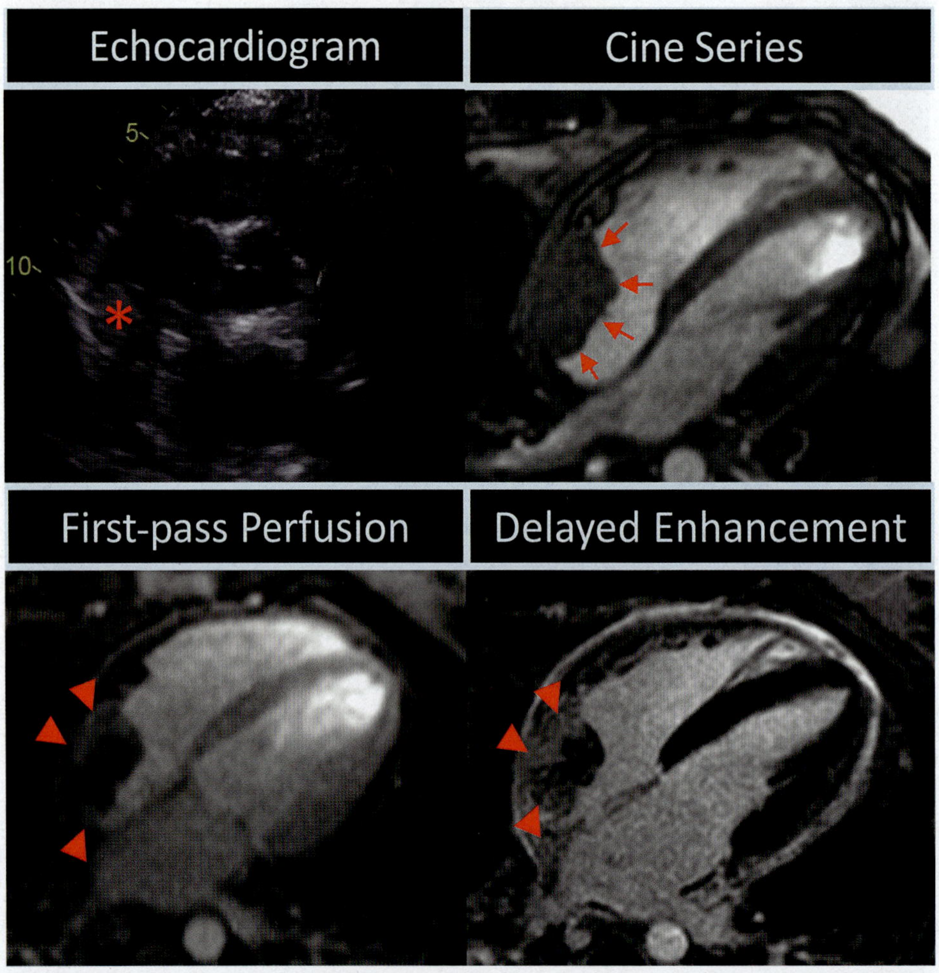

FIG. 31.12 Example of a cardiac mass. A 37-year-old female underwent biopsy for a thoracic spinal lesion, with pathology findings of angiosarcoma of unknown primary source. Transthoracic echocardiography (*top left*) suggested an echogenic structure within the right atrium (*asterisk*); the differential diagnosis included primary malignant tumor versus thrombus. She was referred for cardiovascular magnetic resonance, where cine sequences (*top right*) redemonstrated the right atrial mass (*arrows*), as well as multiple pericardial lesions. First-pass perfusion imaging (*bottom left*) demonstrated heterogeneous peripheral uptake of contrast involving the atrial and pericardial masses (*arrowheads*), with a similar pattern of increased signal intensity on delayed-enhancement imaging (*bottom right*, *arrowheads*). The patient was ultimately diagnosed with right atrial angiosarcoma, thought to be the primary source of her metastatic disease.

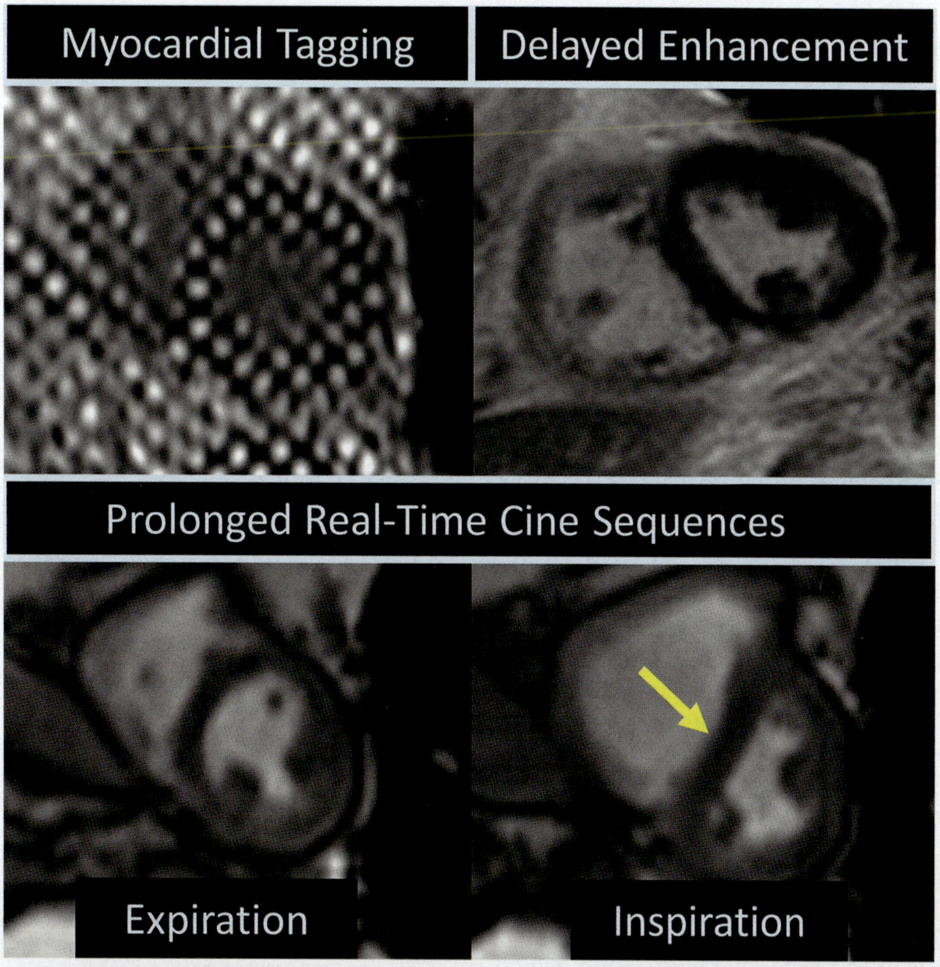

FIG. 31.13 Example of constrictive pericarditis. A 79-year-old male with non-small cell lung carcinoma was treated with carboplatin, paclitaxel, and radiation therapy. Soon after his last treatment cycle he developed exertional dyspnea and was referred for cardiovascular magnetic resonance for evaluation. Cine sequences including those performed with myocardial tagging (*top left*) revealed pericardial thickening with reduced mobility between the visceral and parietal pericardial layers. Postcontrast delayed imaging did not display pericardial enhancement (*top right*). Prolonged real-time cine sequences were performed in the short-axis view while the patient was given instructions to exhale and then deeply inhale (*bottom row*), revealing interventricular septal inversion upon inspiration (*arrow*) suggestive of interventricular dependence of filling (constrictive physiology).

characterization. While there is limited data of the effects of cancer treatment on right ventricular size or function, published reports describe high rates of right ventricular dysfunction in patients who survived pediatric cancers treated with anthracyclines,[23] as well as a temporary increase in right ventricular volumes and decrease in systolic function with trastuzumab therapy even in the absence of overt cardiomyopathy.[24]

Pericardial Disease

Pericardial assessment with CMR is described in depth in another chapter (Chapter 36). In patients who have cancer with metastatic potential, careful inspection of the pericardium with dark-blood structural and cinematic functional imaging is of particular importance to exclude tumor invasion or metastatic involvement. Additionally, patients who have received external beam radiation can be at risk for pericardial inflammation, elevating their risk for chronic pericardial fibrosis.

If either complication occurs, it is important to assess for (1) pericardial thickness, (2) whether there is free movement or adhesions between the visceral and parietal layers (myocardial tagging techniques may assist with this), (3) the presence or absence of a pericardial effusion, (4) pericardial enhancement (if present, it tends to represent an acutely inflamed phase that may be more responsive to antiinflammatory therapy), and (5) the presence or absence of constrictive physiology reflected by ventricular dependence of filling (free breathing real-time cinematic sequences are acquired on deep inspiration, causing abnormal inversion of the interventricular septum toward the LV). An example of constrictive pericarditis is shown in Fig. 31.13.

APPROACHES TO PATIENTS RECEIVING CANCER TREATMENT

Cardiac magnetic resonance imaging can provide highly reproducible anatomic and functional measurements, tissue characterization, and noninvasive assessments of coronary perfusion. Additionally, CMR is the gold standard for assessment of the right ventricle and does not require ionizing radiation. Given these attributes, CMR can provide essential information at every stage of cancer survivorship, from pretreatment through treatment and into long-term survivorship.

Pretreatment

Cardiovascular disease and cancer share risk factors such as tobacco use, increasing age, dietary factors, and physical inactivity. Given the mutual nature of these risk factors, an individual who has been diagnosed with cancer may also be at risk for cardiovascular disease. Conversely, individuals with chronic heart disease are at an increased risk for developing cancer and certain hematologic/oncologic conditions can directly increase the risk for heart disease. As a result, cardiac risk stratification and medical optimization are often an essential step prior to cancer therapy.

Cardiovascular assessment with a recognized risk stratification method is advocated for prior to the initiation of cancer therapy.[25] Individuals with elevated risk may require further cardiovascular assessment with dedicated cardiac imaging. Additionally, cardiac testing is often utilized during bone marrow transplant evaluation, as low LVEF is considered a major risk factor for cardiac toxicity post allogeneic stem cell transplantation. Individuals planning to receive specific cancer therapies, such as HER2 antagonist therapy, may also require serial monitoring of cardiac function.

In these settings, CMR offers a highly reproducible quantitative assessment of cardiac health. Stress CMR can be utilized as a noninvasive method of screening for significant coronary disease, while simultaneously providing an assessment of anatomy and valvular function, which are not readily available with nuclear-based imaging techniques, as well as tissue characterization, which is not available with nuclear or echocardiography-based imaging. Guidelines from the Society for Cardiovascular Magnetic Resonance highlight imaging sequences and reporting strategies to optimize assessment in patients with cancer or suspected cancer treatment–related dysfunction, and are summarized in Table 31.1.

TABLE 31.1 Imaging and reporting recommendations for cancer-related cardiomyopathies.

Imaging Recommendations

- Left ventricular structure and function
- Advanced tissue characterization—optional, although frequently used
- Optional—vasodilator stress-rest perfusion or high-dose dobutamine functional imaging to determine the presence of inducible ischemia
- Late gadolinium enhancement

Reporting recommendations

- Anatomical/structural (all recommended)
  - Left ventricular volumes and mass
    - Left ventricular end diastolic volume, indexed end systolic volume
    - Left ventricular end systolic volume, indexed end diastolic volume
    - Left ventricular mass, indexed mass
  - Wall thickness (preserved, thin-walled, or increased)
  - Right ventricular volumes
    - Right ventricular end diastolic volume, indexed end diastolic volume
    - Right ventricular end systolic volume, indexed end diastolic volume
  - Atrial size
    - Left atrial diameter on 3-chamber view of the left ventricle
    - Left atrial volume
- Functional (recommended)
  - Left ventricular ejection fraction
  - Right ventricular ejection fraction
  - Regional wall motion abnormalities
  - Vasodilator stress perfusion (optional)
  - Pericardial disease (if present)
- Tissue characterization
  - Regional myocardial abnormality by late gadolinium enhancement (presence, extent, location, regional distribution pattern [recommended])
  - Advanced tissue characterization indexes
    - Native T1 for assessed myocardial segments (optional)
    - Location and magnitude of elevation in T1 (recommended)
    - T2 for assessed myocardial segments in patients with troponin rise (optional)
    - Location and magnitude or regional T2 increase in patients with troponin rise (recommended)
    - Extracellular volume in assessed myocardial segments (optional)
    - Global extracellular volume (optional if performed)
    - Location and magnitude (%) of extracellular volume elevation (recommended if performed)
- Other
  - Valvular stenosis (qualitative presence of stenosis, severity of stenosis, mean and peak transvalvular gradients)
  - Mitral regurgitation (central or eccentric, mechanism of regurgitation, quantification of regurgitant volume and fraction)
  - Myocardial masses
    - Cardiac or paracardiac tumor
    - Intraventricular thrombus
    - Size, mobility, location
    - Perfusion (qualitative appearance and heterogeneity of perfusion in 2 orthogonal planes)

Adapted from Kramer, C.M., Barkhausen, J., Bucciarelli-Ducci, C. et al. Standardized cardiovascular magnetic resonance imaging (CMR) protocols: 2020 update. *J Cardiovasc Magn Reson* 22, 17 (2020). https://doi.org/10.1186/s12968-020-00607-1 and Hundley, W.G., Bluemke, D.A., Bogaert, J. et al. Society for cardiovascular magnetic resonance (SCMR) guidelines for reporting cardiovascular magnetic resonance examinations. *J Cardiovasc Magn Reson* 24, 29 (2022). https://doi.org/10.1186/s12968-021-00827-z.

During Cancer Treatment

The goal of the cardio-oncologist is to promote cardiac health among cancer survivors while limiting interruptions in cancer therapy. Given the relative absence of pathognomonic indicators of cancer treatment–related cardiovascular toxicity, often the cardio-oncologist must utilize diagnostic imaging to determine the underlying etiology of cardiovascular disease. An example of a CMR protocol optimized toward this patient population is provided in Table 31.2, along with the illustrative case examples in prior sections that highlight the unique capabilities of CMR in diagnostic or treatment dilemmas. Potential cardiovascular complications of specific cancer therapies with the highest risk of cardiac toxicity are outlined in Table 31.3, with suggested CMR sequences to aid in the evaluation of these patients.

Long-Term Survivorship

An increased long-term risk for cardiovascular disease among individuals diagnosed with cancer has been established, regardless of age at time of cancer diagnosis. In fact, for many individuals, 10 years after cancer diagnosis, the risk of death from heart disease is higher than the risk of death from a primary cancer. While cardiac screening in long-term survivors is still an area of investigation, for survivors

TABLE 31.2 Example protocol for use in patients with cancer or cancer treatment–related cardiovascular dysfunction.

SEQUENCE	PURPOSE
Dark blood/bright blood axial images	Broad anatomical evaluation
Long-axis cines	Cardiac chamber structure and function, longitudinal strain measurement with feature tracking if desired
Short-axis cines (can be performed postcontrast to decrease scanning time if desired)	Volumetric assessment of ventricular volumes, mass, and function, radial or circumferential strain analysis with feature tracking if desired
Native T1 maps	Advanced tissue characterization for assessment of fibrosis, edema, and/or infiltrative disease
Native T2 maps	Advanced tissue characterization for assessment of myocardial edema
Phase-contrast studies (optional)	Assessment of valvular dysfunction (e.g., in patients who previously received thoracic radiation)
Contrast administration	
First-pass perfusion at rest	Assessment of cardiac mass, any resting myocardial perfusion defects
Vasodilator stress perfusion or dobutamine functional imaging (optional)	Assessment for the presence of flow-limiting large vessel epicardial coronary artery disease and/or microvascular dysfunction
Angiography or venography (optional)	Assessment of arterial or venous structures, e.g., if comorbid thoracic aortic aneurysm, atrial fibrillation, etc.
Postcontrast axial images with and without fat suppression	Additional anatomical evaluation, tissue characterization
Postcontrast inversion recovery sequences with long inversion time	Assessment for intracardiac thrombus
Late gadolinium enhancement images	Assessment for focal myocardial scar, pericardial inflammation
Prolonged real-time cinematic sequence with deep inspiration (optional)	Assessment for ventricular interdependence of filling in cases of pericardial disease with concerns for constrictive physiology
Postcontrast T1 maps (optional)	Calculation of extracellular volume fraction (requires recent hematocrit value, ideally within 48 hours)

Example of a standardized cardiovascular magnetic resonance scanning sequence protocol for patients with cancer or cancer treatment–related cardiac dysfunction. Sequences may be added or subtracted based on each patient's clinical context, pretest probability for cardiovascular abnormalities, or unanticipated findings during the study.

diagnosed prior to the age of 40 who have been treated with anthracyclines or radiation fields that can impact the heart, serial screening is supported.[26] Much of this screening is performed with echocardiography however, given its superior precision, the use of CMR has been advocated for among high-risk individuals with an ejection fraction of 50%–59% on two-dimensional echocardiography.[27]

Among individuals with cardiomyopathy after anthracycline therapy, CMR may also provide prognostic information. Indexed left ventricular mass has been found to predict risk for major adverse cardiovascular events over a two-year period.[28] Additionally, CMR has the advantage of superior assessment of biventricular function over other imaging techniques such as echocardiography, which can only provide limited assessment of the right ventricle. This can be beneficial in long-term survivors as there is evidence of an increased incidence of biventricular heart failure compared with ischemic and nonischemic cardiomyopathy.[29]

RESEARCH APPLICATIONS WITHIN CANCER POPULATIONS

Due to the low variability of measures and capability of measuring not only cardiovascular structure and function but also tissue characterization and vascular measures, CMR serves as a critical noninvasive resource in cardio-oncology research. In recent years, CMR has been utilized in both observational and interventional studies for subclinical measurements, leading to early identification of cancer therapy–related cardiovascular dysfunction, as well as for treatment response. As described within this chapter, the platform of standard CMR measures has a strong role in understanding cardiovascular health in cancer patients.

From a research perspective, applications of recent technical developments in the field of CMR are poised to aid in answering cardio-oncology–related questions.[30] These tools include machine learning–based advances such as contrast-free virtual native enhancement and quantitative myocardial perfusion as well as advances in rapid magnetic resonance imaging protocols including multiparametric tissue fingerprinting and real-time exercise CMR with magnetic resonance–compatible ergometers (Fig. 31.14).[31] Finally, new cardio-oncology research is exploring the application of magnetic resonance spectroscopy using multinuclei imaging, hyperpolarized ^{13}C spectroscopy, and even ^{1}H spectroscopy to investigate mechanistic associations of different therapies with CTRCD, which may unveil new mechanistic processes in cardio-oncology that may lead to improved patient surveillance and tailored interventional strategies.

CONCLUSION

Therapeutic options have dramatically broadened over the past several decades for cancer survivors, but alongside improved oncologic outcomes providers have documented a variety of potential cardiovascular complications. Cardiovascular disease can be problematic for treatment planning and optimizing survivor outcomes and quality of life. Given the unique ability of CMR to provide the gold standard of cardiac structural and functional assessment, as well as its capacity for detailed tissue characterization, it has progressively solidified its role in the diagnosis, prognosis, and therapeutic guidance for cardiovascular disease among cancer survivors. Incorporation of CMR into future research and clinical initiatives is certain to maximize the precision of cardiovascular monitoring, provide new insights into cardiac complications, and assist with tailored treatment decisions in the coming years.

TABLE 31.3 Cancer treatments with highest potential for cardiovascular toxicity and targeted cardiovascular magnetic resonance sequences for evaluation.

THERAPY	HYPOTHESIZED MECHANISM OF INJURY	CARDIOVASCULAR MANIFESTATIONS	CMR SEQUENCES
• Anthracyclines, Anthraquinones ○ Doxorubicin ○ Daunorubicin ○ Epirubicin ○ Idarubicin ○ Valrubicin ○ Mitoxantrone	• Primary mechanism thought to be inhibition of topoisomerase 2β, as well as involvement of reactive oxygen species • Acute: inflammatory cell infiltration, interstitial edema, cardiomyocyte damage • Chronic: loss of cardiomyocytes, necrosis, fibrosis, vacuole formation	• LV systolic and diastolic dysfunction • Heart failure • Arrhythmias • Pericarditis • Valvular dysfunction	• Cinematic sequences ○ LV mass ○ Function • Native T1 maps ○ Elevated in acute phase (edema) ○ Elevated in chronic phase (fibrosis) • T2 maps ○ Elevated in acute phase (edema) ○ Normal in chronic phase • Postcontrast T1 maps for ECV ○ ECV elevated in acute phase (edema) ○ ECV remains elevated in chronic phase (fibrosis)
• HER2-Targeted Therapies ○ Trastuzumab ○ Pertuzumab ○ Lapatinib	• Not well understood • HER2 signaling appears implicated in myocardial cell survival pathways	• LV dysfunction (can be reversible or permanent) • Heart failure	• Cinematic sequences ○ LV mass ○ Function • Tissue characteristics can help exclude other contributors ○ T1 maps ○ T2 maps ○ Late gadolinium enhancement ○ ECV quantification
• Fluoropyrimidines ○ Fluorouracil (5-FU) ○ Capecitabine ○ Doxifluridine ○ Tegafur	• Endothelial dysfunction leading to diffuse coronary vasoconstriction or focal coronary artery spasm	• Myocardial infarction • Stress cardiomyopathy • LV dysfunction • Heart failure	• Cinematic sequences ○ LV mass ○ Function • Optional: vasodilator stress perfusion • Late gadolinium enhancement ○ Subendocardial (ischemic) enhancement pattern • T2 maps ○ Elevated in acute infarction or stress cardiomyopathy (edema)
• Immune Checkpoint inhibitors ○ Ipilimumab ○ Nivolumab ○ Pembrolizumab ○ Atezolizumab ○ Avelumab ○ Durvalumab ○ Relatlimab ○ Cemiplimab ○ Tremelimumab	• Not well understood • May trigger myocarditis-like events involving lymphocytic infiltration with development of patchy fibrosis • Accelerated atherosclerosis leading to increased risk of acute coronary syndrome	• Fulminant myocarditis • LV dysfunction • Heart failure • Arrhythmias • Myocardial infarction • Pericarditis	• Cinematic sequences ○ LV mass ○ Function • Optional: vasodilator stress perfusion • Tissue characteristics to establish myocardial inflammation criteria ○ T1 maps ○ Late gadolinium enhancement ○ ECV quantification ○ T2 maps ○ T2-weighted imaging
• Hormone Antagonism Therapy ○ Estrogen Deprivation ▪ Selective estrogen receptor degraders (fulvestrant, elacestrant) ▪ Aromatase inhibitors (letrozole, anastrozole, exemestane) ▪ Ovarian suppression (oophorectomy, goserelin, leuprolide) ○ Androgen Deprivation ▪ GnRH agonists (leuprolide, goserelin, triptorelin, buserelin, histrelin) ▪ GnRH antagonists (degarelix, abarelix) ▪ Androgen receptor inhibitors (flutamide, nilutamide, bicalutamide, enzalutamide, apalutamide) ▪ CYP17 inhibitor (abiraterone) ▪ Orchiectomy	• Hypoestrogen effects: lack of estrogen (particularly 17β-estradiol) leads to lower vasodilatory capacity with acceleration and higher inflammatory composition of atherosclerotic lesions, predisposing to ischemia and acute coronary syndrome • Antiandrogen therapy: testosterone is unable to be converted to 17β-estradiol, thus indirectly promoting atherosclerosis • Worsened metabolic profiles (insulin resistance, dyslipidemia, decrease in muscle mass with increased adiposity)	• Accelerated coronary arterial atherosclerosis • Risk of myocardial infarction	• Cinematic sequences ○ LV mass ○ Function • Optional: vasodilator stress perfusion • Tissue characteristics to establish presence of reactive fibrosis ○ T1 maps ○ Late gadolinium enhancement ○ ECV quantification ○ T2 maps if concern for acute myocardial injury
• Radiation Therapy	• Off-target DNA damage with cell senescence and death • Affects coronary endothelial cells leading to increased vascular permeability, inflammatory cell activation, vascular edema, and thrombosis resulting in large vessel or microvascular flow limitations and eventually ischemia/infarction • Similar inflammatory and fibrotic effects on valvular tissue and pericardial tissue • Expression of osteogenic factors on valvular tissue	• LV systolic and diastolic dysfunction • Heart failure • Acute pericarditis, pericardial effusion, constrictive pericarditis • Valvular stenosis or regurgitation • Accelerated coronary arterial atherosclerosis • Aortopathy • Conduction disease	• Cinematic sequences ○ LV mass ○ Function ○ Valvular anatomy and function ○ Assessment of pericardial adhesions ○ Assessment for ventricular interdependence of filling • Optional: vasodilator stress perfusion • Late gadolinium enhancement • T1 and T2 mapping, ECV assessment • Phase contrast imaging (if concerns for valvular dysfunction)

DNA, Deoxyribonucleic acid; *ECV*, extracellular volume; *LV*, left ventricular.

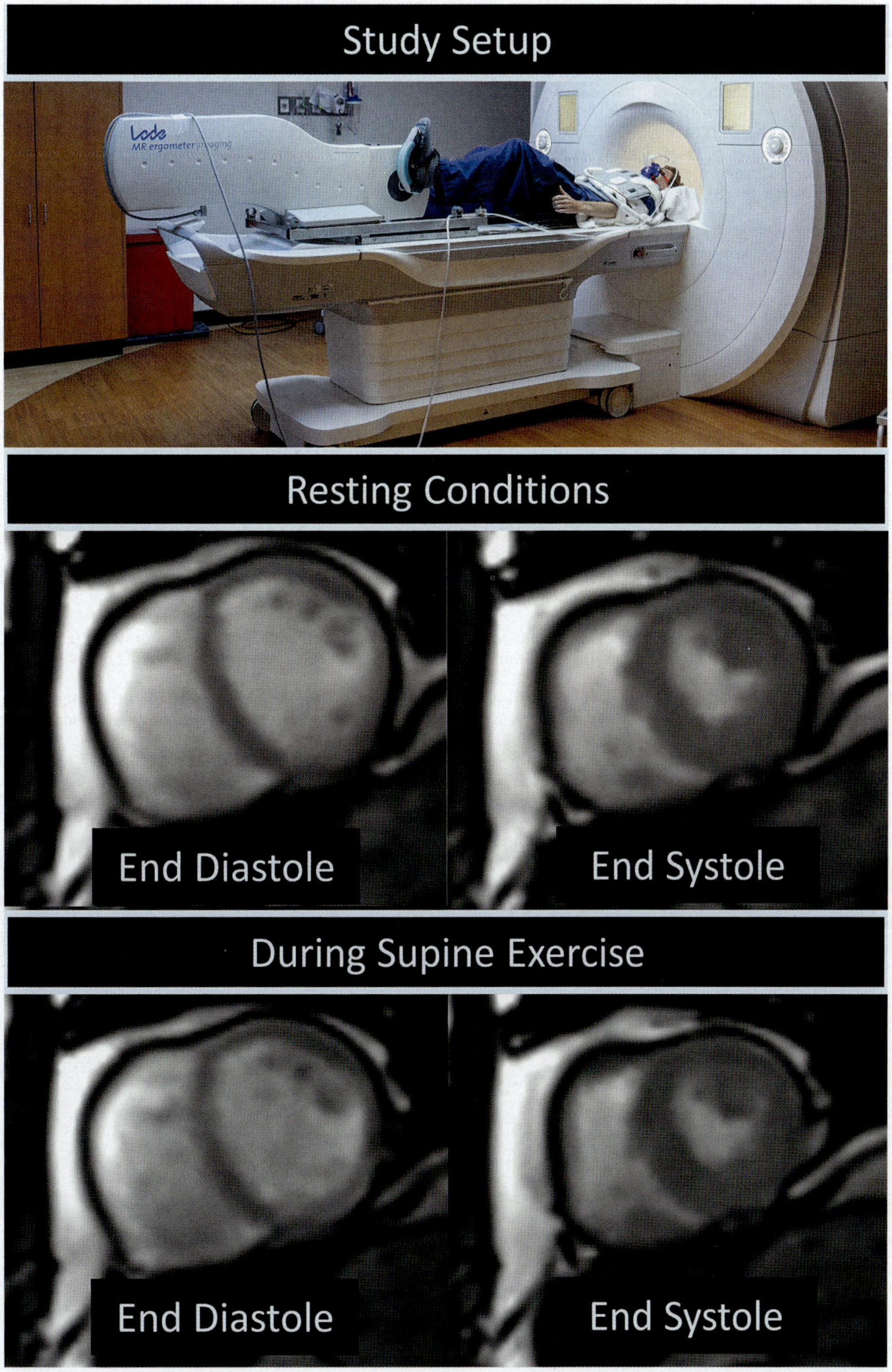

FIG. 31.14 Simultaneous cardiovascular magnetic resonance (CMR) with cardiopulmonary exercise testing. With the use of ergometers that are compatible with the magnetic resonance environment, it is possible to perform exercise stress testing coupled with CMR as the gold standard for wall motion and functional assessment. Additionally, metabolic carts may be modified to allow for gas exchange data for simultaneous cardiopulmonary exercise testing during CMR. These techniques may allow for advanced phenotyping of exertional intolerance in cancer survivors among other patient populations.

REFERENCES

1. Herrmann J. Adverse cardiac effects of cancer therapies: cardiotoxicity and arrhythmia. *Nat Rev Cardiol.* 2020;17(8):474–502. https://doi.org/10.1038/s41569-020-0348-1.
2. Jordan JH, Todd RM, Vasu S, Hundley WG. Cardiovascular magnetic resonance in the oncology patient. *JACC Cardiovasc Imaging.* 2018;11(8):1150–1172. https://doi.org/10.1016/j.jcmg.2018.06.004.
3. Alexander J, Dainiak N, Berger HJ, et al. Serial assessment of doxorubicin cardiotoxicity with quantitative radionuclide angiocardiography. *N Engl J Med.* 1979;300(6):278–283. https://doi.org/10.1056/NEJM197902083000603.
4. Herrmann J, Lenihan D, Armenian S, et al. Defining cardiovascular toxicities of cancer therapies: an International cardio-oncology society (IC-OS) consensus statement. *Eur Heart J.* 2022;43(4):280–299. https://doi.org/10.1093/eurheartj/ehab674.
5. Suerken CK, D'Agostino RB, Jordan JH, et al. Simultaneous left ventricular volume and strain changes during chemotherapy associate with 2-year postchemotherapy measures of left ventricular ejection fraction. *JAHA.* 2020;9(2):e015400. https://doi.org/10.1161/JAHA.119.015400.
6. Battisti NML, Welch CA, Sweeting M, et al. Prevalence of cardiovascular disease in patients with potentially curable malignancies. *JACC CardioOncol.* 2022;4(2):238–253. https://doi.org/10.1016/j.jaccao.2022.03.004.

7. Patel AR, Salerno M, Kwong RY, Singh A, Heydari B, Kramer CM. Stress cardiac magnetic resonance myocardial perfusion imaging. *J Am Coll Cardiol.* 2021;78(16):1655–1668. https://doi.org/10.1016/j.jacc.2021.08.022.
8. Jordan JH, Vasu S, Morgan TM, et al. Anthracycline-associated T1 mapping characteristics are elevated independent of the presence of cardiovascular comorbidities in cancer survivors. *Circ Cardiovasc Imaging.* 2016;9(8):e004325. https://doi.org/10.1161/CIRCIMAGING.115.004325.
9. Haslbauer JD, Lindner S, Valbuena-Lopez S, et al. CMR imaging biosignature of cardiac involvement due to cancer-related treatment by T1 and T2 mapping. *Int J Cardiol.* 2019;275:179–186. https://doi.org/10.1016/j.ijcard.2018.10.023.
10. Toro-Salazar OH, Gillan E, O'Loughlin MT, et al. Occult cardiotoxicity in childhood cancer survivors exposed to anthracycline therapy. *Circ Cardiovasc Imaging.* 2013;6(6):873–880. https://doi.org/10.1161/CIRCIMAGING.113.000798.
11. Kittleson MM, Ruberg FL, Ambardekar AV, et al. 2023 ACC expert consensus decision pathway on comprehensive multidisciplinary care for the patient with cardiac amyloidosis. *J Am Coll Cardiol.* 2023;81(11):1076–1126. https://doi.org/10.1016/j.jacc.2022.11.022.
12. Pereira NL, Grogan M, Dec GW. Spectrum of restrictive and infiltrative cardiomyopathies: part 2 of a 2-part series. *J Am Coll Cardiol.* 2018;71(10):1149–1166. https://doi.org/10.1016/j.jacc.2018.01.017.
13. Muehlberg F, Blaszczyk E, Will K, Wilczek S, Brederlau J, Schulz-Menger J. Characterization of critically ill patients with septic shock and sepsis-associated cardiomyopathy using cardiovascular MRI. *ESC Heart Failure.* 2022;9(4):2147–2156. https://doi.org/10.1002/ehf2.13938.
14. Medina de Chazal H, Del Buono MG, Keyser-Marcus L, et al. Stress cardiomyopathy diagnosis and treatment: JACC state-of-the-art review. *Am Coll Cardiol.* 2018;72(16):1955–1971. https://doi.org/10.1016/j.jacc.2018.07.072.
15. Zaghlol R, Dey AK, Barac A. Takotsubo and cancer. *Eur Heart J.* 2020;41(48):4547–4549. https://doi.org/10.1093/eurheartj/ehaa175.
16. Zhang L, Awadalla M, Mahmood SS, et al. Cardiovascular magnetic resonance in immune checkpoint inhibitor-associated myocarditis. *Eur Heart J.* 2020;41(18):1733–1743. https://doi.org/10.1093/eurheartj/ehaa051.
17. Parr SK, Liang J, Schadler KL, Gilchrist SC, Steele CC, Ade CJ. Anticancer therapy–related increases in arterial stiffness: a systematic review and meta-analysis. *JAHA.* 2020;9(14):e015598. https://doi.org/10.1161/JAHA.119.015598.
18. Jordan JH, Castellino SM, Meléndez GC, et al. Left ventricular mass change after anthracycline chemotherapy. *Circ: Heart Failure.* 2018;11(7):e004560. https://doi.org/10.1161/CIRCHEARTFAILURE.117.004560.
19. Masood IR, Rezvan PH, Lee K, et al. Left ventricle size correlates with peak exercise capacity in pediatric cancer survivors exposed to anthracycline chemotherapy. *Pediatr Cardiol.* 2023;45:1493–1502. https://doi.org/10.1007/s00246-023-03192-z.
20. Tyebally S, Chen D, Bhattacharyya S, et al. Cardiac tumors. *JACC CardioOncology.* 2020;2(2):293–311. https://doi.org/10.1016/j.jaccao.2020.05.009.
21. Shenoy C, Grizzard JD, Shah DJ, et al. Cardiovascular magnetic resonance imaging in suspected cardiac tumour: a multicentre outcomes study. *Eur Heart J.* 2021;43(1):71–80. https://doi.org/10.1093/eurheartj/ehab635.
22. Otto CM, Nishimura RA, Bonow RO, et al. 2020 ACC/AHA guideline for the management of patients with valvular heart disease: a report of the American college of cardiology/American heart association joint committee on clinical practice guidelines. *Circulation.* 2021;143(5):e35–e71. https://doi.org/10.1161/CIR.0000000000000923.
23. Ylänen K, Poutanen T, Savikurki-Heikkilä P, Rinta-Kiikka I, Eerola A, Vettenranta K. Cardiac magnetic resonance imaging in the evaluation of the late effects of anthracyclines among long-term survivors of childhood cancer. *Am Coll Cardiol.* 2013;61(14):1539–1547. https://doi.org/10.1016/j.jacc.2013.01.019.
24. Barthur A, Brezden-Masley C, Connelly KA, et al. Longitudinal assessment of right ventricular structure and function by cardiovascular magnetic resonance in breast cancer patients treated with trastuzumab: a prospective observational study. *J Cardiovasc Magn Reson.* 2017;19(1):44. https://doi.org/10.1186/s12968-017-0356-4.
25. Lyon AR, López-Fernández T, Couch LS, et al. 2022 ESC guidelines on cardio-oncology developed in collaboration with the European hematology association (EHA), the European society for therapeutic radiology and oncology (ESTRO) and the international cardio-oncology society (IC-OS). *Eur Heart J.* 2022;43(41):4229–4361. https://doi.org/10.1093/eurheartj/ehac244.
26. Children's Oncology Group. Long-Term Follow-Up Guidelines for Survivors of Childhood, Adolescent, and Young Adult Cancers Version 6.0. Published online October 2023.
27. Armstrong GT, Plana JC, Zhang N, et al. Screening adult survivors of childhood cancer for cardiomyopathy: comparison of echocardiography and cardiac magnetic resonance imaging. *JCO.* 2012;30(23):2876–2884. https://doi.org/10.1200/JCO.2011.40.3584.
28. Neilan TG, Coelho-Filho OR, Pena-Herrera D, et al. Left ventricular mass in patients with a cardiomyopathy after treatment with anthracyclines. *Am J Cardiol.* 2012;110(11):1679–1686. https://doi.org/10.1016/j.amjcard.2012.07.040.
29. Oliveira GH, Dupont M, Naftel D, et al. Increased need for right ventricular support in patients with chemotherapy-induced cardiomyopathy undergoing mechanical circulatory support. *J Am Coll Cardiol.* 2014;63(3):240–248. https://doi.org/10.1016/j.jacc.2013.09.040.
30. Addison D, Neilan TG, Barac A, et al. Cardiovascular imaging in contemporary cardio-oncology: a scientific statement from the american heart association. *Circulation.* 2023;148(16):1271–1286. https://doi.org/10.1161/CIR.0000000000001174.
31. Canada JM, McCarty J, Jordan JH, et al. Simultaneous exercise stress cardiac magnetic resonance and cardiopulmonary exercise testing to elucidate the Fick components of aerobic exercise capacity: a feasibility and reproducibility study and pilot study in hematologic cancer survivors. *Cardio-Oncology.* 2023;9(1):31. https://doi.org/10.1186/s40959-023-00182-1.

32 Cardiac Thrombus

ANGEL T. CHAN, JONATHAN W. WEINSAFT, AND JIWON KIM

INTRODUCTION

Cardiac thrombus has important implications for clinical decision making, as thrombus provides a substrate for thromboembolic events and a rationale for anticoagulation. Whereas thrombus has traditionally been identified based on its morphologic appearance, this criterion is inherently limited given that thrombus can vary in shape and size as well as ancillary features such as location and mobility. Consistent with this, echocardiography (a technique that identifies thrombus based on morphology and related ancillary features) has yielded conflicting data with respect to the prevalence and magnitude of embolic risk conferred by thrombus. As imaging is widely used to identify cardiac thrombus and its detection markedly impacts clinical care, accurate identification of thrombus is of substantial significance.

Cardiac magnetic resonance (CMR) enables thrombus to be identified based on tissue characteristics: Whereas thrombus can vary in morphology, an intrinsic feature is avascularity—a tissue property that can be discerned on CMR. Given that gadolinium distribution is dependent on vascular supply, lack of gadolinium in a given region provides a robust marker of avascular tissue composition. Using the technique of late gadolinium enhancement (LGE), CMR can identify thrombus based on avascular tissue composition (manifested as lack of gadolinium contrast uptake). LGE-CMR has been shown to provide highly accurate detection of pathology-verified thrombus, improve thrombus identification, and enhance risk stratification for embolic events compared to conventional imaging methods (i.e., echocardiography).[1–3] CMR also enables precise quantification of structural risk factors for thrombus—including myocardial infarct size, contractile function, chamber geometry, and flow velocity; infarct delineation by CMR yields near-exact agreement with histopathology-evidenced myocyte necrosis. Regarding left ventricular (LV) function and remodeling, CMR has been shown to be highly reproducible and to closely agree with necropsy-evidenced LV mass and phantom-verified chamber size. CMR entails no ionizing radiation, making it well suited to serially assess thrombus response to therapeutic interventions, such as resolution or persistence following treatment with anticoagulants.

This chapter provides an overview of CMR for the assessment of thrombus, including identification of thrombus and its predisposing risk factors, diagnostic differentiation from neoplasm, and prediction of clinical prognosis.

IMAGING APPROACH

Late Gadolinium Enhancement—Acquisition

LGE-CMR is widely relied upon as the primary CMR pulse sequence used to identify thrombus. This pulse sequence is predicated on the use of an inversion recovery approach to demonstrate differential T1 recovery times between regions that stem from differences in the distribution of gadolinium (a contrast agent that shortens longitudinal [T1] recovery). Initially used as a tool to characterize viable and infarcted myocardium based on contrast uptake patterns, LGE-CMR can also be used as a tool to detect thrombus. Although contrast uptake is low in viable compared to infarcted myocardium, it is not zero, as is the case with avascular tissue such as thrombus. Thus, on LGE-CMR, thrombus (in which contrast is absent) can be differentiated from viable myocardium (in which contrast distribution is low) as well as blood pool and regions of infarction (in which contrast distribution is high) based on differential T1 recovery times. On conventional LGE-CMR, thrombus has an "etched" appearance with a black border and a central gray zone (reflecting partial T1 recovery) and can be readily identified as a low-signal intensity mass surrounded by high-signal intensity structures such as cavity blood and/or hyperenhanced myocardial infarction.

Differential contrast uptake between viable myocardium and thrombus can be exploited to further improve the conspicuity of thrombus on CMR. To do so, a modified "long inversion time" LGE-CMR sequence can be used in which the inversion time is increased from that needed to null viable myocardium (~300–350 msec) to a fixed time of 600 msec that selectively nulls avascular tissue such as thrombus.[4] With this "long inversion time" (long-TI) sequence, regions with contrast uptake such as viable myocardium increase in image intensity (i.e., appear gray rather than black), thrombus appears homogeneously black, and there is improved delineation of thrombus. Fig. 32.1 provides a schematic illustration of the LGE pulse sequence, inclusive of a conventional application and tailored "long-TI" imaging to selectively null thrombus.

Given that LGE-CMR is a fundamental component of nearly all CMR examinations, it provides a widely available and generalizable approach for the detection of thrombus. Whereas "long-TI" LGE requires a slight pulse sequence modification (i.e., change of inversion time from ~300–350 to 600 msec) and additional imaging, data can be acquired during the (5–10 minute) interval between contrast administration and traditional LGE imaging and thus not add to the time required for the overall CMR examination. Use

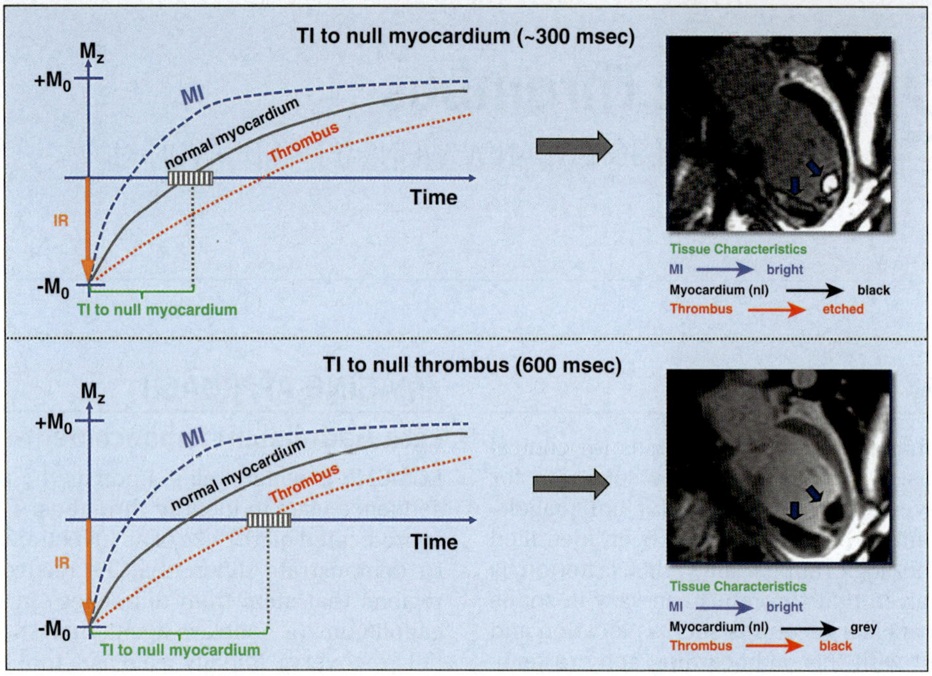

FIG. 32.1 Late gadolinium enhancement (LGE) cardiac magnetic resonance (CMR) pulse sequence. Schematic of LGE pulse sequence as applied conventionally for the purpose of viability/infarct imaging (*top*) and tailored long inversion time long-TI thrombus assessment (*bottom*). Note that thrombus typically appears etched on conventional LGE-CMR—attributable to lack of gadolinium uptake with associated prolonged recovery after initial (180 degrees) inversion pulse. Long-TI LGE imaging entails prolongation of the inversion time (TI: time between inversion pulse and signal acquisition), resulting in tailored "nulling" (*black appearance*) of avascular tissue and improving delineation of thrombus from blood pool and myocardium. *IR*, Inversion recovery; *MI*, myocardial infarction; *TI*, Inversion time.

of accelerated ("single-shot") pulse sequence algorithms for the purpose of long-TI LGE can abbreviate the time required for data acquisition, thus resulting in further time savings and enhancing patient tolerance.

Late Gadolinium Enhancement—Validation

LGE-CMR has been well-validated as an imaging reference for thrombus in relation to both pathology[1,3] and clinical embolic events.[1,5,6] For example, Velangi et al., examined embolic outcomes among a matched case-control cohort inclusive of 157 patients with LGE-CMR–evidenced LV thrombus[5]: During a median follow-up interval of 3.3 years, embolic event rates were >fourfold higher among patients with thrombus compared to those without (3.7% vs. 0.8%). Similarly, among a cohort of 784 patients with LV dysfunction, Weinsaft et al. reported that stratification according to the presence or absence of LV thrombus on LGE-CMR yielded an over sevenfold difference in validated endpoints (Transient Ischemic Attack, Cerebrovascular Accident, or pathology at time of surgical thrombectomy) between patients with and without thrombus (15.1% vs. 2.1%, $P<.0001$), including accurate assessment for thrombus in all patients (8/8) with pathology verification.[1] In comparison, there was only a threefold higher rate of endpoints reached in patients with thrombus identified by cine-CMR (8.6% vs. 2.8%, $P=.06$) even though their anticoagulation (warfarin) treatment was similar to patients grouped by LGE-CMR thrombus. Other studies have similarly shown LGE to provide improved diagnostic utility compared to alternative CMR approaches for thrombus. As evidence of this, direct comparison studies (for which readers were blinded to results of the other pulse sequence) have shown functional (cine) CMR to miss 21%–42% of LV thrombi detected by LGE-CMR.[1,2,7,8]

Thrombus assessment via LGE has also been shown to provide incremental diagnostic utility in other regions of the heart, including both right atrial and left atrial appendage thrombus. For example, among a cohort of 130 cancer patients with central venous catheters, Plodkowski et al. reported that right atrial thrombus detection by cine-CMR yielded a sensitivity of 90% in relation to LGE—the latter of which predicted risk for embolic events at 60-day follow-up (13% vs. 2%; $P=.03$).[9] Similarly, among a cohort of 261 patients with atrial fibrillation (AF) undergoing CMR, Kitkungvan et al. reported that LGE-CMR yielded 100% sensitivity for left atrial/left atrial appendage thrombus in comparison to the reference of transesophageal echocardiography (performed within 7 days of CMR) whereas the sensitivity of cine-CMR and magnetic resonance angiography were lower (both 66.7%).[10] More recently, an outcomes study encompassing cancer patients with cardiac masses (including both thrombus and neoplasm) demonstrated an improved prognostic utility of LGE-CMR compared to perfusion-CMR for the prediction of all-cause mortality, further supporting its use as a reference for diagnosis and risk stratification.[11] Taken together, these data provide evidence of the utility of LGE-CMR as a robust reference standard for tissue characterization–based identification of thrombus.

Ancillary Cardiac Magnetic Resonance Approaches

A major strength of CMR stems from its ability to provide multiparametric assessment of cardiovascular structure, function, and tissue properties within the framework of a single examination. This feature can be leveraged to inform structural and functional risk factors for thrombus, thus providing complementary data to the identification of thrombus itself. For example, myocardial injury, contractile dysfunction, and aneurysm were generally associated with risk for thrombogenesis, but their independent contributions had been challenging to discern in vivo prior to the development of an imaging tool that could directly assess myocardial tissue necrosis, contractile performance, and geometric remodeling near simultaneously, as with LGE and cine-CMR. Moreover, CMR can quantify multiple aspects of flow physiology, including velocity on 2D phase velocity-encoded CMR as well as sophisticated indices such as vorticity and kinetic energy on 4D flow CMR, each of which have been shown to be altered in patients with thrombus.[12] The utility of ancillary CMR indices for defining physiologic indices that predispose to thrombus in different regions of the heart are further detailed below.

CLINICAL APPLICATIONS

Left Ventricular Thrombus—Diagnostic Utility of Late Gadolinium Enhancement Cardiac Magnetic Resonance

The prevalence of LV thrombus is increased among patients with systolic heart failure as well as myocardial infarction—two populations in whom risk for embolic events (stroke) is known to be elevated. Each of these groups has been a major focus of studies concerning the relative utility of LGE-CMR for LV thrombus. Consistent with the above detailed data (see "Late Gadolinium Enhancement—Validation" section), LGE has also been shown to provide improved diagnostic utility in relation to transthoracic echo—the modality that (prior to the development of CMR) had conventionally been used to screen and surveil for thrombus. Among a cross-sectional cohort of 243 patients with LV dysfunction (ejection farction [EF] <50%) undergoing CMR, Weinsaft et al. reported that 10% had LGE-CMR–evidenced LV thrombus and that the overall diagnostic performance of routine transthoracic echo attained for clinical purposes was limited (sensitivity: 33%, specificity: 91%) in relation to the reference of LGE.[2] Echo test performance was improved among patients undergoing testing for the stated indication of LV thrombus assessment, but remained suboptimal (sensitivity 60%, specificity 88%). Fig. 32.2 provides representative examples of thrombus delineation by LGE-CMR, including improved detection of thrombus compared to conventional morphologic assessment as provided by echo and functional (cine) CMR.

To further test the utility of LGE thrombus assessment, Weinsaft et al. prospectively studied 121 patients at high risk for LV thrombus due to prior myocardial infarction and/or LV systolic dysfunction.[8] All patients underwent a standardized multimodality protocol, inclusive of CMR and echo (inclusive of obligate echo contrast use) within a narrow time interval (mean 0.8 ± 1.4 days; maximum 1 week). Consistent with observations derived from the aforementioned clinical studies, data from this rigorous prospective research cohort demonstrated suboptimal performance of echo in relation to LGE-CMR. For example, the diagnostic sensitivity and specificity of noncontrast echo was 33% and 94%, respectively, corresponding to an overall accuracy of 82%. Whereas use of echo contrast improved echo yield, sensitivity (60%) and overall accuracy (92%) remained suboptimal, as did positive and negative predictive values (93% and 91% respectively). LV thrombi detected by LGE-CMR but missed by echo were typically small in size or mural in shape (both $P<.05$), consistent with the notion that identification of LV thrombus based on morphologic appearance (a major criteria used by echo) can be challenging.

The notion that LGE-CMR improves diagnostic assessment of LV thrombus in relation to transthoracic echo has been confirmed in other cohorts. Among a cohort of 110 patients with LGE-evidenced LV thrombus who had echo performed within a 10-day interval (median 2 [interquartile range {IQR} 1–3] days), Velangi et al. reported noncontrast and contrast echo to yield sensitivities of 37% and 54% in comparison to the reference standard of CMR.[5] Among 194 patients undergoing CMR and echo early (2–4 days) after acute ST segment elevation myocardial infarction (STEMI), Delewi et al. reported that LV thrombus was present in 8.8% of patients at initial follow-up and that transthoracic (noncontrast) echo yielded a diagnostic sensitivity and specificity of 24% and 95%, respectively; follow-up results at 4 months yielded similar results (21% and 98% respectively).[13] Similarly, among a cohort of patients with ischemic cardiomyopathy and adverse LV remodeling undergoing ventricular reconstruction surgery in whom the prevalence of pathology-verified LV thrombus was very high (29%), Srichai et al. reported transthoracic echo to yield a suboptimal performance (sensitivity 23 ± 12%, specificity 96 ± 3.6%) that was lower than that of CMR (88 ± 9%, 99 ± 2%) in relation to the reference of pathology-evidenced LV thrombus.[3] Interestingly, whereas the large majority of research has shown LGE-CMR to markedly improve assessment of LV thrombus in relation to echo, some studies have reported discordant results. For example, among a cohort of 100 patients imaged early (median 5.5 [IQR 4.25–6.0] days) after anterior myocardial infarction (MI), Meurin et al. reported transthoracic echo to yield high sensitivity and specificity (94.7% and 98.5%, respectively) for LV thrombus as established by the reference of LGE-CMR.[14] While reasons for the exceptionally high performance of echo in this one study are uncertain, potential explanations include a low incidence of advanced LV remodeling (resulting in improved echo cavity delineation) and/or focus on early post-MI imaging—a time point at which the incidence of laminar thrombus (as is challenging to discern on echo) would be expected to be low.

It should also be noted that some studies have explored the utility of CMR tissue characterization as a tool for assessing thrombus chronicity. For example, Caspar et al. studied the utility of parametric T1 mapping for this purpose among 22 patients with cardiac thrombus—nearly three-quarters of whom (73% [16/22]) had LV thrombus[15]: Among this cohort, the authors reported that cases of recent thrombus (<1 week [n = 6]) had a shorter native T1 than cases of chronic (>1 month)

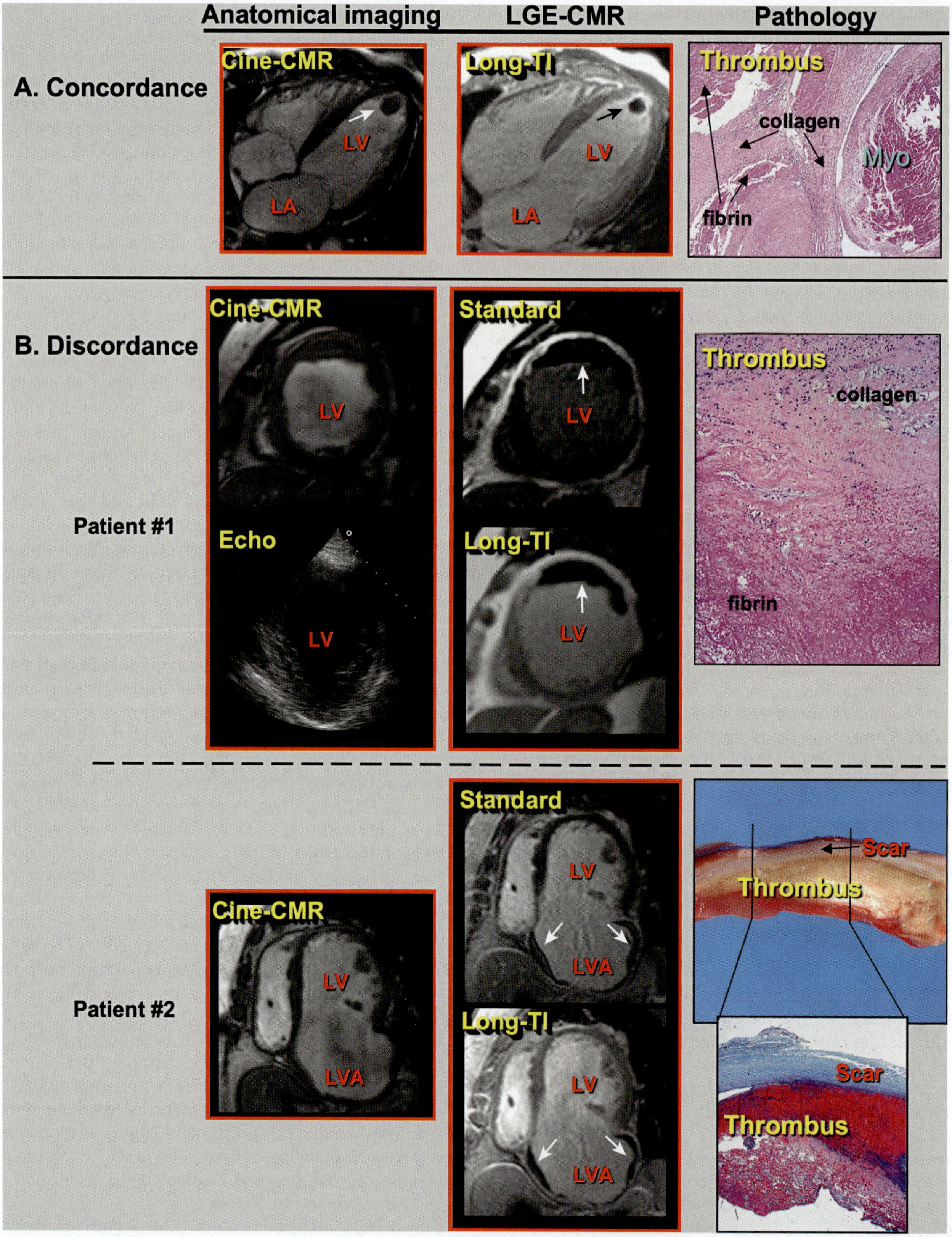

FIG. 32.2 Late gadolinium enhancement (LGE) cardiac magnetic resonance (CMR) compared to conventional imaging for identification of thrombus. (A) Typical images from a patient with concordant findings by anatomical imaging and LGE-CMR. Both techniques show an intracavitary thrombus within the LV apex (4-chamber views). Pathology (hematoxylin and eosin [H & E] stain, low power) confirmed the presence of thrombus with organizing features, including prominent collagen and fibrin content. (B) Images from two patients with discordant findings by anatomical imaging and LGE-CMR. Patient #1 had a large mural thrombus adherent to the LV anterior wall detected by LGE-CMR but missed by cine-CMR and echocardiography (midventricular short-axis views). Patient #2 had a large mural thrombus adherent to an inferior wall aneurysm detected by LGE-CMR but missed by cine-CMR (midventricular short-axis views). In both patients, thrombus was verified by pathology (patient #1: H & E stain, low power; patient #2: gross examination [overlay] and histopathology [inset, Masson trichrome stain]). Note thrombus may have an "etched" appearance with a black border and a central gray zone on standard inversion time (*TI*) LGE-CMR, whereas it appears homogeneously black on long-TI imaging. *LA*, left atrium; *LV*, left ventricle; *LVA*, left ventricular aneurysm; Myo, myocardium. Thrombus denoted by *yellow arrows*. (Modified from Weinsaft JW, Kim HW, Shah DJ, et al., Detection of left ventricular thrombus by delayed-enhancement cardiovascular magnetic resonance: prevalence and markers in patients with systolic dysfunction. *J Am Coll Cardiol*. 2008;52(2):148–157.)

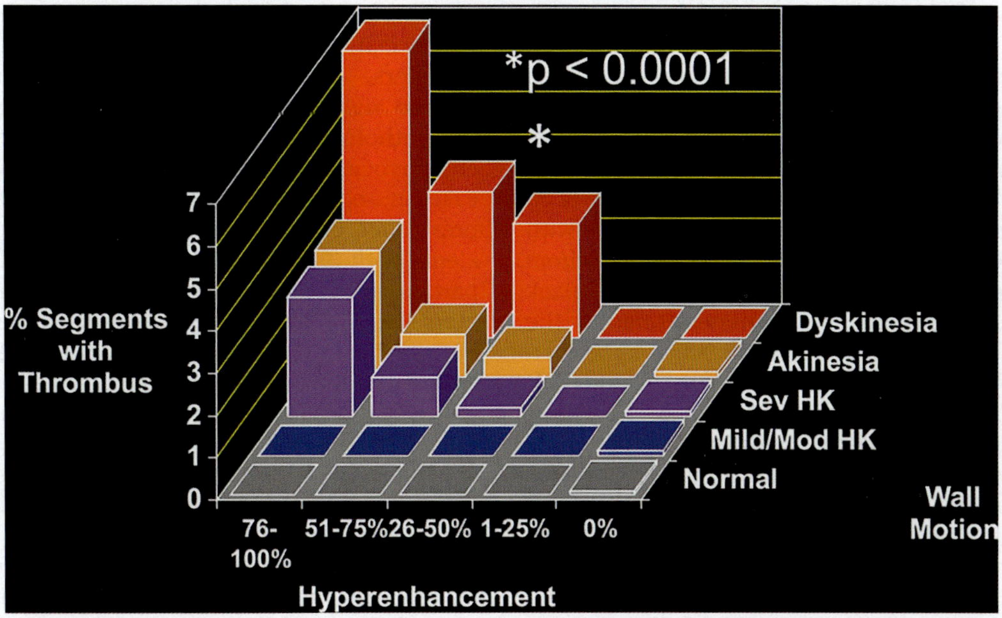

FIG. 32.3 Myocardial infarction and dysfunction as structural markers for LV thrombus. Population-based data derived from dual-center cross-sectional cohort of patients with left ventricular (LV) systolic dysfunction (ejection fraction [EF] <50%) demonstrating stepwise associations between both the extent of transmural myocardial infarction (on late gadolinium enhancement cardiac magnetic resonance [LGE-CMR]) and contractile dysfunction (on cine-CMR) and presence of LV thrombus. Note that both LV dysfunction and extent of transmural infarction were associated with LV thrombus ($P<.001$ for trends), and that independent associations for both dysfunction and infarction with LV thrombus remained significant when both were included in a multivariable model that adjusted for clinical variables (see text for details). *HK*, Hypokinesis. (Modified from Weinsaft JW, Kim HW, Shah DJ, et al., Detection of left ventricular thrombus by delayed-enhancement cardiovascular magnetic resonance: prevalence and markers in patients with systolic dysfunction. *J Am Coll Cardiol*. 2008;52(2):148–157.)

thrombus (911 ± 177 vs. 1169 ± 107 ms, $P=.01$). While promising, larger studies are warranted to further validate this concept.

Left Ventricular Thrombus—Structural Risk Factors as Discerned by Cardiac Magnetic Resonance

In parallel with direct identification of LV thrombus itself, CMR has been shown to provide incremental utility for the characterization of LV remodeling factors associated with thrombogenesis. A major focus in this area has concerned linkage between myocardial infarction (i.e., tissue necrosis) and LV thrombus, including demonstration of independent associations between infarct size and the likelihood of thrombus independent of global or regional impairments in myocardial contractility, as well as the severity of adverse LV geometric remodeling (i.e., global dilation, regional aneurysms). In an initial demonstration of this concept, Weinsaft et al. studied patients with LV dysfunction and demonstrated transmural infarct size on LGE-CMR to be independently associated with LV thrombus (odds ratio [OR] = 1.02 per% LV with transmural infarction [95% confidence interval {CI} 1.002–1.04]; $P=.03$) even after controlling for LV ejection fraction (OR = 0.94 [95% CI 0.92–0.97]; $P<.0001$), as well as clinically documented MI, history of ischemic cardiomyopathy, and age (Fig. 32.3).[1] Consistent with this, the prevalence of LV thrombus was over fivefold higher among patients with ischemic compared to nonischemic cardiomyopathy (9.2% vs. 1.7%; $P=.0002$)—paralleling differential infarct size (larger in patients with ischemic cardiomyopathy) but similar left ventricular ejection fraction (LVEF; both 32%) between groups. This concept was further validated in research by this group among patients at high risk for LV thrombus (83% with prior myocardial infarction), among whom LV thrombus was associated with transmural infarct size (OR = 1.39 per 10% LV myocardium with transmural infarction [95% CI 1.01–1.79]; $P=.04$), even after controlling for LVEF (OR = 1.63 per 10% decrement [95% CI 1.17–2.11]; $P=.007$) and LV aneurysm (OR = 4.43 [95% CI 1.25–15.69]; $P=.02$).[8]

Consistent with the notion that infarct distribution modifies risk for thrombus, a meta-analysis of 2072 patients with STEMI reported the overall incidence of LV thrombus to be 6.3% and that nearly all LV thrombus (96%) occurred among patients with anterior infarction.[16] The prevalence of LV thrombus was 12.2% among patients with anterior STEMI and 19.2% among those with concurrent anterior STEMI and impaired LVEF (<50%). Regarding mechanism, Weinsaft et al. studied a cohort of 201 STEMI patients (of whom 8% had LV thrombus) and reported that thrombus was associated with stepwise decrements in basal-to-apical contractile function, irrespective of whether it was assessed by visual echo wall motion score or quantification of regional endocardial deformation on cine-CMR (both $P=$NS in LV base; $P<.001$ in LV apex).[7] It has also been shown on 4D flow CMR that post-MI patients with LV thrombus have significantly reduced and delayed LV flow wash-in as well as exaggerated decrements in kinetic energy within the distal LV,[12] suggesting that the presence and location of thrombus stems from local perturbations in LV flow physiology.

Left Atrial/Atrial Appendage Thrombus

Left atrial (LA) thrombus typically localizes to the left atrial appendage (LAA), most commonly occurs in patients with AF, and is a risk factor for cardioembolic stroke. Transesophageal echo (TEE) provides excellent delineation of the LAA and is widely used as a reference standard for LAA thrombus, but this modality is invasive and thus not ideal for screening and surveillance of broad unselected cohorts—highlighting the potential utility of noninvasive imaging approaches, which can be provided by CMR.

Several studies have tested CMR as a noninvasive tool to evaluate LAA thrombus, for which results have been promising. For example, Ohyama studied 50 patients with nonrheumatic AF and cardioembolic stroke among whom CMR (using double- and triple-inversion recovery [black blood] pulse sequences) and TEE were performed on the same day.[17] Findings demonstrated good, albeit imperfect, agreement between CMR and TEE (kappa = 0.876), and CMR overestimation of thrombus size in relation to TEE. Other studies focused on LGE-CMR have yielded more favorable results. For example, Rathi et al. studied a retrospective cohort of 97 patients with AF undergoing TEE and CMR prior to pulmonary vein isolation (PVI). CMR included cine, LGE, and 3D magnetic resonance angiography (MRA).[18] When CMR data was examined in aggregate, results demonstrated modalities to be fully concordant with respect to the presence or absence of LAA thrombus. Of note, while the prevalence of LAA thrombus on TEE was extremely low (n = 2), results from this study suggested CMR performance to vary based on pulse sequence—9 (8%) subjects were deemed to be indeterminate for LAA thrombus based on 2D (cine) CMR, and thus required postcontrast imaging to resolve diagnostic uncertainty. Similar results were reported in a subsequent study encompassing 261 patients undergoing CMR for planned PVI who also underwent TEE within 7 (mean 1.3 ± 2.3) days.[10] CMR encompassed distinct components (cine, MRA, long-TI [600 msec] LGE), each of which were interpreted separately. TEE identified thrombus in the LAA on seven examinations (2.7%) and in the LA on two examinations (0.8%). Compared to the reference of TEE, long-TI LGE-CMR had the highest accuracy (99.2%), sensitivity (100%), and specificity (99.2%), followed by contrast-enhanced MRA (accuracy 94.3%, sensitivity 66.7%, and specificity 95.2%) and cine-CMR (91.6%, 66.7%, and 92.5%, respectively). Consistent with this, a meta-analysis encompassing 582 patients from seven papers reported that pooled sensitivity and specificity for cine-CMR (91% and 93%) and MRA (77% and 97%) were lower than that for LGE-CMR (100% and 99%), paralleling higher summary receiver operating characteristics for LGE (0.9938) compared to other CMR methods (cine: 0.9393, MRA: 0.9763).[19] Consistent with this approach, postgadolinium inversion recovery CMR has been used to study LAA thrombus in at-risk populations, including patients with cardiac amyloid, in whom the prevalence of thrombus has been documented to be high (6.2%) in research by Martinez-Naharro et al.[20] These data support the utility of CMR as a noninvasive alternative to TEE for the evaluation of LA/LAA thrombus, and demonstrate that its effectiveness varies in relation to the pulse sequence used for thrombus evaluation, with optimal performance yielded by LGE-CMR.

Right-Sided (Atrial and Ventricular) Thrombus

Thrombus in the right heart (right atrium [RA] or right ventricle [RV]) typically occurs due to transit from the peripheral vasculature (e.g., deep vein thrombosis), or in situ formation on prosthetic materials (e.g., central venous catheters, cardiac devices). Less common etiologies include right ventricular dysfunction/infarction, infiltrative pathologies that impact the right heart (e.g., amyloid, endomyocardial fibrosis), AF, and/or valvular heart disease. In an autopsy study of nearly 24,000 patients, the prevalence of right and left atrial thrombus were equivalent (both 3.1%).[21] One group in which RA thrombus is particularly common is patients with central venous catheters. Despite their widespread use and therapeutic importance for care of patients with cancer and critical illness, catheters can produce localized changes in the right atrial milieu that predispose to thrombus. These include disruptions of intrinsic blood flow patterns (i.e., due to physical impedance of vena caval inflow and tricuspid valve emptying), introduction of foreign material (that differs from native myocardium), and/or atrial wall injury (due to catheter abrasion). The prothrombotic impact of these catheter-induced changes in right heart physiology may be exaggerated in the context of a hypercoagulable milieu that occurs with both cancer and critical illness, resulting in a nidus for thrombus. Given that right atrial thrombus provides a nidus for embolic events such as pulmonary embolism—a potentially life-threatening complication that is potentially preventable with anticoagulation and/or targeted interventions such as thrombolysis and/or catheter removal—imaging tools to identify and surveil thrombus are important for effective care of at-risk populations.

Whereas the majority of CMR research on thrombus has focused on the left heart, available literature supports the notion that it provides utility for right-sided thrombus. The utility of LGE-CMR for native RA and/or RV thrombus has been anecdotally documented in case reports. Broader data exists that demonstrate the value of CMR for catheter-associated RA thrombus. Among a retrospective cohort of 130 cancer patients with central venous catheters, Plodkowski et al. compared the diagnostic performance of CMR and transthoracic echo with respect to RA thrombus.[9] As in prior literature, cine- and LGE-CMR were interpreted independently (blinded to results of the other approach) in order to discern their relative utility. Paralleling its results for LV and LAA thrombus, echo (attained in 64% of the population) demonstrated moderate sensitivity and specificity (75% and 90%, respectively) in relation to LGE-evidenced RA thrombus. Similarly, cine-CMR yielded better performance (sensitivity 90%, specificity 98%) but missed 10% of RA thrombi detected by LGE-CMR. Regarding clinical significance, the presence of pulmonary embolism within 60 days of CMR was significantly associated ($P = .03$) with patients with RA thrombus (13%) vs. patients without RA thrombus (2%), as identified by LGE-CMR.

Differentiation From Neoplasm

A fundamental strength of LGE-CMR assessment of thrombus stems from its ability to identify avascular tissue based on the absence of contrast enhancement. Conversely, the approach can also be used to identify vascularity based on the presence of enhancement within a given region.

Thrombus is intrinsically avascular whereas neoplasms require vascular supply. Leveraging this dichotomy, LGE has been increasingly used as a tool to characterize cardiac masses,[22,23] for which a key clinical need has been the differentiation of thrombus from neoplasm.

In a broad multicenter study testing the utility of CMR for evaluating cardiac masses, Shenoy et al. demonstrated that CMR provides high diagnostic accuracy and prognostic utility.[24] A uniform diagnostic algorithm was employed that distinguished masses from "pseudomasses" (embryonic remnant/anatomic variant or prominent normal structures) based on morphologic appearance on functional (cine) or traditional bright- or dark-blood imaging. Masses were thereafter characterized based on tissue properties on (long-TI) LGE-CMR. As in prior studies detailed above, thrombus was diagnosed based on the absence of contrast uptake (avascular tissue properties). Neoplasms were defined by the presence of enhancement (vascularity) within a given mass and were further characterized as benign or malignant based on ancillary features (e.g., tissue invasion, irregular borders, T1/T2 properties, perfusion). To assess the accuracy of the CMR diagnosis, a 'final diagnosis' for each patient was established using clinical data (including follow-up imaging, pathology data, clinical course [e.g., resolution of thrombus with anticoagulation], and outcomes). The study cohort comprised 903 patients with suspected neoplasm undergoing CMR at four participating institutions. Pathology was available in 226 cases (47% of patients with a CMR diagnosis of benign neoplasm, 60% with a CMR diagnosis of malignant neoplasm). Based on the above algorithm, the CMR diagnosis (25% no mass, 16% pseudomass, 16% thrombus, 17% benign neoplasm, 23% malignant neoplasm) was accurate in 98.4% (889/903) of cases compared against the final diagnosis; only one case (small chaotically mobile lesion) had an incorrect diagnosis of "no mass" on CMR. Follow-up was performed for a median of 4.9 (IQR 1.6–7.3) years, during which patients with pseudomasses and benign neoplasms on CMR had a similar all-cause mortality rate compared to those with no mass, whereas those with thrombus and malignant tumor had increased mortality (both $P<.001$). On Cox proportional hazards regression analysis, CMR diagnosis of thrombus (hazard ratio [HR] = 1.46 [95% CI 1.00–2.11]; $P=.048$) and CMR diagnosis of malignant tumor (HR = 3.31 [95% CI 2.40–4.57]; $P<.001$) were independently associated with mortality even after adjustment for age (HR = 1.09 [CI 1.04–1.13] per 5-year increase), smoking (HR = 1.37 [95% CI 1.11–1.69]), LVEF (HR = 1.05 [95% CI 1.01–1.10] per 5% decrease), and extracardiac malignancy (HR = 2.32 [95% CI 1.81–2.97]; all $P<.05$). CMR-assigned mass classifications yielded incremental prognostic utility among subgroups of patients with and without extracardiac malignancy. Notably, findings from Shenoy et al.[24] align with those of other groups, including studies reporting good performance of LGE-CMR for differentiation of thrombus and neoplasm in both pediatric[25] and adult[26,27] patient populations.

Consistent with data showing its utility in broad cohorts with suspected cardiac masses, one key focus of CMR has been its utility to differentiate thrombus from metastasis in patients with systemic cancer. This application is particularly pertinent given that cardiac metastases (i.e., systemic cancers that metastasize to the heart) are far more common than primary tumors, with a reported 20–40-fold higher incidence. For example, among an autopsy series of 12,485 cases over a 20-year interval, the incidence of primary and secondary cardiac neoplasms was 0.056% and 1.23%, respectively—with the latter varying in both cancer etiology and cardiac location.[28] It is also known that cancer increases systemic hypercoagulability, resulting in an increased proclivity to thrombus formation in the heart and elsewhere. Finally, it should be noted that treatment pathways for cardiac thrombus and metastasis can fundamentally differ, further highlighting the need for accurate diagnosis.

LGE-CMR has been shown to provide prognostic value with respect to differentiating between cardiac metastasis and thrombus among patients with systemic cancer. To test this concept, Chan et al. studied 126 systemic cancer patients undergoing CMR, including patients with cardiac masses (18% thrombus, 32% neoplasm as defined by LGE) and controls (without masses) matched for cancer diagnosis and stage.[29] Mortality during a median follow-up of 2.5 (IQR 1.1–3.8) years was markedly higher among patients with LGE-CMR–defined cardiac metastases compared to those with thrombus (HR = 3.13 [95% CI 1.54–6.39], $P=.002$); prognosis was similar when patients were stratified by lesion size as measured by area (HR = 0.99 per cm2 [95% CI 0.98–1.01], $P=.40$) or maximal diameter (HR = 0.98 per cm [95% CI 0.91–1.06], $P=.61$). Diagnostic differentiation between thrombus and metastasis based on visual interpretation corresponded to quantitative analyses, as evidenced by increased contrast-to-noise (CNR) and signal-to-noise ratios (SNR) (both $P<.01$) for metastases—consistent with tumor requisite vascularity. Fig. 32.4 provides representative examples of neoplasm and thrombus evaluation by CMR, including distinct enhancement patterns in neoplasms and quantitative differences with thrombus.

Regarding quantification, it should be noted that some studies have suggested LGE to be more robust than other CMR tissue characterization metrics for the differentiation of thrombus from neoplasm. For example, among 116 patients undergoing CMR for the evaluation of cardiac masses, Pablo Pazos-López et al. compared an array of CMR approaches, including LGE, perfusion, and quantitative relaxation metrics (T1 and T2).[26] The authors reported that the ability of CMR features to distinguish benign from malignant neoplasms was moderate, with LGE showing the highest accuracy (79%). Regarding differentiation of neoplasm and thrombus, results demonstrated the highest performance to be yielded by inversion recovery pulse sequences, including TI scout (95% accuracy) and LGE-CMR (87% accuracy).

Regarding alternative CMR techniques to differentiate thrombus from neoplasm, Chan et al. compared perfusion to LGE-CMR, with a focus on the prognostic implications of differential performance characteristics.[11] The group studied 462 cancer patients, including patients with cardiac metastases (n = 173) and thrombus (n = 69) classified using the reference standard of LGE-CMR, as well as cancer matched controls. Whereas first-pass perfusion demonstrated metastases to have increased

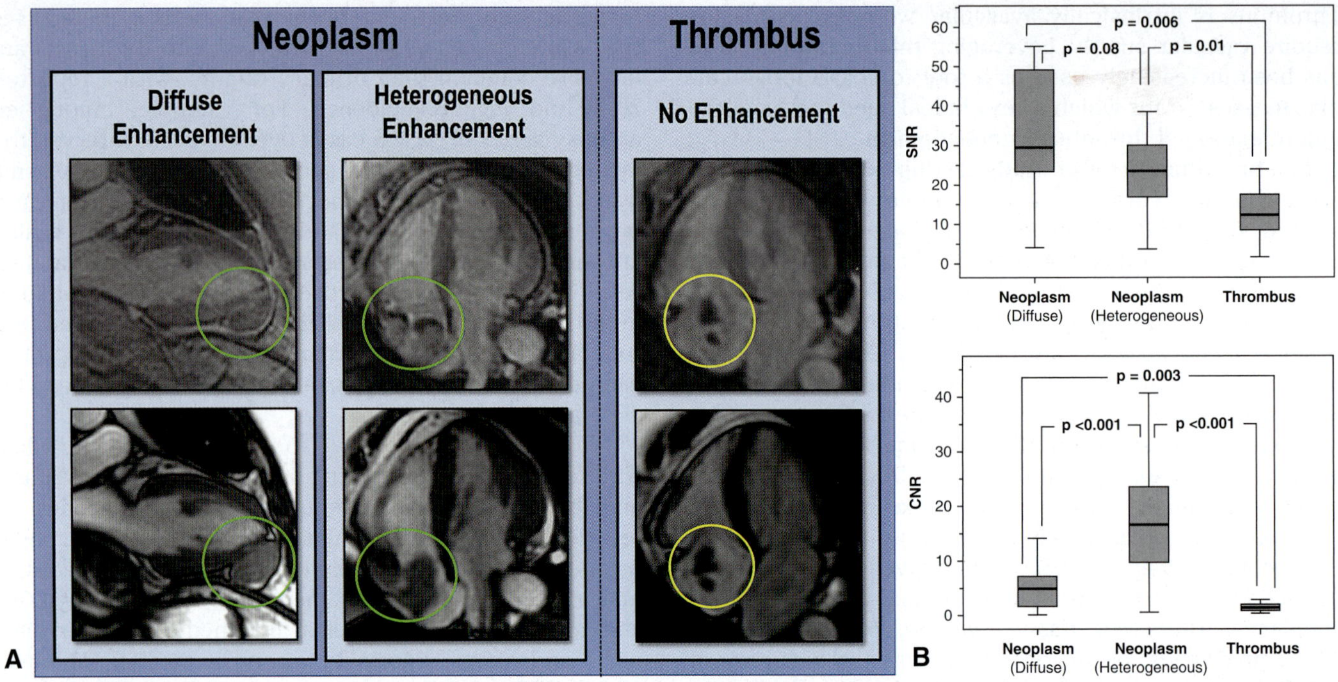

FIG. 32.4 Differentiation of cardiac neoplasm and thrombus by late gadolinium enhancement (LGE) cardiac magnetic resonance (CMR). (A) Two examples of cardiac neoplasms (*left*), for which diagnostic classification was based on the presence of lesion enhancement discerned by LGE-CMR (lesions denoted within *green circles*). Corresponding cine-CMR images shown on bottom for purpose of anatomic localization. Both lesions (diffusely enhancing pericardial lesion adjacent to left ventricle [LV], heterogeneously enhancing right atrial [RA] lesion) identified in patients with melanoma. Conversely, for the patient example on the right, LGE-CMR demonstrated the lesion (*yellow circle*) to be nonenhancing—consistent with avascular composition (*thrombus*). (B) Signal-to-noise ratio (SNR) and contrast-to-noise ratio (CNR) compared between patient groups with cardiac neoplasm and thrombus (data shown as overall distribution [*line bars*] together with 25%–75% distribution [*box*] and median [*central line*]). Note that SNR and CNR were generally higher for C_{NEO}, consistent with contrast enhancement secondary to vascular supply. SNR and CNR comparisons between neoplasm subtypes (diffuse and heterogeneous enhancement) showed increased CNR within heterogeneously enhancing lesions (P<.001 vs. other types), consistent with interspersed regions with and without adequate vascular supply. (Modified from Chan AT, Plodkowski AJ, Pun SC, et al., Prognostic utility of differential tissue characterization of cardiac neoplasm and thrombus via late gadolinium enhancement cardiovascular magnetic resonance among patients with advanced systemic cancer. *J Cardiovasc Magn Reson*. 2017;19(1):76.)

enhancement (consistent with vascularity), perfusion demonstrated modest yield with respect to diagnostic differentiation. Among metrics tested, the perfusion-CMR–evidenced “contrast uptake rate” (defined as slope of signal intensity curve during initial contrast infusion) yielded the highest overall performance (Area Under the Curve [AUC] = 0.93) and accuracy (87%), but its sensitivity (84%) and negative predictive value (71%) were suboptimal, which was attributable to substantial false negatives (n = 27) that typically occurred in the context of metastases with minimal enhancement on LGE. To further test the relative utility of LGE and perfusion, the authors studied a subgroup of 32 patients with LGE-evidenced metastases who had pathology analyses either via surgical excision or biopsy of cardiac and/or contiguous extracardiac tissue, Whereas all had pathology- (and LGE-) evidenced neoplasms, perfusion correctly classified lesions as neoplastic in 75% (24/32). Fig. 32.5 provides examples of perfusion-CMR assessment of cardiac neoplasms for which assessment was impaired in the context of low vascularity lesions, thus confounding differentiation with thrombus.

Mortality in the above study was assessed after CMR (median follow-up duration of 29 [IQR 12.6–48.5] months) to test if perfusion-based diagnostic classification of cardiac metastasis and thrombus conferred a differential prognosis, and if the magnitude of lesion perfusion further differentiated mortality risk. Whereas both CMR methods showed mortality to be increased among patients with cardiac metastases, risk was higher using LGE (HR = 1.52 [95% CI 1.16–2.00]; P = .003) than perfusion (semiquantitative HR = 1.42 [95% CI 1.06–1.90]; P = .02). Regarding thrombus, LGE yielded similar mortality risk between cases and controls (HR = 1.43 [95% CI 0.88–2.32]; P = .15). Conversely, patients with perfusion-CMR–classified thrombus had higher mortality than controls (HR = 1.61 [95% CI 1.07–2.41]; P. 0.02), consistent with the previously noted misclassification of low vascularity (predominantly hypoenhancing) neoplasms.

LGE-CMR has also been compared to metabolic imaging (positron emission tomography [PET]) with regard to its relative diagnostic and prognostic utility among patients with systemic cancer and cardiac masses. Building on prior research, Chan et al. studied 121 cancer patients undergoing CMR and whole-body 18F-fluorodeoxyglucose (18F-FDG) PET[30,31]: Imaging tests were attained within a median interval of 14.8 (IQR 3.9–34.5) days. Consistent with validation literature detailed above, lesion type was defined using the reference standard of LGE (46 neoplasm, 20 thrombus) based on the presence or absence of enhancement; cardiac neoplasm was identified on PET as a discrete lesion with differential FDG uptake from the surrounding blood pool and/or myocardium. All thrombi were nonenhancing on LGE, and none were metabolically active on PET. Among patients with neoplasm, signal-to-noise ratio on LGE CMR moderately correlated with standardized uptake values on PET (r = 0.42–0.49, P < .05). PET yielded reasonable,

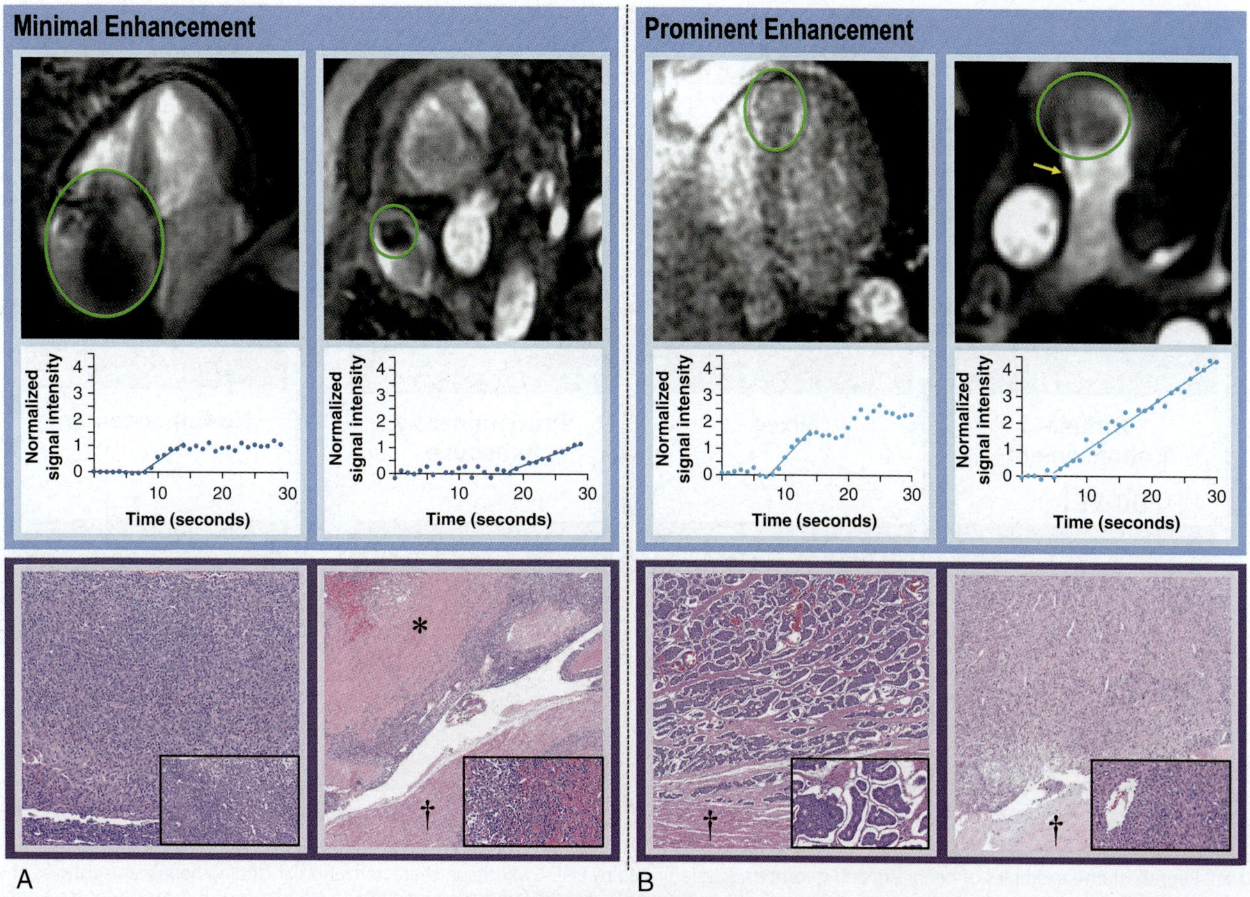

FIG. 32.5 Perfusion cardiac magnetic resonance (CMR) for assessment of pathology-evidenced lesion vascularity. Representative examples of cardiac metastases (C_{MET}) with variable magnitude of perfusion (*top*) together with semiquantitative perfusion CMR analysis (*middle*) and pathology-evidenced lesion vascularity (*bottom*). As shown, variability in contrast kinetics on perfusion CMR paralleled differential vascular and cell density on pathology. (A) Two cases of minimally enhancing C_{MET} on perfusion CMR, including thymoma (*left*), for which pathology demonstrated high tumor cell burden with minimal vascular content, and melanoma (*right*), for which pathology demonstrated scattered vascular content (*melanoma*) with prominent tumor necrosis. (B) Two cases of prominently enhancing C_{MET} on perfusion-CMR (*left*: neuroendocrine, *right*: spindle cell sarcoma), both of which had high vascular density on pathology. *Asterisk*, tumor necrosis; *dagger*, myocardium; *inserts*, high-power views of tumor components (pathology images obtained using hematoxylin and eosin staining). (Modified from Chan AT, Maya TR, Park C, et al., Incremental utility of first-pass perfusion CMR for prognostic risk stratification of cancer-associated cardiac masses. *JACC Cardiovasc Imaging*. 2024;17(2):128–145.)

albeit imperfect, sensitivity (70%–83%) for neoplasm. As shown in Fig. 32.6, diffusely enhancing or mixed lesions were more likely to be detected by PET than were predominantly avascular lesions (87% vs. 63%). Impaired detection of LGE-CMR–evidenced neoplasms impacted the prognostic performance of PET. All-cause mortality was higher among patients with CMR-evidenced neoplasm vs. controls (HR = 1.99 [95% CI 1.1–3.6]; P=.03) despite nonsignificant differences when partitioned via FDG avidity (HR = 1.56 [95% CI 0.85–2.74]; P=.16). Among FDG-positive neoplasms detected concordantly with CMR, mortality risk versus cancer-matched controls was equivalently increased (HR = 2.12 [95% CI 1.01–4.44]; P=.047). Taken together, these findings add to a growing body of data supporting the utility of LGE-CMR as a first-line strategy for the identification and diagnostic differentiation of cardiac neoplasm and thrombus.

FUTURE DIRECTIONS

Evidence-based literature to date has largely focused on the diagnostic and prognostic value of imaging for the identification of thrombus, as well as the differentiation of thrombus from other types of cardiac masses. Whereas thrombus provides a rationale for anticoagulation, therapeutic response is variable. Further research is warranted to test whether CMR tissue characterization via LGE or other methods provides utility for prediction of response to anticoagulation, as well as whether thrombus tissue characteristics on CMR can be used to inform the type and intensity of treatment. It is also known that contrast agents other than gadolinium (as is used for LGE) can be used for CMR. MRI probes that target platelet aggregation[32–34] and fibrin[35] have been tested in experimental animal models but have yet to be used in broad clinical cohorts as a tool to assay the presence and/or chronicity of thrombus. Beyond identification of thrombus at the time of imaging, the predictive value of CMR for future thrombus has yet to be tested; it is also uncertain whether given features of thrombus confer risk for embolism. For example, it has been shown that the extent of myocardial infarction (on LGE) is strongly associated with LV thrombus[1,8] and that patients with LGE-evidenced infarct are at increased risk for stroke even if thrombus is absent at time of CMR.[6] Given this,

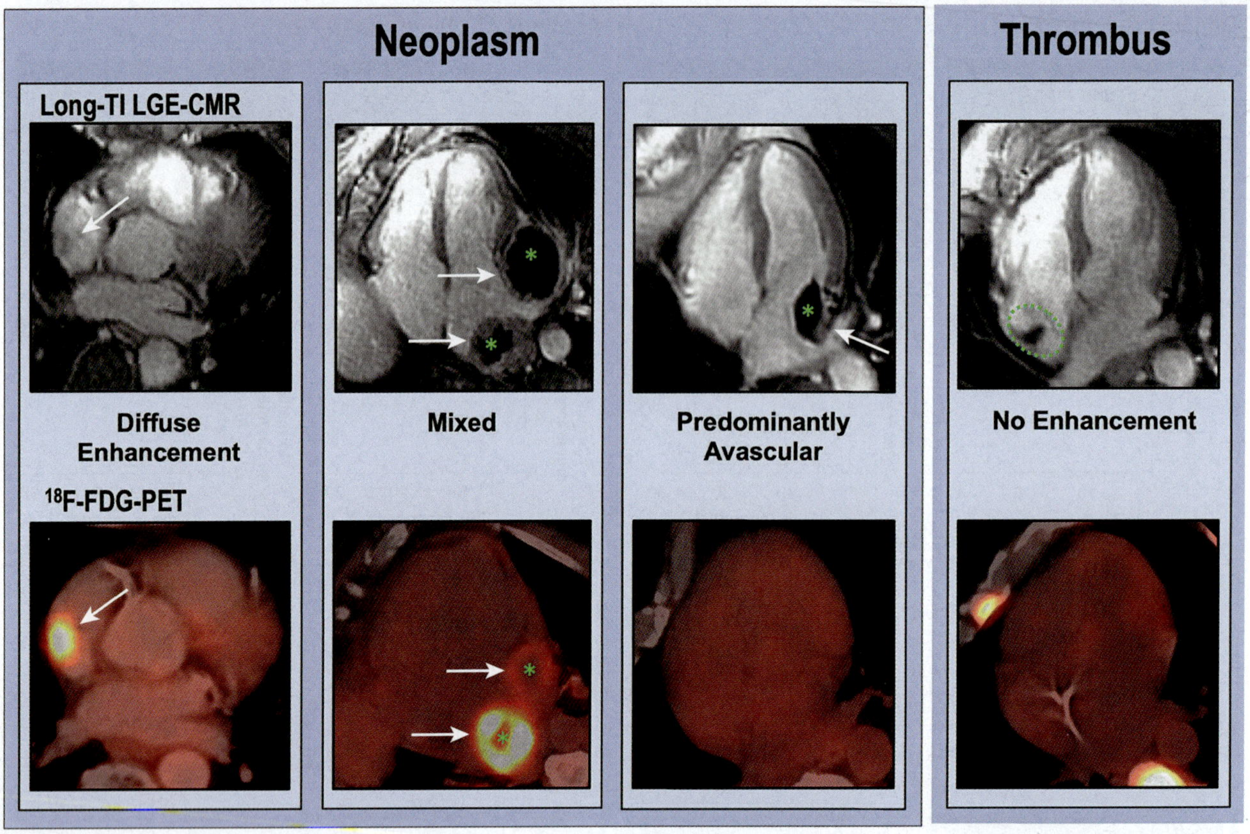

FIG. 32.6 Late gadolinium enhancement-cardiac magnetic resonance (*LGE-CMR*) in positron emission tomography (*PET*) assessment of thrombus and neoplasm. Representative examples of neoplasm and thrombus as established by LGE-CMR tissue characterization, including neoplasm subtypes of diffuse enhancement (*left*), mixed (prominent enhancing and avascular components; *center*), and predominantly avascular (*right*) (*arrows*, contrast-enhancing regions; *asterisks*, avascular regions). Corresponding PET images shown on bottom row: Note prominent fluorodeoxyglucose (*FDG*) avidity corresponding to regions of contrast enhancement and lack of FDG avidity in both predominantly avascular neoplasm as well as thrombus (*far right*). *Long-TI*, long inversion time. (Modified from Chan AT, Fox J, Perez Johnston R, et al., Late Gadolinium enhancement cardiac magnetic resonance tissue characterization for cancer-associated cardiac masses: metabolic and prognostic manifestations in relation to whole-body positron emission tomography. *J Am Heart Assoc*. 2019;8(10):e011709.)

future research is warranted to test whether CMR profiling can be used to predict the development and embolic potential of thrombus so as to rationally inform prophylactic anticoagulation.

SUMMARY

CMR tissue characterization provides a robust and well-validated means for diagnosis and prediction of outcomes among patients with known or suspected cardiac thrombus. Among CMR techniques, LGE—which identifies thrombus based on intrinsic tissue properties stemming from avascularity—has been shown to provide incremental utility vs. conventional imaging methods that identify thrombus based on morphologic appearance, and to perform well in broad clinical cohorts for whom it has demonstrated high diagnostic accuracy and prognostic utility.

REFERENCES

1. Weinsaft JW, Kim HW, Shah DJ, et al. Detection of left ventricular thrombus by delayed-enhancement cardiovascular magnetic resonanceprevalence and markers in patients with systolic dysfunction. *J Am Coll Cardiol*. 2008;52(2):148–157.
2. Weinsaft JW, Kim HW, Crowley AL, et al. LV thrombus detection by routine echocardiography: insights into performance characteristics using delayed enhancement CMR. *JACC Cardiovasc Imaging*. 2011;4(7):702–712.
3. Srichai MB, Junor C, Rodriguez LL, et al. Clinical, imaging, and pathological characteristics of left ventricular thrombus: a comparison of contrast-enhanced magnetic resonance imaging, transthoracic echocardiography, and transesophageal echocardiography with surgical or pathological validation. *Am Heart J*. 2006;152(1):75–84.
4. Shah D, Judd R, Kim RJ. Myocardial viability. In: Edelman RR, Hesselink JR, Zlatkin MB, Crues JV, eds. *Clinical Magnetic Resonance Imaging*. 3rd ed. Elsevier; 2006.
5. Velangi PS, Choo C, Chen KA, et al. Long-term embolic outcomes after detection of left ventricular thrombus by late gadolinium enhancement cardiovascular magnetic resonance imaging: a matched cohort study. *Circ Cardiovasc Imaging*. 2019;12(11):e009723.
6. Merkler AE, Alakbarli J, Gialdini G, et al. Short-term risk of ischemic stroke after detection of left ventricular thrombus on cardiac magnetic resonance imaging. *J Stroke Cerebrovasc Dis*. 2019;28(4):1027–1031.
7. Weinsaft JW, Kim J, Medicherla CB, et al. Echocardiographic algorithm for post-myocardial infarction LV thrombus: a gatekeeper for thrombus evaluation by delayed enhancement CMR. *JACC Cardiovasc Imaging*. 2016;9(5):505–515.
8. Weinsaft JW, Kim RJ, Ross M, et al. Contrast-enhanced anatomic imaging as compared to contrast-enhanced tissue characterization for detection of left ventricular thrombus. *JACC Cardiovasc Imaging*. 2009;2(8):969–979.
9. Plodkowski AJ, Chan AT, Gupta D, et al. Diagnostic utility and clinical implication of late gadolinium enhancement cardiac magnetic resonance for detection of catheter associated right atrial thrombus. *Clin Imaging*. 2020;62:17–22.
10. Kitkungvan D, Nabi F, Ghosn MG, et al. Detection of LA and LAA thrombus by CMR in patients referred for pulmonary vein isolation. *JACC Cardiovasc Imaging*. 2016;9(7):809–818.
11. Chan AT, Maya TR, Park C, et al. Incremental utility of first-pass perfusion CMR for prognostic risk stratification of cancer-associated cardiac masses. *JACC Cardiovasc Imaging*. 2024;17(2):128–145.

12. Garg P, van der Geest RJ, Swoboda PP, et al. Left ventricular thrombus formation in myocardial infarction is associated with altered left ventricular blood flow energetics. *Eur Heart J Cardiovasc Imaging*. 2019;20(1):108–117.
13. Delewi R, Nijveldt R, Hirsch A, et al. Left ventricular thrombus formation after acute myocardial infarction as assessed by cardiovascular magnetic resonance imaging. *Eur J Radiol*. 2012;81(12):3900–3904.
14. Meurin P, Brandao Carreira V, Dumaine R, et al. Incidence, diagnostic methods, and evolution of left ventricular thrombus in patients with anterior myocardial infarction and low left ventricular ejection fraction: a prospective multicenter study. *Am Heart J*. 2015;170(2):256–262.
15. Caspar T, El Ghannudi S, Ohana M, et al. Magnetic resonance evaluation of cardiac thrombi and masses by T1 and T2 mapping: an observational study. *Int J Cardiovasc Imaging*. 2017;33(4):551–559.
16. Bulluck H, Chan MHH, Paradies V, et al. Incidence and predictors of left ventricular thrombus by cardiovascular magnetic resonance in acute ST-segment elevation myocardial infarction treated by primary percutaneous coronary intervention: a meta-analysis. *J Cardiovasc Magn Reson*. 2018;20(1):72.
17. Ohyama H, Hosomi N, Takahashi T, et al. Comparison of magnetic resonance imaging and transesophageal echocardiography in detection of thrombus in the left atrial appendage. *Stroke*. 2003;34(10):2436–2439.
18. Rathi VK, Reddy ST, Anreddy S, et al. Contrast-enhanced CMR is equally effective as TEE in the evaluation of left atrial appendage thrombus in patients with atrial fibrillation undergoing pulmonary vein isolation procedure. *Heart Rhythm*. 2013;10(7):1021–1027.
19. Chen J, Zhang H, Zhu D, Wang Y, Byanju S, Liao M. Cardiac MRI for detecting left atrial/left atrial appendage thrombus in patients with atrial fibrillation: meta-analysis and systematic review. *Herz*. 2019;44(5):390–397.
20. Martinez-Naharro A, Gonzalez-Lopez E, Corovic A, et al. High prevalence of intracardiac thrombi in cardiac amyloidosis. *J Am Coll Cardiol*. 2019;73(13):1733–1734.
21. Ogren M, Bergqvist D, Eriksson H, Lindblad B, Sternby NH. Prevalence and risk of pulmonary embolism in patients with intracardiac thrombosis: a population-based study of 23 796 consecutive autopsies. *Eur Heart J*. 2005;26(11):1108–1114.
22. Hundley WG, Bluemke DA, Finn JP, et al. ACCF/ACR/AHA/NASCI/SCMR 2010 expert consensus document on cardiovascular magnetic resonance. *Circulation*. 2010;121(22):2462–2508.
23. Leiner T, Bogaert J, Friedrich MG, et al. SCMR position paper (2020) on clinical indications for cardiovascular magnetic resonance. *J Cardiovasc Magn Reson*. 2020;22(1):76.
24. Shenoy C, Grizzard JD, Shah DJ, et al. Cardiovascular magnetic resonance imaging in suspected cardiac tumour: a multicentre outcomes study. *Eur Heart J*. 2021;43(1):71–80.
25. Beroukhim Rebecca S, Ghelani S, Ashwath R, et al. Accuracy of cardiac magnetic resonance imaging in diagnosing pediatric cardiac masses. *JACC Cardiovasc Imaging*. 2022;15(8):1391–1405.
26. Pazos-Lopez P, Pozo E, Siqueira ME, et al. Value of CMR for the differential diagnosis of cardiac masses. *JACC Cardiovasc Imaging*. 2014;7(9):896–905.
27. Mousavi N, Cheezum Michael K, Aghayev A, et al. Assessment of cardiac masses by cardiac magnetic resonance imaging: histological correlation and clinical outcomes. *J Am Heart Assoc*. 2019;8(1):e007829.
28. Lam KY, Dickens P, Chan AC. Tumors of the heart. A 20-year experience with a review of 12,485 consecutive autopsies. *Arch Pathol Lab Med*. 1993;117(10):1027–1031.
29. Chan AT, Plodkowski AJ, Pun SC, et al. Prognostic utility of differential tissue characterization of cardiac neoplasm and thrombus via late gadolinium enhancement cardiovascular magnetic resonance among patients with advanced systemic cancer. *J Cardiovasc Magn Reson*. 2017;19(1):76.
30. Chan AT, Fox J, Perez Johnston R, et al. Late gadolinium enhancement cardiac magnetic resonance tissue characterization for cancer-associated cardiac masses: metabolic and prognostic manifestations in relation to whole-body positron emission tomography. *J Am Heart Assoc*. 2019;8(10):e011709.
31. Aghayev A, Cheezum MK, Steigner ML, et al. Multimodality imaging to distinguish between benign and malignant cardiac masses. *J Nucl Cardiol*. 2022;29(4):1504–1517.
32. Klink A, Lancelot E, Ballet S, et al. Magnetic resonance molecular imaging of thrombosis in an arachidonic acid mouse model using an activated platelet targeted probe. *Arterioscler Thromb Vasc Biol*. 2010;30(3):403–410.
33. Duerschmied D, Meißner M, Peter K, et al. Molecular magnetic resonance imaging allows the detection of activated platelets in a new mouse model of coronary artery thrombosis. *Invest Radiol*. 2011;46(10):618–623.
34. von zur Muhlen C, von Elverfeldt D, Moeller JA, et al. Magnetic resonance imaging contrast agent targeted toward activated platelets allows in vivo detection of thrombosis and monitoring of thrombolysis. *Circulation*. 2008;118(3):258–267.
35. Winter PM, Caruthers SD, Yu X, et al. Improved molecular imaging contrast agent for detection of human thrombus. *Magn Reson Med*. 2003;50(2):411–416.

33 CMR of Cardiac Masses

CHETAN SHENOY AND JOHN D. GRIZZARD

INTRODUCTION

Overview

Cardiac masses represent a diverse group of pathologies that include both neoplastic and nonneoplastic entities. The prevalence of cardiac masses varies based on their type. Primary cardiac tumors are rare, with an incidence estimated at 0.001% to 0.03% in autopsy studies. Of these, approximately 75% are benign, with myxomas and papillary fibroelastomas being the most common. The remaining 25% are malignant, with sarcomas representing the most prevalent subtype. In contrast, metastatic cardiac tumors are much more common, with a frequency up to 20–40 times higher than primary tumors. Lung and breast carcinomas, hematologic malignancies, and melanomas are among the most frequent sources of cardiac metastases.

Nonneoplastic masses such as thrombi, vegetations, and inflammatory masses must also be distinguished from true neoplasms, as their clinical management significantly differs. Patients with suspected cardiac masses may also be found to have no mass or a "pseudomass," such as a prominent normal structure (eustachian valve, crista terminalis, etc.), a variant of a normal structure (lipomatous hypertrophy of the interatrial septum, epicardial fat, etc.), or a nonmass pathology (hiatal hernia) that could be mistaken for a cardiac mass. Given their diverse etiology and the potentially life-threatening consequences of a misdiagnosis, accurate identification and characterization of cardiac masses are critical in clinical practice.

Although cardiac masses are relatively uncommon, they are increasingly a source of referrals for cardiovascular magnetic resonance (CMR) imaging, as CMR is now recognized as the gold standard in the detection and characterization of cardiac masses. It is also the gold standard for the detection and characterization of intracardiac thrombus. Moreover, CMR is also the definitive technique for the exclusion of real pathology when normal variants or pseudotumors need to be distinguished from true neoplasms.

Why Cardiovascular Magnetic Resonance?

CMR imaging has emerged as one of the most powerful diagnostic tools for evaluating suspected cardiac masses. Among all the imaging techniques, CMR also has the most robust evidence supporting its use.

Advantages of CMR in the evaluation of a suspected cardiac mass include:

- **Superior Tissue Characterization:** CMR's ability to distinguish between fat, fluid, fibrosis, and tumor tissue is unparalleled. This is particularly valuable in distinguishing benign from malignant tumors or neoplastic from nonneoplastic masses.
- **Functional Assessment:** In addition to anatomical imaging, CMR provides dynamic assessments of mass mobility, cardiac chamber function, and blood flow. This is essential for evaluating the hemodynamic consequences of a mass, such as obstruction of blood flow or interference with valvular function.
- **Noninvasive Nature:** Unlike biopsy or other invasive diagnostic procedures, CMR provides a comprehensive evaluation without exposing the patient to procedural risks or ionizing radiation.
- **Multiplanar Imaging:** CMR's ability to image in multiple planes (axial, sagittal, coronal) and reconstruct three-dimensional images offers an in-depth evaluation of mass size, extent, and relationship to surrounding structures, which is vital for surgical planning.
- **Late Gadolinium Enhancement (LGE):** The use of gadolinium-based contrast agents in CMR provides additional differentiation between tissues based on vascularity and extracellular matrix content, aiding in the identification of avascular structures such as thrombi, and heterogeneous structures such as malignancies.
- **Perfusion Imaging:** Perfusion imaging allows for the assessment of vascularity of a cardiac mass, an important feature useful in its characterization, and also provides important prognostic information.

In summary, CMR's soft tissue characterization, noninvasive nature, ability to perform functional and morphological assessments in a single session, and lack of ionizing radiation make it the imaging technique of choice for patients with suspected cardiac masses. CMR offers unparalleled precision in identifying the presence of a mass, distinguishing pseudomasses from true masses, distinguishing neoplastic from nonneoplastic masses, and distinguishing benign from malignant neoplasms.

CARDIOVASCULAR MAGNETIC RESONANCE TECHNIQUES (TABLE 33.1)

CMR techniques offer a multifaceted approach to assessing cardiac masses, using different software sequences to provide morphological, functional, and tissue characterization data. This section delves into the core CMR techniques used in evaluating cardiac masses, emphasizing

TABLE 33.1 Sequences used and information obtained using CMR for cardiac masses.

IMAGING	SEQUENCE TYPE	IMAGING PLANE	UTILITY IN IMAGING MASSES
Static morphologic images	Bright-blood imaging performed with single-shot SSFP. Dark-blood imaging performed with HASTE	Stack of images obtained usually in the axial plane. Can also obtain sagittal and coronal stacks	Localization of any mass present. Also useful to exclude a true mass or to visualize a pseudomass
Cine SSFP (standard)	Segmented SSFP cine images	Short axis images from base to apex. Two-, three-, and four-chamber long axis views. Also, images tailored to any mass found	Assess overall cardiac function and any functional compromise produced by a mass. Define lesion borders/infiltration
Perfusion imaging	Saturation recovery (T1-weighted) images to evaluate the transit of contrast through the myocardium	Tailored to provide orthogonal images of any mass detected	Determine lesion vascularity
LGE images (standard)	Segmented gradient-echo inversion-recovery images with inversion time chosen to "null" signal of normal myocardium	Exactly matched to cines	Enhancement characteristics very useful in lesion characterization
LGE images (long-TI)	Segmented gradient-echo inversion-recovery images with inversion time of 600 ms	Exactly matched to cines	Useful in determining lesion as avascular—such as thrombus
T1-weighted images/maps	Gated T1 FSE images (may be obtained pre- and post-contrast)	Matched to short-axis cine and LGE images	Assess T1 characteristics of lesion (cystic/fluid containing vs. solid, etc.). Fat suppression can be added
T2-weighted images/maps	Gated T2 FSE or STIR images. Note STIR images intrinsically fat-suppressed	Matched to short-axis cine and LGE images	Assess T2 characteristics of lesion. Sensitive to edema/fluid content. Fat suppression can be added

how each sequence contributes to tissue characterization, mass localization, and distinction of benign from malignant lesions.

Static Steady-State Free Precession (SSFP) (bright-blood)/HASTE (dark-blood): Scanning through the entire chest with static SSFP and HASTE images can be performed rapidly and without breath holding, and provides a comprehensive overview of cardiac and mediastinal anatomy. Typically, these are obtained in the axial plane with supplementary orthogonal imaging of any detected mass. They are also useful in the exclusion of a mass.

- **Examples:**
  - Cardiac masses and mediastinal lesions readily distinguished from normal structures.
  - Invasion of cardiac and vascular structures may be depicted.

SSFP Cine Imaging: This is the cornerstone for assessing cardiac anatomy and function. These sequences provide high-resolution images with excellent contrast between blood, myocardium, and cardiac masses. Cine CMR is primarily used to evaluate the location, size, and mobility of a mass. It is especially valuable for detecting masses that involve the valves (e.g., papillary fibroelastomas), atria (e.g., myxomas), or other mobile structures.

- **Examples:**
  - **Tumors:** Tumors appear as well-circumscribed masses with different contrast compared to the surrounding myocardium or blood pool. The mobility of pedunculated masses, such as atrial myxomas, is readily visualized.
  - **Thrombi:** Cine imaging can demonstrate the absence of mobility in thrombi, aiding in their differentiation from mobile masses such as myxomas or fibroelastomas.
  - **Vegetations:** Although small vegetations are challenging to visualize directly with cine imaging, SSFP sequences can detect associated valvular abnormalities and functional impact, such as regurgitation.

Perfusion Imaging: Perfusion imaging assesses the degree of vascularity in a cardiac mass, differentiating between highly perfused tumors such as hemangiomas and sarcomas, and avascular structures like thrombi.

- **Examples:**
  - **Tumors:** Some benign (such as hemangiomas) and some malignant (such as sarcomas) tumors demonstrate rapid contrast enhancement during first-pass perfusion, reflecting their rich vascular supply.
  - **Thrombi:** Thrombi, which are avascular, show no enhancement during perfusion imaging.

LGE Imaging: Postcontrast LGE imaging detects regions of fibrosis, scarring, or necrosis by capitalizing on the delayed washout of gadolinium in areas with altered extracellular matrix. LGE is pivotal for differentiating between benign and malignant cardiac masses based on the presence of fibrotic or necrotic tissue.

- **Examples:**
  - **Fibromas:** Cardiac fibromas often demonstrate intense, homogeneous LGE, reflecting their fibrous composition.
  - **Malignant Tumors:** Malignant tumors, particularly sarcomas and lymphomas, display heterogeneous LGE, with areas of necrosis appearing nonenhanced. The presence of extensive necrosis often indicates an aggressive tumor.

Long-Inversion Time (TI) LGE Imaging: LGE imaging with an inversion time (TI) of 600 milliseconds to null avascular structures highlights areas of avascularity such as thrombi and foreign bodies.[1]

- **Examples:**
  - **Thrombi:** Unlike tumors, thrombi do not enhance after gadolinium administration, a key feature for distinguishing them from neoplastic masses.
  - **Foreign Bodies and Calcium:** These are also avascular and do not enhance on long-TI LGE imaging.

T1-Weighted Fast Spin Echo Imaging: T1-weighted imaging helps in characterizing the composition of the mass. It is particularly useful for identifying fatty tumors (e.g., lipomas) or tumors with significant necrotic or fibrotic components.

- **Typical findings:**
  - **Fatty Tumors (Lipomas):** Lipomas have high signal intensity on T1-weighted images, distinguishing them from other types of cardiac masses.
  - **Melanomas:** Melanomas may demonstrate characteristic nodular deposits with high signal on T1-weighted images, which is virtually pathognomonic of this diagnosis.

T2-Weighted Fast Spin Echo Imaging: T2-weighted imaging is essential for detecting tumors with high water content, such as cystic lesions, and for identifying edema or necrosis in malignant tumors.

- **Examples:**
  - **Myxomas:** Some myxomas can exhibit high signal intensity on T2-weighted images due to their high water content.
  - **Malignant Tumors:** Malignant tumors such as sarcomas and lymphomas often have heterogeneous T2 signals, reflecting areas of necrosis, hemorrhage, or edema.
  - **Cystic Lesions:** Cysts (e.g., pericardial cysts) demonstrate very high signal intensity on T2-weighted imaging, which helps distinguish them from solid tumors.

Parametric Mapping: T1 and T2 Mapping: T1 and T2 mapping offer objective, quantitative measurements of tissue characteristics, which may aid in the differentiation between benign and malignant masses and the detection of tissue changes such as fibrosis or edema.

- **Examples:**
  - **T1 Mapping:** Elevated T1 values are often seen in malignant tumors due to increased cellularity and extracellular space. Fibrotic tissues, such as those seen in cardiac fibromas, also demonstrate high T1 values.
  - **T2 Mapping:** Increased T2 values are indicative of edema or necrosis, which are frequently present in malignant masses. T2 mapping can help quantify the degree of edema in tumors, thrombi, or surrounding myocardium.

CLASSIFICATION OF CARDIAC MASSES AND CMR APPEARANCES (TABLE 33.2)

Cardiac masses are a diverse group of pathologies with varying origins, behaviors, and implications for patient management. An accurate classification is essential not only for diagnosis but also for determining treatment strategies and prognosis. Broadly, cardiac masses can be classified into primary cardiac tumors, secondary (metastatic) tumors, nonneoplastic masses such as thrombi and vegetations, and pseudomasses. This section explores the various types of cardiac masses, focusing on their clinical features, pathology, and CMR characteristics.

Many of these masses have distinct CMR characteristics, which help distinguish them from one another and guide clinical decision-making.

Primary Cardiac Tumors

Primary cardiac tumors originate from the heart or pericardium itself and can be classified as benign or malignant. Although rare, with an incidence of about 0.001% to 0.03% in autopsy studies, their clinical relevance is profound due to the potential for significant hemodynamic effects, embolic complications, and in the case of malignancies, local invasion and metastasis.

Benign Primary Cardiac Tumors

Benign cardiac tumors account for the majority (approximately 75%) of primary cardiac tumors. Despite their benign nature, these masses can have significant clinical consequences, including obstruction of blood flow, embolization, and interference with valve function. The most common benign cardiac tumors include:

MYXOMA

Prevalence: In most autopsy and surgical series, myxomas (Fig. 33.1) have been found to be the most frequent primary cardiac tumors, representing approximately 50% of all benign heart tumors. The mean age at presentation is 50, with a broad range from childhood to late adulthood. Women make up two-thirds of cases and 90% of cases are sporadic. Ten percent of cases are part of the Carney complex, an autosomal dominant syndrome that includes multiple endocrine neoplasia, pigmented skin and mucosal lesions, and extracardiac mucinous tumors.

Presentation: The most common presenting symptom is dyspnea, in some cases related to valvular obstruction due to prolapse of a large mobile lesion (Fig. 33.2). Peripheral embolization may occur in left atrial lesions, and between 30%–50% of patients may have constitutional symptoms such as fatigue, weight loss, and fever.

Radiology/pathology correlation: Myxomas are found most often (~80% of cases) in the left atrium attached to the fossa ovalis, often by a short fibrous stalk. Between 10%–15% of cases are found in the right atrium, with a small percentage found in the ventricles or straddling the fossa ovalis as a biatrial lesion. They are largely gelatinous in composition, with a myxoid matrix that has a high water content. They most often have a smooth surface, but some have a papillary surface and those are more prone to embolic events. Minimal coating thrombus and internal calcifications are commonly seen.

TABLE 33.2 Cardiac masses and their typical CMR features.

LOCATION	LESION	TYPICAL CMR FEATURES	SPECIFIC FEATURES
Intracavitary	Myxoma	Oval, mobile left atrial lesion, heterogenous enhancement or homogeneous avascular appearance except for an enhancing stalk	Attachment to fossa ovalis
	Thrombus	Left atrium/appendage or ventricles at sites of stasis/infarction	Low-signal (dark) on long-TI LGE imaging
	Vegetations	Irregular nodules or masses arising along valvular surfaces and perivalvular tissues	Signal intensity similar to thrombus. May have associated septic pulmonary emboli
	Metastases	Transvenous extension of tumor	Lesions extend in continuity from primary lesion to heart
Intramyocardial—children	Rhabdomyomas	Multiple masses with signal intensity similar to muscle	Infants and children with tuberous sclerosis
	Fibromas	Solitary mass distorting normal anatomy	Low in signal intensity on T2-weighted images
Intramyocardial—adults	Metastases	Variable—pericardial effusions very common. Typically known late-stage malignancy. Lesions usually enhance	Melanoma metastases may show high signal on T1-weighted images.
	Lipomatous hypertrophy of interatrial septum	Thickening of septum to >2 cm; typically spares fossa ovalis. High signal on T1-weighted images	Signal drop-out on fat-saturation images
	Lipoma	Epicardial/intramural lesion with high signal on T1-weighted images	Signal drop-out on fat-saturation images
	Paraganglioma	Well-defined lesion arising in atrial walls or septum	"Light-bulb bright" on T2-weighted images
Epicardial/pericardial	Metastases	Variable, pericardial metastases more common than myocardial. Large pericardial effusions common	Direct tumor extension; adjacent adenopathy very suggestive
	Pericardial cyst	Well-defined nonenhancing lesion contiguous with pericardium	Signal follows fluid on all sequences
	Hemangioma	Multiloculated enhancing lesions, may involve epicardium and pericardium	High in signal on T1 and T2; slow progressive enhancement
	Lymphangioma	Rare multicystic lesions may be intramural, epicardial, or pericardial	Low in signal on T1-weighted images, high on T2

CMR findings are closely related to the histological findings of a gelatinous tumor often demonstrating a short fibrous stalk of attachment (Fig. 33.1).

- Cine SSFP: The lesion is higher in signal than myocardium, owing to its higher water content. They are often mobile on cine imaging.
- First-pass perfusion: Occasionally the stalk may show minimal uptake; otherwise, no uptake noted.
- LGE images with standard inversion time: Heterogeneous uptake commonly noted.
- LGE images with TI of 600 ms: The attachment site/stalk often shows enhancement, but the gelatinous periphery will be low in signal, mimicking thrombus. However, the higher signal usually seen on cine SSFP helps to distinguish myxomas from thrombus (which are isointense to myocardium on SSFP cine imaging) (Fig. 33.3).
- T1WI: Iso- or hypointense.
- T2WI: Hyperintense.

Differential diagnosis: The most common differential consideration is thrombus, which can be seen in the atria in cases of long-standing atrial stasis from atrial fibrillation or mitral stenosis. As noted above, thrombi are usually isointense to muscle on cine SSFP, different from myxomas. Rarely, atypical papillary fibroelastomas attached to the atrial endocardium may present a confusing appearance on cine imaging but can be distinguished by their significant enhancement on LGE images obtained with a 15–20-minute delay.

Treatment/prognosis: Surgical resection is usually curative, with rare recurrences essentially limited to syndromic myxomas.

PAPILLARY FIBROELASTOMA

Prevalence: In a 2021 statement by the WHO, papillary fibroelastomas (PFEs) were said to be the most common benign primary cardiac tumor, though most other published data suggest that they are the second most common. In addition, they are the most common neoplasm affecting the cardiac valves. The mean age at detection is 60, and some series suggest there is a slight male predominance.

Presentation: Patients are usually asymptomatic, and most are detected incidentally at imaging studies performed for other reasons. When symptoms do occur, they are usually due to embolic events.

Radiology/pathology correlation: PFEs are small (average size 8 mm) rounded to oval endocardial-based lesions most often located on the cardiac valves and attached by a

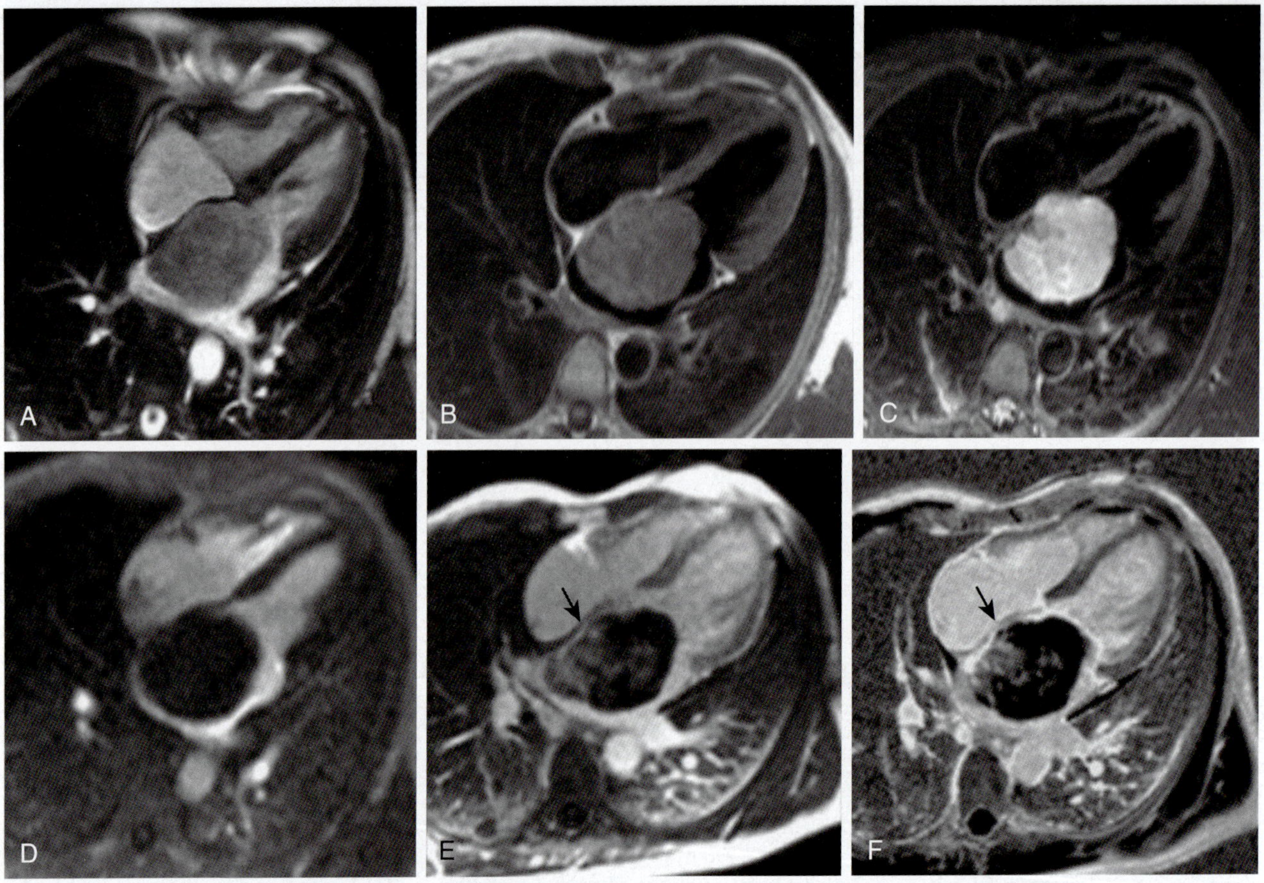

FIG. 33.1 Myxoma: Comprehensive assessment of a left atrial tumor using cardiac magnetic resonance. Four-chamber steady-state free-precession cine image (A) demonstrates a large left atrial myxoma showing the characteristic attachment to the fossa ovalis. Note that the tumor is hyperintense to myocardium on this sequence. T1-weighted image (B) shows that the lesion is isointense to myocardium, but is high in signal on the T2 STIR image (C). First-pass perfusion image (D) shows no uptake by the lesion, while long-TI LGE images (E) and standard LGE images with an inversion time of 300 ms chosen to null signal from normal myocardium (F) show heterogeneous enhancement of the myxoma, predominantly involving the attachment site (*arrows*). Note that the gelatinous periphery of the lesion is high in signal on the T2-weighted image (C), but low in signal on the long-inversion time image (E), in keeping with its jelly-like consistency.

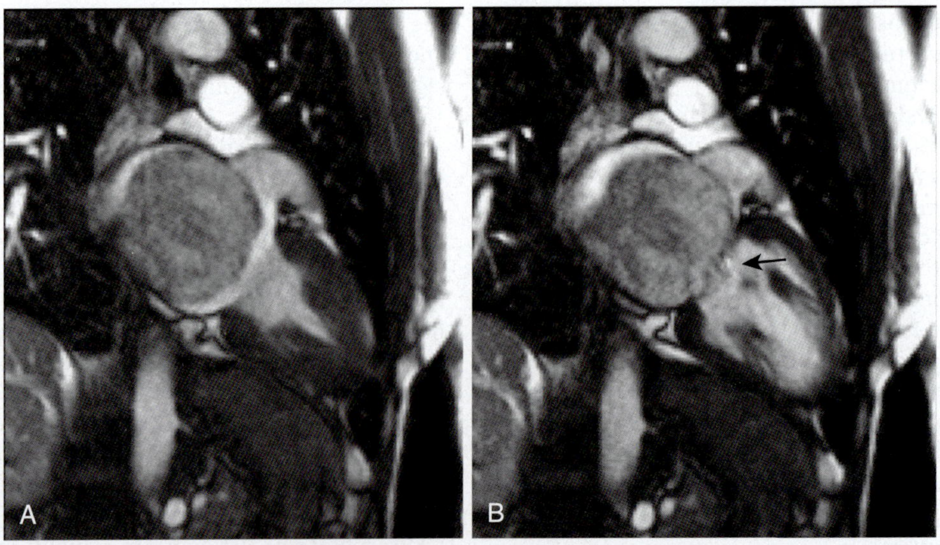

FIG. 33.2 Myxoma obstructing the mitral valve: Two-chamber SSFP cine views in systole (A) and diastole (B) show near-total obstruction of the mitral valve by a large mobile left atrial myxoma, with only a small jet of turbulent flow noted (*arrow* in B).

short stalk. The aortic valve is involved in ~30%, the mitral valve in 25%, pulmonic valve in ~13%, and the tricuspid valve in ~17%. They tend to be on the aortic side of the aortic valve and the left atrial side of the mitral valve. Nonvalvular locations make up the remainder. They are usually slightly removed from the free edge of the valve. Structurally, they are composed of avascular frond-like gelatinous and collagenous material with a surface coating of endothelial cells. The resultant appearance has been likened to that of a sea anemone.

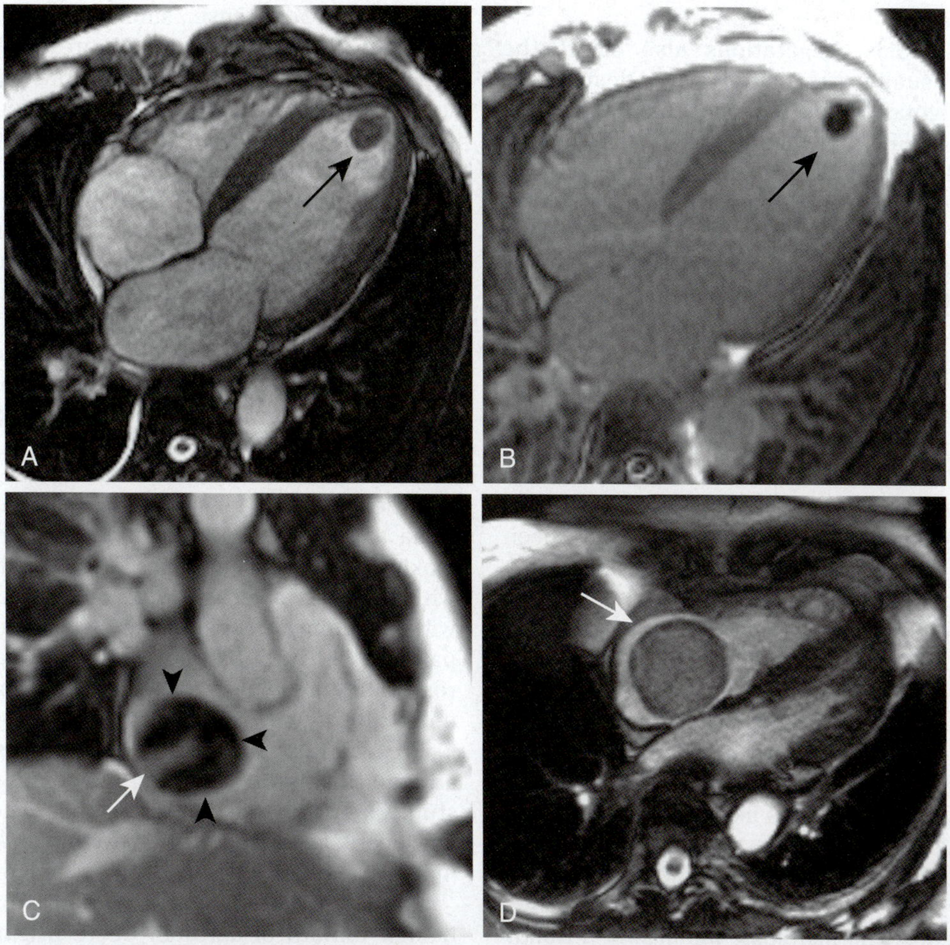

FIG. 33.3 Myxoma vs. thrombus: Four-chamber SSFP cine image (A) shows a polypoid filling defect at the left ventricular apex (*arrow*) that is isointense to LV myocardium. A four-chamber standard LGE image (B), a long-TI LGE image, shows the lesion to have low signal intensity, consistent with an avascular thrombus. For comparison, consider the right ventricular (RV) two-chamber LGE image (C), a long-TI LGE image, demonstrating a small stalk of enhancement (*arrow*) with a large peripheral low signal component (*arrowheads*). Although this appearance could be mistaken for a large thrombus coating a small myxoma, review of the cine SSFP image (D) in this patient shows that the lesion (*arrow*) is higher in signal than myocardium. Therefore, this should be recognized as a myxoma and not a thrombus, which would be isointense to myocardium on SSFP cine images as noted in (A).

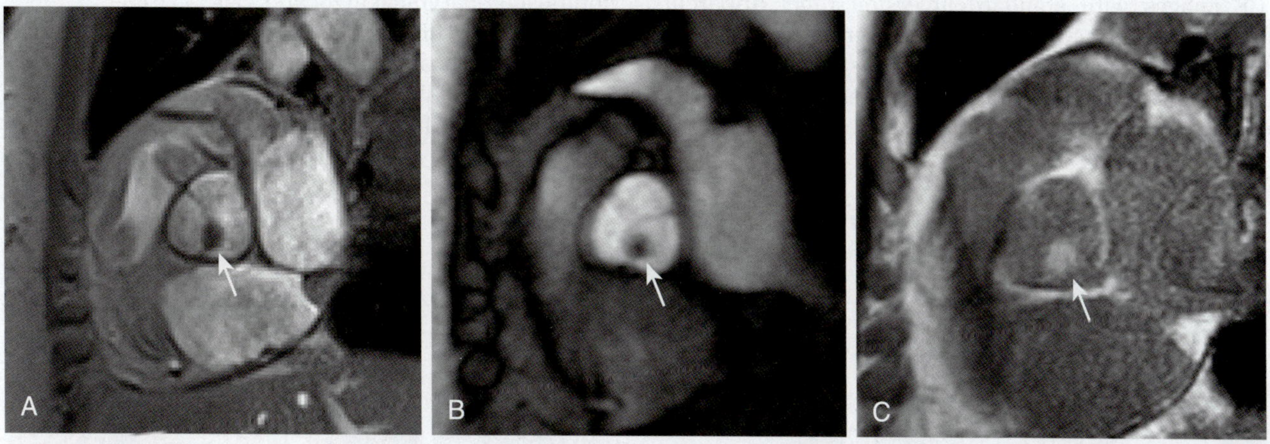

FIG. 33.4 Papillary fibroelastoma: Cine gradient echo aortic valve view (A) shows a rounded low-signal lesion representing a surgically proven papillary fibroelastoma attached to the noncoronary cusp. A first-pass perfusion image (B) shows no uptake by the lesion. An LGE image (C) obtained with a 20-minute delay post contrast shows clear enhancement of the papillary fibroelastoma.

CMR findings reflect the histologic findings of a small, gelatinous and fibrous lesion usually attached to a cardiac valve (Fig. 33.4).

- Cine SSFP: Small, rounded low-signal mobile lesion attached to a valve.
- First-pass perfusion: No uptake.
- LGE images with standard inversion time: Hyperenhancement is usually noted but may require delayed imaging to 15–20 minutes post-contrast.
- T1WI: Iso- or hypointense.

- T2WI: Hyperintense.

Differential diagnosis: Vegetations also affect the valves but are usually associated with destructive changes and valvular incompetence. Lambl excrescences may mimic PFEs, but usually occur at the valve leaflet edges and have a simple architecture without a frond-like appearance. Myxomas rarely involve the valves primarily.

Treatment/prognosis: Surgical resection is usually advised for left-sided lesions to prevent embolic events and is curative.

LIPOMA

Prevalence: These are rare benign tumors that are usually found in adults but may be seen in all age groups.

Presentation: Patients are usually asymptomatic, and most are detected incidentally at imaging studies performed for other reasons. They have occasionally been associated with arrhythmias, and large lesions may obstruct the intracardiac blood flow.

Radiology/pathology correlation: Lipomas are neoplasms composed of mature adipocytes which are encapsulated. They tend to be subendocardial in ~50% of cases, subepicardial in ~25%, and intramyocardial in ~25%. The left ventricle and right atrium are most often affected. Their size is variable ranging from a few millimeters to over 10 cm, with epicardial lesions likely to be larger than other locations. Histologically, they are well-defined fatty tumors with a discernible capsule and without invasion of normal tissue.

CMR findings reflect the histologic findings of a tumor composed of fat cells (Fig. 33.5).

- Cine SSFP: High signal is noted in the lesion that is similar in signal intensity to subcutaneous fat. An "etching artifact" is noted at the interface of the lesion with normal myocardium or the blood pool.
- First-pass perfusion: No uptake.
- LGE images with standard inversion time: Apparent enhancement is actually due to the intrinsic short T1 of the fatty tumor, and not due to contrast uptake.
- T1WI: Hyperintense, similar to fat elsewhere in the image. Suppresses on fat-suppressed images.
- T2WI: Hyperintense, similar to fat elsewhere in the image. Suppresses on fat-suppressed images.

Differential diagnosis: Lipomatous hypertrophy of the interatrial septum may occasionally mimic a lipoma, particularly atypical cases that extend beyond the septum. However, these are not neoplasms but rather represent hyperplasia of unencapsulated fat cells. Epicardial lipomas may be mimicked by teratomas, but teratomas are composed of multiple tissue types. Liposarcomas, when well differentiated, may resemble lipoma but will demonstrate uptake of contrast and infiltrating margins.

Treatment/prognosis: Surgical resection is usually curative. Occasionally, proximity to the coronary arteries limits the resection, but regrowth is uncommon.

RHABDOMYOMA

Prevalence: This benign tumor may represent a hamartoma and is the most common pediatric cardiac tumor, making up over 90% of cases. They are strongly associated with tuberous sclerosis, with 50% of patients presenting with rhabdomyoma being affected. In addition, virtually all patients with multiple rhabdomyomas have tuberous sclerosis. They are usually diagnosed in infancy, with few cases noted after the age of 6.

Presentation: Affected infants are usually asymptomatic, and many are detected incidentally at fetal imaging studies performed for other reasons. They have occasionally been associated with arrhythmias, and large lesions may cause obstruction of left ventricular outflow.

Radiology/pathology correlation: Rhabdomyomas are benign tumors of cardiomyocyte origin and are usually well circumscribed. They tend to involve the septum and the left ventricular free-wall myocardium, where they appear as intramural masses. At pathology they appear as nodules composed of rounded atypical myocytes termed "spider" cells.

CMR findings reflect the histologic findings of a tumor composed of atypical myocytes (Fig. 33.6).

- Cine SSFP: The lesions are similar in signal intensity to normal myocardium, and often appear as poorly contractile mass-like foci.
- First-pass perfusion: No uptake.

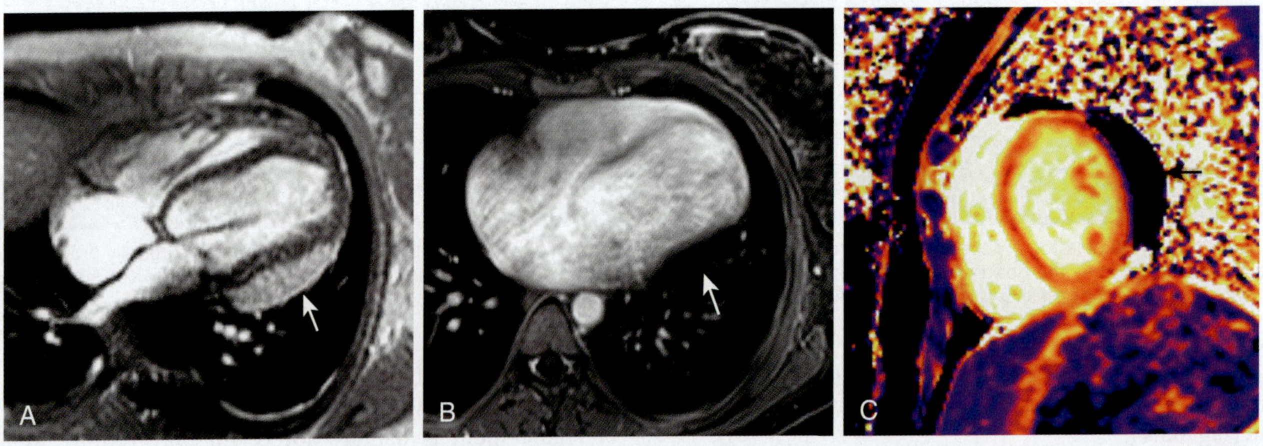

FIG. 33.5 Lipoma: Axial cine SSFP image (A) demonstrates high signal in a lipoma along the lateral epicardial margin of the left ventricle (*arrow*), which shows decreased signal on a T1-weighted image with fat-suppression (B). Short-axis T1 mapping color-coded image (C) confirms the short T1 of the lesion (T1 = 318 ms).

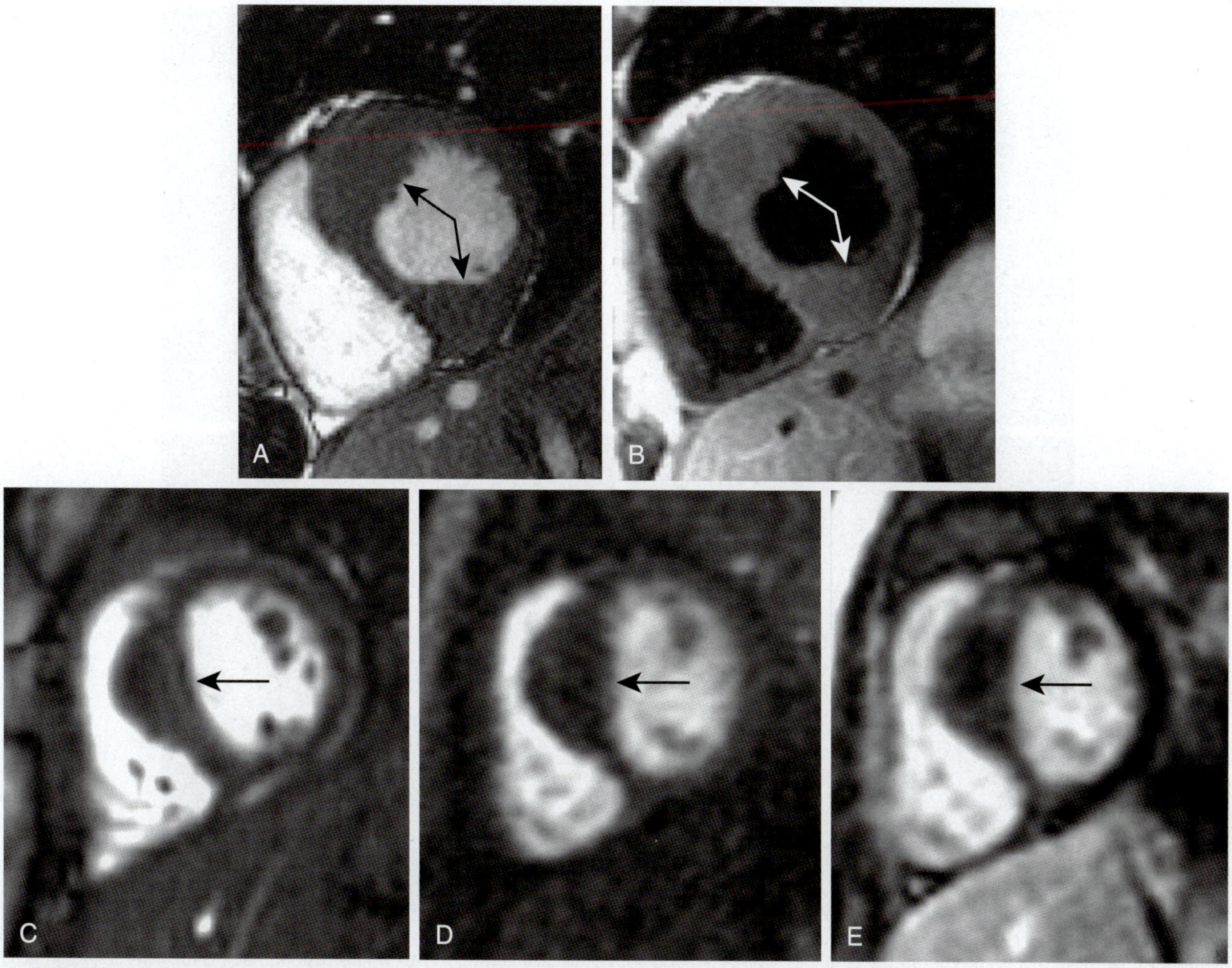

FIG. 33.6 Rhabdomyoma: Short-axis cine SSFP (A) and T1-weighted (B) images show rhabdomyomas (*arrows*) involving the anteroseptum and inferior wall in this patient with tuberous sclerosis. In another patient note the solitary rhabdomyoma (*arrow*) involving the septum on the short-axis SSFP cine (C), first-pass perfusion (D), and LGE (E) images. Note that the lesion is isointense to myocardium on the cine image (C), and does not show uptake of contrast on perfusion imaging (D). Importantly, it does not show significant enhancement different from the myocardium on the LGE image (E). This helps to distinguish this lesion from fibroma, which would show marked enhancement on LGE imaging.

- LGE images with standard inversion time: The lesions "null" like normal myocardium. (This is in marked contrast to fibromas, which show intense hyperenhancement.)
- T1WI: Isointense to normal myocardium.
- T2WI: Minimally hyperintense.

Differential diagnosis: Fibroma is the main differential diagnostic consideration. Its appearance and location can closely mimic rhabdomyoma. However, fibromas are solitary (not multiple) lesions and demonstrate intense hyperenhancement on LGE imaging.

Treatment/prognosis: Spontaneous regression is very common in these lesions, and surgical resection is reserved for cases of significant obstruction to blood flow or intractable arrhythmias.

FIBROMA

Prevalence: This benign tumor also likely represents a hamartoma and is the second most common pediatric cardiac tumor. Eighty percent of cases are seen in children, with 20% seen in adolescents and adults. The mean age at diagnosis is 13. They are occasionally seen with Gorlin syndrome, a premalignant condition with multisystem involvement, but only 4% of patients have this syndrome.

Presentation: One-third of patients present with arrhythmias or syncope, one-third with heart failure, and one-third are asymptomatic.

Radiology/pathology correlation: Fibromas are benign tumors of fibroblasts and collagen and are not encapsulated. They often are observed to interdigitate with normal myocardium, a finding that may explain the propensity of the lesions to cause arrhythmias. Like rhabdomyomas, they tend to be intramural tumors affecting the interventricular septum and the ventricular free walls. At pathology they are noted to have variable cellularity that decreases with advancing patient age. Internal calcifications are frequent.

CMR findings reflect the histologic findings of a tumor composed largely of collagen and variable amounts of fibroblasts (Fig. 33.7).

- Cine SSFP: The lesions are similar in signal intensity to normal myocardium, and often appear as poorly contractile mass-like foci.
- First-pass perfusion: No uptake.
- LGE images with standard inversion time: The lesions show intense hyperenhancement, sometimes with a dark central core that may fill-in over time.
- T1WI: Isointense to normal myocardium.

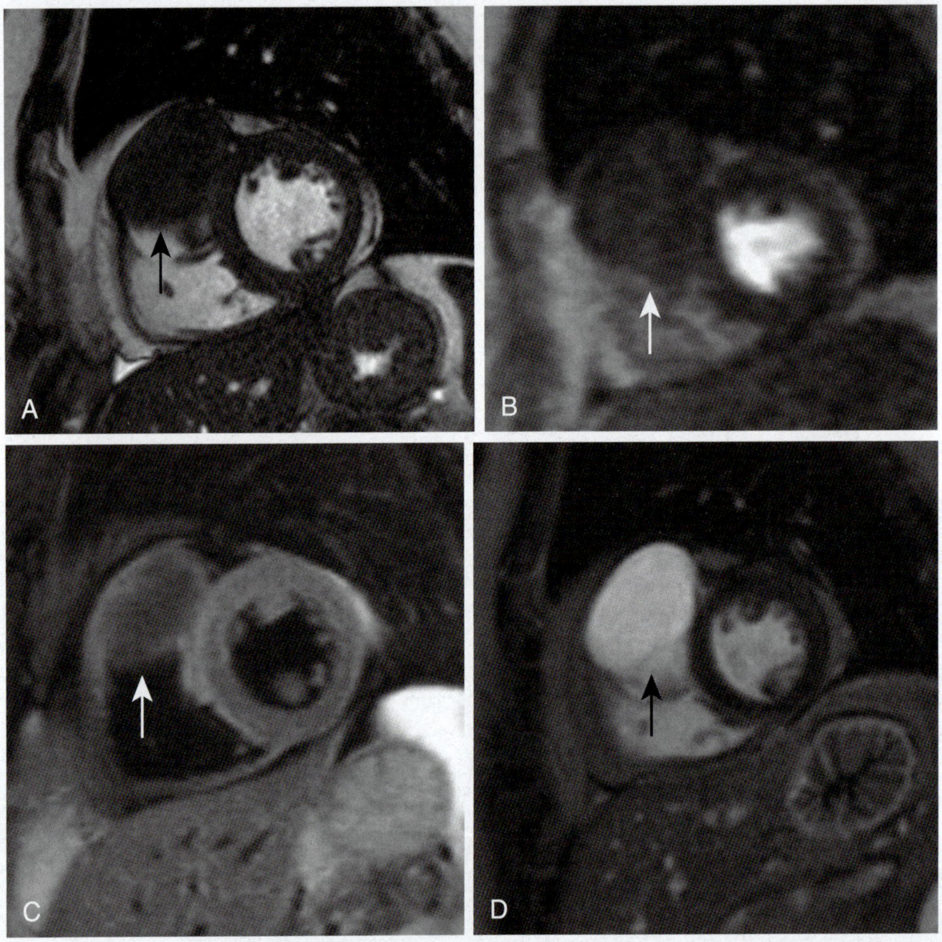

FIG. 33.7 Fibroma: Short-axis cine (A), first-pass perfusion (B), T2-weighted image (C), and LGE (D) images show a solitary fibroma (*arrows*) in the anterior wall of the right ventricle. It is isointense on the cine SSFP image (A) and shows no uptake of contrast on perfusion imaging (B). The T2-weighted image (C) shows that the lesion is low in signal intensity relative to myocardium, and the lesion shows marked enhancement on the LGE image (D). The low T2 signal is characteristic of fibroma, and is uncommon in other masses. In addition, the marked LGE enhancement clearly distinguishes fibroma from the other common childhood tumor, rhabdomyoma, which does not show hyperenhancement on LGE.

- T2WI: In adults, the lesions may be *hypointense*, a finding uncommon in any other cardiac mass. This is likely due to its fibrous composition in adults. However, in children the tumors are often more cellular and may therefore be mildly hyperintense.

Differential diagnosis: Rhabdomyoma is the main differential diagnostic consideration. Its appearance and location can closely mimic fibroma. However, rhabdomyomas are often multiple and do not demonstrate intense hyperenhancement on LGE imaging. Hypertrophic cardiomyopathy may occasionally result in a mass-like appearance of the anterior septum. While foci of hypertrophic cardiomyopathy may enhance, they are not as markedly hyperintense as fibromas.

Treatment/prognosis: Surgical resection is usually curative, even when incomplete.

HEMANGIOMA

Prevalence: These are rare, benign tumors of vascular endothelial cells and have a wide age distribution. The make up approximately 5%–10% of benign cardiac tumors and account for 2.8% of all primary cardiac masses.

Presentation: Most patients are asymptomatic, and the lesions are picked up as incidental findings. When symptomatic, dyspnea on exertion and shortness of breath are common symptoms. Rarely they may be associated with Kasabach–Merritt syndrome with recurrent thrombocytopenia.

Radiology/pathology correlation: Hemangiomas can involve any chamber. They may be subdivided into cavernous, capillary, or arteriovenous types, with cavernous histology being most common (50%), and often intramural or epicardial in location. Capillary types make up ~25% of cases and are often endocardial in location and protrude intraluminally. Arteriovenous lesions are often intramural in location.

CMR findings reflect the histologic findings of a tumor composed of vascular endothelium with variable degrees of increased vascularity (Fig. 33.8).

- Cine SSFP: The lesions are higher in signal intensity compared to normal myocardium. Septations may be seen but are more evident on T2 imaging.
- First-pass perfusion: Variable increased uptake that may be quite brisk with arteriovenous malformation–type lesions, but more commonly is slowly progressive and nodular in appearance.
- LGE images with standard inversion time: The lesions are heterogeneous, with areas of clear hyperenhancement.

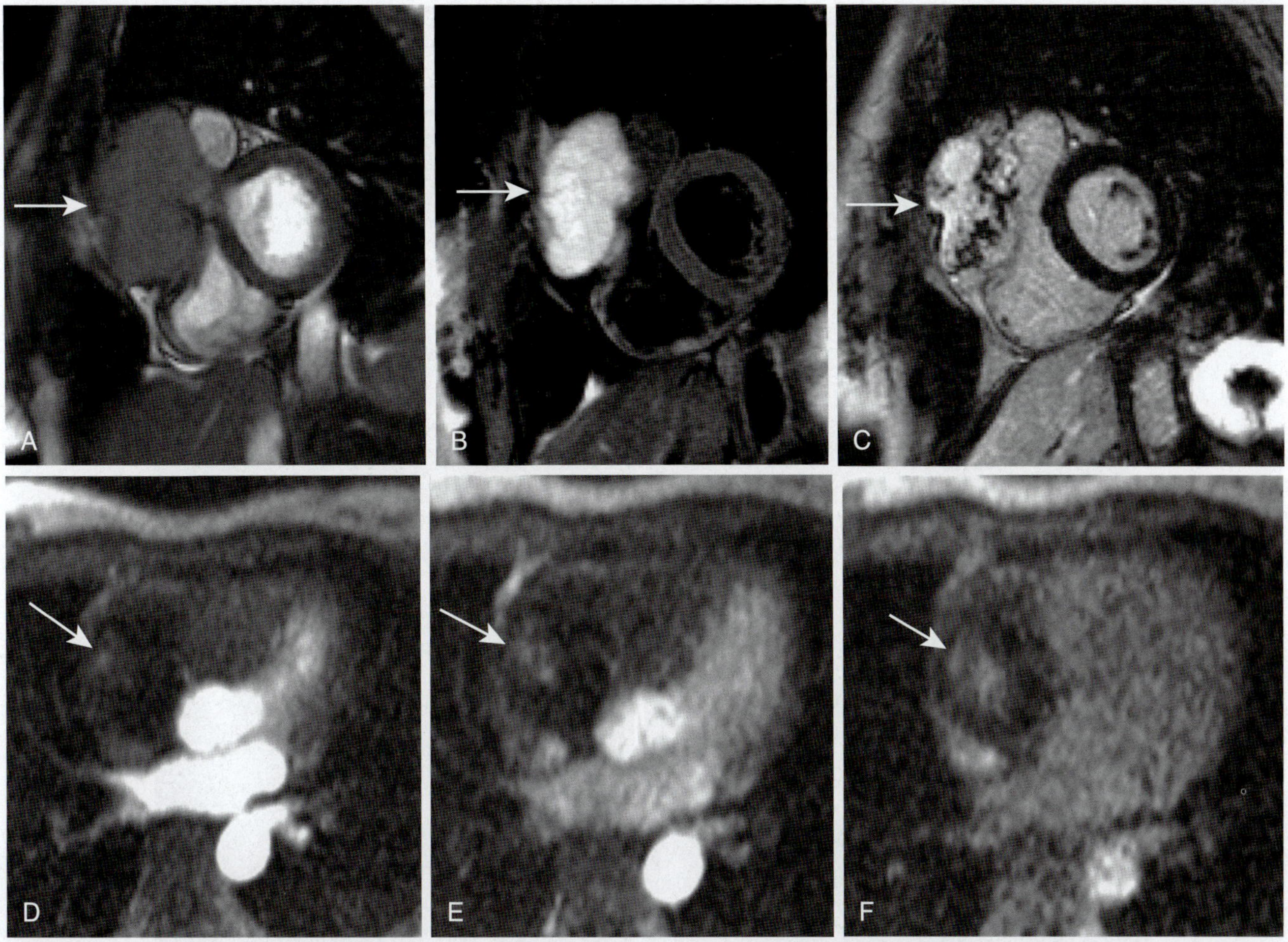

FIG. 33.8 Hemangioma: Short-axis cine SSFP (A), T2-weighted STIR (B), and LGE (C) images show a hemangioma (*arrows*) involving the anterior right ventricle and aortic root. Note that the lesion is mildly hyperintense on cine SSFP. It is quite bright on the STIR image and shows internal septations, as is commonly seen with hemangiomas. The LGE image (C) shows the usual heterogeneous enhancement. The images in the lower row (D–F) are axial first-pass perfusion images showing slow, progressive enhancement of the lesion with faint contrast seen on the early-phase image (*arrow* in D) becoming more evident on the middle- (E) and late-phase (F) images.

- T1WI: Isointense to mildly hyperintense to normal myocardium.
- T2WI: Hyperintense, similar to hemangiomas occurring elsewhere. Septations are commonly seen on T2 and STIR images.

Differential diagnosis: Small intracavitary capillary-type lesions may be mistaken for an atypical myxoma. Larger, hypervascular lesions must be distinguished from primary or secondary cardiac malignancies, but hemangiomas are usually more well-defined and less infiltrative in appearance. Paragangliomas are also hypervascular primary lesions, and are very high in signal on T2 images, similar to hemangiomas. They tend to enhance even more avidly than hemangiomas on perfusion imaging.

Treatment/prognosis: Surgery may be necessary if the diagnosis is uncertain, or the lesion is thought to be symptomatic. However, most remain asymptomatic and require no specific therapy.

PARAGANGLIOMA

Prevalence: These are extremely rare benign tumors of chromaffin origin that are usually seen in adults, with a wide age distribution and a mean age of 40. Cardiac paragangliomas account for ~2% of all paragangliomas. They are usually sporadic and not part of a multiple endocrine neoplasia syndrome.

Presentation: The range of reported functional lesions with clinical manifestations of catecholamine excess ranges from 31%–79%. Nonsecretory lesions are largely asymptomatic and are detected on imaging performed for other reasons.

Radiology/pathology correlation: Paragangliomas usually arise along the sites of cardiac autonomic paraganglia, such as the roof of the left atrium, along the atrioventricular grooves, and near the roots of the great vessels. Histologically, they are like paragangliomas occurring elsewhere, with nests of paraganglial cells surrounded by sustentacular cells. They are usually markedly hypervascular.

CMR findings reflect the histologic findings of a hypervascular tumor composed of a population of uniform paraganglial cells of chromaffin origin (Fig. 33.9).

- Cine SSFP: The lesions are higher in signal intensity than normal myocardium. Typically, they are well-circumscribed lesions.
- First-pass perfusion: Marked intense enhancement is present throughout the lesion.

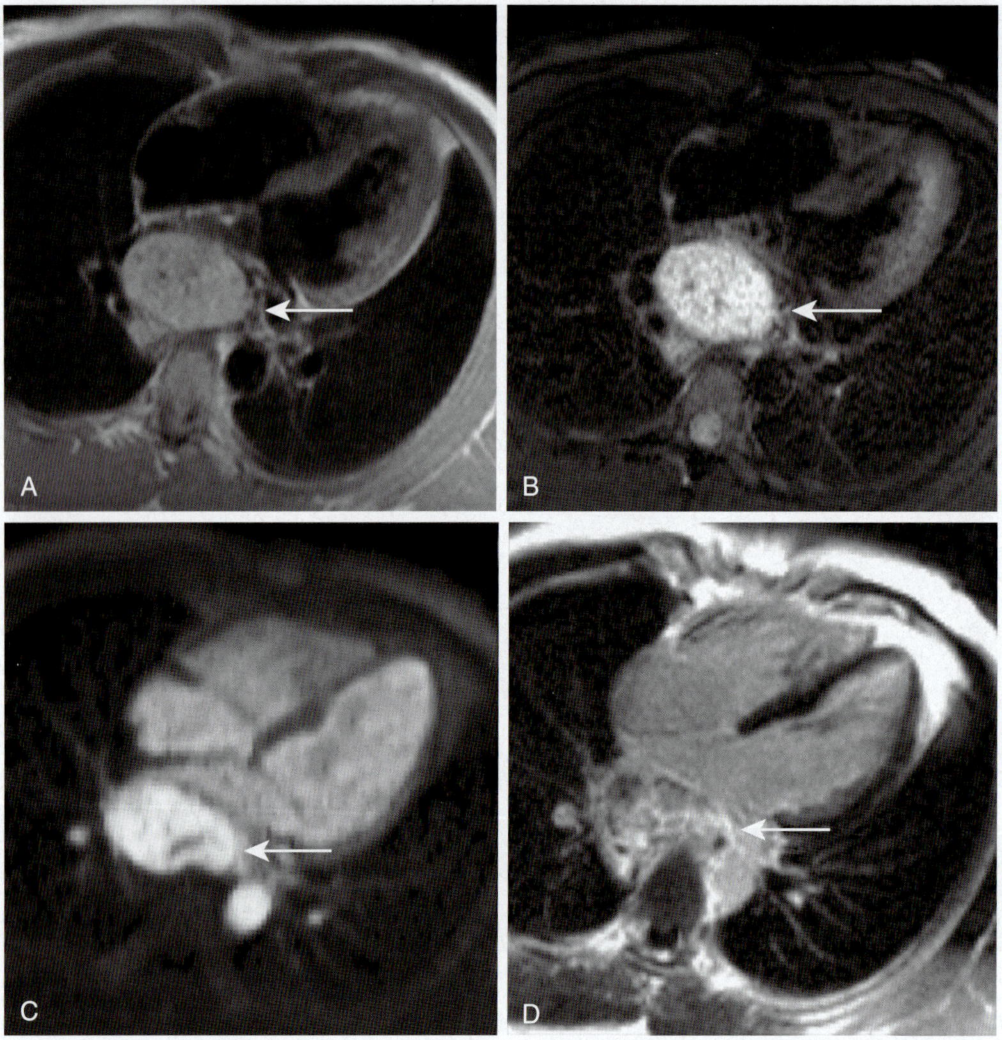

FIG. 33.9 Paraganglioma: Four-chamber T1-weighted (A), T2-weighted (B), first-pass perfusion (C), and LGE (D) images show a paraganglioma (*arrows*) involving the posterior margin of the left atrium. It is isointense on T1 imaging (A), but markedly hyperintense on the fat-suppressed T2 image (B), characteristic of these tumors. Note the intense enhancement of the lesion on first-pass perfusion imaging (C), and the heterogeneous appearance on the LGE image (D). Paragangliomas—along with hemangiomas—are one of the few benign tumors demonstrating these latter two characteristics, which may result in a misdiagnosis of a more aggressive neoplasm.

- LGE images with standard inversion time: The lesions are mildly heterogeneous, with the majority showing discernible hyperenhancement.
- T1WI: Isointense to normal myocardium. Typically, are well-circumscribed lesions. "Salt-and-pepper" appearance of the lesion may be noted.
- T2WI: Very hyperintense ("light-bulb bright") on T2 and STIR images. "Salt-and-pepper" appearance of the lesion may be noted.

Differential diagnosis: In cases with secretory function, the diagnosis is usually quite clear and can be confirmed with catecholamine measurements. Nonsecretory lesions may be mimicked by hemangiomas, but hemangiomas typically enhance in a slow, progressive fashion rather than the early and complete enhancement seen with paragangliomas. Primary and secondary malignancies may show avid enhancement, but usually have infiltrative features lacking in paragangliomas.

Treatment/prognosis: Rare instances of recurrence and even metastatic disease have been reported, but surgery is usually curative, with a low risk of recurrence.

ANGIOSARCOMA

Prevalence: These are the most common primary cardiac malignancy, accounting for ~40% of cases. They are aggressive infiltrating malignancies that tend to occur in adults, with a peak in the fourth and fifth decades.

Presentation: As they most commonly involve the right atrium, symptoms tend to reflect impaired right ventricular filling and occasionally tamponade related to complicating hemorrhage.

Radiology/pathology correlation: Angiosarcomas have a distinct predilection to involve the right atrial wall, with or without pericardial involvement. This is in contradistinction to virtually all other cardiac sarcomas that have a left atrial predominance. They are typically bulky, infiltrating masses that may protrude into the atrial cavity and often have areas of internal hemorrhage. They are composed of malignant vascular endothelial cells that form irregular sinusoids.

CMR findings reflect the histologic findings of a hypervascular tumor infiltrating the right atrial wall (Fig. 33.10).

- Cine SSFP: Poor border definition and infiltration of the right atrial wall by a large, heterogeneous mass is apparent.

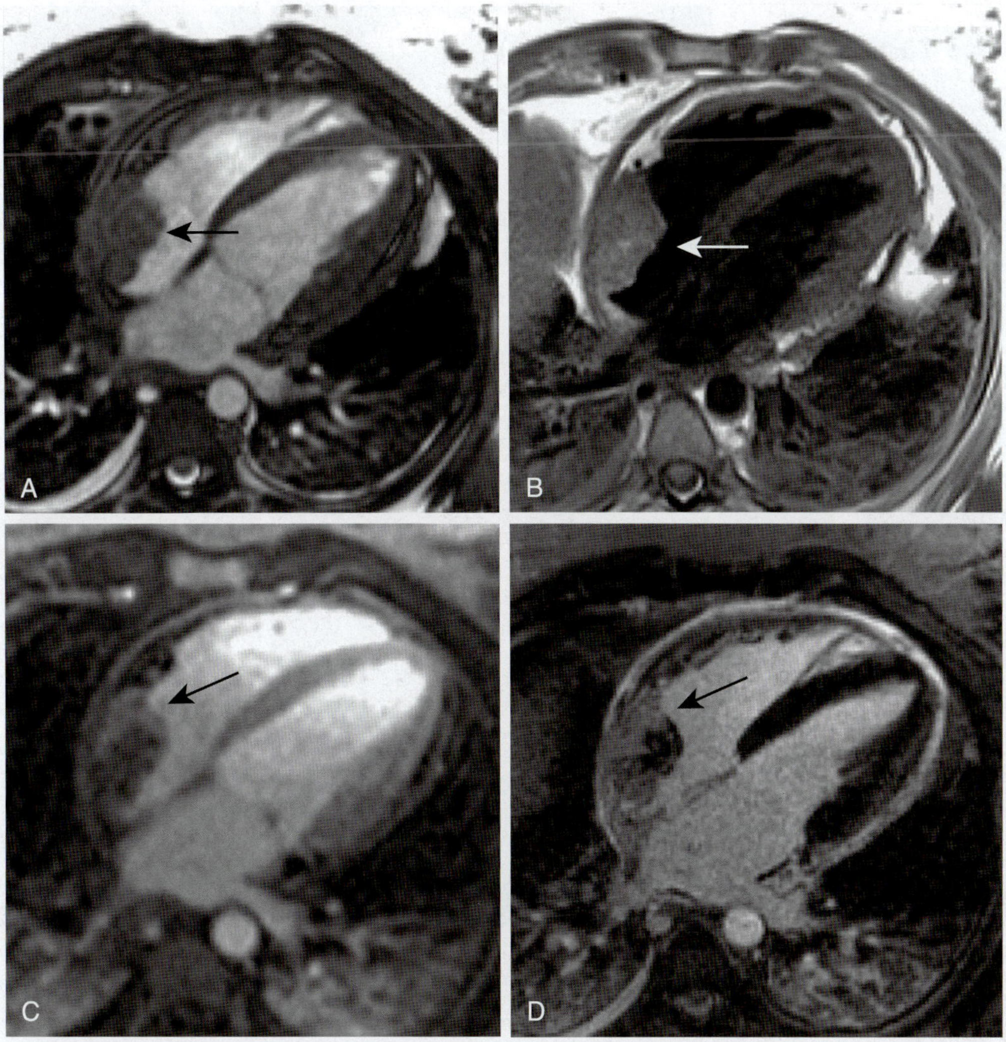

FIG. 33.10 Angiosarcoma: Four-chamber cine SSFP (A), T1-weighted turbo spin-echo (B), first-pass perfusion (C), and LGE (D) images demonstrate a bulky angiosarcoma (*arrows*) infiltrating the right atrial wall. Pericardial thickening is also apparent, signifying pericardial involvement as frequently seen with this tumor. Note the small areas of internal high signal within the lesion on the T1-weighted image, consistent with small foci of internal hemorrhage. First-pass perfusion images show areas of irregular enhancement, greatest along the periphery of the lesion (*arrow* in C). The lesion demonstrates heterogeneous enhancement on LGE imaging (*arrow* in D), commonly seen in malignant lesions.

- First-pass perfusion: Heterogeneous low-grade enhancement is usually present, reflecting areas of necrosis intermixed with viable tumor.
- LGE images with standard inversion time: The lesions are markedly heterogeneous, reflecting areas of necrosis intermixed with viable tumor.
- T1WI: Predominantly isointense, but areas of internal hemorrhage may be hyperintense.
- T2WI: Heterogeneously hyperintense.

Differential diagnosis: Metastatic disease is the main differential diagnostic consideration, as they can result in bulky right atrial lesions, but metastatic disease most often occurs in patient with known malignancy. Rarely, hemangiomas involving the right atrial wall may mimic angiosarcoma.

Treatment/prognosis: Surgical resection when possible is recommended, but the overall prognosis is bleak, with an average life expectancy of less than a year.

Other sarcomas: Multiple other mesenchymal tissues can be associated with a sarcoma, including pleomorphic sarcoma, fibrosarcoma, osteosarcoma, leiomyosarcoma, and rhabdomyosarcoma. Most of these occur in the left atrium, but otherwise are similar to angiosarcoma in their imaging appearances. Other than rhabdomyosarcoma, which tends to involve children, there is no way to reliably distinguish between them.

PRIMARY CARDIAC LYMPHOMA

Prevalence: These are rare as isolated primary lesions, making up 1% of primary cardiac tumors and 0.5% of extranodal lymphomas. The average age at diagnosis is 60, and there is a 2:1 male predominance. They are more frequent in immunocompromised patients, including those with HIV.

Presentation: Many lesions are asymptomatic, but dyspnea, chest pain, and arrhythmias may be seen in those with symptoms. A diagnosis of primary cardiac lymphoma requires that there is no substantial extracardiac disease.

Radiology/pathology correlation: Primary cardiac lymphoma may involve any cardiac chamber and/or the pericardium and is frequently accompanied by pericardial effusion. The right atrium is most frequently involved, and encasement of the adjacent right coronary artery is commonly seen. Histologically, they may appear as sheet-like infiltration of the myocardium, or as multiple infiltrating

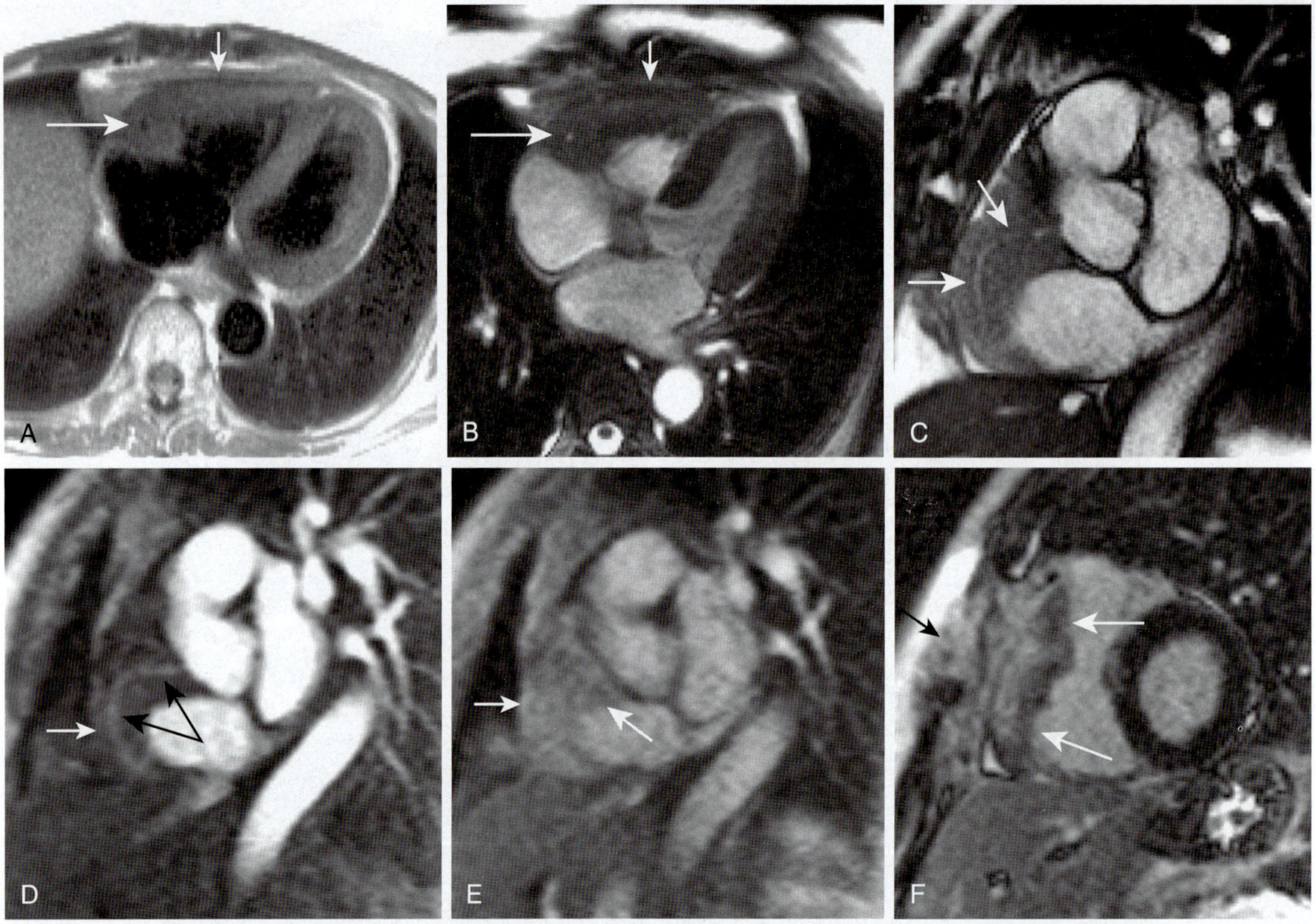

FIG. 33.11 Lymphoma: Four-chamber HASTE image (A) and cine SSFP image (B) demonstrate a soft-tissue mass representing lymphoma infiltrating the anterior right ventricular wall (*short arrows*) and encasing the right coronary artery (RCA) (*long arrows*). Note also the extension of abnormal soft-tissue into the anterior mediastinal fat (*short arrows*). Short-axis images in the plane of the atrioventricular groove confirm the RCA encasement (*arrows*) on the cine SSFP image (C) and the early-phase perfusion image (D). Note that on the later perfusion image (E), the lymphomatous tissue (*arrows*) has enhanced, obscuring the encased RCA. The short-axis LGE image (F) demonstrates heterogeneous enhancement of the infiltrating neoplasm (*arrows*).

nodules. Most often, they are a subtype of B-cell non-Hodgkin lymphoma.

CMR findings are diverse, reflecting the varied distribution of these lesions, with findings suggestive of malignancy apparent (Fig. 33.11).

- Cine SSFP: Poor border definition and infiltration of the myocardium is apparent, most often involving the right atrial wall. Encasement of the right coronary artery is commonly seen in such cases.
- First-pass perfusion: Diffuse enhancement is usually present.
- LGE images with standard inversion time: The lesions are usually heterogeneous, but often with more uniform enhancement than sarcomas or metastatic lesions.
- T1WI: Isointense.
- T2WI: Hyperintense.

Differential diagnosis: Metastatic disease is the main differential diagnostic consideration, as they are more common than primary cardiac malignancies of any type. The clinical history is often useful as metastatic lesions are usually seen in patients with known malignancy. Angiosarcomas can mimic primary cardiac lymphoma, and differentiation may be difficult on imaging alone, but in general, sarcomas tend to have a more heterogeneous internal architecture than do lymphomas.

Treatment/prognosis: Chemotherapy is the usual treatment of choice, and immunotherapies are also used. Treatment has improved the prognosis, and presently 3-year survival has improved to 60%.

PERICARDIAL MESOTHELIOMA

Prevalence: Although extremely rare, they are the most common primary malignancy of the pericardium. Unlike pleural mesotheliomas, a definite link to asbestos exposure is not as well defined.

Presentation: Patients usually present at a mean age of 57 with symptoms related to associated pericardial effusions and/or constrictive symptoms related to filling of the pericardium with bulky tumor nodules.

Radiology/pathology correlation: At pathology, most commonly numerous confluent tumor nodules are seen throughout the pericardial space, accompanied by pericardial thickening and fluid. A more focal nodular form is distinctly less common.

CMR findings are diverse, reflecting the above-described appearance, with multiple intrapericardial tumor nodules seen studding the cardiac surface, accompanied by pericardial fluid and thickening (Fig. 33.12).

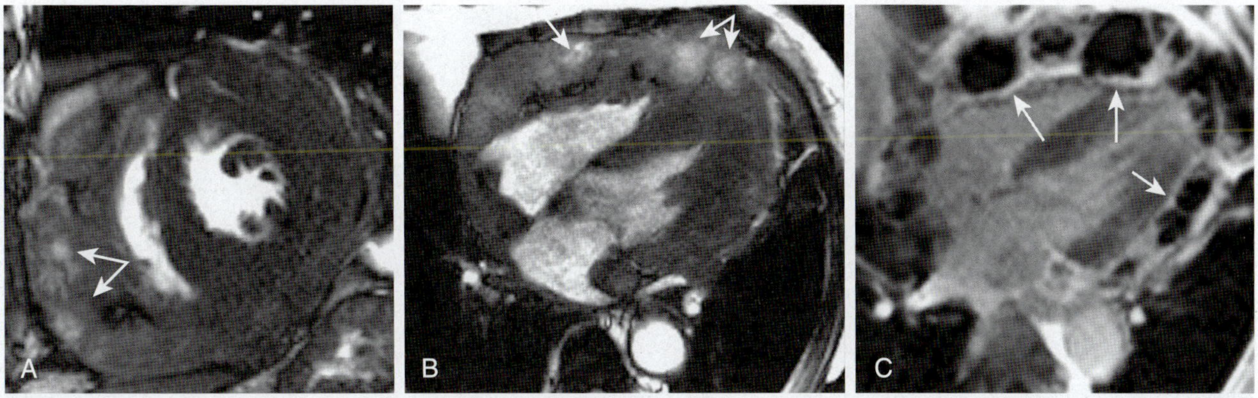

FIG. 33.12 Pericardial mesothelioma: Short-axis (A) and four-chamber (B) cine SSFP images demonstrate that the heart is encased by nodular thickening of the pericardium due to an extensive pericardial mesothelioma. These nodules of neoplastic pericardial tumor are low in signal on the LGE four-chamber image (C), with diffuse enhancement of the thickened pericardium evident (*arrows* in C).

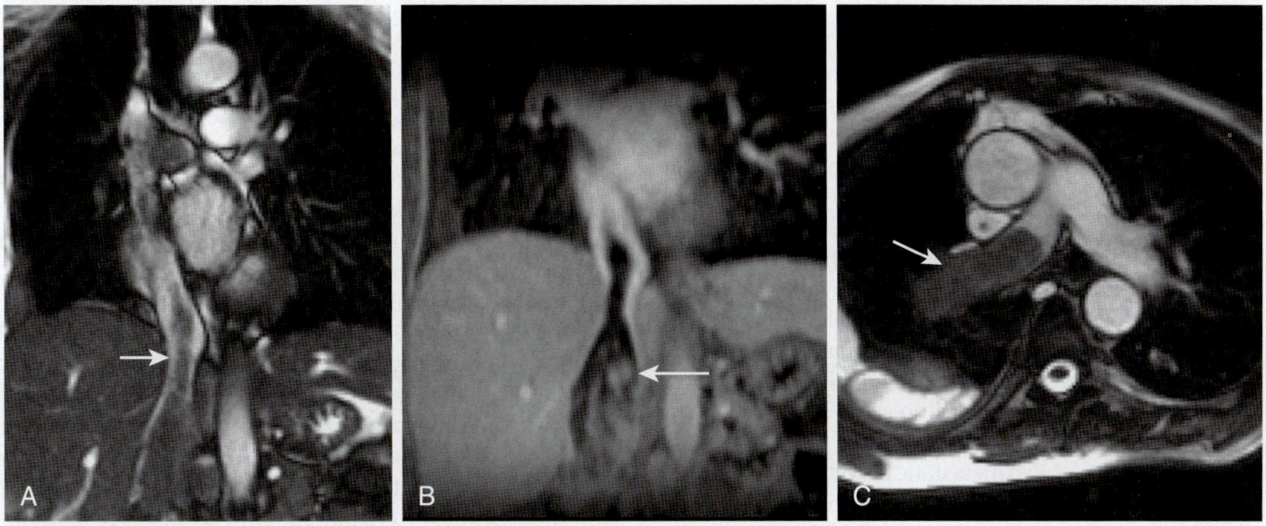

FIG. 33.13 Transvenous tumor spread: Coronal cine SSFP (A) and postcontrast fat-suppressed T1-weighted gradient-echo (B) images demonstrate a large soft-tissue filling defect in the inferior vena cava (*arrow*). The IVC lesion shows irregular enhancement (*arrow* in B), indicating that this represents tumor extension and not simply bland thrombus. In addition, the cine SSFP image at the level of the pulmonary artery bifurcation (C) shows a filling defect in the right pulmonary artery (*arrow* in C) that is nearly occlusive. The detection of both the IVC tumor extension and the embolization to the right pulmonary artery in this patient with urothelial carcinoma was made possible by the large field of view provided by CMR.

- Cine SSFP: Multiple high signal tumor nodules are seen along the margins of the heart. Abnormal septal motion may be noted if RV filling is impaired.
- First-pass perfusion: Pericardial enhancement is sometimes seen; nodules do not usually enhance significantly.
- LGE images with standard inversion time: The lesions are usually heterogeneous, and nodules may show little enhancement.
- T1WI: Isointense pericardial thickening with variable nodule signal.
- T2WI: Inhomogeneously hyperintense.

Differential diagnosis: Metastatic disease is the main differential diagnostic consideration, as they are significantly more common than primary pericardial malignancies.

Treatment/prognosis: The prognosis is quite poor, with median survival of ~6 months reported, but with occasionally longer survival with chemotherapeutic regimens.

METASTATIC DISEASE

Prevalence: Autopsy data indicate that ~10% of patients dying with cancer will have cardiac metastases, but far fewer are detected clinically during life. When noted, they are often seen in patients with advanced malignancy, and seldom are the presenting manifestation. They are at least 40 times more common than primary cardiac malignancy with the most common primary sites being the lung (36%), followed by leukemia/lymphoma (20%). Cardiac involvement is seen in 10%–12% of breast cancer patients, and in up to 56% of melanoma patients.

Presentation: 50% of patients are asymptomatic, but frequent pericardial involvement at presentation (70%) often leads to the development of pericardial effusions and sometimes tamponade. New arrhythmia developing in a patient with known malignancy may signify myocardial involvement.

Radiology/pathology correlation: Metastases may reach the heart via direct invasion, via hematogenous spread, via lymphatic extension from involved mediastinal lymph nodes, and via transvenous spread. This latter mechanism is commonly seen with extension to the right heart from primary carcinomas of the kidneys, adrenals, and the liver (Fig. 33.13). Extension to the left atrium via the pulmonary veins is usually

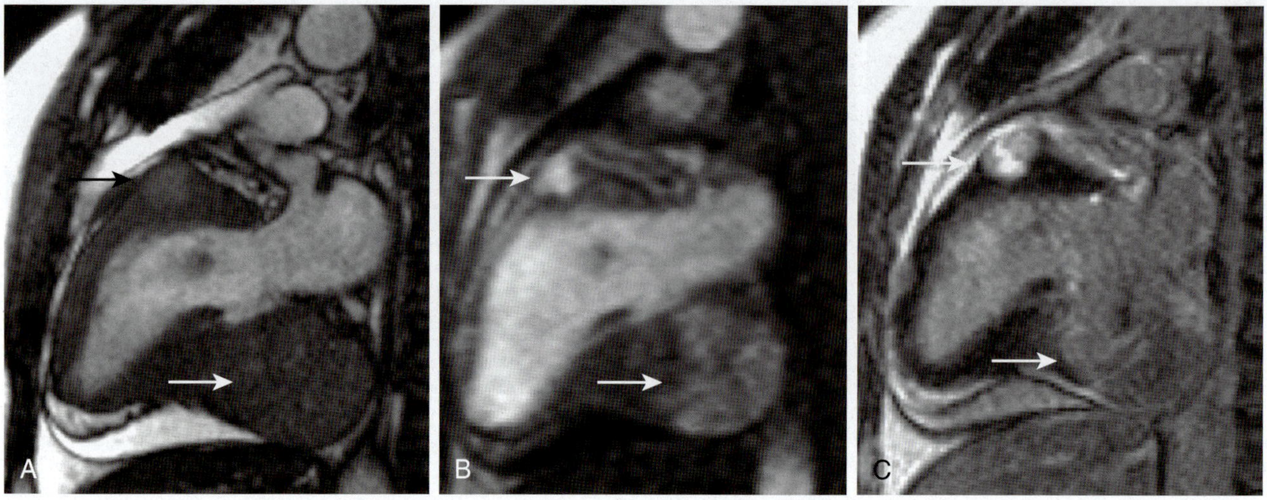

FIG. 33.14 Hematogenous metastatic disease: Two-chamber cine SSFP (A), first-pass perfusion (B), and LGE (C) images show hypervascular metastatic deposits in the anterior and inferior walls (*arrows*) in this patient with metastatic renal cell carcinoma. Note the brisk enhancement of the lesions on the perfusion image (B). The intramyocardial location and the multiplicity of lesions are consistent with hematogenous spread of malignancy.

due to lung cancer. Findings at pathologic exam vary with the mode of spread; direct invasion and transvenous spread are usually readily apparent. Spread via the lymphatics often results in pericardial involvement. The presence of multiple infiltrating nodules involving primarily the myocardium is commonly seen in cases of hematogenous spread.

CMR findings are diverse, reflecting the varied nature of these lesions, with findings suggestive of malignancy (such as multiple infiltrating nodules or masses) apparent (Fig. 33.14).

- Cine SSFP: Poor border definition of the lesions and infiltration of the myocardium is often seen. Pericardial effusions and nodularity may be evident.
- First-pass perfusion: Most metastatic lesions will show some enhancement. Certain hypervascular lesions such as renal cell carcinoma metastases will show marked enhancement.
- LGE images with standard inversion time: The lesions are usually heterogeneous in appearance.
- T1WI: Isointense in general; however, T1 hyperintensity may be seen in melanomas due to the T1 shortening effect of their melanin content. Areas of internal hemorrhage may also be high on T1WI images.
- T2WI: Hyperintense.

Differential diagnosis: Primary cardiac sarcomas are the main differential diagnostic consideration, but are far less common than metastatic disease, and are usually solitary lesions. The clinical history is often useful as metastatic lesions are usually seen in patients with known malignancy. Hypervascular benign lesions such as hemangiomas and paragangliomas can occasionally be mistaken for metastatic disease on imaging, but clinically are usually distinct.

Treatment/prognosis: Given that cardiac metastatic lesions are usually seen in the setting of known advanced malignancy, it is not surprising that the prognosis is grim. A variety of treatment options including chemotherapy, radiotherapy, and immunotherapy are available and are the subject of clinical trials.

Nonneoplastic Masses

Nonneoplastic masses are entities that mimic tumors on imaging but are distinct in their etiology and treatment. These include thrombi, vegetations, and inflammatory masses.

Thrombus

Thrombi are the most common nonneoplastic mass seen in the heart, particularly in patients with atrial fibrillation, ventricular dysfunction, or post-MI. Thrombi are critical to distinguish from tumors, as their management often involves anticoagulation rather than surgery.

On CMR, thrombi appear as low signal intensity masses on both T1- and T2-weighted images. However, the pathognomonic feature is avascularity and homogeneously low signal on long-TI LGE imaging (Fig. 33.15). This helps distinguish them from neoplastic masses. In our multicenter study, we found that long-TI LGE imaging was highly accurate (98.7%) in distinguishing thrombus from tumor.[2] The few inaccuracies were almost entirely in cases of myxomas mistaken for thrombi, or vice versa, because of the overlap in rare cases of imaging findings common to both.

Further details regarding the critical role of CMR for the evaluation of patients with thrombus are provided in Chapter 34 ("Cardiac Thrombus").

Vegetations

Vegetations are masses of fibrin, platelets, and microorganisms that form on valve leaflets during infective endocarditis. They can lead to embolic events or destruction of valve tissue. Large vegetations can be seen attached to the valves. Smaller and irregularly mobile vegetations may be difficult to see with CMR due to the segmented sequences used for standard cine and LGE imaging. CMR can also help distinguish vegetations from valve tumors such as fibroelastomas.

Cystic Lesions

Pericardial cysts and other cystic lesions such as hydatid cysts can mimic tumors (Fig. 33.16). These are benign but may cause symptoms depending on their size and location.

Cystic lesions have well-defined borders, are fluid-filled, and appear hyperintense on T2-weighted images. They do not enhance with gadolinium, helping distinguish them from neoplastic lesions.

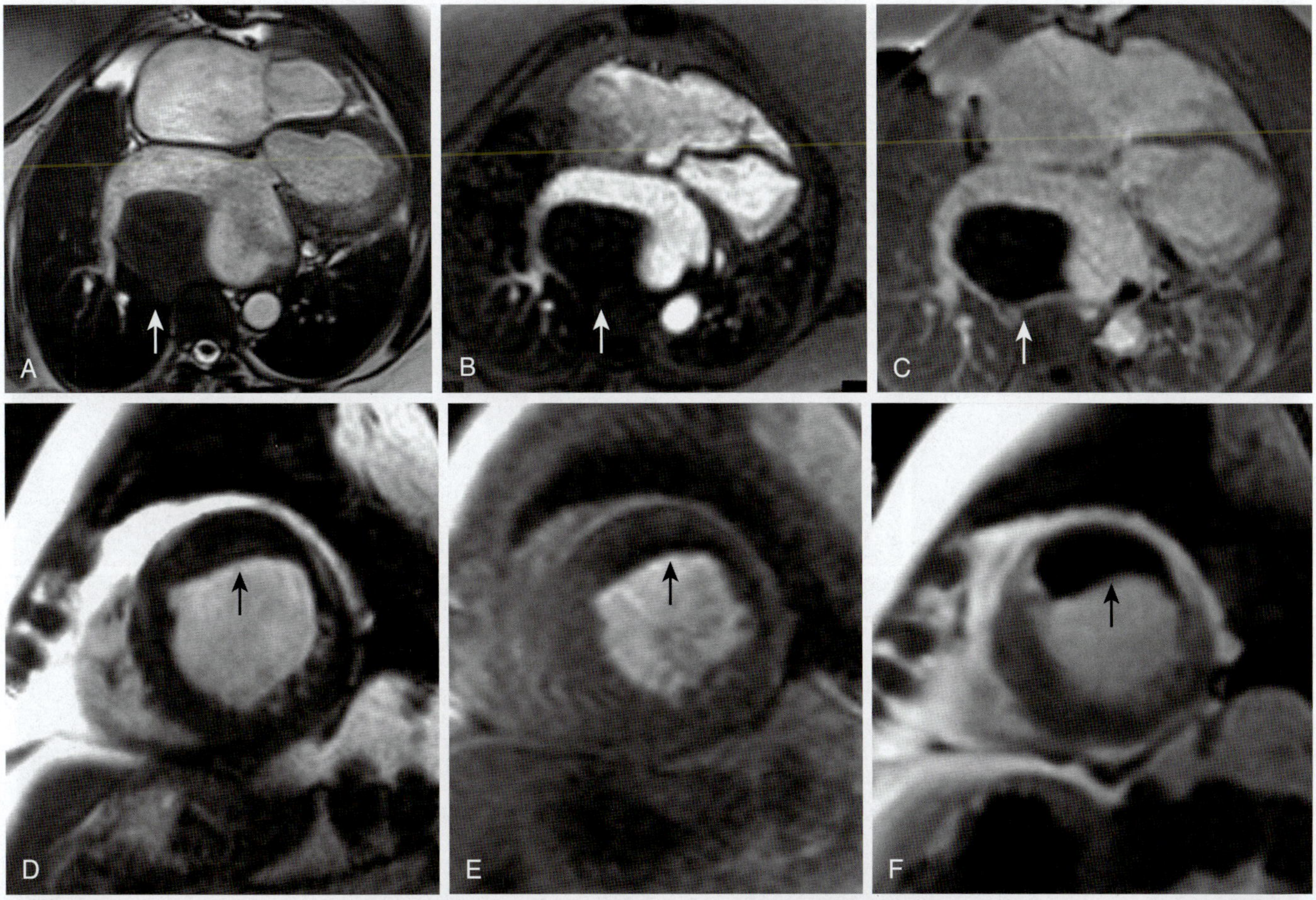

FIG. 33.15 Thrombus: Four-chamber cine SSFP (A), first-pass perfusion (B), and long-TI LGE (C) images show a large left atrial thrombus (*arrows*) along the posterior wall of the left atrium in a patient with mitral valve disease and long-standing atrial fibrillation. Short-axis (*bottom row*) cine SSFP (D), first-pass perfusion (E), and long-TI LGE (F) images show a large nonenhancing mural thrombus along the anterior wall of the left ventricle. Note that the thrombi are isointense to muscle on cine SSFP images (A, D) and do not show contrast uptake on perfusion images (B, E). Note also the homogeneous low-signal on LGE images obtained with an inversion time of 600 ms (C, F).

Pseudomasses

A pseudomass is a prominent normal structure (eustachian valve, crista terminalis, etc.), a variant of a normal structure (lipomatous hypertrophy of the interatrial septum, epicardial fat, etc.), or a nonmass pathology (hiatal hernia) that could be mistaken for a cardiac mass (Fig. 33.16). Other common normal structures that could be mistaken for cardiac masses include the Chiari network, moderator band, and prominent papillary muscles.

CLINICAL RELEVANCE OF CMR IN CARDIAC MASS DIAGNOSIS

Diagnostic Accuracy

CMR has emerged as a pivotal tool in the diagnosis of cardiac masses, providing comprehensive insights into their nature, location, and potential implications. Its high-resolution images and advanced sequences enable precise differentiation between various cardiac masses, including benign and malignant tumors, thrombi, and other nontumoral masses. Using tissue characteristics from T1-weighted, T2-weighted, long-TI LGE, standard LGE, and perfusion imaging the composition of a cardiac mass can be seen, which is critical in distinguishing the different types of cardiac masses. This ability to characterize the tissue composition noninvasively enhances diagnostic accuracy, allowing clinicians to make informed decisions regarding management strategies.

In a large multicenter study of 903 patients, we demonstrated that the CMR diagnosis was accurate in 98.4% of patients when compared with the final diagnosis determined after follow-up using all available data.[2] Similarly, Aghayev et al. showed a sensitivity of 98% and specificity of 84% for CMR to distinguish between benign and malignant cardiac masses.[3] Most recently, Paolisso and Bergamaschi et al. showed that CMR has an area under the curve of 0.976 to distinguish between benign and malignant cardiac masses.[4]

Impact on Clinical Decision-Making

The accurate characterization of cardiac masses via CMR significantly impacts clinical decision-making processes. For instance, in cases where a mass is identified as a myxoma, surgical intervention may be warranted due to the risk of obstruction or embolization. Conversely, if a mass is characterized as a benign lipoma or a nonthrombotic mass without hemodynamic compromise, a conservative approach may be appropriate.

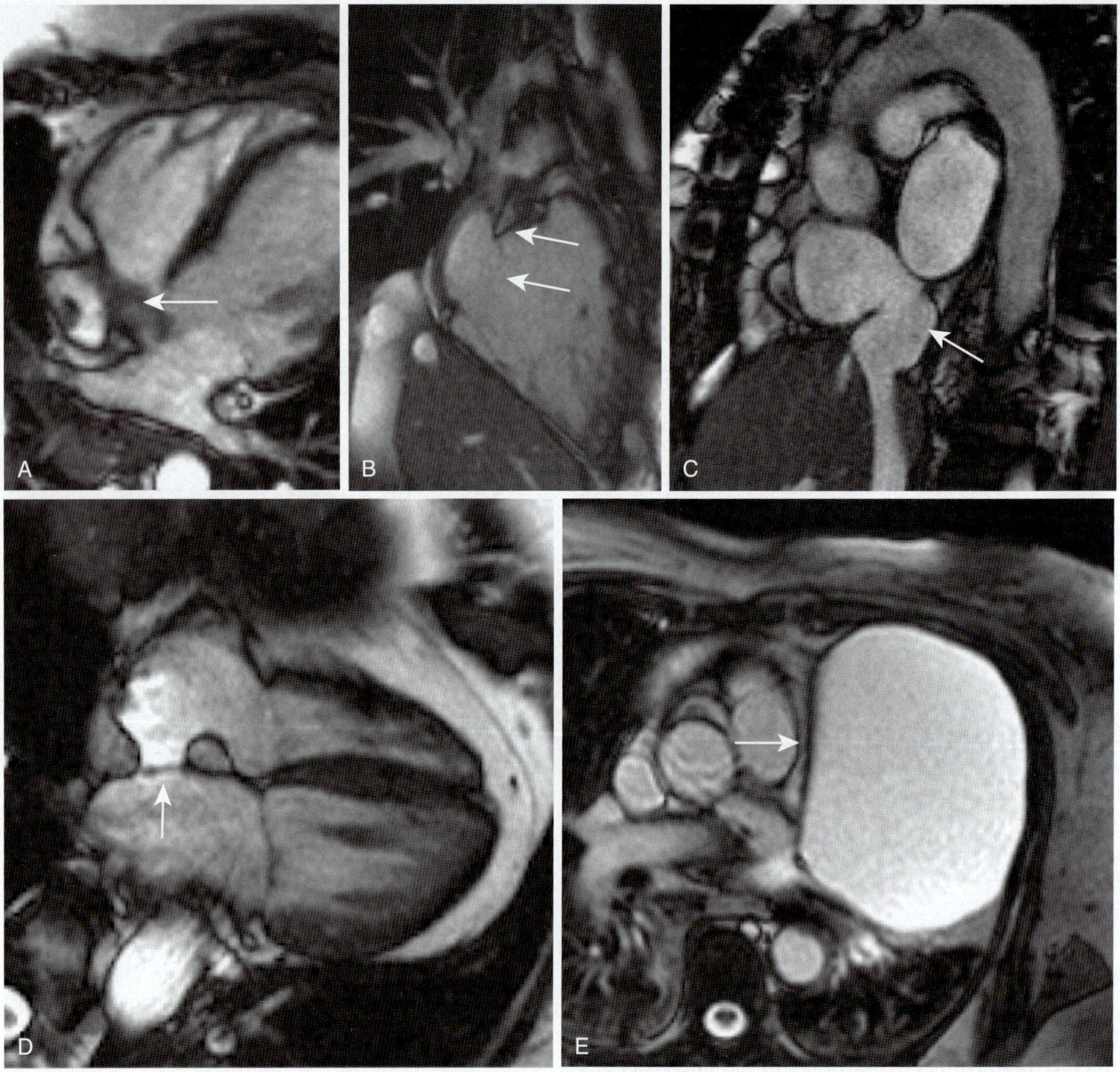

FIG. 33.16 Pseudomasses: Four-chamber (A) and oblique coronal (B) cine SSFP images demonstrate a prominent crista terminalis (*arrows*), a normal variant. A short-axis cine SSFP image (C) of the right atrial/IVC junction shows a prominent eustachian valve (*arrow*). This is a prominent normal variant as well. Four-chamber cine SSFP image (D) shows lipomatous hypertrophy of the interatrial septum, showing the usual sparing of the fossa ovalis (*arrow*), a common finding. Axial T2-weighted image (E) shows a large pericardial cyst, atypical in location.

Furthermore, CMR can assist in monitoring the growth of cardiac masses over time, aiding in the determination of whether surgical intervention is necessary. Regular follow-up imaging using CMR can inform decisions regarding the need for intervention, particularly in cases where the mass exhibits concerning features such as increased size, changes in morphology, or significant hemodynamic effects.

Risk Stratification

CMR's capability to identify the specific type of mass is critical for effective risk stratification. In our study, patients with CMR diagnoses of pseudomass and benign tumor had similar mortality to those with no mass, whereas those with malignant tumor [hazard ratio (HR) 3.31 (2.40–4.57)] and thrombus [HR 1.46 (1.00–2.11)] had greater mortality.[2] The CMR diagnosis provided incremental prognostic value over clinical factors including left ventricular ejection fraction, coronary artery disease, and history of extracardiac malignancy ($P < .001$).[2]

Chan et al. demonstrated that perfusion CMR provides prognostic value complementary to LGE CMR in cancer patients with cardiac masses. Among patients with cardiac metastatic tumors identified by LGE CMR, the extent of hypoperfusion of the tumor on perfusion imaging was associated with mortality.[5]

Identifying High-Risk Masses Based on CMR Features

Mobility is a particularly important characteristic in assessing the risk associated with cardiac masses. For instance, a large, mobile myxoma poses a higher risk for embolization compared to a sessile one. CMR can accurately quantify mass mobility and provide insights into associated risks, enabling clinicians to stratify patients based on their need for surgical intervention versus conservative management.

Additionally, the presence of hemodynamic obstruction, detected through flow imaging and functional assessment techniques, allows for further stratification. Masses that obstruct blood flow can lead to significant clinical consequences, including heart failure or arrhythmias, underscoring the importance of timely intervention.

Role of Multimodality Imaging

The high accuracy of CMR to identify the presence of a cardiac mass and to distinguish between benign and malignant cardiac masses in multiple studies indicates that CMR alone should be sufficient for evaluating patients with cardiac masses, and a multimodality approach is not necessary, except perhaps in very rare cases.

Aghayev et al. demonstrated that combining CMR and ^{18}F-fluorodeoxyglucose positron emission tomography (FDG-PET) resulted in a worse performance (sensitivity of 85% and specificity of 88%) compared to using CMR alone (sensitivity of 98% and specificity of 84%).[3] D'Angelo et al. studied 60 patients who received cardiovascular computed tomography (CCT) and PET for evaluation of cardiac masses over a 19-year period starting from 2000, and concluded that there was a role for CCT and PET, but they did not demonstrate an incremental value of these imaging techniques over CMR.[6]

Guiding Interventions

CMR can guide the decision between biopsy and surgical resection of a cardiac mass to determine the specific histologic subtype. For instance, if a mass has features consistent with malignancy—such as significant necrosis, rapid growth, or infiltrative patterns—a surgical approach may be prioritized. Conversely, if imaging suggests a benign process, a biopsy may be performed to confirm the diagnosis before proceeding with invasive interventions.

For patients who undergo surgical resection, CMR aids surgeons in surgical planning, minimizing complications and optimizing outcomes by providing precise localization and detailed information on mass involvement with surrounding structures.

SUGGESTED APPROACH TO THE INTERPRETATION OF CMR FOR SUSPECTED CARDIAC MASS (FIG. 33.17)

An algorithm of our suggested approach to interpretation of CMR for suspected cardiac mass is given in Fig. 33.17. The interpretation is based on conventional imaging features described earlier. However, we emphasize a stepwise approach with certain diagnoses more dependent on specific CMR techniques than others.

In our experience, some CMR techniques (such as cine CMR and LGE CMR) are much more valuable than others (T1-weighted CMR and T2-weighted CMR) for the evaluation of suspected cardiac masses. For example, distinguishing thrombus from tumor (e.g., Fig. 33.17 "Step 2") should be based on long-TI LGE images. Exclusion of a cardiac mass ("no mass") requires the absence of a mass or any structure that could have been mistaken for a mass on prior imaging. A "pseudomass" is diagnosed when a prominent normal structure (eustachian valve, crista terminalis, etc.), a variant of a normal structure (lipomatous hypertrophy of the interatrial septum, epicardial fat, etc.), or a nonmass pathology (hiatal hernia) that could have been mistaken for a cardiac mass on prior imaging is noted. A thrombus is diagnosed based on its location within the cardiac cavity, and tissue characteristics consistent with a homogeneous, avascular mass. This determination is made on postcontrast LGE images obtained with a long TI showing a homogeneously dark mass with no contrast uptake. A tumor is diagnosed and determined to be benign or malignant, based on general features such as location (intracavitary, intramural, or epicardial), morphology (rounded, irregular), border definition at the interface with the normal myocardium (well-defined, infiltrating), perfusion characteristics (hypoperfused, hypervascular), and late contrast uptake (homogeneous, heterogeneous), as well as sequence-specific characteristics, suggesting that the mass was composed of fat (fat suppression sequences) or cystic fluid (T1 and/or T2 weighting consistent with fluid).

In our study, we used this approach to obtain an accuracy of 98.4% when compared with the final diagnosis determined after follow-up using all available data.[2]

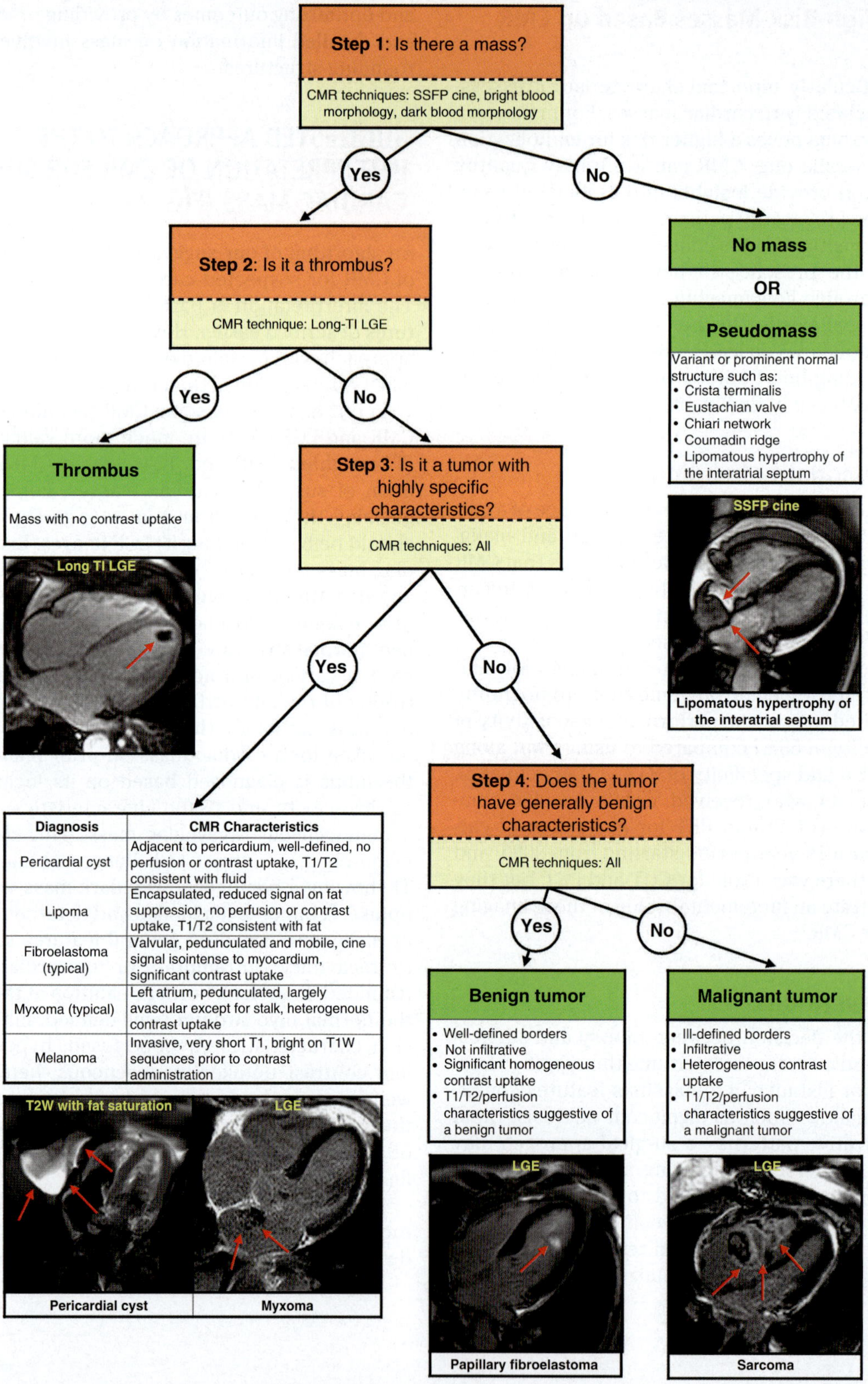

FIG. 33.17 Stepwise algorithm used for CMR interpretation of patients with suspected cardiac tumors. (Reproduced from Shenoy C, et al. Cardiovascular magnetic resonance imaging in suspected cardiac tumour: a multicentre outcomes study. *Eur Heart J*. 2021;43:71–80 (Figure 1).)

CONCLUSION

In conclusion, CMR has firmly established itself as an indispensable tool in the evaluation and management of cardiac masses. This chapter has outlined the role of CMR in identifying the presence of a mass, distinguishing between tumors, nonneoplastic masses, and pseudomasses, and in patients with tumors, distinguishing between benign and malignant tumors. The diagnostic accuracy of CMR is complemented by its high prognostic power to risk-stratify patients based on the CMR diagnosis of the type of cardiac masses.

REFERENCES

1. Weinsaft JW, Kim HW, Shah DJ, et al. Detection of left ventricular thrombus by delayed-enhancement cardiovascular magnetic resonance. *J Am Coll Cardiol*. 2008;52:148–157.
2. Shenoy C, Grizzard JD, Shah DJ, et al. Cardiovascular magnetic resonance imaging in suspected cardiac tumour: a multicentre outcomes study. *Eur Heart J*. 2021;43:71–80.
3. Aghayev A, Cheezum MK, Steigner ML, et al. Multimodality imaging to distinguish between benign and malignant cardiac masses. *J Nucl Cardiol*. 2022;29:1504–1517.
4. Paolisso P, Bergamaschi L, Angeli F, et al. Cardiac magnetic resonance to predict cardiac mass malignancy: the CMR mass score. *Circ Cardiovasc Imaging*. 2024;17:e016115.
5. Chan AT, Maya TR, Park C, et al. Incremental utility of first-pass perfusion CMR for prognostic risk stratification of cancer-associated cardiac masses. *JACC, Cardiovasc Imaging*. 2024;17:128–145.
6. D'Angelo EC, Paolisso P, Vitale G, et al. Diagnostic accuracy of cardiac computed tomography and 18-F fluorodeoxyglucose positron emission tomography in cardiac masses. *JACC, Cardiovasc Imaging*. 2020;13:2400–2411.

34 The Pericardium: Anatomy, Function, and Disease

SIMRAT KAUR, ALLAN L. KLEIN, AND DEBORAH KWON

PERICARDIAL ANATOMY AND FUNCTION

The pericardium is a dual-layered membrane comprised of visceral and parietal pericardium surrounding the heart as well as origins of the great vessels.[1] The visceral pericardium composed of mesothelial cells is adherent to the epicardium of the heart. The parietal pericardium is acellular with collagen and elastin fibers and is normally 2 mm in thickness. It has elastic properties which help retain the cardiac shape and volume maintaining a constant position in the mediastinum. The pericardial space normally accommodates around 15–50 mL of serous fluid which minimizes friction between the two layers.

The pericardium reflects over the base of the aorta and pulmonary trunk and at the insertions of the superior and inferior vena cava as well as the four pulmonary veins.[2] The pericardial cavity also has further interconnecting sinuses.[3] The transverse sinus is the space between two pericardial layers superior to the left atrium (LA) and posterior to the aorta and pulmonary artery. The oblique sinus is a cul-de-sac at the inferior border of the vena cava and four pulmonary veins lying posterior to the LA.[2] The pericardium also helps in assisting atrial filling by creating negative suction during systole. It provides an appropriate milieu for balancing ventricular compliance as well as decreasing friction with other mediastinal structures. It also helps in assisting diastolic interaction and ventricular interdependence. The parietal pericardium is relatively avascular but well innervated, resulting in chest pain in the setting of inflammation.

IMAGING MODALITIES

Three imaging modalities are commonly used for evaluation of pericardial pathologies and their hemodynamic effects, including echocardiography, cardiac computed tomography (CT), and cardiac magnetic resonance imaging (CMRI).[4] Echocardiography is typically the first-line imaging modality. Two-dimensional transthoracic echocardiography (TTE) is a readily available portable imaging tool which can detect pericardial pathologies including any hemodynamic compromise.[5] Real-time TTE along with a respirometer can detect respirophasic changes across mitral and tricuspid inflows as well as septal motion with excellent temporal resolution. Pericardial cysts or masses can also be diagnosed on TTE. This can help discern constrictive as well as tamponade physiology. Pericardial thickness, however, is not reliably assessed by TTE, and focal areas of calcification can be difficult to discern. The acoustic windows are often limited by body habitus, chest deformities, and parenchymal lung diseases, and definitive diagnoses are often challenging by echocardiography in isolation. Advanced imaging modalities such as cardiac CT and CMRI provide important complementary imaging assessment, particularly when echocardiographic assessment is limited.[5]

Both cardiac CT and CMR provide direct visualization of pericardium as well as surrounding mediastinal structures.[6,7] Both can also identify extracardiac pathologies such as tumors which could be contributing to presentation (Table 34.1). For diagnosis of cardiac pathologies, ECG gating is recommended for both modalities to minimize motion artifact.[6,7] Cardiac CT can identify pericardial calcification which is often present in cases of constrictive pericarditis and is difficult to discern with CMR. Limitations of cardiac CT include limited functional assessment, limited assessment of pericardial inflammation, and exposure to ionizing radiation, which is of concern particularly in younger individuals with pericarditis requiring sequential imaging. While four-dimensional (4D) CT can provide functional assessment, this requires significant incraese in ionizing radiation and also requires intravenous iodinated contrast, which can be limited by renal function.[5]

CMR provides comprehensive anatomical, functional, and hemodynamic assessment of the pericardium without utilizing ionizing radiation (Fig. 34.1).[8] CMR can also uniquely characterize pericardial pathologies including effusions, pericarditis, and pericardial masses through the use of T1-, T2-weighted as well as post-gadolinium contrast imaging. The presence of constrictive physiology can also be accurately assessed on real-time free-breathing sequences.[8] Basic knowledge of MRI techniques have been discussed in prior chapters and is briefed discussed below in their applications to pericardial assessment.

Steady-State Free Precession (SSFP)

Steady-state free precession is the most widely used bright blood cine sequence and is dependent on the T2/T1 magnetic properties of tissue. It produces images of high spatial and temporal resolution due to its excellent blood/tissue interface. It allows for accurate assessment of anatomy and volume quantification of cardiac chambers and vascular anatomy by delineating the blood pool.[9] It also enables the assessment of pericardial effusions as well as the impact of pericardial disease on cardiac physiology, manifested by the presence of a diastolic bounce and respirophasic shift involving the interventricular

TABLE 34.1 Pericardial tumors and specific tissue characterization on CMR.

	CARDIAC MASSES	T1 WEIGHTED	T2 WEIGHTED	LGE
Benign	Pericardial Cyst	Hypo	Hyper	No uptake
	Lipoma	Hyper	Hyper	No uptake
	Hemangioma	Iso	Hyper	Homo/Heterogeneous
	Teratoma	Iso or Hypo	Hyper	Heterogeneous
	Fibroma	Iso	Hypo	Increased uptake or no uptake
Malignant	Mesothelioma	Iso	Hyper	Increased uptake
	Sarcoma	Iso	Hyper	Heterogeneous
	Lymphoma	Iso	Hyper	No uptake
	Metastasis	Iso[a]	Hyper	Heterogeneous

[a]Except melanoma.

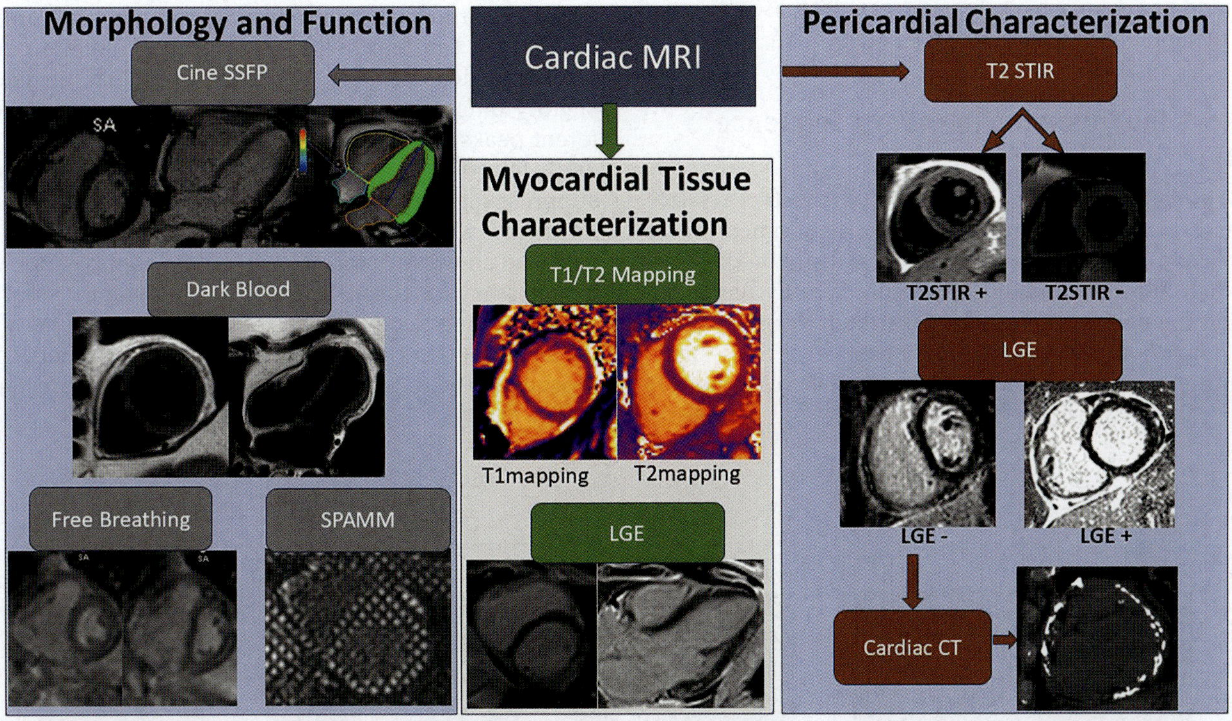

FIG. 34.1 Comprehensive evaluation of cardiac MRI for pericardial assessment. Cine SSFP sequences provide quantitative assessment of ventricular volumes, function, deformation, and assessment of ventricular interdependence physiology. Black blood sequences (fast spin echo/double-inversion recovery T1-weighted imaging) best delineate pericardial thickness and anatomy. Free-breathing and SPAMM sequences allow for identification of constrictive physiology. Myocardial tissue characterization with T1/T2 mapping and LGE enables the ability to determine the presence of concomitant myocarditis, or infiltration of pericardial masses. Pericardial characterization via a T2 STIR sequence provides the ability to identify pericardial edema, and LGE assessment provides the ability to determine the presence of inflammation and neovascularization. In cases of burnt-out pericarditis, T2 STIR and LGE become negative, and calcification of the pericardium often occurs. CMR does not allow reliable identification of calcification, and cardiac CT is often required to confirm the presence and extent of pericardial calcium.

septum, conical deformities of ventricles, and tethering of the cardiac chambers in the setting of constrictive physiology.[8]

Endocardial and epicardial borders are commonly traced along the short-axis stack of the left ventricle and endocardial borders of the right ventricle to measure end-diastolic and systolic volumes, ejection fraction, stroke volume, cardiac mass, as well as output. Feature tracking software can be used to measure strain on CMR and may also help distinguish constrictive pericarditis from restrictive cardiomyopathies. Spatial modulation of magnetization (SPAMM) by using radiofrequency saturation pulses also offers a unique and effective manner for diagnosing constrictive physiology.[10]

Black Blood Imaging

Electrocardiogram-gated fast spin-echo double-inversion recovery T1-weighted sequences are utilized for properly nulled blood pool signal which appears black and allows sharp delineation of the tissue contrast between myocardium, epicardium, pericardium, and mediastinum.[9] Pericardial thickness ≥3 mm signifies pathologic pericardial thickening and the evaluation of the presence and severity of pericardial thickness is best determined on this imaging sequence due to the absence of chemical shift/India ink artifacts that obscure more precise assessment with SFFP imaging.

Real-Time Free-Breathing Sequences

Free-breathing sequences are taken over at least two complete respiratory cycles where patients are asked to inspire and expire deeply to determine the presence of interventricular dependence. Typically, a single short-axis midventricular slice is acquired. Respirophasic septal flattening during inspiration has been shown to be pathognomonic for constrictive physiology, with prior studies quoting 80% sensitivity and 100% specificity.[11,12] However, the presence of RV pressure/volume overload states, such as tricuspid regurgitation and pulmonary hypertension, can decrease the specificity of septal flattening to identify constriction.

T2 Short Tau Inversion Recovery Sequence (STIR)

The STIR sequence provides the ability to detect relative increases in water. An inversion prepulse is timed for fat suppression resulting in nulled epicardial and mediastinal fat, which allows the ability to readily identify enhanced signal in the pericardium and myocardium to signify areas of inflammation and edema. The absence of STIR signal in the pericardium is consistent with the following: (1) absence of active inflammation, (2) response to treatment, or (3) progression to a burnt-out phase of pericarditis based on clinical scenario.[9]

Late Gadolinium Enhancement (LGE)

Images are typically acquired 10–15 minutes after intravenous gadolinium contrast administration to identify areas where gadolinium has entered into interstitial spaces, which are identified with high T1-weighted signal. Pericardial inflammation and fibrosis can lead to abnormal retention of gadolinium within the pericardium that can also be seen in recurrent and chronic cases when T2 STIR sequences can be negative. Burnt out pericarditis cases, however, usually lack LGE. Because epicardial fat also appears bright, pericardial enhancement can be difficult to accurately identify, particularly in the presence of prominent epicardial fat. Therefore, fat suppression prepulse techniques can improve discernment of definite pericardial enhancement (Fig. 34.2). Water and fat resonate at slightly different frequencies of precession and have different peaks with a frquence difference of ~220 Hz at 1.5 T and ~440 Hz at 3T. An adiabatic inversion pulse is used to suppress fat signals is SPAIR (Spectral Adiabatic Inversion Recovery) which is less prone to variations of the magnetic field and allows for more consistent fat suppression which is necessary for these cases. SPIR (Spectral Presaturation with Inversion Recovery) sequence is less commonly used in cardiac MRI because it's more sensitive to B_0 and B_1 inhomogeneities with inadequate epicardial fat suppresion.

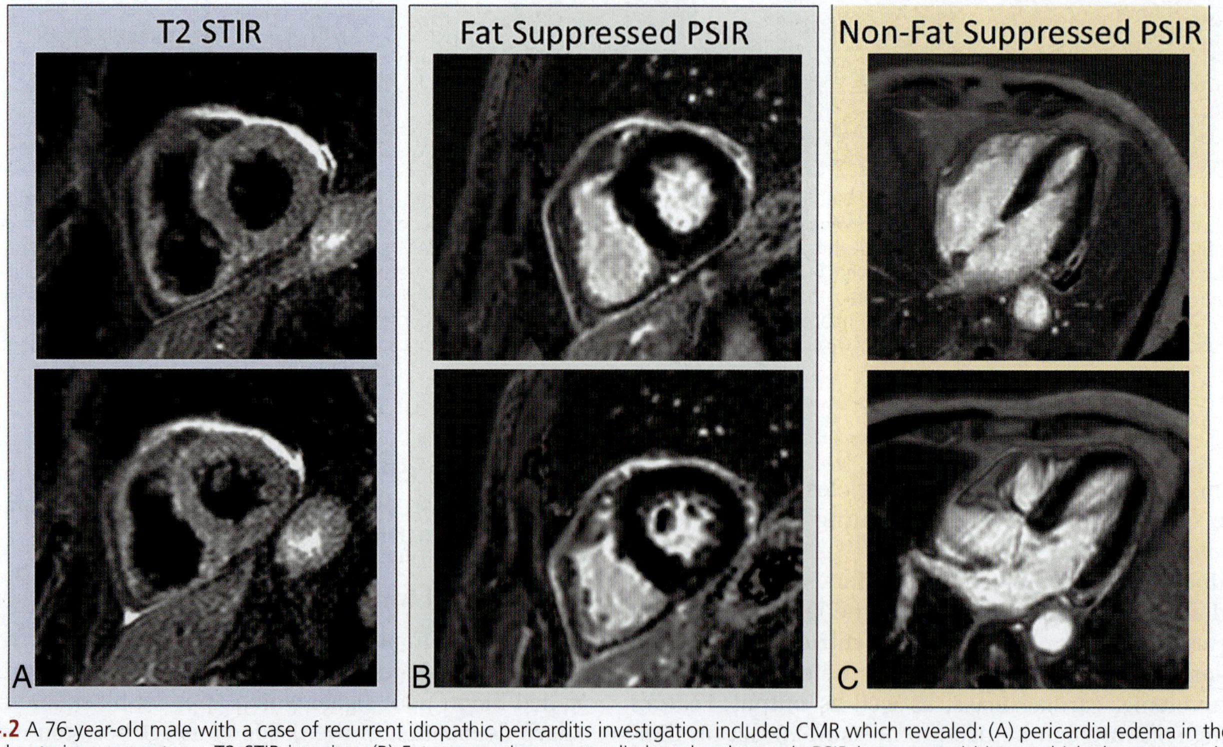

FIG. 34.2 A 76-year-old male with a case of recurrent idiopathic pericarditis investigation included CMR which revealed: (A) pericardial edema in the basal and mid-anterior segments on T2 STIR imaging. (B) Fat suppression was applied to the short-axis PSIR image acquisitions, which demonstrated >50% circumferential extent of LGE with >3 mm thickness along the mid and apical segments. (C) Non-fat suppressed PSIR imaging in this same patient, demonstrates heterogenous LGE uptake on long-axis imaging that is not distinct from the adjacent epicardial and mediastinal fat.

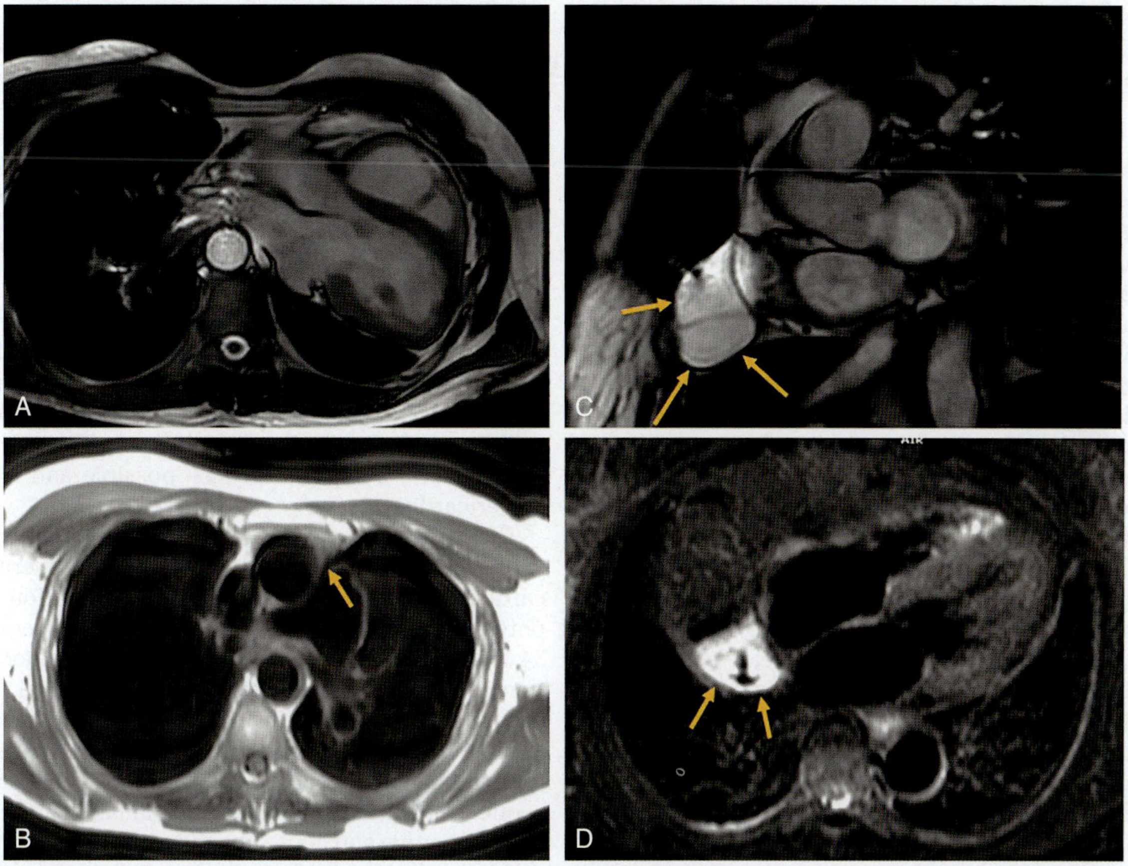

FIG. 34.3 Congenital deformities of pericardium. (A) SSFP sequence demonstrating levopositioning of the heart and posterolateral displacement on LV apex consistent with congenital absence of pericardium. (B) Black blood sequence with lung interposed between the great vessels seen in cases of congenital absence of pericardium. (C) SSFP sequence depicting well-defined pericardiac cystic lesion adjacent to right atrium with high signal intensity. (D) T2 STIR sequence showing a large 9.2 × 3.4. 4 cm cystic lesion with high signal intensity consistent with pericardial cyst.

Phase Velocity Mapping

Phase velocity mapping (PVM) is used for the assessment of valvular abnormalities and quantifying blood flow and velocity assessment. The presence of >25% decrease and >40% increase in velocities of mitral and tricuspid inflow velocities during inspiration respectively can signify pericardial constriction or tamponade physiology.

T1 and T2 Mapping

T1 and T2 image mapping are increasingly utilized techniques that enable quantitative measurements of T1/T2 times and extracellular volume fraction (ECV) of the myocardium. These techniques can improve the sensitivity of identify myocardial inflammation consistent with myopericarditis. T2 mapping can be performed using a T2 preparation module or with a gradient spin echo sequences. Native T1 mapping can also be utilized to discern transudative from exudative effusions with longer T1 time of >3103 ms in exudative effusions.[13]

Tissue Tagging with Spatial Modulation of Magnetization (SPAMM)

Radiofrequency saturation pulses can be placed in grids on the heart to follow the spatial modulation of epicardial/pericardial motion throughout the cardiac cycle.[14,15] Normally, discontinuous tag lines are visualized due to rapid slippage in the setting of a normal pericardium. However, persistence of the tag lines can indicate tethering seen with constriction.

PERICARDIAL DISEASES

Congenital Abnormalities

1. *Congenital Absence of Pericardium:* Congenital absence of pericardium is a rare spectrum of disorders ranging from small defects to complete bilateral absence of pericardium (Fig. 34.3). Left-sided partial defects are most common, with rare reports of right-sided defects.[16] A study from Mayo Clinic reported the prevalence to be around 0.044%.[17] Association with other abnormalities such as patent ductus arteriosus, tetralogy of Fallot, mitral stenosis, pectus excavatum, bronchogenic cysts, and diaphragmatic hernia has been reported.[16] Most patients are asymptomatic and are often diagnosed after incidental chest or cardiac imaging.[16] In rare cases it can lead to herniation and entrapment of cardiac tissue necessitating surgical management.

CMR provides complete visualization of the pericardium and its absence, along with a wide field of view of the chest and any associated abnormalities.[6,7] The leftward orientation of the heart with leftward rotation and entrapment of lung tissue between the aorta and pulmonary artery or the heart and hemidiaphragm are some identifiable clues to congenital absence of pericardium (Fig. 34.3). Unrestrained movement of cardiac apex on cine images can also suggest congenital absence of pericardium.

2. *Pericardial Cysts:* Pericardial cysts are congenital fluid collections in the pericardium developing from embryological pericardial remnants, and the cyst walls are lined with a single layer of mesothelial cells.[18] The cysts are thin-walled, unilocular, and filled with clear transudative fluids (Fig. 34.3). They can be found anywhere along the pericardium, but a common location is at the right followed by the left cardiophrenic angle.

Pericardial cysts are usually asymptomatic and diagnosed incidentally on chest imaging. In rare circumstances larger cysts can lead to compressive symptoms such as chest pain, dyspnea, and cough requiring aspiration or surgical removal.[19]

Pericardial cysts can be seen occasionally on echocardiography, although they are not always clearly visualized. On CMR, pericardial cysts are seen as nonenhancing, well-circumscribed, thin-walled, encapsulated cysts without any septations or heterogeneous imaging properties. Due to their water content, they are seen as hypointense on T1-weighted images and homogeneous high signal on T2-weighted images. Pericardial cysts are avascular and thus do not demonstrate any gadolinium uptake on perfusion sequences. They demonstrate simple water characteristics on LGE imaging, and do not enhance.[3,5] In rare cases, pericardial cyst can contain exudative fluid and will be seen as high intensity on T1-weighted images.

Pericarditis

1. *Acute Pericarditis:* Acute pericarditis occurs due to pericardial inflammation and is a common etiology for chest pain with rates increasing post COVID-19 pandemic.[20] The most common causes include idiopathic or postviral with post cardiac injury syndromes increasing with cardic procedures. Other etiologies include drug toxicity, post-myocardial infarction, post-vaccination, trauma, infection, neoplasm, radiation, and autoimmune disorders.[21] Typically, these episodes are self-limiting and improve within 4–6 weeks. Clinical presentation, the presence of pericardial effusion and/or thickened pericardium on echocardiography, along with elevated serum biomarkers (erythrocyte sedimentation rate and C-reactive protein) are often diagnostic.[21] The 2025 ACC expert consensus document outlines a new diagnostic criteria for diagnosis which includes pericarditic chest pain in addition to pericardial rub, ECG changes, pericardial effusions, elevated inflammatory markers and imaging findings of pericarditis on CT or MRI with a score of 0 being unlikely, 1 - possible and 2 + definite pericarditis.[22]

CMR provides powerful and unique tissue characterization of pericardium, delineation of the severity of pericardial inflammation, as well as prognostication, including potential concomitant myocardial involvement (Fig. 34.1). T1-weighted sequences with black blood preparation are utilized for assessment of pericardial thickening and assessment of effusion.[23] Pericardial thickening of >3 mm is commonly associated with pericarditis. Pericardial enhancement on a T2-weighted STIR fat-suppressed sequence identifies significant inflammation and edema and signifies active and acute inflammation. Significant pericardial inflammation leads to pericardial neovascularization, leading to enhancement on late gadolinium imaging with extremely high sensitivity (94%–100%).[24] Acute pericarditis is characterized by pericardial enhancement with both T2STIR and LGE imaging. On the other hand, lack of T2STIR enhancement in the setting of significant pericardial LGE is associated with subacute pericarditis. Lack of pericardial enhancement on T2STIR and/or LGE should suggest an alternative etiology for the patient's symptoms.[25]

CMR also provides the unique ability to identify associated myopericarditis, which is present in 15%–24% of patients presenting with pericarditis, and is characterized

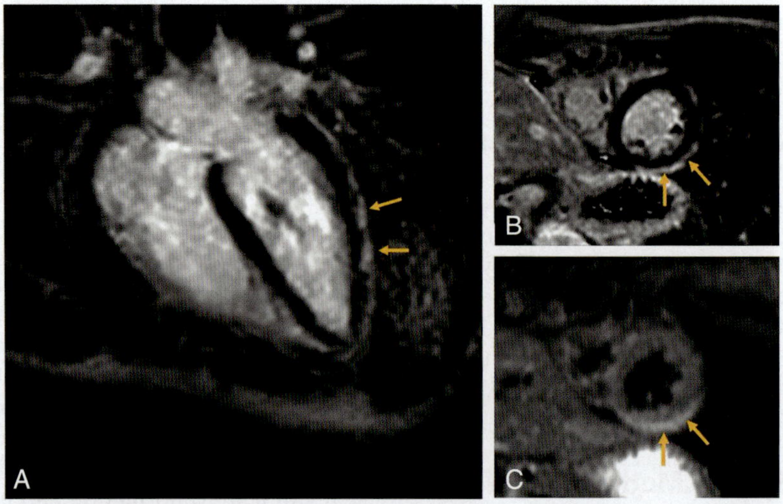

FIG. 34.4 Case of a 22-year-old male with persistent chest pain post COVID-19 infection. (A) Mild pericardial LGE as well as mild epicardial myocardial enhancement along the lateral wall on the four-chamber phase sensitive inversion recovery LGE imaging. (B) Short axis with LGE in the mid-distal inferolateral wall involving the subepicardial aspect of the myocardium and the pericardium. (C) T2 STIR image depicting hyperintense signal in the same area consistent with acute inflammation and edema demonstrating acute focal myopericarditis.

by associated myocardial delayed enhancement in a mid-myocardial or epicardial distribution (Fig. 34.4).[8,23] T1/T2 mapping may also increase the diagnostic accuracy in identifying concurrent myocardial inflammation.[26] Recent 2025 ESC guidelines provide a class 1 indication for cardiac MRI in patients with suspected myocpericardial syndrome and a class 1 recommendation for a follow up CMR within 6 months of symptom onset for onhoing risk statification and tailoring therapy.[27]

2. *Recurrent Pericarditis:* Recurrent pericarditis is defined as recurrence of symptoms after a latency of about 6 weeks. It the most common complication and can occur in 15%–30% of patients with acute pericarditis. About half of patients having one episode of recurrence will continue to have subsequent episodes. CMR is essential to identify ongoing pericardial inflammation and assessment of progression after intensification of therapy. Prominent LGE in the absence of increased signal on T2 STIR imaging is suggestive of subacute pericarditis. A multicenter study of patients with idiopathic recurrent pericarditis found that pericardial edema seen on T2STIR imaging (79.5%) and LGE (75.3%) on CMR was identified within 2 weeks of symptoms.[28] The presence of both pericardial edema and LGE had a sensitivity of 73% and specificity of 99% in this study.[28]
3. *Incessant/Chronic Pericarditis:* Chronic pericarditis occurs if persistence of symptoms occurs beyond 3 months. Though symptoms may be significant, serologic inflammatory markers may not accurately reflect active inflammation due to ongoing antiinflammatory therapy. Hence, imaging assessment is crucial. Follow-up CMR enables the ability to determine the severity of pericardial inflammation and to guide therapeutic decision-making to determine the need for escalation of therapy, and appropriate timing for tapering therapy (Fig. 34.5).
4. *Constrictive Pericarditis:* Constrictive pericarditis can be considered a late presentation in the disease spectrum of pericarditis, due to progressive inflammation. This results in ongoing interventricular dependence and eventually right heart failure. The pericardium becomes thickened due to intense inflammation, resulting in diastolic restraint. When pericardial inflammation is inadequately mitigated, fibrin deposition/fibrosis, or calcification ensue, thus leading to irreversible impairment of diastolic filling of cardiac chambers. CMR provides the unique ability to discern two distinct underlying etiologies of constrictive pericarditis: (1) transient constriction due to significant acute pericarditis; or (2) fibrosed or calcified chronic constriction due to burnt-out pericarditis. A study by Bolen et al published a decision tree algorithm for prediction of constrictive pericarditis which included a septal excursion of ≥12% and a pericardial thickness of ≥3 mm and in those with a septal excursion of ≤12 and pericardial thickness of <3 mm a septal excursion of ≥6.3% is considered significant for constrictive pericarditis.[29] While echocardiography is the initial test of choice to detect evidence of constrictive physiology,[6,7] it cannot reliably discern between transient and burnt-out constrictive pericarditis. Recently published reports have also shown the utility of parametric mapping such as extracellular volume measurement in the liver that can detect congestive hepatopathy due to constriction.[30] Cardiac CT is often used to assess the presence and extent of pericardial calcification; however, CMR is the

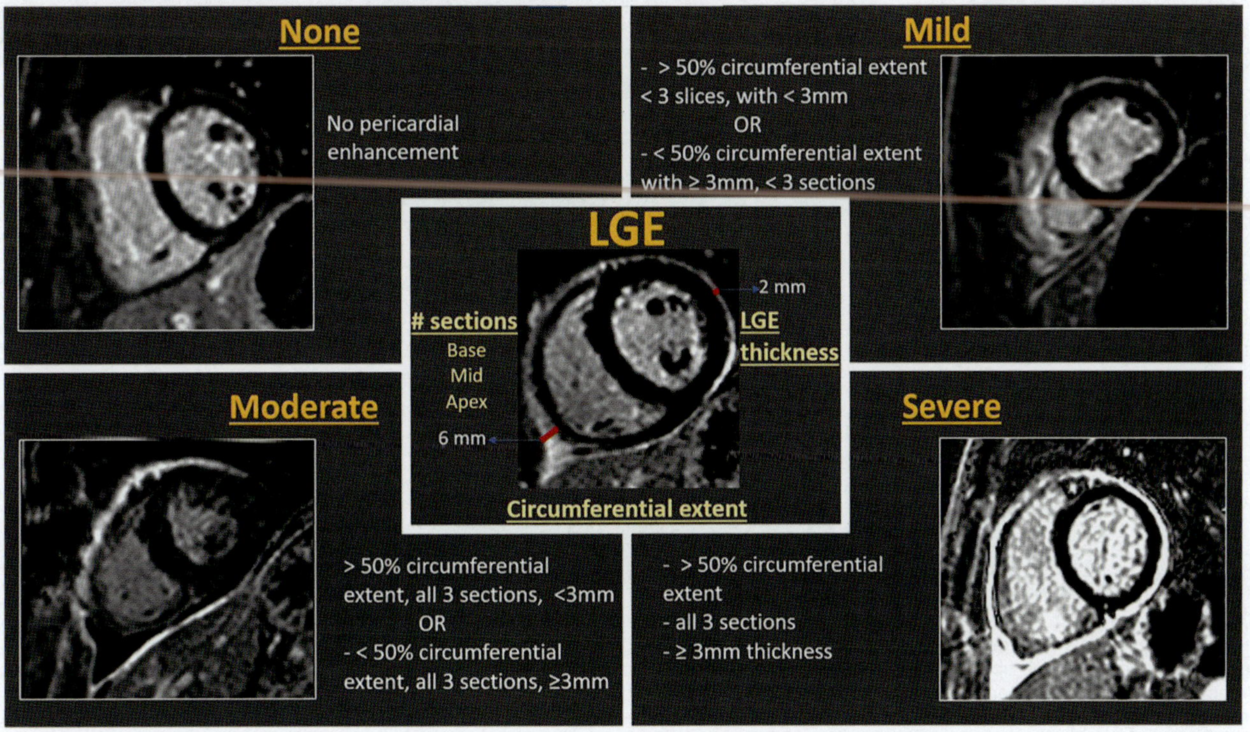

FIG. 34.5 Grading of late gadolinium enhancement depending of severity of pericarditis. Semiquantitative grading can be performed by determining the areas with LGE thickness ≥3 mm, circumferential extent, and extent through the base, mid, and apical sections. This can best be determined on the LGE short-axis stack. Semiquantitative criteria for none, mild, moderate, and severe are provided.

test of choice to discern pericardial inflammation and should be included for comprehensive assessment in patients with suspected constriction.[5,29]

CMR features of constrictive physiology include: thickened pericardium, conical deformity of both ventricles, prominent diastolic bounce, and respirophasic septal flattening on free-breathing sequences.[8] In addition, CMR radiofrequency tagging sequences can be utilized to evaluate the degree of pericardial myocardial tethering.[8] Similar to echocardiography, respirophasic variations across mitral and tricuspid valves can be assessed over 10 seconds during real-time phase contrast sequences and values exceeding 25% and 45%, respectively, are considered abnormal.

As outlined above, CMR enables the ability to provide important tissue characterization to identify transient constriction due to acute pericarditis versus burnt-out constriction. Enhancement of the pericardium on T2 STIR imaging and LGE in the setting of morphologic and functional ventricular assessment consistent with constriction suggests transient constriction due to acute pericarditis. Identifying inflammation as the underlying etiology of constrictive physiology significantly impacts therapeutic decision-making, as patients with significant pericardial enhancement on T2STIR and LGE imaging are likely to respond with intensive antiinflammatory medications, with potential resolution of constrictive physiology.[31]

On the other hand, the absence of enhancement on either T2 imaging or LGE indicates progression to the burnt-out phase of constriction.[5,8,23] Patients with little or no pericardial LGE in the setting of constrictive physiology are less likely to respond antiinflammatory medications, and are likely best suited for pericardiectomy. CMR can also guide planning strategies for cardiac decompression at the time of pericardiectomy, based on RV volumes/function and pericardial anatomy to decrease the risk of postoperative complications.[32]

Effusive constriction is another subtype of constrictive pericarditis in the presence of a significant pericardial effusion, which is defined as failure of a fall in right atrial pressure by 50% or less than 10 mm Hg after pericardiocentesis (Fig. 34.6). Treatment of effusive constrictive physiology is dictated by the presence and severity of pericardial enhancement on T2STIR and LGE imaging. Effusive constrictive physiology due to acute pericarditis may improve and potentially resolve with aggressive antiinflammatory therapy. However, radical pericardiectomy is often required for burnt-out chronic pericarditis leading to constriction (Fig. 34.7).[31,33]

Pitfalls: The disadvantages of CMR include inability to discern pericardial calcification from fibrosis for which CCT (cardiac computed tomography) is indicated (Fig. 34.8). Cardiac and respiratory gating can be challenging

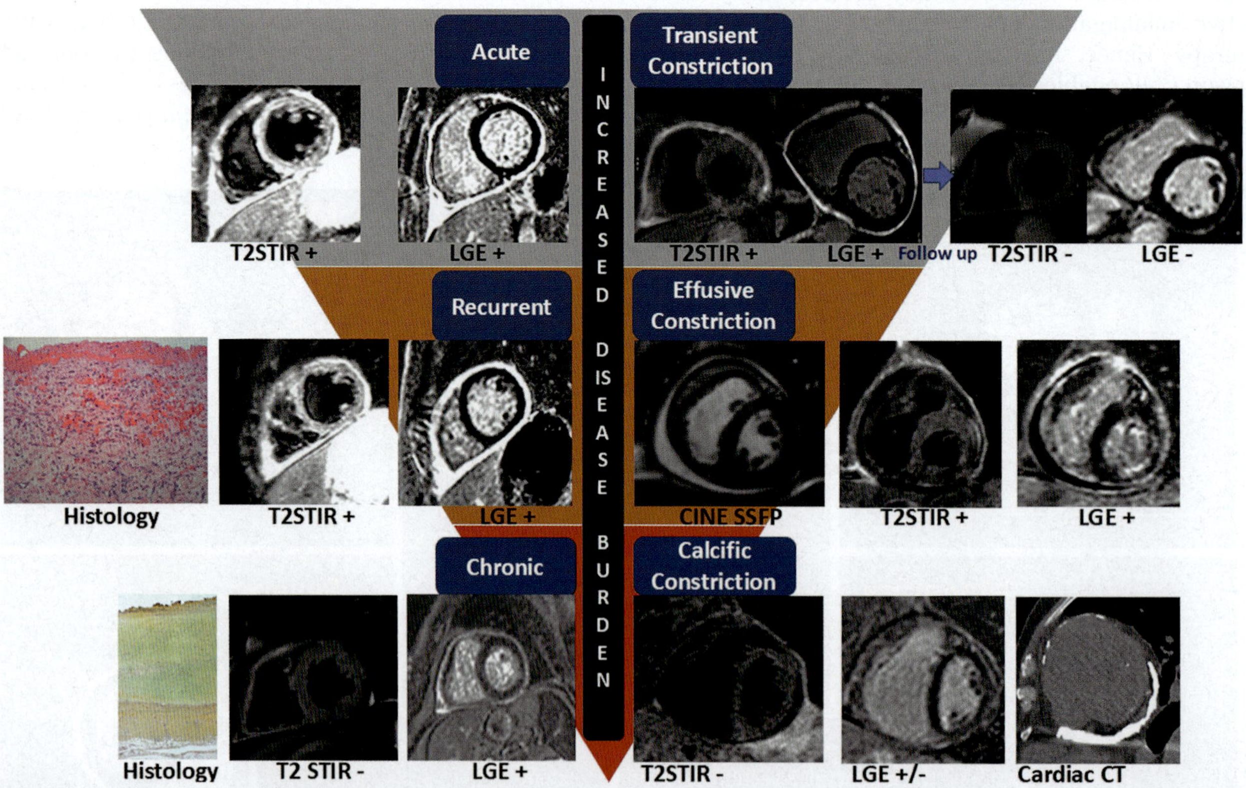

FIG. 34.6 Disease spectrum of pericarditis with acute cases showing hyperintense T2 STIR and late gadolinium enhancement without constrictive physiology. Recurrent pericarditis often results in significant neovascularization, and fibrosis of the pericardium can also develop. This can progress into the chronic phase, where significant irreversible thickening/fibrosis of the pericardium can occur in the setting of chronic inflammation. Gross pericardiectomy specimen demonstrates significant pericardial thickening with histology showing marked fibrosis and mild chronic inflammation. Constrictive physiology can occur in the setting of significant pericardial inflammation, presence of a pericardial effusion, fibrous thickened pericardium, and significant calcification. Transient pericarditis can resolve after treatment and intensive antiinflammatory medications. Effusive constrictive pericarditis, findings are often similar to transient constriction, but with the presence of a significant effusion on SSFP imaging. Burnt-out constriction often occurs with the presence of calcification. Calcified areas appear hypo-intense on cine SSFP and T2 STIR sequences, but are best confirmed with cardiac CT.

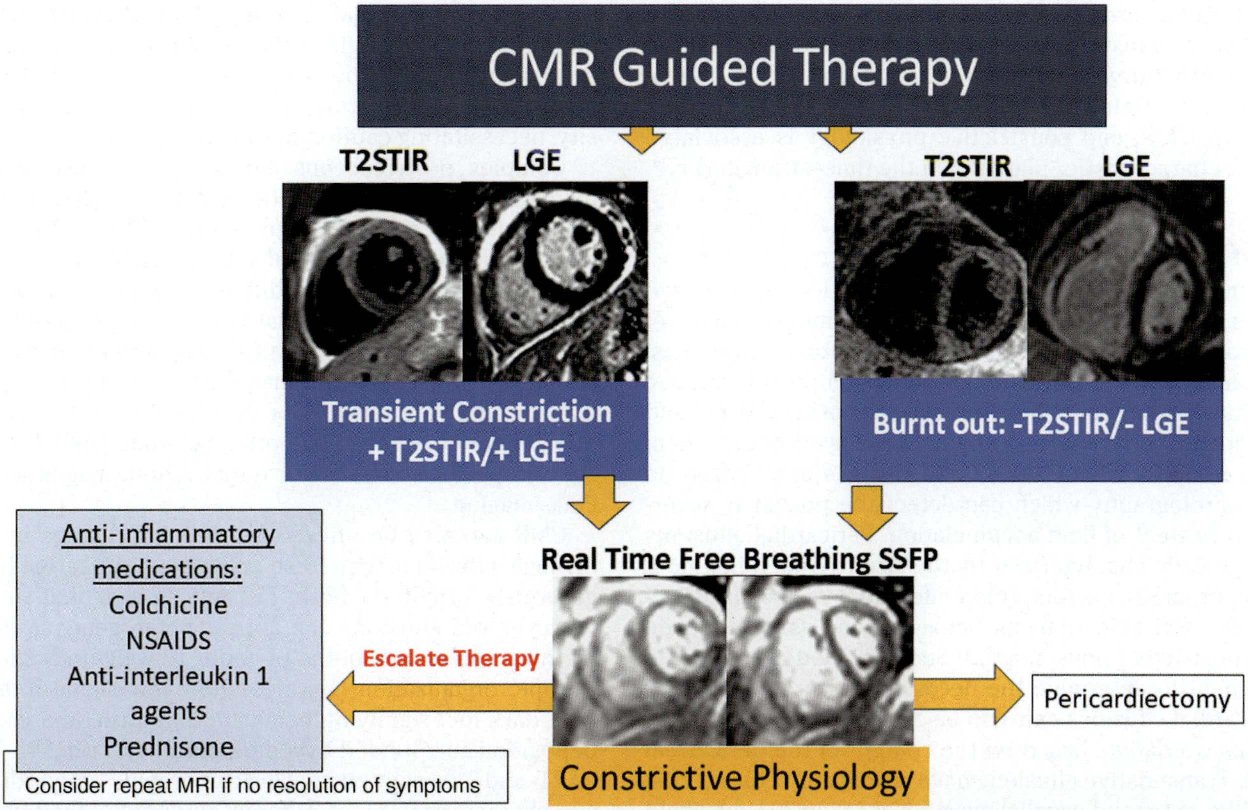

FIG. 34.7 Contemporary management of recurrent/incessant pericarditis. Pericarditis should be classified based on the presence or absence of constrictive physiology. Patients with acute/subacute pericarditis, but without constriction, are treated with antiinflammatory medications, and the intensity of the antiinflammatory regimen and cadence of tapering can be dictated by the severity of inflammation on CMR. CMR should be repeated if there is no resolution of symptoms after 3–6 months of therapy to guide decisions regarding intensification of antiinflammatory medications. Patients with constrictive physiology, but no evidence of active inflammation, should be referred for pericardectomy. On the other hand, the presence of significant pericardial inflammation in patients with constrictive physiology identifies an inflammatory etiology which can resolve with an intensive antiinflammatory therapeutic regimen. CMR should be repeated if there is no resolution of symptoms after 3–6 months of therapy to guide decisions regarding intensification of antiinflammatory medications. Patients who experience significant continued symptoms despite maximal medical therapy or progress to burnt-out constriction should be referred for pericardectomy.

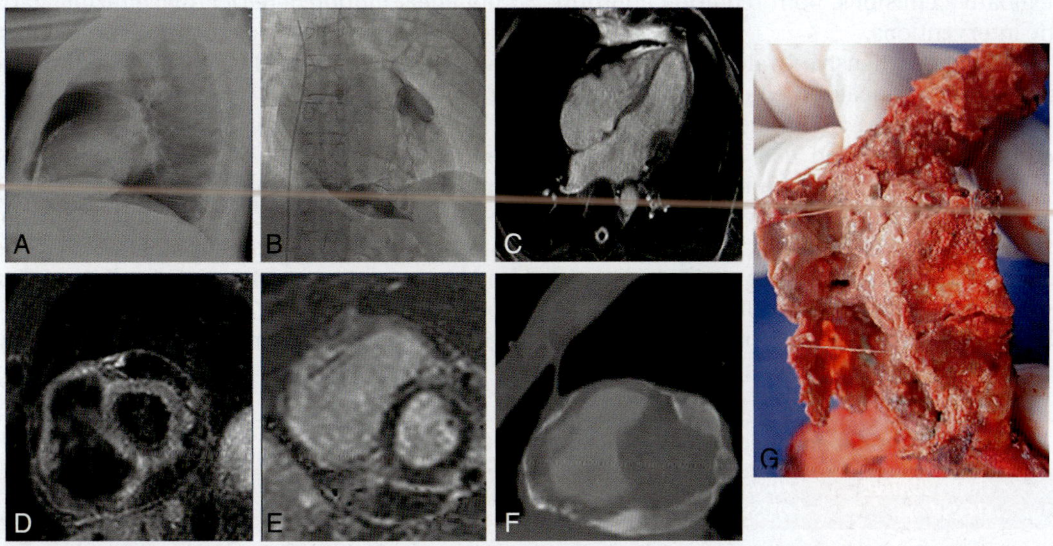

FIG. 34.8 (A) Diffuse severe thick pericardial calcification noted on lateral chest x-ray. (B) Fluoroscopic image of the heart depicting dense anterior and inferior pericardial calcification. (C) Cine SSFP sequence with circumscribed areas of hypointense signal in the basal anterolateral and inferior wall which is also seen on (D) T2 STIR and (E) LGE sequence without any delayed enhancement. (F) CT scan showing near circumferential dense calcification of the pericardium. (G) Gross specimen demonstrating thickened and calcified pericardium with areas of liquefaction.

in cases of supraventricular arrhythmias and in patients unable to tolerate prolonged breath hold due to persistent dyspnea.[34] Fat-suppression sequences are utilized to differentiate pericardial inflammation from adjacent epicardial fat; however, the fat suppression prepulse may not provide uniform suppression, posing interpretation challenges.[4]

Novel applications: Feature-tracking assessment of global longitudinal strain can be performed to discern constriction versus restriction, with restrictive myocardial disease demonstrating significantly blunted deformation mechanics (area under the curve [AUC] 0.84).[35] A diastolic time–strain curve can also be derived from feature-tracking CMR, and constrictive physiology is associated with a characteristic "plateau" on the time–strain curve.[36]

Pericardial Effusion

Accumulation of excess fluid in the pericardial sac can be simple, bloody, or chylous (rare). Common causes of pericardial effusions include: inflammatory processes, post-myocardial infarction, infectious/post-infectious, trauma, aortic dissection, uremia, hypothyroidism, and malignancy. However, no clear underlying etiology is identified in up to 50% of cases.[37] Diagnosis is often based on echocardiography which can detect the presence, severity, and extent of fluid accumulation. Pericardial effusions are typically characterized by the size (trivial, mild, moderate, or large), location (circumferential vs. localized/loculated), and hemodynamic impact (none vs. tamponade vs. constrictive physiology).[38] Such detailed assessments also help to determine the need for pericardiocentesis.[34] Pericardial effusions can also be classified as transudative versus exudative, based on the content of the pericardial fluid. Transudative effusions have attenuation characteristics like water and usually measure less than 20 Hounsfield units (HU), while more complex effusive or hemorrhagic effusions demonstrate higher HU.[5] Noninflammatory idiopathic effusions are also typically transudative, and transudative effusions can also develop in the setting of increased venous pressure in congestive heart failure or pulmonary hypertension, and decreased absorption rate. Chylous pericardial effusions and purulent effusions are examples of exudative effusions, both requiring appropriate therapeutic interventions.

CMR provides a comprehensive evaluation of pericardial effusions, particularly localized effusions that can be missed by echocardiography. SSFP cine sequences best identify pericardial effusions and can provide accurate assessment of their size, complexity, and clues regarding transudative versus exudative based on differential signal intensity of the fluid. A multislice approach can allow precise quantification of the volume of pericardial fluid with the following size definitions: small (<1 cm), moderate (1–2 cm), and large (>2 cm). Transudative effusions have bright signal intensity due to their water content on T2-weighted imaging and low signal intensity of T1-weighted imaging, and often appear brighter than epicardial fat on gradient echo sequences.[8,39] However, in patients with smaller effusions, nonlaminar cardiac motion may alter signal intensity, necessitating caution during interpretation.

Complex proteinaceous effusions show low to intermediate signal intensity on T2-weighted imaging and high signal intensity on T1-weighted imaging. It can also clearly demonstrate the presence of septa, debris, or loculation. LGE imaging is essential to differentiate localized pericardial effusions from pericardial tumors. On phase-sensitive inversion recovery (PSIR) LGE assessment, pericardial effusions enhance on the magnitude images, but appear black on the PSIR image. However, pericardial tumors frequently either enhance on both magnitude and PSIR imaging, or appear iso-intense or dark on both magnitude and PSIR imaging.

CMR can also be utilized for defining the age in hemorrhagic effusions, with fresh collections appearing homogeneously bright on both T1- and T2-weighted images, however, old effusions can appear heterogeneous due to methemoglobin on both T1- and T2-weighted imaging. Chronic organization can also show low signal intensity with dark foci signifying hemosiderin, fibrin, and calcium deposition surrounded by a dark peripheral rim.[8,39]

T1- and T2-weighted imaging can provide pericardial tissue characterization, as different underlying fluid characteristics exhibit different T1 and T2 relaxation times (Table 34.2). Typically, pericardial effusions appear bright on T2-weighted and SSFP cine imaging. Native T1 mapping may also provide further quantitative classification of pericardial fluid assessment, as a threshold of 3013 ms can classify exudative versus transudative with a high degree of accuracy (94% sensitivity and 79% specificity).[40] However, nonlinear motion of pericardial effusion, particularly in the setting of larger effusion, can cause an inhomogeneous T1-weighted signal, which can lead to inaccurate quantitative T1 measurements.

Cardiac tamponade occurs due to hemodynamic compromise in the setting of pericardial effusion. Rapidly accumulating effusions can lead to tamponade physiology at relatively low volumes, however, slowly accumulating effusions require accumulation of large effusions for hemodynamic compromise. Diagnosis is often made clinically with bedside echocardiography, and the patients require emergent treatment with drainage either percutaneously or surgically. CCT and CMR are not indicated in these patients.

TABLE 34.2 Pericardial effusions and fluid characteristics seen on CMR.

	TRANSUDATIVE EFFUSION	EXUDATIVE EFFUSION	HEMOPERICARDIUM	PROTEINACEOUS EFFUSION	FIBRINOUS EFFUSION	PURULENT
T1-weighted imaging	Decreased signal	Isointense	Decrease signal (early phase, >15 days) Bright (3–15 days)	Bright (heterogeneous)	Decreased signal	Decreased signal
T2-weighed imaging	Bright	Isointense	Decrease signal (early phase, >15 days) Bright (3–15 days)	Decreased signal	Bright	High signal
Native T1 mapping	<3013 ms	>3013 ms				

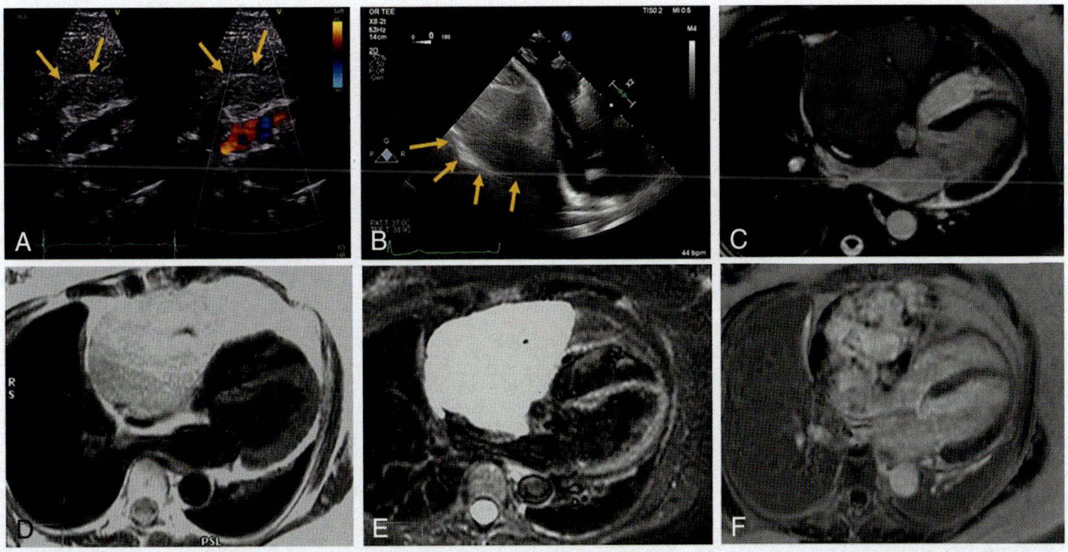

FIG. 34.9 (A) Large right-sided pericardial mass with compression of the right atrium and the ventricle visualized on the subcostal sequence of transthoracic echocardiogram. (B) Transesophageal echocardiogram redemonstrating large heterogeneous mass present lateral to the right atrium and ventricle causing compression of the right heart chambers. (C) SSFP imaging demonstrates hypo-intense mass compressing the right atrium. (D) T2 turbospin echo sequence with a hyperintense signal intensity and (E) T2 STIR sequence also demonstrating high signal intensity causing significant compression of RA. (F) Predominant heterogeneous enhancement of the mass with small focal nonenhancing areas seen on late gadolinium enhancement. Surgical resection of this mass confirmed an intrapericardial hemangioma causing significant right-sided chamber compression.

Pericardial Tumors

Pericardial tumors can be classified into primary versus secondary tumors. While primary tumors can be either benign or malignant, secondary most commonly reflect metastasis of malignant neoplasms. CMR provides comprehensive assessment of the pericardial tumor location, size, assessment of invasive properties, tissue characterization, and hemodynamic impact. SSFP imaging, black blood imaging, fat-saturated T2-weighted imaging, as well as T1-/T2-weighted imaging and late gadolinium enhancement can be utilized to differentiate the signal intensity of the tumor in relation to the healthy myocardium. Assessment of the vascularity of the pericardial tumor can also be determined by rest perfusion imaging. Representative pericardial tumors and their respective tissue properties are listed in Table 34.2.

1. *Primary Benign Pericardial Tumors*: Primary tumors of the pericardium are rare. Benign etiologies include lipomas, teratomas, neuromas, fibromas, and hemangiomas, and are often diagnosed on echocardiography.[41] Pericardial lipomas demonstrate bright signal on T1- and T2-weighted image sequences due to the fatty contents, with suppressed signal intensity on fat-saturated imaging sequences. Lipomas also show a unique "India-ink artifact," which leads to peripheral signal drop out in voxels containing both fat and nonfat components and is seen on out-of-phase T1-weighted imaging.[41,42]

   Teratomas are often detected in pediatric patients and appear as heterogeneous masses on echocardiography and CMR. Visualization of calcium, suggested by loss of signal on all imaging sequences, intermingled with fat within pericardial masses, can suggest its presence.[41] Hemangiomas characteristically demonstrate intermediate T1 and high signal intensity T2 images because of its hypervascularity and are hyperintense during as well as following contrast administration (Fig. 34.9). Pericardial fibromas can appear homogeneous with hypo- to iso-intense on T1-weighted imaging with low signal intensity on T2-weighted imaging and may or may not depict contrast enhancement.[42]
2. *Primary Malignant Pericardial Tumors*: Primary malignant pericardial tumors are rare and far less common than secondary pericardial tumors. Most common malignant primary pericardial tumors include mesothelioma, thymoma, sarcoma, lymphoma, and liposarcoma. Malignant pericardial tumors can be seen invading the myocardium and mediastinum, and are also typically associated with a pericardial effusion and lymphadenopathy.

   Primary mesothelioma is the most common pericardial malignancy, which can present with pericardial plaques, hemorrhagic effusion, or constriction. On CMR it appears isointense to myocardium on T1-weighted imaging, bright on T2-weighted imaging, with intense late gadolinium enhancement (Fig. 34.10).[42]

   Various subtypes of pericardial sarcoma can exist including, but not limited, to angiosarcoma, fibrosarcoma, liposarcoma, rhabdomyosarcoma, leiomyosarcoma, and synovial sarcomas.[41] Angiosarcoma is the most frequently described associated with hemorrhage and necrosis, hence appearing heterogeneous and hyperintense on T2-weighted imaging, but isointense on T1-weighted imaging with significant LGE, which is often heterogeneous.[42] Contrast administration can show enhancement, and the appearance has been described as like a "sun ray."[43] Liposarcomas can present with similar signal characteristics as lipoma, but demonstrate invasive properties.

   Lymphomas, on the other hand, present hypointense on T1 imaging and iso-hyperintense on T2 imaging, with minimal LGE.[43] Thymomas can sometimes be mistaken for pericardial cysts, as the location of these tumors is in a typical location for pericardial cysts. However, tissue characteristics other than simple water characteristics should

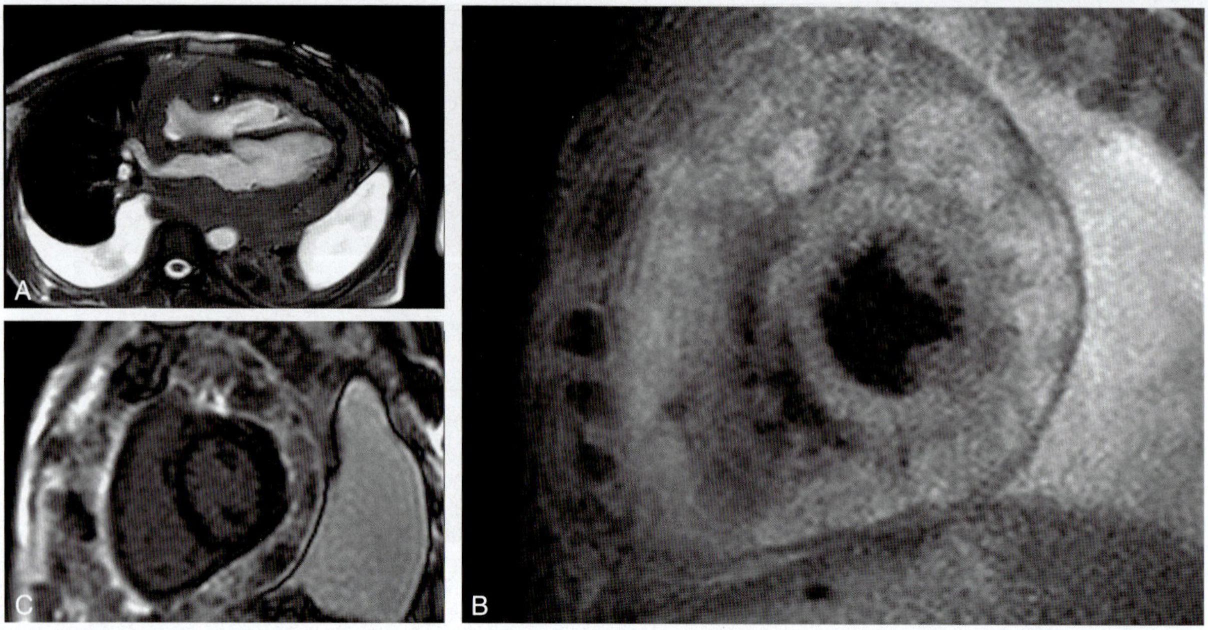

FIG. 34.10 A 46-year-old female with malignant mesothelioma. (A) SSFP cine sequence showing hypointense lobulated circumferential, infiltrative pericardial mass, with loss of epicardial fat margins along the lateral wall and atria associated with myocardial invasion. (B) T2 STIR sequence again demonstrating lobulated infiltrating mass with high signal intensity. (C) LGE imaging demonstrates heterogeneous enhancement with areas of enhancement.

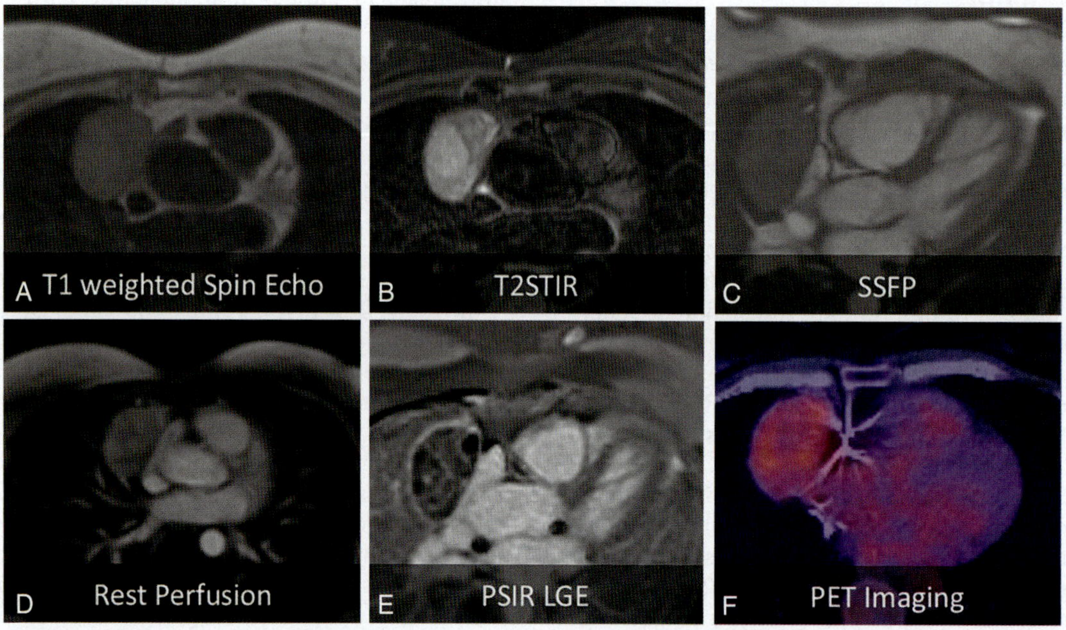

FIG. 34.11 A 50-year-old female with a known bicuspid aortic valve who was noted to have a mediastinal mass that was initially reported as a pericardial cyst. Cardiac MRI at that time revealed a 4.5 × 3.1 cm structure which appeared intrapericardial and hypointense on T1-weighted spin echo (A) and hyperintense on T2 STIR images (B). However, the mass appears somewhat heterogeneous, and appears hypointense on SSFP imaging (C). Furthermore, the mass demonstrated heterogeneous perfusion (D) and LGE (E), which would not be expected for a simple pericardial cyst. The patient was sent for PET imaging (F), and demonstrated marked metabolic activity. The patient underwent CT-guided biopsy, and histopathology was consistent with thymoma.

raise suspicion for an alternative differential diagnosis (Fig. 34.11).

3. *Secondary Pericardial Metastasis:* Metastasis to the pericardium is the most common site of involvement in the heart occurring due to direct spread, hematogenous, or lymphatic dissemination. Common cancers involving the pericardium include lung, breast, or esophageal malignancies, or melanomas, leukemias, and lymphomas. Detection of pericardial involvement often occurs because of pericardial effusion, which can become hemodynamically significant and require drainage. Rarely, patients can also present with symptoms of pericarditis or constrictive physiology. Often, pericardial cytology can be the first diagnosis of cancer and hemorrhagic pericardial effusions are strongly associated with cancers.[42,43]

CMR can show nodular pericardial thickening, effusion, and extension of the masses, which typically enhance with late gadolinium. Metastatic pericardial tumors are typically hypointense on T1-weighted images and with bright signal on T2-weighted images, and variable heterogeneous LGE.[42] Metastatic melanoma can be characterized by similar tissue properties, except that it is hyperintense of T1-weighted imaging. Comprehensive CMR assessment can provide important guidance regarding the feasibility of surgical resection.

Clinical Implications and Impact

CMR provides unique assessment of pericardial disease, and provides an important impact on clinical and therapeutic decision-making as it has been shown to be associated with decreased recurrence and decreased steroid use.[44] Quantitative assessment of the severity of pericardial enhancement provides important guidance for therapy and the appropriate intensity of antiinflammatory therapy.[4] Nonetheless, the presence of pericardial inflammation is typically reported as a binary finding: present/absent. However, CMR enables important determination of the intensity of active pericardial inflammation and is more accurate than plasma serologies such as erythrocyte sedimentation rate and C-reactive protein. This is due to the fact that inflammatory serologies are not specific to the pericardium and can be suppressed in the setting of antiinflammatory treatment, even when active pericardial inflammation is present. Furthermore, patients with severe pericarditis may have prolonged clinical courses, and accurate determination of the response to antiinflammatory therapeutic strategies can dictate when more aggressive biologic therapy is indicated.[33] Semiquantitative assessment of pericardial severity can provide a simple and clinically realistic standardized approach for grading pericardial enhancement to guide therapeutic decision-making, which is outlined in Fig. 34.5.

However, interpretation of pericardial enhancement should be assessed in the clinical context and inflammatory markers. For instance, interval improvement of symptoms in the setting of continued pericardial enhancement on LGE assessment may reflect resolving pericarditis, which lagging imaging features. Presumably pericardial enhancement on LGE imaging may be present in patients with significant resolving pericarditis or recurrent pericarditis that are in remission, presumably due to the development of fibrosis versus persistent neovascularization in the pericardium, which may take several months to years to resolve. Serial CMR imaging may be used in certain situations, such as refractory response to therapy.

Repeat CMR can provide further guidance in the setting of severe cases, refractory symptoms, or unclear therapeutic management, based on clinical assessment alone. Antiinflammatory treatment includes nonsteroidal antiinflammatory drugs (NSAIDs) plus colchicine. Rilonacept plus colchicine is an alternative first-line strategy in patients with significant pericardial enhancement presenting with fever and elevated serologies (inflammatory phenotype).[28] On the other hand, patients presenting with significant pericardial enhancement, but normal serologies and afebrile (noninflammatory) may be better managed with steroids. Noninflammatory patients with continued symptoms on corticosteroids may benefit from azathioprine and intravenous immunoglobulins.[45]

A schematic diagram for the CMR-guided management of patients with suspected pericarditis and/or constrictive pericarditis is provided in Fig. 34.7.

CONCLUSIONS

CMR provides comprehensive evaluation of pericardial disease and provides an important complimentary role to echocardiography and CT. CMR evaluation is particularly important in patients with suspected constrictive pericarditis, and can dictate appropriate management in regard to the initiation of antiinflammatory medications versus referral for surgical pericardiectomy. Standardized grading of pericardial inflammation may help to guide determination of the intensity and duration of antiinflammatory medications, including new biologic medications. Further studies and treatment guidelines are needed to develop standardized CMR-guided treatment protocols.

ACKNOWLEDGMENTS

We would like to thank Dr. Jay S. Leb and Dr. Susie N. Hong for their contributions to this chapter in the previous edition. We would also like to thank Deborah Agler for her support and assistance with providing figures for this chapter.

REFERENCES

1. Rodriguez ER, Tan C. Structure and Anatomy of the Human Pericardium. *Prog Cardiovasc Dis*. 2017;59:327–430.
2. Vesely TM, Cahill DR. Cross-sectional anatomy of the pericardial sinuses, recesses, and adjacent structures. *Surg Radiol Anat: SRA*. 1986;8:221–227.
3. Mori S, Bradfield Jason S, Peacock Warwick J, Anderson Robert H, Shivkumar K. Living anatomy of the pericardial space. *JACC: Clin Electrophysiol*. 2021;7:1628–1644.
4. Chetrit M, Xu B, Kwon DH, et al. Imaging-guided therapies for pericardial diseases. *JACC Cardiovasc Imaging*. 2020;13:1422–1437.
5. Chetrit M, Xu B, Verma BR, Klein AL. Multimodality imaging for the assessment of pericardial diseases. *Curr Cardiol Rep*. 2019;21:41.
6. Cosyns B, Plein S, Nihoyanopoulos P, et al. European association of cardiovascular imaging (EACVI) position paper: multimodality imaging in pericardial disease. *Eur Heart J - Cardiovasc Imaging*. 2014;16:12–31.
7. Klein AL, Abbara S, Agler DA, et al. American society of echocardiography clinical recommendations for multimodality cardiovascular imaging of patients with pericardial disease: endorsed by the society for cardiovascular magnetic resonance and society of cardiovascular computed tomography. *J Am Soc Echocardiogr: Off Publ Am Soc Echocardiogr*. 2013;26:965–1012. e15.
8. Wang TKM, Ayoub C, Chetrit M, et al. Cardiac magnetic resonance imaging techniques and applications for pericardial diseases. *Circ: Cardiovasc Imaging*. 2022;15:e014283.
9. Kramer CM, Barkhausen J, Bucciarelli-Ducci C, Flamm SD, Kim RJ, Nagel E. Standardized cardiovascular magnetic resonance imaging (CMR) protocols: 2020 update. *J Cardiovasc Magn Reson: Off J Soc Cardiovasc Magn Reson*. 2020;22:17.
10. Power JA, Thompson DV, Rayarao G, Doyle M, Biederman RWW. Cardiac magnetic resonance radiofrequency tissue tagging for diagnosis of constrictive pericarditis: a proof of concept study. *J Thorac Cardiovasc Surg*. 2016;151:1348–1355.
11. Francone M, Dymarkowski S, Kalantzi M, Rademakers FE, Bogaert J. Assessment of ventricular coupling with real-time cine MRI and its value to differentiate constrictive pericarditis from restrictive cardiomyopathy. *Eur Radiol*. 2006;16:944–951.
12. Kusunose K, Dahiya A, Popović ZB, et al. Biventricular mechanics in constrictive pericarditis comparison with restrictive cardiomyopathy and impact of pericardiectomy. *Circ Cardiovasc Imaging*. 2013;6:399–406.
13. Antonopoulos AS, Vrettos A, Androulakis E, et al. Cardiac magnetic resonance imaging of pericardial diseases: a comprehensive guide. *Eur Heart J Cardiovasc Imaging*. 2023;24:983–998.
14. Aldweib N, Farah V, Biederman RWW. Clinical utility of cardiac magnetic resonance imaging in pericardial diseases. *Curr Cardiol Rev*. 2018;14:200–212.

15. Kojima S, Yamada N, Goto Y. Diagnosis of constrictive pericarditis by tagged cine magnetic resonance imaging. *New Engl J Med.* 1999;341:373–374.
16. Shah AB, Kronzon I. Congenital defects of the pericardium: a review. *Eur Heart J - Cardiovasc Imaging.* 2015;16:821–827.
17. Van Son JA, Danielson GK, Schaff HV, Mullany CJ, Julsrud PR, Breen JF. Congenital partial and complete absence of the pericardium. *Mayo Clin Proc.* 1993;68:743–747.
18. Najib MQ, Chaliki HP, Raizada A, Ganji JL, Panse PM, Click RL. Symptomatic pericardial cyst: a case series. *Eur J Echocardiogr.* 2011;12:E43.
19. Khayata M, Alkharabsheh S, Shah NP, Klein AL. Pericardial cysts: a contemporary comprehensive review. *Curr Cardiol Rep.* 2019;21:64.
20. Patone M, Mei XW, Handunnethti L, et al. Risks of myocarditis, pericarditis, and cardiac arrhythmias associated with COVID-19 vaccination or SARS-CoV-2 infection. *Nat Med.* 2022;28:410–422.
21. Little WC, Freeman GL. Pericardial disease. *Circulation.* 2006;113:1622–1632.
22. Imazio M, Venturelli F, Tomat MC, Savonitto G, Stolfo D, Collini V. Pericarditis at the crossroads: unlocking the next wave of therapies. *IJC Heart Vasc.* 2025;61:101841.
23. Bogaert J, Francone M. Cardiovascular magnetic resonance in pericardial diseases. *J Cardiovasc Magn Reson.* 2009;11:14.
24. Taylor AM, Dymarkowski S, Verbeken EK, Bogaert J. Detection of pericardial inflammation with late-enhancement cardiac magnetic resonance imaging: initial results. *Eur Radiol.* 2006;16:569–574.
25. Chiabrando JG, Bonaventura A, Vecchié A, et al. Management of acute and recurrent pericarditis. *J Am Coll Cardiol.* 2020;75:76–92.
26. Ferreira VM, Schulz-Menger J, Holmvang G, et al. Cardiovascular magnetic resonance in nonischemic myocardial inflammation: expert recommendations. *J Am Coll Cardiol.* 2018;72:3158–3176.
27. Schulz-Menger J, Collini V, Gröschel J, Adler Y, Brucato A, et al. 2025 ESC Guidelines for the management of myocarditis and pericarditis: Developed by the task force for the management of myocarditis and pericarditis of the European Society of Cardiology (ESC) Endorsed by the Association for European Paediatric and Congenital Cardiology (AEPC) and the European Association for Cardio-Thoracic Surgery (EACTS). *Eur Heart J.* 2025;46(40):3952–4041.
28. Imazio M, Pivetta E, Palacio Restrepo S, et al. Usefulness of cardiac magnetic resonance for recurrent pericarditis. *Am J Cardiol.* 2020;125:146–151.
29. Bolen MA, Rajiah P, Kusunose K, et al. Cardiac MR imaging in constrictive pericarditis: multiparametric assessment in patients with surgically proven constriction. *Int J Cardiovasc Imaging.* 2015;31:859–866. https://doi.org/10.1007/s10554-015-0616-z.
30. Bogaert J, Dresselaers T, Imazio M, Sinnaeve P, Tassetti L, Masci PG, et al. Noninvasive assessment of congestive hepatopathy in patients with constrictive pericardial physiology using MR relaxometry. *Int J Cardiol.* 2021;338:265–273.
31. Feng D, Glockner J, Kim K, et al. Cardiac magnetic resonance imaging pericardial late gadolinium enhancement and elevated inflammatory markers can predict the reversibility of constrictive pericarditis after antiinflammatory medical therapy: a pilot study. *Circulation.* 2011;124:1830–1837.
32. Azzu A, Morosin M, Antonopoulos AS, Capoccia M, Rosendahl U, Mohiaddin R. Cardiac decompression by pericardiectomy for constrictive pericarditis: multimodality imaging to identify patients at risk for prolonged inotropic support. *J Cardiovasc Imaging.* 2021;29:361–372.
33. Cremer PC, Tariq MU, Karwa A, et al. Quantitative assessment of pericardial delayed hyperenhancement predicts clinical improvement in patients with constrictive pericarditis treated with anti-inflammatory therapy. *Circ Cardiovasc Imaging.* 2015;8.
34. Ariyarajah V, Jassal DS, Kirkpatrick I, Kwong RY. The utility of cardiovascular magnetic resonance in constrictive pericardial disease. *Cardiol Rev.* 2009;17:77–82.
35. Amaki M, Savino J, Ain DL, et al. Diagnostic concordance of echocardiography and cardiac magnetic resonance-based tissue tracking for differentiating constrictive pericarditis from restrictive cardiomyopathy. *Circ Cardiovasc Imaging.* 2014;7:819–827.
36. Yang Z, Wang H, Chang S, et al. Left ventricular strain-curve morphology to distinguish between constrictive pericarditis and restrictive cardiomyopathy. *ESC Heart Fail.* 2021;8:4863–4872.
37. Imazio M. Pericardial involvement in systemic inflammatory diseases. *Heart (Br Card Soc).* 2011;97:1882–1892.
38. Permanyer-Miralda G. Acute pericardial disease: approach to the aetiologic diagnosis. *Heart (Br Card Soc).* 2004;90:252–254.
39. Cremer PC, Kwon DH. Multimodality imaging of pericardial disease. *Curr Cardiol Rep.* 2015;17:24.
40. Rosmini S, Seraphim A, Knott K, et al. Non-invasive characterization of pleural and pericardial effusions using T1 mapping by magnetic resonance imaging. *Eur Heart J Cardiovasc Imaging.* 2022;23:1117–1126.
41. Restrepo CS, Vargas D, Ocazionez D, Martínez-Jiménez S, Cuellar SLB, Gutierrez FR. Primary pericardial tumors. *Radiographics.* 2013;33:1613–1630.
42. Motwani M, Kidambi A, Herzog BA, Uddin A, Greenwood JP, Plein S. MR imaging of cardiac tumors and masses: a review of methods and clinical applications. *Radiology.* 2013;268:26–43.
43. Tyebally S, Chen D, Bhattacharyya S, et al. Cardiac tumors. *JACC: CardioOncol.* 2020;2:293–311.
44. Alraies MC, AlJaroudi W, Yarmohammadi H, et al. Usefulness of cardiac magnetic resonance-guided management in patients with recurrent pericarditis. *Am J Cardiol.* 2015;115:542–547.
45. Avondo S, Andreis A, Casula M, Biondi-Zoccai G, Imazio M. Pharmacologic treatment of acute and recurrent pericarditis: a systematic review and meta-analysis of controlled clinical trials. *Panminerva Medica.* 2021;63:314–323.

35 Assessment of Valvular Heart Disease Using Cardiac Magnetic Resonance Imaging

K. CARLOS EL-TALLAWI, MAAN MALAHFJI, AND DIPAN J. SHAH

GENERAL INTRODUCTION

Cardiovascular magnetic resonance (CMR) offers a number of unique advantages over echocardiography, which remains the first-line modality used in the evaluation of valvular heart disease. From an acquisition standpoint, CMR provides unrivaled versatility with free choice of anatomic planes and freedom from limitations related to suboptimal acoustic windows. Some specific strengths of CMR in the assessment of valvular heart disease include the following:

- Depiction by cine imaging of valve motion and jet flow in various planes and orientations.
- Measurement of ventricular volumes and mass by multislice cine imaging.
- Measurement of blood flow across various major vessels and outflow tracts using phase contrast imaging.

Although CMR is generally regarded as a second-line imaging modality after echocardiography for the assessment of heart valve disease,[1] it can add important contributions toward decision-making in regard to the timing and nature of surgical intervention, particularly in cases in which there have been inconclusive or conflicting findings on echocardiography.[2,3] Before embarking on this chapter and discussing the major methods and advantages in assessing valve disease using CMR, it is important to recognize some potential weaknesses and pitfalls:

- CMR images are not usually acquired in real time but are reconstructed from data gathered over several heart cycles during a breath-hold. Therefore, valve leaflets are not always well seen, especially in the setting of arrhythmia. This also renders CMR ineffective at visualizing the smaller, highly mobile structures such as flail valve segments or vegetations in endocarditis.
- Since CMR is a tomographic imaging modality, it is helpful to depict a valve and jet structure by cine imaging in several planes and orientations since appearances and, potentially, interpretation can differ between images of a particular valve acquired in different planes. Contiguous stacks of cine images are valuable for covering all parts of the mitral or tricuspid valves, especially when depicting a lesion mechanism.
- The accuracy of phase velocity mapping cannot be always taken for granted.[4] For jet velocity mapping, the dimensions of the voxels can be large in relation to the size and shape of a narrow or fragmented jet, leading to possible inaccuracies because of signal loss, partial volume averaging, and other artifacts. Therefore, we typically place the phase contrast plane in zones with laminar flow to reduce those errors. Another way to mitigate such errors and improve flow measurements is through baseline correction against stationary tissues.[5]
- Measurements of biventricular volume and function can be less reliable in cases when there is arrhythmia or metallic artifact owing to intracardiac or intrathoracic hardware. The methods of acquisition and analysis need to be specified appropriately for comparisons over time or between patients.

Keeping those remarks in consideration, the purpose of this chapter is to outline key concepts and direct users toward CMR methods that we and other experts have deemed valuable in assessing the various presentations of valvular heart disease.

Basic and general principles related to CMR physics, its interaction with valvular lesions and jets, and the tools employed to assess the valves are described first. Stenotic and regurgitant lesions of each heart valve are detailed later. An overview of measures of the severity of valve dysfunction is given in Table 35.1, which reflects the recommendations of the American Society of Echocardiography/Society of Cardiovascular Magnetic Resonance and the American College of Cardiology/American Heart Association Guidelines for the Management of Patients with Valvular Heart Disease.[1,6]

BASIC PRINCIPLES

Slice Thickness and the Visualization of Thin Structures

The CMR approach to visualization of heart valves and associated blood flow generally involves imaging of two-dimensional (2-D) slides. A typical CMR slice thickness, such as 5–6 mm, is substantially thicker than the dimensions of an individual pixel, which range from 1.0 to 2.0 mm. Consequently, the resulting image comprises a layer of elongated, narrow voxels, as depicted in Fig. 35.1. The resulting anisotropic voxels mean that a relatively thin

TABLE 35.1 Classification of the severity of valvular regurgitation and stenosis.

		MILD	MODERATE	SEVERE
Mitral regurgitation	Regurgitant volume (mL)	<30 mL	30–59 mL	≥60 mL
	Regurgitant fraction (%)	<30%	30%–49%	≥50%
	Additional parameters	• Orifice area typically <0.2 cm^2 • No/slightly visible jet core • Narrow orifice jet • Central, quickly dissipating jet	• Orifice area 0.2–0.4 cm^2 • Bright jet core with normal size or mildly enlarged LV and LA	• Orifice area >0.40 cm^2 • Wall-hugging jet with significant swirling in the LA cavity • Dilated LV, LA, and pulmonary veins • Hypercontractile LV with relatively reduced systemic flow • Flail mitral valve (especially with large flail width and gap)
Aortic regurgitation	Regurgitant volume (mL)	<30 mL	30–59 mL	≥60 mL
	Regurgitant fraction (%)	<30%	30%–49%	≥50%
	Additional parameters	• Orifice area <0.19 cm^2[a] • Faint central jet with narrow origin and limited extension into the LV • Absent diastolic flow reversal in the descending thoracic aorta • No significant primary AV abnormality or aortic root dilation	• Orifice area approximately 0.2–0.28 cm^2 • Mild/moderately dilated LV • Bulging of the interventricular septum toward the RV in diastole	• Orifice area >0.28 cm^2[a] • Cusp prolapse/flail with bright eccentric jet extending occupying the LVOT and extending into the LV • Holodiastolic flow reversal in the descending thoracic aorta • Severely dilated LV • Bulging of the interventricular septum toward the RV in diastole
Tricuspid regurgitation	Regurgitant volume (mL)	<30 mL	30–44 mL	≥45 mL
	Regurgitant fraction (%)	<30%	30%–49%	≥50%
	Additional parameters	• No/slightly visible jet core • Narrow orifice jet • Central, quickly dissipating jet • Normal-size RA and RV (in the absence of other right-sided lesions)	• Visible TR jet without significant extension into the RA cavity • Mildly enlarged RA/RV	• Jet origin cross-sectional area >0.20 cm^2[b] • Prominent TR jet with significant swirling in the RA cavity • Moderately/severely dilated RV, RA; significantly dilated IVC • Significantly dilated TV annulus with leaflets malcoaptation
Pulmonic regurgitation	Regurgitant volume (mL)	<30 mL	30–40 mL	>40 mL
	Regurgitant fraction (%)	<20%	20%–40%	>40% (ASE/SCMR guidelines)
	Additional parameters	• Faint jet on phase contrast imaging • Normal RV size (in the absence of other right sided lesions)	–	• Leaflets prolapse/flail • Significantly dilated RV
Aortic stenosis	Valve orifice area (cm^2)	>1.5 cm^2	1.0–1.5 cm^2	<1.0 cm^2
	Peak jet velocity (m/s)[c]	<3 m/s	3–4 m/s	>4 m/s
	Additional parameters	–	• No significant AV thickening/calcifications • No/mild concentric LV hypertrophy	• Significant aortic valve thickening/calcifications • Concentric LV hypertrophy • LV myocardial replacement fibrosis • Evidence of "metastatic AS" with LA enlargement, MR, or RV impairment.
Mitral stenosis	Valve orifice area (cm^2)	>2.5 cm^2	1.5–2.5 cm^2	≤1.5 cm^2
	Additional parameters	–	• No significant mitral leaflets thickening/calcifications • Nonsevere LA enlargement	• Significant mitral leaflets and annulus thickening/calcifications • Severely dilated LA; dilated pulmonary arteries; RV dilation and impairment
Tricuspid stenosis	Valve orifice area (cm^2)			<1 cm^2
	Additional parameters			Significantly dilated RA and IVC

TABLE 35.1 Classification of the severity of valvular regurgitation and stenosis.—cont'd

		MILD	MODERATE	SEVERE
Pulmonic stenosis	Valve orifice area (cm^2)			<1.0 cm^2
	Peak jet velocity (m/s)	<3 m/s	3–4 m/s	>4 m/s
	Additional parameters	–	–	• RV hypertrophy; poststenotic dilatation of the pulmonary arteries • Subpulmonary and pulmonary artery stenosis should be excluded

[a]Goffinet et al. "Comprehensive assessment of the severity and mechanism of aortic regurgitation using multidetector CT and MR." *European Radiology* 20 (2010): 326–336.
[b]Medvedofsky, Diego et al. "Multi-parametric quantification of tricuspid regurgitation using cardiovascular magnetic resonance: A comparison to echocardiography." *European Journal of Radiology* 86 (2017): 213–220.
[c]In the setting of normal flow conditions (stroke volume index >35 mL/m^2).

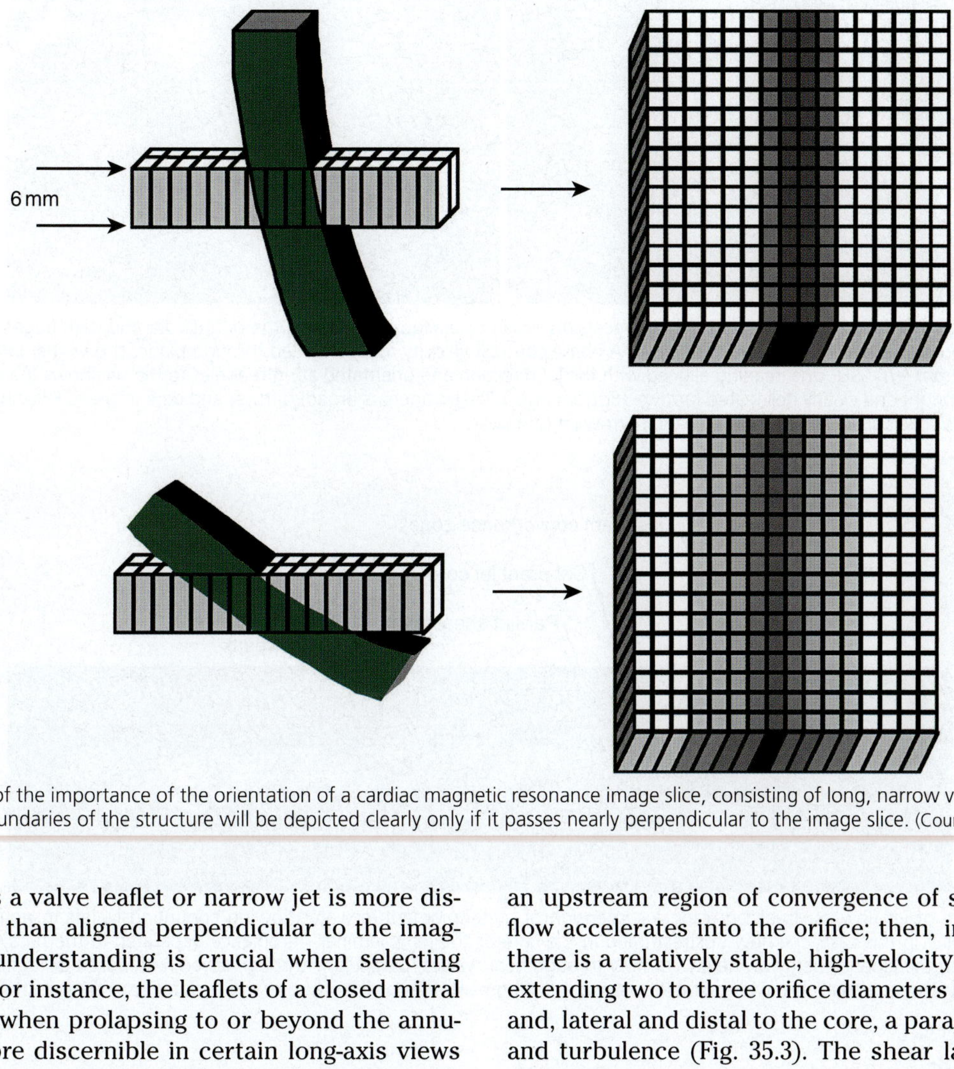

FIG. 35.1 Illustration of the importance of the orientation of a cardiac magnetic resonance image slice, consisting of long, narrow voxels, with respect to a thin structure. The boundaries of the structure will be depicted clearly only if it passes nearly perpendicular to the image slice. (Courtesy of Robert Merrifield.)

structure such as a valve leaflet or narrow jet is more distinctly visualized than aligned perpendicular to the imaging plane. This understanding is crucial when selecting imaging planes. For instance, the leaflets of a closed mitral valve, especially when prolapsing to or beyond the annular plane, are more discernible in certain long-axis views rather than short-axis planes. Similarly, a flat jet through a narrow orifice is most distinct when the imaging plane intersects perpendicularly to the jet, as shown in Fig. 35.2.

Visualization and Planimetry of Jets by Cine Imaging

Stenosis or regurgitation of a diseased heart valve is associated with jet formation and consequent dissipation of energy through shear and turbulence. Appreciation of the structure of jet flow is fundamental to the interpretation of jet appearances on cine images. Jet flow is associated with an upstream region of convergence of streamlines where flow accelerates into the orifice; then, in most situations, there is a relatively stable, high-velocity jet core, typically extending two to three orifice diameters beyond the orifice and, lateral and distal to the core, a parajet region of shear and turbulence (Fig. 35.3). The shear layer is the region with the most extreme spatial gradients of velocity, and this is where much of the turbulence of a jet originates and where there is likely to be most loss of signal in cine acquisitions and potential inaccuracies in phase velocity maps. Each of the characteristic zones of a jet may be identifiable on cine images, but the appearances depend not only on jet shape and structure but also on the nature of the acquisition—the slice thickness, pixel dimensions and orientation, sequence design, and echo time[7]—and, importantly, on the location of the image slice relative to the jet.

Steady-state free precession (SSFP) imaging has become widely used in CMR because of the strong image contrast

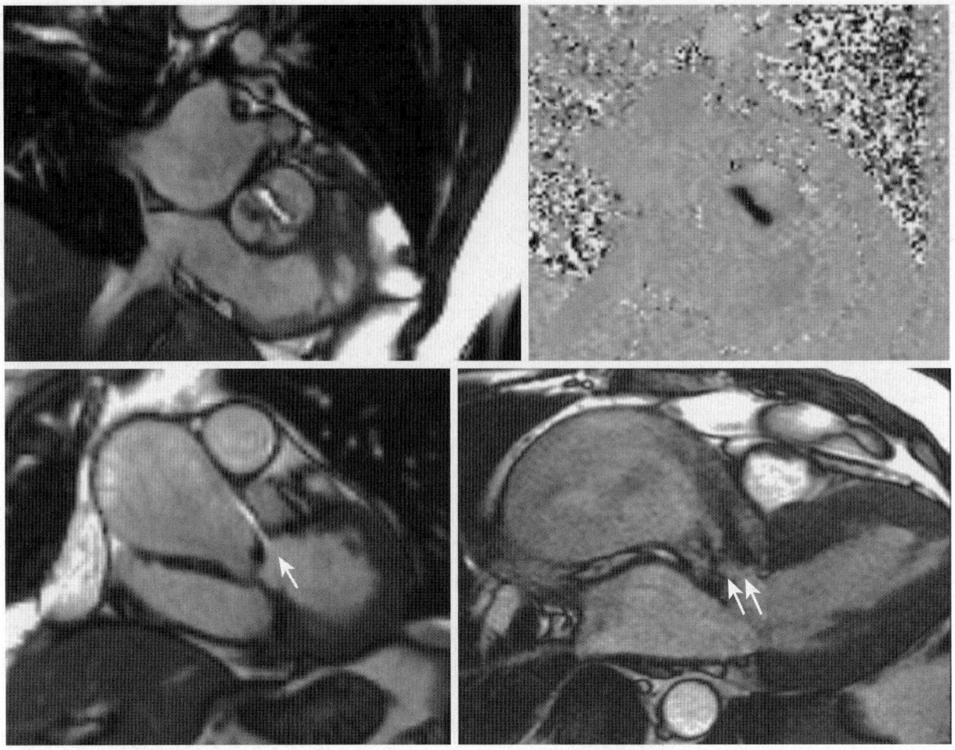

FIG. 35.2 (*Top left*) A systolic frame of a steady-state free precession (SSFP) cine acquisition shows the bright core and dark edges of the jet through the slit-like orifice of a stenosed bicuspid aortic valve. (*Top right*) A phase contrast velocity map, encoded through-plane, shows the dark jet, recording a peak velocity of 4.2 m/s. (*Bottom left*) SSFP cine imaging aligned with the jet direction and orientated at right angles to the slit shows the narrower dimension of the jet, which appears bright and clearly delineated (*arrow*). (*Bottom right*) The jet appears broad, diffuse, and dark in the SSFP cine, which is aligned with the length of the slit, its voxels spanning the width of the narrow jet (*arrows*).

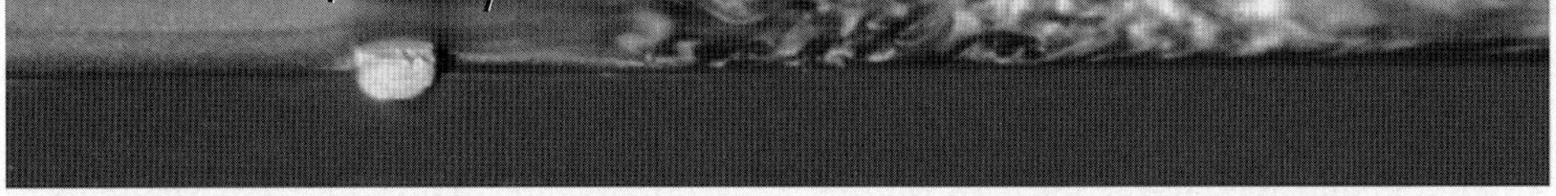

FIG. 35.3 The structure of jet flow as visualized using a suspension of metal pigment in water flowing continuously, left to right, in an open channel indented by a "stenosis." In this case, the flow upstream and in the core of the jet is laminar. Turbulence generated in the parajet shear layer is swept downstream, dissipating the kinetic energy of the jet. Jet flow through heart valves, particularly through severely stenosed or regurgitant orifices, is likely to be more complex in structure than this, with possible splaying and fragmentation of the jet core and possible asymmetric attachment to one wall or valve leaflet.

it provides between blood and adjacent tissues. Its properties also make it suitable for the delineation of flow jets, but appearances differ somewhat from those of gradient echo imaging. The echo times used for SSFP imaging are usually very short (e.g., 2 ms), thus minimizing signal loss because of the higher orders of motion associated with turbulence.

Under optimal conditions, however, typical appearances of a jet on SSFP imaging include a relatively bright jet core, clearly delineated on either side by dark lines that represent the shear layers (Figs. 35.2 and 35.4). However, this is the case only if there is a coherent core and the image plane is aligned with it. The same jet may appear dark, with no bright core, if the imaging plane is displaced slightly to one side, tangential to the shear layer. For this reason, careful alignment of planes, sequentially cross-cutting one cine acquisition with another and then another, is important in the assessment of heart valve disease by CMR. Each jet should be imaged in multiple planes (Fig. 35.2), to fully assess the size, shape, and functional significance of a jet. In cases where substantial artifacts occur from SSPF cine sequences (e.g., patients with implanted devices or when using high-field-strength scanners) a gradient recalled echo (GRE) cine sequence can be used.

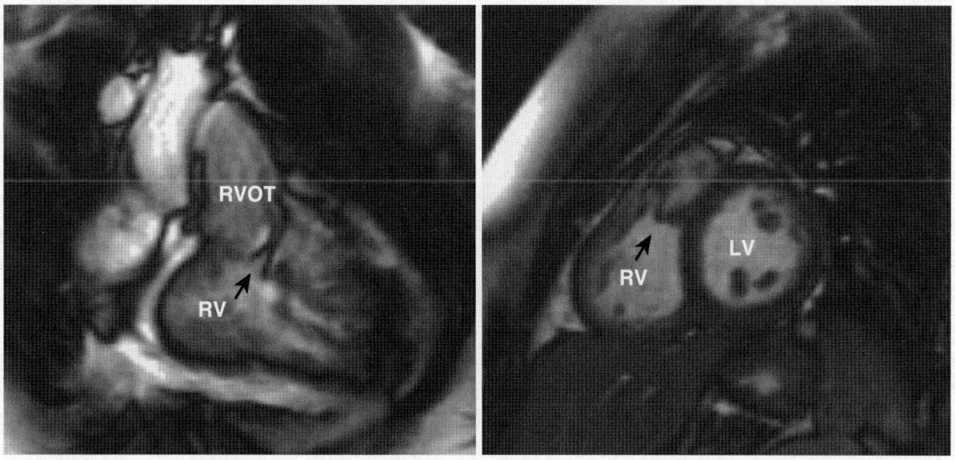

FIG. 35.4 Double-chambered right ventricle, or subinfundibular stenosis, shown by steady-state free precession cine imaging in oblique coronal (*left*) and short-axis (*right*) planes, with the systolic jet from the hypertrophied lower part of the RV into the outflow tract arrowed. The pulmonary valve was not stenosed in this patient. *LV*, Left ventricle; *RVOT*, right ventricular outflow tract.

Phase Contrast Velocity Mapping

The principles of phase contrast velocity mapping are explained in Chapter X. In brief, one or more of the directional components of velocity are encoded in the phase of the signal in each voxel of the image for each phase of the cardiac cycle.[8] Velocity can be encoded either in-plane (in the X- or Y-direction) or through-plane (Z-direction). In-plane encoding is useful for visualization of the jet but cannot be utilized for measurement of flow. Through-plane encoding in the Z-direction on the other hand is employed in phase contrast velocity mapping for measurement of flow across an area of interest. As with Doppler flow measurement, phase contrast velocity mapping is represented by shifts of phase and so is subject to aliasing. To avoid this, an appropriate velocity-encoding range (Venc) should be chosen before acquiring velocity data in a particular cavity or vessel. An appropriate Venc exceeds the peak expected velocity by 20% to 50%, meaning that 180 degrees of phase contrast corresponds to 120%–150% of the expected peak velocity. If the Venc is too low, set below the level of the peak velocity, the result is aliasing, in which case the acquisition should be repeated with the Venc increased appropriately. Too high a Venc, however, reduces the sensitivity of velocity mapping by reducing the amount of velocity-related phase shifts relative to background noise or other artifact-related phase shifts.[9] Velocity mapping is used clinically for jet velocity measurements and for volume flow measurements. Each can be subject to artifacts, generally of distinct kinds in each case, and these can give misleading clinical results if they are not recognized and, if possible, corrected.

Phase contrast velocity mapping is able to measure velocities in pixels throughout the plane of acquisition, which can be acquired in any chosen orientation. An advantage of this is that the volume of flow passing through an image plane can be calculated. This is done by multiplying the cross-sectional area of a vessel, for example, the aorta or pulmonary trunk, by the mean through-plane component of velocity in that area for each phase of the cardiac cycle, after delineating the area of the vessel in every frame of the acquisition. In this way, CMR is able to measure the volumes of forward or reversed flow in a large vessel. Through-plane flow measurements are subject to particular kinds of inaccuracy, however, especially when used for regurgitant or shunt flow rather than total flow measurements.[5] Background phase offset errors can cause slight inaccuracies of velocity measurement across the whole field of view and through the whole cardiac cycle, typically increasing with distance from the isocenter of the magnet. Most CMR vendors currently allow the phase contrast sequence to move the patient table so that the set imaging plane remains at the isocenter, minimizing phase offset errors. These errors have been identified as being mainly a result of concomitant Maxwell gradients, which can be calculated and corrected by using appropriate software, and to eddy currents in hardware components, which are harder to predict and eliminate.[4] The result can be an upward or downward shift of the baseline of the flow curve, which can significantly affect the calculation of a regurgitant fraction. The amount of the shift of the flow curve depends not only on the underlying cause of the artifact but also on the Venc that is chosen (the higher the Venc, the greater the error), and on the cross-sectional area of the vessel measured (the larger the area, the greater the error). A further source of inaccuracy can be movement of the plane of a regurgitant valve itself relative to the plane of acquisition. Because such movements, for example, of the aortic valve in diastole or of the mitral valve in systole, displace a volume of blood in the direction opposite that of the regurgitant flow, they cause underestimation of the regurgitation measured, the error increasing with the amount of valve movement and the cross-section of the flow area measured. It is an error that can be overcome by appropriately implemented motion tracking,[10] although this is not yet available on most systems. Both manufacturers and users need to be aware of these potential sources of inaccuracy and work together toward the optimization of systems and sequences.

Jet Velocity Mapping for the Assessment of Stenoses

In jet flow, measurement of the peak velocity of the jet and the rates of change of the peak velocity through time or use of the velocity time integral[11] may contribute to the assessment of the severity of stenosis or possibly regurgitation.

Recovery of signal is a prerequisite for calculation of velocity, so it is necessary for voxels to lie sufficiently within the coherent core of a jet to measure its velocity accurately. If a jet is narrow and fragmented, this condition may be difficult to fulfill because there may not be a core of sufficient dimensions. Initial breath-hold cine acquisitions should be used to decide whether it is worth trying to measure jet velocity by CMR. These, possibly followed by a preliminary in-plane breath-hold velocity map, can then be used to locate a through-plane breath-hold velocity map to measure the velocities of the core of the jet. Breath-hold sequences are recommended because their echo time will be short and so will minimize several potential artifacts,[5] and any respiratory motion of the jet will also be avoided. What may be harder to avoid is movement of the valve related to cardiac motion. The plane chosen should therefore be located at the phase of peak flow, or, better still, a moving plane is located by using a motion-tracking method of acquisition, if available.[10] In spite of these precautions, velocity maps, particularly of a narrow jet, may give misleading values. Of particular concern, voxels in the shear layer at the edge of a jet are subject to signal loss and possible phase errors caused by abrupt deceleration. Apparent velocities of edge pixels should therefore be treated with suspicion if they differ from those in the core of the jet, and they may degrade attempts to measure volume flow at or downstream of a narrow orifice. These problems explain why CMR velocity mapping is generally less suitable than Doppler echocardiography for the assessment of right ventricular or pulmonary artery pressures by direct measurement of the velocities of relatively narrow tricuspid or pulmonary regurgitant jets.

In echocardiography, it became routine for jet velocity measurements to be converted to estimated differences of pressure, often referred to as gradients, in units (mm Hg) that were familiar from the use of catheterization. This conversion relies on assumptions that may not always be applicable (e.g., that all of the jet or stream reaches a uniform peak velocity and that virtually all of its kinetic energy is dissipated in turbulence). It is advisable that peak velocities measured at specific locations, by either CMR or Doppler echocardiography, are quoted as such without conversion to presumed differences of pressure. Finally, it is important to note that the velocity of a jet through an orifice is, of course, affected by the rate of flow as well as by the degree of narrowing, so a low flow rate because of ventricular dysfunction, for instance, will reduce the degree of elevation of velocity through a stenosed outflow valve.

VALVULAR REGURGITATION

General Principles

In regurgitant heart valve disease, the optimal time for surgical intervention depends on a balanced assessment of when valve dysfunction is sufficiently severe to warrant the short- and long-term risks of intervention but before the heart muscle sustains irreversible damage. The form, structure, and mobility of regurgitant valve leaflets, particularly mitral and tricuspid, should be characterized considering the potential plan for a surgical repair. Owing to the slice thickness of acquisitions, this may not be easy by CMR in certain scenarios, such as a flail segment or valve damage from endocarditis, for instance. The need for intervention is determined partly by the presence of symptoms and objective clinical indices such as oxygen consumption and exercise capacity, but the measurements of regurgitant volume or regurgitant fraction and ventricular function are a crucial step. Regurgitant volume quantification may occasionally be challenging with current echocardiographic and angiographic techniques—in which case several CMR methods can be employed to assess the severity of valvular regurgitation.

Some fundamental flow principles are worth mentioning here before proceeding into more details:

1. In the absence of shunt or regurgitation, flow in all cardiac chambers should be equal—e.g., LV stroke volume = aortic flow = RV stroke volume = PA flow.
2. Ventricular stroke volume (LV or RV) can have up to four components: systemic stroke volume, great vessel regurgitation (AR or PR), atrioventricular valve regurgitation (MR or TR), and intracardiac shunt flow.
3. Understanding and employing those concepts is key to solving complex multilesion scenarios and their respective individual contributions.

Regurgitation of any single heart valve, if isolated and uncomplicated by the presence of an intracardiac shunt, may be calculated by comparison of the total LV and RV stroke volumes measured by planimetry from a standard multislice short-axis volume acquisition, preferably using software that can combine short-axis data with information on the locations and movements of the mitral and tricuspid valve planes in long-axis acquisitions. The ventricle with the regurgitating valve will have excess stroke volume that represents the regurgitant volume. This method is advantageous in cases with beat-to-beat variability (atrial fibrillation, frequent ectopy) where matching the left and right ventricular stroke volumes is important. The accuracy of this approach is dependent on the image quality and accuracy of planimetry. Hypertrophy and deformity of the right ventricle (e.g., in congenital heart disease) can present some challenges to planimetry of the right ventricle. Standardized approaches need to be taken to the inclusion or exclusion of myocardial trabeculations in the case of the RV, and the papillary muscles in the case of the LV.

A probably more robust method used for assessing regurgitation of the atrioventricular valves is by measuring the total ventricular stroke volumes using multislice planimetry, and aortic or pulmonic stroke volumes using phase contrast flow measurements. In order to calculate regurgitation of the respective inflow valve, the systolic flow measured in the great vessel is subtracted from the stroke volume of the corresponding ventricle (e.g., mitral regurgitant volume equals the LV stroke volume minus systolic aortic flow).[12]

Table 35.2 summarizes the methodologies, formulas, along with the advantages and disadvantages of regurgitant lesions assessment using CMR.

MITRAL REGURGITATION ASSESSMENT

Mechanism and Etiologies

Mitral regurgitation (MR) can be broadly categorized into two primary mechanistic groups: primary (or degenerative), and functional (or secondary). The distinction

TABLE 35.2 Valvular regurgitation assessment methods' advantages and disadvantages.

LESION	METHOD	FORMULA/ACQUISITION	ADVANTAGES	DISADVANTAGES
Mitral regurgitation	Orifice area	Stack of slightly overlapping slices, shifting gradually from upstream to immediately downstream of the orifice	• Direct parameter of MR assessment • Relatively straightforward parameter to trace when properly captured en face	• Can be dynamic throughout systole, leading to overestimation of MR (e.g., in MVP) • Orifice could be tilted relative to mitral annulus plane and therefore difficult to capture en-face
	Regurgitant volume—Method 1	Mitral regurgitant volume = Total LV stroke volume – Aortic stroke volume	• Practical and reproducible • Wealth of studies • Can be used even with coexistent AR	• Can lead to inaccuracies in the setting of arrhythmias (AF, frequent ectopy) • Depends on high-resolution LV short-axis slices and high-quality aortic phase contrast acquisitions
	Regurgitant volume—Method 2	Mitral regurgitant volume = Total LV stroke volume – Net pulmonary stroke volume	Useful when aortic SV is inaccurate due to LV outflow turbulence (subaortic stenosis, MV systolic anterior motion)	• Net pulmonary SV should be used (i.e., existing significant PR or shunt need to be excluded) • Aortic SV is within 5% of net pulmonic stroke volume
	Regurgitant volume—Method 3	Mitral regurgitant volume = Total LV stroke volume – Total RV stroke volume	• Can be useful in scenarios with significant beat-to-beat variability (AF, frequent ectopy) • Can be used when flows are inaccurate or not feasible	• Prone to inaccuracies since the RV SV can be less accurate due to the extensive RV trabeculations • Any significant concomitant regurgitant lesion or shunt would invalidate this method
	Regurgitant fraction	Mitral regurgitant fraction (%) = Mitral regurgitant volume/Mitral stroke volume	–	–
Aortic regurgitation	Orifice area	Stack of slightly overlapping slices, shifting gradually from upstream to immediately downstream of the orifice	• Direct parameter of AR assessment • Relatively easy to obtain and trace in central AR • Might represent AR severity independent from hemodynamic fluctuations (HR and BP)	• Can be challenging to obtain and trace in primary AR such as in bicuspid or calcified AV • Not very well studied
	Regurgitant volume – Direct method	Through-plane velocity-mapping plane prescribed to transect the STJ	• Direct parameter of AR assessment • Single acquisition variable (less prone to compounded errors) • Useful when the aortic or pulmonic forward stroke volumes are inaccurate or nonfeasible	• Diastolic upward recoil of the aorta could lead to AR underestimation • Phase contrast background baseline shift can lead to inaccuracies • Setting the velocity encoding too high might affect the sensitivity of the measurement
	Regurgitant volume – Indirect method 1	Aortic regurgitant volume = Aortic forward stroke volume – Net pulmonic stroke volume	• Relatively easy to acquire and apply • Can be used in the majority of cases • Useful when direct method suffers from baseline shift errors or oblique transection of the STJ	• Can lead to AR underestimation when significant PR or left-to-right shunt present, which must be accounted for
	Regurgitant volume – Indirect method 2	Aortic regurgitant volume = LV Total stroke volume – RV stroke volume	• Particularly useful when the aortic or pulmonic forward stroke volumes are inaccurate or nonfeasible • Can be used in cases of AF with significant beat-to-beat variability	• Can be used only with isolated AR • Prone to RV tracing errors (trabeculations)

Continued

TABLE 35.2 Valvular regurgitation assessment methods' advantages and disadvantages.—cont'd

LESION	METHOD	FORMULA/ACQUISITION	ADVANTAGES	DISADVANTAGES
	Regurgitant fraction	Regurgitant fraction (%) = Aortic regurgitant volume/Aortic stroke volume	–	–
Tricuspid regurgitation	Regurgitant volume—Method 1	Tricuspid regurgitant volume = Total RV stroke volume – Pulmonic stroke volume	• More practical and reproducible than the other methods • Applies even in the presence of significant PR	• Can lead to inaccuracies in the setting of arrhythmias (AF, frequent ectopy) • Depends on high-resolution RV short-axis slices (trabeculations) and high-quality aortic phase contrast acquisitions
	Regurgitant volume—Method 2	Tricuspid regurgitant volume = Total RV stroke volume – Net aortic stroke volume	Useful in patients with pulmonic stenosis or turbulence in the RV outflow tract (e.g., subvalvular stenosis)	• Net aortic SV should be used (i.e., existing significant AR needs to be excluded) • Aortic SV is within 5% of net pulmonic stroke volume
	Regurgitant volume—Method 3	Tricuspid regurgitant volume = Total RV stroke volume – Total LV stroke volume	• Can be useful in setting of atrial fibrillation with significant beat-to-beat variability • Can be used when flows are inaccurate or not feasible	• RV stroke volume less reproducible due to extensive trabeculations of RV • Significant concomitant regurgitant lesions invalidate this method's use
	Regurgitant fraction	Regurgitant fraction (%) = TR regurgitant Volume/(RV stroke volume – PR)	–	–
Pulmonic regurgitation	Regurgitant volume – Direct method	Through-plane velocity-mapping plane prescribed to transect the pulmonary trunk	• Direct parameter of PR assessment • Single acquisition variable (less prone to compounded errors) • Useful when the aortic or pulmonic forward stroke volumes are inaccurate or nonfeasible	• Phase contrast background baseline shift can lead to inaccuracies • Setting the velocity encoding too high might affect the sensitivity of the measurement
	Regurgitant volume – Indirect method	Pulmonary regurgitant volume = Pulmonic forward stroke volume – Net aortic stroke volume	• Relatively easy to acquire and apply • Can be used in the majority of cases	Can lead to PR underestimation or overestimation when significant AR or left-to-right shunt present, respectively; both must be accounted for
	Regurgitant fraction	Regurgitant fraction (%) = Pulmonic regurgitant volume/Pulmonic stroke volume	–	–

between primary and secondary MR is important from both a diagnostic and therapeutic standpoint since clinical outcomes can be different.[13] Primary MR is characterized by an intrinsic abnormality of the mitral valve leaflets such as myxomatous degeneration (i.e., mitral valve prolapse) in highly developed countries, and rheumatic valve disease in developing countries.[14] In contrast, in functional MR, the leaflets are visually normal (it is known that the leaflets can be biologically abnormal[15,16]), with malcoaptation and regurgitation resulting from alteration and tethering of one or more of the components of the MV apparatus, typically due to one or a combination of left ventricular, left atrial, and/or annular remodeling. For instance, in cases of global LV dilation or regional dysfunction following an inferior or inferolateral infarct, there is displacement of the papillary muscles with resultant tethering of the chordae tendinae and tenting of the mitral valve leaflets. This, in addition to possible preexisting annular dilation, leads to suboptimal leaflets coaptation and resultant functional MR. Fig. 35.5 provides example cases of various MR mechanisms depicted on CMR.

More recently there has been a growing interest in LA remodeling and the resultant MR—labeled as atrial functional MR. This entity appears to coexist in patients with chronic atrial fibrillation and a history of heart failure with preserved ejection fraction.[17] The mechanism of atrial functional MR is incompletely understood, however, the prevailing theory behind it appears to describe an atriogenic posterior pull of the posterior annulus and leaflet behind the crest of the LV myocardium at that location, with resultant leaflets malcoaptation.[18,19] Also, a characteristic anatomical aspect of this entity is the inward bending

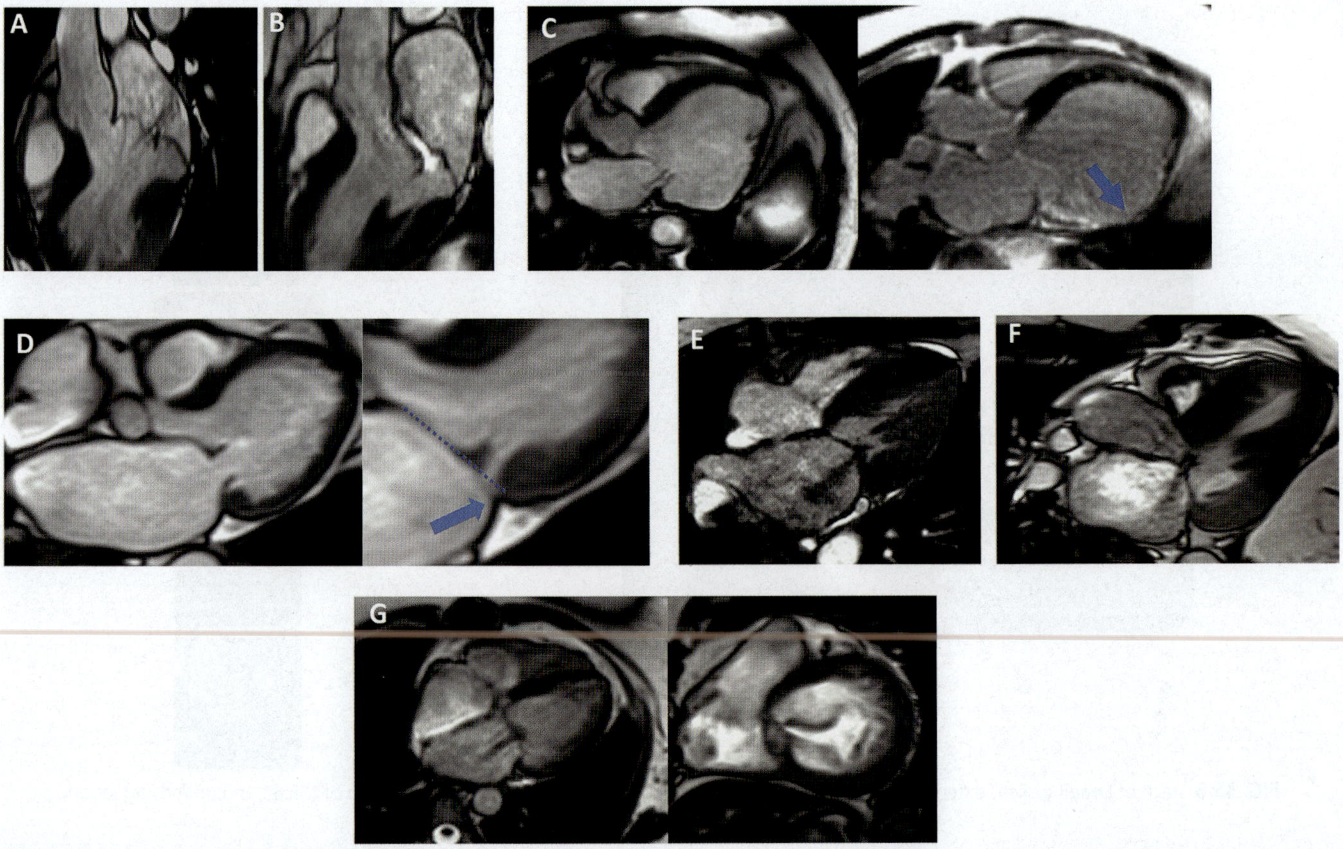

FIG. 35.5 Examples of MR mechanisms. (A) A case of bileaflet mitral valve prolapse (Barlow disease). (B) A case of posterior leaflet flail (P2 scallop) with severe MR. (C) A case of ischemic MR due to posterior leaflet tethering (*left*) due to a large lateral infarct (*right*; *blue arrow* showing transmural LGE). (D) A case of atrial functional MR with a dilated atrium and normal LV size and regional and global function (*left*). Notice the flat leaflets coaptation plane in systole (*right*; *dashed blue line*), along with the posterior atriogenic tethering of the posterior leaflet relative to the crest of the muscle (*blue arrow*). (E) Calcified mitral valve with primary calcific MR. (F) Systolic anterior motion of the anterior mitral leaflet leading to posteriorly directed MR. (G) A case of central MR (*left*) depicted to be due to a cleft anterior leaflet upon visualization of the mitral valve on short axis imaging plane.

of the basal posterior LV wall which is exacerbated in diastole and paradoxically moves outward in systole. It is theorized that this finding is a result of the mass effect from the enlarging left atrium, and that the paradoxical systolic outward motion of the basal posterior wall increases posterior leaflet tension and worsens coaptation, leading to more significant MR[18] (Fig. 35.5D). The forces and underlying anatomical variants driving the posterior migration of the posterior leaflet are still unknown and probably require longitudinal studies to better elucidate this. Do those patients have underlying prominent mitral annular disjunction which allows for the annulus to migrate behind the crest of the LV myocardium? Finally, it is important to recognize that this dichotomy of primary versus functional MR is not mutually exclusive as both types can coexist (i.e., mixed etiology of MR) in a single patient.

Cardiac magnetic resonance imaging provides adequate spatial and temporal resolution of the mitral apparatus and left heart chambers, facilitating precise evaluation of mitral pathology and underlying MR mechanism in most scenarios (Fig. 35.5). Stork et al.[20] found that CMR and transesophageal echocardiography (TEE) share comparable accuracy, approximately 90%, in identifying the mechanisms underlying primary MR. In addition, CMR excels in identifying wall motion abnormalities, scarring from prior infarction, and accurately measuring the dimensions of the mitral annulus dimensions, and quantifying left ventricular and atrial volumes. These are key factors in assessing functional MR mechanisms.

The thickness of CMR slices can make the assessment of valve structure problematic in some cases, and obtaining cine acquisitions in multiple slices is important for adequate visualization of the dynamic morphology of the valve and its suspensory apparatus. To achieve this, a contiguous stack of 5- or 6-mm thick cine slices is recommended to give comprehensive coverage of all scallops of the mitral valve, starting at the anterolateral commissure and extending down to the inferomedial commissure. The stack is oriented parallel to an oblique LV outflow tract (LVOT) long-axis plane, orthogonal to the central part of the valve, progressing down from the superior commissure through each scallop of the valve (A1 to P1, A2 to P2, A3 to P3) so that any regurgitant jet, prolapse, or tethering of part of the valve can be visualized and located with a view to possible surgical repair (Fig. 35.6).

MR SEVERITY ASSESSMENT

Jet Characteristics

Valvular regurgitation typically results in jet formation and consequent dissipation of that flow energy through shear and turbulence. Appreciation and understanding of the jet structure and direction/trajectory are key to the interpretation

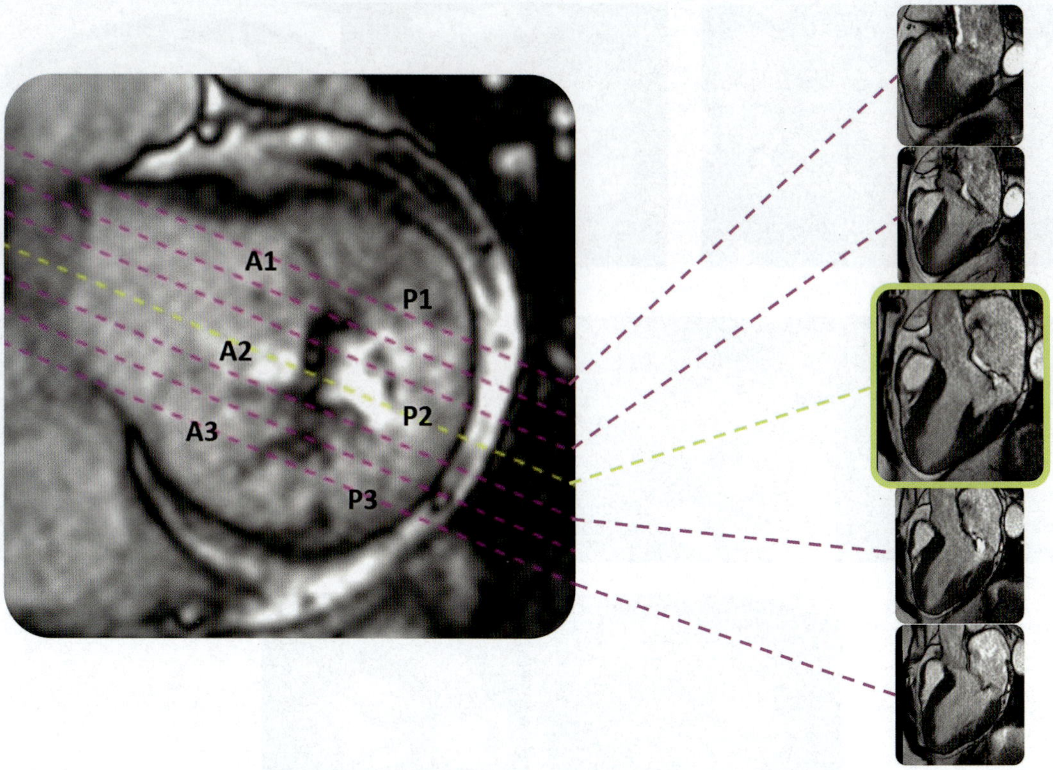

FIG. 35.6 Stack of imaging slices extending from anterolateral to inferomedial commissure for localization of MR jet and underlying lesion.

of MR severity and, more importantly, its mechanism. The MR jet is associated with an upstream region of flow convergence (the basis of the PISA method on echocardiography) where the blood accelerates into the orifice. The flow then contracts and assumes its highest velocity in an area located immediately distal to the anatomic orifice (the vena contracta). The jet travels distally in a trajectory determined by the mechanism and location of the underlying pathology. As the jet travels further into the left atrium, friction dissipates its kinetic energy as heat, with the fluid losing its turbulence and momentum as it travels further downstream. It is important to note that eccentric wall-hugging jets characteristic of mitral prolapse and flail tend to lose their momentum and kinetic energy more rapidly due to friction with the nearby surface of the mitral leaflet or the atrial wall. This makes the qualitative assessment of severity solely based on the jet reach more prone to underestimation, a fact well known in the echocardiography sphere. Ideally, an MR lesion should be imaged in multiple planes before the operator can be reasonably confident that the size, shape, and functional significance of a jet have been adequately depicted to reflect the underlying mechanism and extent of MR more closely. It is for those reasons that the regurgitant jet should ideally be employed as a screener—as opposed to a grading parameter—of MR. Importantly, screening for an MR jet (or any other regurgitant lesion for that matter) should be the initial step in its assessment and should serve as the anchor point for further quantitative assessment. If a comprehensive set of velocity-encoded images covering the mitral space fails to show any significant jet formation or dissipation into the left atrium, then it should be fairly accurate to assume the absence of significant MR.

Regurgitant Orifice Area

As noted earlier in the Basic Principles section, when planimetry is attempted, it is advisable to acquire a stack of slightly overlapping slices, shifting gradually from upstream to immediately downstream of the orifice, in approximately 3-mm steps, to ensure that the smallest anatomic regurgitant orifice area is captured and visualized en face (Fig. 35.7). This approach is most accurate when the orifice is relatively simple in shape and the jet core is coherent. It is not likely to be accurate if the orifice is irregularly deformed or is a narrow slit, giving rise to a fragmented, splayed, or fan-like jet.[4] Two important points regarding the MR anatomic regurgitant area need to be addressed for a full understanding of planimetry, and its strengths and weaknesses. First, the orifice area is dynamic and can vary throughout systole. This is best exemplified in cases of mitral valve prolapse and late systolic MR where the orifice area is maximal in late systole, but for a relatively brief time period, yielding a less pronounced total volume of regurgitation. Second, the MR orifice can occasionally be tilted relative to the mitral annulus such as in cases of MR due to single leaflet prolapse or flail, where the orifice plane is situated at an angle compared to the mitral annular plane (Fig. 35.7B). In those scenarios, one has to be prudent, and calculating the mitral regurgitant volume may provide a more comprehensive assessment of the MR along with its loading effect on the left heart chambers. In a study by Buchner et al., a CMR-derived anatomic orifice area >0.40 cm^2 had a 94% sensitivity and specificity for identification of Sellers angiographic grade 3 or 4 mitral regurgitation.[21]

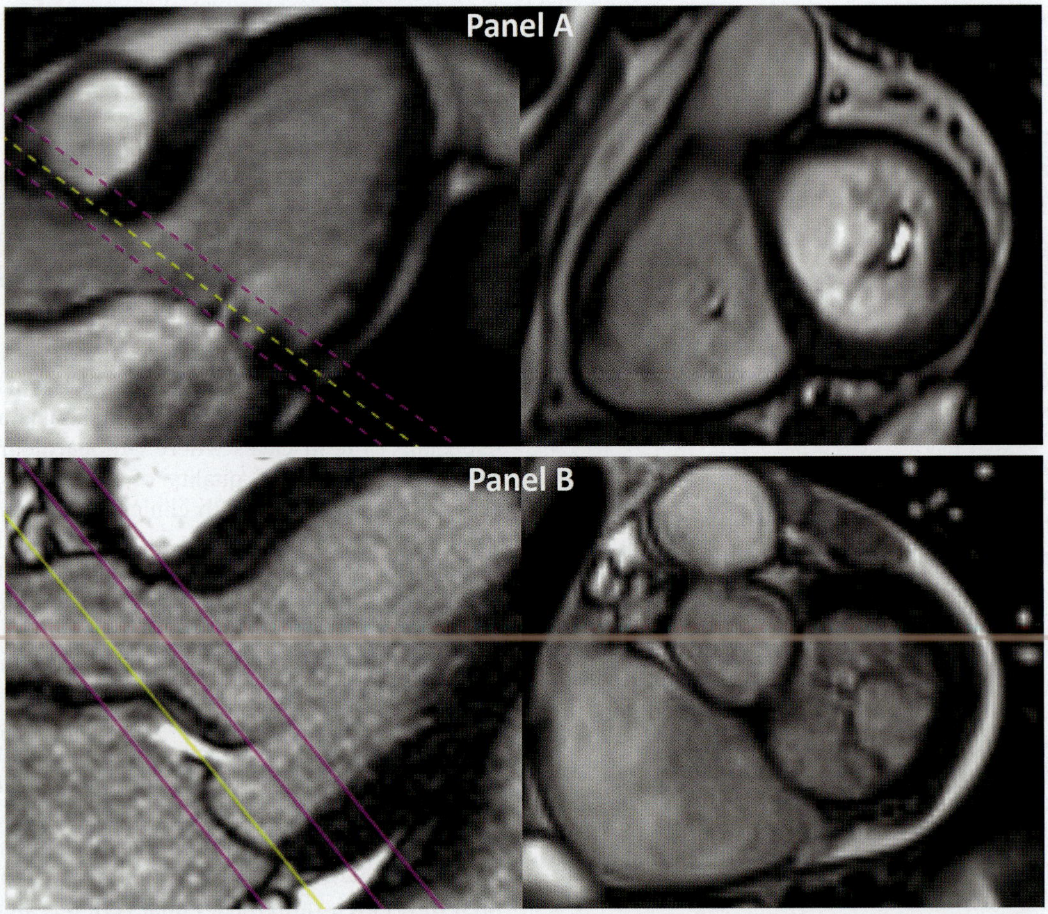

FIG. 35.7 Depiction of regurgitant orifice area in a central (A) versus eccentric MR (B). Notice that in primary MR due to prolapse or flail the orifice lies at an angle compared to the mitral annulus which makes it difficult to depict and assess the anatomic orifice area.

Mitral Regurgitant Volume and Fraction

Several approaches to the quantification of mitral regurgitation can be employed using various combinations of the previously described methodologies involving ventricular volumes, and aortic and pulmonary flows. Each of those methods has inherent advantages and disadvantages which need to be weighed and applied according to the clinical and imaging scenarios and constraints.

Method 1: Mitral Regurgitant Volume
= Total LV stroke volume – Aortic forward stroke volume

This method constitutes the "workhorse" of volumetric regurgitation assessment in contemporary laboratories. It is more practical and more reproducible than the other methods listed below, and it also applies even in the presence of concomitant aortic, pulmonic, or tricuspid regurgitation without additional adjustments to the basic formula. The method is based on the knowledge that, in the presence of MR, the total LV stroke volume can be deconstructed into its volume constituents which are the systemic forward flow (aortic stroke volume) and the mitral regurgitant volume. Since the total LV stroke volume can be measured using planimetry of end-diastolic and end-systolic multislice short-axis volume acquisitions, the mitral regurgitant volume would be calculated as the difference of the total LV stroke volume and the aortic forward flow. In the setting of concomitant AR, the aortic regurgitant volume component would be included in both [total LV stroke volume] and the [aortic forward stroke volume], which would then cancel out as follows:

$$\text{MR} = \text{LVSV} - \text{Aortic SV} = \underbrace{[\cancel{\text{Systemic SV}} + \text{MR} + \cancel{\text{AR}}]}_{\text{LVSV}} - \underbrace{[\cancel{\text{Systemic SV}} + \cancel{\text{AR}}]}_{\text{Aortic SV}} = \text{MR}.$$

Of note, it is advisable to acquire both aortic and LVOT level flow planes for cases of MR assessment to increase the yield and minimize errors in estimating MR. This is particularly true in cases of valvular or supravalvular aortic stenosis where turbulence in the aortic root and proximal ascending aorta would affect the accuracy of flow measurement at that location. In such cases we advise utilizing the LVOT flow for forward stroke volume.

Method 2: Mitral Regurgitant Volume
= Total LV stroke volume – Net Pulmonary stroke volume

When the aortic stroke volume is deemed inaccurate or not feasible due, for instance, to outflow turbulence from subaortic stenosis and flow turbulence (e.g., with MV systolic anterior motion or subaortic membrane), which could render both the LVOT and aortic flow measurements inaccurate, the pulmonary stroke volume could be used as a surrogate for aortic flow. It is, however, crucial here to realize that since the *net* pulmonary stroke volume should be used this means that any existing significant pulmonic regurgitation volume or left-to-right shunt volume needs to be quantified and excluded from the measured total systolic pulmonary flow in order to obtain the net stroke volume that would make its way to the left heart.

$$\textit{Method 3: Mitral Regurgitant Volume} = \textit{Total LV stroke volume} - \textit{Total RV stroke volume}$$

Finally, when the previously mentioned methods cannot be employed, one can estimate the mitral regurgitant volume from the stroke volume difference between the LV and RV. This method is more prone to inaccuracies, especially since the RV stroke volume can be less accurate and reproducible due to the extensive trabeculations of the RV. Also, any significant concomitant regurgitant lesion or intracardiac shunt would invalidate this method's use since the additional lesion volume will be incorporated in either the LV or the RV total stroke volume. It should be noted that a clinical scenario with concomitant MR and AR could still be reportable with the difference in stroke volume between the LV and RV representing the total LV regurgitant load (MR + AR). Finally, this method could be useful in the setting of atrial fibrillation with significant beat-to-beat variability where there could be a temporal mismatch between the aortic outflow and the LV stroke volume which are obtained from different heart beats. Therefore, comparing LV and RV stroke volumes that are inherently derived from the same set of cardiac cycles could favor this approach in the setting of atrial fibrillation.

Regurgitant Fraction

$$\textit{Mitral regurgitant fraction}\,(\%) = \textit{Mitral regurgitant volume}/\textit{Mitral Forward Stroke Volume}$$

By definition, the regurgitant fraction represents the ratio of the regurgitant volume over the total forward volume (stroke volume) across a given cardiac valve. For the mitral valve, the regurgitant volume can be calculated using the methods listed earlier. As for the mitral stroke volume (the denominator), this can theoretically be measured directly using a phase contrast plane placed at the level of mitral annulus and planimetry of the diastolic flow at that location. However, given the significant motion of the mitral annulus during the cardiac cycle, this direct measurement can be prone to errors of underestimation of the total stroke volume unless motion-tracking software is available. However, since the volume constituents of the mitral forward stroke volume (MR + systemic stroke volume) are the same as those of the total LV stroke volume, the latter parameter can be employed as a more practical surrogate of the underlying mitral inflow volume for estimating mitral regurgitant fraction. Importantly, when AR coexists with MR, the additional AR volume component becomes part to the LV stroke volume (MR + systemic stroke volume + AR), which no longer reflects the mitral stroke volume. In such a scenario, the AR will need to be measured and subtracted from the LV stroke volume in order to obtain the mitral forward stroke volume and ultimately the mitral regurgitant fraction:

$$\textit{Mitral regurgitant fraction}\,(\%) = \textit{Mitral regurgitant volume}/(\textit{LV Stroke Volume} - \mathrm{AR})$$

What is Severe Mitral Regurgitation? When is Intervention Indicated?

Determination of mitral regurgitation severity using CMR has become generally widely accepted as a reliable measure upon which clinical decision-making is built.[1,2] This is especially true in cases where echocardiography is nonfeasible (i.e., reduced quality of 2D or Doppler parameters) or a discordance with clinical symptoms or physical examination. Several studies have evaluated the optimal thresholds of severe mitral regurgitation using various echocardiographic and clinical parameters as a reference standard. Gelfand et al. published one of the earlier studies on this subject and proposed mitral regurgitant fraction of 26%–48% for moderate-severe, and >48% for severe.[22] However, their study used echocardiography as a reference standard where MR was assessed by estimating the ratio of the regurgitant jet area to the area of the left atrium, along with systolic flow reversal in the pulmonary veins, which was used as a requirement to diagnose severe MR. We now know that 50% of patients with an elevated jet area to LA area ratio have nonsevere MR, and that 25% of patients with pulmonary veins systolic flow reversal have nonsevere MR.[23] The MR jet can be affected by many hemodynamic factors (jet momentum) which can lead to MR overestimation. Also, eccentric jets in primary MR tend to lose their kinetic energy due to friction with the walls of the receiving chamber, leading to underestimation of the regurgitation based on the jet characteristics alone.

Myerson et al.[24] studied 109 asymptomatic patients with echocardiographic moderate or severe mitral regurgitation who had a baseline CMR and were followed-up for up to 8 years. Their results demonstrated a significant association between CMR quantified mitral regurgitation and clinical outcomes, which was superior to echocardiographic grading of regurgitation based on the 2003 ASE guidelines. In their study, 91% of subjects with CMR regurgitant volume ≤55 mL survived to 5 years without surgery compared with only 21% with regurgitant volume >55 mL ($P < .0001$). A similar separation was observed for regurgitant fraction ≤40% and >40%. Penicka et al.[25] similarly showed a significantly better discriminative ability of CMR at predicting events compared to echocardiography in 258 asymptomatic patients followed up for a median of 5.0 years. A clinically relevant finding of their study was that most of the discordances between CMR and echocardiography grading of MR severity occurred in the setting of late systolic, multiple, or eccentric MR jets. This is of great importance because it informs us as to which patients are the ones who would benefit the most from a CMR study following the index echocardiogram. Additionally, the study shows that an MR severity cut-off of ≥45 mL had an 85% sensitivity and 66% specificity for predicting mortality and mitral intervention, whereas a cut-off of ≥60 mL had an inverse predictability with a reduced 67% sensitivity and a higher 85% specificity for those same outcomes. As can be concluded from those studies, the threshold for severe MR should be considered as a continuum of risk with values above 50–55 mL as more specific for severe and those below as more sensitive. It is up to the clinician to place the values obtained with CMR or other imaging in the correct clinical context along with other parameters to make the decision that benefits the patient the most. With the understanding of the abovementioned studies, it is important to be guided by the ASE/SCMR[2] and ACC/AHA[1] guidelines when clinically managing mitral regurgitation. The guidelines share the same thresholds for both primary and secondary mitral regurgitation as follows: mild (<30 mL, <30%), moderate (30–59 mL, 30%–49%) [mild-moderate 30–44 mL, 30%–40%; moderate-severe 45–59 mL, 40%–49%], severe (≥60 mL; ≥50%).

These categories for grading severity are not modality specific and we suggest using similar categories for CMR. It is important to note that there are certain situations where regurgitant volume and fraction are not concordant and fall in different categories. The optimal way to approach such scenarios is discussed in the "Special Scenarios of Valvular Regurgitation" section.

AORTIC REGURGITATION ASSESSMENT

Mechanism and Etiologies

Aortic regurgitation (AR) can be broadly categorized into three types based on the Carpentier classification originally adapted for the mitral valve (Fig. 35.8).[26] It is essential to identify the mechanism for AR as this has implications pertaining to aortic valve repair, along with extravalvular disease such as aortic aneurysm and coarctation in bicuspid aortic valves. The Carpentier system classifies AR mechanism based on the size, mobility, and morphology of the aortic root and aortic leaflets. Type I is associated with normal leaflet motion. It is subdivided into type Ia with dilatation of the sino-tubular junction (STJ) and ascending aorta, type Ib with dilatation of the sinuses of Valsalva and the STJ, and type Ic with dilatation of aortic annulus. Type Id included cusp perforation with preserved leaflets motion, such as in a case of endocarditis for example. Type II aortic regurgitation includes cusp prolapse as seen in cases of bicuspid aortic valve. Finally, type III includes cases with cusps and leaflets restriction such as in cases of significant valve calcification and rheumatic or other inflammatory valve diseases. For a more unified categorization of regurgitation mechanisms among the aortic and mitral valves, one can think of the Carpentier types Id, II, and III as akin to *primary AR* (similar to primary MR due to prolapse, flail, calcifications, or endocarditis), whereas types Ia, Ib, and Ic are thought of as *secondary AR* (similar to secondary MR due to annular and ventricular remodeling). CMR provides a large field of view imaging with adequate spatial and temporal resolution to permit for the accurate assessment of the aorta and aortic valve morphology, pathology, and underlying AR mechanisms. In this regard CMR can serve as a one-stop-shop for this multifaceted entity, especially since some of those cases can be suboptimally visualized using the narrow field of view characteristic of ultrasound imaging, not to mention the occasional inability to confidently determine cusp morphology or AR severity.

AR SEVERITY ASSESSMENT

Regurgitant Orifice Area

As noted earlier in the Basic Principles section, when planimetry is attempted, it is advisable to acquire a stack of slightly overlapping slices, shifting gradually from upstream to immediately downstream of the orifice, in approximately 3-mm steps, to ensure that the proper AROA (anatomic regurgitant orifice area) is captured and visualized (Fig. 35.9). One study found that an AROA of 0.28 cm^2 had a 91% sensitivity and 90% specificity for severe AR as determined by echocardiography. The authors also found a good correlation (r = 0.75) between AROA and CMR-derived aortic regurgitant volume.[27] Planimetry for AR assessment is probably more reliable in secondary AR when the orifice is central and relatively simple in shape. It is likely to be

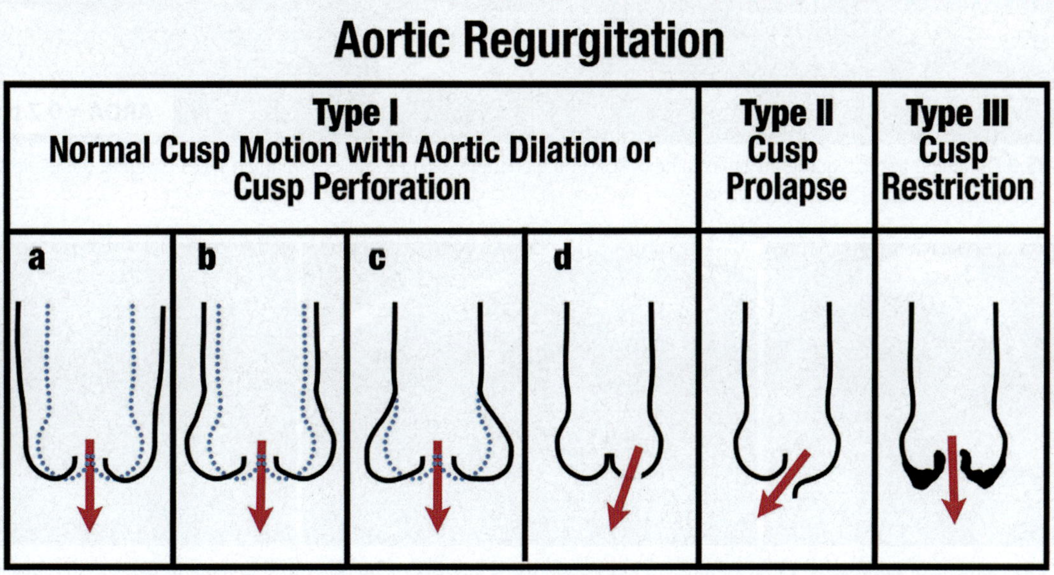

FIG. 35.8 Carpentier classification of AR. (From https://doi.org/10.1016/j.echo.2017.01.007)

challenging however, if the orifice is situated at an angle with the aortic annulus such as in primary AR with leaflet prolapse/flail, or with irregularly shaped orifices in calcific AR. An important point to understand is that the AROA is an anatomic measure of AR severity (as opposed to the traditional volumetric parameters). Hence, the aortic regurgitant orifice area is a relatively fixed parameter that is devoid of the hemodynamic factors that govern the aortic regurgitant volume. For example, changes in blood pressure or heart rate are known to modify the regurgitant volume with virtually no expected effect on the AROA. While one can view this as a weakness of this parameter, it could also be viewed as a purer descriptor of AR severity that is independent of the changing hemodynamics.

Direct Volumetric Method

Direct aortic regurgitant volume assessment is a relatively straightforward measure achieved using through-plane velocity mapping, with the imaging plane prescribed to orthogonally transect the aortic root just above the valve plane in diastole (Fig. 35.10). In the absence of valvular or outflow stenosis, it is advisable to set the velocity encoding (Venc) at approximately 2 m/s. Setting the Venc too high might affect the sensitivity of the measurement and too low would resulting in an aliasing artifact. Therefore, mixed stenotic and regurgitant valve disease present a challenge, requiring a higher Venc in the systolic phase and a lower one for the diastolic phase to capture the relatively low-velocity regurgitant flow. This is achieved with a set of Vencs with higher velocity used for the systolic frames only, and another set with lower more sensitive Venc used for diastole. An important issue to recognize when using this direct method is the aspect of translational motion of the section of aortic root beneath the velocity mapping plane throughout the cardiac cycle. This motion is related to the compliance of the aorta and more importantly to left ventricular contraction—with the aortic root pulled downward and expanding during systole, then recoiling through the plane of acquisition in diastole when aortic regurgitation is being measured. This upward movement of the root through the imaging plane is detected as a slight diastolic forward flow by velocity mapping, and could thus cause underestimation of the regurgitant volume/fraction in some cases with AR. The underestimation error is small if the root is small and relatively immobile (e.g., after previous surgery), but can be of more significance if the root is enlarged (i.e., larger area of detected flow) and ventricular function is preserved. One way to avoid this underestimation is to use motion-tracking software during the velocity flow mapping acquisition.[10] Whenever this is not available, the approximate volume of underestimation can be calculated by multiplying the root cross-sectional area by the distance of valve plane movement (volume of a cylinder). Additionally, one must be careful of the background baseline shift when using the direct method as such a shift could affect the diastolic flow curve used to calculate the AR. In such cases, the proper baseline shift could be identified and corrected so that the STJ forward flow curve stroke volume matches the total LV stroke volume (in the absence of significant MR), after which the diastolic tracing could be used to estimate the direct AR.

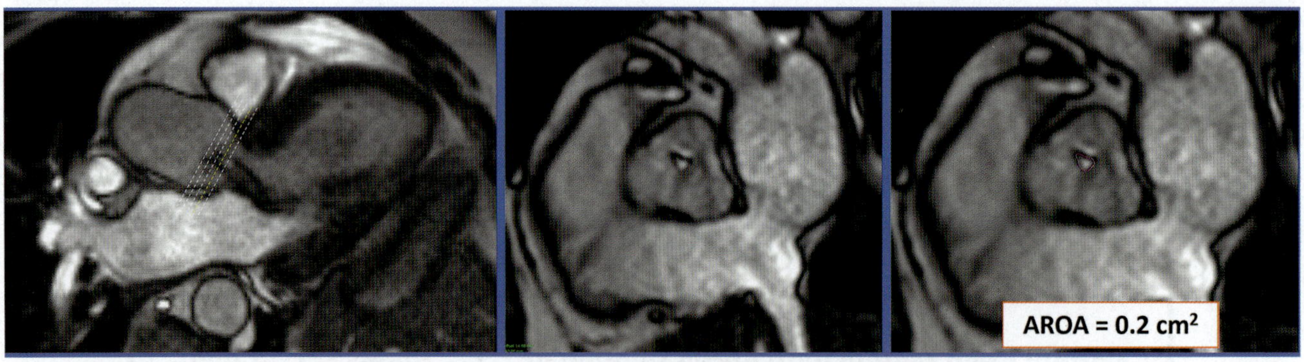

FIG. 35.9 Obtaining aortic regurgitant orifice area (*AROA*) via planimetry using a stack of imaging slices covering the leaflets' tip.

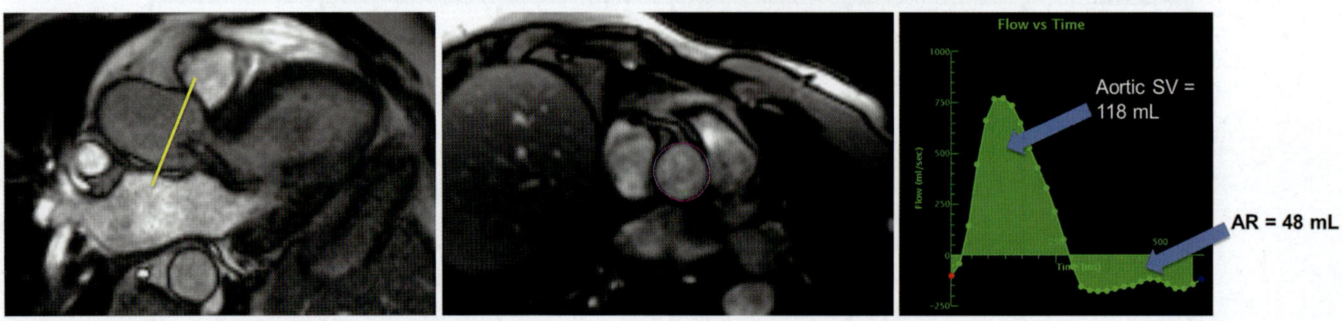

FIG. 35.10 Direct assessment of aortic regurgitant volume using through-plane velocity mapping with the imaging plane orthogonally transecting the aortic root immediately above the valve plane.

Indirect Volumetric Method

There are also indirect methods of AR measurement which could be routinely used. The most common of these is by subtracting the pulmonary flow from the aortic forward flow (Fig. 35.11). This method, however, can lead to underestimation of AR in cases where there is significant additional volume, such as significant pulmonic regurgitation or left-to-right shunt, which must be accounted for to calculate the *net* pulmonary flow. Pulmonic regurgitation volume needs to be assessed directly (as will be explained in the following chapters) and omitted from the systolic pulmonary flow in order to obtain the *net* pulmonary stroke volume. The same applies for left-to-right shunt occurring proximal to the semilunar valves whereby direct shunt flow needs to be measured and omitted from the systolic pulmonary flow in order to obtain the net pulmonary stroke volume. Finally, in the absence of other significant regurgitant lesions or intracardiac shunt, one can estimate AR by subtracting the total RV stroke volume from that of the LV. Note that, in cases of concomitant aortic stenosis and regurgitation (e.g., bicuspid aortic valve), it is advisable to use the LVOT stroke volume for estimation of total forward flow since flow turbulence distal to the aortic valve can affect the accuracy of this parameters and ultimately the AR.

AR CALCULATION FORMULAS

Indirect Methods

- Aortic Regurgitant Volume = Aortic Forward Stroke Volume – *Net* Pulmonic Stroke Volume
- Aortic Regurgitant Volume = LV Total Stroke Volume – RV Stroke Volume (applies only with isolated AR; prone to RV tracing errors; can be used in cases of atrial fibrillation with significant beat-to-beat variability)

Regurgitant Fraction

As noted earlier, by definition, the regurgitant fraction represents the ratio of the regurgitant volume over the total forward volume (stroke volume) across a given cardiac valve (Fig. 35.11). For the aortic valve, the forward stroke volume and regurgitant volume can both be calculated using the same flow acquisition (as the STJ) or using separate flows (i.e., STJ for the AR and LVOT for the forward stroke volume). Since both forward and regurgitant flow are acquired directly at the level of the aortic root this formula would apply even in the presence of concomitant valve regurgitant lesions such as MR. As mentioned earlier, the regurgitant fraction parameter is more resistant to hemodynamic changes compared to the regurgitant volume itself. In tachycardia, for instance, there would be a reduction in both forward stroke volume and AR (reduced diastolic time), while the opposite occurs in bradycardia. Since those changes almost cancel out on the numerator and denominator, the regurgitant fraction itself does not vary significantly.[28]

Regurgitant Fraction (%)
= *Aortic Regurgitant Volume/Aortic Stroke Volume*

What is Severe Aortic Regurgitation? When is Intervention Indicated?

Optimal timing of aortic valve replacement in patients with significant aortic valve regurgitation is crucial. Current criteria for surgery in patients with significant AR concentrate on symptoms and LV dilatation or impairment, on a background of severe regurgitation based on similar cut-offs as those used for MR (mild <30 mL, <30%; moderate 30–59 mL, 30%–49%; severe ≥60 mL, ≥50%).[1] This approach could be problematic because prognosis is already reduced by the time the patients are symptomatic or have LV dysfunction. Therefore, there has been an accumulation of data favoring lower cut-offs for significant AR for earlier identification of patients that would benefit from valve intervention. Myerson et al.[29] studied 113 patients with echocardiographic moderate or severe AR who were followed for up to 9 years after a CMR scan, and their progression to symptoms or other indications for surgery were monitored. A regurgitant fraction of 33% identified with high accuracy

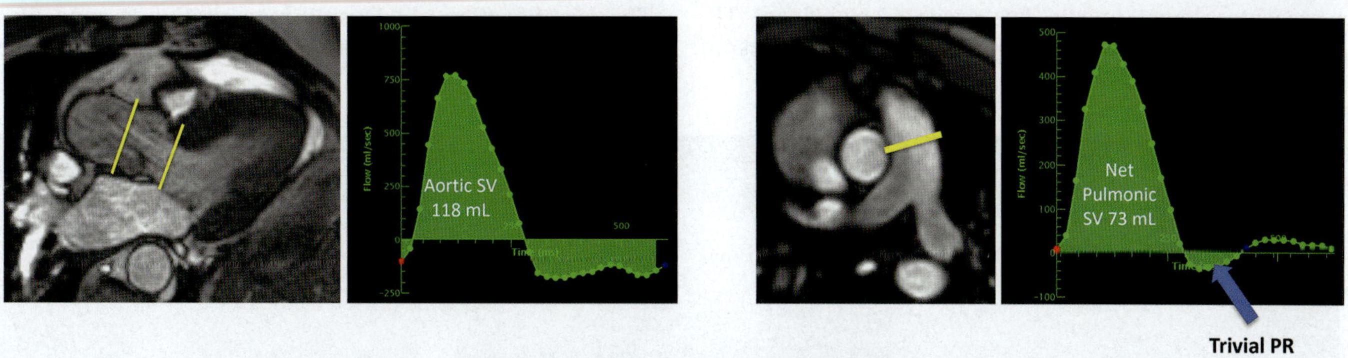

$$\text{Aortic SV} - \text{Net Pulmonic SV}$$
$$118 - 73 = \mathbf{45\ mL}$$

$$\text{Regurgitant Fraction (\%)} = \frac{\text{Aortic Rergurgitant Volume}}{\text{Aortic SV}} = \frac{45}{118} = \mathbf{38\%}$$

FIG. 35.11 An example depicting the method of *indirect* assessment of aortic regurgitant volume.

those patients who progressed to require surgery (mostly within 3 years). A similar regurgitant fraction cut-off was also found to be associated with worse outcomes by Kammerlander et al.[30] More recently, Vejpongsa et al.[31] found, in a large series of AR patients, that a regurgitant volume >38 mL and regurgitant fraction >35% had high sensitivity and specificity (89%–89% and 86%–88%, respectively) for identifying patients who required aortic valve intervention. Finally, in a multicenter study by Malahfji et al.[32] including 458 asymptomatic patients with AR, aortic regurgitant volume and fraction of 47 mL and 43%, respectively, provided the optimal thresholds for association with the primary outcome consisting of symptoms, LVEF reduction, surgery, or death. Those studies highlight the fact that the recommended thresholds in current guidelines[1,2] may be too specific for severe AR, and a lowering of those values to identify more patients who would benefit from intervention is anticipated in the upcoming revision of the guidelines. An important factor aiding toward a move in this direction is the recent advancement in transcatheter aortic valve interventions for AR. The lower risk pertaining to those procedures compared to open surgical replacement should assist with the decision-making around treating this lesion.

TRICUSPID REGURGITATION ASSESSMENT

Mechanism and Etiologies

Mild degrees of tricuspid regurgitation (TR) are common in healthy individuals. More severe grades of TR can occur due to a primary leaflet abnormality (primary TR), or to alterations in the tricuspid apparatus and/or the right ventricular and atrial geometry (secondary TR), leading to failure of leaflet coaptation. Secondary TR is the most common form of regurgitation, accounting for approximately 80% of cases[33] and usually occurs due to annular dilation and/or RV dysfunction in the setting of pulmonary hypertension from left-sided disease or primary pulmonary pathologies. Right-sided leads (pacemakers, defibrillators) also represent a common etiology for more than mild TR. Primary TR, on the other hand, represents almost one in five cases of significant TR. Example cases include tricuspid valve prolapse, tricuspid valve endocarditis, carcinoid disease, or Ebstein anomaly. Tricuspid valve prolapse (TVP) is a relatively less known entity compared to mitral valve prolapse (MVP). It has been defined recently by Guta et al. using CMR imaging as atrial leaflet displacement of ≥2 mm for the anterior and posterior leaflets and ≥3 mm for the septal leaflet. TVP was found almost exclusively in conjunction with MVP, with double the prevalence in bileaflet MVP compared to single-leaflet MVP, likely indicative of advanced myxomatous degeneration when present. Finally, patients with TVP were more likely to have severe MR and severe TR.[34] In Ebstein anomaly, parts of the tricuspid valve, usually the septal and mural leaflets, are displaced toward the apex with "atrialization" of the basal and inferior parts of the RV. This is commonly associated with severe tricuspid regurgitation and, in some cases, an atrial septal defect or pulmonary valve dysfunction.

TR SEVERITY ASSESSMENT

Jet Characteristics

If the tricuspid regurgitant jet is not visible in a standard four-chamber view, a contiguous stack of transaxial cines can be acquired to visualize all parts of the tricuspid valve and right ventricle and to locate the regurgitant signal. If pulmonary resistance is normal or nearly normal, the pressure difference propelling the jet of tricuspid regurgitation is low in comparison with regurgitant lesions of the left heart, and through-plane velocity mapping, encoded through a plane transecting the tricuspid regurgitant jet, is a very useful way of determining the size and shape of the regurgitant orifice (Fig. 35.12). The Venc that is chosen is likely to be in the range of 2–3 m/s, depending on relative RV systolic and atrial pressures. The relationship between orifice area and severity is not straightforward, but one study showed that a TR jet origin cross-sectional area >20 mm^2 has good accuracy for severe tricuspid regurgitation.[35]

Tricuspid Regurgitant Volume and Fraction

The quantification of tricuspid regurgitation is conceptually similar to that of mitral regurgitation, with the same

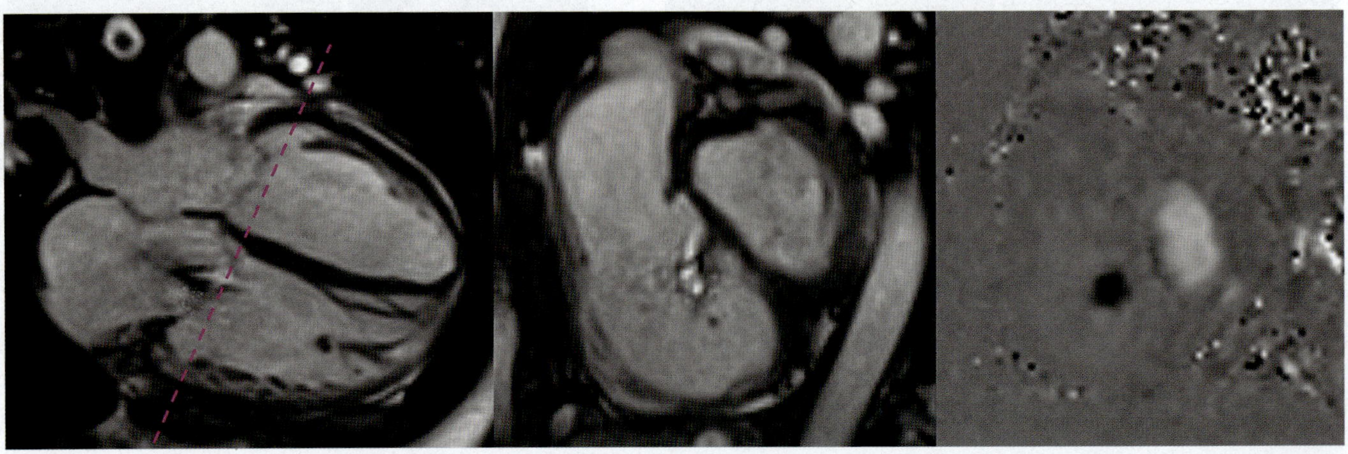

FIG. 35.12 Short-axis stack of the tricuspid valve for AROA measurement.

caveats as previously described. Several formulas and approaches for the quantification of tricuspid regurgitant volume and fraction can be employed, and each has its own advantages and disadvantages which need to be weighed and applied according to the clinical and imaging constraints:

Method 1: TR Volume
= Total RV stroke volume − Pulmonic stroke volume

More practical and reproducible than the other methods.

Applies even in the presence of significant PR.

Method 2: TR Volume
= Total RV stroke volume − Net Aortic stroke volume

Useful in patients with pulmonic stenosis or turbulence in the RV outflow tract (e.g., subvalvular stenosis).

Method 3: TR Volume
= Total RV stroke volume − Total LV stroke volume

RV stroke volume less reproducible due to extensive trabeculations of RV.

Significant concomitant regurgitant lesions invalidate this method's use.

Can be useful in setting of atrial fibrillation with significant beat-to-beat variability.

Regurgitant Fraction: Regurgitant Fraction(%)
= TR Regurgitant Volume/(RV stroke volume − PR)

What Is Severe Tricuspid Regurgitation? When Is Intervention Indicated?

As per the most current guidelines from the ASE/SCMR and ACC/AHA,[1,2] the partition values for TR severity are as follows: mild <30 mL; moderate 30–44 mL; severe ≥45 mL. The reason the cut-off values for severe are lower than in MR is because the systolic pressure gradient between the RV and RA is generally significantly lower than that of the LV and LA. Therefore, for the same orifice size/area, the tricuspid regurgitant volume is expected to be lower than the mitral regurgitant volume during the same systolic time. Although the guidelines do not specifically mention tricuspid regurgitant fraction, a study by Zhan et al. involving a large cohort of functional (secondary) TR found that a regurgitant volume of ≥45 mL or fraction ≥50% had increased likelihood or mortality (adjusted hazard ratios 2.26 and 2.60, respectively) after adjustment for multiple clinical and imaging variables including right ventricular ejection fraction.[36] With the recent advancement in transcatheter tricuspid valve interventions, it has been noted in clinical trials that patients with very advanced grades of TR with EROA >0.8 cm^2 (severe is EROA ≥0.4 cm^2) have been deriving quality-of-life improvements post-intervention despite a reduction in TR from "severe" (EROA 0.85 ± 0.22 mm^2) to "severe" (0.63 ± 0.29 mm^2).[37] Thus, an expansion of the severe TR grade to encompass "massive" TR (RVol 60–74 mL) and "torrential" TR (RVol ≥75 mL) categories had been proposed.[38] The ACC/AHA guidelines recommend surgical intervention for severe TR mostly when left-sided valve surgery is indicated. However, isolated tricuspid surgery (replacement or repair) can be attempted to reduce symptoms and recurrent hospitalizations in symptomatic patients on optimal medical therapy.[1]

Pulmonary Regurgitation Assessment

Although significant pulmonary regurgitation is relatively uncommon as an isolated or acquired lesion, it is commonly found as a residual lesion following repair of tetralogy of Fallot[39,40] or valvotomy for congenital pulmonary stenosis. Pulmonary regurgitation, even if wide open, meaning that there is effectively absent valve function, is usually well tolerated for decades, but late morbidity and mortality can ensue, due to eventual deterioration of RV function and the onset of potentially fatal arrhythmias.[41,42] Despite the wide-open nature of a PR lesion following a congenital repair, for instance, the pulmonary regurgitant volumes and fractions can remain relatively low and considerably less than would be expected on the systemic side of the heart. *Regurgitant fractions of 35%–45% are usually seen with free pulmonary regurgitation in our experience.* Higher values may be attributable to additional factors such as an unusually capacitant right ventricle on the upstream side and, on the downstream side, large and compliant pulmonary arteries, raised pulmonary vascular resistance at the branch arterial or microvascular level, or combinations of those factors.[43] In other words, the pulmonary regurgitant fraction, above a level of about 30%, reflects other aspects of right-sided pathophysiology, which should be assessed, as much as dysfunction of the valve itself. We suggest use of the terms *free* or *almost free* rather than *severe* pulmonary regurgitation when there is not an effective valve and a regurgitant fraction below 40%. If the pulmonary regurgitant fraction exceeds 40%, however, it should be called *severe*,[2] and the contributory factors should be considered: for example, unusually compliant pulmonary arteries and/or elevated pulmonary vascular resistance.

For pulmonary flow measurement, a suitable velocity-mapping plane transects the pulmonary trunk, or the ventriculopulmonary conduit, above expected valve level and proximal to the bifurcation (Fig. 35.13). Viewing RVOT cines in sagittal and oblique cross-cut orientations should help to determine the most appropriate level in a particular patient. A Venc of 2 m/s is usually sufficient to measure systolic and diastolic velocities, but a higher Venc will be needed if there is a degree of stenosis. Direct pulmonary regurgitant volume is determined by the integral of retrograde flow within the diastolic component of the flow curve, with regurgitant fraction calculated as the ratio of the regurgitant volume to the forward flow on that same curve. Pulmonary regurgitant volume can also be measured indirectly by subtracting the *net* aortic stroke volume (i.e., after calculating and excluding existing AR) from the total forward pulmonic stroke volume. Caution, however, should be applied in cases when an intracardiac shunt is present (which is not uncommon in the typically congenital cases with significant PR). It is important to note that PR will be overestimated with this approach

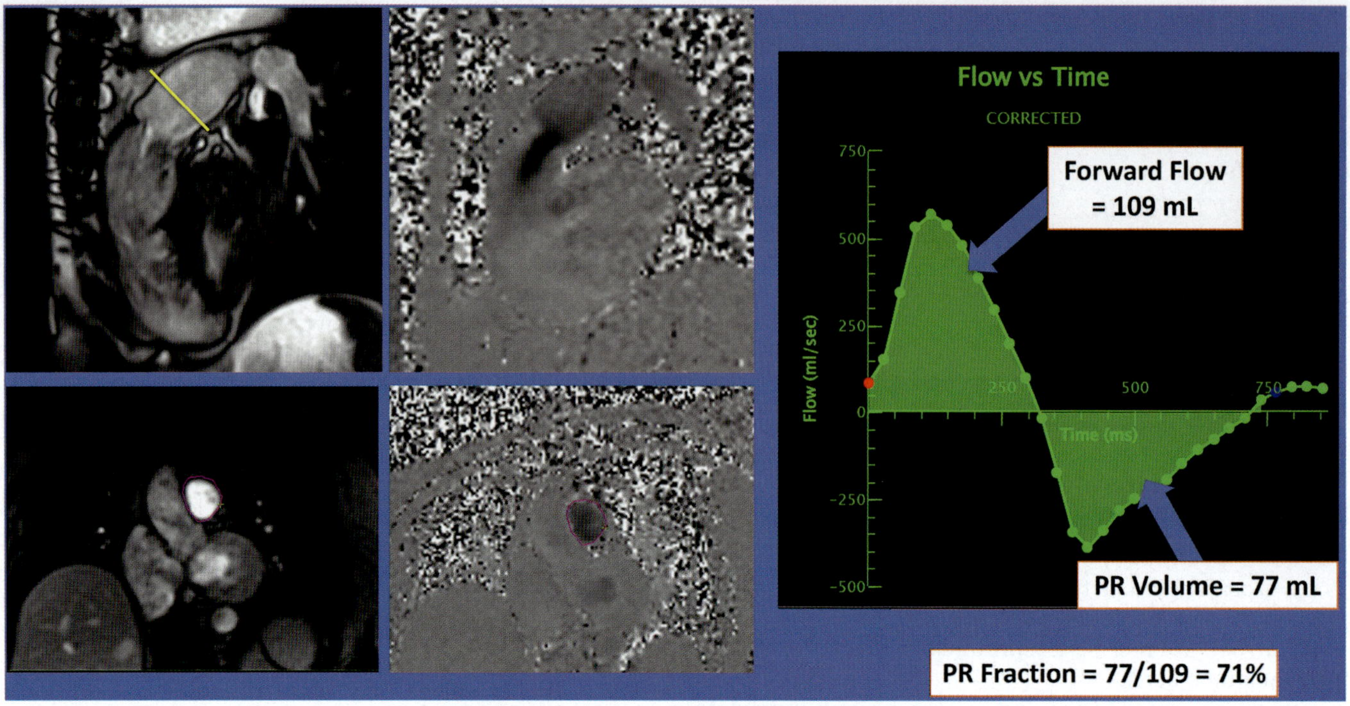

FIG. 35.13 Example of significant PR on phase contrast.

in the setting of a left-to-right shunt. In this scenario the shunt needs to be calculated and accounted for. Finally, pulmonary regurgitant fraction is calculated as the percentage ratio of regurgitant volume over the pulmonic forward stoke volume.

VALVULAR STENOSIS

Aortic Valve Stenosis

Aortic valve stenosis can be a result of congenital malformation of the valve (e.g., bicuspid or unicuspid aortic valve), age-related degeneration (i.e., calcific stenosis), rheumatic heart disease, or radiation induced. Transthoracic echocardiography (TTE) remains the modality of choice for assessment of aortic stenosis, however, there are certain scenarios where assessment becomes challenging, and a direct anatomic assessment of the aortic valve area (AVA) is required. Such scenarios include patients with challenging acoustic windows, difficulty in continuous-wave Doppler alignment with the jet, inaccuracies and assumptions pertaining to LVOT diameter and area estimation, subvalvular aortic stenosis (from concomitant mitral valve SAM or subaortic membrane), and discordance in gradients and aortic valve area (e.g., AVA $<1\,cm^2$ with mean gradient <40 mm Hg, especially in normal flow conditions). In such scenarios, other modalities can be employed to resolve the true grade of aortic stenosis. These include direct planimetry with transesophageal echocardiography (TEE) or cardiac computed tomography (CCT), and catheter-based assessment of the LV-aorta gradients and estimation of the aortic valve area (Gorlin formula). CMR represents a noninvasive, radiation-free, and iodinated contrast-free tool which can offer clinically useful parameters pertaining to aortic stenosis assessment and consequences on the LV myocardium such as LV mass, wall thickness, and interstitial and replacement fibrosis, which can be critical in decision-making in AS. Ranges of measurements reflecting different severities of aortic stenosis (AS) and other valve lesions are shown in Table 35.1.

DIRECT PLANIMETRY

Several prior publications on CMR quantification of AS have used planimetry of the orifice to make direct estimates of orifice area.[44–47] A recent meta-analysis looking at studies evaluating aortic stenosis by CMR found a comparable anatomic area estimate versus TEE, but an AVA that is on average 10.7% (mean area difference $+0.14\,cm^2$ [0.07–$0.21\,cm^2$]) larger than that calculated using TTE, with the vast majority of those studies conducted on 1.5 Tesla scanners using SSFP acquisitions.[48] It must be emphasized that the area assessed by CMR (or CCT and TEE) represents the *anatomic* valve area (Fig. 35.14), as opposed to the *effective* valve area derived using the continuity equation on TTE. The echocardiographic effective valve area is generally smaller than the anatomic valve area because: (1) it is measured at the point of maximal flow velocity immediately distal to the valve orifice where the jet contracts to its narrowest (vena contracta) and (2) the effective valve area is calculated using the velocity–time integral (VTI) throughout systole, which reflects the mean orifice area of the valve during systole, as opposed to the peak orifice area captured on anatomic imaging. CMR-based *effective* orifice area can be calculated and will be discussed in the following paragraph.

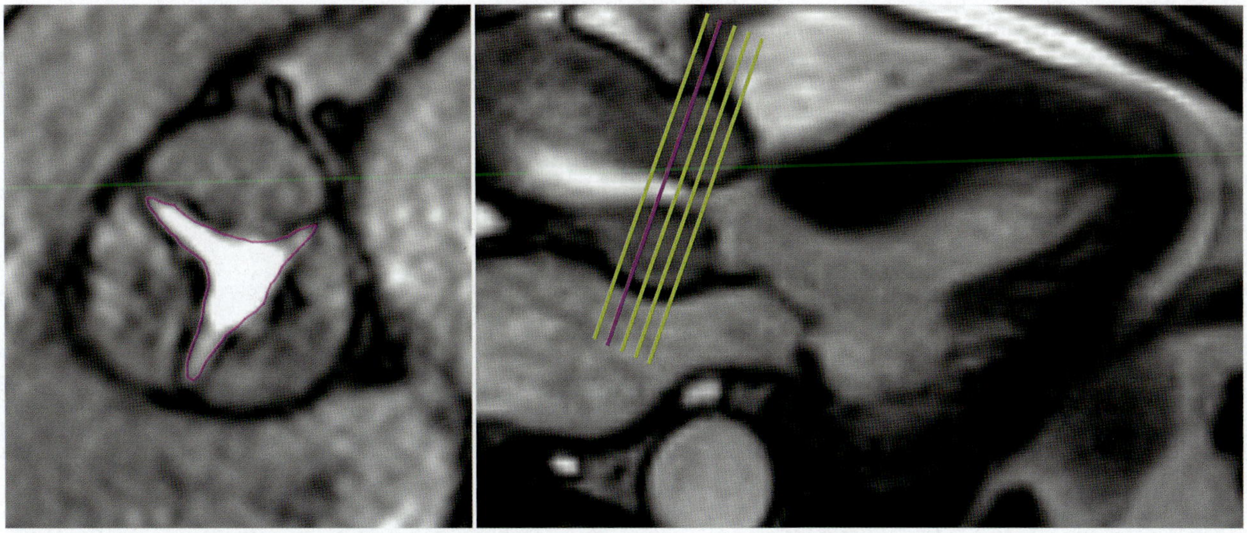

FIG. 35.14 An example depicting anatomic AVA measurement.

For direct planimetry of the valve orifice, high-resolution breath-hold GRE or SSFP imaging in a stack of about five slices, shifting 3 mm at a time from immediately upstream to just downstream of the orifice, should be acquired. The best cine, which is probably the one that shows the smallest, most clearly delineated cross-section of the jet, should then be used for direct planimetry. It is important to mention that the planimetry method of a stenotic aortic valve can be prone to measurement errors, especially if the aortic orifice is curved (nonplanar), or with severe calcifications, which can cause signal void and render border discrimination of the valve leaflets challenging. A stenosed bicuspid aortic valve generally has a slit-like nonplanar orifice (Fig. 35.2), whereas calcified valves can have irregular or three-pointed orifices, and the considerations described earlier regarding jet shape and the locations of image slices are important in those scenarios. A direct planimetry area that is $<1.0\,cm^2$ is generally consistent with severe stenosis, and an area that is $>1.5\,cm^2$ is consistent with a nonsevere stenosis. One cannot make a strong conclusion as to the severity of the stenosis when AVA is $1–1.4\,cm^2$ since the absolute difference versus TTE can be $+0.14\,cm^2$ ($0.07–0.21\,cm^2$).[48] This is important since clinical decision-making is guided by guidelines based on TTE measurements, especially when CMR AVA lacks a validated prognostic threshold.

VELOCITY AND GRADIENTS ASSESSMENT

Peak stenotic jet velocity and mean jet velocity are possible approaches to the assessment of the severity of stenosis, which can be complimentary to planimetry, or alternative parameters when planimetry may be unsatisfactory. Jet velocities depend on the flow rate as well as stenosis severity. Jet velocity and gradient estimation can be used in two ways: (1) to assess the peak velocity and mean gradient across the valve, and (2) to calculate an effective aortic valve area using the continuity equation. To acquire the peak jet velocity, cine imaging is first used to show the location and direction of the jet core. In-plane breath-hold velocity mapping with the direction of velocity encoding aligned with that of the jet can be helpful to visualize the jet, but it is likely to underestimate peak velocity if the jet is narrow. The above acquisitions should then be used to align a velocity-mapping slice to transect the jet core, with the velocity of an appropriate range (Venc) encoded through the image plane. The velocity of the jet should be analyzed with caution in the resulting image, particularly if the stenosis is severe. Signal loss can allow background noise or other artifacts to contribute spurious phase shifts, particularly in the shear region at the edge of a jet, so peak jet velocity should be measured in a region of good signal recovery within the core of the jet. Importantly, since the velocity encoding plane needs to horizontally transect the jet core at the highest velocity region (vena contracta), any slight movement in either direction of the plane relative to jet core (e.g., even minimal respiratory motion) would result in underestimation of the maximal velocity. Another factor that could lead to underestimation compared to TTE is the lower temporal resolution on CMR. Therefore, a recorded CMR peak jet velocity of $>4.0\,m/s$ is confidently in favor of severe AS. Jet velocity assessment can also be used in prosthetic aortic valves where the associated artifacts can limit planimetry and area estimation.

Garcia et al. compared the effective orifice area calculated using Doppler echocardiography and CMR. Interestingly, they found that the LVOT area is underestimated on TTE versus CMR due to its elliptical nature (TTE LVOT area $3.84 \pm 0.80\,cm^2$ vs. CMR LVOT area $4.78 \pm 1.05\,cm^2$). On the other hand, LVOT VTI was overestimated on TTE versus CMR (21 ± 4 vs. 15 ± 4 cm), and good concordance was found for the aortic jet VTI (61 ± 22 vs. 57 ± 20 cm). Ultimately, TTE- and CMR-derived effective orifice areas had good correlation and concordance (1.53 ± 0.67 vs. $1.59 \pm 0.73\,cm^2$, $r = 0.92$).[49]

IMPACT ON THE LV MYOCARDIUM

An important strength of CMR is the assessment of the consequences of valve lesions on the affected cardiac chambers. This will be covered in more detail in the subsequent Chapter 36 on Valvular Heart Disease: Assessment of Cardiac Remodeling.

TABLE 35.3 Suggested cardiovascular magnetic resonance protocol for transcatheter aortic valve replacement planning.

MRI SEQUENCE	SEQUENCE PLANNING	PARAMETERS PERTINENT TO TAVR PLANNING
Noncontrast, ECG-triggered, navigator-gated, free-breathing three-dimensional acquisition using a steady-state free precession sequence	• Cubic three-dimensional volume set-up to cover the range between the LVOT and the ascending aorta • Sequence obtained in systole (aortic annulus measurements) and in diastole (aortic root measurements)	• Aortic annulus size (area, circumference, diameters) • Aortic root (sinus of Valsalva, ST junction) size • Coronary arteries origins and height relative to the annulus plane • Ascending aorta–annulus angle • Significant LVOT calcifications (increased risk of root rupture)
3D Gradient echo gadolinium contrast MRA	• Sequence obtained pre- and post-IV administration of gadolinium contrast • MRA acquisition volume extends from the aortic arch vessels cranially to the femoral arteries caudally	• Thoraco-abdominal aorta dimensions and plaque/thrombus assessment • Aortic arch vessels patency and anatomy (can serve as secondary access vessels in the case of femoral arteries or aorta stenoses) • Distal access arteries patency and tortuosity (femoral and iliac arteries)

Role of CMR in TAVI Planning and Follow-Up

Transcatheter aortic valve implantation (TAVI) is an effective alternative to surgical aortic valve replacement in patients with higher surgical risk or who are deemed inoperable.[50,51] Cardiac imaging plays an essential role for assessment of the severity of aortic valve stenosis and for selecting anatomically suitable patients for this procedure. A number of imaging modalities are often used for this purpose, including echocardiography, CCT, and CMR. Each imaging method has its advantages and limitations.[52] The use of CMR in patients undergoing, or being considered for, TAVI is likely to expand. CMR provides several important pieces of structural information before consideration for TAVI; in addition to accurate quantification of ventricular volumes, mass, and function, aortic valve planimetry can be performed to accurately determine valve area, and late gadolinium enhancement (LGE) can show areas of myocardial scarring related to aortic stenosis.[53,54] Importantly, CMR-guided TAVI planning can be utilized in cases where CT is not available or iodinated LV contrast is deemed inappropriate. In a recent randomized trial involving 248 patients, CMR-guided TAVI planning was shown to be non-inferior to CT-guided planning in terms of device implantation success.[55] Table 35.3 summarizes a suggested TAVR acquisition protocol utilizing CMR.[55,56]

Additionally, magnetic resonance angiography (MRA) of the peripheral vasculature can be performed to assess access routes (Fig. 35.15). Following TAVI, CMR can be employed to assess ventricular remodeling, with studies showing an expected reduction in LV mass, diastolic volume, and systolic volume, and increase in LVEF, within 6–15 months following TAVI.[57] The joint ASE/SCMR guidelines also now recognize CMR as an important tool to quantify paravalvular regurgitation severity after TAVI, which can be challenging to echocardiography.[58] In a study by Ribeiro et al.,[59] CMR performed a median of 40 days after TAVI had a greater association with adverse clinical events (mortality and heart failure rehospitalization) compared with early post-TAVI echocardiography. Importantly, a CMR RF >30% was the best predictor of poor outcomes, with regurgitant volume failing to predict adverse events. This can be explained by the fact that post-TAVI AR is a form of acute regurgitation in an often hypertrophied, small, and stiff left ventricle which was dealing with preexisting AS. Therefore, small regurgitant volumes may correspond to a large regurgitant fraction, with a significant effect on outcomes.

Ultimately, unless any postprocedural CMR-specific measurements can be shown to lead to treatment changes affecting prognosis, it will remain highly debatable whether it is worth the time and expense to perform CMR on a routine basis after TAVI, as echocardiography may be sufficient in the majority of cases. But in the longer term, a role may arise for percutaneous valve interventions such as TAVI to be completely MRI guided.

Subaortic Stenosis

There are important anatomic differences between the left and right ventricular outflow tracts, resulting in distinct types of subvalvular stenotic lesion. Two types of subaortic stenosis need to be distinguished. One that is typical of hypertrophic cardiomyopathy is caused by narrowing in the proximal part of the outflow tract between the hypertrophied basal part of the septum and the septal leaflet of the mitral valve. Because the valve leaflet is mobile, its tip can be drawn still closer to the septum by the low pressure of the jet, a fluid dynamic phenomenon known as the Venturi effect, causing systolic anterior motion of the mitral valve, with probable vibration of the leaflet. Velocity mapping on CMR tends to be unsuccessful when this type of stenosis is significant, whereas Doppler echocardiography is probably more reliable. This is because the relatively modest temporal resolution of CMR velocity mapping is typically unreliable at capturing the short-duration late-systolic peak velocity characteristic of dynamic LVOT. Such stenoses tend to become more severe on exertion, owing to enhancement of the Venturi effect with rapid ejection, and may be associated with eccentric posteriorly directed mitral regurgitation. Because administration of pharmacologic stress agents can be risky in such cases, with the patient lying in the bore of a magnet, echocardiography with exercise stress is a more appropriate approach for the assessment of severity. CMR is nevertheless valuable, giving good views of all parts of the ventricle and of any associated pathology of the mitral apparatus (e.g., long anterior mitral leaflet, reduced aorto-mitral angle),

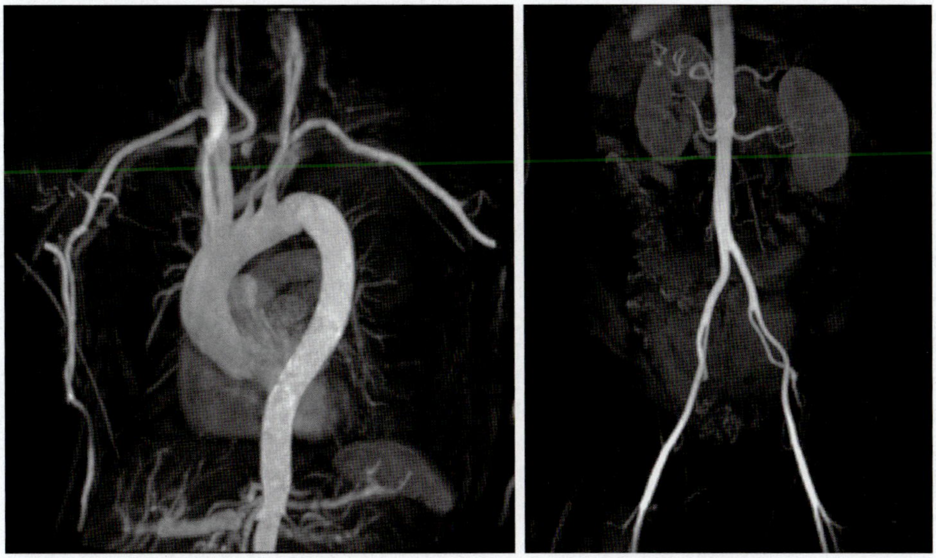

FIG. 35.15 MRA for access vessels assessment as part of TAVI planning.

or the ventricle (e.g., sigmoid septum or hypertrophic cardiomyopathy).

A second type of subaortic stenosis is caused by a subvalvular ridge or membrane, usually only a few millimeters below the level of the valve. It is advisable here, as elsewhere, to acquire cine images of jet flow in several orientations, especially as it can be hard to distinguish subvalvular from valvular stenosis. In-plane velocity mapping can help to establish the level of flow acceleration, followed by velocity mapping through two planes, each clearly labeled, immediately below and above the level of the valve. If subvalvular stenosis is present, the aortic valve leaflets, even if normal, cannot be expected to open fully, owing to the Venturi effect, so assessment of the aortic valve has to remain cautious when subvalvular stenosis is present unless it is clear that there is additional, more severe stenosis at the level of the valve itself.

Pulmonary and Other Stenoses of the Right Ventricular Outflow Tract

Stenosis of the pulmonary valve generally presents as a congenital condition early in life, either isolated or associated with other abnormalities of the RVOT and pulmonary arteries, as in tetralogy of Fallot. Transcatheter or surgical relief of pulmonary stenosis is typically recommended when there are peak-to-peak transpulmonary catheter pressure differences of 40 mm Hg, or 30 mm Hg in symptomatic patients. This probably translates into peak velocity measurements of the order of 3–4 m/s by CMR jet velocity mapping, but as was outlined earlier, jet velocity mapping can be subject to errors, particularly if acquisitions are not perfectly located. The strength of CMR in this setting is in the evaluation of associated pathophysiology, particularly of RV hypertrophy and dysfunction, and possible additional levels of stenosis, including the branch pulmonary arteries. RV to pulmonary artery conduits are also readily evaluated by CMR, although ferromagnetic valve rings or sternal wires may cause localized artifacts.

Isolated pulmonary valve stenosis can also present later in life, although a more common progressive lesion in the adult population is double-chambered right ventricle, which can also be called subinfundibular stenosis (Fig. 35.4).[60] Double-chambered right ventricle is a diagnosis that can be misinterpreted on echocardiography as a ventricular septal defect, which frequently coexists, or as stenosis at the infundibular or pulmonary valve level. The distinction is important and is usually clear on CMR imaging because subinfundibular stenosis is treatable, if necessary, by transatrial surgical resection of the obstructing muscle bands without the need for pulmonary valve replacement. It is important to use the excellent access provided by CMR to visualize the level and nature of any RVOT stenosis as clearly as possible. RV to pulmonary artery conduits and the function of their valves can also be evaluated very effectively by CMR cine imaging and velocity mapping.

Mitral and Tricuspid Valve Stenosis

Methods of assessment of stenosis are fairly similar for the mitral and tricuspid valves. Both can usually be adequately assessed by 2D and Doppler echocardiography, and more recently by area planimetry using 3D echocardiography, which can contribute additional useful morphologic information. The cross-sectional shape and area of the stenotic orifice can generally be seen and measured on CMR short-axis cine acquisitions and phase velocity maps, oriented to transect the jet at right angles to or very close to the orifice on the downstream side. Motion tracking should be used if available. Comparative studies between CMR and both transthoracic and transesophageal echocardiography showed excellent agreement between CMR planimetered area and echocardiographic calculated and planimetered mitral valve areas.[61,62] ACC/AHA guidelines define severe mitral stenosis when the area is ≤1.5 cm^2, with no labeled cut-offs for mild and moderate.[1] The ASE guidelines for the evaluation of rheumatic heart disease further categorized mild and moderate mitral stenosis as an area of >2.5 cm^2 and 1.5–2.5 cm^2, respectively.[63]

Not only the area and velocity of the jet but also the time course of jet flow is important, with loss of the normal biphasic mitral flow pattern and prolonged elevation of velocity as stenosis increases in severity. The slope of the decline in the maximum velocity has been used to estimate the pressure half-time (the time it takes until the initial pressure difference across the orifice is halved).[64] The time curve of pulmonary venous flow, with marked atrial systolic reversal, can also be informative.[65] An important contribution of CMR is in the assessment of associated pathophysiology such as the degree of atrial dilatation, and possible changes of the pulmonary veins, pulmonary arteries, and RV if pulmonary hypertension has developed secondary to mitral stenosis.

Special Scenarios of Valvular Regurgitation

DISCREPANT MITRAL REGURGITANT VOLUME AND FRACTION

There are certain clinical scenarios where regurgitant volume and fraction parameters are not concordant and fall in different grading categories (e.g., RV of 25 mL and RF 35% or RV of 65 mL and RF 45%). We propose the following approach in those scenarios. (1) When one parameter is in the mild grade while the other is in the moderate grades it is reasonable to use the label "mild-moderate" since it is unlikely for this to be an actionable lesion and will only require regular follow-up. (2) When MR is more significant (e.g., one parameter in the moderate grade and one in the severe grades) and possibly contributing to clinical symptoms, we suggest placing more weight on the volume versus the fraction components based on the underlying mechanism of the MR. In other words, patients with primary MR tend to have a hypercontractile left ventricle with a high total stroke volume, making them occasionally achieve the volume threshold of severe (≥60 mL) before the fraction exceeds the threshold (≥50%).[66] A flail mitral valve with 65 mL regurgitant volume and 45% fraction is most likely severe and portrays a poor outcome if left untreated (as mentioned in earlier studies). On the contrary, in secondary MR there is usually a low total stroke volume state which may lead to a regurgitant fraction achieving the severe threshold while regurgitant volume may not (e.g., 40 mL and 60%). In such a case the fraction is probably more representative of the loss of forward flow in this low-flow state and reflects a severe lesion. However, more study is still warranted to determine how best to approach secondary regurgitant lesions.

MIXED MITRAL AND AORTIC REGURGITATION

Concomitant valve lesions can pose a quantitative and clinical challenge; therefore, it is essential to assess and report those cases accurately and clearly. Dealing with a "double moderate" scenario can be especially challenging. In terms of quantification, we usually begin by calculating the aortic regurgitant volume and fraction using either the indirect or direct AR methods available (as described in the "Aortic Regurgitation Assessment" section). This is followed by calculation of the MR load. As mentioned before, the volumetric method of MR calculation (method 1) performs well irrespective of coexisting AR severity, thus it can be employed accurately to calculate the mitral regurgitant volume. In this case, calculating the mitral regurgitant fraction is done as follows: *Mitral regurgitant fraction (%) = Mitral regurgitant volume/(LV stroke volume – AR).* When reporting the final results, it is essential to assert the following aspects: (1) aortic and mitral regurgitant volumes; (2) *total volume load* "seen" by the LV—that is the combined AR + MR regurgitant volumes; and (3) the dominant lesion in the particular scenario (i.e., the one leaning closer to the severe range). This information would assist the clinician in appreciating the gravity of the combined lesions, along with tailoring and prioritizing the treatment approach.

MITRAL PROLAPSE VOLUME

Classic mitral valve prolapse (Barlow disease) is characterized by myxomatous degeneration of the mitral leaflets secondary to the accumulation of proteoglycans and degradation of matrix proteins, resulting in large, thick, and redundant leaflets usually combined with a dilated annulus and elongated chords. The bileaflet multisegment prolapse characteristic of Barlow disease leads to the formation of a dome-shaped three-dimensional volume—the prolapse volume—at end-systole. The prolapse volume is bordered by the prolapsing leaflets' surface basally and the mitral annular plane apically. Depending on the prolapse extent, surface area of the leaflets, and annulus circumference, the dome-like prolapse volume can harbor a significant quantity of blood at end-systole. Current practice focuses on the transvalvular MR as the main loading volume of the left heart chambers in patients with mitral valve disease. The prolapse volume, on the other hand, crosses the mitral annulus without traversing the mitral leaflets during systole, being retained underneath in a "ventricularized" portion of the left atrium and may represent an important contributor to LV volume overload in diastole (Fig. 35.16A). We have studied a spectrum of prolapse volumes in single- versus bileaflet prolapse cases and shown that the prolapse volume is part of the total volume load exerted on the LV during the cardiac cycle, as evidenced by the parallel increase in LV size with increasing prolapse volumes (Fig. 35.16B). This could help explain the disproportionate LV enlargement relative to MR severity historically noted in Barlow disease. In our laboratory, we report bileaflet MVP cases using the following rationale and methods. (1) We manually calculate the prolapse volume using the methodology described in our paper[67] (2) When tracing the end-systolic LV endocardium (where the prolapse volume is present) on short-axis slices, the most basal LV slice is chosen based on the crest of the LV myocardium (as is typically performed in non-MVP cases). (3) The resultant total LV stroke volume (end-diastolic minus end-systolic volumes) would therefore include three volume parts: [systemic forward flow] + [transvalvular MR] + [prolapse volume]. (4) We then subtract the calculated phase-contrast calculated systemic forward flow from the total LV stroke volume to obtain the *total regurgitant volume load* (transvalvular

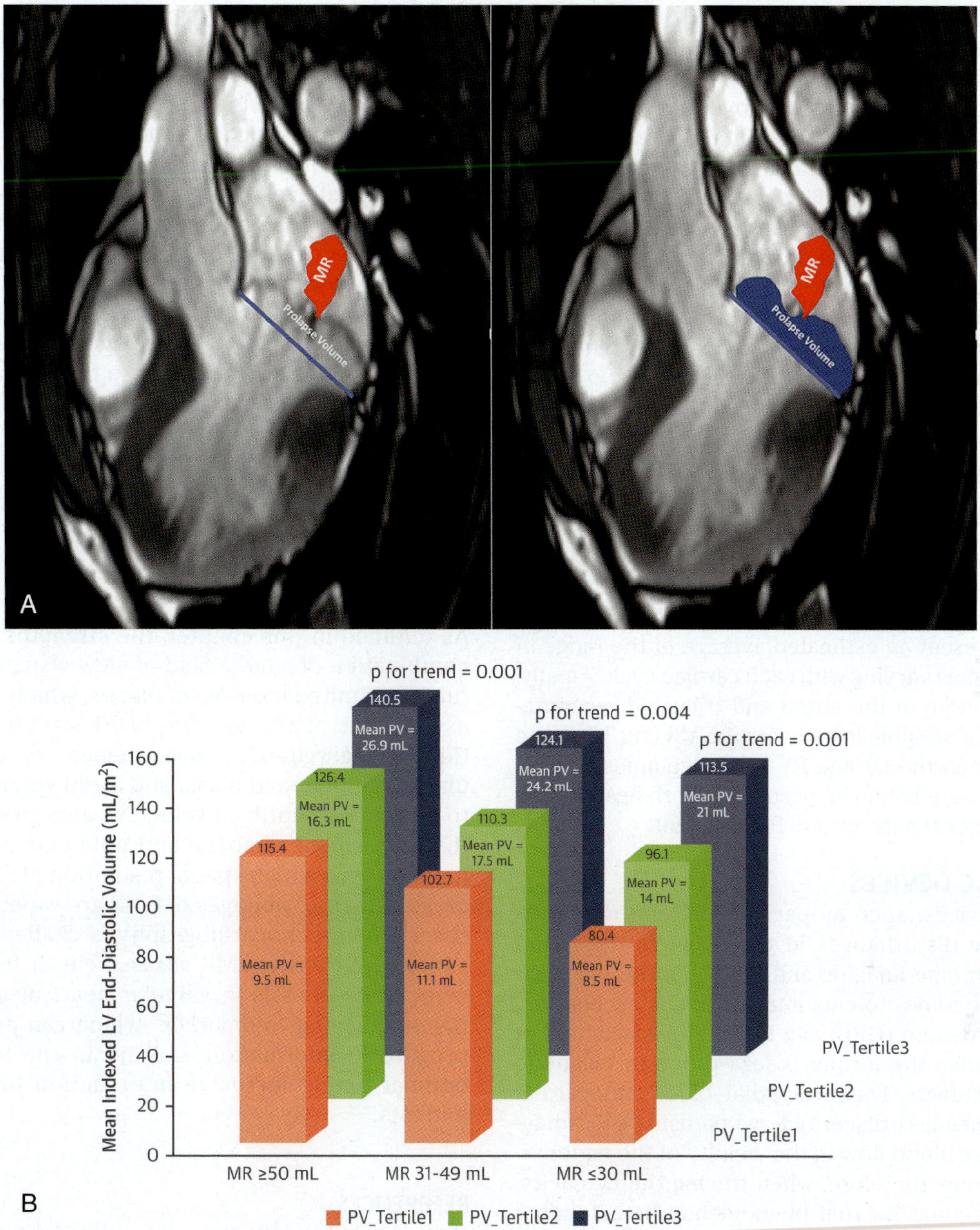

FIG. 35.16 (A) Schematic representation of the anatomy and borders of the prolapse volume in a case of bileaflet mitral valve prolapse. (B) A three-dimensional bar chart illustrating how left ventricular end-diastolic volume (*indexed*) progressively increases along two dimensions: From right to left as mitral regurgitation severity increases across tertiles, and within each MR tertile from front to back as valve prolapse volume increases across its own tertiles. (From https://doi.org/10.1016/j.jcmg.2020.08.029.)

MR + prolapse volume). (5) Finally, we report the traditional transvalvular MR, and supplement it with the prolapse volume and total volume load. This approach is made easier when the transvalvular MR is already in the severe range, where the additional prolapse volume won't exert a major effect on decision-making. However, the dilemma occurs in those cases when the prolapse volume elevates the MR grade when accounted for, which we found in approximately 50% of cases.[67] In cases when the transvalvular MR is moderate and the total MR volume is severe, it is important to be as clear and descriptive in the report as possible. Occasionally, it is advisable to directly communicate with the clinician when evident signs of ventricular remodeling or dysfunction are noted, especially when the lesion is potentially actionable.

MITRAL REGURGITATION AND SYSTOLIC ANTERIOR MOTION (SAM)

Mitral valve SAM is a known cause of mitral regurgitation. However, the flow turbulence commonly seen in the LVOT and proximal ascending aorta due to the dynamic LVOT obstruction and flow acceleration can lead to inaccuracies in measuring the aortic outflow stroke volume essential to calculating MR. In such scenarios, we advise using the net pulmonary arterial stroke flow as a surrogate and subtracting that volume from the total LV stroke volume to obtain the MR. One has to be careful about the presence of significant PR or left-to-right shunts, which will have to be independently calculated and omitted from the pulmonary outflow stroke volume to obtain the net volume ultimately making its way to the LVOT.

ATRIAL FIBRILLATION AND VALVE REGURGITATION

Atrial fibrillation (AF) can present a multilevel challenge during a CMR study acquisition and interpretation. Since cine CMR acquisition is achieved over several cardiac cycles, stability of the heart position in the chest from one cycle to the next is key to maintaining a high-quality image. The irregular cardiac contractility in AF exemplifies such a scenario, however, multiple strategies are usually employed to overcome this challenge and optimize the image (e.g., triggering adjustment, multi-beat acquisition, real-time imaging). Another challenge emerges when quantification is attempted, since the irregularity affects both volumetric and flow measurements. It is key to realize that no single parameter we typically measure is constant when the heart is in AF. The ejection fractions, ventricular stroke volumes, outflow stroke volumes, all vary with every cardiac cycle. Expecting fixed numbers of such parameters is therefore unrealistic. However, since chamber volumes and flows are typically acquired using a strategy reflecting an average R-R interval (using triggering and multi-beat acquisition, respectively), one can therefore expect the resultant regurgitant volumes to represent an estimated average of the range of regurgitant volumes varying with each cardiac cycle. Finally, as mentioned before in the mitral and tricuspid regurgitation sections, it is possible to estimate the MR and TR as the difference between the LV and RV stroke volumes using a single multislice acquisition incorporating both heart chambers, assuming nonsignificant AR, PR, or shunt.

INTRACARDIAC DEVICES

Intracardiac devices, such as pacemakers and defibrillators, can create disturbances in the magnetic field that can render both cine imaging and flow quantitation challenging. When it comes to cine imaging in such scenarios, gradient recalled echo (GRE) can be employed instead of SSFP imaging since the former is less prone to magnetic susceptibility artifacts. The myocardial–blood endocardial interface becomes less discernible when using GRE imaging due to slower blood flow in the vicinity of the endocardial trabeculations, therefore, when tracing the LV cavity, one needs to account for that phenomenon by extending the drawn line more outward into the LV by approximately 1–2 mm. The flow measurements can also be affected by magnetic susceptibility artifacts, more commonly the pulmonic outflow from our experience, likely due to its closer proximity to the device generator and its associated metallic artifact. When there is a significant discrepancy in flow measurements between the aortic and pulmonic outflow volumes, we typically use the flow curve that appears more physiological and the one that yields flow volumes which match our LV/RV stroke volumes in the setting of minimal or no regurgitation or shunt.

Future Directions

Many improvements in CMR have occurred over the past few decades, several of which are now part of the daily clinical routine and are outlined in this chapter. However, existing and new areas of CMR technology continue advancing and emerging. Examples include free-breathing sequences[68] for more rapid and convenient acquisitions, along with potentially prognostic tools such as ventricular strain evaluation.[69] Perhaps more pertinent to this chapter are the novel ways in assessing stenotic and regurgitant valvular diseases using 4D flow. This technique is based on 3D phase-contrast acquisitions (as opposed to the current 2D planar acquisitions) which provide three-dimensional time-resolved velocity information encompassing the entire heart.[70,71] Four-dimensional flow is still hindered by long acquisition times, however, improvements in hardware power and image reconstruction have made its appearance on the clinical stage more tangible. This tool is particularly useful in cases with multivalvular pathologies or complex flows such as in congenital heart disease patients (see consensus statement on 4D flow[72]). Additionally, its ability to visualize jet vortices can offer important insight into the effect of the jets besides the volumetric quantification, such as in bicuspid aortic valves with aortic aneurysms.[73]

Conclusion

As outlined in this chapter, the strengths of CMR lie in a combination of a large field-of-view visualization with virtually unlimited freedom of planes, which allows accurate assessment of the various heart structures, quantification of regurgitation, measurement of ventricular volumes, function, and mass, and atrial volumes. The ability to measure stenotic jet velocities also gives CMR a role in the assessment of aortic and pulmonic stenosis, in conjunction with a high spatial resolution planimetry of valve areas. Those advantages of CMR are especially of value in cases where echocardiography is challenging or nonfeasible. Importantly, CMR assessment of focal and diffuse myocardial fibrosis in valvular heart disease presents a unique imaging "biomarker" which can provide valuable prognostic information and aid in the identification of optimal timing for valve intervention in asymptomatic patients.

REFERENCES

1. Otto CM, Nishimura RA, Bonow RO, et al. 2020 ACC/AHA guideline for the management of patients with valvular heart disease: executive summary: a report of the American college of cardiology/American heart association joint committee on clinical practice guidelines. *J Am Coll Cardiol.* 2021;77(4):450–500.
2. Zoghbi WA, Adams D, Bonow RO, et al. Recommendations for noninvasive evaluation of native valvular regurgitation. *J Am Soc Echocardiogr.* 2017;30(4):303.
3. Myerson SG. Heart valve disease: investigation by cardiovascular magnetic resonance. *J Cardiovasc Magn Reson.* 2012;14:1–23.
4. Kilner PJ, Gatehouse PD, Firmin DN. Flow measurement by magnetic resonance: a unique asset worth optimising. *J Cardiovasc Magn Reson.* 2007;9(4):723–728.
5. Chernobelsky A, Shubayev O, Comeau CR, Wolff SD. Baseline correction of phase contrast images improves quantification of blood flow in the great vessels. *J Cardiovasc Magn Reson.* 2007;9(4):681–685.
6. Zoghbi WA, Adams D, Bonow RO, et al. Recommendations for noninvasive evaluation of native valvular regurgitation: a report from the american society of echocardiography developed in collaboration with the society for cardiovascular magnetic resonance. *J Am Soc Echocardiogr.* 2017;30(4):303–371.
7. Kilner P, Firmin DN, Rees RS, et al. Valve and great vessel stenosis: assessment with MR jet velocity mapping. *Radiology.* 1991;178(1):229–235.
8. Mohiaddin RH, Longmore DB. Functional aspects of cardiovascular nuclear magnetic resonance imaging. Techniques and application. *Circulation.* 1993;88(1):264–281.
9. Lotz J, Meier C, Leppert A, Galanski M. Cardiovascular flow measurement with phase-contrast MR imaging: basic facts and implementation. *Radiographics.* 2002;22(3):651–671.

10. Kozerke S, Schwitter J, Pedersen EM, Boesiger P. Aortic and mitral regurgitation: quantification using moving slice velocity mapping. *J Magn Reson Imaging: Off J Int Soc Magn Reson Med*. 2001;14(2):106–112.
11. Yap S, Geuns R, Meijboom FJ, et al. A simplified continuity equation approach to the quantification of stenotic bicuspid aortic valves using velocity-encoded cardiovascular magnetic resonance. *J Cardiovasc Magn Reson*. 2007;9(6):899–906.
12. Kon MW, Myerson SG, Moat NE, Pennell DJ. Quantification of regurgitant fraction in mitral regurgitation by cardiovascular magnetic resonance: comparison of techniques. *J Heart Valve Dis*. 2004;13(4):600–607.
13. Dziadzko V, Clavel M, Dziadzko M, et al. Outcome and undertreatment of mitral regurgitation: a community cohort study. *Lancet*. 2018;391(10124):960–969.
14. Iung B, Vahanian A. Epidemiology of valvular heart disease in the adult. *Nat Rev Cardiol*. 2011;8(3):162–172.
15. Grande-Allen KJ, Barber JE, Klatka KM, et al. Mitral valve stiffening in end-stage heart failure: evidence of an organic contribution to functional mitral regurgitation. *J Thorac Cardiovasc Surg*. 2005;130(3):783–790.
16. Marsit O, Clavel M, Côté-Laroche C, et al. Attenuated mitral leaflet enlargement contributes to functional mitral regurgitation after myocardial infarction. *J Am Coll Cardiol*. 2020;75(4):395–405.
17. Mesi O, Gad MM, Crane AD, et al. Severe atrial functional mitral regurgitation: clinical and echocardiographic characteristics, management and outcomes. *Cardiovasc Imaging*. 2021;14(4):797–808.
18. Silbiger JJ. Mechanistic insights into atrial functional mitral regurgitation: far more complicated than just left atrial remodeling. *Echocardiography*. 2019;36(1):164–169.
19. Zoghbi WA, Levine RA, Flachskampf F, et al. Atrial functional mitral regurgitation: a JACC: cardiovascular imaging expert panel viewpoint. *Cardiovasc Imaging*. 2022;15(11):1870–1882.
20. Stork A, Franzen O, Ruschewski H, et al. Assessment of functional anatomy of the mitral valve in patients with mitral regurgitation with cine magnetic resonance imaging: comparison with transesophageal echocardiography and surgical results. *Eur Radiol*. 2007;17:3189–3198.
21. Buchner S, Debl K, Poschenrieder F, et al. Cardiovascular magnetic resonance for direct assessment of anatomic regurgitant orifice in mitral regurgitation. *Circ: Cardiovasc Imaging*. 2008;1(2):148–155.
22. Gelfand EV, Hughes S, Hauser TH, et al. Severity of mitral and aortic regurgitation as assessed by cardiovascular magnetic resonance: optimizing correlation with Doppler echocardiography. *J Cardiovasc Magn Reson*. 2006;8(3):503.
23. Uretsky S, Animashaun IB, Sakul S, et al. American society of echocardiography algorithm for degenerative mitral regurgitation: comparison with CMR. *Cardiovasc Imaging*. 2022;15(5):747–760.
24. Myerson SG, D'arcy J, Christiansen JP, et al. Determination of clinical outcome in mitral regurgitation with cardiovascular magnetic resonance quantification. *Circulation*. 2019;133(23):2287.
25. Penicka M, Vecera J, Mirica DC, Kotrc M, Kockova R, Van Camp G. Prognostic implications of magnetic resonance–derived quantification in asymptomatic patients with organic mitral regurgitation. *Circulation*. 2018;137(13):1349.
26. Carpentier A. Cardiac valve surgery—the "French correction." *J Thorac Cardiovasc Surg*. 1983;86(3):323–337.
27. Goffinet C, Kersten V, Pouleur A, et al. Comprehensive assessment of the severity and mechanism of aortic regurgitation using multidetector CT and MR. *Eur Radiol*. 2010;20:326–336.
28. Firth BG, Dehmer GJ, Nicod P, et al. Effect of increasing heart rate in patients with aortic regurgitation: effect of incremental atrial pacing on scintigraphic, hemodynamic and thermodilution measurements. *Am J Cardiol*. 1982 June;49(8):1860–1867.
29. Myerson SG, D'arcy J, Mohiaddin R, et al. Aortic regurgitation quantification using cardiovascular magnetic resonance. *Circulation*. 2012;126(12):1452.
30. Kammerlander AA, Wiesinger M, Duca F, et al. Diagnostic and prognostic utility of cardiac magnetic resonance imaging in aortic regurgitation. *JACC: Cardiovasc Imaging*. 2019;12(8):1474.
31. Vejpongsa P, Xu J, Quinones MA, Shah DJ, Zoghbi WA. Differences in cardiac remodeling in left-sided valvular regurgitation. *JACC: Cardiovasc Imaging*. 2022;15(10):1730.
32. Malahfji M, Crudo V, Kaolawanich Y, et al. Influence of cardiac remodeling on clinical outcomes in patients with aortic regurgitation. *J Am Coll Cardiol*. 2023;81(19):1885–1898.
33. Nishimura RA, Otto CM, Bonow RO, et al. 2014 AHA/ACC guideline for the management of patients with valvular heart disease: a report of the American college of cardiology/American heart association task force on practice guidelines. *Circulation*. 2014;129(23):e521–e643.
34. Guta AC, El-Tallawi KC, Nguyen DT, et al. Prevalence and clinical implications of tricuspid valve prolapse based on magnetic resonance diagnostic criteria. *J Am Coll Cardiol*. 2023;81(9):882.
35. Medvedofsky D, Jiménez JL, Addetia K, et al. Multi-parametric quantification of tricuspid regurgitation using cardiovascular magnetic resonance: a comparison to echocardiography. *Eur J Radiol*. 2017;86:213–220.
36. Zhan Y, Debs D, Khan MA, et al. Natural history of functional tricuspid regurgitation quantified by cardiovascular magnetic resonance. *J Am Coll Cardiol*. 2020;76(11):1291.
37. Hahn RT, Meduri CU, Davidson CJ, et al. Early feasibility study of a transcatheter tricuspid valve annuloplasty: SCOUT trial 30-day results. *J Am Coll Cardiol*. 2017;69(14):1795–1806.
38. Go YY, Dulgheru R, Lancellotti P. The conundrum of tricuspid regurgitation grading. *Front Cardiovasc Med*. 2018;5:164.
39. Rebergen SA, Chin JG, Ottenkamp J, Van der Wall EE, De Roos A. Pulmonary regurgitation in the late postoperative follow-up of tetralogy of Fallot. Volumetric quantitation by nuclear magnetic resonance velocity mapping. *Circulation*. 1993;88(5):2257–2266.
40. Chaturvedi RR, Redington AN. Pulmonary regurgitation in congenital heart disease. *Heart*. 2007;93(7):880–889.
41. Gatzoulis MA, Balaji S, Webber SA, et al. Risk factors for arrhythmia and sudden cardiac death late after repair of tetralogy of Fallot: a multicentre study. *Lancet*. 2000;356(9234):975–981.
42. Shinebourne EA, Babu-Narayan SV, Carvalho JS. Tetralogy of Fallot: from fetus to adult. *Heart*. 2006;92(9):1353–1359.
43. Kilner PJ, Balossino R, Dubini G, et al. Pulmonary regurgitation: the effects of varying pulmonary artery compliance, and of increased resistance proximal or distal to the compliance. *Int J Cardiol*. 2009;133(2):157–166.
44. Reant P, Lederlin M, Lafitte S, et al. Absolute assessment of aortic valve stenosis by planimetry using cardiovascular magnetic resonance imaging: comparison with transoesophageal echocardiography, transthoracic echocardiography, and cardiac catheterisation. *Eur J Radiol*. 2006;59(2):276–283.
45. Debl K, Djavidani B, Seitz J, et al. Planimetry of aortic valve area in aortic stenosis by magnetic resonance imaging. *Invest Radiol*. 2005;40(10):631–636.
46. Kupfahl C, Honold M, Meinhardt G, et al. Evaluation of aortic stenosis by cardiovascular magnetic resonance imaging: comparison with established routine clinical techniques. *Heart*. 2004;90(8):893.
47. John AS, Dill T, Brandt RR, et al. Magnetic resonance to assess the aortic valve area in aortic stenosis: how does it compare to current diagnostic standards? *J Am Coll Cardiol*. 2003;42(3):519–526.
48. Woldendorp K, Bannon PG, Grieve SM. Evaluation of aortic stenosis using cardiovascular magnetic resonance: a systematic review & meta-analysis. *J Cardiovasc Magn Reson*. 2020;22:1–9.
49. Garcia J, Kadem L, Larose E, Clavel M, Pibarot P. Comparison between cardiovascular magnetic resonance and transthoracic Doppler echocardiography for the estimation of effective orifice area in aortic stenosis. *J Cardiovasc Magn Reson*. 2011;13:1–9.
50. Smith CR, Leon MB, Mack MJ, et al. Transcatheter versus surgical aortic-valve replacement in high-risk patients. *N Engl J Med*. 2011;364(23):2187–2198.
51. Carabello BA. Transcatheter aortic-valve implantation for aortic stenosis in patients who cannot undergo surgery. *Curr Cardiol Rep*. 2011;13:173–174.
52. Zamorano JL, Gonçalves A, Lang R. Imaging to select and guide transcatheter aortic valve implantation. *Eur Heart J*. 2014;35(24):1578–1587.
53. Dweck MR, Joshi S, Murigu T, et al. Midwall fibrosis is an independent predictor of mortality in patients with aortic stenosis. *J Am Coll Cardiol*. 2011;58(12):1271.
54. Barone-Rochette G, Piérard S, De Meester de Ravenstein C, et al. Prognostic significance of LGE by CMR in aortic stenosis patients undergoing valve replacement. *J Am Coll Cardiol*. 2014;64(2):144–154.
55. Reindl M, Lechner I, Holzknecht M, et al. Cardiac magnetic resonance imaging versus computed tomography to guide transcatheter aortic valve replacement: a randomized, open-label, noninferiority trial. *Circulation*. 2023;148(16):1220–1230.
56. Klug G, Reinstadler S, Troger F, et al. Cardiac magnetic resonance imaging versus computed tomography to guide transcatheter aortic valve replacement: study protocol for a randomized trial (TAVR-CMR). *Trials*. 2022;23(1):726.
57. Mehdipoor G, Chen S, Chatterjee S, et al. Cardiac structural changes after transcatheter aortic valve replacement: systematic review and meta-analysis of cardiovascular magnetic resonance studies. *J Cardiovasc Magn Reson*. 2020;22:1–10.
58. Zoghbi WA, Asch FM, Bruce C, et al. Guidelines for the evaluation of valvular regurgitation after percutaneous valve repair or replacement. *J Am Soc of Echocardiogr*. 2019;32(4):431.
59. Ribeiro HB, Orwat S, Hayek SS, et al. Cardiovascular magnetic resonance to evaluate aortic regurgitation after transcatheter aortic valve replacement. *J Am Coll Cardiol*. 2016;68(6):577–585.
60. Kilner PJ, Sievers B, Meyer GP, Yen Ho S. Double-chambered right ventricle or sub-infundibular stenosis assessed by cardiovascular magnetic resonance. *J Cardiovasc Magn Reson*. 2002;4(3):373–379.
61. Helvacioglu F, Yildirimturk O, Duran C, et al. The evaluation of mitral valve stenosis: comparison of transthoracic echocardiography and cardiac magnetic resonance. *Eur Heart J–Cardiovasc Imaging*. 2014;15(2):164–169.
62. Uygur B, Celik O, Ustabasioglu FE, Akinci O, Erturk M. Three-dimensional transesophageal echocardiography vs cardiac magnetic resonance in the assessment of planimetric mitral valve area in rheumatic mitral stenosis. *Echocardiography*. 2018;35(10):1621–1625.
63. Pandian NG, Kim JK, Arias-Godinez JA, et al. Recommendations for the use of echocardiography in the evaluation of rheumatic heart disease: a report from the American society of echocardiography. *J Am Soc Echocardiogr*. 2023;36(1):3–28.
64. Lin SJ, Brown PA, Watkins MP, et al. Quantification of stenotic mitral valve area with magnetic resonance imaging and comparison with Doppler ultrasound. *J Am Coll Cardiol*. 2004;44(1):133–137.
65. Mohiaddin RH, Amanuma M, Kilner PJ, Pennell DJ, Manzara C, Longmore DB. MR phase-shift velocity mapping of mitral and pulmonary venous flow. *J Comput Assist Tomogr*. 1991;15(2):237–243.
66. Shah DJ, El-Tallawi KC. Not all flails are created equal. *J Am Coll Cardiol*. 2021;78(25):2547–2549.

67. El-Tallawi KC, Kitkungvan D, Xu J, et al. Resolving the disproportionate left ventricular enlargement in mitral valve prolapse due to Barlow disease: insights from cardiovascular magnetic resonance. *Cardiovasc Imaging*. 2021;14(3):573–584.
68. Moghari MH, Komarlu R, Annese D, Geva T, Powell AJ. Free-breathing steady-state free precession cine cardiac magnetic resonance with respiratory navigator gating. *Magn Reson Med*. 2015;73(4):1555–1561.
69. Zhuang B, Yu S, Feng Z, et al. Left ventricular strain derived from cardiac magnetic resonance can predict outcomes of pulmonary valve replacement in patients with repaired tetralogy of Fallot. *Front Cardiovasc Med*. 2022;9:917026.
70. Pelc NJ, Bernstein MA, Shimakawa A, Glover GH. Encoding strategies for three-direction phase-contrast MR imaging of flow. *J Magn Reson Imaging*. 1991;1(4):405–413.
71. Wigström L, Sjöqvist L, Wranne B. Temporally resolved 3D phase-contrast imaging. *Magn Reson Med*. 1996;36(5):800–803.
72. Dyverfeldt P, Bissell M, Barker AJ, et al. 4D flow cardiovascular magnetic resonance consensus statement. *J Cardiovasc Magn Reson*. 2015;17(1):1–19.
73. Lorenz R, Bock J, Barker AJ, et al. 4D flow magnetic resonance imaging in bicuspid aortic valve disease demonstrates altered distribution of aortic blood flow helicity. *Magn Reson Med*. 2014;71(4):1542–1553.

36 Cardiac Remodeling and Implications of Valvular Heart Disease

MAAN MALAHFJI, K. CARLOS EL-TALLAWI, AND DIPAN J. SHAH

INTRODUCTION

Cardiac magnetic resonance (CMR) is the gold standard for the evaluation of ventricular volumes, mass, and ejection fraction, which are the principal parameters used to characterize and quantify ventricular remodeling related to valvular heart disease (VHD). The advantages of CMR in cardiac remodeling assessment stem from its ability to image the heart in all imaging planes, accurate and reproducible calculation of ventricular volumes and mass, and reliable assessment of flow volumes and velocities. Tissue characterization techniques have led to important insights into the cellular and extracellular remodeling that occurs with VHD. In this chapter, we review the principles of cardiac remodeling assessment in VHD using CMR and outline relevant CMR studies that furthered our understanding of cardiac cavity and tissue remodeling in VHD.

EVALUATION OF CARDIAC REMODELING

The hemodynamic load of VHD can be characterized as an increase in preload, afterload, or both. Compensatory morphologic changes in the left ventricle (LV) are typically characterized by LV dilatation, increased LV mass, and geometric shape remodeling. Ventricular remodeling has been considered to be initially adaptive to compensate for increased wall stress, and to later transition to "maladaptive" remodeling after a varied period of time. The traditional patterns of increased LV mass include concentric hypertrophy and eccentric hypertrophy. In addition, patterns of concentric remodeling (increased mass to volume ratio) and preserved normal geometry are also observed (dilatation with normal indexed LV mass). Typically, left-sided VHD is characterized by increased afterload in aortic stenosis (AS), increased preload in mitral regurgitation (MR), and combined increase in afterload and preload in aortic regurgitation (AR).[1] Analogous right ventricular (RV) characterizations were observed with pulmonic stenosis (PS), pulmonic regurgitation (PR), and tricuspid regurgitation (TR). Isolated stenosis of the atrioventricular valves (mitral stenosis [MS] and tricuspid stenosis [TS]) does not lead to significant ventricular remodeling and its burden is reflected primarily in the atria in the early stages of disease, while pulmonary valve disease and associated remodeling most often occur in the context of congenital heart disease. The remodeling changes in patients with mixed or multiple VHD lesions have not been as well characterized as isolated VHD, and patients usually incur combined effects of the two or more valve lesions they have. For the purposes of reviewing the CMR evaluation of cardiac remodeling in VHD, we will focus the discussion in this chapter on AS, AR, MR, and TR.

Evaluation of cardiac remodeling has traditionally relied on echocardiography. Although echocardiography remains the first-line study to evaluate VHD, it is not without limitations. The use of LV dimensions and wall thickness to quantify remodeling may not fully reflect the extent and pattern of LV remodeling.[2,3] Two-dimensional echocardiographic evaluation of LV volumes and mass requires geometric assumptions that may be particularly jeopardized in VHD.[4,5] Additionally, right ventricular assessment using echocardiography can also be fraught by increased interobserver and intraobserver variability.[2] Suboptimal echocardiographic windows, the presence of mixed valve lesions, and limited imaging planes can also limit the reliability of echocardiographic quantitation of VHD severity and related cardiac remodeling. The use of 3D echocardiography eliminates the need for geometric assumptions, but LV volumes by 3D assessment are generally underestimated compared with CMR or cardiac computed tomography.[6,7]

The use of CMR circumvents many of the challenges faced by echocardiography. Cardiac magnetic resonance has become the noninvasive gold standard in evaluating ventricular volumes, mass, and ejection fraction, with excellent accuracy against reference standards including pathologic specimens.[8] As a result, CMR is well positioned to study the patterns and extent of cardiac remodeling in VHD and their prognostic implications. In addition, tissue characterization with CMR using techniques such as late gadolinium enhancement (LGE) and T1 mapping has led to new insights into the myocardial tissue alterations in VHD, which previously were evaluated only on selective biopsy samples at the time of surgery. Reference values for ventricular volumes, mass, and ejection fraction by CMR are well established and should be used to determine the presence and extent of ventricular remodeling.[9] In addition, age- and sex-specific reference ranges should be incorporated into the assessment. It should be noted that ventricular and atrial volumes are underestimated on echocardiography compared to CMR, and caution should be applied not to use echocardiographic reference values to evaluate ventricular and atrial parameters on CMR studies. Left ventricular end-diastolic and end-systolic diameters are measured on CMR as well, traditionally using the three-chamber view at the mitral leaflet tips, but these approaches can suffer from increased interobserver and intraobserver variability and may not be reflective of the

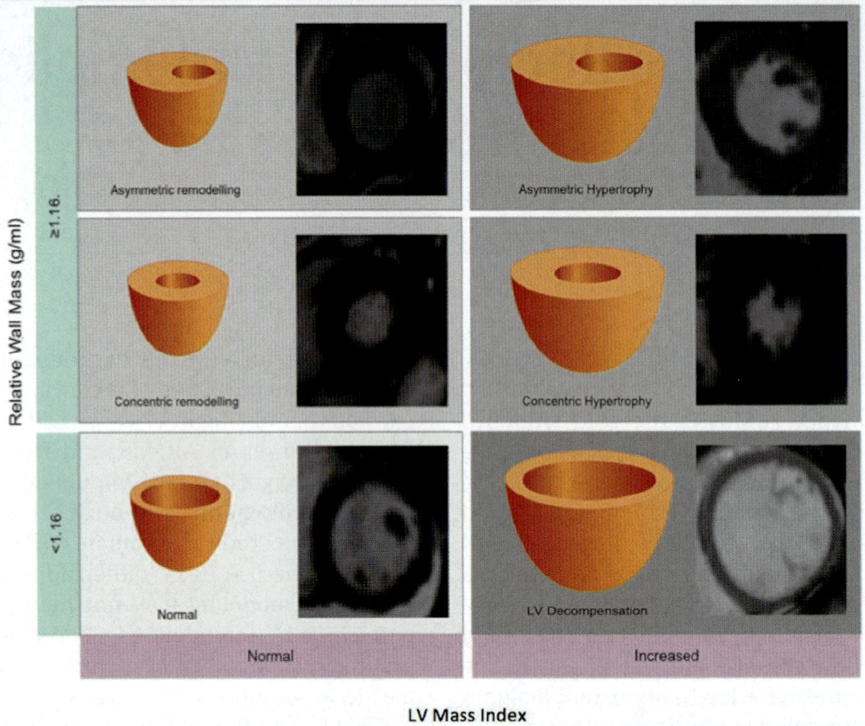

	LV Mass Index	Indexed LVEDV	M/V	Asymmetric wall thickening	Ejection Fraction
Normal	=	=	=	✖	=
Concentric Remodeling	=	↓	↑	✖	=/↑
Asymmetric Remodeling	=	↓	↑	✔	=/↑
Concentric Hypertrophy	↑	=	↑	✖	=/↓
Asymmetric Hypertrophy	↑	=	↑	✔	=/↓
LV Decompensation	↑	↑	=	✖	↓

FIG. 36.1 Overview of left ventricular (*LV*) remodeling patterns in aortic stenosis. Determination of remodeling pattern relies first on evaluating the LV mass index and mass to volume (*M/V*) ratio (relative wall mass). (Figure available at: https://jcmr-online.biomedcentral.com/articles/10.1186/1532-429X-14-50/figures/1.)

extent of ventricular dilatation. This can be the case particularly in AR and MR cases with a spherical-shaped ventricle, in which the midventricular diameter is significantly larger than the basal diameter. Due to these limitations, CMR approaches for assessing ventricular dilation should be based upon measurement of ventricular volumes as opposed to linear dimensions.

AORTIC STENOSIS

Assessment of Cardiac Remodeling by Cardiac Magnetic Resonance

AS is considered the classic lesion of LV pressure overload. With progressive narrowing of the aortic valve, LV hypertrophy ensues to a varied degree and pattern. The increased LV wall thickness and mass are considered to be an initial adaptive mechanism to normalize wall stress according to the Laplace equation, and patients will remain asymptomatic for a variable period. Maladaptive changes also occur, including inappropriate hypertrophy, fibrosis, dilatation, and contractile impairment. Eventually, decompensation occurs with development of symptoms and/or overt LV dysfunction.

CMR studies highlight the significant variability in the extent and pattern of LV hypertrophy in AS. In one study of 91 patients with isolated moderate or severe AS and no coronary artery disease (CAD), LV hypertrophy was investigated using indexed LV mass index, indexed LV volumes, and the LV mass/volume ratio (Fig. 36.1).[10] The LV mass/volume ratio (M/V) is calculated by dividing the left ventricular mass by the LV end diastolic volume. Conceptually, it is similar to the relative wall thickness formula on echocardiography, but it is superior as it uses direct planimetry of the LV mass without geometric assumptions, as is the case with echocardiography. Using healthy volunteer data,

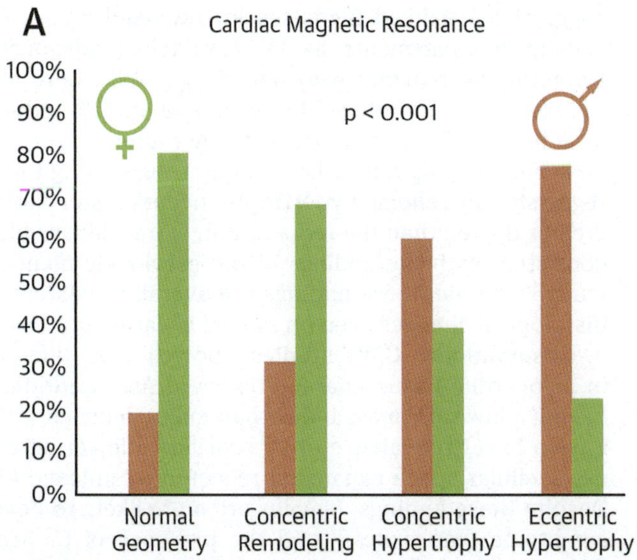

FIG. 36.2 Overview of cardiac remodeling patterns by sex in patients with aortic stenosis. Sex differences in the patterns of remodeling in males (*green bars*) vs. females (*red bars*) were demonstrated by cardiac magnetic resonance but not by echocardiography. Panel A shows findings of cardiac remodeling patterns demonsrated on CMR. Panel B shows findings of remodeling demonstrated on echocardiography. (Available at: https://www.sciencedirect.com/science/article/pii/S1936878X17309075?via%3Dihub.)

the abnormal value for the M/V ratio was found to be 1.16. Patients with normal indexed LV mass but abnormal M/V ratio would be categorized as having concentric remodeling. Six patterns of LV adaptation were observed: normal ventricular geometry (12%), concentric remodeling (12%), asymmetric remodeling (12%), concentric hypertrophy (37%), asymmetric hypertrophy (16%), and LV decompensation (11%). The severity of AS was unrelated to the degree and pattern of LV hypertrophy, albeit the study was relatively small in sample size. A follow-up study from the same group also showed that the asymmetric wall-thickening pattern (regional wall thickening ≥13 mm and >1.5-fold the thickness of the opposing myocardial segment) to be associated with increased myocardial injury, left ventricular decompensation, and adverse events.[11]

Sex differences have also been described in AS-related cardiac remodeling. In a study of 168 patients (55% male, similar AS severity between males and females),[12] CMR demonstrated sex differences in LV remodeling that were not apparent using echocardiography. Normal geometry (82% female) and concentric remodeling (60% female) dominated in females, while concentric hypertrophy (71% male) and eccentric hypertrophy (76% male) dominated in males (Fig. 36.2). Males also had a higher prevalence of LV decompensation and higher levels of myocardial injury biomarkers (high-sensitivity troponin T and N-terminal pro-brain natriuretic peptide). In a larger multicenter prospective study of 674 patients with severe AS (425 males and 249 females), males also demonstrated more advanced cardiac remodeling than females for a similar AS severity.[13] There are also potential sex differences in the prevalence and extent of myocardial fibrosis related to AS, which are further described below. Overall, the pattern of LV hypertrophy should be noted in AS patients, incorporating indexed LV mass, M/V ratio, and ventricular volumes. The correlation between AS severity and indexed LV mass is rather modest and appears to predominate in males only. Whether patterns of LV remodeling should be incorporated into decision making for intervention beyond current parameters is largely unknown and warrants further study.

Assessment of Subclinical Ventricular Dysfunction in Aortic Stenosis

Beyond LV ejection fraction, deformation analysis and strain parameters can be evaluated in AS patients to detect LV contractile impairment. The most studied parameter is global longitudinal strain (GLS) using speckle-tracking echocardiography. Longitudinal LV function is driven primarily by the subendocardial layer of fibers and is the most sensitive for detecting myocardial disease. Impaired GLS can be present in asymptomatic AS patients with preserved LV ejection fraction, which is associated with an increased risk of adverse outcomes and need for intervention.[14] Myocardial tagging techniques with CMR can evaluate LV strain parameters in the longitudinal, radial, and circumferential direction, but they require specialized acquisitions and postprocessing, which may be time consuming. Feature-tracking CMR now allows the evaluation of global and regional strain values using cine sequences, without the need for additional acquisitions.[15] Global longitudinal strain on CMR was shown to correlate with LV mass regression after surgery.[16,17] There is also a moderate correlation between GLS and measures that can infer diffuse fibrosis on CMR (indexed extracellular volume) as well as LV scar, which are further detailed below.[18]

Tissue Characteristics by Cardiac Magnetic Resonance in Aortic Stenosis

AS is known to lead to myocardial histological changes beyond cellular hypertrophy. Myocardial fibrosis in AS has been shown in LV biopsy samples at the time of surgery, and the occurrence of fibrosis and myocyte death has been linked to the progression to heart failure in AS.[19] Myocardial replacement fibrosis or scar can be detected by the LGE technique on CMR, and its usual patterns include midwall scar in the interventricular septum, patchy noncoronary distribution scar, and subendocardial scar. The prevalence and extent of LV scar in AS has varied among published reports, and has been seen in about a third to more than half of significant AS patients.[20–23] Left ventricular scar has universally been found to be irreversible after aortic valve replacement, and to be associated with adverse outcomes.[20–22,24,25] In a large multicenter prospective study (674 patients with severe AS), LV scar was present in 51% of patients (18% infarct pattern, 33% noninfarct pattern). The presence and extent of LV scar was independently associated with overall mortality and cardiovascular death, even after aortic valve replacement (AVR).[20] The extent of LV scar was inversely associated with LV functional improvement after AVR. A randomized clinical trial is ongoing to evaluate early AVR vs routine care in asymptomatic severe AS patients with LGE.[26]

Extracellular volume fraction (ECV) is derived from T1 mapping before and after administration of gadolinium contrast (which is extracellular). It measures the percent of the myocardium that is extracellular compartment, thus inferring interstitial fibrosis not detected by the LGE technique. The ECV fraction and planimetered LV end-diastolic volume can be used to derive the absolute volume of the cellular and extracellular compartments. The indexed ECV or "indexed matrix volume" can be calculated as (indexed ECV = ECV × indexed LV end-diastolic myocardial volume), and the cellular compartment volume can be derived as well (cell volume = indexed LV end-diastolic myocardial volume × [1 − ECV]). Both ECV fraction and indexed ECV measures have demonstrated good correlation with diffuse fibrosis on biopsy, and were shown to be associated with mortality and adverse remodeling in AS, independent of LV scar assessment (Fig. 36.3).[27–30]

While LV scar is irreversible after surgery, ECV fraction and indexed ECV can change postoperatively. A CMR study of 181 severe AS patients incorporated pre and postoperative comprehensive assessments and confirmed that LGE does not resolve after AVR, while measures of interstitial fibrosis and the cellular volume regress.[25] These changes were accompanied by improvement in diastolic function, N-terminal pro–B-type natriuretic peptide, 6-min walk test results, and New York Heart Association functional class. However, changes in indexed ECV suggest that cellular hypertrophy regressed to a greater degree by 1 year after AVR compared to the inferred interstitial fibrosis. As a result, ECV fraction was found to increase postoperatively (Fig. 36.4).

Another study evaluated the natural history of cardiac cavity and tissue remodeling in AS.[31] The study included the spectrum of AS severity and incorporated serial imaging with CMR and echocardiography. In asymptomatic patients (43% mild, 34% moderate, and 23% severe AS), significant increases in peak aortic-jet velocity, indexed LV mass, indexed ECV, and LV scar burden mass were observed after 2.1 ± 0.7 years, with the most rapid progression in those with the most severe stenosis. Patients with baseline LGE demonstrated particularly rapid increases in scar burden (78% increase in LGE mass per year). The indexed ECV increased over time, suggesting progressive expansion of the extracellular compartment and possible increases in diffuse interstitial fibrosis. The ECV fraction did not demonstrate any evidence of progression, suggesting balanced increases in the cellular and extracellular compartments as LV remodeling advances. In symptomatic patients who underwent AVR, there was a 19% reduction in indexed LV mass and an 11% reduction in indexed ECV volume 0.9 ± 0.3 years after surgery, with an accompanying rise in ECV fraction, suggesting that the regression in cellular hypertrophy occurs faster and to a greater degree than the reduction in extracellular volume, consistent with the findings of the previously mentioned study.[25] Of note, these findings are overall consistent with histological changes seen on biopsy in earlier studies.[32]

Observational CMR studies showed sex differences in myocardial tissue characteristics in AS. In addition to having a lower LV mass index than males, females with AS have a lower prevalence of LV scar and a lower extent of extracellular space expansion reflected by indexed ECV.[12] Despite these findings, females are more likely to develop symptoms than males,[33] and the presence of LV scar is associated with poor outcomes in females as well.

Machine learning approaches in the CMR evaluation of AS have also been used. In a multinational study of severe AS patients undergoing AVR, a machine learning model incorporating clinical and CMR variables (29 total variables) showed that the four most predictive CMR markers of post-AVR death were ECV fraction, LV scar, indexed left ventricular end-diastolic volume (iLVEDV), and right ventricular ejection fraction (RVEF).[24] The addition of CMR variables improved the predictability of outcomes, and the findings were validated in an external cohort. Finally, cardiac amyloidosis can coexist with AS, particularly in older adults,[34] and evaluation of CMR tissue characteristics is critical to screen for amyloidosis in AS patients.

In conclusion, CMR studies have led to important and novel findings with regard to cavity and tissue remodeling assessment of AS. There is significant heterogeneity in the extent and pattern of LV remodeling, and the presence of adverse remodeling markers by CMR such as LGE and ECV have a strong and independent association with outcomes in AS. Whether CMR-guided treatment of AS, particularly based on LV scar, can improve patient outcomes will be evaluated in ongoing randomized clinical trials.[26]

AORTIC REGURGITATION

Assessment of Cardiac Cavity Remodeling in Aortic Regurgitation

AR results in a combined LV pressure and volume overload state. The natural history of AR has been characterized by progressive LV dilatation and hypertrophy in response to the hemodynamic load on the ventricle, with increased wall stress and eventual manifestation of LV dysfunction and symptoms.[35–37] CMR can evaluate the morphology of the aortic valve and the mechanism of AR can often be delineated, although highly mobile small structures such as vegetations may not be well visualized or missed. High-resolution steady-state free precession sequences can be incorporated into the scanning protocol of AR patients to further evaluate the aortic valve morphology and mechanism of AR using a small field of view and thin slices.

FIGURE 2 iECV as a Marker of Extracellular Expansion in the Myocardium

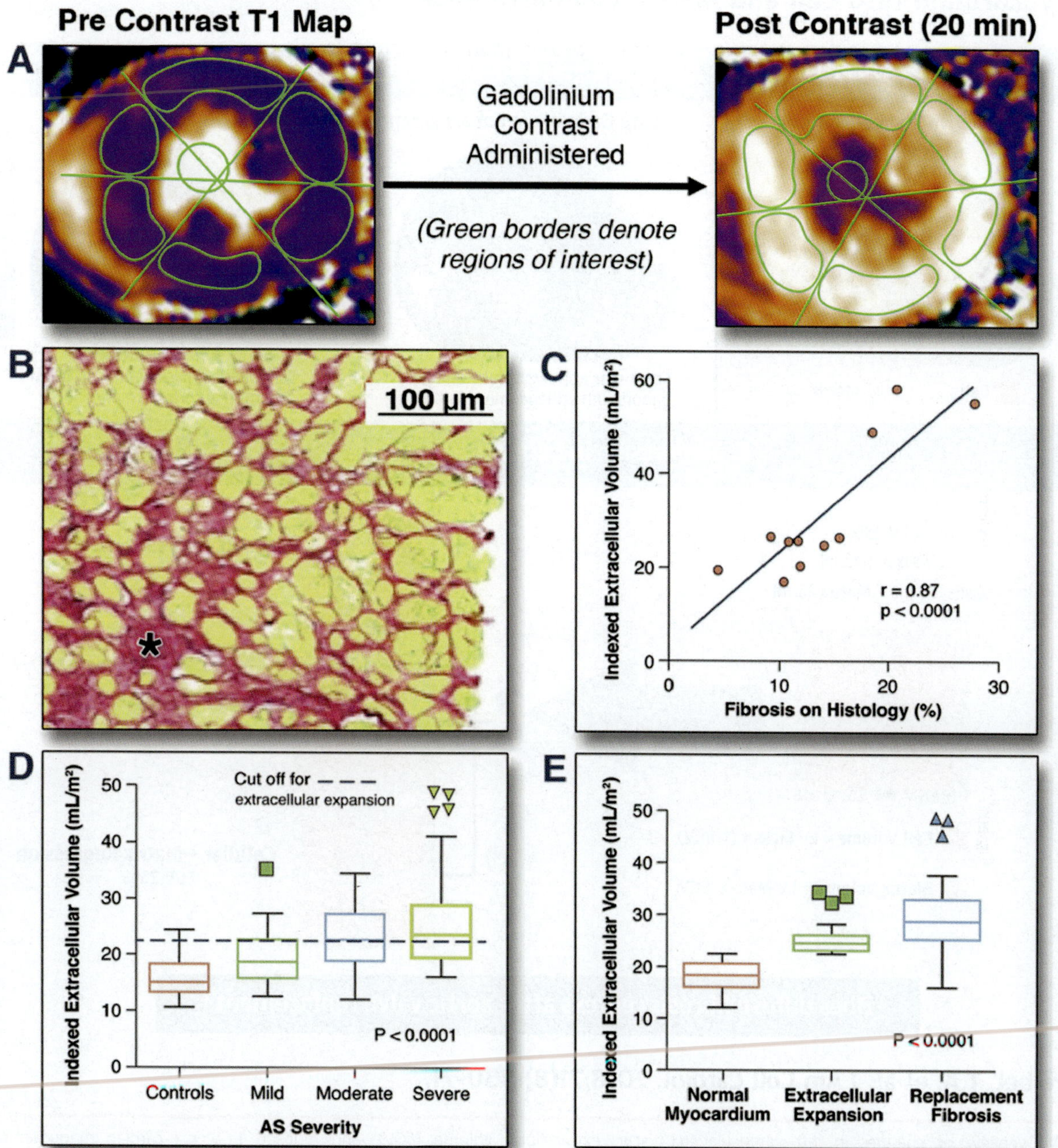

(A) Regions of interest manually drawn onto native and post-contrast T1 maps are used to calculate indexed extracellular volume (iECV). **(B)** Histology from a patient with aortic stenosis (AS) with areas of diffuse fibrosis stained with picrosirus red. **(C)** Excellent correlation between iECV and diffuse myocardial fibrosis on histology. **(D)** iECV provided good discrimination between disease states. **(E)** iECV values were higher in patients with replacement fibrosis than patients with normal myocardium or extracellular expansion.

FIG. 36.3 Overview of indexed extracellular volume assessment in aortic stenosis (*AS*) by cardiac magnetic resonance (A), its histologic correlates (B, C), relationship against AS severity (D), and progressive increases in normal myocardium, intermediate stages of extracellular expansion, and those with left ventricular scar (E). (Available at: https://www.sciencedirect.com/science/article/pii/S1936878X16309020?via%3Dihub.)

Measures of AR severity include the regurgitant volume (RVol) and regurgitant fraction (RF), which are calculated from phase-contrast sequences. Other indirect and semi-quantitative measures include the presence of diastolic flow reversal in the descending aorta, the extent of LV dilatation in chronic AR, and the anatomic regurgitant orifice area.[38,39] Evaluation of AR severity by CMR is highly reproducible and associated with clinical outcomes and the need for AVR.[40–45] In addition, CMR measurement of RVol does not require geometric assumptions and is more reproducible than echocardiographic quantitation.[45] Given the previously outlined strengths of CMR in myocardial

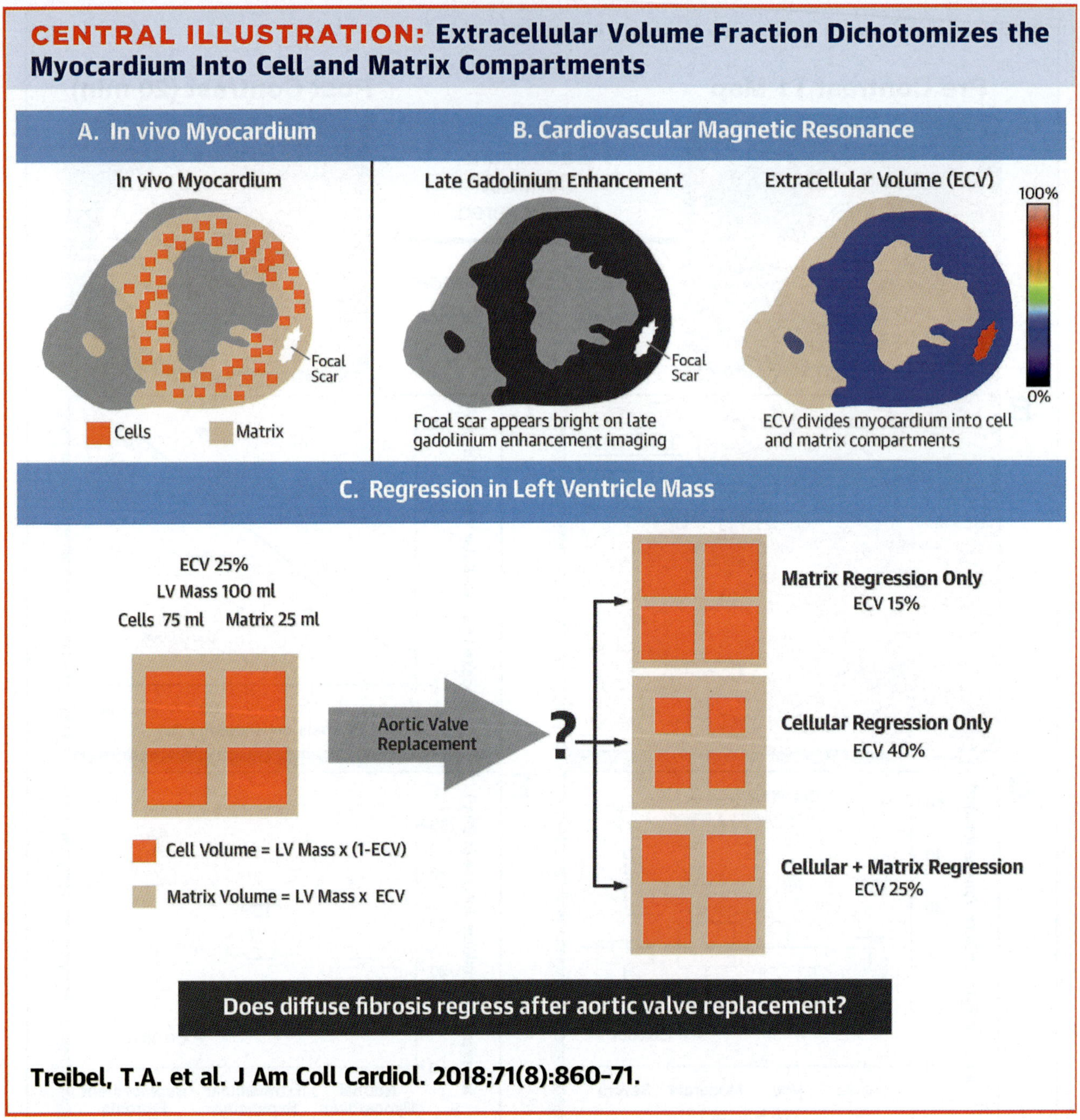

FIG. 36.4 Overview of changes in left ventricular (*LV*) scar, extracellular volume (*ECV*), and indexed ECV on cardiac magnetic resonance after aortic valve replacement (AVR) for aortic stenosis. LV scar does not regress after AVR. The indexed ECV and derived volumes of the cellular and extracellular compartments regress at different rates, leading to apparent increase in ECV fraction (%) after AVR. (Available at: https://www.sciencedirect.com/science/article/pii/S0735109717420377?via%3Dihub.)

remodeling assessment, it is well suited for a comprehensive evaluation of AR and for use in serial monitoring of patients to detect progressive changes in LV volume and function. It should be noted that LV diameters can particularly underestimate the extent of LV dilatation as the ventricle enlarges.[3] This is of particular importance in AR patients, who often develop severe LV dilatation prior to the onset of symptoms, and where the extent of LV dilatation beyond certain thresholds is an indication for intervention.

There is a strong and linear relationship between the extent of LV dilatation and severity of chronic AR. The first CMR study to evaluate this relationship included 34 isolated AR patients and 23 MR patients.[46] In both lesions, ventricular volumes were shown to have a stronger correlation with RVol than linear dimensions, which had a poor correlation with regurgitation severity. AR led to greater LV enlargement and hypertrophy than MR for the same regurgitation severity. These findings were corroborated in other CMR studies.[44,47] In a study of 240 isolated AR patients and 424 isolated primary MR patients covering the spectrum of regurgitation severity, similar findings were observed for iLVEDV, indexed left ventricular end-systolic volume (iLVESV), and indexed LV mass. There was a proportional increase in each parameter with increasing regurgitation severity, and AR was associated with greater

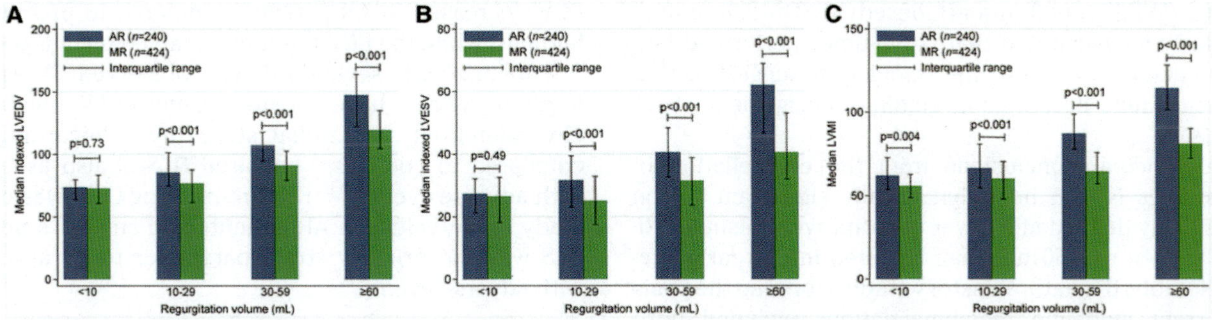

FIG. 36.5 Differences in indexed left ventricular end-diastolic volume (Panel A), indexed left ventricular end-systolic volume (Panel B), and indexed LV mass (Panel C) between aortic regurgitation (*AR*) and mitral regurgitation (*MR*) patients at increasing degrees of regurgitation. (Available at: https://www.ahajournals.org/doi/10.1161/CIRCIMAGING.122.014684.)

LV dilatation and hypertrophy than MR (Fig. 36.5). In addition, patterns of LV remodeling were defined according to indexed LV mass and the LV M/V ratio (Fig. 36.6), similar to prior AS studies.

AR and MR are traditionally considered to cause eccentric hypertrophy, but the pattern of "myocardial thinning" is also observed in MR, causing a thin, enlarged, and compliant ventricle.[1] The myocardial thinning pattern in the aforementioned study[47] was defined based on a low M/V ratio (lower than 2 standard deviations below normal volunteer mean M/V ratio data) and normal indexed mass. In patients with ≥moderate AR or MR, AR patients had a higher prevalence of eccentric hypertrophy (58.3% vs. 17.5% in MR), whereas MR patients most often had normal geometry (56.7%), followed by the myocardial thinning phenotype (18.4%). The patterns of eccentric hypertrophy and myocardial thinning were more common in symptomatic AR and MR patients as well. Whether treatment decisions and timing need to incorporate the LV remodeling patterns warrants further study.

ASSESSMENT OF AORTIC REGURGITATION SEVERITY BY CARDIAC MAGNETIC RESONANCE AND SEX DIFFERENCES IN CARDIAC REMODELING

The degree of regurgitant volume, fraction, and LV remodeling that constitute hemodynamically significant AR has been a focus of recent research. Earlier studies that investigated regurgitation severity thresholds in AR patients—and formed the basis for the guidelines[48]—had a relatively small sample size and were based on angiographic assessment. In addition, evidence from contemporary outcome studies has raised concern over the optimal timing for surgical intervention in patients with chronic AR and that current guideline thresholds may lead to surgery referrals later than ideal.[49–51]

Recent studies using CMR quantitation suggest that the quantitative thresholds for hemodynamically significant AR may be lower than in the current guidelines,[40,41,43,52–54] and may be different than MR thresholds. A prospective CMR study[40] found an RF >33% to be associated with developing indications for aortic valve surgery. In another study that included 418 isolated AR patients, an RF threshold of >35% had high sensitivity (86%) and specificity (88%) for identifying patients who underwent valve surgery. The traditional cutoffs of RF of 50% and RVol of 60 mL were highly specific (99.1% and 98.1%) but poorly sensitive (24.7% and 53.4%) for identifying a clinical indication for surgery.[52] An additional study evaluated 178 patients with ≥moderate AR by echocardiography who underwent CMR and showed that a threshold of RF of ≥32% and iLVESV ≥45 mL/m² was associated with adverse outcomes.[41] Most recently, a multicenter study of asymptomatic chronic AR patients with preserved LV function and significant AR (RVol ≥30 mL and/or RF ≥ 30%) found the thresholds associated with adverse outcomes to be an RVol ≥47 mL, RF ≥ 43%, indexed LVEDV ≥109 mL/m², and indexed LVESV ≥43 mL/m². Similar to what was observed in echocardiographic studies, the LV diameters associated with outcomes were lower than currently recommended in the guidelines, at an LV end-systolic

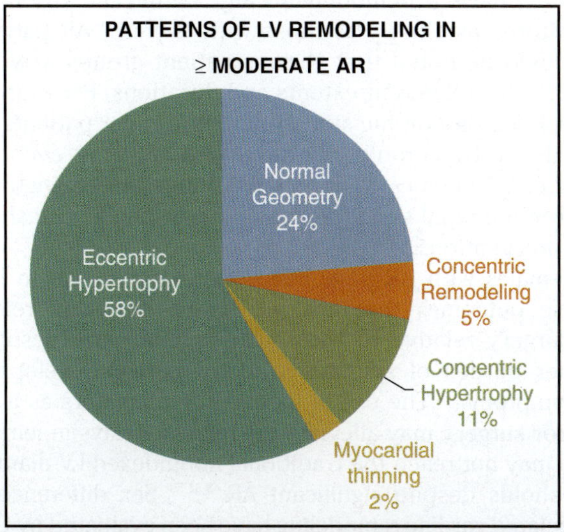

Pattern	LV mass	Mass/Volume ratio
Normal geometry	Normal	Normal
Myocardial thinning	Normal	↓
Concentric remodeling	Normal	↑
Concentric hypertrophy	↑	↑
Eccentric hypertrophy	↑	Normal

FIG. 36.6 Overview of the observed cardiac remodeling patterns by cardiac magnetic resonance in patients with ≥moderate aortic regurgitation (*AR*), and the determination of patterns of remodeling. *LV*, Left ventricular. (Available at: https://www.ahajournals.org/doi/10.1161/CIRCIMAGING.122.014684.)

diameter (LVESD) of 4.0 cm and indexed LVESD of 2.0 cm/m^2.[43] This study further noted that LV volumes performed better than diameters in outcome association, suggesting that the former may be better at guiding management of AR patients.

The principal conclusions from the constellation of CMR studies is that hemodynamically significant AR on CMR is likely defined at a lower quantitative threshold (RF of ~40%; RVol ~45–50 mL) than is stated in current guidelines. Notably, the natural history studies forming the basis for current guideline recommendations included both moderate-severe and severe AR patients, indicating that CMR findings do not significantly differ. However, patients classified as having "moderate-severe" should be considered to have a hemodynamically significant lesion and monitored as closely as those with "severe" AR patients. It should be noted that various patient groups may "tolerate" AR to different extents and durations. For example, an echocardiographic study found that older patients and females with chronic AR developed adverse events at smaller LV volumes compared to younger males, highlighting the potential need for sex- and age-specific thresholds for intervention.[55]

Females with AR have been previously shown to have worse outcomes than males,[56,57] with delays in referral to surgery relative to their male counterparts despite a higher burden of symptoms and/or earlier development of symptoms.[58] The use of indexed LV diameters as a trigger for surgery may alleviate the referral delays in females, who may not reach the traditional nonindexed LV diameter thresholds despite significant AR.[49,51,58] Sex differences in AR-related cardiac remodeling have been evaluated by CMR-based studies. One study evaluated the CMR findings of 243 patients (24% female) with ≥moderate chronic AR (although AR severity was determined by echocardiography and not matched between males and females).[59] Significant sex differences in LV remodeling emerged on CMR. Females demonstrated significantly smaller iLVEDV and iLVESV and blunted LV dilation in the setting of increasing AR severity. Two other studies were consistent overall and showed that indexing to body surface area did not "correct" for the LV dilatation extent between males and females.[60,61]

Reduction of LV volumes (reverse remodeling) after AVR is an important parameter of AR assessment, since patients with persistent dilatation have worse outcomes.[62,63] There are a few CMR studies on reverse remodeling after AVR. One CMR study of 29 patients with severe AR showed a significant reduction of LV volumes and mass after AVR, with 24% of patients having persistent LV dilatation and 45% exhibiting persistent elevation of indexed LV mass at a mean of approximately 7 months after surgery. Left ventricular end-diastolic volume was a significant independent predictor of favorable remodeling after AVR, whereas echocardiography measures were not.[64] Another study of aortic valve disease patients included 32 patients with severe AR (and 67 with AS), and evaluated pre and postoperative CMR findings,[65] including assessments of LGE, ECV fraction, and indexed ECV. Extracellular volume fraction and indexed ECV were significantly higher among patients with AR than in the AS group. As shown in AS studies, LV scar did not change in AR patients' postsurgery. The indexed ECV decreased in AR patients compared to preoperative findings, while the ECV fraction remained unchanged.

Patients with severe AR and preserved LV ejection fraction can also have impaired values of LV longitudinal, circumferential, and radial strain by echocardiography compared to controls.[66] Impaired GLS is also associated with adverse events.[67,68] Feature-tracking CMR was used to study strain values in AR patients in a smaller study, and GLS was the primary strain parameter to be associated with adverse events.[69]

Assessment of Tissue Characteristics in Aortic Regurgitation by Cardiac Magnetic Resonance

Tissue characteristics on CMR have also been studied in AR. The initial LV remodeling of AR with myocyte hypertrophy and fiber elongation compensates for increased wall stress. However, myocardial fibrosis and cell death occur in AR as in AS and have been described in histopathology studies. In addition, increased interstitial fibrosis has been reported via an increase in fibronectin and noncollagen components.[70] Myocardial fibrosis is also associated with adverse remodeling and dysfunction.[71–73] The prevalence of LV scarring by LGE on CMR was evaluated in a study of 392 patients with AR (RVol≥30 mL or RF≥30%).[74] Myocardial scar was present in a third of the patients, and the presence of LV scar (both infarction and noninfarction scar) was independently associated with a 2.5-fold increase in mortality (Fig. 36.7). Among patients with myocardial scar, AVR was independently associated with a lower risk of mortality even after adjustment for confounders. In another study of 177 patients with isolated chronic AR including the full spectrum of regurgitation severity, the indexed ECV was also associated with adverse events (death or need for AVR), more closely than ECV fraction or LV scar.[75]

In conclusion, CMR is a powerful modality to evaluate the cardiac cavity and tissue remodeling in AR. Quantitation of AR severity and LV volumes is key in the assessment and follow-up of AR patients, and CMR can be an optimal test for many patients. Tissue characteristics on CMR are associated with outcomes in AR as in AS but have not been as extensively evaluated. Whether CMR abnormalities such as LV scar or extracellular expansion parameters can help in decision making for intervention is an active area of investigation.

MITRAL REGURGITATION

MR can be broadly categorized into primary MR due to leaflet abnormalities and functional MR due to ventricular and/or atrial remodeling. Two of the main strengths of CMR in MR assessment are the "indirect" method of quantifying MR severity by subtracting the aortic forward stroke volume from the planimetered LV stroke volume, which does not rely on jet characteristics to quantify MR, and the highly reproducible ventricular cavity and tissue characterization.

Chronic primary MR is characterized by volume overload that leads to progressive cardiac remodeling, manifesting as ventricular enlargement and eventual myocardial

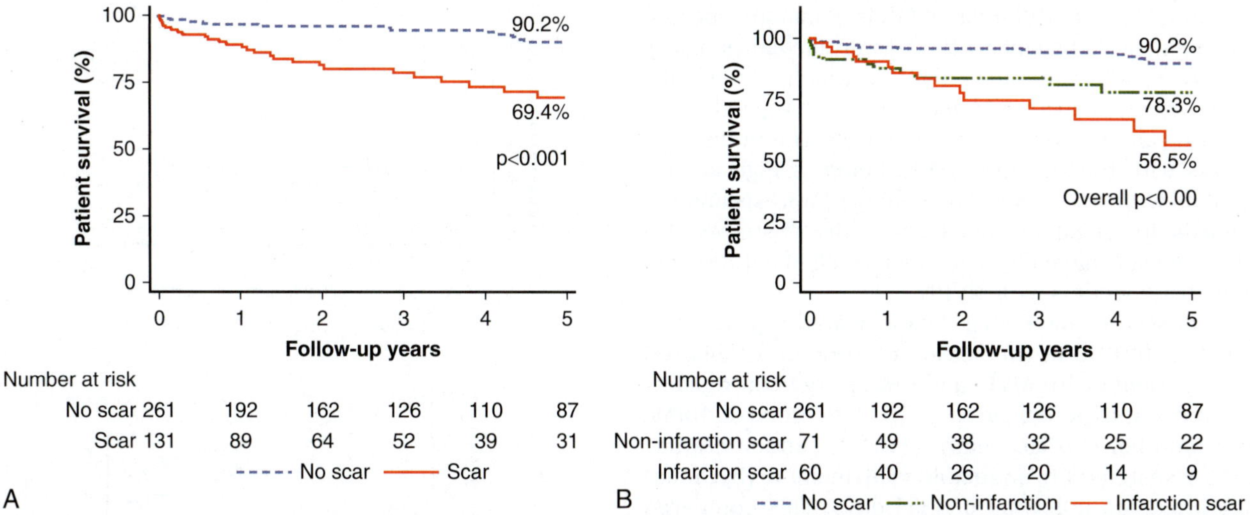

FIG. 36.7 Kaplan-Meier curves for survival by presence of scar (A) and scar type (B) in patients with ≥moderate aortic regurgitation by cardiac magnetic resonance. (Available at: https://www.ahajournals.org/doi/full/10.1161/JAHA.120.018731.)

systolic dysfunction and symptom development. Thus, patients with severe MR can be asymptomatic for an extended period of time, and there is a need for reliable early noninvasive markers of maladaptive cardiac remodeling, which could represent triggers for mitral valve intervention in the asymptomatic patient before the occurrence of irreversible damage.[76] If correction of MR is pursued too late in the disease course, historical data demonstrate that irreversible cardiac changes can occur by the time of symptom development, which will lead to suboptimal long-term outcomes.

Current guidelines incorporate measures of LV ejection fraction and chamber size as triggers of mitral intervention in primary MR.[77] CMR is a well-established method for quantifying LV ejection fraction with high reproducibility and obviating the need for geometric assumptions. Linear dimensions may not be the optimal method for assessment of the LV in primary MR due to the spherical remodeling process that occurs in MR. Instead, LV volumes are a more reliable marker. Assessment of LV volumes is more accurate and reproducible with CMR than with echocardiography, and CMR is well positioned as a result for the determination of timing of surgery in asymptomatic patients based on LV remodeling extent. It should be noted, however, that the accurate quantitation of MR severity is the first key step in the evaluation of patients with MR. Confirmation of a hemodynamically significant lesion should then be followed by assessment of the extent of remodeling to decide on the timing of surgery in an asymptomatic patient. Quantitation of MR severity is more reproducible with CMR than with echocardiography and predicts postoperative LV remodeling to a higher extent.[45,78–82] In a study of 109 asymptomatic patients with moderate or severe MR on echo, CMR quantification of MR severity and LV volumes accurately identified patients who progressed to symptoms or other indications for surgery, demonstrating an iLVEDV threshold of <100 mL/m2 to confer a 90% rate of surgery-free survival at five years.[81] In a separate series of asymptomatic MR patients, CMR-derived indexed LVESV demonstrated a higher area under the curve than echo-derived LV end-systolic diameter for survival free of mitral surgery.[82] The expected pattern of LV remodeling in MR has been eccentric hypertrophy traditionally, but the aforementioned study, which included 424 primary MR patients, demonstrated significant heterogeneity in the patterns of observed remodeling (Fig. 36.8).[47] In patients with moderate or greater MR, the majority (57%) had normal LV mass and normal LV M/V ratio, while 18% had eccentric hypertrophy. Another important pattern is the myocardial thinning pattern (which was observed in 18% of patients), which is characterized by normal LV mass but a low M/V ratio (2 standard deviations below healthy volunteer reference values), reflecting a dilated thinned walled ventricle.

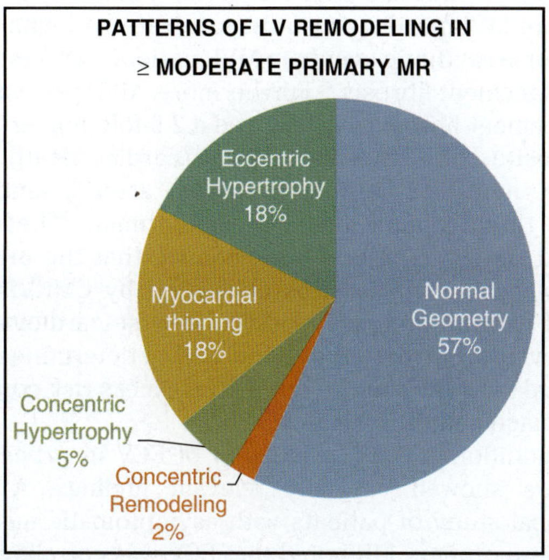

FIG. 36.8 Overview of the observed cardiac remodeling patterns by cardiac magnetic resonance in patients with ≥moderate mitral regurgitation (*MR*). *LV*, Left ventricular. (Available at: https://www.ahajournals.org/doi/10.1161/CIRCIMAGING.122.014684.)

Replacement myocardial fibrosis or LV scarring as evidenced by LGE has been observed in the setting of primary MR, primarily due to mitral valve prolapse (MVP). In a study of 356 primary MR patients (177 MVP and 179 non-MVP), the presence of LGE was more prevalent in the MVP group than the non-MVP group (36.7% vs. 6.7%; *P*<.001).[83]

LGE in patients with MVP-related MR is commonly located in the segments adjacent to the posteromedial papillary muscle (e.g., inferolateral or inferior walls), is typically small in extent, occurring in midwall striae or patchy patterns, and can be subendocardial as well. The prevalence increases with the severity of MR, being as high as 50% in patients with severe MR. The finding of fibrosis and the propensity for segments adjacent to the posteromedial papillary muscle have also been confirmed in autopsies of sudden death victims with MVP.[84]

Several studies have also demonstrated a prognostic implication of LGE in the setting of MVP. In a US-based series,[83] patients with MVP- and CMR-evidenced replacement fibrosis experienced a 7.7% rate of arrhythmic events (sudden cardiac death, aborted sudden cardiac arrest, or sustained or inducible ventricular arrhythmia) during a median follow-up of 1354 days. This compared to an arrhythmic rate of 2.7% for MVP patients without replacement fibrosis and 0.6% for the group of primary MR due to non-MVP etiology (in which the prevalence of replacement fibrosis was very low). Similarly, a French study of MVP patients also demonstrated a higher likelihood of arrhythmic events in MVP patients with evidence of replacement fibrosis.[85] Furthermore, MVP patients with replacement fibrosis experienced a 2.6-fold higher rate of composite cardiovascular events (cardiac death, heart failure, new-onset atrial fibrillation, arterial embolism, or life-threatening ventricular arrhythmia). These data extend the growing body of evidence that the presence of replacement fibrosis, as evidenced by CMR, is associated with an increased risk of adverse cardiovascular (CV) events. Further study is needed to determine if early surgical intervention can lessen the excess risk conferred by replacement fibrosis in MVP.

In addition to LGE, evaluation of ECV in primary MR patients showed clinically relevant findings. A cross-sectional study of patients with asymptomatic moderate or severe primary MR noted that ECV was correlated with total exercise time, metabolic equivalent, and peak volume of oxygen (VO2).[86] In a large study of patients with chronic primary MR, ECV was higher in patients with symptomatic MR.[87] Furthermore, when followed longitudinally, patients with an ECV ≥30% experienced a higher likelihood of death or need for mitral valve surgery.[87,88] While still an emerging marker, the current evidence suggests that ECV may represent a marker of maladaptive remodeling and subclinical decompensation in chronic primary MR. Further study is needed to determine if this may serve as a trigger for early mitral valve intervention.

In functional MR, evaluation of LV remodeling and tissue characteristics by CMR achieves multiple goals: accurate assessment of systolic function and extent of LV dilatation; identification of myocardial scar presence, extent, and viability; quantitation of degree of MR; and a further description of mechanism (e.g., MR due to ischemia, annular dilatation, atrial functional MR and mixed etiology MR.). In a study of 578 patients with ischemic cardiomyopathy,[89] the extent of myocardial scarring and ischemic functional MR had a significant interaction, which provided risk stratification beyond LV volumes and clinical parameters. Concomitant significant MR (regurgitant fraction ≥35%) and

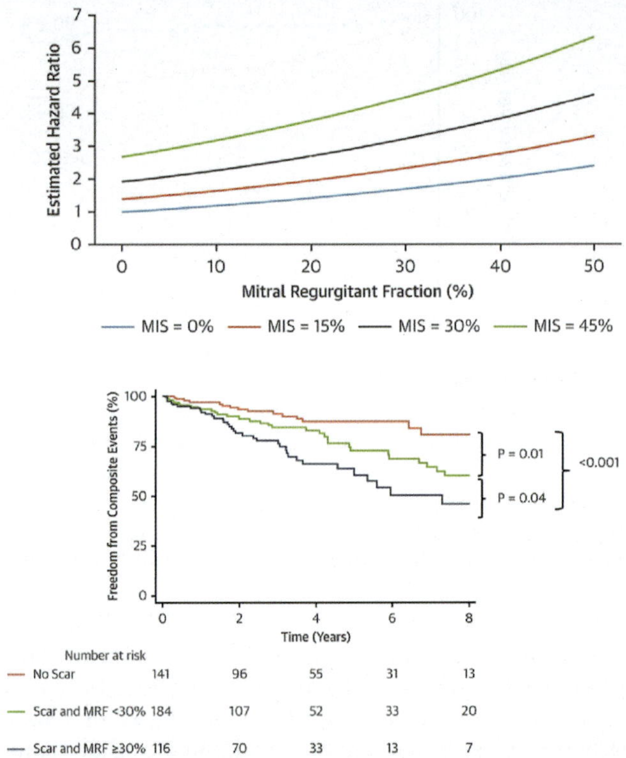

FIG. 36.9 Interactions of mitral regurgitation (MR) severity and extent of left ventricular (LV) scarring in patients with functional MR. Top panel shows adjusted hazard ratios for adverse outcomes as a function of MR severity in patients with increasing scar extent. Bottom panel shows survival curves of patients with no scar, lesser degrees of MR with LV scar vs significant MR and LV scar. *MIS,* myocardial infarct size; *MRF,* mitral regurgitant fraction. (Available at: https://www.sciencedirect.com/science/article/pii/S1936878X19310265?via%3Dihub.)

large scar extent (≥30% of LV mass) had the highest risk for adverse events (Fig. 36.9).

In another study of 441 patients with ischemic and nonischemic cardiomyopathy,[90] MR fraction ≥30% was associated with increased risk of adverse events. When stratified by presence or absence of scar, MR fraction ≥30% was associated with events only among patients with scar but not among patients without scar. On further classification of patients with scar, the prognostic significance of functional MR was observed primarily among patients with intermediate scar burden.

Evaluation of myocardial ischemia by stress CMR plays a role in the evaluation of patients with ischemic functional MR. In a multicenter study of 2647 patients with coronary artery disease, 34% had functional MR and 7% had ≥moderate functional MR. The prevalence of functional MR was associated with the presence and extent of ischemia and infarction in the LV segments subtending the mitral valve apparatus (Fig. 36.10), highlighting the advantages of CMR in providing a comprehensive evaluation of functional MR patients.

Overall, the extent of MR by CMR quantitation that is associated with adverse outcomes is lower with functional MR than with primary MR, but the treatment decisions of patients with functional MR are much more complex with the interplay of medical therapy for heart failure, revascularization, resynchronization therapy, and others. Selection of patients for transcatheter MR repair based on CMR

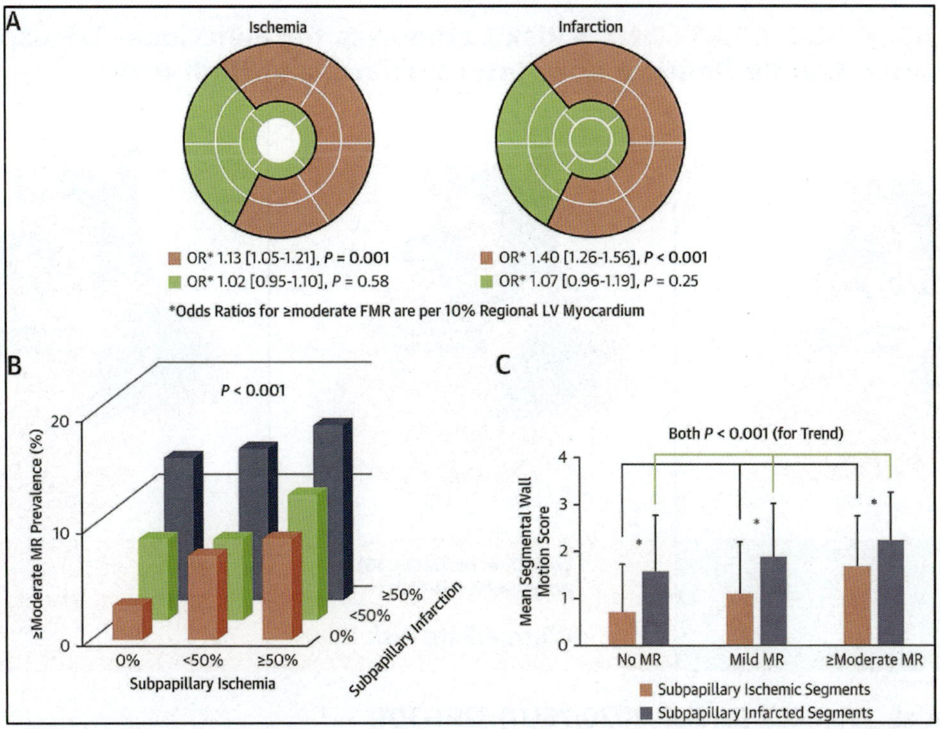

FIG. 36.10 Evaluation of ischemic and left ventricular (LV) infarction by cardiac magnetic resonance in segments subtending the papillary muscles and mitral valve apparatus (*red segments*) vs remote areas of the LV (*green segments*), (A). The prevalence of ≥moderate functional mitral regurgitation (*MR*) increases with increased prevalence of subpapillary muscle ischemia and infarction (B), and extent of wall motion abnormalities (C). *FMR,* functional mitral regurgitation. (Available at: https://www.sciencedirect.com/science/article/pii/S1936878X22001796?via%3Dihub.)

findings requires further study. Whether the presence or extent of LV scar should influence management decisions also requires study.

TRICUSPID REGURGITATION

TR results in volume overload of the RV leading to RV dilatation and eventual systolic dysfunction. The anatomy and hemodynamics of the RV are significantly different than the LV, and functional TR is much more common than primary TR (~90–95% of patients). CMR evaluation of TR severity is analogous to MR evaluation, and the natural history of TR involves progressive right heart chamber dilatation, with eventual systolic dysfunction and right heart failure. The CMR quantification of TR is reproducible and does not require the assessment of multiple frequently discordant parameters, as is the case with echocardiography.

Recent outcome studies provided further validation to the assessment of TR severity by CMR. In a large study of 547 patients with functional TR undergoing CMR, measurement of tricuspid RVol and RF was independently associated with all-cause mortality. Patients in the highest-risk strata of RVol ≥45 mL or RF ≥50% had the worst prognosis, and patients with RVol of 30–44 mL or RF 30%–49% had an intermediate risk, while patients with lower grades of TR (RVol <30 mL, RF <30%) had low risk (Fig. 36.11).

TR severity is well correlated to the extent of RV dilatation parameters (RV end-diastolic volume and end-systolic volume), and measures of TR severity are associated with adverse outcomes independent of RV function (RVEF). However, it is unknown whether specific RV dilatation parameters should be used to guide decision making in patients with hemodynamically significant TR, particularly since most patients are referred late for intervention or surgery, after significant RV remodeling has taken place. It is likely that RV systolic function is the more important parameter. In a CMR study of 79 patients undergoing transcatheter tricuspid valve repair,[91] 18 (23%) presented with RVEF ≤45% and 40 (51%) presented with longitudinal RV dysfunction (reduced tricuspid annular plane systolic excursion [TAPSE] as measured on echo). Only RVEF by CMR but not TAPSE was associated with the outcome of all-cause death or heart failure hospitalization. Feature-tracking CMR also evaluates RV free wall strain, which has shown promise in further evaluation of RV systolic function. In a multicenter study of patients with severe functional TR,[92] 544 were followed for a median of 6 years and RV free wall strain was measured from cine CMR. Patients with free wall strain ≥ the median (-16%) had significantly reduced event-free survival compared with those with free wall strain < the median ($P<.001$). By multivariable modeling, RV free wall strain was associated with increased risk of death after adjustment for clinical and imaging risk factors, including RV size and ejection fraction (Fig. 36.12).

Whether parameters of RV function and the extent of RV remodeling should be incorporated into decision making for intervention—and whether they predict outcomes after intervention—will require further research.

A summary of various cardiac cavity and tissue remodeling findings by CMR across various VHD conditions is provided in Table 36.1.

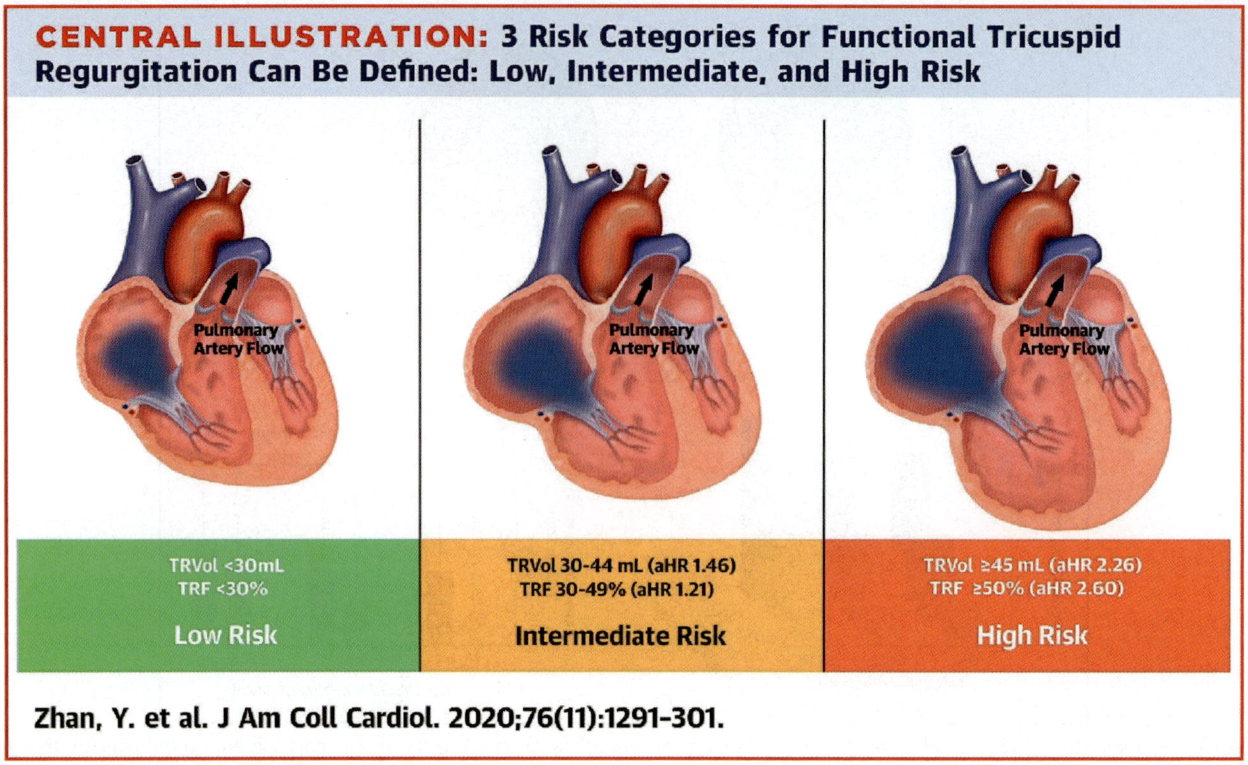

FIG. 36.11 Overview of functional tricuspid regurgitation (TR) quantitation by cardiac magnetic resonance and outcomes according to TR severity assessment. *TRVol,* tricuspid regurgitant volume; *TRF,* tricuspid regurgitant fraction. (Available at: https://www.sciencedirect.com/science/article/pii/S0735109720360356?via%3Dihub.)

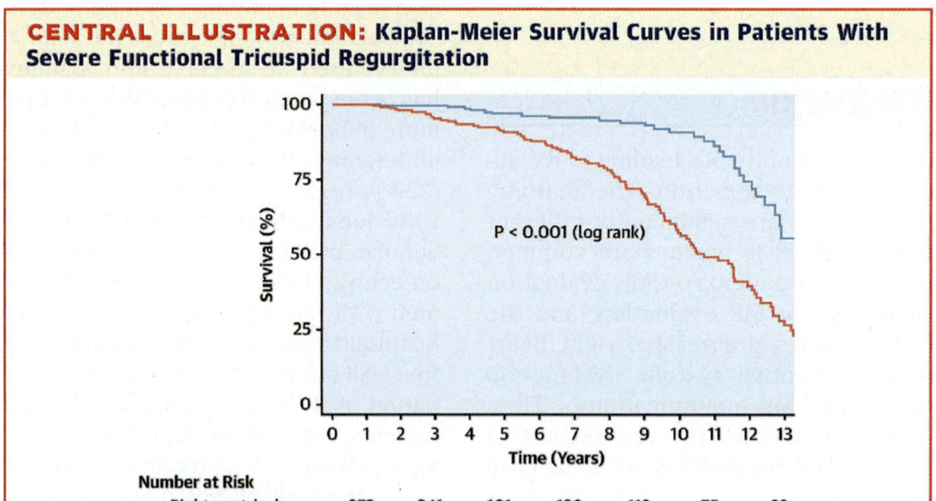

FIG. 36.12 Outcomes of patients with severe functional tricuspid regurgitation according to right ventricular free wall strain measured by feature-tracking cardiac magnetic resonance. (Available at: https://www.sciencedirect.com/science/article/pii/S1936878X21001832?via%3Dihub.)

TABLE 36.1 Overview of Cardiac Remodeling and Tissue Characteristics by Cardiac Magnetic Resonance in Individual Valvular Lesions.

VALVE LESION	AORTIC STENOSIS	AORTIC REGURGITATION	MITRAL REGURGITATION	TRICUSPID REGURGITATION
Hemodynamic load	Pressure overload	Pressure and volume overload	Volume overload	Volume overload
Primary chamber involvement	Left ventricle	Left ventricle	Left atrium and left ventricle	Right atrium and right ventricle
Pattern of cardiac chamber remodeling	Concentric hypertrophy	Eccentric hypertrophy (plus mildly increased LV wall thickness)	Eccentric hypertrophy and dilated ventricle with thin walls, left atrial dilatation	Right ventricle dilatation and right atrial dilatation
Sex differences	• Males: predominance of concentric hypertrophy and increased LV mass • Females: predominance of concentric remodeling and normal geometry (may not be related to AS severity)	Males appear to develop greater ventricular dilation and hypertrophy then females, indexed LV parameters may not fully correct for sex differences	Uncertain if sex differences are present with regards to cavity remodeling in response to MR	Uncertain if sex differences are present with regards to cavity remodeling in response to TR
Tissue Characteristics				
LGE	• LV scar present in ~30–50% of severe AS patients • Various patterns present including non-CAD midwall scar • Independently associated with adverse outcomes • Irreversible after surgery	• LV scar present in ~15–30% of ≥ moderate AR patients • Independently associated with adverse outcomes • Aortic valve replacement may alleviate the risk in patients with scar	• LV fibrosis/scar primarily in MVP patients, increases with MR severity • Predominates in segments of mechanical stretch related to MVP (basal inferior/lateral wall and papillary muscle • Related to arrhythmic events, uncertain outcomes after MV surgery	• Unknown if significant TR with RV remodeling leads to RV scarring
T1 mapping findings	• ECV % increases with AS severity and associated with adverse outcomes independent of LGE • Indexed ECV also associated with outcomes and may decrease after surgery to lesser extent than cellular compartment volume>>patients may have increased ECV % after surgery	• ECV% does not appear to be associated with AR severity or adverse outcomes • Limited data suggested indexed ECV to be associated with adverse events (death or need for surgery)	• ECV % increases with MR severity and is independently associated with adverse outcomes (death or developing surgery indications)	• T1 mapping of the right ventricle is challenging and no outcome data are available in patients with TR

AR, aortic regurgitation; *AS*, aortic stenosis; *CAD*, coronary artery disease; *ECV*, extracellular volume; *LV*, left ventricle; *MVP*, mitral valve prolapse; *RV*, right ventricle; *TR*, tricuspid regurgitation.

CONCLUSION

CMR provides a comprehensive evaluation of cardiac chamber and tissue remodeling in VHD. Due to its high reproducibility and direct calculation of ventricular volumes and mass, there is now a wealth of descriptive and prognostic CMR studies in VHD, with clinically relevant findings in aortic and mitral valve disease. Prospective studies are needed—and some are ongoing—to study the value of CMR in decision making for intervention in VHD.

REFERENCES

1. Carabello BA. The relationship of left ventricular geometry and hypertrophy to left ventricular function in valvular heart disease. *J Heart Valve Dis*. 1995;4:S132–S138.
2. Lang RM, Badano LP, Victor MA, et al. Recommendations for cardiac chamber quantification by echocardiography in adults: an update from the American society of echocardiography and the European association of cardiovascular imaging. *J Am Soc Echocardiogr*. 2015;28(1):1–39. https://doi.org/10.1016/J.ECHO.2014.10.003.
3. Dujardin KS, Enriquez-Sarano M, Rossi A, Bailey KR, Seward JB. Echocardiographic assessment of left ventricular remodeling: are left ventricular diameters suitable tools? *J Am Coll Cardiol*. 1997;30(6):1534–1541. https://doi.org/10.1016/S0735-1097(97)00329-X.
4. Zoghbi WA, Asch FM, Bruce C, et al. Guidelines for the evaluation of valvular regurgitation after percutaneous valve repair or replacement: a report from the American Society of echocardiography developed in collaboration with the society for cardiovascular angiography and interventions. *J Am Soc Echocardiogr*. 2019;32(4):431–475. https://doi.org/10.1016/j.echo.2019.01.003.
5. Baumgartner H, Hung J, Bermejo J, et al. Recommendations on the echocardiographic assessment of aortic valve stenosis: a focused update from the European association of cardiovascular imaging and the American society of echocardiography. *Eur Heart J Cardiovasc Imaging*. 2017;18(3):254–275. https://doi.org/10.1093/ehjci/jew335.
6. Mor-Avi V, Jenkins C, Kühl HP, et al. Real-time 3-dimensional echocardiographic quantification of left ventricular volumes: multicenter study for validation with magnetic resonance imaging and investigation of sources of error. *JACC Cardiovasc Imaging*. 2008;1(4):413–423. https://doi.org/10.1016/J.JCMG.2008.02.009.
7. Sugeng L, Mor-Avi V, Weinert L, et al. Quantitative assessment of left ventricular size and function. *Circulation*. 2006;114(7):654–661. https://doi.org/10.1161/CIRCULATIONAHA.106.626143.
8. Rehr RB, Malloy CR, Filipchuk NG, Peshock RM. Left ventricular volumes measured by MR imaging. *Radiology*. 1985;156(3):717–719. https://doi.org/10.1148/RADIOLOGY.156.3.4023232.
9. Kawel-Boehm N, Hetzel SJ, Ambale-Venkatesh B, et al. Reference ranges ("normal values") for cardiovascular magnetic resonance (CMR) in adults

and children: 2020 update. *J Cardiovasc Magn Reson*. 2020;22(1). https://doi.org/10.1186/S12968-020-00683-3.

10. Dweck MR, Joshi S, Murigu T, et al. Left ventricular remodeling and hypertrophy in patients with aortic stenosis: Insights from cardiovascular magnetic resonance. *J Cardiovasc Magn Reson*. 2012;14(1):50. https://doi.org/10.1186/1532-429X-14-50.
11. Kwiecinski J, Chin CWL, Everett RJ, et al. Adverse prognosis associated with asymmetric myocardial thickening in aortic stenosis. *Eur Heart J Cardiovasc Imaging*. 2018;19(3):347. https://doi.org/10.1093/EHJCI/JEX052.
12. Treibel TA, Kozor R, Fontana M, et al. Sex dimorphism in the myocardial response to aortic stenosis. *JACC Cardiovasc Imaging*. 2018;11(7):962–973. https://doi.org/10.1016/j.jcmg.2017.08.025.
13. Singh A, Musa T Al, Treibel TA, et al. Original research article: sex differences in left ventricular remodelling, myocardial fibrosis and mortality after aortic valve replacement. *Heart*. 2019;105(23):1818. https://doi.org/10.1136/HEARTJNL-2019-314987.
14. Vollema EM, Sugimoto T, Shen M, et al. Association of left ventricular global longitudinal strain with asymptomatic severe aortic stenosis: natural course and prognostic value. *JAMA Cardiol*. 2018;3(9):839. https://doi.org/10.1001/JAMACARDIO.2018.2288.
15. Hor KN, Baumann R, Pedrizzetti G, et al. Magnetic resonance derived myocardial strain assessment using feature tracking. *J Vis Exp*. 2011;48:2356. https://doi.org/10.3791/2356.
16. Kim MY, Park EA, Lee W, Lee SP. Cardiac magnetic resonance feature tracking in aortic stenosis: exploration of strain parameters and prognostic value in asymptomatic patients with preserved ejection fraction. *Korean J Radiol*. 2020;21(3):268–279. https://doi.org/10.3348/KJR.2019.0441.
17. Hwang JW, Kim SM, Park SJ, et al. Assessment of reverse remodeling predicted by myocardial deformation on tissue tracking in patients with severe aortic stenosis: a cardiovascular magnetic resonance imaging study. *J Cardiovasc Magn Reson: Off J Soc Cardiovasc Magn Reson*. 2017;19(1):80. https://doi.org/10.1186/S12968-017-0392-0.
18. Spath NB, Gomez M, Everett RJ, et al. Global longitudinal strain analysis using cardiac MRI in aortic stenosis: comparison with left ventricular remodeling, myocardial fibrosis, and 2-year clinical outcomes. *Radiol Cardiothorac Imaging*. 2019;1(4):e190027. https://doi.org/10.1148/RYCT.2019190027.
19. Hein S, Arnon E, Kostin S, et al. Progression from compensated hypertrophy to failure in the pressure-overloaded human: Heart structural deterioration and compensatory mechanisms. *Circulation*. 2003;107(7):984–991. https://doi.org/10.1161/01.CIR.0000051865.66123.B7.
20. Musa TA, Treibel TA, Vassiliou VS, et al. Myocardial scar and mortality in severe aortic stenosis: data from the BSCMR valve consortium. *Circulation*. 2018;138(18):1935–1947. https://doi.org/10.1161/CIRCULATIONAHA.117.032839.
21. Azevedo CF, Nigri M, Higuchi ML, et al. Prognostic significance of myocardial fibrosis quantification by histopathology and magnetic resonance imaging in patients with severe aortic valve disease. *J Am Coll Cardiol*. 2010;56(4):278–287. https://doi.org/10.1016/j.jacc.2009.12.074.
22. Dweck MR, Joshi S, Murigu T, et al. Midwall fibrosis is an independent predictor of mortality in patients with aortic stenosis. *J Am Coll Cardiol*. 2011;58(12):1271–1279. https://doi.org/10.1016/J.JACC.2011.03.064.
23. Barone-Rochette G, Piérard S, De Meester De Ravenstein C, et al. Prognostic significance of LGE by CMR in aortic stenosis patients undergoing valve replacement. *J Am Coll Cardiol*. 2014;64(2):144–154. https://doi.org/10.1016/J.JACC.2014.02.612.
24. Kwak S, Everett RJ, Treibel TA, et al. Markers of myocardial damage predict mortality in patients with aortic stenosis. *J Am Coll Cardiol*. 2021;78(6):545–558. https://doi.org/10.1016/J.JACC.2021.05.047/SUPPL_FILE/MMC1.DOCX.
25. Treibel TA, Kozor R, Schofield R, et al. Reverse myocardial remodeling following valve replacement in patients with aortic stenosis. *J Am Coll Cardiol*. 2018;71(8):860–871. https://doi.org/10.1016/j.jacc.2017.12.035.
26. Bing R, Everett RJ, Tuck C, et al. Rationale and design of the randomized, controlled early valve replacement guided by biomarkers of left ventricular decompensation in asymptomatic patients with severe aortic stenosis (EVOLVED) trial. *Am Heart J*. 2019;212:91–100. https://doi.org/10.1016/J.AHJ.2019.02.018.
27. Chin CWL, Everett RJ, Kwiecinski J, et al. Myocardial fibrosis and cardiac decompensation in aortic stenosis. *JACC Cardiovasc Imaging*. 2017;10(11):1320–1333. https://doi.org/10.1016/j.jcmg.2016.10.007.
28. Everett RJ, Treibel TA, Fukui M, et al. Extracellular myocardial volume in patients with aortic stenosis. *J Am Coll Cardiol*. 2020;75(3):304–316. https://doi.org/10.1016/J.JACC.2019.11.032.
29. Kockova R, Kacer P, Pirk J, et al. Native T1 relaxation time and extracellular volume fraction as accurate markers of diffuse myocardial fibrosis in heart valve disease - comparison with targeted left ventricular myocardial biopsy. *Circ J*. 2016;80(5):1202–1209. https://doi.org/10.1253/CIRCJ.CJ-15-1309.
30. De Meester De Ravenstein C, Bouzin C, Lazam S, et al. Histological validation of measurement of diffuse interstitial myocardial fibrosis by myocardial extravascular volume fraction from modified look-locker imaging (MOLLI) T1 mapping at 3 T. *J Cardiovasc Magn Reson*. 2015;17(1):1–11. https://doi.org/10.1186/s12968-015-0150-0.
31. Everett RJ, Tastet L, Clavel MA, et al. Progression of hypertrophy and myocardial fibrosis in aortic stenosis: a multicenter cardiac magnetic resonance study. *Circ Cardiovasc Imaging*. 2018;11(6):e007451. https://doi.org/10.1161/CIRCIMAGING.117.007451.
32. Krayenbuehl HP, Hess OM, Monrad ES, Schneider J, Mall G, Turina M. Left ventricular myocardial structure in aortic valve disease before, intermediate, and late after aortic valve replacement. *Circulation*. 1989;79(4):744–755. https://doi.org/10.1161/01.CIR.79.4.744.
33. Singh A, Chan DCS, Greenwood JP, et al. Symptom onset in aortic stenosis: relation to sex differences in left ventricular remodeling. *JACC Cardiovasc Imaging*. 2019;12(1):96–105. https://doi.org/10.1016/j.jcmg.2017.09.019.
34. Treibel TA, Fontana M, Gilbertson JA, et al. Occult transthyretin cardiac amyloid in severe calcific aortic stenosis. *Circ Cardiovasc Imaging*. 2016;9(8). https://doi.org/10.1161/CIRCIMAGING.116.005066.
35. Carabello BA. Aortic regurgitation. A lesion with similarities to both aortic stenosis and mitral regurgitation: editorial comment. *Circulation*. 1990;82(3):1051–1053. https://doi.org/10.1161/01.CIR.82.3.1051.
36. Wisenbaugh T, Spann JF, Carabello BA. Differences in myocardial performance and load between patients with similar amounts of chronic aortic versus chronic mitral regurgitation. *J Am Coll Cardiol*. 1984;3(4):916–923. https://doi.org/10.1016/S0735-1097(84)80349-6.
37. Bonow RO, Lakatos E, Maron BJ, Epstein SE. Serial long-term assessment of the natural history of asymptomatic patients with chronic aortic regurgitation and normal left ventricular systolic function. *Circulation*. 1991;84(4):1625–1635. https://doi.org/10.1161/01.CIR.84.4.1625.
38. Bolen MA, Popovic ZB, Rajiah P, et al. Cardiac MR assessment of aortic regurgitation: holodiastolic flow reversal in the descending aorta helps stratify severity. *Radiology*. 2011;260(1):98–104. https://doi.org/10.1148/RADIOL.11102064/ASSET/IMAGES/LARGE/102064T04.JPEG.
39. Debl K, Djavidani B, Buchner S, et al. Assessment of the anatomic regurgitant orifice in aortic regurgitation: a clinical magnetic resonance imaging study. *Heart*. 2008;94(3). https://doi.org/10.1136/HRT.2006.108720.
40. Myerson SG, D'arcy J, Mohiaddin R, et al. Aortic regurgitation quantification using cardiovascular magnetic resonance: association with clinical outcome. *Circulation*. 2012;126(12):1452–1460. https://doi.org/10.1161/CIRCULATIONAHA.111.083600.
41. Hashimoto G, Enriquez-Sarano M, Stanberry LI, et al. Association of left ventricular remodeling assessment by cardiac magnetic resonance with outcomes in patients with chronic aortic regurgitation. *JAMA Cardiol*. 2022;7(9):924–933. https://doi.org/10.1001/JAMACARDIO.2022.2108.
42. Honda N, Machida K, Hashimoto M, et al. Aortic regurgitation: quantitation with MR imaging velocity mapping. *Radiology*. 1993;186(1):189–194. https://doi.org/10.1148/radiology.186.1.8416562.
43. Malahfji M, Crudo V, Kaolawanich Y, et al. Association of cardiac remodeling with aortic regurgitation outcomes: the AR consortium of the SCMR registry. *J Am Coll Cardiol*. 2023;81(19):1885–1898. https://doi.org/10.1016/J.JACC.2023.03.001.
44. Harris AW, Krieger EV, Kim M, et al. Cardiac magnetic resonance imaging versus transthoracic echocardiography for prediction of outcomes in chronic aortic or mitral regurgitation. *Am J Cardiol*. 2017;119(7):1074–1081. https://doi.org/10.1016/j.amjcard.2016.12.017.
45. Cawley PJ, Hamilton-Craig C, Owens DS, et al. Prospective comparison of valve regurgitation quantitation by cardiac magnetic resonance imaging and transthoracic echocardiography. *Circ Cardiovasc Imaging*. 2013;6(1):48–57. https://doi.org/10.1161/CIRCIMAGING.112.975623.
46. Uretsky S, Supariwala A, Nidadovolu P, et al. Quantification of left ventricular remodeling in response to isolated aortic or mitral regurgitation. *J Cardiovasc Magn Reson*. 2010;12(1):32. https://doi.org/10.1186/1532-429X-12-32.
47. Malahfji M, Kitkungvan D, Senapati A, et al. Differences in myocardial remodeling and tissue characteristics in chronic isolated aortic and mitral regurgitation. *Circ Cardiovasc Imaging*. 2023;16:e014684. https://doi.org/10.1161/CIRCIMAGING.122.014684.
48. Zoghbi WA, Adams D, Bonow RO, et al. Recommendations for noninvasive evaluation of native valvular regurgitation: a report from the American society of echocardiography developed in collaboration with the society for cardiovascular magnetic resonance. *J Am Soc Echocardiogr*. 2017;30(4):303–371. https://doi.org/10.1016/j.echo.2017.01.007.
49. Yang LT, Michelena HI, Scott CG, et al. Outcomes in chronic hemodynamically significant aortic regurgitation and limitations of current guidelines. *J Am Coll Cardiol*. 2019;73(14):1741–1752. https://doi.org/10.1016/j.jacc.2019.01.024.
50. de Meester C, Gerber BL, Vancraeynest D, et al. Do guideline-based indications result in an outcome penalty for patients with severe aortic regurgitation? *JACC Cardiovasc Imaging*. 2019;12(11P1):2126–2138. https://doi.org/10.1016/j.jcmg.2018.11.022.
51. Mentias A, Feng K, Alashi A, et al. Long-term outcomes in patients with aortic regurgitation and preserved left ventricular ejection fraction. *J Am Coll Cardiol*. 2016;68(20):2144–2153. https://doi.org/10.1016/j.jacc.2016.08.045.
52. Vejpongsa P, Xu J, Quinones MA, Shah DJ, Zoghbi WA. Differences in cardiac remodeling in left-sided valvular regurgitation: implications for optimal definition of significant aortic regurgitation. *Cardiovasc Imaging*. 2022;15(10):1730–1741. https://doi.org/10.1016/J.JCMG.2022.05.006.
53. Gabriel RS, Renapurkar R, Bolen MA, et al. Comparison of severity of aortic regurgitation by cardiovascular magnetic resonance versus transthoracic echocardiography. *Am J Cardiol*. 2011;108(7):1014–1020. https://doi.org/10.1016/j.amjcard.2011.05.034.
54. Kammerlander AA, Wiesinger M, Duca F, et al. Diagnostic and prognostic utility of cardiac magnetic resonance imaging in aortic regurgitation. *JACC Cardiovasc Imaging*. 2019;12(8):1474–1483. https://doi.org/10.1016/J.JCMG.2018.08.036.
55. Emmanuel A, Yoshihito S, Lorenzo B, et al. Impact of age and sex on left ventricular remodeling in patients with aortic regurgitation. *J Am Coll Cardiol*. 2023;81(15):1474–1487. https://doi.org/10.1016/j.jacc.2023.02.037.
56. Klodas E, Enriquez-Sarano M, Tajik AJ, Mullany CJ, Bailey KR, Seward JB. Surgery for aortic regurgitation in women: contrasting indications and

outcomes compared with men. *Circulation*. 1996;94(10):2472–2478. https://doi.org/10.1161/01.CIR.94.10.2472.

57. Klodas E, Enriquez-Sarano M, Tajik AJ, Mullany CJ, Bailey KR, Seward JB. Optimizing timing of surgical correction in patients with severe aortic regurgitation: role of symptoms. *J Am Coll Cardiol*. 1997;30(3):746–752. https://doi.org/10.1016/S0735-1097(97)00205-2.
58. Yang LT, Enriquez-Sarano M, Pellikka PA, et al. Sex differences in outcomes of patients with chronic aortic regurgitation: closing the mortality gap. *Mayo Clin Proc*. 2021;96(8):2145–2156. https://doi.org/10.1016/J.MAYOCP.2020.11.033.
59. Tower-Rader A, Mathias IS, Obuchowski NA, et al. Sex-based differences in left ventricular remodeling in patients with chronic aortic regurgitation: a multi-modality study. *J Cardiovasc Magn Reson*. 2022;24(1):1–13. https://doi.org/10.1186/S12968-022-00845-5/FIGURES/7.
60. Kammerlander AA, Donà C, Nitsche C, et al. Sex differences in left ventricular remodeling and outcomes in chronic aortic regurgitation. *J Clin Med*. 2020;9(12):4100. https://doi.org/10.3390/JCM9124100.
61. Malahfji M, Senapati A, Debs D, et al. Sex differences in myocardial remodeling and extracellular volume in aortic regurgitation. *Sci Rep*. 2023;13(1). https://doi.org/10.1038/S41598-023-37444-Y.
62. Kumpuris AG, Quinones MA, Waggoner AD, Kanon DJ, Nelson JG, Miller RR. Importance of preoperative hypertrophy, wall stress and end-systolic dimension as echocardiographic predictors of normalization of left ventricular dilatation after valve replacement in chronic aortic insufficiency. *Am J Cardiol*. 1982;49(5):1091–1100. https://www.sciencedirect.com/science/article/pii/0002914982900327. Accessed May 14, 2022. Accessed.
63. Gaasch W, Carroll J, Levine HJ, Criscitiello MG. Chronic aortic regurgitation: prognostic value of left ventricular end-systolic dimension and end-diastolic radius/thickness ratio. *J Am Coll Cardiol*. 1983;1(3):775–782. https://www.sciencedirect.com/science/article/pii/S0735109783801909. Accessed May 14, 2022. Accessed.
64. Seldrum S, de Meester C, Pierard S, et al. Assessment of left ventricular reverse remodeling by cardiac MRI in patients undergoing repair surgery for severe aortic or mitral regurgitation. *J Cardiothorac Vasc Anesth*. 2019;33(7):1901–1911. https://doi.org/10.1053/j.jvca.2018.11.013.
65. Pires LT, Rosa VEE, Morais TC, et al. Postoperative myocardial fibrosis assessment in aortic valvular heart diseases—a cardiovascular magnetic resonance study. *Eur Heart J Cardiovasc Imaging*. 2023;24(7):851–862. https://doi.org/10.1093/EHJCI/JEAD041.
66. Ewe SH, Haeck MLA, Ng ACT, et al. Detection of subtle left ventricular systolic dysfunction in patients with significant aortic regurgitation and preserved left ventricular ejection fraction: speckle tracking echocardiographic analysis. *Eur Heart J Cardiovasc Imaging*. 2015;16(9):992–999. https://doi.org/10.1093/EHJCI/JEV019.
67. Alashi A, Khullar T, Mentias A, et al. Long-term outcomes after aortic valve surgery in patients with asymptomatic chronic aortic regurgitation and preserved lvef: impact of baseline and follow-up global longitudinal strain. *JACC Cardiovasc Imaging*. 2020;13(1 Pt 1):12–21. https://doi.org/10.1016/J.JCMG.2018.12.021.
68. Alashi A, Khullar T, Mentias A, et al. Long-term outcomes after aortic valve surgery in patients with asymptomatic chronic aortic regurgitation and preserved LVEF: impact of baseline and follow-up global longitudinal strain. *JACC Cardiovasc Imaging*. 2020;13(1):12–21. https://doi.org/10.1016/j.jcmg.2018.12.021.
69. Fernández-Golfín C, Hinojar-Baydes R, González-Gómez A, et al. Prognostic implications of cardiac magnetic resonance feature tracking derived multidirectional strain in patients with chronic aortic regurgitation. *Eur Radiol*. 2021;31(7):5106–5115. https://doi.org/10.1007/S00330-020-07651-6.
70. Borer JS, Truter S, Herrold EM, et al. Myocardial fibrosis in chronic aortic regurgitation molecular and cellular responses to volume overload. *Circulation*. 2002;105(15):1837–1842. https://doi.org/10.1161/01.CIR.0000014419.71706.85.
71. Liu SK, Magid NR, Fox PR, Goldfine SM, Borer JS. Fibrosis, myocyte degeneration and heart failure in chronic experimental aortic regurgitation. *Cardiology*. 1998;90(2):101–109. https://doi.org/10.1159/000006827.
72. Olsen NT, Dimaano VL, Fritz-Hansen T, et al. Hypertrophy signaling pathways in experimental chronic aortic regurgitation. *J Cardiovasc Transl Res*. 2013;6(5):852–860. https://doi.org/10.1007/S12265-013-9503-Y.
73. Taniguchi K, Kawamaoto T, Kuki S, et al. Left ventricular myocardial remodeling and contractile state in chronic aortic regurgitation. *Clin Cardiol*. 2000;23(8):608–614. https://doi.org/10.1002/CLC.4960230812.
74. Malahfji M, Senapati A, Tayal B, et al. Myocardial scar and mortality in chronic aortic regurgitation. *J Am Heart Assoc*. 2020;9(23):e018731. https://doi.org/10.1161/jaha.120.018731.
75. Senapati A, Malahfji M, Debs D, et al. Regional replacement and diffuse interstitial fibrosis in aortic regurgitation: prognostic implications from cardiac magnetic resonance. *JACC Cardiovasc Imaging*. 2021;14(11):2170–2182. https://doi.org/10.1016/J.JCMG.2021.04.028.
76. Enriquez-Sarano M, Sundt TM. Early surgery is recommended for mitral regurgitation. *Circulation*. 2010;121(6):804–811. https://doi.org/10.1161/CIRCULATIONAHA.109.868083.
77. Otto CM, Nishimura RA, Bonow RO, et al. 2020 ACC/AHA guideline for the management of patients with valvular heart disease: a report of the American college of cardiology/American heart association joint committee on clinical practice guidelines. *J Am Coll Cardiol*. 2021;77(4):e25–e197. https://doi.org/10.1016/j.jacc.2020.11.018.
78. Uretsky S, Argulian E, Narula J, Wolff SD. Use of cardiac magnetic resonance imaging in assessing mitral regurgitation. *J Am Coll Cardiol*. 2018;71(5):547–563. https://doi.org/10.1016/j.jacc.2017.12.009.
79. Uretsky S, Argulian E, Supariwala A, et al. A comparative assessment of echocardiographic parameters for determining primary mitral regurgitation severity using magnetic resonance imaging as a reference standard. *J Am Soc Echocardiogr*. 2018;31(9):992–999. https://doi.org/10.1016/j.echo.2018.04.006.
80. Uretsky S, Gillam L, Lang R, et al. Discordance between echocardiography and MRI in the assessment of mitral regurgitation severity: a prospective multicenter trial. *J Am Coll Cardiol*. 2015;65(11):1078–1088. https://doi.org/10.1016/j.jacc.2014.12.047.
81. Myerson SG, D'Arcy J, Christiansen JP, et al. Determination of clinical outcome in mitral regurgitation with cardiovascular magnetic resonance quantification. *Circulation*. 2016;133(23):2287–2296. https://doi.org/10.1161/CIRCULATIONAHA.115.017888.
82. Penicka M, Vecera J, Mirica DC, Kotrc M, Kockova R, Van Camp G. Prognostic implications of magnetic resonance-derived quantification in asymptomatic patients with organic mitral regurgitation: comparison with doppler echocardiography-derived integrative approach. *Circulation*. 2018;137(13):1349–1360. https://doi.org/10.1161/CIRCULATIONAHA.117.029332.
83. Kitkungvan D, Nabi F, Kim RJ, et al. Myocardial fibrosis in patients with primary mitral regurgitation with and without prolapse. *J Am Coll Cardiol*. 2018;72(8):823–834. https://doi.org/10.1016/j.jacc.2018.06.048.
84. Basso C, Perazzolo Marra M, Rizzo S, et al. Arrhythmic mitral valve prolapse and sudden cardiac death. *Circulation*. 2015;132(7):556–566. https://doi.org/10.1161/CIRCULATIONAHA.115.016291.
85. Constant Dit Beaufils AL, Huttin O, Jobbe-Duval A, et al. Replacement myocardial fibrosis in patients with mitral valve prolapse: relation to mitral regurgitation, ventricular remodeling, and arrhythmia. *Circulation*. 2021;143(18):1763–1774. https://doi.org/10.1161/CIRCULATIONAHA.120.050214.
86. Edwards NC, Moody WE, Yuan M, et al. Quantification of left ventricular interstitial fibrosis in asymptomatic chronic primary degenerative mitral regurgitation. *Circ Cardiovasc Imaging*. 2014;7(6):946–953. https://doi.org/10.1161/CIRCIMAGING.114.002397.
87. Kitkungvan D, Yang EY, El Tallawi KC, et al. Extracellular volume in primary mitral regurgitation. *JACC Cardiovasc Imaging*. 2021;14(6):1146–1160. https://doi.org/10.1016/J.JCMG.2020.10.010.
88. Kitkungvan D, Yang EY, El Tallawi KC, et al. Prognostic implications of diffuse interstitial fibrosis in asymptomatic primary mitral regurgitation. *Circulation*. 2019;140(25):2122–2124. https://doi.org/10.1161/CIRCULATIONAHA.119.043250.
89. Cavalcante JL, Kusunose K, Obuchowski NA, et al. Prognostic impact of ischemic mitral regurgitation severity and myocardial infarct quantification by cardiovascular magnetic resonance. *Cardiovasc Imaging*. 2020;13(7):1489–1501. https://doi.org/10.1016/J.JCMG.2019.11.008.
90. Tayal B, Debs D, Nabi F, et al. Impact of myocardial scar on prognostic implication of secondary mitral regurgitation in heart failure. *JACC Cardiovasc Imaging*. 2021;14(4):812–822. https://doi.org/10.1016/j.jcmg.2020.11.004.
91. Kresoja KP, Rommel KP, Lücke C, et al. Right ventricular contraction patterns in patients undergoing transcatheter tricuspid valve repair for severe tricuspid regurgitation. *JACC Cardiovasc Interv*. 2021;14(14):1551–1561. https://doi.org/10.1016/J.JCIN.2021.05.005.
92. Romano S, Dell'atti D, Judd RM, et al. Prognostic value of feature-tracking right ventricular longitudinal strain in severe functional tricuspid regurgitation: a multicenter study. *JACC Cardiovasc Imaging*. 2021;14(8):1561–1568. https://doi.org/10.1016/J.JCMG.2021.02.009.

37 Pulmonary Vein Angiography and Left Atrial Fibrosis Imaging

THOMAS H. HAUSER AND DANA C. PETERS

MAGNETIC RESONANCE ANGIOGRAPHY OF THE PULMONARY VEINS AND LEFT ATRIUM

The pulmonary veins can be identified using standard anatomic and functional magnetic resonance imaging (MRI) sequences, such as cine and black-blood fast spin echo. Contrast-enhanced magnetic resonance angiography (MRA) is usually used for a volumetric 3D understanding of the intricate pulmonary venous anatomy. A 3D spoiled gradient echo sequence is acquired during the first-pass of gadolinium contrast. Clinical protocols vary but have mainly common elements.[1] The technique uses short repetition times (2–5 ms), a high flip angle (25–60 degrees), and fractional echoes, all of which provide T1 weighting and minimal flow artifacts. The spatial resolution typically ranges from 1–2 × 1–2 mm in-plane with 2–4 mm slices, before interpolation. A single 3D volume requires a 10–20 second breath-hold to suppress ventilatory motion, but scan time can be shortened using smaller fields of view, shorter repetition times, partial Fourier, lower spatial resolution, parallel imaging, or compressed sensing. Deep learning reconstructions are being tested for rapid undersampled MRA.[2] For the pulmonary veins, ECG-triggering is not employed, although it is recognized that the position and shape of the pulmonary veins changes throughout the cardiac cycle.[3] Images obtained with this ungated method appear to reflect the pulmonary veins at their maximal size.[4] Axial or coronal slabs are usually acquired using either sequential or centric k-space filling. For the pulmonary vasculature, the arterial-venous transit time is very short (4–7 seconds) and therefore artery-vein separation is highly challenging and generally not attempted. Contrast is injected at a dose of 0.1 to 0.2 mmol/kg at a rate of 1–2 mL/sec, followed by a saline flush. A precontrast mask can be acquired, although mask subtraction is not essential for pulmonary venography since the background signal in the lungs is very low. Timing of the acquisition to the first pass of contrast through the pulmonary veins is critical and is achieved using either a bolus timing scan or fluoroscopic triggering, or by acquiring two or more timeframes during the first pass to ensure acquisition during peak contrast. For all methods, optimal imaging begins with the appearance of contrast in the left atrium. Contrast agents that are either partly intravascular (e.g., gadobenate dimeglumine, gadofosveset trisodium) or fully intravascular (ferumoxytol)[5] are available to extend the duration of shortened blood T1 and improve quality, and have been studied for pulmonary MRA.[6] They will reduce the contrast between blood and scar/fibrosis if late gadolinium enhancement (LGE) is later acquired.

NONCONTRAST MAGNETIC RESONANCE ANGIOGRAPHY OF THE PULMONARY VEINS AND LEFT ATRIUM

Noncontrast methods to image the pulmonary veins are also available and can be valuable for patients in whom contrast administration is not advisable due to prior allergic reaction to MRI contrast or severe renal insufficiency. While 3D cine balanced steady state free precession (SSFP) does not visualize the left atrium and pulmonary veins well due to off-resonance and flow, *single phase* ECG-triggered and respiratory-compensated free-breathing methods can be used to image the pulmonary veins and left atrium, with balanced SSFP contrast and fat saturation to improve contrast, as is performed for coronary MRA. Additionally, an inversion recovery magnetization transfer contrast[7,8] preparation pulse improves contrast between blood and tissues by suppressing myocardium but not blood signal.

MRA has advantages compared to computed tomography angiography (CTA), in that it does not require ionizing radiation and gadolinium has a lesser risk of nephrotoxicity compared to CT contrast agents. This is especially important for congenital heart disease patients who are younger and atrial fibrillation patients who are imaged frequently. MRI also has the capability of measuring functional values, such as flows and shunt volumes, and performing tissue characterization, which CT lacks. CT is a faster examination and has superior resolution, which is not necessary for angiography but might be useful, for example, in measuring left atrial wall thickness.[9]

Magnetic Resonance Angiography of the Pulmonary Veins and Left Atrium: Image Display

Once the 3D MRA dataset is obtained, the images can be transferred to a workstation for further manipulation and analysis (Fig. 37.1). This includes dynamically viewing 2D slices within the 3D dataset in the axial, coronal, and sagittal planes. The axial images usually provide a good overview of the pulmonary veins and their relationship to the left atrium, but the coronal and sagittal images are frequently required to determine specific anatomic findings, such as a left common or anomalous pulmonary vein. Maximal intensity projection and 3D reconstructions displayed as shaded surface or volume-rendered images take full advantage of the 3D dataset and provide particularly good summary images. By convention, the left

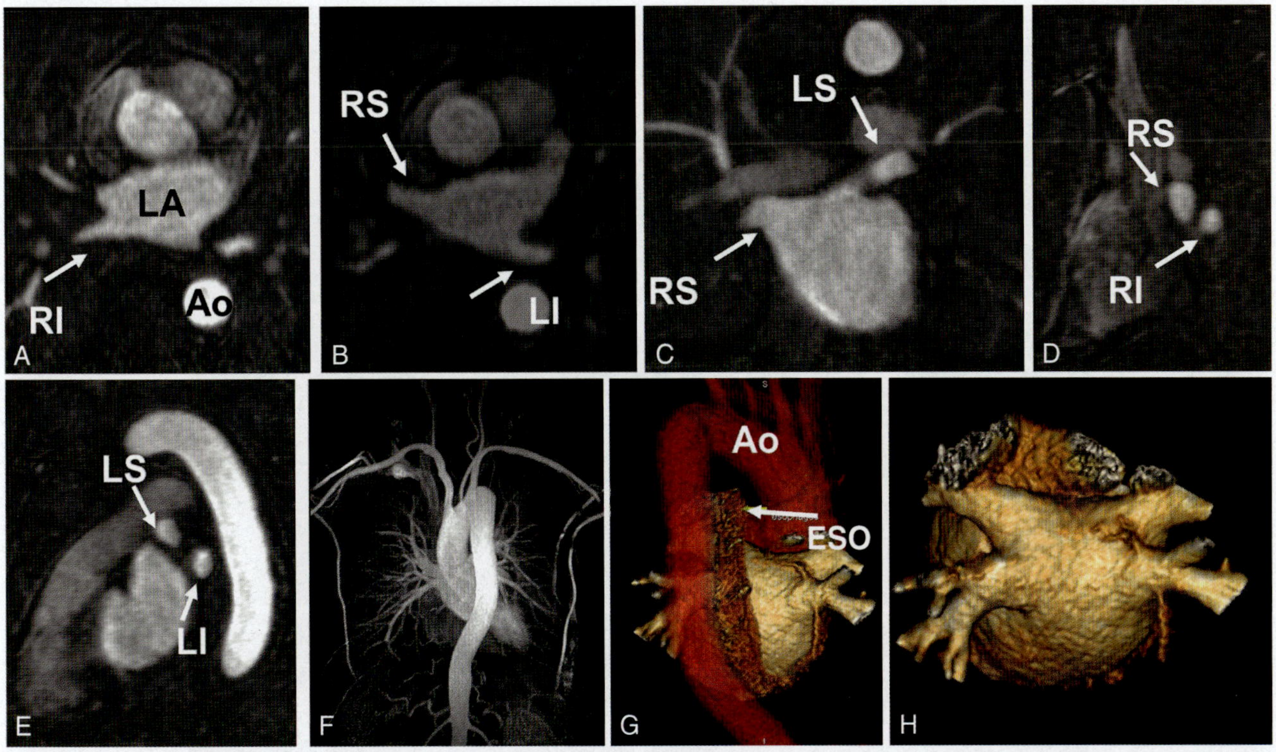

FIG. 37.1 Normal anatomy and quantification of pulmonary vein size. These images show the normal complement of four pulmonary veins, along with left atrium (*LA*) and descending aorta (*Ao*). The right inferior (*RI*), right superior (*RS*), and left inferior (*LI*) pulmonary veins are shown in the axial plane (A and B). The left superior (*LS*) and right superior pulmonary veins are shown in the coronal plane from the posterior-anterior orientation (C). The right-sided (D) and left-sided (E) pulmonary veins are shown in the sagittal plane (anterior to the left). All pulmonary veins are shown in the axial maximal intensity projection (F) and posterior-anterior volume-rendered (G–H) images. By removing the aortic and esophageal structures, the visualization is clearer (H).

atrium and pulmonary veins are viewed in the posterior-anterior orientation. Images that are 3D-rendered can also be rotated to better appreciate the anatomy. Because the aorta is directly posterior to the left-sided pulmonary vein, it frequently obscures them from view in the maximal intensity projection images and should be excluded. Direct anatomic measurements should not be obtained from these postprocessed images but from the 2D slices instead.

Normal and Variant Pulmonary Venous Anatomy

There are usually four pulmonary veins that enter the left atrium: the right superior, right inferior, left superior, and left inferior (Fig. 37.1). Each of the veins is directed laterally, with the inferior veins directed posteriorly and the superior veins directed anteriorly. The left superior pulmonary vein frequently has a cranial angulation and may appear to arise from the superior portion of the left atrium. Variant, nonpathologic pulmonary vein anatomy is very common, present in approximately 40% of patients.[10] Although numerous variations have been described, the most common variations in the usual anatomy are the presence of a single left common pulmonary vein or an additional right middle pulmonary vein (Fig. 37.2).[11] These variations occur more or less due to incorporation of the primitive common pulmonary vein into the left atrium during embryologic development (Fig. 37.3); they have not yet been identified as a cause of pathology.

Left Atrial and Left Atrial Appendage Morphology

Increased left atrial (LA) “sphericity” (how closely the left atrial shape resembles a sphere) has been demonstrated to be a marker of poor prognosis[12] related to atrial fibrillation recurrence after ablation, and more predictive than LA volume. Additionally, the left atrial appendage (LAA) morphology may help risk stratify patients for thromboembolic events,[13] with “chicken wing” morphologies predicting fewer events. MRA can also be used in preprocedural planning for percutaneous closure of the LAA[14] and in detecting LAA thrombus.[15] Beyond these applications, left atrial volume, ejection fraction, and strain are important early indicators of subclinical heart failure, as described in Chapter 20.

CONGENITAL PULMONARY VENOUS ANOMALIES

Imaging has an important role in the evaluation of congenital pulmonary venous anomalies.[16] Congenital pulmonary venous anomalies account for up to 3% of all congenital heart disease and approximately 2% of all deaths from congenital heart disease in the first year of life.[17] The congenital anomalies that affect pulmonary veins are atresia, stenosis, and anomalous connections, which can be total or partial. These conditions occur when the normal connections of the primitive pulmonary venous system form abnormally or if embryologic connections to the

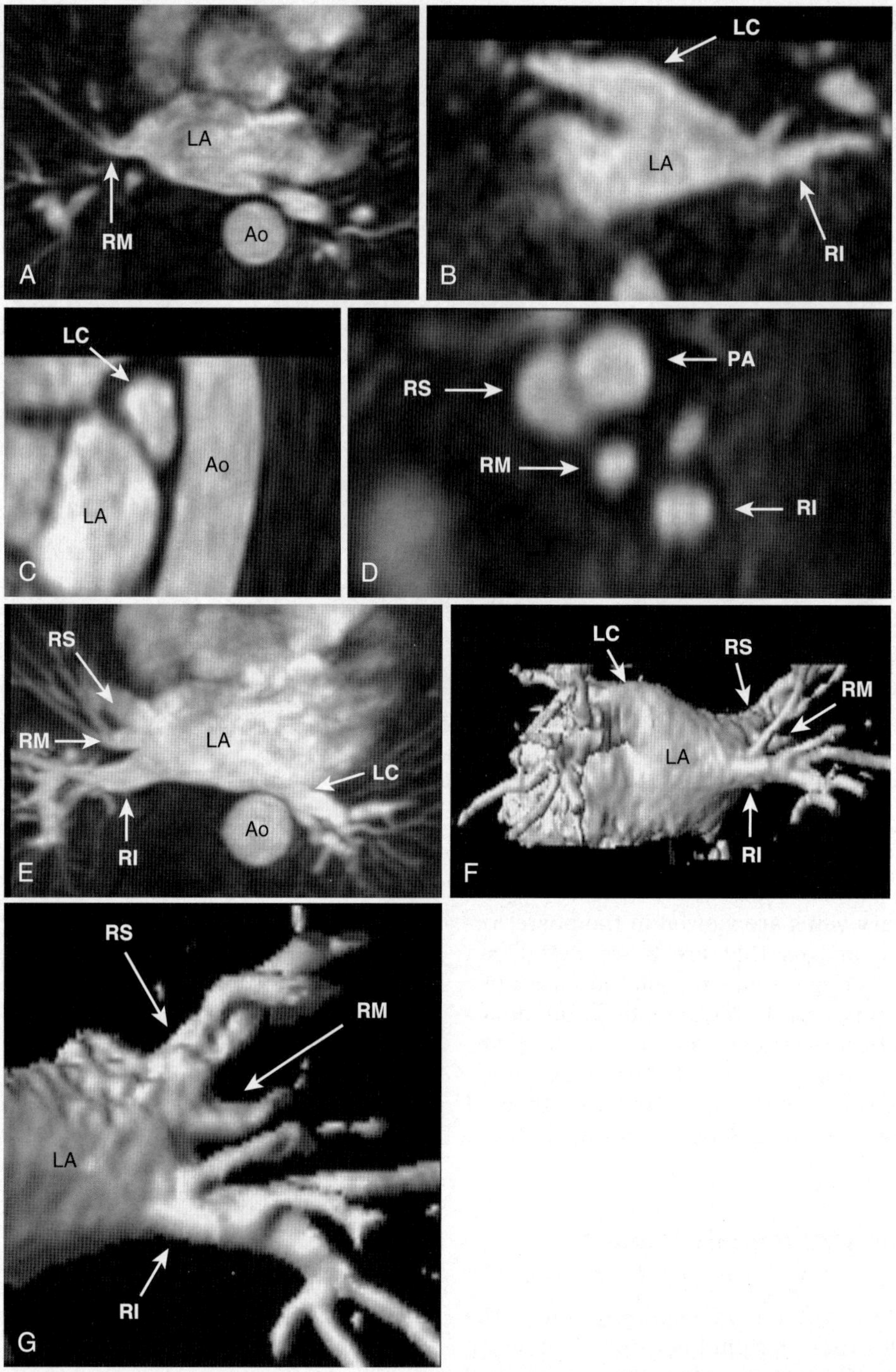

FIG. 37.2 Variant pulmonary venous anatomy. These images were obtained from a patient with right middle and left common pulmonary veins. The right middle (*RM*) pulmonary vein is shown in the axial plane (A). The left common (*LC*) pulmonary vein is shown in the coronal plane from the posterior-anterior orientation (B). The single left common (C) and all three right pulmonary veins (D) are shown in the sagittal plane (anterior to the left) along with the pulmonary artery (*PA*) immediately adjacent to the right superior pulmonary vein. All of the pulmonary veins are shown in the axial maximal intensity projection (E) and posterior-anterior volume-rendered (F) images. The aorta has been removed from the volume-rendered image. The right middle pulmonary vein is obscured by the right inferior pulmonary vein and is best seen with cranial angulation (G). It is frequently necessary to manipulate the point of view to see all of the pulmonary veins.

cardinal vein or umbilicovitelline systems persist, and are frequently associated with other major congenital cardiac anomalies.[18]

Anomalous pulmonary venous connections are the most common congenital anomaly.[17] In total anomalous pulmonary venous connection, there is no connection of the pulmonary veins to the left atrium such that all of the pulmonary venous drainage enters the right atrium directly or via a systemic vein. This anomaly is necessarily associated with an atrial right-to-left shunt. Pulmonary venous hypertension is common due to twists in the artery or compression from adjacent vascular structures,[19] while small atrial septal defects restrict systemic blood flow.[20] These conditions results in cyanosis and congestive heart failure. Although the mortality rate for symptomatic infants is 80% at 1 year,[17] surgical repair is usually feasible and reduced the mortality rate in one study to 14%.[21] MRI has a role in the evaluation[22] and is

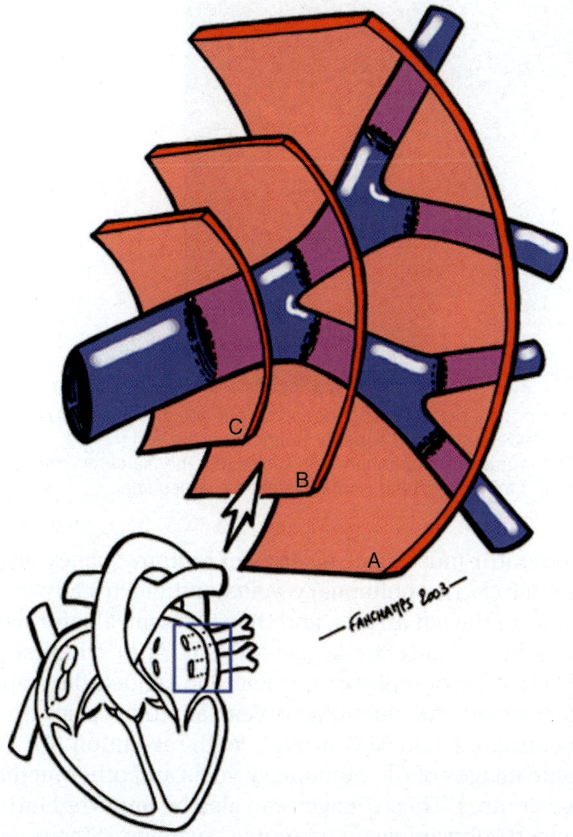

FIG. 37.3 Incorporation of the primitive common pulmonary vein into the left atrium. The incorporation of the primitive common pulmonary vein is variable and results in nonpathological variations in the normal anatomy. The most common pattern is two left-sided pulmonary veins (plane B). With less incorporation of the common pulmonary vein into the left atrium, there is only a single left common pulmonary vein (plane C). With more incorporation, there are additional pulmonary veins (plane A). (From Haissaguerre M, Jais P, Shah DC, et al. Spontaneous initiation of atrial fibrillation by ectopic beats originating in the pulmonary veins. *N Engl J Med.* 1998;339(10):659–666.)

superior to CT because it can quantify shunt fraction and does not use ionizing radiation. In partial anomalous pulmonary venous return, one or more pulmonary veins, but not all, enter the right atrium or a systemic vein. The physiology of this anomaly is similar to that of an atrial septal defect and depends on the magnitude of the left-to-right shunt and the presence of increased pulmonary vascular resistance.[18] Patients are often asymptomatic if the shunt is relatively small and the pulmonary vascular resistance is normal, and the diagnosis may not be made until adulthood. The scimitar syndrome, named after the characteristic chest radiograph finding, is a specific form of partial anomalous pulmonary venous connection in which all of the venous drainage from the right lung enters the inferior vena cava (Fig. 37.4). This rare syndrome is also associated with anomalous arterial supply of the right lower lobe from the aorta, dextroposition of the heart, and hypoplasia of the right lung.[23]

Congenital pulmonary vein atresia is defined as the absence of any connection of the pulmonary veins to either the left atrium or any other vascular structure. This is a very rare condition that is not compatible with life, although infants may survive for a short period of time due to small connections between the pulmonary veins and esophageal or brachial veins.[18]

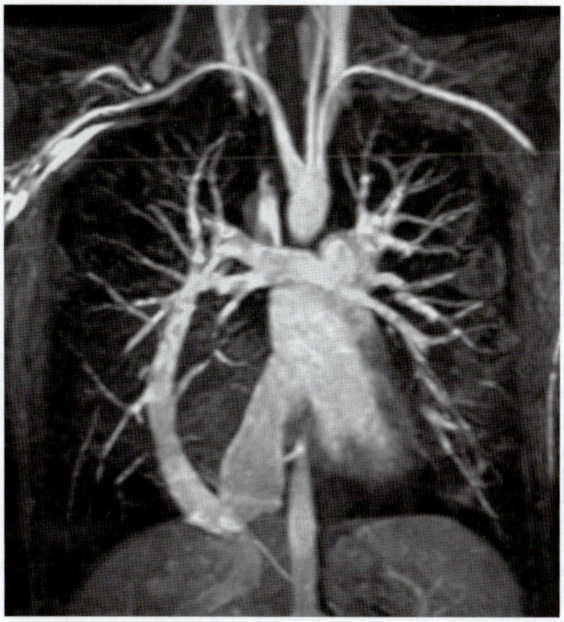

FIG. 37.4 Scimitar syndrome. This coronal maximal intensity projection image in the anterior-posterior orientation shows the typical findings of the scimitar syndrome. The single right pulmonary vein (RPV) enters the inferior vena cava (IVC). The right atrium (RA) and descending aorta (AoD) are also shown. (From Greil GF, Powell AJ, Gildein HP, Geva T. Gadolinium-enhanced three-dimensional magnetic resonance angiography of pulmonary and systemic venous anomalies. *J Am Coll Cardiol.* 2002 Jan 16;39(2):335–41. https://doi.org/10.1016/s0735-1097(01)01730-2. PMID: 11788228.)

Congenital pulmonary vein stenosis can involve a focal segment of one or more pulmonary veins or more diffusely involve an entire pulmonary vein and is usually associated with other congenital cardiac malformations. Severe stenosis frequently results in cyanosis, congestive heart failure, and death, although surgical repair is possible if only focal stenosis is present.[18]

PULMONARY VEINS AND THE PATHOPHYSIOLOGY OF ATRIAL FIBRILLATION

Atrial fibrillation is the most common sustained cardiac arrhythmia and is a global epidemic affecting more than 33 million people.[24] Atrial fibrillation affects more than 6 million people in the United States, a figure that is expected to increase to 12 million by 2030, and is a major cause of morbidity and mortality, accounting for more than 400,000 hospitalizations each year[25] in the United States and increasing the risk of death by 40% to 90%, with a higher risk for females. Atrial fibrillation increases the risk of stroke by 400% 500%, with twice the risk of stroke in females compared to males.[25] The costs associated with the treatment of atrial fibrillation was estimated at more than $28 billion in 2016 in the United States alone.[25]

Evidence has shown that the pulmonary veins play a critical role in the pathophysiology of atrial fibrillation.[26] The pulmonary veins and left atrium are both derived from the primitive common pulmonary vein and therefore both have smooth-walled electrically active myocardium.[27] Myocardium in the pulmonary veins is frequently discontinuous and fibrotic. Proarrhythmic reentrant beats and sustained focal activity can be easily induced.[28] Radiofrequency

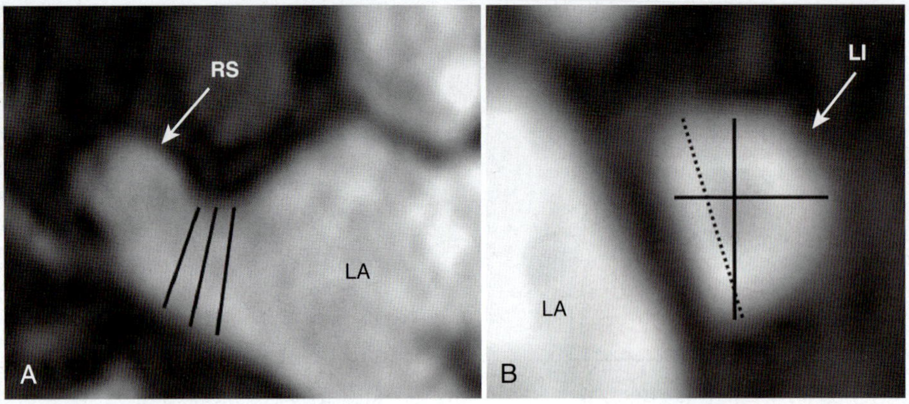

FIG. 37.5 Difficulty in measurement of pulmonary vein diameters. These images show a right superior (RS) pulmonary vein in the axial plane (A) and a left inferior (LI) pulmonary vein in the sagittal plane (B). There is no clear anatomic border between the right superior pulmonary vein and the left atrium (LA) (A) such that several potential diameter measurements are possible (*solid lines*). The left inferior (LI) pulmonary vein is oval (B). The diameters measured in the axial plane (*horizontal line*) and coronal plane (*vertical line*) differ from each other and from the true maximal diameter (*dashed line*).

ablation of these foci can result in complete suppression of atrial fibrillation in a majority of patients.

The mechanisms that sustain atrial fibrillation are still not known. Proposed mechanisms include triggers and an abnormal left atrial substrate. Triggers potentially include regions with ectopic electrical activity or atrial rotors. The presence of an enlarged left atrium, by itself and with associated electrical, metabolic, and structural remodeling (e.g., fibrosis),[29,30] comprise the abnormal substrate that may sustain atrial fibrillation.

Based on these early studies,[26] several related procedures were developed for the treatment of atrial fibrillation, usually involving encircling the pulmonary veins with ablation lesions. These procedures use radiofrequency ablation to electrically isolate the pulmonary veins from the left atrium, with or without additional ablation within the left atrium. Cryoablation is also used for pulmonary vein isolation.[31] While the CABANA trial showed that ablation does not reduce mortality or morbidity[32] compared to medical therapy (except for those with heart failure[33,34]), multiple studies have consistently shown a reduced recurrence of atrial fibrillation and significant symptomatic improvement after ablation.[35] The EAST-AFNET4 study showed a significant reduction in adverse cardiovascular events with early rhythm control (including atrial fibrillation ablation) in patients with new-onset atrial fibrillation.[36] Recent guidelines now recommend atrial fibrillation ablation for many patients with atrial fibrillation, including first-line therapy in younger patients with symptomatic paroxysmal atrial fibrillation.[35]

IMAGING BEFORE AND AFTER ATRIAL FIBRILLATION ABLATION

Imaging can be performed before atrial fibrillation ablation to determine the pulmonary vein anatomy. Important aspects include the size of the left atrium, number of PVs, the ostial sizes, the presence of venous variants, evaluation of the foramen ovale, and identification of the presence of a lipomatous atrial septum.[37] The accurate determination of pulmonary vein anatomy is valuable for the planning and execution of atrial fibrillation ablation. To achieve success, the operator must place a series of radiofrequency lesions that encircle the pulmonary veins and electrically isolate them from the left atrium, and thus anatomical information is valuable.[38] Centers can use MRA, CTA, or transesophageal echocardiography or intracardiac echocardiography[39] to determine the pulmonary vein anatomy prior to the procedure. CT and MRI provide high-resolution 3D tomographic images of the pulmonary veins and other mediastinal structures. These images can also be imported into the 3D electrophysiological mapping systems. Single-center experience with image integration has been associated with shorter procedure times and improved outcome after ablation for atrial fibrillation,[40] but randomized trials and a subsequent meta-analysis showed no benefit.[41] The accurate measurement of pulmonary vein size is needed for preprocedural planning. Most investigators have measured pulmonary vein diameters in a specified plane, usually at the ostia. These measurements tend to have poor reproducibility (Fig. 37.5) because there is no clear anatomic border between them, the pulmonary vein ostia are not round,[10,42] and there are variations over the cardiac cycle.[43] A simple method for determining pulmonary vein size in the sagittal plane is highly reproducible (Fig. 37.1).[42]

It is also important to identify the relationship of the pulmonary veins to other mediastinal structures to avoid complications from the procedure. This includes the esophagus to avoid atrial-esophageal fistula, a rare (<0.25% of procedures) but catastrophic complication caused by excessive heating of the left atrial wall and the adjacent esophagus (Fig. 37.6).[44] Indeed, the esophagus often appears enhanced on postablation LGE, even in the absence of symptoms.[45] The esophagus and its relationship to the left atrium can be readily identified on standard anatomic MRI sequences and on LGE. The esophagus is usually closer to the left-sided pulmonary veins, but the location is highly variable[46–48] and is mobile even during the procedure.[49]

The pulmonary veins can be imaged after the procedure to screen for pulmonary vein stenosis caused by the ablation, although this is not commonly performed. Pulmonary vein stenosis is an uncommon but severe complication of atrial fibrillation ablation (Fig. 37.7). Severe stenosis was found by careful surveillance to occur in 0.5% of patients

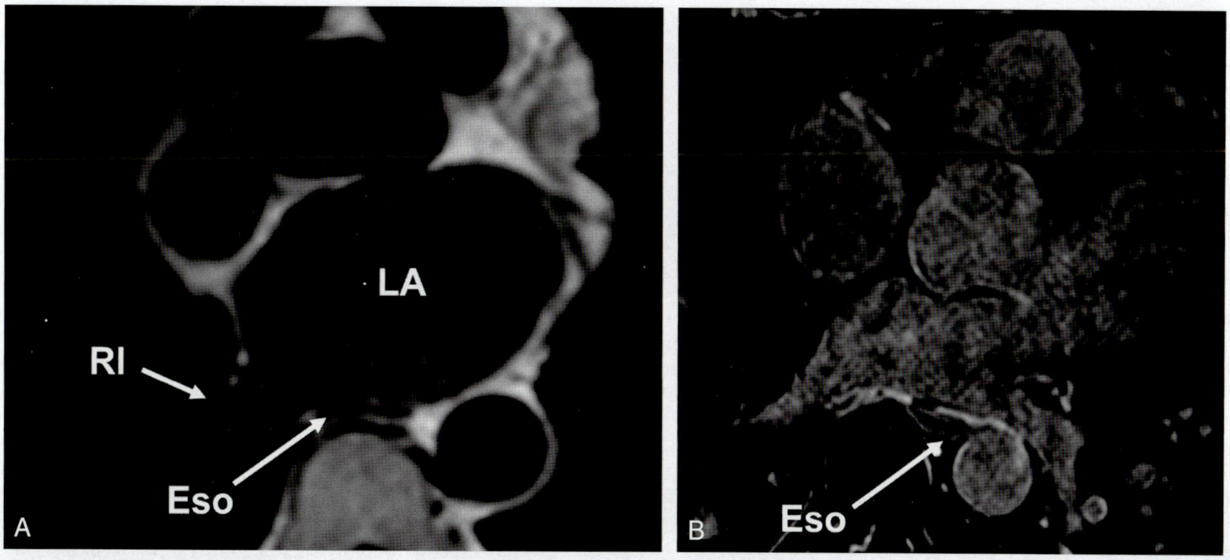

FIG. 37.6 Anatomic relationship of the esophagus to the pulmonary veins and left atrium (LA). (A) This T1-weighted black-blood fast spin echo image shows the esophagus (*Eso*) immediately posterior to the left atrium and adjacent to the right inferior pulmonary vein. The esophagus is compressed between the enlarged left atrium and spinal column. (B) In a different subject, postablation late gadolinium enhancement image also shows the esophagus, adjacent to a region of ablation. *LI*, left inferior pulmonary vein; *RI*, right inferior pulmonary vein.

following ablation in a large study,[50] but was more common with earlier ablation techniques that placed ablations further into the pulmonary vein trunk.[51–53] Mild stenosis still commonly occurs.

Late Gadolinium Enhancement of the Left Atrium and Pulmonary Veins

Fibrosis and ablation scar imaging using LGE has the potential to noninvasively assess both the extent of left atrial remodeling (fibrosis) associated with atrial fibrillation, and the completeness of ablation lines after pulmonary vein isolation. LGE may have applications in both risk stratifying patients for ablation and in periprocedural or real-time guidance of an ablation to ensure minimal gaps. A modified LGE technique[54] is used for atrial imaging: a T1-weighted inversion recovery gradient echo sequence with imaging acquired 15 to 30 minutes after the injection of gadolinium contrast.[55] To detect scar in the left atrium, the LGE method is modified to include fat suppression (since the atrium is covered in fat, Fig. 37.5A), and to achieve higher spatial resolution ($1.3 \times 1.3 \times 3\text{–}5\,mm^3$) by acquiring a 3D volume during free breathing with ventilatory motion–compensated imaging (Fig. 37.8).[56] Fig. 37.9 describes potential pitfalls in atrial LGE imaging, including the importance of fat suppression (requires centric acquisition), TI choice, phase-encoding direction choice (should be right left), and the appearance of artifacts due to poor fat suppression and arrhythmia. A recent study[57] regarding optimization of 3D LGE found that 4mm is an optimal slice thickness, 1.5T outperformed 3.0T, and imaging later postinjection (20 to 30 minutes) provided better quality. Recent improvements in atrial LGE have included increased spatial resolution and acceleration,[58,59] and dark-blood LGE[60,61] to achieve dark-blood contrast. Theoretically, dark-blood LGE is important, delineating diffuse fibrosis on the LA wall from blood pool. However, its capability has not been fully demonstrated. Another improvement uses Dixon LGE to obtain fat-water–separated images, which also permits noncentric acquisition order[62,63] and more effective fat saturation for improved LGE quality. With all of these improvements as well as better motion compensation, the 3D LGE image quality still ranges from excellent to mediocre, and an approach that provides consistently high quality 3D LA LGE is needed.

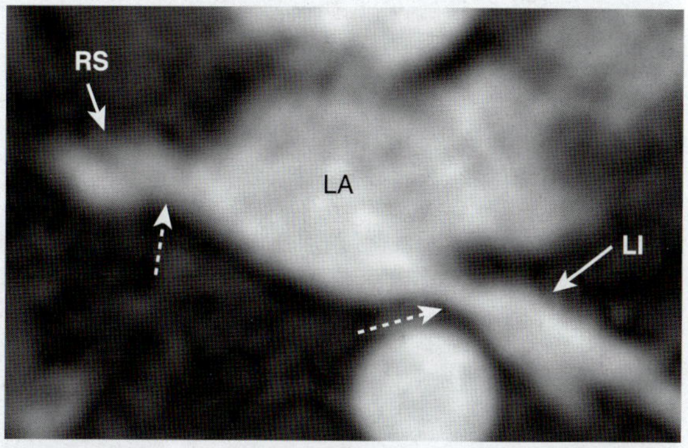

FIG. 37.7 Pulmonary vein stenosis. There is severe stenosis of the left inferior (LI) pulmonary vein and moderate stenosis of the right superior (RS) pulmonary vein, indicated by the *dashed arrows*. There is pre-stenotic dilation of the left inferior pulmonary vein. *LA,* left atrium.

Scar and Fibrosis Measurement

Like LGE in the left ventricle, scar can be segmented by carefully drawn region of interest (ROIs) and thresholding (Fig. 37.10). First, a blood pool ROI and atrial wall ROI are constructed, from which scar is segmented using a threshold. Fibrosis extent is measured by segmenting the LGE-enhanced atrial myocardium volume, and normalizing it by the total atrial myocardial volume, which is approximately equal to the atrial wall surface area × 2 mm (mean atrial wall thickness).[64] Such segmentations can be visualized in 3D, and the percentage of the wall that is enhanced can be quantified. This type of analysis is time intensive and has moderate reproducibility.[65] The concept of normalizing the volume of scar or fibrosis by the left

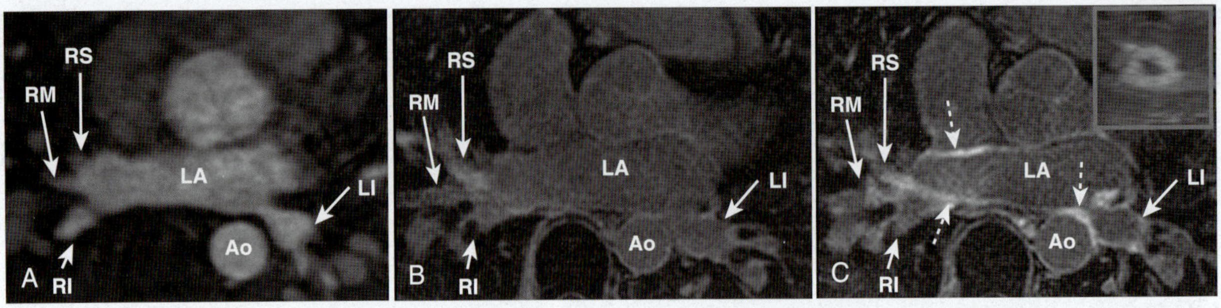

FIG. 37.8 Late gadolinium enhancement imaging. These images show the pulmonary vein anatomy (A) in a patient who underwent delayed enhancement imaging before (B) and 6 weeks after (C) atrial fibrillation ablation. There is variant anatomy with an additional right middle (RM) pulmonary vein (A). Prior to ablation (B) there is no delayed enhancement of the pulmonary veins. There is increased signal in the right superior (RS) and right middle pulmonary veins due to artifact from the ventilatory compensation technique. After ablation (C) there is evidence of pulmonary vein scar (*dashed arrows*). The inset shows a reformatted image of the left inferior (LI) pulmonary vein that shows circumferential scar. *LA*, left atrium; *Ao*, aorta.

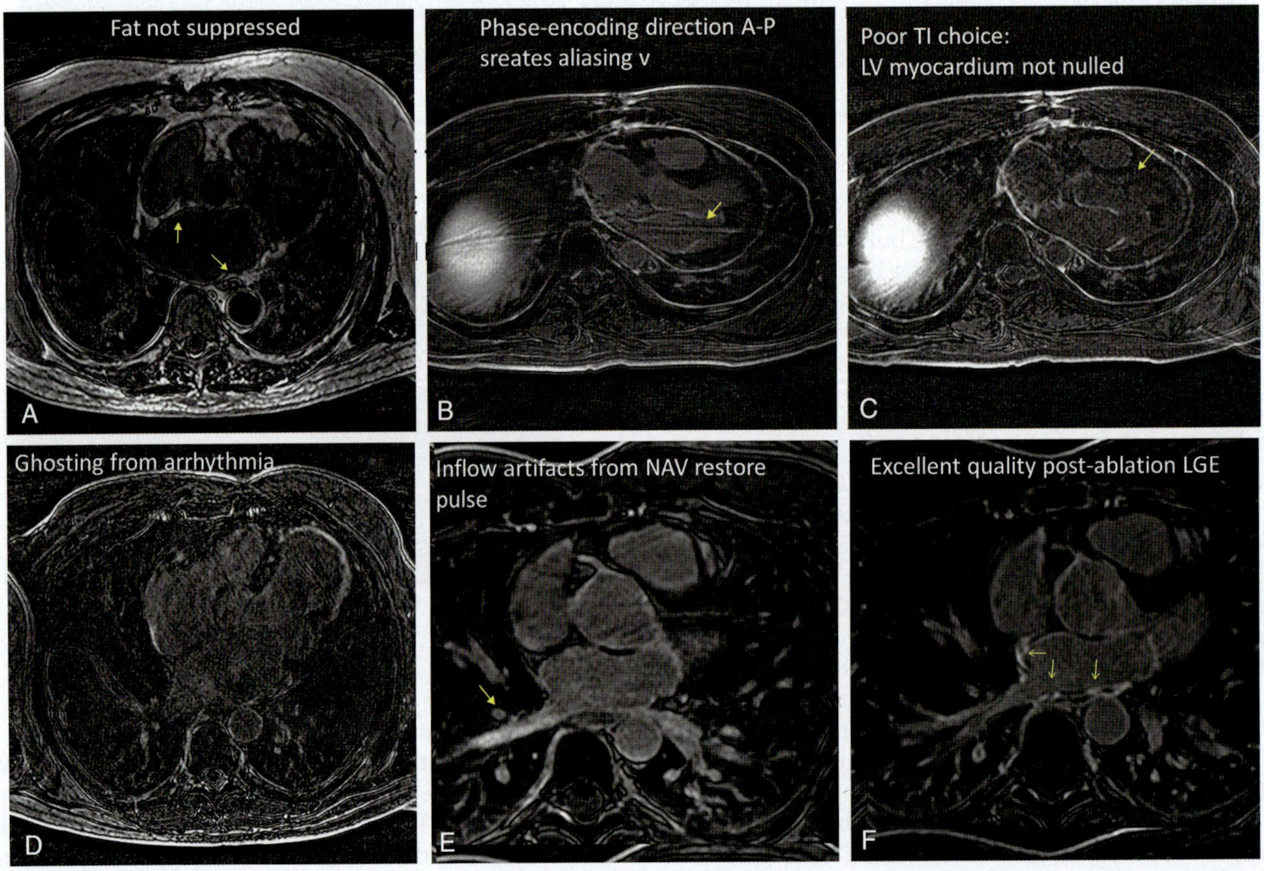

FIG. 37.9 Examples of late gadolinium enhancement (*LGE*) imaging atrial fibrosis and scar. (A–E) Preablation LGE. (A) Poor fat suppression (see *arrows*) with poor *TI* choice, which nulls blood. The fat that surrounds the left atrium is visible. (B) Phase-encoding direction should be right-left. *Arrows* show respiratory motion artifact. (C) The same subject and slice as in (B), except phase-encoding direction is now right-left instead of anterior-posterior (AP); the TI was too short so the left ventricle (LV) is not nulled. (D) Patient with arrhythmia, showing ghosted, poor quality images. (E) Good quality image, with inflow artifact in the right inferior pulmonary vein (*arrow*). This can be reduced using a navigator (NAV) pulse at the end of the data acquisition. (F). Excellent quality postablation image, with evident scar (*arrows*).

atrial myocardial volume, while scientifically rigorous and commonly employed, is in some sense counterproductive, since these two metrics themselves are known to vary in a positive linear fashion (large left atria have more fibrosis). The choice of a signal threshold for atrial fibrosis and scar determines the sensitivity and specificity of method. Often the threshold is defined by signal-to-blood contrast to noise ratio (CNR) (CNR >2 to 3, with standard deviation [SD] measured in the blood pool[66]) or by signal-to-blood intensity ratio (IIR) of 1.2 to 1.5. Using an IIR threshold instead of a CNR threshold has value since it is less sensitive to the underlying blood SNR of the scan. However, if a specific IIR corresponds to a low CNR (enhanced signal to blood), the result is that many pixels isointense with blood will be inadvertently classified as scar (low specificity). Therefore, when choosing an IIR threshold, the corresponding CNR must be considered. A low IIR/CNR (e.g., IIR of 1.2), which is advocated to best identify low voltage regions,[67] may be more sensitive but less specific and likely less accurate than a higher IIR. For identifying enhanced pixels, some have advocated Otsu thresholding.[68] It is known that the optimal choice of threshold (IIR or CNR based)

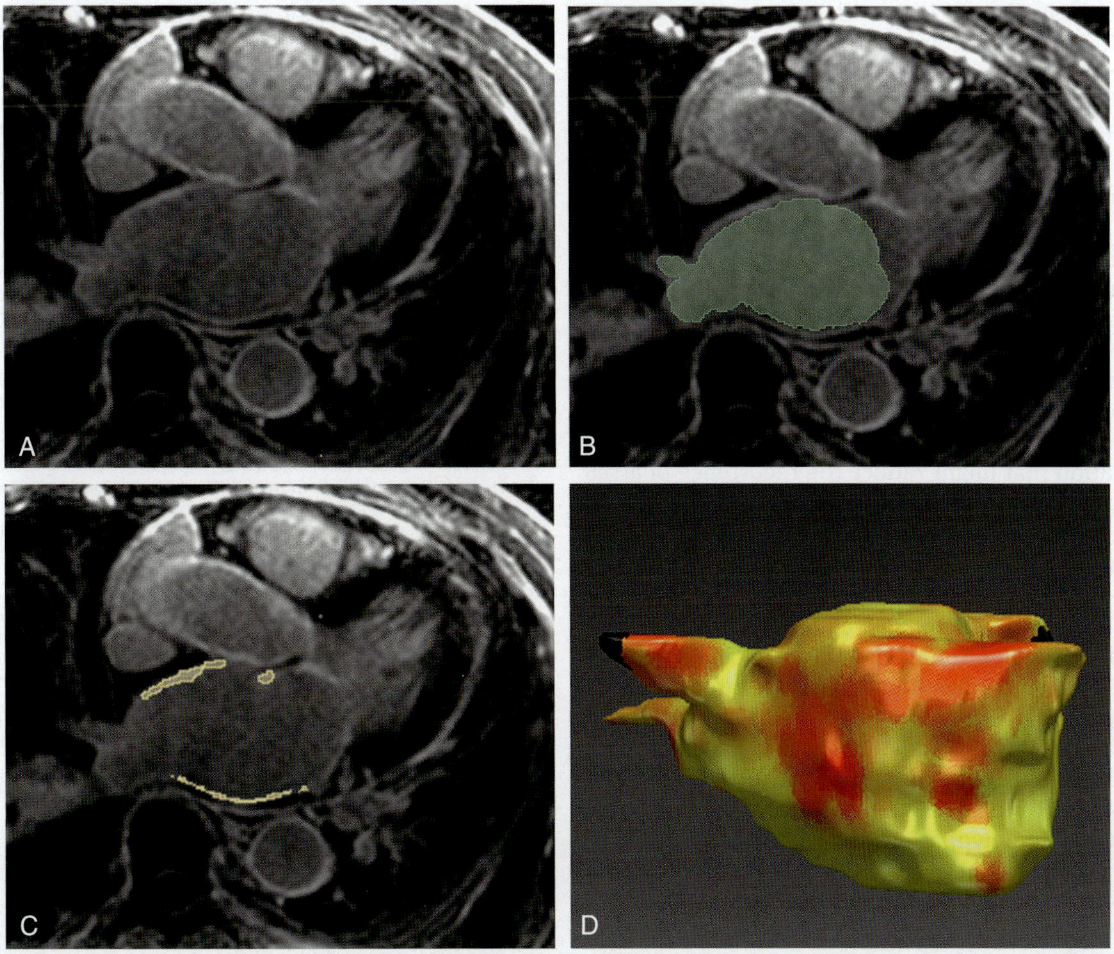

FIG. 37.10 Segmenting fibrosis or scar from the left atrial (LA) late gadolinium enhancement (LGE). (A) A patient presenting with myocarditis exhibits extensive atrial LGE. (B) The LA cavity is segmented. The LA myocardial wall is considered to consist of a thin (~2 mm) perimeter surrounding the LA cavity. (C) The enhanced signal, based on thresholding, within the LA wall is identified as fibrosis or scar. Careful attention is needed to avoid including enhancement from the mitral valve and aorta. After segmenting the LA wall and scar/fibrosis in each slice, the percentage of the atrial wall that is enhanced can be measured. (D) Here, a maximum intensity projection of the highest signal within the atrial wall is displayed by volume-rendering using CemrgApp.[73] (With help of Steven Williams and Irun Kotadia). Razeghi O, Sim I, Roney CH, et al. Fully Automatic Atrial Fibrosis Assessment Using a Multilabel Convolutional Neural Network *Circ Cardiovasc Imaging*. 2020;13(12):e011512 www.cemrgapp.com.)

depends on the time postinjection, and using the same IIR or CNR will provide a different scar volume depending on time postinjection.[57,69] Preprocessing of the LGE volume is valuable to remove surface coil–induced signal variations that prevent use of a single threshold value. This sometimes can be performed within the pulse sequence.

Automated segmentation is also possible, with many tools developed. These generally include traditional or deep learning segmentation of the left atrial cavity[70–72] followed by defining the atrial wall as a thin perimeter (e.g., 2 mm) around the cavity. Then a threshold is chosen and segmentation is performed. Commercial products for atrial segmentation include Galgo Medical's Adas3D and Marrek (Merisight), and other methods are freely available,[70,73] some now interactive, e.g. in ITKSNAP, based on nnU-net. The deep learning methods have shown excellent results—and many are available and include training sets– but might be less accurate for out-of-domain data sets. Challenges exist for atrial LGE segmentation, with no consistent practice regarding inclusion or exclusion of pulmonary vein sleeves or optimal threshold choice for LGE, and there is not uncommonly inadvertent inclusion of enhanced mitral valve and aortic structures in publications.

Postablation Assessments of Atrial Scar

Radiofrequency ablation for the treatment of atrial fibrillation results in scarring of the pulmonary vein and left atrium.[74] Several studies have found increased ablation scar or an increased number of fully ablated veins in subjects without recurrence.[75,76] Other groups have worked toward the goal of identifying gaps in the ablation lines around individual pulmonary veins using LGE, with mixed success. In studies of patients undergoing repeat ablations, some studies found no correlation between sites of electrical reconnection and minimal ablation-induced LGE[77,78] while others found a relationship. Likely, improved LGE quality and interpretation is required before LGE can guide reablation. MRI to guide ablation in real time has employed both T2- or T1-weighted images[79] and LGE.

Atrial Fibrosis by Late Gadolinium Enhancement to Predict Atrial Fibrillation Recurrence Postablation

It has long been known by pathology that patients with atrial fibrillation have fibrotic atria.[80] A series of studies beginning with Oakes et al.[30,66] have developed evidence for the hypothesis that patients with more significant atrial fibrosis prior to ablation are more prone to atrial fibrillation recurrence after ablation. The DECAAF I trial, a large multicenter study,[81] used careful monitoring of recurrence post-PVI and classified fibrosis extent into four categories. Few (15%) patients with the least fibrosis and many (51%) patients with the most fibrosis had atrial fibrillation recurrence. The majority of studies linking recurrence and pre-procedural atrial LGE are from a single group. Finally, it is critical to note that atrial fibrosis imaging by LGE has not yet been correlated with pathology due to a lack of animal models of atrial fibrosis, although these models are in development.[82]

The subsequent DECAAF II[83] trial attempted to build on the results of DECAAF I by targeting regions of fibrosis for further ablation that might reduce the recurrence of atrial fibrillation, but no additional benefit was observed.

Furthermore, effort has been made to correlate LA voltage mapping with fibrosis, with the goal of establishing one-to-one correspondence between low voltage and LA enhancement as a surrogate validation. These studies find decreased bipolar voltage in regions of LGE enhancement.[66,67,77,84] These studies found LGE vs. voltage correlations ranging from strong to weak and were mainly in mixed pre and post-PVI populations.

Importantly, patients with other cardiovascular diseases (beyond AF) also exhibit atrial fibrosis, including hypertrophic cardiomyopathy,[85] amyloid,[86] and others.[87,88] Recently it has been observed that atrial fibrosis is a predictor for the development of new atrial arrythmias[87] and a greater burden of arrhythmia, even using rigorous loop recorders to define arrhythmias.[89] Greater atrial LGE is found in patients with embolic strokes of undetermined source.[90] This type of evidence and more has led to the concept of an atrial myopathy (electrical and structural remodeling of the atrium) independent of AF.[91]

Controversy and skepticism exist regarding the accuracy of atrial LGE, partly due to the challenges of obtaining good quality atrial fibrosis images and the correct observation that the walls of major arteries and valvular apparatus enhance on LA LGE, which makes the enhancement seem nonspecific. These structures contain elastin and collagen and thus do exhibit LGE enhancement at high resolution. Skepticism is partly warranted due to the lack of validation using an animal model. However, data in humans show that LA LGE correlates with voltage mapping, age, LA volumes, LA strain, and LA function and predicts AF recurrence after ablation and new onset of arrythmia, which is increased in specific cardiomyopathies and clinical conditions. Nevertheless, greater accuracy (sensitivity and specificity to the presence of fibrosis in left atrial myocardium) is still needed.

REFERENCES

1. Schonberger M, Usman A, Galizia M, Popescu A, Collins J, Carr JC. Time-resolved MR venography of the pulmonary veins precatheter-based ablation for atrial fibrillation. *J Magn Reson Imaging*. 2013;37(1):127–137.
2. Haji-Valizadeh H, Shen D, Avery RJ, et al. Rapid reconstruction of four-dimensional MR angiography of the thoracic aorta using a convolutional neural network. *Radiol Cardiothorac Imaging*. 2020;2(3):e190205.
3. Lickfett L, Dickfeld T, Kato R, et al. Changes of pulmonary vein orifice size and location throughout the cardiac cycle: dynamic analysis using magnetic resonance cine imaging. *J Cardiovasc Electrophysiol*. 2005;16(6):582–588.
4. Hauser TH, Yeon SB, Kissinger KV, Josephson ME, Manning WJ. Variation in pulmonary vein size during the cardiac cycle: implications for non-electrocardiogram-gated imaging. *Am Heart J*. 2006;152(5):974.e1–974.e6. https://doi.org/10.1016/j.ahj.2006.05.018. PMID: 17070170.
5. Camren GP, Wilson GJ, Bamra VR, Nguyen KQ, Hippe DS, Maki JH. A comparison between gadofosveset trisodium and gadobenate dimeglumine for steady state MRA of the thoracic vasculature. *Biomed Res Int*. 2014;2014:625614.
6. Knobloch G, Colgan T, Schiebler ML, et al. Comparison of gadolinium-enhanced and ferumoxytol-enhanced conventional and UTE-MRA for the depiction of the pulmonary vasculature. *Magn Reson Med*. 2019;82(5):1660–1670.
7. Ginami G, Lopez K, Mukherjee RK, et al. Non-contrast enhanced simultaneous 3D whole-heart bright-blood pulmonary veins visualization and black-blood quantification of atrial wall thickness. *Magn Reson Med*. 2019;81(2):1066–1079.
8. Dohy Z, Kiss M, Suhai FI, et al. Feasibility and image quality of bright-blood and black-blood phase-sensitive inversion recovery (BOOST) sequence in clinical practice using for left atrial visualization in patients with atrial fibrillation. *Eur Radiol*. 2023;34(4):2689–2698.
9. Karim R, Blake LE, Inoue J, et al. Algorithms for left atrial wall segmentation and thickness—evaluation on an open-source CT and MRI image database. *Med Image Anal*. 2018;50:36–53.
10. Wittkampf FH, Vonken EJ, Derksen R, et al. Pulmonary vein ostium geometry: analysis by magnetic resonance angiography. *Circulation*. 2003;107(1):21–23.
11. Hassani C, Saremi F. Comprehensive cross-sectional imaging of the pulmonary veins. *Radiographics*. 2017;37(7):1928–1954.
12. Bisbal F, Alarcon F, Ferrero-de-Loma-Osorio A, et al. Left atrial geometry and outcome of atrial fibrillation ablation: results from the multicentre LAGO-AF study. *Eur Heart J Cardiovasc Imaging*. 2018;19(9):1002–1009.
13. Lupercio F, Carlos Ruiz J, Briceno DF, et al. Left atrial appendage morphology assessment for risk stratification of embolic stroke in patients with atrial fibrillation: a meta-analysis. *Heart Rhythm*. 2016;13(7):1402–1409.
14. Bertsche D, Metze P, Luo E, et al. Cardiac magnetic resonance imaging for preprocedural planning of percutaneous left atrial appendage closure. *Front Cardiovasc Med*. 2023;10:1132626.
15. Kitkungvan D, Nabi F, Ghosn MG, et al. Detection of LA and LAA thrombus by CMR in patients referred for pulmonary vein isolation. *JACC Cardiovasc Imaging*. 2016;9(7):809–818.
16. Dillman JR, Yarram SG, Hernandez RJ. Imaging of pulmonary venous developmental anomalies. *AJR Am J Roentgenol*. 2009;192(5):1272–1285.
17. Krabill KA, Lucas RV. Abnormal pulmonary venous connections. In: Emmanouilides GC, Riemenschneider TA, Allen HD, et al, eds. *Moss and Adams' Heart Disease in Infants, Children and Adolescents*. 5th ed. Williams and Wilkins; 1995:838.
18. Friedman WF, Silverman N. Congenital heart disease in infancy and childhood. In: Braunwald E, Zipes DP, Libby P, eds. *Heart Disease*. 6th ed. W. B. Saunders Company; 2001:1552.
19. Wang JK, Lue HC, Wu MH, Young ML, Wu FF, Wu JM. Obstructed total anomalous pulmonary venous connection. *Pediatr Cardiol*. 1993;14(1):28–32.
20. Ward KE, Mullins CE, Huhta JC, Nihill MR, McNamara DG, Cooley DA. Restrictive interatrial communication in total anomalous pulmonary venous connection. *Am J Cardiol*. 1986;57(13):1131–1136.
21. Husain SA, Maldonado E, Rasch D, et al. Total anomalous pulmonary venous connection: factors associated with mortality and recurrent pulmonary venous obstruction. *Ann Thorac Surg*. 2012;94(3):825–831; discussion 831-822.
22. Robinson BL, Kwong RY, Varma PK, Wolfe M, Couper G. Magnetic resonance imaging of complex partial anomalous pulmonary venous return in adults. *Circulation*. 2014;129(1):e1–e2.
23. Gao YA, Burrows PE, Benson LN, Rabinovitch M, Freedom RM. Scimitar syndrome in infancy. *J Am Coll Cardiol*. 1993;22(3):873–882.
24. Linz D, Gawalko M, Betz K, et al. Atrial fibrillation: epidemiology, screening and digital health. *Lancet Reg Health Eur*. 2024;37:100786.
25. Martin SS, Aday AW, Almarzooq ZI, et al. 2024 Heart disease and stroke statistics: a report of US and global data from the American heart association. *Circulation*. 2024;149(8):e347–e913.
26. Haissaguerre M, Jais P, Shah DC, et al. Spontaneous initiation of atrial fibrillation by ectopic beats originating in the pulmonary veins. *N Engl J Med*. 1998;339(10):659–666.
27. Hassink RJ, Aretz HT, Ruskin J, Keane D. Morphology of atrial myocardium in human pulmonary veins: a postmortem analysis in patients with and without atrial fibrillation. *J Am Coll Cardiol*. 2003;42(6):1108–1114.
28. Arora R, Verheule S, Scott L, et al. Arrhythmogenic substrate of the pulmonary veins assessed by high-resolution optical mapping. *Circulation*. 2003;107(13):1816–1821.
29. De Jong AM, Maass AH, Oberdorf-Maass SU, Van Veldhuisen DJ, Van Gilst WH, Van Gelder IC. Mechanisms of atrial structural changes caused by stretch occurring before and during early atrial fibrillation. *Cardiovascular Research*. 2011;89(4):754–765.
30. Oakes RS, Badger TJ, Kholmovski EG, et al. Detection and quantification of left atrial structural remodeling with delayed-enhancement magnetic resonance imaging in patients with atrial fibrillation. *Circulation*. 2009;119(13):1758–1767.
31. Yacoub M, Sheppard RC. *Cryoballoon Pulmonary Vein Catheter Ablation of Atrial Fibrillation*. StatPearls. Treasure Island (FL) ineligible companies. Disclosure: Robert Sheppard declares no relevant financial relationships with ineligible companies. 2024.
32. Packer DL, Mark DB, Robb RA, et al. Effect of catheter ablation vs antiarrhythmic drug therapy on mortality, stroke, bleeding, and cardiac arrest among patients with atrial fibrillation: the CABANA randomized clinical trial. *JAMA*. 2019;321(13):1261–1274.

33. Marrouche NF, Brachmann J, Committee C-AS. Catheter ablation versus standard conventional treatment in patients with left ventricular dysfunction and atrial fibrillation (CASTLE-AF)—study design. *Pacing Clin Electrophysiol*. 2009;32(8):987–994.
34. Packer DL, Piccini JP, Monahan KH, et al. Ablation versus drug therapy for atrial fibrillation in heart failure: results from the CABANA trial. *Circulation*. 2021;143(14):1377–1390.
35. Writing Committee M, Joglar JA, Chung MK, et al. 2023 ACC/AHA/ACCP/HRS guideline for the diagnosis and management of atrial fibrillation: A Report of the American College of Cardiology/American Heart Association Joint Committee on Clinical Practice Guidelines. *J Am Coll Cardiol*. 2024;83(1):109–279.
36. Kirchhof P, Camm AJ, Goette A, et al. Early rhythm-control therapy in patients with atrial fibrillation. *N Engl J Med*. 2020;383(14):1305–1316.
37. Quintana RA, Dong T, Vajapey R, et al. Preprocedural multimodality imaging in atrial fibrillation. *Circ Cardiovasc Imaging*. 2022;15(10):e014386.
38. Marine JE, Dong J, Calkins H. Catheter ablation therapy for atrial fibrillation. *Prog Cardiovasc Dis*. 2005;48(3):178–192.
39. Minciuna IA, Puiu M, Cismaru G, et al. The role of intracardiac echocardiography in reducing radiation exposure during atrial fibrillation ablation. *Med Ultrason*. 2021;23(4):424–429.
40. Bertaglia E, Bella PD, Tondo C, et al. Image integration increases efficacy of paroxysmal atrial fibrillation catheter ablation: results from the cartomerge Italian registry. *Europace*. 2009;11(8):1004–1010.
41. Mammadli A, Demirtola AI, Diker E. Impact of image integration on clinical and procedural outcomes of radiofrequency catheter ablation of atrial fibrillation: a meta-analysis of randomized controlled trials. *J Arrhythm*. 2021;37(3):550–555.
42. Hauser TH, Yeon SB, McClennen S, et al. A method for the determination of proximal pulmonary vein size using contrast-enhanced magnetic resonance angiography. *J Cardiovasc Magn Reson*. 2004;6(4):927–936.
43. Syed MA, Peters DC, Rashid H, Arai AE. Pulmonary vein imaging: comparison of 3D magnetic resonance angiography with 2D cine MRI for characterizing anatomy and size. *J Cardiovasc Magn Reson*. 2005;7(2):355–360.
44. Kapur S, Barbhaiya C, Deneke T, Michaud GF. Esophageal injury and atrioesophageal fistula caused by ablation for atrial fibrillation. *Circulation*. 2017;136(13):1247–1255.
45. Meng J, Peters DC, Hsing JM, et al. Late gadolinium enhancement of the esophagus is common on cardiac mr several months after pulmonary vein isolation: preliminary observations. *Pace*. 2010;33(6):661–666.
46. Lemola K, Sneider M, Desjardins B, et al. Computed tomographic analysis of the anatomy of the left atrium and the esophagus: implications for left atrial catheter ablation. *Circulation*. 2004;110(24):3655–3660.
47. Tsao HM, Wu MH, Higa S, et al. Anatomic relationship of the esophagus and left atrium: implication for catheter ablation of atrial fibrillation. *Chest*. 2005;128(4):2581–2587.
48. Cury RC, Abbara S, Schmidt S, et al. Relationship of the esophagus and aorta to the left atrium and pulmonary veins: implications for catheter ablation of atrial fibrillation. *Heart Rhythm*. 2005;2(12):1317–1323.
49. Good E, Oral H, Lemola K, et al. Movement of the esophagus during left atrial catheter ablation for atrial fibrillation. *J Am Coll Cardiol*. 2005;46(11):2107–2110.
50. Raeisi-Giglou P, Wazni OM, Saliba WI, et al. Outcomes and management of patients with severe pulmonary vein stenosis from prior atrial fibrillation ablation. *Circ Arrhythm Electrophysiol*. 2018;11(5):e006001.
51. Holmes Jr DR, Monahan KH, Packer D. Pulmonary vein stenosis complicating ablation for atrial fibrillation: clinical spectrum and interventional considerations. *JACC Cardiovasc Interv*. 2009;2(4):267–276.
52. Kluge A, Dill T, Ekinci O, et al. Decreased pulmonary perfusion in pulmonary vein stenosis after radiofrequency ablation: assessment with dynamic magnetic resonance perfusion imaging. *Chest*. 2004;126(2):428–437.
53. Arentz T, Weber R, Jander N, et al. Pulmonary haemodynamics at rest and during exercise in patients with significant pulmonary vein stenosis after radiofrequency catheter ablation for drug resistant atrial fibrillation. *Eur Heart J*. 2005;26(14):1410–1414.
54. Kim RJ, Wu E, Rafael A, et al. The use of contrast-enhanced magnetic resonance imaging to identify reversible myocardial dysfunction. *N Engl J Med*. 2000;343(20):1445–1453.
55. Simonetti OP, Kim RJ, Fieno DS, et al. An improved MR imaging technique for the visualization of myocardial infarction. *Radiology*. 2001;218(1):215–223.
56. Peters DC, Wylie JV, Kissinger KV, et al. Detection of pulmonary vein ablation with high resolution MRI. *Soc Cardiovasc Magn Reson*. 2006.
57. Chubb H, Aziz S, Karim R, et al. Optimization of late gadolinium enhancement cardiovascular magnetic resonance imaging of post-ablation atrial scar: a cross-over study. *J Cardiovasc Magn Reson*. 2018;20(1):30.
58. Gunasekaran S, Haji-Valizadeh H, Lee DC, et al. Accelerated 3D left atrial late gadolinium enhancement in patients with atrial fibrillation at 1.5 T: technical development. *Radiol Cardiothorac Imaging*. 2020;2(5):e200134.
59. Basha TA, Akcakaya M, Liew C, et al. Clinical performance of high-resolution late gadolinium enhancement imaging with compressed sensing. *J Magn Reson Imaging*. 2017;46(6):1829–1838.
60. Jenista ER, Wendell DC, Kim HW, et al. Comparison of magnetization transfer-preparation and T2-preparation for dark-blood delayed-enhancement imaging. *NMR Biomed*. 2020;33(11):e4396.
61. Si D, Wu Y, Xiao J, et al. Three-dimensional high-resolution dark-blood late gadolinium enhancement imaging for improved atrial scar evaluation. *Radiology*. 2023;307(5):e222032.
62. Shaw JL, Knowles BR, Goldfarb JW, Manning WJ, Peters DC. Left atrial late gadolinium enhancement with water-fat separation: the importance of phase-encoding order. *J Magn Reson Imaging*. 2014;40(1):119–125.
63. Skoda I, Henningsson M, Stenberg S, Sundin J, Carlhall CJ. Simultaneous assessment of left atrial fibrosis and epicardial adipose tissue using 3D late gadolinium enhanced dixon MRI. *J Magn Reson Imaging*. 2022;56(5):1393–1403.
64. Whitaker J, Karady J, Karim R, et al. Standardised computed tomographic assessment of left atrial morphology and tissue thickness in humans. *Int J Cardiol Heart Vasc*. 2021;32:100694.
65. Karim R, Housden RJ, Balasubramaniam M, et al. Evaluation of current algorithms for segmentation of scar tissue from late gadolinium enhancement cardiovascular magnetic resonance of the left atrium: an open-access grand challenge. *J Cardiovasc Magn Reson*. 2013;15(1):105.
66. Malcolme-Lawes LC, Juli C, Karim R, et al. Automated analysis of atrial late gadolinium enhancement imaging that correlates with endocardial voltage and clinical outcomes: a 2-center study. *Heart Rhythm*. 2013;10(8):1184–1191.
67. Benito EM, Carlosena-Remirez A, Guasch E, et al. Left atrial fibrosis quantification by late gadolinium-enhanced magnetic resonance: a new method to standardize the thresholds for reproducibility. *Europace*. 2017;19(8):1272–1279.
68. Kamali R, Schroeder J, DiBella E, et al. Reproducibility of clinical late gadolinium enhancement magnetic resonance imaging in detecting left atrial scar after atrial fibrillation ablation. *J Cardiovasc Electrophysiol*. 2020;31(11):2824–2832.
69. Hopman L, Bhagirath P, Mulder MJ, et al. Quantification of left atrial fibrosis by 3D late gadolinium-enhanced cardiac magnetic resonance imaging in patients with atrial fibrillation: impact of different analysis methods. *Eur Heart J Cardiovasc Imaging*. 2022;23(9):1182–1190.
70. Li L, Zimmer VA, Schnabel JA, Zhuang X. Medical image analysis on left atrial LGE MRI for atrial fibrillation studies: a review. *Med Image Anal*. 2022;77:102360.
71. Xiong Z, Xia Q, Hu Z, et al. A global benchmark of algorithms for segmenting the left atrium from late gadolinium-enhanced cardiac magnetic resonance imaging. *Med Image Anal*. 2021;67:101832.
72. Bai JY, Qiu RY, Chen JY, et al. A two-stage method with a shared 3D U-net for left atrial segmentation of late gadolinium-enhanced MRI images. *Cardiovasc Innov App*. 2023;8(1).
73. Razeghi O, Sim I, Roney CH, et al. Fully automatic atrial fibrosis assessment using a multilabel convolutional neural network. *Circ Cardiovasc Imaging*. 2020;13(12):e011512. www.cemrgapp.com.
74. Taylor GW, Kay GN, Zheng X, Bishop S, Ideker RE. Pathological effects of extensive radiofrequency energy applications in the pulmonary veins in dogs. *Circulation*. 2000;101(14):1736–1742.
75. Peters DC, Wylie JV, Hauser TH, et al. Recurrence of atrial fibrillation correlates with the extent of post-procedural late gadolinium enhancement: a pilot study. *JACC Cardiovasc Imaging*. 2009;2(3):308–316.
76. Badger TJ, Daccarett M, Akoum NW, et al. Evaluation of left atrial lesions after initial and repeat atrial fibrillation ablation: lessons learned from delayed-enhancement MRI in repeat ablation procedures. *Circ Arrhythm Electrophysiol*. 2010;3(3):249–259.
77. Harrison JL, Sohns C, Linton NW, et al. Response to letter from Bisbal et al regarding, "Repeat left atrial catheter ablation: cardiac magnetic resonance prediction of endocardial voltage and gaps in ablation lesion sets." *Circ Arrhythm Electrophysiol*. 2015;8(3):754–755.
78. Spragg DD, Khurram I, Zimmerman SL, et al. Initial experience with magnetic resonance imaging of atrial scar and co-registration with electroanatomic voltage mapping during atrial fibrillation: success and limitations. *Heart Rhythm*. 2012;9(12):2003–2009.
79. Guttman MA, Tao S, Fink S, et al. Acute enhancement of necrotic radio-frequency ablation lesions in left atrium and pulmonary vein ostia in swine model with non-contrast-enhanced T(1)-weighted MRI. *Magn Reson Med*. 2020;83(4):1368–1379.
80. Thiedemann KU, Ferrans VJ. Left atrial ultrastructure in mitral valvular disease. *American Journal of Pathology*. 1977;89(3):575–604.
81. Marrouche NF, Wilber D, Hindricks G, et al. Association of atrial tissue fibrosis identified by delayed enhancement MRI and atrial fibrillation catheter ablation: the DECAAF study. *JAMA*. 2014;311(5):498–506.
82. Schwarzl M, Alogna A, Zweiker D, et al. A porcine model of early atrial fibrillation using a custom-built, radio transmission-controlled pacemaker. *J Electrocardiol*. 2016;49(2):124–131.
83. Marrouche NF, Wazni O, McGann C, et al. Effect of MRI-guided fibrosis ablation vs conventional catheter ablation on atrial arrhythmia recurrence in patients with persistent atrial fibrillation: the DECAAF II randomized clinical trial. *JAMA*. 2022;327(23):2296–2305.
84. Khurram IM, Beinart R, Zipunnikov V, et al. Magnetic resonance image intensity ratio, a normalized measure to enable interpatient comparability of left atrial fibrosis. *Heart Rhythm*. 2014;11(1):85–92.
85. Latif SR, Nguyen VQ, Peters DC, et al. Left atrial fibrosis correlates with extent of left ventricular myocardial delayed enhancement and left ventricular strain in hypertrophic cardiomyopathy. *Int J Cardiovasc Imaging*. 2019;35(7):1309–1318.

86. Vergaro G, Aimo A, Rapezzi C, et al. Atrial amyloidosis: mechanisms and clinical manifestations. *Eur J Heart Fail*. 2022;24(11):2019–2028.
87. Quail M, Grunseich K, Baldassarre LA, et al. Prognostic and functional implications of left atrial late gadolinium enhancement cardiovascular magnetic resonance. *J Cardiovasc Magn Reson*. 2019;21(1):2.
88. Cochet H, Mouries A, Nivet H, et al. Age, atrial fibrillation, and structural heart disease are the main determinants of left atrial fibrosis detected by delayed-enhanced magnetic resonance imaging in a general cardiology population. *J Cardiovasc Electrophysiol*. 2015;26(5):484–492.
89. Bertelsen L, Diederichsen SZ, Haugan KJ, et al. Left atrial late gadolinium enhancement is associated with incident atrial fibrillation as detected by continuous monitoring with implantable loop recorders. *JACC Cardiovasc Imaging*. 2020;13(8):1690–1700.
90. Kuhnlein P, Mahnkopf C, Majersik JJ, et al. Atrial fibrosis in embolic stroke of undetermined source: a multicenter study. *Eur J Neurol*. 2021;28(11):3634–3639.
91. Shen MJ, Arora R, Jalife J. Atrial myopathy. *JACC Basic Transl Sci*. 2019;4(5):640–654.

38 Cardiovascular Magnetic Resonance Angiography: Carotids, Aorta, and Peripheral Vessels

LIISA L. BERGMANN, JITKA STAREKOVA, AND CHRISTOPHER FRANCOIS

INTRODUCTION

Magnetic resonance imaging (MRI) of the vessels, or magnetic resonance angiography (MRA) and venography (MRV), is an important imaging modality for the diagnosis of vascular pathology and its management.[1,2] One benefit of magnetic resonance (MR) is the elimination of patient exposure to ionizing radiation, in line with the "Image Wisely" and "Image Gently" pledges made available by numerous radiologic and radiology technician societies.[3,4] An additional benefit of vascular MR results from MRI's high soft tissue contrast: MRA characterizes the vessel wall, including atherosclerotic plaque, in addition to the lumen. MRI's ability to demonstrate the vessel wall was first noted in 1995, when Skinner et al. described the characterization of atherosclerotic plaque in rabbits in *Nature Medicine*; Dr. Peter Libby, in his associated commentary "Lesion versus Lumen," then noted that low-density atherosclerotic plaque was associated with a higher risk of embolization and myocardial infarction even when there is less luminal stenosis relative to high-density plaque.[1,5,6]

This chapter consists of two sections: state-of-the-art and emerging vascular MR techniques followed by the application of some of these techniques in peripheral arteries. We have chosen to introduce the acronym VMR for vascular magnetic resonance because, as you will soon understand, with some MR sequences and contrast agents, MRA and MRV are obtained sequentially or even simultaneously.

In the first section, we will discuss the technical aspects of VMR. We will begin by discussing contrast-enhanced VMR (CE-VMR). We will use the acronym CE-VMR when including both arterial and venous imaging, and CE-MRA and CE-MRV when discussing MR angiography and MR venography, respectively. We will update the reader regarding contrast media, including gadolinium-based contrast agents (GBCAs) and one alternative, and their safety profiles. We will then discuss noncontrast enhanced vascular MR (NE-VMR). Similarly, we will use the acronym NE-VMR when including both arterial and venous imaging, and again, more specifically NE-MRA and NE-MRV in regard to noncontrast-enhanced angiography and venography, respectively.

Second, we will discuss vascular MR of various anatomy, including the carotid arteries, abdominal aorta, renal arteries, peripheral arteries, and veins.

Contrast-Enhanced Vascular Magnetic Resonance Technique

CE-VMR is probably the most commonly performed VMR technique.[2] CE-VMR demonstrates the vessel lumen by intensifying the signal of intraluminal blood, creating high contrast with the vessel walls and other surrounding soft tissues, and offers detailed three-dimensional (3D) visualization of vessels within the selected anatomical region.[7] This is typically achieved with the help of GBCAs, which shorten the longitudinal or T1 relaxation time of blood, enhancing its signal intensity. On T1-weighted imaging, blood vessels appear brighter on MR images compared to their surrounding tissues. GBCA-enhanced CE-VMR offers a significant advantage over noncontrast techniques by relying primarily on T1 relaxation for contrast, making it relatively independent of flow velocity. This allows for clear visualization of vessels regardless of flow variations or the direction of flow within the vessels, making CE-MRA valuable for accurate diagnosis across diverse vascular pathologies.[1]

Despite their generally safe profile, the use of GBCAs have come under scrutiny in the last 2 decades due to their association with nephrogenic systemic fibrosis (NSF) and gadolinium deposition in tissues.[8] Consequently, there is an increased interest in alternative contrast agents including superparamagnetic particles of iron oxide. While their use as MRI contrast agents remains off-label at the time of this writing, one ultrasmall superparamagnetic iron oxide has been Food and Drug Administration (FDA)-approved for iron deficiency anemia therapy in patients, including those with impaired kidney function and pregnant patients, creating an exciting alternative.

GADOLINIUM-BASED CONTRAST AGENTS

GBCAs are the most commonly used contrast agents in VMR. They are typically readily available, and can be rapidly administered intravenously. This allows for early-phase CE-MRA as well as time-resolved VMR. Major vendors currently have commercially available time-resolved VMR sequences, including TRAQ (Time-Resolved AcQuisition, Philips), TRICKS (Time-Resolved Imaging of Contrast KineticS, GE), and TWIST (Time-resolved imaging WIth Stochastic Trajectories, Siemens). Time-resolved sequences allow for the visualization of vessels at numerous time-points. The kidneys rapidly excrete GBCAs, which makes the timing of vascular MR critical, as well as the consideration of GBCA dosing, in particular for VMR. Please see Fig. 38.1, which shows multiple phases of MRA of the abdomen and pelvis.

In its trivalent form, the gadolinium ion (Gd^{3+}) possesses seven unpaired outer shell electrons that exhibit Curie paramagnetism—in other words, when in a magnetic field, trivalent gadolinium ions effectively become tiny magnets. This makes gadolinium highly effective at decreasing protons' time required for T1 relaxation, also known as longitudinal relaxation and spin-lattice relaxation. Shorter T1 relaxation times result in an increased signal intensity in T1-weighted images.[9]

The quantity of T1 relaxation time shortening is related to the concentration of gadolinium in the vessel of concern. The arterial concentration of gadolinium is proportionately related to injection rate and inversely related to cardiac output[2] in a linear fashion, as follows:

$$[\mathrm{Gd}]_{\mathrm{arterial}}\ (\mathrm{mol}/L) = \frac{\text{injection rate (mol/}s)}{\text{cardiac output }(L/s)}$$

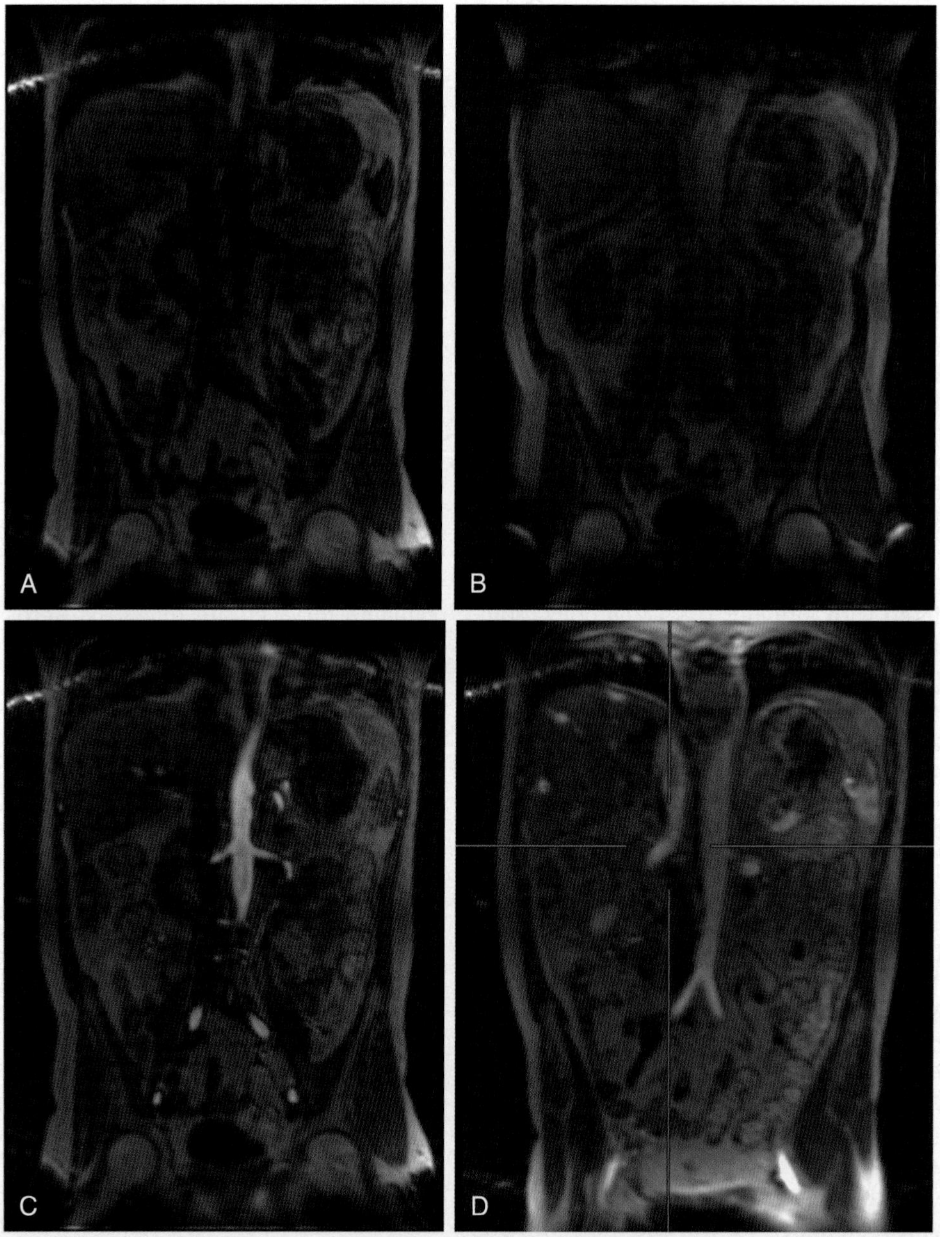

FIG. 38.1 Multiphasic vascular magnetic resonance (VMR) of the abdomen and pelvis in a single patient, during the same magnetic resonance (MR) imaging. (A). Coronal T1-weighted MR abdomen, precontrast. (B). Coronal T1-weighted VMR abdomen. This coronal slice was imaged repeatedly in short succession, with a high temporal resolution, until this final image demonstrating sufficiently high signal intensity in the abdominal aorta, due to sufficiently high concentration of gadolinium-based contrast agent. Once signal intensity becomes sufficiently high in the abdominal aorta, VMR of the full volume of the region of interest are obtained. This may not be respiratory gated, as was the case in this examination, with visualized motion artifact. (C). Coronal T1-weighted VMR abdomen, arterial phase, showing the abdominal aorta and proximal bilateral renal arteries. (D). Three-dimensional multiplanar reformatting was used to create this obliqued-coronal "second pass" VMR abdomen, showing decreased signal intensity in the abdominal aorta, with signal hyperintensity in the suprarenal inferior vena cava, with inflow of contrast from the right renal vein to the inferior vena cava (IVC). The infrarenal IVC is hypointense in sigla, with some flow artifact superior to the right renal vein, where nonenhanced blood in the infrarenal IVC flows into the suprarenal IVC.

The GBCA concentration in the arteries is higher with faster injection rates and decreased cardiac output. The T1 relaxation time is then shortened by a GBCA in relation to that agent's T1 relaxivity in addition to its concentration in the blood, according to the following equation:

$$(1/T1_{\text{observed}}) = (1/T1_{\text{blood}}) + R * [\text{Gd}]$$

where $T1_{blood}$ is 1500 ms in a 1.5 T field, R is the relaxivity of the contrast agent in units $mol^{-1}sec^{-1}$, and [Gd] is the gadolinium concentration in mol.[2,10,11] This equation may be easier to conceptualize in rates, given its multiple components with time in the denominator—when near a high concentration of a high-relaxivity GBCA, proton precessions longitudinally relax more quickly. Different GBCAs have different T1 relaxivities, and any GBCA's T1 relaxivity increases with increasing field strength.[12,13] In summary, assuming all other parameters are kept constant, the T1 times observed in the arteries in CE-MRA are shorter with higher field strengths, higher-relaxivity GBCA, and higher concentration of the GBCA. In the simplest terms possible, higher-relaxivity GBCA, which is more highly concentrated in the blood vessel of interest, results in that blood vessel having higher signal intensity on T1-weighted imaging.

Because signal intensity on T1-weighted CE-MRA is so dependent on the concentration of GBCA, the timing of image acquisition is critical. Ideally, image acquisition will occur during peak gadolinium concentration, particularly data acquisition for the center of *k*-space, which is most important for image contrast. This is relative to peripheral *k*-space, which is more important for spatial resolution.[2] This is also important in peripheral vessels, for example, MRA of the lower extremities for peripheral artery disease (PAD).[14,15]

In MRI, longitudinal magnetization is conventionally defined as the *z*-axis in-line with the magnet bore and in line with the strongest magnetic field of the magnet that is always on, typically 1.5 T or 3 T. Hydrogen atoms in water in the human body precess in line with the field, effectively making any patient in the bore a magnet, also. When energy is added to the bore via a radiofrequency pulse, the protons in the patient begin to precess out of line with the field, the bore, and the *z*-axis; these precessions create transverse magnetization in the *xy* plane. With time, the system loses energy, arguably from the spinning or precessing protons into the adjacent tissues or the lattice. The protons' precessions lose their *xy* transverse component and begin to realign with the *z*-axis, the strongest field, and the magnet bore. T1 times are when approximately 63% of the initial, maximum, longitudinal magnetization has been regained. The 63% is calculated using the formula $(1-(1/e))$.

Gd^{3+} is toxic in its free ionic form, so prior to its use as a GBCA, it is chelated to organic ligands—linear or macrocyclic—which can be either nonionic or ionic, depending on their net charge.[16] Chelation facilitates the rapid elimination of GBCAs, thereby reducing the possibility of unwanted biotransformation and interaction of free gadolinium with tissues.[17]

The overall chemical stability of a GBCA is determined by its thermodynamic and kinetic stability. Thermodynamic stability refers to how much Gd^{3+} is released under defined, stable conditions.[17] Kinetic stability refers to the rate of Gd^{3+} release (dissociation rate) and extent of Gd^{3+} release from the body (elimination rate).[17] The combination of a fast dissociation rate with a slow elimination rate can potentiate the release of free Gd^{3+} in vivo, for example, through transmetalation, when another ion replaces the gadolinium in the GBCA, ultimately resulting in gadolinium retention in the body.[8,17] Although all GBCAs are remarkably stable, there are some differences, with a general trend toward higher stability among macrocyclic GBCAs.[18] From a clinical perspective, all approved GBCAs currently used clinically bind gadolinium tightly and are considered stable, safe, and effective.[18]

GBCAs can be categorized based on their distribution in tissue after intravenous administration as extracellular or intravascular.[18] The majority of GBCAs are designed to be extracellular. After intravascular administration, extracellular GBCAs rapidly diffuse through the capillary walls of blood vessels into the extravascular space and are eventually eliminated through the kidneys via glomerular filtration, as well as through the liver for some GBCAs with dual excretion pathways.[18] The timing of image acquisition is crucial in CE-MRA with extracellular GBCA to reduce signal from gadolinium in the extravascular space and avoid venous enhancement. Therefore, CE-MRA with these agents is limited to dynamic or first-pass arterial studies.

In contrast, gadofosveset (Ablavar, Lanthaneus Medical Imaging, Billerica), a vascular GBCA approved by the FDA in 2008, was designed to enhance visualization of small blood vessels by binding to plasma proteins and remaining in the bloodstream longer.[19] Despite its benefits, gadofosveset was discontinued in 2017, leading to the current lack of commercially available, FDA-approved gadolinium-based blood pool contrast agents.

Every GBCA administration requires careful consideration of both the potential benefits and risks, like any medication. Major safety considerations with GBCAs are acute allergic-like reactions. However, these occur less commonly than with iodinated contrast agents (0.1%–0.4% vs. 0.73%) and are predominantly mild.[20–23] Beyond allergic-like reactions, there are three distinct safety-related entities described in the literature. A rare but well-accepted risk associated with the administration of GBCA in patients with kidney impairment is NSF, a scleroderma-like fibrosing condition that can be progressive and sometimes fatal.[24] In 2007, the FDA issued a boxed warning about the risk of NSF in patients with kidney disease, 1 year after the association between NSF and GBCA was first reported.[25] In response, precautions and guidelines have been issued by numerous medical societies in the United States and worldwide, which has led to a dramatic decrease in the incidence of NSF.[16,26] The American College of Radiology (ACR) classifies GBCAs into three groups based on *"reported associations with NSF in vulnerable patients."*[26] Group I are those GBCAs associated with the greatest number of cases of NSF; group II are those GBCAs associated with few, if any, cases of NSF; and group III GBCAs are those with insufficient data to conclude the real risk of NSF. Due to their strong association with NSF in patients with poor kidney function, group I GBCAs are contraindicated in acute kidney injury (AKI) and chronic kidney disease (CKD) stages 4 and 5 (estimated glomerular filtration rate [eGFR] $<$ 30 mL/

min/1.73 m²). In the light of an improved understanding of NSF, group II GBCAs are considered safe to use regardless of kidney function, including in AKI and stages 4 and 5 CKD, and the ACR ceased to recommend mandatory kidney function screening by 2018.[27] According to recent literature, the risk of developing NSF after exposure to group II GBCAs in patients with kidney impairment is exceedingly small, with the 95% confidence interval (CI) of risk ranging from 0.07% to 0.81%.[18,28] Nonetheless, the FDA maintains a black box warning on all GBCAs as a precautionary measure.[29] With the ACR's publication of the 2024 Manual on Contrast Media, the evidence was sufficient to regroup gadoxetate disodium (Eovist, Bayer) into group II, leaving zero group III agents at the time of this writing.[26,30]

Unrelated to NSF, considerable evidence has demonstrated the deposition of trace amounts of gadolinium in the brain and other organs after repeated GBCA administration.[8,18] Gadolinium deposition occurs with all agents, but linear agents tend to deposit more compared to macrocyclic agents.[17,18] There is currently no evidence in the peer-reviewed scientific literature to support that gadolinium deposition in patients with normal kidney function is associated with any adverse clinical outcomes.[8,18]

While research continues, organizations like the National Institutes of Health, Radiological Society of North America, and ACR emphasize the need to determine definitively whether gadolinium retention causes harm.[8] To support this effort, the ACR recently introduced the term "Symptoms Associated with Gadolinium Exposure (SAGE)," aiming to create a standardized way for researchers and clinicians to describe symptoms potentially associated with gadolinium exposure.[31]

ALTERNATIVES TO GADOLINIUM-BASED CONTRAST AGENTS

Ferumoxytol (Feraheme, AMAG Pharmaceuticals) is an iron-based medication that is FDA-approved for the parenteral treatment of iron-deficiency anemia, including in renal failure and during pregnancy.[32] Due to its highly favorable T1-time foreshortening and pharmacokinetics, ferumoxytol is increasingly being used off-label as a blood pool contrast agent in MRI.[33–35] At the time of writing, ferumoxytol has variable availability at US and UK institutions, and it is very challenging to obtain even for research use in some nations. Evidence-based best safety practices require ferumoxytol to be infused over 15 minutes, which may create challenges in obtaining time-resolved VMR sequences depending on the policies and MR-safe administration devices of an institution. The superparamagnetic ultrasmall iron oxide particles in ferumoxytol have a prolonged intravascular half-life of over 14 hours[34,36] and markedly shorten T1 or longitudinal relaxation times.[36,37] Ferumoxytol nanoparticles are relatively large compared to other contrast agents. Due to its size, ferumoxytol remains confined within the intravascular space after injection, leading to high contrast between vessels and surrounding tissues. This permits for image acquisition over an extended temporal window after infusion, during which time all vascular systems will demonstrate uniformly hyperintense signal on T1-weighted imaging without the need for additional contrast injections (Fig. 38.2). These characteristics make ferumoxytol a particularly valuable blood pool contrast agent for MRA.

Ferumoxytol is safe for administration in patients with CKD, is biodegradable, and carries no potential risk of NSF. It shows no long-term retention in human tissue when administered at the FDA-approved therapeutic doses used for iron-deficiency anemia (single infusion of 1020 mg, or two infusions of 510 mg at 3–8-day intervals). Therapeutic doses are substantially higher than doses typically used for diagnostic MRI (1–7.3 mg/kg, typically ~3 mg/kg, with maximum dose of 510 mg).[18,32,33,35,38–40]

Ferumoxytol is generally considered to have an excellent safety profile, but early use with undiluted bolus injections sparked concerns due to rare anaphylactic-like reactions.[25,41,42] These reactions are thought to be linked to the interaction between a rapidly infused, high concentration of the iron and mast cells in the vascular wall. Due to a number of fatal instances, the FDA issued a boxed warning in 2015. To minimize the risk of reaction, based on the published literature and a 2015 communication,[32,41] ferumoxytol should be diluted and infused slowly over a minimum of 15 minutes. For VMR purposes, dilution factors of 4 and 5 in saline have been reported.[40,42] Standard precautions with regard to adverse reactions and blood pressure monitoring are recommended for a minimum period of 30 minutes following ferumoxytol administration.[32,40]

Ferumoxytol, as an off-label blood pool agent, allows for the visualization of both arteries and veins in a single VMR scan.[42–45] By eliminating the need for precise timing and contrast boluses, it has shown promise in pediatric imaging.[35] In adults, there is considerable literature and evidence supporting off-label use in vascular imaging.[44] Ferumoxytol is safe for CKD patients and provides greater detail of kidney vasculature, enabling not only morphologic but also quantitative assessment.[42,46] Recently, ferumoxytol-enhanced VMR has shown promise as an imaging alternative for pregnant females suspected of pulmonary embolism; with an appropriate field of view, the VMR can simultaneously show pulmonary embolism and deep venous thrombus.[40] In comparison to GBCAs, primate studies have demonstrated that ferumoxytol does not cross the placenta and deposit in fetal tissues.[47,48] Despite the lack of controlled studies in human pregnancy, the increasing therapeutic and off-label imaging use of ferumoxytol in pregnant females is providing preliminary evidence of its potential safety.[39,49] Finally, ferumoxytol has shown to be an attractive option for venous imaging, with results that are comparable to contrast-enhanced imaging with gadofosveset and superior to noncontrast time of flight.[50]

CONTRAST-ENHANCED VASCULAR MAGNETIC RESONANCE PULSE SEQUENCES AND ARTIFACTS

In CE-VMR, T1-weighted, fast, 3D spoiled gradient-echo (GRE) sequences are used, with a short repetition time (TR) of 3 to 8 ms, a short echo time (TE) of 1 to 3 ms, and a flip angle of 20 to 40 degrees, to achieve optimal T1 weighting. These sequences fill *k*-space in variable orders; however, central *k*-space is typically filled first. As noted above, it is preferable that central *k*-space be acquired synchronously with peak GBCA concentration in the vessels of interest,

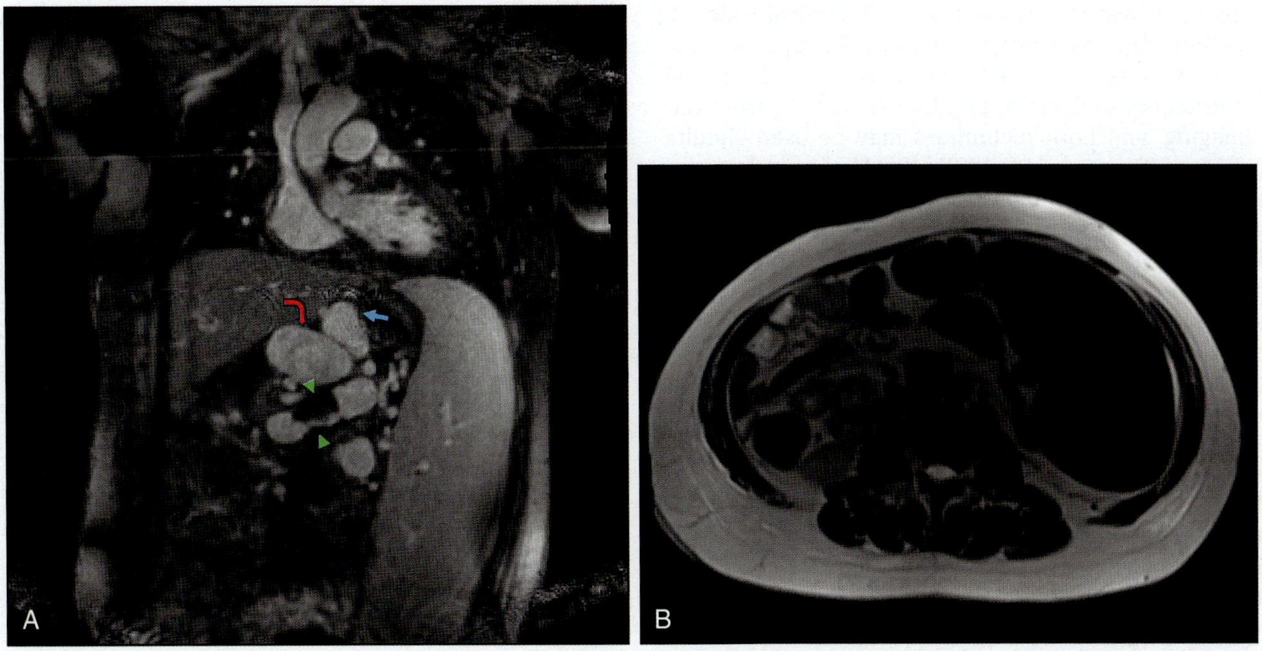

FIG. 38.2 Ferumoxytol-enhanced vascular magnetic resonance (Fe-VMR). (A). Coronal T1-weighted Fe-VMR demonstrates pathology in multiple vascular systems that enhance simultaneously. In the context of splenomegaly, there is also splenic artery aneurysm (*red curved arrow*), nonocclusive splenic vein thrombus (*green arrow heads*) extending into the portal vein, and extrahepatic portosystemic collateral coursing superiorly toward the chest (*blue straight arrow*). Ferumoxytol is Food and Drug Administration–approved for intravenous therapy for iron-deficiency anemia, including in patients with renal failure and who are pregnant. It is the only available blood-pool magnetic resonance contrast agent in the United States, when used off-label, with an intravascular half-life of over 14 hours. Current safety data suggests that slow infusion over 15 minutes is safest for patients. (B). Axial T2-weighted imaging in the same patient following ferumoxytol infusion. T2-weighting is created using long repetition and echo times, with hyperintense signal resulting from proton precessions' maintenance of transverse component. Hypointense signal in both the abdominal aorta and the inferior vena cava (IVC) on T2-weighted imaging is secondary to the iron oxide in the blood pool causing blood pool protons' precessions' to lose its transverse component quickly.

as central *k*-space is most important to image contrast; this timing is critical to eliminate artifacts. Image acquisition slightly earlier than peak contrast concentration can cause the appearance of ringing, or Maki artifact[51]; this is an apparent filling defect in the artery that can mimic dissection flap or nonocclusive thrombus.

Additional artifacts in CE-VMR include low GBCA resulting from turbulence, which is most commonly seen just distal to a stenosis with high flow velocity; this results in signal loss just distal to the stenosis, creating the appearance that the stenotic segment is longer than it actually is. Vessel tortuosity in combination with slice thickness can also mimic stenosis, particularly when the vessel courses just along the edge, or just outside of the field of view. Vessels with high signal intensity can have a parallel "ghost" vessel.[52] Image acquisition begun too late will result in contrast enhancement in the veins, called "venous contamination" this can lead to challenges in diagnosis. Patient motion between "mask" imaging and CE-VMR imaging can result in subtraction artifacts. Of course, the same artifacts that plague all MRI can also be found in CE-VMR, including susceptibility artifacts and whole-patient motion, respiratory motion, cardiac motion, and pulsation artifacts.

Subsampling techniques like parallel imaging significantly reduce acquisition time, allowing for the acquisition of larger 3D data volumes within a single breath-hold. Advanced *k*-space sampling techniques (e.g., spiral, keyhole, echo planar imaging) may also be used to achieve faster acquisition. There are several evolving techniques in CE-VMR that are pushing the boundaries such as compressed sensing, deep learning, and advanced reconstruction algorithms.[53,54]

Three-dimensional datasets can be postprocessed to create multiplanar reformats (MPR), which allow for viewing in nonconventional anatomic orientations. MPR postprocessing benefits from thin slices, preferably a 3 mm slice thickness or less. Three-dimensional datasets can also be used to create maximum intensity projection (MIP) images, which can also be rotated. Sometimes, 8–10 mm thick slices are sufficient for MIPs without rotation, and of course this also decreases the total number of slices obtained, as well as image acquisition time, even down to 1 second.

NONCONTRAST-ENHANCED VASCULAR MAGNETIC RESONANCE TECHNIQUES AND ARTIFACTS

Vascular MR can be and has been performed without contrast, at least since the 1990s. Since then, clinical MR hardware and software improvements have made NE-VMR more clinically feasible, including increased implementation of parallel imaging. Despite the name "parallel imaging" making it sound like it is an imaging acquisition sequence, parallel imaging is in fact a reconstruction technique from data that is intentionally undersampled to speed acquisition time, with the undersampled data obtained via multiple receiver coils so that spatial resolution can be maintained with the appropriate reconstruction.[55] Parallel imaging acronyms you may be familiar with include SENSE (SENSitivity Encoding) and ASSET (Array coil Spatial Sensitivity Encoding). A technical sidenote to hopefully improve clarity: "compressed sensing" is an additional technique to decrease image acquisition time via semirandom undersampling that is distinct from parallel imaging, and both techniques may be used simultaneously (e.g., Compressed SENSE).[56–59] Many vendors now have commercially available options that include parallel imaging, compressed sensing, and some form of artificial intelligence (AI)[60]; although outside of the scope of this chapter, these are particularly helpful in decreasing image acquisition time in the heart and in particular the coronaries, whether with and without contrast.

Unlike CE-VMR, NE-VMR techniques are sensitive to blood flow, which can result in artifacts that do not occur when you use contrast.[2] Then why elect NE-VMR? One consideration is the environment. Gadolinium is a "rare earth metal," which means that it does not exist in nature in an ore like gold and copper, and that the mined earth requires processing in order for gadolinium to be purified. Quantities of gadolinium in the Earth's crust are not low. Currently, gadolinium is mined predominantly in northern China, and was previously predominantly mined in California; it is found on multiple other continents. By eliminating the use of contrast agents, NE-VMR is arguably more environmentally sustainable, because it decreases mining.

Interest in NE-VMR also stems from NSF; however, no unconfounded cases of NSF have been found in numerous studies in patients with decreased renal function.[61–63] Another motivation to perform NE-VMR is due to known gadolinium deposition in the human body. Some gadolinium disassociates from its chelate, and this freed gadolinium deposits in the brain where calcium also tends to deposit, and also in bone, liver, and skin.[64–68] As of the time of this writing, there is not convincing evidence in the peer-reviewed literature that gadolinium deposition has any long-term negative health effects, and many research questions remain unanswered.[8]

NE-VMR techniques include black-blood, bright-blood, and 4D flow visualization. The authors have elected to maintain this section from the first edition with minimal changes, due to its excellent physics explanations.

Black-Blood Imaging

Black-blood imaging of blood vessels uses double-inversion recovery to null the signal of flowing blood.[69] This technique is flow sensitive. Two 180 degree inversion recovery prepulses are applied to null the signal of flowing blood: the first prepulse inverts the longitudinal magnetization vector in the entire body, whereas the second inversion prepulse inverts the magnetization in the selected imaging slice back to its original orientation. The signal of blood entering the imaging slice after the second prepulse has undergone reinversion and will appear dark in the images. Electrocardiogram (ECG)-gated partial Fourier fast spin echo (FSE) is the sequence of choice,[70,71] using a slice thickness of 6 to 8 mm stacked in the transverse plane of the chest or in a double-oblique sagittal view of the aorta, often called "candy-cane" view). Single-shot FSE sequences are much faster than basic FSE sequences and allow for acquisition of the entire imaging stack in a single breath-hold. Fat

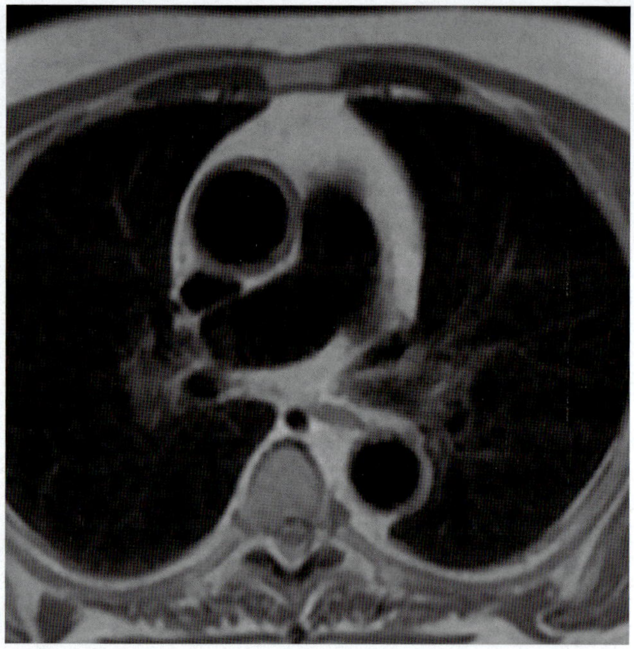

FIG. 38.3 A 74-year-old female with giant cell arteritis with thickened ascending aorta wall on T1-weighted dark blood magnetic resonance imaging (*arrows*).

saturation is recommended to increase the conspicuity of aortic wall hematoma.[72] Despite being an established technique, black-blood imaging is prone to artifacts because inadequate nulling of blood signal may occur by slow flow, or when in-plane blood flow is present. Black-blood imaging can be most useful in visualizing intramural hematoma, a type of acute aortic syndrome (Fig. 38.3).

BRIGHT-BLOOD IMAGING: TIME OF FLIGHT

Time of flight (TOF) imaging is also flow dependent. In the selected imaging volume, the longitudinal magnetization from the background tissue is suppressed by multiple radiofrequency (RF) excitations, so that the background tissue protons' magnetic precessions do not have sufficient time to fully regain their longitudinal magnetization; in other words, the stationary background tissues will be "saturated" and demonstrate hypointense signal on T1-weighted imaging sequences, creating contrast with the relatively higher signal intensity within the blood vessels. Saturation of background signal will reach a steady state determined by the flip angle, repetition time, and the T1 of the background tissue. The bright signal intensity of flowing blood is the consequence of the continuous inflow of blood into the imaging slice that was not included in the selected imaging volume that had its signal intensity saturated.[73] This effect is known as flow-related enhancement,[74] and can be maximized by using sequences with a short TR. Ideally, the imaging slice should be thin and oriented perpendicular to the direction of flow. ECG gating can be used to optimize the synchronization of acquisition to the blood flow during the cardiac cycle and consequently to the signal present in the artery of interest.

TOF techniques may be two-dimensional (2D) or 3D. Two-dimensional TOF with consecutive slices stacked together can produce excellent contrast in the vessels when the imaging slices are planned perpendicular to the vessels of interest. When in-plane flow occurs, the longitudinal magnetization of blood will become saturated, and signal is progressively lost. Slow arterial flow and poststenotic turbulent flow can also result in signal intensity loss within the blood vessels, an artifact that may appear to be stenosis. Venous signal may also be suppressed with presaturation slabs, positioned parallel and next to the imaging slices, to saturate the longitudinal magnetization of blood flowing into the imaging slice from the opposite side of arterial blood flow. Resolution of 2D TOF is often limited by the slice thickness used. Thin slice acquisitions are possible, but signal-to-noise ratio (SNR) will decrease with decreasing slice thickness, and acquisition time will increase with the increased number of slices required to cover the vasculature.

Three-dimensional TOF may be performed with isotropic voxel sizes of 1 mm^3. High resolution is essential to visualize small branch vessels, stenosis, and to provide a clear delineation of tortuous vessels. Three-dimensional TOF must deal with the saturation effects of arterial blood flow, especially slow flow. On the other hand, the SNR will be increased by using 3D imaging. Decreasing the flip angle may reduce excessive saturation effects. TOF, in particular 3D TOF, is used very frequently to perform NE-MRA of the head (Fig. 38.4).

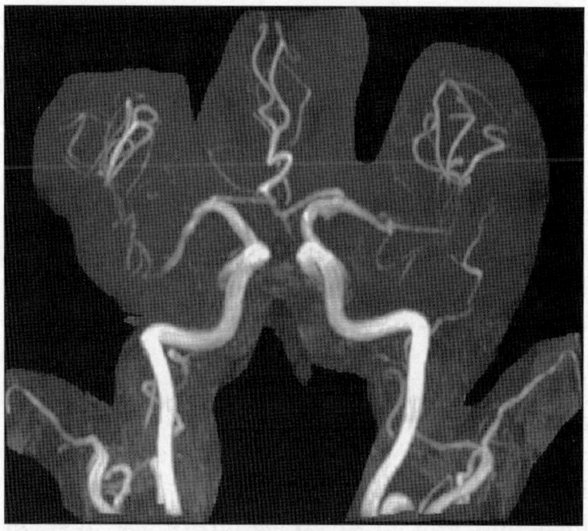

FIG. 38.4 Noncontrast enhanced magnetic resonance angiography of the circle of Willis, using 3D time-of-flight sequence, and reconstructed maximum intensity projection.

BRIGHT-BLOOD IMAGING: PHASE-CONTRAST ANGIOGRAPHY

In phase-contrast angiography (PCA), the contrast between flowing blood and the surrounding stationary tissue is generated by the flow-induced phase shift in the transverse magnetization of the moving blood. As the magnetic field strength and precession frequency of spins are linearly related, the precession frequency will increase when spins move along a positive gradient in the magnetic field. Compared with spins that remain fixed in position (i.e., in stationary tissue), moving spins (i.e., in flowing blood) will accumulate phase in the transverse magnetization. This phase shift is proportional to its velocity and the gradient strength.[75] In addition to this velocity-sensitive acquisition, a velocity-compensation acquisition is defined that uses a bipolar gradient with equal positive and negative effects to achieve no difference in net phase shift between spins moving with uniform velocity. PCA uses the subtraction of both velocity-sensitive and velocity-compensation acquisitions to visualize moving spins. The velocity can be directly quantified from the resultant phase images. A priori to the acquisition, the velocity sensitivity needs to be determined by choosing the velocity-encoding range (Venc), that is, the outer limit of the velocity range that is encoded by the phase shift of +180 degrees and −180 degrees. If the Venc upper limit velocity is set below the maximum velocity, then there is resultant aliasing artifact.

TOF and PCA, two conventional bright-blood NE-MRA techniques, are highly time consuming and, moreover, suffer from artifacts caused by turbulence and in-plane saturation. In a meta-analysis,[76] the sensitivity and specificity for the detection of significant stenosis (>50% luminal reduction) for 2D TOF ranged from 64% to 100% and 68% to 96%, compared with 92% to 100% and 91% to 99%, respectively, for CE-MRA. Such limitations resulted in declining interest for TOF and PCA in favor of CE-MRA. Interest was revived when concern for NSF increased; however, there is now sufficient data showing that use of a class II GBCA poses almost zero risk of NSF, even in AKI and CKD stages 4 and 5.[26] Interest has again increased in NE-VMR due to an increased commitment to environmental sustainability, and due to gadolinium depositing in the human body (despite having no convincing evidence of related risks), crossing the human placenta, and causing teratogenicity in animal models.

Bright-Blood Imaging: Steady-State Free Precession

Steady-state free precession (SSFP) produces high signal intensity for blood because of the inherently T2/T1-weighted image contrast, which is high for all fluids, independent of inflow effects. ECG-gated cine acquisitions with balanced SSFP (bSSFP) are used to visualize the anatomy of thoracic and abdominal aorta with breath-hold sequences. Aneurysms, coarctations, stenoses, and dissection flaps can be visualized using this approach.

The aortic root is best evaluated in multiple planes, including long-axis planes of the left ventricular outflow tract. The remainder of the thoracic aorta is best evaluated with images in the axial plane of the chest and in the double-oblique sagittal "candy-cane" view. bSSFP sequences are susceptible to magnetic field inhomogeneity, which are particularly present at high field strength. Off-resonance artifacts may result in nondiagnostic images in bSSFP, especially at higher field strengths. Dedicated shimming algorithms may aid in minimizing these off-resonance artifacts.

Bright-Blood Imaging: Dixon

Another relatively new bright-blood approach relies on an old MR technique based on the chemical shift between both water and fat. Dixon's water-fat separation[77] uses the phase shift from the water-fat resonance frequency and carefully chosen multiple echo times to achieve excellent separation between water and fat in four distinct images:

separate water and fat images as well as images with signal from both tissues in and out of phase. The Dixon technique may be applied for noncontrast MRA purposes, and its application may be promising for imaging of the coronaries as well as the thoracic aorta.[60,78]

Four-Dimensional Flow Visualization

Phase-contrast imaging enables quantitation of blood flow velocity in the direction of a magnetic field gradient. In addition to conventional through-plane one-directional velocity-encoding, advanced 3D time-resolved imaging is possible with velocity encoding in all three directions, providing the temporal distribution of a velocity vector field and representing the flow of blood inside a 3D volume (i.e., so-called 4D flow data).[79] Tools for visualizing streamlines, pathlines, and wall shear stress have been developed to display this data and to segment blood vessels of interest from their surrounding tissue. The usability of this technique has been shown in the aorta, pulmonary arteries, carotid arteries, and abdominal circulation as well as the circulation in the brain. This technique is still being translated from a research application to regular clinical use.[80,81] The additional hemodynamic information (e.g., wall shear stress, stenotic pressure drop, pulse wave velocity, viscous energy dissipation), which becomes available with 4D flow CMR in combination with the excellent 3D visualization possibilities of complex vascular structures and pathologies, will likely develop 4D flow as a clinically viable application. Of note, although 4D flow MR does not require use of contrast, some institutions do use ferumoxytol and/or GBCA for increased intravascular signal intensity in 4D flow imaging, in particular in infants undergoing evaluation for congenital cardiac disease.[82]

MAGNETIC RESONANCE ANGIOGRAPHY OF EXTRACRANIAL CAROTID ARTERIES

Stroke is a major health concern worldwide. Atherosclerosis of the extracranial carotid arteries is an important cause of stroke, and is estimated to cause approximately 8% of ischemic strokes.[83,84] The annual incidence of stroke in the United States is approximately 800,000, including ~610,000 first-stroke patients and 185,000 patients with recurrent stroke.[85] In 2017–20, the estimated prevalence of stroke among US residents age 20 years and older was approximately 9.4 million, which is approximately 3.3%.[85] A full discussion of the epidemiology of stroke in the United States is well beyond the scope of this chapter; however, it is imperative to mention that there are geographic variations within the United States, and there are significant and well-researched sex, ethnic, and socioeconomic disparities in stroke; for example, the demographic with the expected greatest increase in stroke by 2030 is Hispanic males. In contrast, the research on stroke disparities remains nascent in transgender patients.[86,87] Stroke accounts for approximately 1 of every 21 deaths in the United States.[85] Nonfatal stroke can lead to significant disability; the total cost attributed to stroke in 2019–20 was estimated to have been greater than $56 billion in the United States alone,[85] and this may not account for nonremunerated care provided by family members. Carotid atherosclerosis is a significant factor for risk stratification. Plaque area in the highest quartile is associated with approximately 60% and 70% increased risk of first-ever ischemic stroke in females and males, respectively,[88] and following transient ischemic attack, carotid atherosclerosis is associated with more than a doubling in the stroke risk.[89] Accurate evaluation of the extracranial carotid artery is essential.

For evaluating the severity of carotid stenosis, fluoroscopic digital subtraction angiography (DSA) is the standard of reference. The spatial resolution of angiography is high; however, the invasiveness of this imaging approach is associated with a small risk of stroke, estimated at 0.5% to 4%,[90] and it also requires the use of ionizing radiation and iodinated contrast. Therefore, noninvasive imaging techniques are now considered most appropriate in the routine assessment of patients with suspected carotid artery stenosis.[91] Techniques such as duplex Doppler ultrasound (DUS), computed tomography angiography (CTA), CE-MRA, and NE-MRA are the most appropriate and widely available and have largely replaced invasive cervical arteriography in daily clinical routine.

When compared with DSA, noninvasive imaging techniques are generally less accurate for low-degree carotid artery stenoses. For 50%–69% stenosis of the internal carotid artery, a meta-analysis showed a sensitivity and specificity for DUS of 36% and 91%, for CE-MRA of 77% and 97%, for CTA of 67% and 79%, and for NE-MRA of 37% and 91%, respectively.[92] For high-grade 70%–99% stenosis, the same meta-analysis found that noninvasive techniques had higher sensitivity and specificity: for DUS 89% and 84%, for CE-MRA 94% and 93%, for CTA 77% and 95%, and for NE-MRA 99% and 84%, respectively.

DUS is widely available, easily accessible, cost effective, and often used as a first-line investigation in standardized protocols assessing carotid artery disease.[93] In experienced hands it is an accurate test; however, it has higher interobserver variability and lower sensitivity and specificity when compared with CE-MRA and CTA.

When DUS detects a significant stenosis (>70%), it is useful to evaluate the severity by performing MRA or CTA. For assessing carotid artery stenosis, CE-MRA shows a comparable accuracy.

However, CTA has important limitations. It employs potentially harmful ionizing radiation and the administration of a higher volume of iodinated contrast. Moreover, plaque calcification may hamper stenosis gradation. The development of commercially available photon-counting computed tomography (CT) does decrease calcium blooming artifact, improving evaluation of vessel stenosis; however, exposure to ionizing radiation may be eliminated using DUS as a first-line screening modality followed by CE-MRA for gradation of carotid stenosis.

CE-MRA is the MRA technique of choice to evaluate carotid artery disease (Fig. 38.5). Typically, 3D CE-MRA data are acquired in the coronal plane. Bolus timing is essential, because venous return in the veins of the neck is quite fast. Spatial resolutions of 0.71 mm^3 at 1.5 T and 0.54 mm^3 at 3 T are recommended.[90]

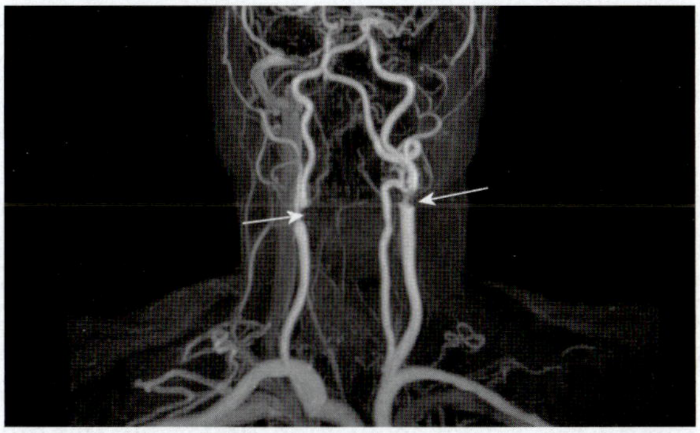

FIG. 38.5 Neck contrast-enhanced magnetic resonance angiography demonstrating a severe bilateral stenoses of the proximal internal carotid arteries (*arrows*). (Previously FIG. 44.1 in the first edition.)

Generally, a single dose (0.1 mmol/kg) of a GBCA is sufficient to achieve excellent image quality and resolution at 1.5 T. Several studies have shown that dose reduction to half a dose (0.05 mmol/kg) is feasible at 3 T without compromising SNR and spatial resolution.[94,95]

In several studies, TOF NE-MRA (Fig. 38.4) showed good sensitivity and specificity in detecting stenosis of the carotid bifurcation.[96,97] However, CE-MRA offers high-resolution imaging of a larger field of view in shorter acquisition times,[98,99] and therefore has replaced TOF MRA in many clinical practices.

The development of new NE-MRA sequences shows promising results and could have the potential to become an alternative imaging approach for evaluating carotid artery disease. Zhoa et al.[100] showed that 3D black-blood CMR imaging provided high agreement for stenosis measurements compared with DSA. Three-dimensional black-blood CMR imaging depicted longer lesion length than DSA because of its ability to define vessel wall morphology and the distribution of plaque. When compared with CE-MRA, 3D black-blood MRA shows accurate measurement of carotid stenosis[101] and sensitivity and specificity comparable to CTA.[102]

Other vascular diseases of the carotid artery can also be diagnosed by CE-MRA. Fibromuscular dysplasia is a nonatherosclerotic, noninflammatory arteriopathy with segmental involvement of small- and medium-sized arteries. The etiology is unknown and the extracranial carotid, vertebral, and renal arteries are most frequently affected. The so-called string-of-beads sign of the involved arteries is a classic pattern seen in fibromuscular dysplasia, but also other imaging findings are described such as aneurysm, fusiform arterial ectasia, and vascular loops. Fibromuscular dysplasia can accurately be diagnosed using CE-MRA; however, a negative result on CE-MRA does not exclude fibromuscular dysplasia. In this case, DSA is still recommended in patients with high clinical suspicion of fibromuscular dysplasia in the carotid arteries, or alternatively, noninvasive assessment of the renal arteries is an appropriate next step.[103–106]

Carotid artery dissection is one of the most common causes of stroke in young patients. Dissection may occur after trauma or may arise spontaneously. In patients suspected to have carotid artery dissection, CE-MRA is the imaging modality of choice.[107,108] Mural hematoma can be visualized by performing additional axial T1-weighted images with fat suppression. Although DSA is the reference standard for the evaluation of the lumen of the carotid artery, it does not provide details of the arterial wall. In suspected cases, it is important to acquire high-resolution isovolumetric voxels and then reformat them in axial thin slices to depict an intimal flap.

AORTIC MAGNETIC RESONANCE ANGIOGRAPHY

Diseases of the thoracic and abdominal aorta can be examined by several imaging modalities. Over the last decade, noninvasive imaging techniques have improved significantly, and therefore the need for DSA as an imaging tool in clinical practice has decreased. With noninvasive techniques, the risks of arterial catheterization and the use of iodinated contrast medium can be avoided.

A wide spectrum of vascular diseases affecting the thoracic and abdominal aorta can be evaluated by angiographic imaging, including aortic aneurysm, suspected aortic dissection, penetrating atherosclerotic ulcer, atherosclerotic arterial occlusive disease, genetic diseases (e.g., Marfan syndrome), and congenital abnormalities such as coarctation of the aorta. For imaging the thoracic aortic lumen, current established noninvasive techniques such as transthoracic echocardiography (TTE), transesophageal echocardiography (TEE), MRA, and CTA are able to provide additional information about the aortic wall and the relationship of vascular disease to the surrounding tissue. TTE is the most common first-line imaging modality, but MRA and CTA are widely used. The abdominal aorta is most typically imaged by ultrasound, MRA, and CTA,[109] whereas TTE is the most frequently used imaging modality for evaluating the aortic root and proximal ascending aorta.

In a standardized TTE examination, the thoracic aorta is routinely assessed.[110] Despite the fact that TTE is limited in assessing the complete thoracic aorta, it still permits adequate assessment of several aortic segments, especially when monitoring aortic root diameters.[111] Moreover, TTE can be used as a screening tool for proximal ascending aorta dilatation, but it is not sensitive for detection of aortic dissection, particularly beyond the proximal ascending aorta; however, TTE is quite useful in assessing for associated complications of type A dissections (e.g., aortic valve disruption/regurgitation, hemopericardium).

Because of the proximity of the esophagus to the thoracic aorta, TEE is often used in thoracic aorta assessment and overcomes several of the limitations of TTE. TEE reveals high resolution images and, unlike TTE, allows gradual assessment of the thoracic aorta from the aortic root to the descending aorta.[112,113] However, if TTE and/or TEE reveal inconclusive information or abnormalities are present, another imaging modality is required for confirmation/further evaluation.

CTA is an important imaging technique in vascular diseases of the thoracic and abdominal aorta. In particular, in acute aortic syndrome (i.e., aortic dissection, intramural

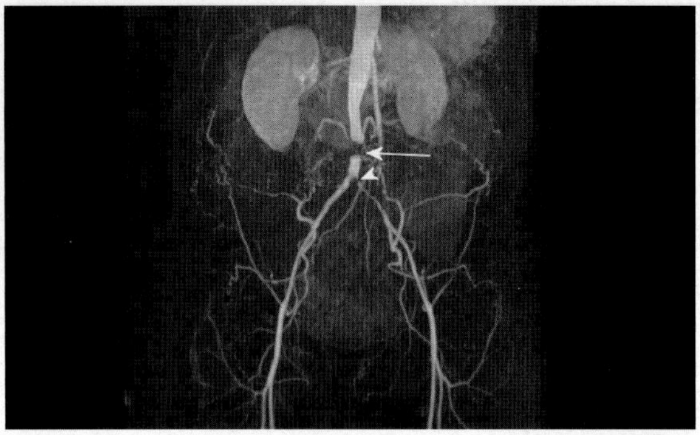

FIG. 38.6 Abdominal-pelvic contrast–enhanced magnetic resonance angiography shows a short distal aortic occlusion (*arrow*) and a significant stenosis of the proximal left common iliac artery (*arrowhead*). (FIG. 44.2 in the first edition)

hematoma, penetrating atherosclerotic ulcer, and contained aortic rupture), CTA plays a key role and is the preferred primary imaging technique because of its speed, wide availability, and high spatial resolution. As a result, CTA has essentially replaced invasive DSA. The diagnostic accuracy of CTA for the detection of dissection and traumatic injury is excellent. The sensitivity and specificity for the detection of dissection are 100%.[114] Steenburg et al.[115] reported a sensitivity of 96%, a specificity of 99.8%, and accuracy of 99.8% for multislice CTA compared with DSA in patients with acute thoracic aortic injury. False positives have been described with CTA if ECG gating is not performed.[116]

MRA in the evaluation of acute aortic syndrome is appropriate in stable patients, per the ACR Appropriateness Guidelines.[117] Monitoring acute, unstable patients in the CMR scanner is more complicated and acquisition times are longer. However, MRA has several advantages over CTA, such as the previously mentioned radiation-free nature of the imaging modality, in which the need for iodinated contrast medium is avoided. Therefore, MRA is highly suitable for the evaluation of aortic disease in young patients and for follow-up studies.[118]

CE-MRA has emerged as the preferred MRA technique for the evaluation of thoracic and abdominal vascular pathology independent of blood flow. High-resolution 3D image acquisition permits multiplanar and MIP reconstructions in any desired plane for detailed image evaluation (Fig. 38.6). Three-dimensional CE-MRA acquisition does not require ECG triggering and can be performed during a single breath-hold of 15 to 20 seconds.

For optimizing SNR, surface phased array coils are used for imaging the thoracic and abdominal aorta, although sufficient image quality can often be achieved with the body coil. Positioning of the surface phased array coil in thoracic aorta imaging is important because the volume stack should include the proximal brachiocephalic arteries. When imaging the abdominal aorta, positioning of the 3D volume is essential so that the acquired volume contains the proximal course of major arterial branches, such as the celiac trunk, superior mesenteric artery, renal arteries, and iliac arteries.

For both the thoracic and abdominal aortic CE-MRA, patients are routinely imaged in the supine position. The imaging protocol of the thoracic aorta consists of a survey or localizer sequence, bSSFP cine imaging, contrast bolus timing sequence (test bolus or fluoroscopic real-time imaging), 3D CE-MRA sequence precontrast and postcontrast, and, depending on vascular disease, a T1-weighted postcontrast sequence to rule out, for example, aortitis (Fig. 38.3). Single-shot FSE or bSSFP acquired during breath-holding can serve as a localizer sequence in three directions. For optimal planning and positioning of the 3D CE-MRA imaging volume, it is essential that the survey scan is performed in the same breath-holding position as used for the 3D CE-MRA acquisition. Preferably, this breath-holding is during end expiration because it is more reproducible compared with end inspiration.[119] bSSFP images are acquired with ECG triggering and during breath-holding. Preferably, two directions (axial and parasagittal planes) are acquired. bSSFP images provide additional information about the vessel wall and surrounding tissue.

The precontrast 3D scan is acquired to verify proper positioning of the 3D volume and to exclude possible aliasing artifacts. For 3D CE-MRA, 0.1 to 0.2 mmol/kg body weight gadolinium contrast is administered. The 3D dataset can be obtained in the coronal, sagittal, or parasagittal plane. Covering the thoracic aorta in a coronal plane requires a larger volume and, consequently, longer breath-holding to maintain high spatial resolution. Therefore, in clinical practice, the sagittal or parasagittal plane is favored. Typically, the field of view ranges from 30 to 40 cm. Usually, the abdominal aorta is imaged in the coronal plane and a field of view of 35 to 40 cm. For both thoracic and abdominal CE-MRA, spatial resolution of at least 1 to 1.5 mm is recommended.[120] In CE-MRA of the thoracic and abdominal aorta, optimally two postcontrast datasets are obtained. Large aneurysms or false lumen in aortic dissection may have slow flow and therefore require a longer time interval between contrast injection and 3D image acquisition to become fully enhanced. As a consequence, they may be only fully established during the second 3D volume acquisition. Moreover, slow flow and therefore potential nonfilling with contrast of the lumen can be better distinguished from thrombus.

Additionally, ECG-triggered T1-weighted images with fat suppression can be acquired to analyze the aortic wall. Phase-contrast sequences can be performed to quantify flow.

NE-MRA of the thoracic aorta can also provide additional information about the aortic wall and surrounding tissue, and therefore this acquisition is an important sequence within the standard MRA imaging protocol. NE-MRA by bSSFP may serve as a useful alternative for the evaluation and follow-up of aortic disease compared with CE-MRA in patients with contraindications to gadolinium use or with poor intravenous access. bSSFP showed high diagnostic accuracy for aortic dimensions and vascular pathology and similar reader confidence compared with CE-MRA.[121,122] For the detection of aortic disease, free-breathing 3D SSFP MRA with navigator gating showed a 100% diagnostic accuracy with CE-MRA serving as reference standard.[123] Furthermore, bSSFP showed significantly higher image quality of the aortic root, whereas non-ECG–gated CE-MRA images may suffer motion artifacts in this region, hindering diagnostic image evaluation.

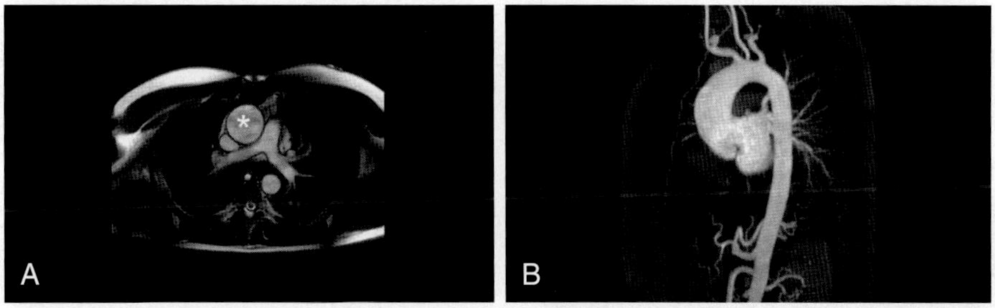

FIG. 38.7 (A) Axial, bright-blood balanced steady-state free precession axial image shows a fusiform aneurysm of the ascending aorta (*). (B) Contrast-enhanced magnetic resonance angiography (sagittal maximum intensity projection) of the same patient. (Previously FIG. 44.3.)

For CE-MRA, postprocessing of the acquired 3D dataset is essential. On MPR and MIP reconstructions, aortic vascular pathology can be assessed in relation to the origin of branching vessels. For serial follow-up examinations in patients with aortic dilatation, the consistency and accuracy of aortic diameter measurements are critical because an increase in diameter may have an important impact on risk stratification and planning of the surgical intervention.[124,125] The maximal diameter should be measured perpendicular to the axis of flow: double oblique or so-called centerline reconstruction.[126] Double oblique measurements of aortic diameter provided better agreement with the reference standard of planimetry than axial measurements and, therefore, may have a potentially important impact on surgical decision making.[127]

An aneurysm of the thoracic aorta is often an incidental finding during TTE for another indication or on chest x-ray in asymptomatic patients. Aortic aneurysm may lead to aortic rupture or aortic dissection. These acute events may be rapidly fatal in a large proportion of patients[128]; therefore, serial follow-up examinations in this patient population are vital. CE-MRA is a robust, accurate, and reproducible imaging modality for evaluation of the entire aorta and is therefore favorable for long-term monitoring examinations because it does not employ ionizing radiation or iodinated contrast (Fig. 38.7).

Reports have shown a high accuracy for the detection of thoracic and abdominal aneurysms with a sensitivity of 100% and specificity of 100%, respectively, compared with surgery or DSA.[10,129]

Atherosclerosis more often causes aneurysm formation in the descending and abdominal aorta, whereas dilatation of the ascending aorta more frequently occurs in aortic valvular disease, as in aortic valvular regurgitation, and in patients with bicuspid valves. Other causes of aortic aneurysm are connective tissue diseases (e.g., Marfan, Ehlers-Danlos, and Loeys-Dietz syndromes) (Fig. 38.8), Turner syndrome, inflammatory disease, trauma, chronic dissection (Figs. 38.9 and 38.10), and aortic surgery. Hypertension, smoking, hypercholesterolemia, and low high-density lipoprotein cholesterol levels are also significantly associated with aortic dilatation.[130,131]

Aneurysms can be classified as true or false aneurysms. A true aneurysm retains all three layers of the aortic wall—the intima, media, and adventitia. In a so-called false aneurysm, a disruption in the arterial wall causes blood leakage and the aneurysm is contained by only the adventitia or surrounding tissue. The disruption may be caused by trauma, iatrogenic origin (e.g., percutaneous or surgical procedures), or inflammation. Risk of aneurysm rupture is much higher in a false aneurysm compared with true aneurysms.[132]

Morphologically, two types of aneurysms can be recognized: fusiform (see Fig. 38.7) and saccular. A fusiform aneurysm is concentric and involves dilatation of the full circumference of the aortic wall. A saccular aneurysm is eccentric and consists of an asymmetric outpouching of a part of the aortic wall.

Bacterial infections of the aortic wall can cause the formation of mycotic aneurysms. The most common infecting organisms are *Staphylococcus aureus* and *Salmonella*. Mycotic aneurysms are usually saccular and are more prone to rupture. For optimal treatment, early diagnosis is essential. Normally, patients present with signs of infection, including fever or sometimes sepsis. Bacteremia is often present; however, negative blood cultures do not exclude a mycotic aneurysm.[133] Therefore, imaging is crucial for diagnosis. Besides the saccular aneurysm, CE-MRA can demonstrate additional perivascular inflammatory changes such as soft tissue inflammation, edema, gas, and irregularity of the aortic wall, leading to the diagnosis of mycotic aneurysm.

In aortic dissection (Figs. 38.9 and 38.10), intraluminal blood penetrates into the media layer of the aortic wall through a tear in the intima, thereby dissecting the aortic wall. The proximal ascending aorta and the descending aorta distal to the origin of the left subclavian artery are the two most common initiating sites for the intimal tear. The bleeding between the dissected layers of the aortic wall forms the false lumen and may propagate proximally or distally. Distention of the false lumen may narrow and compress the true lumen. Bleeding within the medial layer of the aortic wall can also cause the formation of a localized intramural hematoma and facilitate the development of an intimal tear.

Currently, three classification systems— the Stanford, DeBakey, and Society of Thoracic Surgeons (STS)/Society for Vascular Surgery (SVS) classifications—are most frequently used for aortic dissection.[117,134] The Stanford classification differentiates only type A and type B aortic dissection. Stanford type A dissection involves the ascending aorta and may also involve the arch and descending thoracic aorta. Stanford type B aortic dissection does not involve the ascending aorta. If not surgically intervened upon emergently, patients with acute Stanford type A aortic dissection have a very high mortality of 50% within the first 48 hours[135]; therefore, surgery is the treatment of choice. Hemodynamically stable patients with type B dissection are often treated medically with close surveillance to identify possible progression of the dissection, which is an indication for procedural intervention. The DeBakey classification subdivides aortic dissection into types I, II, and III. A DeBakey type I aortic dissection involves the ascending and descending thoracic aorta; in type II DeBakey, only the ascending aorta and aortic arch are involved; and in type III, only the descending aorta is involved. The STS/SVS classification system is the newest of the three, published in 2020, and is only applicable to Stanford type B dissections.[136]

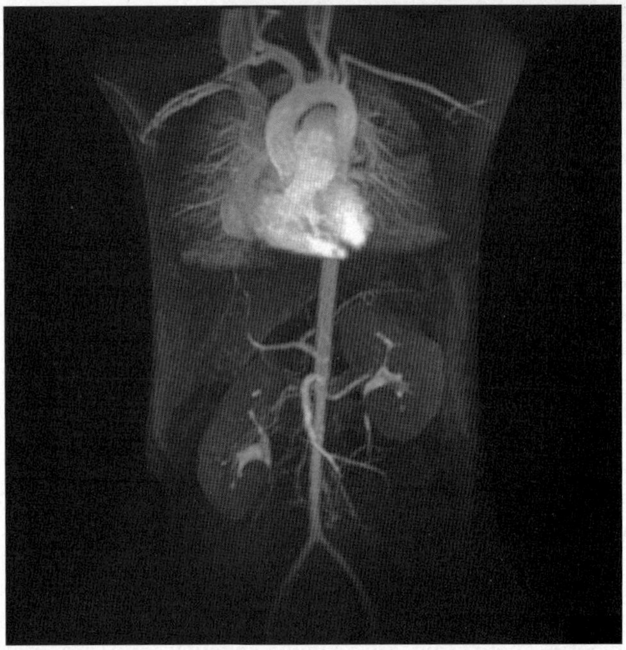

FIG. 38.8 A 4-year-old with Loeys-Dietz syndrome. Maximum intensity projection image from contrast-enhanced magnetic resonance angiography of the entire chest and abdomen.

For patients with suspected aortic dissection, imaging of the thoracic and, if necessary, abdominal aorta is essential. CTA is the imaging technique of choice in most patients with suspected aortic dissection in the acute setting because of the availability of CT in the emergency department. CE-MRA is an excellent technique for multiple follow-up examinations, with no ionizing radiation or use of iodinated contrast, and NE-MRA may also be considered.[117] For MR, high sensitivity and specificity, both 98%, in the diagnosis of aortic dissection were reported.[134,137]

CE- and NE-MRA are also helpful in characterizing coarctation, including midaortic syndrome (Fig. 38.11).

T1-weighted imaging can determine blood in the aortic wall and additional T2-weighted imaging can further help to analyze the blood compounds, characteristics, and age of intramural hemorrhage. CE-MRA clearly reveals the extent of aortic dissection and possible extension into arterial side branches. Moreover, branching arteries originating from the true or false lumen can be evaluated. Both bSSFP images and CE-MRA can clearly visualize the intimal

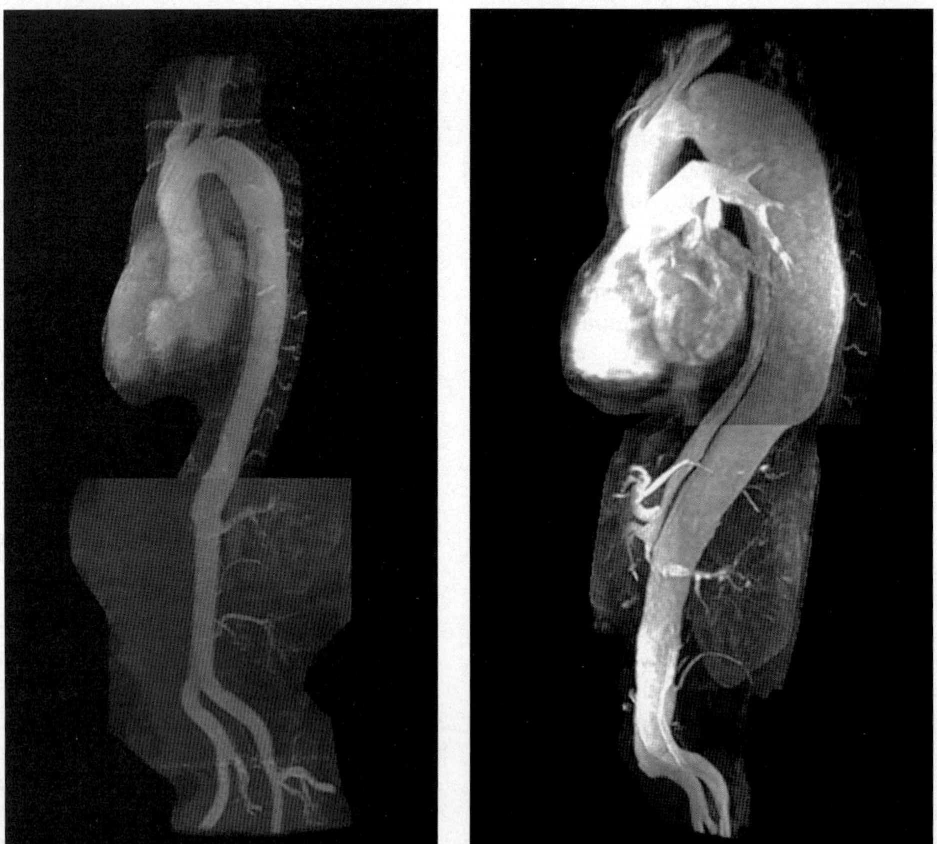

FIG. 38.9 A 67-year-old with a history of aortic dissection. The descending aorta grew substantially between baseline magnetic resonance angiography (MRA) (A) and MRA done 4 years later (B).

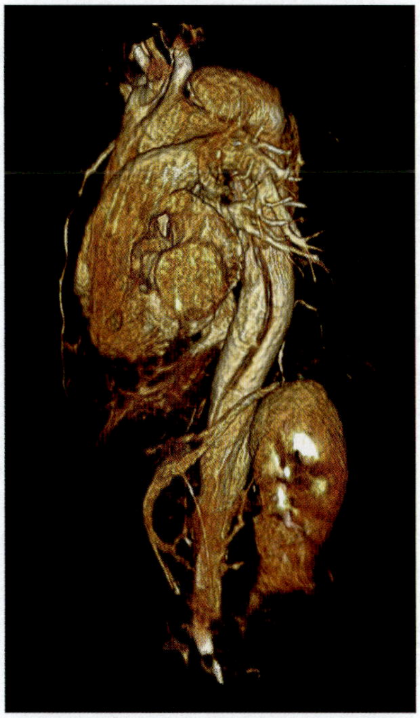

FIG. 38.10 A 45-year-old with a history of aortic dissection. Volume-rendered image from contrast-enhanced magnetic resonance angiography shows the dissection flap (*arrows*), true lumen, and false lumen.

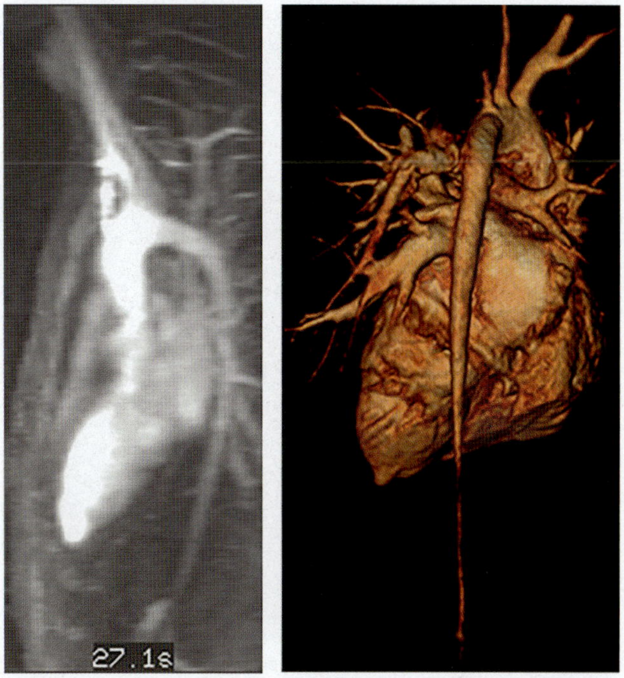

FIG. 38.11 Female in her mid-20s with Williams syndrome including supravalvular aortic stenosis and left pulmonary hypoplasia. Sagittal maximum intensity projection of time-resolved magnetic resonance angiography and posterior 3D reformatted image showing middle aortic syndrome.

flap. However, MIP images may obscure the intimal flap and dissection may be missed. Therefore, it remains important to review both source images of the CE-MRA sequence, together with bSSFP images and MPR, in patients with suspicion of or known aortic dissection. It is not advisable to make a diagnosis based solely on the projection images.

RENAL ARTERY MAGNETIC RESONANCE ANGIOGRAPHY

Renal artery stenosis is characterized by the narrowing of the renal artery lumen, which impairs blood flow to the kidneys. It encompasses a broad spectrum of pathophysiology, and is associated with major clinical syndromes including hypertension, ischemic nephropathy, CKD, and destabilizing cardiac syndromes.[138] Atherosclerotic disease and fibromuscular dysplasia are the most common causes of renal artery stenosis, with atherosclerosis accounting for the majority of cases.

Atherosclerotic renal artery disease is a progressive disease characterized by increasing narrowing of the renal arteries and eventual occlusion, with wider significant consequences in regard to organ function as well as patient prognosis[138] (Fig. 38.12). While studies suggest a 1%–5% prevalence in the general population, this increases to 22%–89% in high-risk groups, such as those with peripheral or coronary artery disease.[138–140] Renal artery stenosis is often bilateral,[141,142] with the most common sites including the proximal third of the artery, the ostium, and the perirenal aorta.[138] Luminal diameter narrowing of more than 50% is considered hemodynamically significant.[139]

Fibromuscular dysplasia is an idiopathic, noninflammatory, segmental disease of the arterial wall (with predominant involvement of the media) that can lead to stenosis, aneurysm, and dissection and/or occlusion of small- to medium-sized arteries, including the carotid arteries, as discussed above (Fig. 38.13). It predominantly occurs in premenopausal females, often with low burden of atherosclerotic risk factors; in contrast to atherosclerosis, the distal two-thirds of the renal artery are the most common location affected by fibromuscular dysplasia.[138] Also unlike atherosclerotic disease, fibromuscular dysplasia is generally associated with a good prognosis.

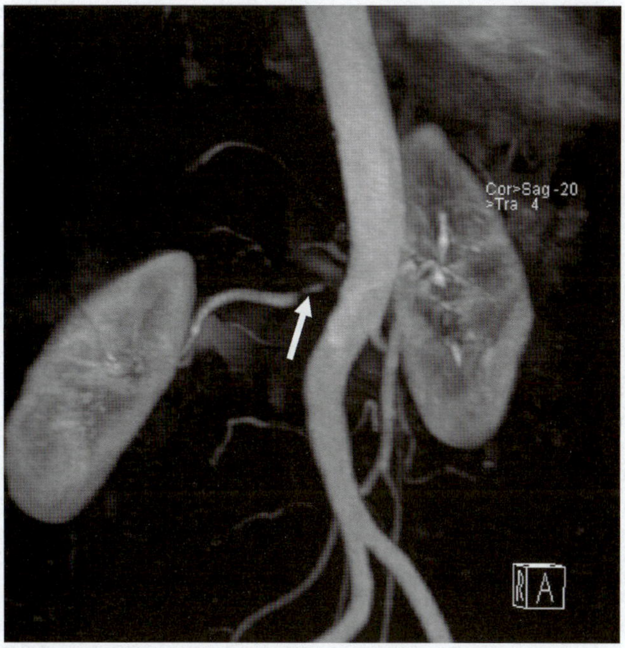

FIG. 38.12 A 76-year-old female with renovascular hypertension due to severe right renal artery stenosis (*arrow*).

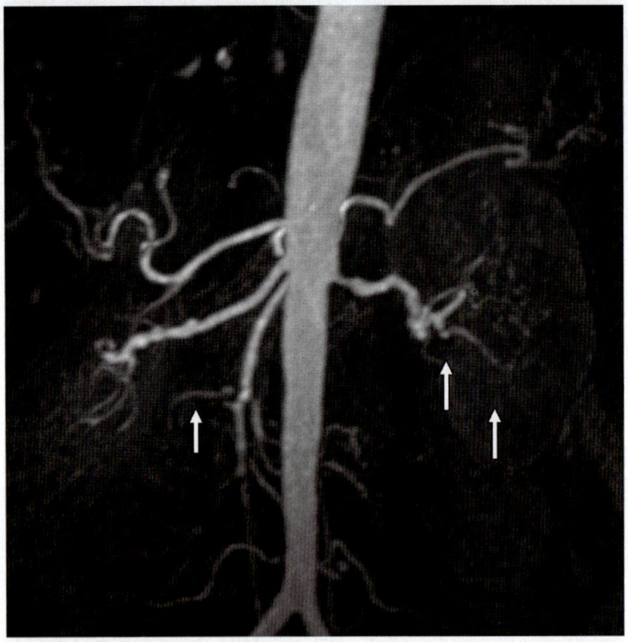

FIG. 38.13 A 68-year-old female with renovascular hypertension due to fibromuscular dysplasia. Maximum intensity projection image shows beading of the renal arteries bilaterally (*arrows*).

The 2013 American College of Cardiology (ACC)/American Heart Association (AHA) (class I, level of evidence B) and 2017 European Society of Cardiology (ESC) guidelines largely agree on diagnosing renal artery stenosis: both recommend duplex ultrasonography (ESC as primary method of choice), CTA, and MRA as diagnostic methods.[118] When the results of noninvasive test are inconclusive, catheter angiography or DSA is recommended.[118,143] While ultrasonography is often the first imaging test for renal artery stenosis, it has drawbacks such as technical limitations related to the acoustic window, operator dependence, and a limited ability to detect accessory renal arteries. CTA provides accurate and detailed visualization of renal arteries; however, its use can be limited in some patients due to concerns about radiation exposure and contrast-induced kidney injury.

Like CTA, MRA also reliably demonstrates the renal artery lumens. Benefits of MRA are that it also demonstrates the renal artery walls and provides additional insights into functional parameters related to renal arterial flow. Among MRA techniques, CE-MRA is the preferred method for visualization of the renal arteries,[144] because of its high diagnostic accuracy for renal artery stenosis, with a reported median sensitivity and specificity of 96% and 93%, respectively, compared to conventional angiography.[145] The most frequently employed technique is 3D GRE imaging, which provides high-resolution images of the renal arteries with excellent spatial and contrast resolution.[145] For assessing blood flow dynamics and the hemodynamic significance of stenosis, 3D PCA and 2D cine PCA are used.[145] Additionally, dynamic contrast-enhanced MRI is used for its time-resolved capability, allowing for the evaluation of renal perfusion and function by tracking the contrast agent's distribution over time.[145]

When selecting GBCAs for patients with impaired kidney function, it is important to consider the risk of NSF. The ACR recommends using group II GBCAs for these patients due to their very low risk of NSF, making routine kidney function assessment before administration optional.[26] Despite the FDA's black box warning on all GBCAs, group II agents are generally considered safer alternatives for patients with impaired kidney function[18,26] and, according to ACR guidelines, routine kidney function screening prior to their use is not necessary. In contrast, it is recommended that patients be screened for kidney failure and related risk factors before administering ACR group III GBCAs, and laboratory testing may be necessary. Notably, no GBCAs are currently classified under group III according to the latest ACR guidelines update.[26] GBCA I contrast agents are contraindicated in patients with impaired kidney function.[26]

Other MRI alternatives are now available that do not require the use of GBCAs. Nonenhanced MRA (NE-MRA) has been reexplored as a promising alternative to CE-MRA for assessing renal arteries using 3D bSSFP sequences.[139,146,147] SSFP is a GRE-based sequence with T2/T1-weighted image contrast, enabling high signal intensity of blood with little reliance on inflow. Three-dimensional acquisition allows angiographic images with a high SNR to be produced. Cardiac and respiratory triggering can be implemented to avoid motion artifacts.[139] The image quality of NE-MRA has improved drastically, making it comparable to CE-MRA.[147] In fact, the visualization of intraparenchymal arteries has been reported to be superior with NE-MRA, which is particularly useful for diagnosing conditions such as fibromuscular dysplasia or vasculitis.[147] Using CE-MRA or DSA as the reference standard, the accuracy for detecting renal artery stenosis has been reported to be 94%, and the sensitivity and specificity of NE-MRA ranged between 72%–100% and 82%–99%, respectively.[146,147] NE-MRA can sometimes overestimate stenosis, however.[139,147] NE-MRA is particularly advantageous for patients who are at risk for NSF or for those who may have undergone multiple MRIs, for whom concerns about gadolinium deposition in the body arise.

Another nongadolinium-based alternative for visualizing renal artery stenosis is ferumoxytol-enhanced MRA.[42,46] Ferumoxytol, an iron oxide nanoparticle MRA contrast agent (off label), offers a promising alternative to gadolinium-based agents, especially for patients with impaired kidney function or concerns about NSF. It provides high-resolution images with improved safety profiles and extended intravascular persistence, enhancing the visualization of renal arteries.

MAGNETIC RESONANCE ANGIOGRAPHY OF THE MESENTERIC ARTERIES

Atherosclerotic vascular disease of the mesenteric arteries is the leading cause of chronic mesenteric ischemia. In a population-based prevalence study, significant mesenteric arterial disease (i.e., a stenosis of more than 70% or an occlusion) was reported in 18% of asymptomatic older adult patients.[148] However, significant mesenteric arterial stenosis does not necessarily indicate the presence of mesenteric ischemia clinically.[149] The reason for this is that the mesenteric arterial circulation contains an extensive collateral circulation between the celiac artery, superior mesenteric artery, and inferior mesenteric artery. Therefore, involvement of atherosclerosis in the mesenteric arteries in patients with generalized atherosclerosis infrequently leads to symptoms of chronic mesenteric ischemia. The collateral pathways of the mesenteric arterial circulation include the pancreatico-duodenal arcade, arc of Riolan, arc of Buhler, arc of Barkow, and the marginal artery of Drummond. In general, in patients with symptoms of chronic mesenteric ischemia, two of the three mesenteric arteries show significant stenosis or occlusion.[150,151] Mostly, patients with stenosis of one of the three mesenteric arteries do not present chronic mesenteric ischemia symptoms.[152] However, chronic mesenteric ischemia has been reported in isolated mesenteric arterial stenosis.[153]

In patients with chronic mesenteric ischemia, mesenteric arterial stenosis or occlusion compromises the blood flow to the intestine, leading to postprandial abdominal pain, so-called angine abdominale. Typically, this pain starts within 30 minutes of eating and can last for several hours. This may lead to avoidance of food and significant weight loss. Patients may also present with atypical symptoms such as nausea, vomiting, diarrhea, constipation, or colitis. In the majority of patients, diagnosis of chronic mesenteric ischemia is established in an advanced stage of the disease.

The incidence of chronic mesenteric ischemia increases with age and is more prevalent in females and patients with risk factors for atherosclerotic vascular disease such as history of smoking, hypertension, and hyperlipidemia.[154] Less commonly, chronic mesenteric ischemia occurs in young patients with fibromuscular dysplasia, Takayasu vasculitis, polyarteritis nodosa, arterial dissection, abdominal aortic aneurysm, or postradiation therapy.

The clinical diagnosis of chronic mesenteric ischemia is established based on clinical symptoms and consistent imaging characteristics. Identification of stenotic arterial mesenteric disease without associated clinical symptoms is not diagnostic of chronic mesenteric ischemia.

For diagnosing chronic mesenteric ischemia, conventional DSA remains the reference standard. Advantageously, an endovascular therapeutic procedure can be performed at the time of diagnosis of mesenteric arterial stenosis. However, DSA is an invasive procedure with the already mentioned disadvantages such as exposure to radiation, nephrotoxic iodinated contrast, and the associated complications of the invasive procedure.[155] In common clinical practice, MRA and CTA have replaced DSA as an imaging tool in the workup of patients suspected for chronic mesenteric ischemia.

In patients suspected of chronic mesenteric ischemia, DUS is useful for screening and is the preferred initial imaging modality. Visualization of high-grade stenoses in the celiac artery or superior mesenteric artery associated with chronic mesenteric ischemia may be technically challenging, especially because of overlying bowel gas or patient habitus. When compared with angiography, the celiac and superior mesenteric arteries are accurately visualized in more than 80% and 90% of patients, respectively.[156] The inferior mesenteric artery can rarely be evaluated by DUS because of its anatomical location.[157,158] Peak systolic velocity has been widely used for evaluating celiac and superior mesenteric arterial disease with a sensitivity and specificity for diagnosing hemodynamically significant stenosis of 92% and 96%, and 87% and 80%, respectively.[159]

Van Petersen et al.[160] showed that stenosis in the celiac or superior mesenteric artery results in an increase of flow velocities in the other mesenteric arteries. The increase in flow was correlated with the presence of collateral vessels. This may lead to overgrading or mimicking of stenosis in the other mesenteric artery. Therefore, DUS should be used only as an initial screening imaging tool, and in case of demonstrated arterial stenosis further evaluation with MRA or CTA is required.

CTA is considered the first-line alternative to diagnostic DSA for the evaluation of chronic mesenteric ischemia.[157] Especially in the emergency situation of suspicion of acute mesenteric ischemia, CTA is the most appropriate imaging modality. It is a fast, noninvasive imaging technique and is widely available. Acquired 3D data sets can be postprocessed in varying planes and other causes for abdominal pain can be evaluated. For stenosis grading of mesenteric arteries, a high sensitivity and specificity of 100% and 95%, respectively, were reported with DSA as the reference standard.[161] However, the diagnostic value of CTA may be limited with the presence of extensive calcifications. Other known drawbacks include the use of radiation and iodinated contrast; therefore CE-MRA is an accurate and reliable alternative noninvasive imaging tool for diagnosing chronic mesenteric ischemia. Three-dimensional CE-MRA has a high sensitivity and specificity, ranging from 92% to 100% and 95% to 100%, respectively.[161–163] CE-MRA has, however, a limited role in the evaluation of distal mesenteric arteries and depicting stenosis in the inferior mesenteric artery.[164,165]

Routinely, 3D CE-MRA is acquired with the patient in the supine position using a surface phased-array coil for optimizing SNR. As with other previously described 3D CE-MRA protocols, the mesenteric arteries are evaluated with a protocol that comprises a survey or localizer sequence, a contrast bolus timing sequence (test bolus or fluoroscopic real-time imaging), and a 3D CE-MRA sequence precontrast and postcontrast. Spatial resolution and slice thickness should be tailored to the individual patient such that the 3D volume can be imaged in one single breath-hold. The same breath-holding position is used for the survey scan and the 3D CE-MRA acquisition. The precontrast 3D scan can be used to check correct positioning of the 3D volume and rule out aliasing artifacts, as was discussed previously. The 3D CE-MRA sequence is performed after intravenous administration of gadolinium contrast (0.1–0.2 mmol/kg body weight). The 3D volume slab is positioned in the sagittal plane if the primary clinical indication is to determine arterial disease of the mesenteric arteries, which occurs mostly proximal in the course of the mesenteric arteries. Also, the coronal plane can be used to include the aorta and portal vein. In addition to the arterial phase, the sequence can be repeated to obtain the portal and systemic venous phase. Typically, images are required with an in-plane resolution of approximately 1 to 2 mm and a slice thickness of 1 to 2 mm, resulting in a breath-hold of 10 to 20 seconds.[166]

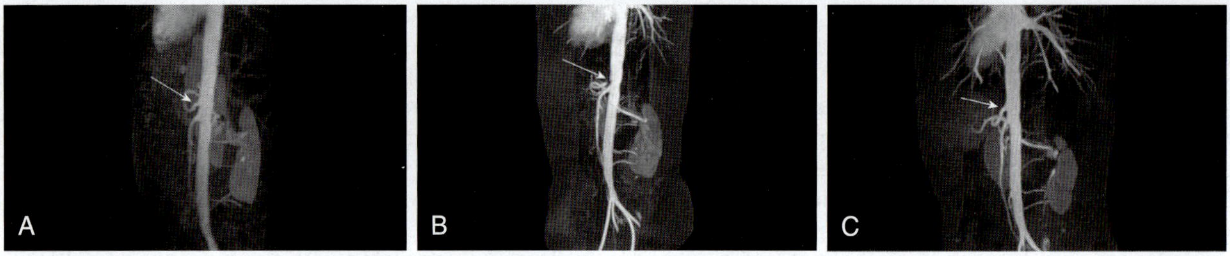

FIG. 38.14 A patient diagnosed with the arcuate ligament syndrome shows significant narrowing of the celiac artery (*arrow*) on contrast-enhanced magnetic resonance angiography (CE-MRA) (maximum intensity projection) (A) during expiration, (B) disappearing with inspiration (*arrow*), and (C) CE-MRA during inspiration after surgical release of the median arcuate ligament (*arrow*).

CE-MRA should be performed in both inspiration and expiration when median arcuate ligament syndrome is suspected (Fig. 38.14). In median arcuate ligament syndrome, the celiac artery is compressed by the central tendon of the diaphragm crura. The classical finding is a smooth narrowing of the proximal celiac artery in expiration, diminishing or disappearing in inspiration. With inspiration, the celiac artery moves inferiorly and more vertically, alleviating the compression of the ligamentous band. By performing 3D CE-MRA in both inspiration and expiration, the diagnosis can be obtained and differentiated from atherosclerotic arterial disease.

NE-MRA such as TOF and PCA are flow-dependent CMR techniques and may suffer from decreased sensitivity and specificity because of slow flow and artifacts from turbulence overestimating stenosis. bSSFP techniques demonstrated superior visualization of the inferior mesenteric artery compared with CE-MRA[167] and may play a role in patients with contraindications to intravenous administration of gadolinium-based or iodinated contrast media.

MAGNETIC RESONANCE ANGIOGRAPHY OF THE PERIPHERAL ARTERIES

Peripheral arterial disease is a common clinical manifestation of atherosclerosis and is—together with coronary artery disease and stroke— one of the leading causes of atherosclerotic cardiovascular morbidity.[168] It has been estimated that around 8.5 million people in the United States are affected by peripheral arterial disease over the age of 40 years.[169] Because of raised life expectancy, the prevalence of peripheral arterial disease increased over the last few decades by more than 20% and it has become a global problem affecting more than 200 million people worldwide,[168] causing a global increase in the morbidity and mortality associated with peripheral arterial disease.[170] Prevalence rates increase with age, and the prevalence in males and females is similar.[171] However, in the last decades females experienced a more dramatic increase in morbidity and mortality from peripheral arterial disease compared with males.[170] Risk factors significantly associated with the incidence of peripheral arterial disease include smoking, diabetes mellitus, hypertension, hypercholesterolemia, and CKD.[172] Markers of inflammation and thrombosis are also associated with peripheral arterial disease.[173] Intermittent claudication is the classic symptom in peripheral arterial disease, however it is only described in about 10% of patients[174]; men are more likely to have classic symptoms of claudication. The large majority of patients show a wide range of leg symptoms or are even asymptomatic.

Peripheral arterial disease is associated with increased risk for cardiac and cerebral events[175,176] and, moreover, several reports have shown an up to 6 times higher risk for mortality from cardiovascular causes and a 2.5 times higher overall mortality rate in patients with symptomatic peripheral arterial disease.[171,177] Therefore, assessment of risk factors for risk stratification in patients with peripheral arterial disease is very relevant.[178] Assessment of risk factors such as hypertension, diabetes mellitus, body mass index, levels of triglyceride and high-density lipoprotein in blood plasma samples, and ankle-brachial index is essential when risk factor reduction is pursued. Moreover, the usefulness of noninvasive imaging for risk assessment in cardiovascular disease is recognized[179]; for example, the assessment of CMR imaging biomarkers such as mean MRA stenosis and pulse wave velocity showed prognostic value for all-cause mortality and cardiac events in patients with symptomatic peripheral arterial disease.[180]

Clinically, symptoms in patients with peripheral arterial disease can be staged according to the Fontaine or Rutherford classification. The Fontaine classification[171,181] is divided into four different stages: stage I, asymptomatic; stage IIa, intermittent claudication after more than 200 m of pain-free walking; stage IIb, intermittent claudication after less than 200 m of walking; stage III, rest pain or nocturnal pain; and stage IV, ischemic ulcers or gangrene.

The Rutherford classification[171,182] is divided into three grades: (1) grade I comprises category 0: asymptomatic, category 1: mild claudication, category 2: moderate claudication, and category 3: severe claudication; (2) grade II comprises category 4: ischemic rest pain, and category 5: minor tissue loss, nonhealing ulcer, or focal gangrene; and (3) grade III comprises category 6: major, severe ischemic ulcers or gangrene. Both the Fontaine and the Rutherford classifications may be used routinely in clinical practice or in research settings.

For the evaluation of patients with symptomatic peripheral arterial disease, several noninvasive tests such as segmental blood pressure, pulse volume recording, DUS, and ankle-brachial index are widely available. These inexpensive techniques are easily repeatable and commonly used in the initial screening to analyze the presence and location of atherosclerotic arterial disease of the run-off arteries.[183,184] However, DUS is highly operator dependent[185] and has several other drawbacks, such as hampered evaluation

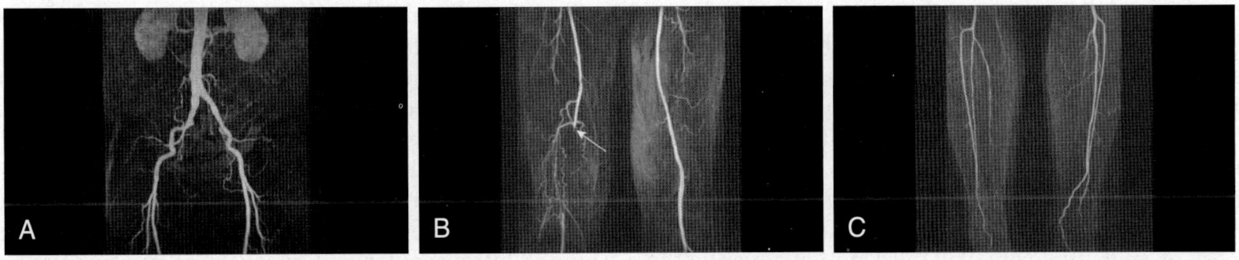

FIG. 38.15 (A) Contrast-enhanced magnetic resonance angiography of the distal aorta and common iliac arteries. (B) Peripheral arteries show an occlusion of the right superficial femoral artery (*arrow*). (C) Run-off arteries.

of peripheral arteries in obese patients and difficulty obtaining consistent, high image quality in the run-off vessels distal to the popliteal artery. The ankle-brachial index is commonly used as a first-line diagnostic imaging tool in clinical practice. A normal ankle-brachial index ranges from 1 to 1.4, and an abnormal value is defined as ≤0.9.[186] Ankle-brachial index values of 0.91 to 0.99 are regarded "borderline," and values >1.4 are an indication of noncompressible arteries. Moreover, several studies reported ankle-brachial index to predict all-cause mortality and cardiovascular events in cardiovascular disease.[187–189] A low ankle-brachial index is a strong indicator of the presence of peripheral arterial disease; however, because of false-negative rates, a normal ankle-brachial index does not exclude peripheral arterial disease,[190] and the ankle-brachial index may underestimate the prevalence of atherosclerotic arterial disease of the lower extremities compared with CE-MRA.[191]

DSA is still considered a standard reference for the evaluation of stenosis in peripheral arteries. However, because of its invasive character and the risk of possible complications, DSA is generally not used as a diagnostic imaging tool. Moreover, because of technical developments in noninvasive imaging techniques such as CTA and MRA, DSA is consequently indicated only in patients with symptomatic peripheral arterial disease for whom percutaneous revascularization is planned or in patients with contraindications to performing a CTA or MRA examination.

For further workup and planning of revascularization in patients with symptomatic peripheral arterial disease, CTA and MRA are widely available and used in clinical practice. CTA is an accurate technique for evaluating stenosis severity in patients with peripheral arterial disease. Modern multislice CT scanners allow rapid acquisition of high-resolution, thin CT images. Accurate timing of the data acquisition during maximal iodinated arterial contrast enhancement provides detailed imaging of the run-off arteries. A meta-analysis estimated a sensitivity and specificity for CTA of 96% and 95%, respectively. However, CTA employs potentially harmful radiation and requires the use of iodinated contrast material, as stated before. Moreover, arterial wall calcification may compromise diagnostic image quality and hamper stenosis evaluation, especially in patients with diabetes mellitus and renal failure.[192]

For the detection of peripheral arterial disease, CE-MRA is superior to conventional NE-MRA techniques such as 2D TOF or PCA. These conventional and older NE-MRA techniques were quite lengthy. Moreover, they suffered from artifacts caused by turbulence and in-plane saturation. In a meta-analysis,[76] the sensitivity and specificity for the detection of significant stenosis (>50% luminal reduction) for 2D TOF ranged from 64% to 100% and 68% to 96%, and for CE-MRA from 92% to 100% and 91% to 99%, respectively.

In CE-MRA, the run-off vessels are imaged during the arterial first pass of gadolinium-based contrast material after intravenous injection (Fig. 38.15). As with CTA, precise bolus timing is essential for high-quality CE-MRA. Starting the acquisition too early, when the contrast bolus is still arriving in the vessels of interest, can cause ringing or Maki artifacts.[51,193] Starting the acquisition too late can cause venous enhancement, hampering image quality, especially in the lower legs. Arterial imaging is thus performed in the time window between arterial and venous enhancement. This time window depends on the rate of contrast agent injection and will be patient specific.[14] Arterial enhancement must coincide with data readout of the central k-lines and, for improved arterial/venous differentiation, the central k-lines have to be sampled before venous return.[194]

To cover the whole region of the distal abdominal aorta and the run-off vessels, two methods are clinically used: the single-injection, three-station, moving-table (bolus-chase) technique and the multistation/multiinjection method. In both methods, imaging is performed in a coronal orientation, usually with three stations with overlapping fields of view, covering the complete anatomic region. Typically, the first station covers the distal abdominal aorta and pelvic region, the second station the upper legs, and the third station the lower legs. The quadrature body coil or phased-array surface coils are used for signal transmission and reception. In both techniques, 3D volumes are planned on acquired 2D TOF survey images. Thereafter, precontrast mask images are acquired in all stations. Subtraction of the precontrast mask images from the contrast-enhanced images will suppress surrounding tissue.[195]

In the bolus-chase technique, a biphasic contrast material injection protocol is typically used. The first half of the contrast bolus is administered at a flow rate of 1.0 to 1.2 mL/s and the remaining half at 0.5 to 0.6 mL/s. Contrast injection is followed by a saline flush at 0.5 to 0.6 mL/s. Modern commercially available 1.5 and 3 T CMR scanners allow acquisition of CE-MRA of the run-off vessels with a bolus-chase technique with excellent diagnostic performance.[196]

In the multistation/multiinjection approach, the three regions of the leg stations are acquired sequentially with two or three separate bolus injections of contrast medium.[197] Gadolinium-based contrast is injected at a rate of 1 to 1.5 mL/s, resulting in high signal intensity in the arteries.

A disadvantage of this approach is that it is more time consuming compared with the bolus-chase technique. However, in patients with multiple risk factors, adequate arterial enhancement with minimal venous enhancement can be obtained with this technique.[198] The first station covering the distal abdominal aorta and pelvic region is acquired during breath-holding and the acquired resolution of the first two stations is 1.3 × 1.3 mm with a slice thickness of 3 mm, typically. The third station covering the lower leg scan be acquired with a submillimeter voxel size, allowing accurate diagnostic evaluation.[199]

Acquired high-resolution image data can be postprocessed using multiplanar reconstructions or MIPs; however, for obtaining an adequate diagnosis, evaluation of 2D source images is essential. Furthermore, the role of CE-MRA in the evaluation of possible restenosis in (metallic) stents is limited because of dephasing of CMR signal, causing signal void. New developments in CMR imaging technology have provided a large homogeneous field of view at 3 T, revealing robust CE-MRA of the complete vascular tree of the run-off vessels and allowing accurate clinical evaluation of patient on high-field 3-T scanners.[196] Moreover, two-point Dixon fat suppression allows subtractionless CE-MRA, avoiding possible misregistration artifacts between precontrast mask dataset and contrast-enhanced images.[200] Furthermore, new techniques such as three-station bolus-chase MRA with real-time fluoroscopic tracking and precise triggering of table motion can provide high-resolution imaging of the run-off vessels. These new developments can potentially reduce contrast material dose and examination time.[201]

Conclusion and Future Directions

Throughout this chapter, we have discussed several themes of peripheral VMR that are relevant to all anatomy. Although angiography remains the established "gold standard" and allows for concurrent diagnosis and intervention, it is decreasingly used as a first-line diagnostic tool, arguably due to its invasiveness and because of patient exposure to higher doses of ionizing radiation and iodinated IV contrast. Technical advances in MRI have resulted in improved spatial resolution in commercially available systems and the option to decrease the time of image acquisition, so that MR is an increasingly strong contender for consideration in clinical use, relative to CTA. NE-MRA and ferumoxytol VMR also eliminate the use of gadolinium-based contrasts, however we would like to reiterate the current ACR recommendations that class II GBCAs are safe, even in AKI and CKD stages 4 and 5, because they have resulted in no unconfounded cases of NSF in over 15 years.

Four-dimensional flow MR sequences have also increased since the publication of the first edition of this chapter.[80] Flow is measured in the *x*-, *y*-, and *z*-dimensions over time. This sequence requires that the tech place a large, rectangular-prism–shaped volume region of interest, then the data is obtained in approximately 10–20 minutes. This sequence potentially decreases patient table time, thereby increasing individual patient comfort and improving all patients' MR access. Once all data is successfully obtained, it requires postprocessing in any one of several commercially available software applications, which can be time consuming.

Looking to the future, the concept of MR-guided interventions has been written about for over 20 years.[202] MR-guided biopsy is common in breast imaging, with a recent increase in MR-guided biopsy and MR-guided therapeutic intervention in the prostate. Additionally, MR guidance can be used for tumor ablation in the liver and lung.[203] Intravascular and intracardiac interventions using "MR fluoro" are increasing, arguably in congenital cardiac patients in particular,[204] and now there are published references regarding how to establish a program with low-field strength, MR-guided congenital cardiac procedures.[205]

ACKNOWLEDGMENTS

The authors wish to acknowledge support from GE Healthcare and Bracco Diagnostic who provide research support to the University of Wisconsin. Additionally, the authors wish to acknowledge here, in addition to citation below, the authors of the first edition of this chapter: Harrie van den Bosch, Jos J.M. Westenberg, and Albert de Roos.
Conflicts of interest: No authors have any relevant conflicts.

REFERENCES

1. Yuan C, Hatsukami TS, Mossa-Basha M, eds. *Vessel Based Imaging Techniques: Diagnosis, Treatment, and Prevention*. Elsevier; 2019.
2. van den Bosch HW, Westenberg JJM, de Roos A. Cardiovascular magnetic resonance angiography: carotids, aorta, and peripheral vessels. In: Manning WJP, Pennell DJ, eds. *Cardiovascular Magnetic Resonance: A Companion to Braunwald's Heart Disease*. Elsevier; 2019:518–528.e5.
3. AAPM, A.R.A. Image Wisely. 2024. Available from: https://www.imagewisely.org.
4. ASRT, T.S.f.P.R.A.A. Image Gently. 2014. Available from: http://www.imagegently.org.
5. Skinner MP,Yuan C, Misumori L, Hayes CE, Raines EW, Nelson JA, Ross R. Serial magnetic resonance imaging of experimental atherosclerosis detects lesion fine structure, progression and complications in vivo. *Nature Medicine*. 1995;1(1):69–73.
6. Libby P. Lesion versus lumen. *Nature Medicine*. 1995;1(1):17–18.
7. Riederer SJ, et al. Recent advances in 3D time-resolved contrast-enhanced MR angiography. *J Magn Reson Imaging*. 2015;42(1):3–22.
8. McDonald RJ, et al. Gadolinium retention: a research roadmap from the 2018 NIH/ACR/RSNA workshop on gadolinium chelates. *Radiology*. 2018;289(2):517–534.
9. Wahsner J, et al. Chemistry of MRI contrast agents: current challenges and new frontiers. *Chem Rev*. 2019;119(2):957–1057.
10. Prince MR. Gadolinium-enhanced MR aortography. *Radiology*. 1994;191(1):155–164.
11. Cheng YN, Haacke EM. Magnetic resonance angiography. *Current Protocols in Magnetic Resonance Imaging*. 2002;7(1):B7.3.1-B7.3.1.
12. Shen Y, et al. T1 relaxivities of gadolinium-based magnetic resonance contrast agents in human whole blood at 1.5, 3, and 7 T. *Invest Radiol*. 2015;50(5):330–338.
13. Szomolanyi P, et al. Comparison of the relaxivities of macrocyclic gadolinium-based contrast agents in human plasma at 1.5, 3, and 7 T, and blood at 3 T. *Invest Radiol*. 2019;54(9):559–564.
14. Prince MR, et al. Contrast material travel times in patients undergoing peripheral MR angiography. *Radiology*. 2002;224(1):55–61.
15. Wang Y, et al. Bolus arterial-venous transit in the lower extremity and venous contamination in bolus chase three-dimensional magnetic resonance angiography. *Invest Radiol*. 2002;37(8):458–463.
16. Weinreb JC, et al. Use of intravenous gadolinium-based contrast media in patients with kidney disease: consensus statements from the American College of radiology and the national kidney foundation. *Radiology*. 2021;298(1):28–35.
17. Davies J, et al. Gadolinium: pharmacokinetics and toxicity in humans and laboratory animals following contrast agent administration. *Arch Toxicol*. 2022;96(2):403–429.
18. Starekova J, Pirasteh A, Reeder SB. Update on gadolinium based contrast agent safety, from the AJR special series on contrast media. *AJR Am J Roentgenol*. 2024;223(3):e2330036.

19. Goyen M. Gadofosveset-enhanced magnetic resonance angiography. *Vasc Health and Risk Manag*. 2008;4(1):1–9.
20. Behzadi AH, et al. Immediate allergic reactions to gadolinium-based contrast agents: a systematic review and meta-analysis. *Radiology*. 2018;286(2):471–482.
21. Cha MJ, et al. Hypersensitivity reactions to iodinated contrast media: a multicenter study of 196 081 patients. *Radiology*. 2019;293(1):117–124.
22. Ahn YH, et al. Allergic-like hypersensitivity reactions to gadolinium-based contrast agents: an 8-year cohort study of 154 539 patients. *Radiology*. 2022;303(2):329–336.
23. McDonald JS, et al. Acute reactions to gadolinium-based contrast agents in a pediatric cohort: a retrospective study of 16,237 injections. *AJR Am J Roentgenol*. 2021;216(5):1363–1369.
24. Attari H, et al. A systematic review of 639 patients with biopsy-confirmed nephrogenic systemic fibrosis. *Radiology*. 2019;292(2):376–386.
25. US Food and Drug Administration. FDA drug safety communication: FDA warns that gadolinium-based contrast agents (GBCAs) are retained in the body; requires new class warnings. *US Food and Drug Administration*. 2018.
26. ACR Committee on Drugs and Contrast Media. *ACR Manual on Contrast Media*. American College of Radiology; 2024.
27. ACR Committee on Drugs and Contrast Media. *ACR Manual On Contrast Media*. American College of Radiology; 2018. Version 10.3.
28. Woolen SA, et al. Risk of nephrogenic systemic fibrosis in patients with stage 4 or 5 chronic kidney disease receiving a group II gadolinium-based contrast agent: a systematic review and meta-analysis. *JAMA Intern Med*. 2020;180(2):223–230.
29. U.S., Food and Drug Administration. FDA warns that gadolinium-based contrast agents (GBCAs) are retained in the body; requires new class warnings. *Drug Safety Communications*. 2017.
30. ACR Committee on Drugs and Contrast Media. *ACR Manual on Contrast Media*. American College of Radiology; 2026.
31. McDonald RJ, Weinreb JC, Davenport MS. Symptoms associated with gadolinium exposure (SAGE): a suggested term. *Radiology*. 2022;302(2):270–273.
32. U.S., Food and Drug Administration. FERAHEME (Ferumoxytol Injection), Full prescribing information. 2018.
33. Huang Y, et al. Repurposing ferumoxytol: diagnostic and therapeutic applications of an FDA-approved nanoparticle. *Theranostics*. 2022;12(2):796–816.
34. Bashir MR, et al. Emerging applications for ferumoxytol as a contrast agent in MRI. *J Magn Reson Imaging*. 2015;41(4):884–898.
35. Adams LC, et al. Ferumoxytol-enhanced MRI in children and young adults: state of the art. *AJR Am J Roentgenol*. 2023;220(4):590–603.
36. Knobloch G, et al. Comparison of gadolinium-enhanced and ferumoxytol-enhanced conventional and UTE-MRA for the depiction of the pulmonary vasculature. *Magn Reson Med*. 2019;82(5):1660–1670.
37. Knobloch G, et al. Relaxivity of ferumoxytol at 1.5 T and 3.0 T. *Invest Radiol*. 2018;53(5):257–263.
38. Theruvath AJ, et al. Brain iron deposition after ferumoxytol-enhanced MRI: a study of Porcine brains. *Nanotheranostics*. 2020;4(4):195–200.
39. Gerb J, et al. Ferumoxytol for the treatment of iron deficiency and iron-deficiency anemia of pregnancy. *Ther Adv Hematol*. 2021;12:20406207211018042.
40. Starekova J, et al. Pulmonary MRA during pregnancy: early experience with ferumoxytol. *J Magn Reson Imaging*. 2023;57(6):1815–1818.
41. Starekova J, et al. Ferumoxytol-enhanced pulmonary MRA in pregnancy: evaluation of initial safety and image quality. *Int Soc Magn Reson Med*. 2021. https://cds.ismrm.org/protected/21MProceedings/PDFfiles/0186.html.
42. Stoumpos S, et al. Ferumoxytol-enhanced magnetic resonance angiography for the assessment of potential kidney transplant recipients. *Eur Radiol*. 2018;28(1):115–123.
43. Hope MD, et al. Vascular imaging with ferumoxytol as a contrast agent. *AJR Am J Roentgenol*. 2015;205(3):W366–W373.
44. Lehrman ED, et al. Ferumoxytol-enhanced MRI in the peripheral vasculature. *Clin Radiol*. 2019;74(1):37–50.
45. Toth GB, et al. Current and potential imaging applications of ferumoxytol for magnetic resonance imaging. *Kidney Int*. 2017;92(1):47–66.
46. Timms L, et al. Ferumoxytol-enhanced ultrashort TE MRA and quantitative morphometry of the human kidney vasculature. *Abdom Radiol (NY)*. 2021;46(7):3288–3300.
47. Nguyen KL, et al. Multicenter safety and practice for off-label diagnostic use of ferumoxytol in MRI. *Radiology*. 2019;293(3):554–564.
48. Zhu A, et al. Quantitative ferumoxytol-enhanced MRI in pregnancy: a feasibility study in the nonhuman primate. *Magn Reson Imaging*. 2020;65:100–108.
49. Pavord S, et al. UK guidelines on the management of iron deficiency in pregnancy. *Br J Haematol*. 2020;188(6):819–830.
50. Oliveira IS, et al. Blood pool contrast agents for venous magnetic resonance imaging. *Cardiovasc Diagn Ther*. 2016;6(6):508–518.
51. Maki JH, Prince MR, Chenevert TC. Optimizing three-dimensional gadolinium-enhanced magnetic resonance angiography. Original investigation. *Invest Radiol*. 1998;33(9):528–537.
52. Mitsuzaki K, et al. Delineation of simulated vascular stenosis with Gd-DTPA-enhanced 3D gradient echo MR angiography: an experimental study. *J Comput Assist Tomogr*. 2000;24(1):77–82.
53. Fu Q, et al. Subtractionless compressed-sensing-accelerated whole-body MR angiography using two-point Dixon fat suppression with single-pass half-reduced contrast dose: feasibility study and initial experience. *J Cardiovasc Magn Reson*. 2023;25(1):41.
54. Riederer SJ, Stinson EG, Weavers PT. Technical aspects of contrast-enhanced MR angiography: current status and new applications. *Magn Reson Med Sci*. 2018;17(1):3–12.
55. Deshmane A, et al. Parallel MR imaging. *J Magn Reson Imaging*. 2012;36(1):55–72.
56. Kocaoglu M, et al. Quantitative assessment of velocity and flow using compressed SENSE in children and young adults with adequate acquired temporal resolution. *J Cardiovasc Magn Reson*. 2021;23(1):113.
57. Kocaoglu M, et al. Breath-hold and free-breathing quantitative assessment of biventricular volume and function using compressed SENSE: a clinical validation in children and young adults. *J Cardiovasc Magn Reson*. 2020;22(1):54.
58. King KF. Combining compressed sensing and parallel imaging. *Int Soc Magn Reson Med*. 2008. https://cds.ismrm.org/protected/08MProceedings/PDFfiles/01488.pdf.
59. Zhang Y, et al. 3D whole-heart noncontrast coronary MR angiography based on compressed SENSE technology: a comparative study of conventional SENSE sequence and coronary computed tomography angiography. *Insights Imaging*. 2023;14(1):35.
60. Wu X, et al. Accelerated 3D whole-heart non-contrast-enhanced mDIXON coronary MR angiography using deep learning-constrained compressed sensing reconstruction. *Insights Imaging*. 2024;15(1):224.
61. Bruce R, et al. Incidence of nephrogenic systemic fibrosis using Gadobenate Dimeglumine in 1423 patients with renal insufficiency compared with Gadodiamide. *Invest Radiol*. 2016;51(11):701–705.
62. Nandwana SB, et al. Gadobenate Dimeglumine administration and nephrogenic systemic fibrosis: is there a real risk in patients with impaired renal function? *Radiology*. 2015;276(3):741–747.
63. Reeder SB, Rowley HA, Sadowski EA. *Updated NSF Screening Procedure at the University of Wisconsin*. University of Wisconsin School of Medicine and Public Health: Department of Radiology; 2016:1.
64. Kanda T, et al. High signal intensity in dentate nucleus on unenhanced T1-weighted MR images: association with linear versus macrocyclic gadolinium chelate administration. *Radiology*. 2015;275(3):803–809.
65. Kanda T, et al. High signal intensity in the dentate nucleus and globus pallidus on unenhanced T1-weighted MR images: relationship with increasing cumulative dose of a gadolinium-based contrast material. *Radiology*. 2014;270(3):834–841.
66. Murata N, et al. Macrocyclic and other non-group 1 gadolinium contrast agents deposit low levels of gadolinium in brain and bone tissue: preliminary results from 9 patients with normal renal function. *Invest Radiol*. 2016;51(7):447–453.
67. Murata N, et al. Gadolinium tissue deposition in brain and bone. *Magn Reson Imaging*. 2016;34(10):1359–1365.
68. Wang YX, et al. Total gadolinium tissue deposition and skin structural findings following the administration of structurally different gadolinium chelates in healthy and ovariectomized female rats. *Quant Imaging Med Surg*. 2015;5(4):534–545.
69. Simonetti OP, et al. "Black blood" T2-weighted inversion-recovery MR imaging of the heart. *Radiology*. 1996;199(1):49–57.
70. Miyazaki M, Akahane M. Non-contrast enhanced MR angiography: established techniques. *J Magn Reson Imaging*. 2012;35(1):1–19.
71. Miyazaki M, Lee VS. Nonenhanced MR angiography. *Radiology*. 2008;248(1):20–43.
72. Holloway BJ, Rosewarne D, Jones RG. Imaging of thoracic aortic disease. *Br J Radiol*. 2011;84(Spec No 3):S338–S354.
73. Axel L. Blood flow effects in magnetic resonance imaging. *AJR Am J Roentgenol*. 1984;143(6):1157–1166.
74. Bradley Jr WG, Waluch V. Blood flow: magnetic resonance imaging. *Radiology*. 1985;154(2):443–450.
75. Lotz J, et al. Cardiovascular flow measurement with phase-contrast MR imaging: basic facts and implementation. *Radiographics*. 2002;22(3):651–671.
76. Nelemans PJ, et al. Peripheral arterial disease: meta-analysis of the diagnostic performance of MR angiography. *Radiology*. 2000;217(1):105–114.
77. Korosec FR, Mistretta CA. MR angiography: basic principles and theory. *Magn Reson Imaging Clin N Am*. 1998;6(2):223–256.
78. Nezafat M, et al. Coronary MR angiography at 3T: fat suppression versus water-fat separation. *MAGMA*. 2016;29(5):733–738.
79. Calkoen EE, et al. Cardiovascular function and flow by 4-dimensional magnetic resonance imaging techniques: new applications. *J Thorac Imaging*. 2014;29(3):185–196.
80. Bissell MM, et al. 4D Flow cardiovascular magnetic resonance consensus statement: 2023 update. *J Cardiovasc Magn Reson*. 2023;25(1):40
81. Dyverfeldt P, et al. 4D flow cardiovascular magnetic resonance consensus statement. *J Cardiovasc Magn Reson*. 2015;17(1):72.
82. Kollar SE, et al. Impact of ferumoxytol vs gadolinium on 4D flow cardiovascular magnetic resonance measurements in small children with congenital heart disease. *J Cardiovasc Magn Reson*. 2022;24(1):58.
83. Inzitari D, et al. The causes and risk of stroke in patients with asymptomatic internal-carotid-artery stenosis. North American Symptomatic Carotid Endarterectomy Trial Collaborators. *N Engl J Med*. 2000;342(23):1693–1700.
84. Flaherty ML, et al. Carotid artery stenosis as a cause of stroke. *Neuroepidemiology*. 2013;40(1):36–41.
85. Martin SS, et al. 2024 heart disease and stroke statistics: a report of US and global data from the American heart association. *Circulation*. 2024;149(8):e347–e913.

86. Connelly PJ, et al. Gender-affirming hormone therapy, vascular health and cardiovascular disease in transgender adults. *Hypertension*. 2019;74(6):1266–1274.
87. Ignacio KHD, et al. Stroke in male-to-female transgenders: a systematic review and meta-analysis. *Can J Neurol Sci*. 2022;49(1):76–83.
88. Mathiesen EB, et al. Carotid plaque area and intima-media thickness in prediction of first-ever ischemic stroke: a 10-year follow-up of 6584 men and women: the Tromso Study. *Stroke*. 2011;42(4):972–978.
89. Amarenco P, et al. One-year risk of stroke after transient ischemic attack or minor stroke. *N Engl J Med*. 2016;374(16):1533–1542.
90. Hankey GJ, Warlow CP, Sellar RJ. Cerebral angiographic risk in mild cerebrovascular disease. *Stroke*. 1990;21(2):209–222.
91. Expert Panel on Neurological Imaging, I, Pannell JS, Corey AS, et al. ACR appropriateness criteria(R) cerebrovascular diseases-stroke and stroke-related conditions. *J Am Coll Radiol*. 2024;21(6S):S21–S64.
92. Wardlaw JM, et al. Non-invasive imaging compared with intra-arterial angiography in the diagnosis of symptomatic carotid stenosis: a meta-analysis. *Lancet*. 2006;367(9521):1503–1512.
93. Arous EJ, et al. National variation in preoperative imaging, carotid duplex ultrasound criteria, and threshold for surgery for asymptomatic carotid artery stenosis. *J Vasc Surg*. 2015;62(4):937–944.
94. Dehkharghani S, et al. Dose reduction in contrast-enhanced cervical MR angiography: field strength dependency of vascular signal intensity, contrast administration, and arteriographic quality. *AJR Am J Roentgenol*. 2015;204(6):W701–W706.
95. Tomasian A, et al. Supraaortic arteries: contrast material dose reduction at 3.0-T high-spatial-resolution MR angiography-feasibility study. *Radiology*. 2008;249(3):980–990.
96. Townsend TC, et al. Contrast material-enhanced MRA overestimates severity of carotid stenosis, compared with 3D time-of-flight MRA. *J Vasc Surg*. 2003;38(1):36–40.
97. Patel MR, et al. Preoperative assessment of the carotid bifurcation. Can magnetic resonance angiography and duplex ultrasonography replace contrast arteriography? *Stroke*. 1995;26(10):1753–1758.
98. De Marco JK, et al. Contrast-enhanced carotid MR angiography with commercially available triggering mechanisms and elliptic centric phase encoding. *AJR Am J Roentgenol*. 2001;176(1):221–227.
99. Wright VL, et al. Assessment of CE-MRA for the rapid detection of supra-aortic vascular disease. *Neurology*. 2005;65(1):27–32.
100. Zhao H, et al. Assessment of carotid artery atherosclerotic disease by using three-dimensional fast black-blood MR imaging: comparison with DSA. *Radiology*. 2015;274(2):508–516.
101. Mihai G, et al. Assessment of carotid stenosis using three-dimensional T2-weighted dark blood imaging: initial experience. *J Magn Reson Imaging*. 2012;35(2):449–455.
102. Jiang L, et al. Role of transthoracic lung ultrasonography in the diagnosis of pulmonary embolism: a systematic review and meta-analysis. *PLoS One*. 2015;10(6):e0129909.
103. Varennes L, et al. Fibromuscular dysplasia: what the radiologist should know: a pictorial review. *Insights Imaging*. 2015;6(3):295–307.
104. Furie DM, Tien RD. Fibromuscular dysplasia of arteries of the head and neck: imaging findings. *AJR Am J Roentgenol*. 1994;162(5):1205–1209.
105. Zhou X, Huang C. Multifocal fibromuscular dysplasia involving the coronary arteries. *Radiology*. 2024;313(1):e241283.
106. Expert Panels on Vascular, I, Francois CJ, Skulborstad EP, et al. ACR appropriateness criteria((R)) nonatherosclerotic peripheral arterial disease. *J Am Coll Radiol*. 2019;16(5S):S174–S183.
107. Debette S, Leys D. Cervical-artery dissections: predisposing factors, diagnosis, and outcome. *Lancet Neurol*. 2009;8(7):668–678.
108. Ben Hassen W, et al. Imaging of cervical artery dissection. *Diagn Interv Imaging*. 2014;95(12):1151–1161.
109. Wang D, et al. ACR Appropriateness Criteria® Pulsatile abdominal mass, suspected abdominal aortic aneurysm. *J Am Coll Radiol*. 2023;20(11S):S513–S520.
110. American College of Cardiology Foundation Appropriate Use Criteria Task F, et al. ACCF/ASE/AHA/ASNC/HFSA/HRS/SCAI/SCCM/SCCT/SCMR 2011 Appropriate Use Criteria for Echocardiography. A Report of the American College of Cardiology Foundation Appropriate Use Criteria Task Force, American Society of Echocardiography, American Heart Association, American Society of Nuclear Cardiology, Heart Failure Society of America, Heart Rhythm Society, Society for Cardiovascular Angiography and Interventions, Society of Critical Care Medicine, Society of Cardiovascular Computed Tomography, and Society for Cardiovascular Magnetic Resonance Endorsed by the American College of Chest Physicians. *J Am Coll Cardiol*. 2011;57(9):1126–1166.
111. Evangelista A, et al. Echocardiography in aortic diseases: EAE recommendations for clinical practice. *Eur J Echocardiogr*. 2010;11(8):645–658.
112. Flachskampf FA, et al. Recommendations for transoesophageal echocardiography: update 2010. *Eur J Echocardiogr*. 2010;11(7):557–576.
113. Flachskampf FA, et al. Guidelines from the Working Group. Recommendations for performing transesophageal echocardiography. *Eur J Echocardiogr*. 2001;2(1):8–21.
114. Sommer T, et al. Aortic dissection: a comparative study of diagnosis with spiral CT, multiplanar transesophageal echocardiography, and MR imaging. *Radiology*. 1996;199(2):347–352.
115. Steenburg SD, Ravenel JG. Acute traumatic thoracic aortic injuries: experience with 64-MDCT. *AJR Am J Roentgenol*. 2008;191(5):1564–1569.
116. Freeman LA, et al. CT and MRI assessment of the aortic root and ascending aorta. *AJR Am J Roentgenol*. 2013;200(6):W581–W592.
117. Allen BD, Bergmann LL. Current concepts in acute aortic syndrome. *Advances in Clinical Radiology*. 2021;3(September 2021):139–151.
118. Erbel R, et al. 2014 ESC guidelines on the diagnosis and treatment of aortic diseases: document covering acute and chronic aortic diseases of the thoracic and abdominal aorta of the adult. The Task Force for the Diagnosis and Treatment of Aortic Diseases of the European Society of Cardiology (ESC). *Eur Heart J*. 2014;35(41):2873–2926.
119. Plathow C, et al. Assessment of reproducibility and stability of different breath-hold maneuvres by dynamic MRI: comparison between healthy adults and patients with pulmonary hypertension. *Eur Radiol*. 2006;16(1):173–179.
120. Kramer CM, et al. Standardized cardiovascular magnetic resonance imaging (CMR) protocols, society for cardiovascular magnetic resonance: board of trustees task force on standardized protocols. *J Cardiovasc Magn Reson*. 2008;10(1):35.
121. Lim RP, et al. Highly accelerated single breath-hold noncontrast thoracic MRA: evaluation in a clinical population. *Invest Radiol*. 2013;48(3):145–151.
122. Krishnam MS, et al. Image quality and diagnostic accuracy of unenhanced SSFP MR angiography compared with conventional contrast-enhanced MR angiography for the assessment of thoracic aortic diseases. *Eur Radiol*. 2010;20(6):1311–1320.
123. Srichai MB, et al. Non-gadolinium-enhanced 3-dimensional magnetic resonance angiography for the evaluation of thoracic aortic disease: a preliminary experience. *Tex Heart Inst J*. 2010;37(1):58–65.
124. Hiratzka LF, et al. 2010 ACCF/AHA/AATS/ACR/ASA/SCA/SCAI/SIR/STS/SVM Guidelines for the diagnosis and management of patients with thoracic aortic disease. A Report of the American College of Cardiology Foundation/American Heart Association Task Force on Practice Guidelines, American Association for Thoracic Surgery, American College of Radiology, American Stroke Association, Society of Cardiovascular Anesthesiologists, Society for Cardiovascular Angiography and Interventions, Society of Interventional Radiology, Society of Thoracic Surgeons,and Society for Vascular Medicine. *J Am Coll Cardiol*. 2010;55(14):e27–e129.
125. Cozijnsen L, et al. What is new in dilatation of the ascending aorta? Review of current literature and practical advice for the cardiologist. *Circulation*. 2011;123(8):924–928.
126. Svensson LG, et al. Aortic valve and ascending aorta guidelines for management and quality measures. *Ann Thorac Surg*. 2013;95(6 Suppl):S1–S66.
127. Mendoza DD, et al. Impact of image analysis methodology on diagnostic and surgical classification of patients with thoracic aortic aneurysms. *Ann Thorac Surg*. 2011;92(3):904–912.
128. Landenhed M, et al. Risk profiles for aortic dissection and ruptured or surgically treated aneurysms: a prospective cohort study. *J Am Heart Assoc*. 2015;4(1):e001513.
129. Arlart IP, et al. [MR angiography using Gd-DTPA in staging of abdominal aortic aneurysm: a correlation with DSA and CT]. *Rofo*. 1997;167(3):257–263.
130. Singh K, et al. Prevalence of and risk factors for abdominal aortic aneurysms in a population-based study : The Tromso Study. *Am J Epidemiol*. 2001;154(3):236–244.
131. Forsdahl SH, et al. Risk factors for abdominal aortic aneurysms: a 7-year prospective study: the Tromso Study, 1994-2001. *Circulation*. 2009;119(16):2202–2208.
132. Tessier DJ, et al. Clinical features and management of splenic artery pseudoaneurysm: case series and cumulative review of literature. *J Vasc Surg*. 2003;38(5):969–974.
133. Deipolyi AR, et al. Diagnosis and management of mycotic aneurysms. *Clin Imaging*. 2016;40(2):256–262.
134. Nienaber CA, et al. The diagnosis of thoracic aortic dissection by noninvasive imaging procedures. *N Engl J Med*. 1993;328(1):1–9.
135. Chiappini B, et al. Early and late outcomes of acute type A aortic dissection: analysis of risk factors in 487 consecutive patients. *Eur Heart J*. 2005;26(2):180–186.
136. Lombardi JV, et al. Society for vascular surgery (SVS) and society of thoracic surgeons (STS) reporting standards for type B aortic dissections. *J Vasc Surg*. 2020;71(3):723–747.
137. Shiga T, et al. Diagnostic accuracy of transesophageal echocardiography, helical computed tomography, and magnetic resonance imaging for suspected thoracic aortic dissection: systematic review and meta-analysis. *Arch Intern Med*. 2006;166(13):1350–1356.
138. Weber BR, Dieter RS. Renal artery stenosis: epidemiology and treatment. *Int J Nephrol Renovasc Dis*. 2014;7:169–181.
139. Angeretti MG, et al. Non-enhanced MR angiography of renal arteries: comparison with contrast-enhanced MR angiography. *Acta Radiol*. 2013;54(7):749–756.
140. Harding MB, et al. Renal artery stenosis: prevalence and associated risk factors in patients undergoing routine cardiac catheterization. *J Am Soc Nephrol*. 1992;2(11):1608–1616.
141. Rimmer JM, Gennari FJ. Atherosclerotic renovascular disease and progressive renal failure. *Ann Intern Med*. 1993;118(9):712–719.
142. Courand PY, et al. Resistant hypertension and atherosclerotic renal artery stenosis: effects of angioplasty on ambulatory blood pressure. a retrospective uncontrolled single-center study. *Hypertension*. 2019;74(6):1516–1523.
143. Anderson JL, et al. Management of patients with peripheral artery disease (compilation of 2005 and 2011 ACCF/AHA guideline recommendations): a report of the American College of Cardiology Foundation/American heart association Task Force on practice guidelines. *Circulation*. 2013;127(13):1425–1443.
144. Attenberger UI, et al. Assessment of the kidneys: magnetic resonance angiography, perfusion and diffusion. *J Cardiovasc Magn Reson*. 2011;13(1):70.

145. Zhang HL, et al. Renal artery stenosis: imaging options, pitfalls, and concerns. *Prog Cardiovasc Dis.* 2009;52(3):209–219.
146. Sebastia C, et al. Accuracy of unenhanced magnetic resonance angiography for the assessment of renal artery stenosis. *Eur J Radiol Open.* 2016;3:200–206.
147. Lal H, et al. Non-contrast MR angiography versus contrast enhanced MR angiography for detection of renal artery stenosis: a comparative analysis in 400 renal arteries. *Abdom Radiol (NY).* 2021;46(5):2064–2071.
148. Hansen KJ, et al. Mesenteric artery disease in the elderly. *J Vasc Surg.* 2004;40(1):45–52.
149. Roobottom CA, Dubbins PA. Significant disease of the celiac and superior mesenteric arteries in asymptomatic patients: predictive value of Doppler sonography. *AJR Am J Roentgenol.* 1993;161(5):985–988.
150. Parameshwarappa SK, et al. Chronic mesenteric ischemia and therapeutic paradigm of mesenteric revascularization. *Indian J Gastroenterol.* 2014;33(2):169–174.
151. Matsumoto AH, et al. Percutaneous transluminal angioplasty of visceral arterial stenoses: results and long-term clinical follow-up. *J Vasc Interv Radiol.* 1995;6(2):165–174.
152. Brandt LJ, Boley SJ. AGA technical review on intestinal ischemia. American Gastrointestinal Association. *Gastroenterology.* 2000;118(5):954–968.
153. Carrick RP, et al. Chronic mesenteric ischemia resulting from isolated lesions of the superior mesenteric artery–a case report. *Angiology.* 2005;56(6):785–788.
154. Cangemi JR, Picco MF. Intestinal ischemia in the elderly. *Gastroenterol Clin North Am.* 2009;38(3):527–540.
155. Balduf LM, et al. Complication rates of diagnostic angiography performed by vascular surgeons. *Vasc Endovascular Surg.* 2002;36(6):439–445.
156. Moneta GL, et al. Mesenteric duplex scanning: a blinded prospective study. *J Vasc Surg.* 1993;17(1):79–84; discussion 85–86.
157. Oliva IB, et al. ACR Appropriateness Criteria (R) imaging of mesenteric ischemia. *Abdom Imaging.* 2013;38(4):714–719.
158. Expert Panels on Vascular I, et al. ACR Appropriateness Criteria((R)) Imaging of Mesenteric Ischemia. *J Am Coll Radiol.* 2018;15(11S):S332–S340.
159. Moneta GL. Screening for mesenteric vascular insufficiency and follow-up of mesenteric artery bypass procedures. *Semin Vasc Surg.* 2001;14(3):186–192.
160. van Petersen AS, et al. Mesenteric stenosis, collaterals, and compensatory blood flow. *J Vasc Surg.* 2014;60(1):111–119, 119 e1–2.
161. Schaefer PJ, et al. Comparison of noninvasive imaging modalities for stenosis grading in mesenteric arteries. *Rofo.* 2013;185(7):628–634.
162. Meaney JF, et al. Gadolinium-enhanced MR angiography of visceral arteries in patients with suspected chronic mesenteric ischemia. *J Magn Reson Imaging.* 1997;7(1):171–176.
163. Holland GA, et al. Breath-hold ultrafast three-dimensional gadolinium-enhanced MR angiography of the aorta and the renal and other visceral abdominal arteries. *AJR Am J Roentgenol.* 1996;166(4):971–981.
164. Jaster A, et al. Anatomic and radiologic review of chronic mesenteric ischemia and its treatment. *Clin Imaging.* 2016;40(5):961–969.
165. Laissy JP, Trillaud H, Douek P. MR angiography: noninvasive vascular imaging of the abdomen. *Abdom Imaging.* 2002;27(5):488–506.
166. Hagspiel KD, et al. Computed tomography angiography and magnetic resonance angiography imaging of the mesenteric vasculature. *Tech Vasc Interv Radiol.* 2015;18(1):2–13.
167. Iozzelli A, et al. The value of true-FISP sequence added to conventional gadolinium-enhanced MRA of abdominal aorta and its major branches. *Eur J Radiol.* 2009;72(3):489–493.
168. Fowkes FG, et al. Comparison of global estimates of prevalence and risk factors for peripheral artery disease in 2000 and 2010: a systematic review and analysis. *Lancet.* 2013;382(9901):1329–1340.
169. Allison MA, et al. Ethnic-specific prevalence of peripheral arterial disease in the United States. *Am J Prev Med.* 2007;32(4):328–333.
170. Sampson UK, et al. Global and regional burden of death and disability from peripheral artery disease: 21 world regions, 1990 to 2010. *Glob Heart.* 2014;9(1):145–158e21.
171. Norgren L, et al. Inter-Society Consensus for the Management of Peripheral Arterial Disease (TASC II). *J Vasc Surg.* 2007;45(Suppl S):S5–67.
172. Eraso LH, et al. Peripheral arterial disease, prevalence and cumulative risk factor profile analysis. *Eur J Prev Cardiol.* 2014;21(6):704–711.
173. Khawaja FJ, Kullo IJ. Novel markers of peripheral arterial disease. *Vasc Med.* 2009;14(4):381–392.
174. Hirsch AT, et al. Peripheral arterial disease detection, awareness, and treatment in primary care. *JAMA.* 2001;286(11):1317–1324.
175. Criqui MH, et al. Progression of peripheral arterial disease predicts cardiovascular disease morbidity and mortality. *J Am Coll Cardiol.* 2008;52(21):1736–1742.
176. Araki Y, et al. Prevalence and risk factors for cerebral infarction and carotid artery stenosis in peripheral arterial disease. *Atherosclerosis.* 2012;223(2):473–477.
177. Sigvant B, Lundin F, Wahlberg E. The risk of disease progression in peripheral arterial disease is higher than expected: a meta-analysis of mortality and disease progression in peripheral arterial disease. *Eur J Vasc Endovasc Surg.* 2016;51(3):395–403.
178. Goff Jr DC, et al. 2013 ACC/AHA guideline on the assessment of cardiovascular risk: a report of the American College of Cardiology/American Heart Association Task Force on Practice Guidelines. *J Am Coll Cardiol.* 2014;63(25 Pt B):2935–2959.
179. Greenland P, et al. 2010 ACCF/AHA guideline for assessment of cardiovascular risk in asymptomatic adults: a report of the American College of Cardiology Foundation/American Heart Association Task Force on Practice Guidelines. *J Am Coll Cardiol.* 2010;56(25):e50–103.
180. van den Bosch H, et al. Prognostic value of cardiovascular MR imaging biomarkers on outcome in peripheral arterial disease: a 6-year follow-up pilot study. *Int J Cardiovasc Imaging.* 2016;32(8):1281–1288.
181. Dormandy J, Heeck L, Vig S. The natural history of claudication: risk to life and limb. *Semin Vasc Surg.* 1999;12(2):123–137.
182. Dormandy JA, Rutherford RB. Management of peripheral arterial disease (PAD). TASC Working Group. TransAtlantic Inter-Society Consensus (TASC). *J Vasc Surg.* 2000;31(1 Pt 2):S1–S296.
183. Hirsch AT, et al. ACC/AHA 2005 Practice Guidelines for the management of patients with peripheral arterial disease (lower extremity, renal, mesenteric, and abdominal aortic): a collaborative report from the American Association for Vascular Surgery/Society for Vascular Surgery, Society for Cardiovascular Angiography and Interventions, Society for Vascular Medicine and Biology, Society of Interventional Radiology, and the ACC/AHA Task Force on Practice Guidelines (Writing Committee to Develop Guidelines for the Management of Patients With Peripheral Arterial Disease): endorsed by the American Association of Cardiovascular and Pulmonary Rehabilitation; National Heart, Lung, and Blood Institute; Society for Vascular Nursing; TransAtlantic Inter-Society Consensus; and Vascular Disease Foundation. *Circulation.* 2006;113(11):e463–e654.
184. Rooke TW, et al. 2011 ACCF/AHA Focused Update of the Guideline for the Management of Patients With Peripheral Artery Disease (updating the 2005 guideline): a report of the American College of Cardiology Foundation/American Heart Association Task Force on Practice Guidelines. *J Am Coll Cardiol.* 2011;58(19):2020–2045.
185. O'Keeffe ST, Persson AV. Use of noninvasive vascular laboratory in diagnosis of venous and arterial disease. *Cardiol Clin.* 1991;9(3):429–442.
186. Ankle Brachial Index C, et al. Ankle brachial index combined with Framingham Risk Score to predict cardiovascular events and mortality: a meta-analysis. *JAMA.* 2008;300(2):197–208.
187. Newman AB, et al. Ankle-arm index as a predictor of cardiovascular disease and mortality in the Cardiovascular Health Study. The Cardiovascular Health Study Group. Arterioscler Thromb Vasc. *Biol.* 1999;19(3):538–545.
188. McDermott MM, et al. The ankle-brachial index as a predictor of survival in patients with peripheral vascular disease. *J Gen Intern Med.* 1994;9(8):445–449.
189. McKenna M, Wolfson S, Kuller L. The ratio of ankle and arm arterial pressure as an independent predictor of mortality. *Atherosclerosis.* 1991;87(2–3):119–128.
190. Doobay AV, Anand SS. Sensitivity and specificity of the ankle-brachial index to predict future cardiovascular outcomes: a systematic review. *Arterioscler Thromb Vasc Biol.* 2005;25(7):1463–1469.
191. Wikstrom J, et al. Ankle brachial index <0.9 underestimates the prevalence of peripheral artery occlusive disease assessed with whole-body magnetic resonance angiography in the elderly. *Acta Radiol.* 2008;49(2):143–149.
192. Meyer BC, et al. Do the cardiovascular risk profile and the degree of arterial wall calcification influence the performance of MDCT angiography of lower extremity arteries? *Eur Radiol.* 2010;20(2):497–505.
193. Maki JH, et al. The effects of time varying intravascular signal intensity and k-space acquisition order on three-dimensional MR angiography image quality. *J Magn Reson Imaging.* 1996;6(4):642–651.
194. Altaha MA, et al. Non-contrast-enhanced MR angiography in critical limb ischemia: performance of quiescent-interval single-shot (QISS) and TSE-based subtraction techniques. *Eur Radiol.* 2017;27(3):1218–1226.
195. Ho KY, et al. Peripheral vascular tree stenoses: detection with subtracted and nonsubtracted MR angiography. *Radiology.* 1998;206(3):673–681.
196. van den Bosch HC, et al. Peripheral arterial occlusive disease: 3.0-T versus 1.5-T MR angiography compared with digital subtraction angiography. *Radiology.* 2013;266(1):337–346.
197. Watanabe Y, et al. Dynamic subtraction contrast-enhanced MR angiography: technique, clinical applications, and pitfalls. *Radiographics.* 2000;20(1):135–152; discussion 152–153.
198. Dinter DJ, et al. Peripheral bolus-chase MR angiography: analysis of risk factors for nondiagnostic image quality of the calf vessels–a combined retrospective and prospective study. *AJR Am J Roentgenol.* 2009;193(1):234–240.
199. Bezooijen R, et al. Peripheral arterial disease: sensitivity-encoded multiposition MR angiography compared with intraarterial angiography and conventional multiposition MR angiography. *Radiology.* 2004;231(1):263–271.
200. Leiner T, et al. Subtractionless first-pass single contrast medium dose peripheral MR angiography using two-point Dixon fat suppression. *Eur Radiol.* 2013;23(8):2228–2235.
201. Johnson CP, et al. Three-station three-dimensional bolus-chase MR angiography with real-time fluoroscopic tracking. *Radiology.* 2014;272(1):241–251.
202. Barkhausen J, et al. White paper: interventional MRI: current status and potential for development considering economic perspectives, Part 1: general application. *Rofo.* 2017;189(7):611–623.
203. Winkelmann MT, Kubler J, Hoffmann R. Magnetic resonance-guided procedures: consensus on rationale, techniques, and outcomes. *Tech Vasc Interv Radiol.* 2023;26(3):100914.
204. Valverde I, Hussain T, Razavi R. Novel imaging techniques for the diagnosis and treatment of congenital heart defects: MR-guided interventions and beyond. *Future Cardiol.* 2012;8(2):149–152.
205. Amin EK, Campbell-Washburn A, Ratnayaka K. MRI-guided cardiac catheterization in congenital heart disease: how to get started. *Curr Cardiol Rep.* 2022;24(4):419–429.

39 Thoracic Aortic Disease

CHRISTOPH A. NIENABER AND XUN YUAN

The anatomic and functional characteristics of the aorta, which may at first glance appear relatively straightforward, are now recognized to be complex. Recent insights from both modern imaging technology and a better understanding of the hydraulic principles associated with the variety of aortic diseases have helped the medical community realize the multiple facets of in vivo aortic pathology as well as its varied clinical presentation.

Diagnostic modalities such as transesophageal echocardiography (TEE), cardiovascular magnetic resonance imaging (CMR), and spiral computed tomography (CT) have all been shown to be useful in interrogating the aorta in both chronic disease and acute aortic syndromes. X-ray contrast angiography, the former gold standard in acute and chronic aortic syndromes, has been relegated to a secondary role after the emergence of noninvasive techniques, most importantly CMR, with their high sensitivity, specificity, and practical advantages.[1–5] However, none of the diagnostic modalities listed above are ideal for all patients, and for a given individual, knowledge of both accuracy and limitations in the presenting clinical scenario are required.[4–7] While the information content of CMR may greatly overlap with established methods such as echocardiography, CT, and angiography, the technique is more comprehensive and offers more options including four-dimensional (4D) functional magnetic resonance imaging (MRI).

Besides images with high soft tissue contrast without any radiation, MRI can demonstrate and quantify functional parameters beyond anatomic depiction. Combining anatomical and functional information in a single acquisition means that MRI can potentially provide a more comprehensive evaluation of thoracic aortic disease including aortic valve morphology and function. Magnetic resonance (MR) is an ideal imaging modality for surveillance in a relatively young patient population requiring long-term or even lifelong follow-up care.[8–10] Although the cost effectiveness of CMR has not been proven in all areas,[11] it is the preferred modality in both acquired aortic diseases, including aneurysm, dissection, and its precursors, and in congenital and inherited heart diseases. This chapter focuses on emerging advantages of CMR with respect to a spectrum of aortic pathologies.

PRINCIPLES OF CARDIOVASCULAR MAGNETIC RESONANCE IN AORTIC IMAGING

Spin Echo Cardiovascular Magnetic Resonance Imaging

Spin echo T1-weighted imaging provides the anatomic detail of the aortic wall and pathologic conditions such as atheromatous plaques, intimal flaps, and intramural hemorrhage and is still the basis of any aortic study while T2-weighted images (repetition time: 2/3R-R; echo time: 80 to 100 msec) can be used in tissue characterization of the aortic wall or blood components. Electrocardiographic (ECG) triggering is essential for minimizing motion and pulsatility artifacts. A slice thickness of 3 to 8 mm and an echo time (TE) of 20 to 30 msec are standard, while repetition time (TR) is determined from the R-R interval of the ECG. A shorter acquisition time can be achieved with fast spin echo pulse sequences whereby a long train of echoes is acquired by using a series of 180 degree radiofrequency (RF) pulses; washout effects are even more substantial than in conventional spin echo techniques. A superior black-blood effect is achieved using preparatory pulses[12] (such as presaturation, dephasing gradients, and preinversion) with one or more additional RF pulses outside the plane to suppress the signal intensity of inflowing blood and nullify the blood signal (Fig. 39.1). Therefore, "black-blood" fast T1- and T2-weighted spin echo sequences have improved image quality, and constitute the method of choice for morphologic assessment of the thoracic aorta. Images are acquired in axial and additional planes depending on the anatomy and diagnostic problems to define the extent of the disease in three-dimensional (3D) space.

Gradient Echo Cardiovascular Magnetic Resonance Imaging and Flow Mapping

Gradient echo techniques provide dynamic and functional information, although with fewer details of the vessel wall. The bright signal of the blood pool on gradient echo images results from flow-related enhancement obtained by applying RF pulses to saturate a volume of tissue. With a short TR (4 to 8 msec) and low flip angle (20 degrees to 30 degrees), maximal signal is emitted by blood flowing in the voxel, and ECG-gated acquisition provides a high degree of temporal resolution throughout the cardiac cycle (up to 20 to 25 frames) to be displayed in cine format. Flow-related enhancement is produced by inflow of unsaturated blood exposed to only one RF pulse. As a result, the laminar moving blood displays a bright signal in contrast to stationary tissues. The signal can be reduced if the flow is low, as in aortic aneurysms. Mural thrombi can be identified by persistent low-signal intensity in different phases of the cardiac cycle. Turbulent flow produces rapid spin dephasing and results in a signal void, providing additional information in many pathologic conditions such as coarctation, aortic valve insufficiency, aortic aneurysm, and dissection.[13] Particularly in aortic dissection, the detection of entry and reentry sites is a special capability of functional CMR that can be helpful in planning both surgical and endovascular therapy. Accurate quantitative information on blood flow is obtained from modified gradient echo sequences with parameter reconstruction from the phase rather than the amplitude of the MR signal; this is also known as flow mapping or phase-contrast or velocity-encoded cine CMR (Fig. 39.2).[14] In each pixel of velocity images, the phase of the signal is related to the velocity component in the direction of a bipolar velocity phase-encoding gradient. In the phase image, the velocity of blood flow can be determined for any site of the vascular system. Flow velocity is calculated using a formula in which velocity is proportional to the change in the phase angle of protons in motion. MR maps of flow velocity are obtained two-dimensionally, which is particularly important in a profile of nonuniform flow, such as that in the great vessels. Quantitative data on flow velocity and flow volume are obtained from the velocity maps through a region of interest. The mean blood flow is estimated by multiplying the spatial mean velocity and the cross-sectional area of the vessel. Vector mapping has been used to describe flow patterns in different aortic diseases (e.g., hypertension, aneurysms, dissection, Marfan syndrome, coarctation).[15,16]

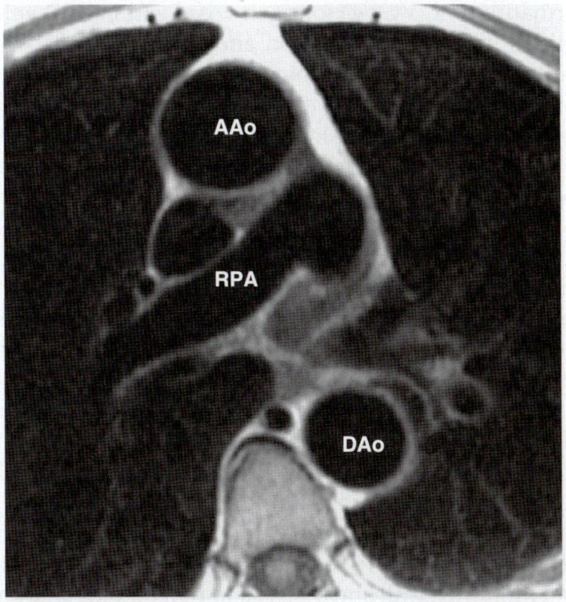

FIG. 39.1 Black-blood vascular imaging of the aorta obtained with cardiac gating and breath-holding. Axial image shows the ascending (*AAo*) and descending (*DAo*) aorta at the level of the right pulmonary artery (*RPA*). Note the excellent suppression of the luminal blood signal and demonstration of the vessel wall.

Magnetic Resonance Angiography

A variety of magnetic resonance angiography (MRA) techniques, including various pulse sequences, methods of data acquisition, and postprocessing, have been developed, but first-pass 3D contrast-enhanced MRA constitutes the method of choice for evaluation of the aorta.[8,17,18] The technique relies on the contrast-induced T1-shortening effects of Gadolinium-diethylenetriamine penta-acetic acid (Ga-DTPA) whereby saturation problems with slow flow or turbulence-induced signal voids are avoided. During the short intravascular phase, the paramagnetic contrast agent provides a precise signal in the arterial or venous system, enhancing the vessel-to-background contrast-to-noise ratio irrespective of flow patterns and velocity, which not only delineates the dissection lamella, but also the

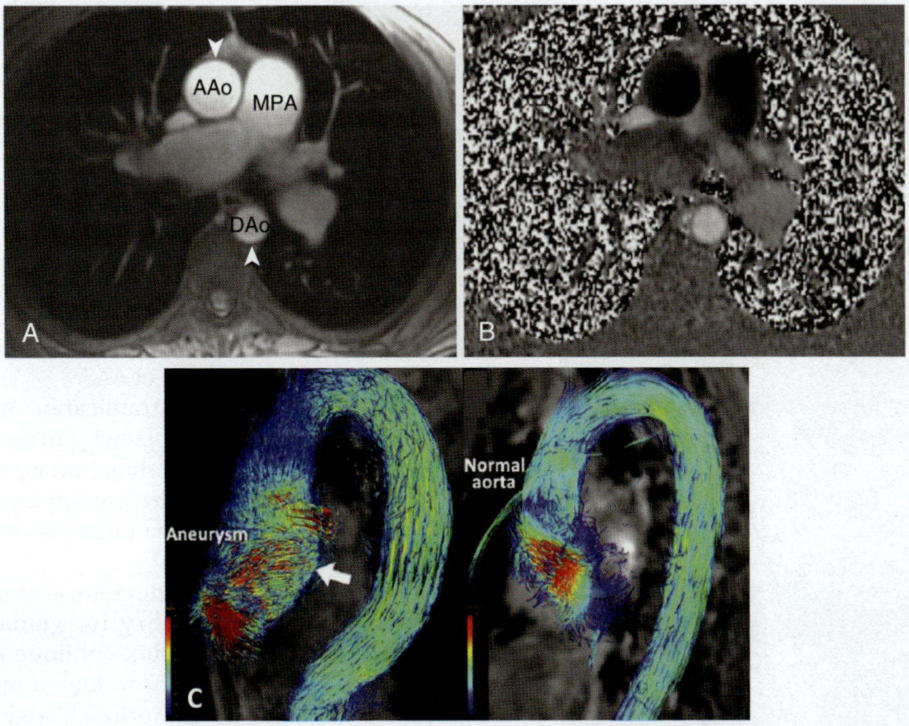

FIG. 39.2 Phase-contrast imaging of the aorta. Magnitude (A) and phase (B) axial images show the ascending (*AAo*) and descending (*DAo*) aorta at the level of the main pulmonary artery (*MPA* in panel A). On the phase image (B), the ascending aorta and main pulmonary artery appear black, and the descending aorta appears white, owing to the opposite directions of flow in these arteries. The 3D pathline images (C) show an aneurysm of the ascending aorta with abnormal helical flow (*left*) as opposed to a normal laminar flow pattern in a normal ascending aorta (*right*).

filling of critical side branches. Intravenous bolus timing is necessary to ensure peak enhancement during the middle of CMR acquisition, and not exceeding the acquisition time.[19] Improved gradient systems allow a considerable reduction of the minimum TRs and TEs and the acquisition of complex 3D datasets within a breath-hold interval of under 30 seconds. With the support of maximum intensity projection (MIP) images and 3D multiplanar reformation, this technique delineates all the morphologic details of the aorta and its side branches in any plane in a 3D format; the more conventional imaging modality in daily practice, however, is the use of a CT angiogram with 3D reconstruction (Fig. 39.3).

Some caution must be exercised in patients with poor renal function both when using classic iodine-based contrast material and gadolinium as well with MRI, as MR contrast agents have been associated with the development of nephrogenic systemic fibrosis in several cases. From a technical point of view, blood pool imaging can be acquired without the use of a contrast agent using an ECG-gated and respiratory-navigated balanced steady state-free precession acquisition. After an intervention, first-pass contrast-enhanced angiography is instrumental to assess the success of the procedure and to quantify false lumen thrombosis, a well-established prognostic indicator. The image acquisition is timed according to the arrival of the contrast bolus in the proximal unaffected aorta and thrombosis is assumed to be present when there is no contrast agent in the false lumen. However, recent studies have shown that the flow rates in the false lumen are highly variable and often very slow,[20–22] encouraging the use of a new MR technique using gadofosveset trisodium blood pool agent in an equilibrium state.[20,21]

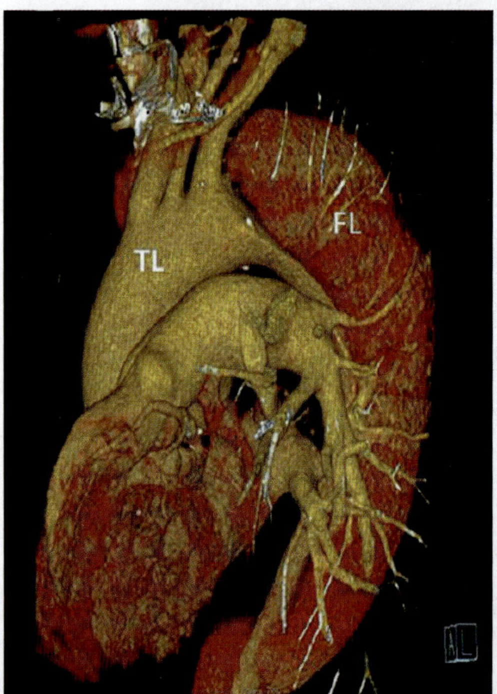

FIG. 39.3 Contrast-enhanced three-dimensional reconstruction of a computed tomography image of a type B aortic dissection with clear delineation of the true and false lumen.

Four-Dimensional Flow Magnetic Resonance Imaging

Phase-contrast sequences (or time-resolved 3D phase contrast or 4D flow MRI) are used to assess blood flow and velocity. This imaging technique adds complementary information to diagnostic imaging and provides flow-related parameters in each lumen of the aorta for prognostic assessment of a given patient.[22] This 3D velocity information (Vx, Vy, Vz) for each voxel within a 3D volume provides valuable information and the potential to study complex aortic flow dynamics in vivo, flow patterns, and derived vessel wall parameters such as wall shear stress.[23] This evolving MRI modality shows promise for preventative management of aortic conditions[24] and stratification of patients according to their risk of developing late aneurysmal degeneration (Fig. 39.4).[21]

In healthy subjects, 4D flow analysis detects changes with aging or as a result of heart failure and stroke volume reduction.[25] The contrast-enhanced MR angiography technique 4D-TRAK can acquire multiple time-resolved 3D volumes over time using image acceleration techniques[26] to acquire several phases of contrast distribution, including both arterial and venous phases, and is thus clinically useful for characterizing flow-related phenomena such as false lumen thrombus distribution and endoleak.[21,26]

In vitro flow studies using computational fluid dynamics have shown promising results for calculating a consistent correlation with wall shear stress in real patient anatomy,[27] introducing the concept of instantaneous human aorta stress mapping.[28] Importantly, in the ascending aorta, segmental increases in wall shear stress (now automatically subjected to deep learning algorithms) are associated with extracellular matrix degeneration and thinning of elastic fibers in aortopathy as a result of a bicuspid aortic valve.[29,30]

ACUTE AORTIC SYNDROME

Acute aortic syndrome (AAS) comprises a spectrum of life-threatening conditions from classic aortic dissection to limited focal dissection and intramural hematoma to symptomatic penetrating atherosclerotic ulcers of the aortic wall. Imaging with CTA or MR angiographic techniques is the gold standard for establishing these granular diagnoses within the spectrum of AAS.

Imaging-based risk stratification metrics (or parameters) such as maximum diameter in defined locations along the aorta, entry site location and size, and most recently flow velocity metrics drive contemporary recommendations for the type and the timing of open surgery or endovascular intervention.

Accurate and reproducible measurements of aortic dimensions are necessary for guidance and therapeutic decision making; double-oblique reformatted images perpendicular to the aortic lumen in short-axis orientation or automated centerline-based measurements are most reliable; if an aortic lumen appears oval-shaped the shorter diameter is usually more accurate. The size of the aorta can be overestimated if the outer-to-outer

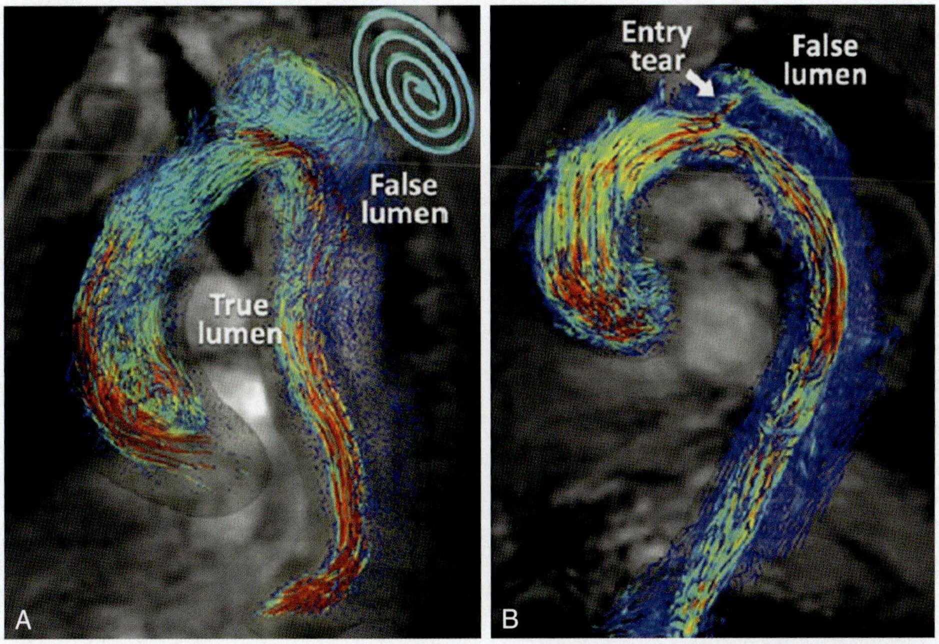

FIG. 39.4 Visualization of 3D flow (*pathline*) magnetic resonance images in a case of type B aortic dissection with a tear near the left subclavian artery; a vortexlike flow pattern is seen in the proximal false lumen (A), and high blood flow velocity is demonstrated at the entry tear to the false lumen (B).

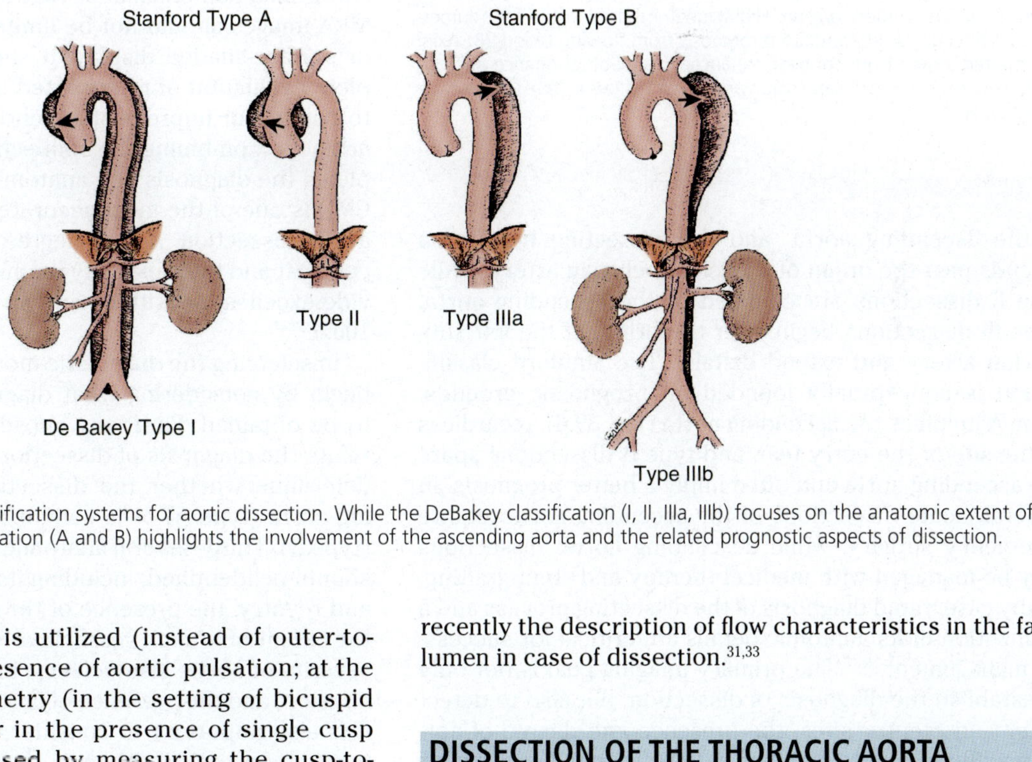

FIG. 39.5 Commonly used classification systems for aortic dissection. While the DeBakey classification (I, II, IIIa, IIIb) focuses on the anatomic extent of the dissection, the Stanford classification (A and B) highlights the involvement of the ascending aorta and the related prognostic aspects of dissection.

edge of the aortic wall is utilized (instead of outer-to-inner edge) or in the presence of aortic pulsation; at the aortic root level asymmetry (in the setting of bicuspid aortic valve anatomy or in the presence of single cusp prolapse) can be assessed by measuring the cusp-to-commissure diameter in all cusps separately rather than just recording and documenting the maximal dimension of the root.[31,32]

A comprehensive MRI analysis should ideally include the type of AAS; the location and extent of the involved aortic segment (best using the TEM (type, entry and malperfusion) classification system); the maximum aortic diameter at prespecified locations; the extent of the dissection to branch vessels and potential signs of end-organ malperfusion, patency, or thrombus in the false lumen; the suspicion of rupture and extraaortic blood collection; and most recently the description of flow characteristics in the false lumen in case of dissection.[31,33]

DISSECTION OF THE THORACIC AORTA

Acute aortic dissection is a life-threatening medical emergency requiring prompt diagnosis and treatment. The 14-day period after onset has been designated as an acute phase because the rates of morbidity and mortality are highest during this period.[34,35] The two most frequently used classifications (DeBakey and Stanford) are based on the anatomic location and extent of the intimal flap (Fig. 39.5). DeBakey's nomenclature is based on the anatomic site of the intimal tear and the extent of the resulting dissection. In a type I dissection, the intimal tear originates

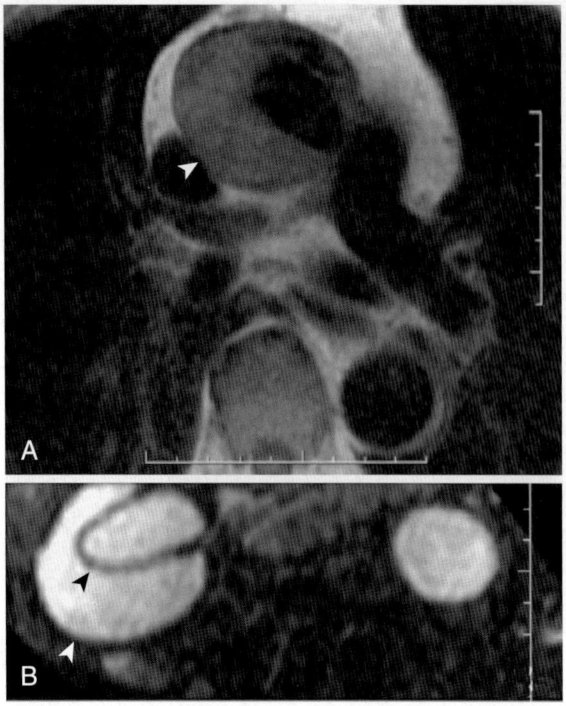

FIG. 39.6 Stanford type A aortic dissection. (A) Axial T1-weighted black-blood image shows nearly circumferential compression of the true aortic lumen by a false lumen (*arrow*). High signal intensity in the false lumen makes it difficult to differentiate thrombosis from flowing blood. (B) Axial reformatted image from contrast enhanced magnetic resonance angiography shows an intimal flap (*black arrow*) with flow in the false lumen (*white arrow*).

in the ascending aorta, and the dissecting hematoma extends past the origin of the left subclavian artery, while type II dissections are confined to the ascending aorta. Type III dissections begin after the origin of the left subclavian artery and extend distally. The Stanford classification is conceptually founded on prognostic grounds. Type A involves the ascending aorta (Fig. 39.6), regardless of the site of the entry tear, and type B dissections spare the ascending aorta and often imply a better prognosis. In general, acute dissections of the ascending aorta require emergency surgery, while descending aortic dissections may be managed with medical therapy and stent-grafting; in any case, rapid diagnosis of the dissecting process and a delineation of its anatomic details are critical for successful management.[36,37] The primary imaging goal is not only to establish the diagnosis of dissection, but also to detect entry and reentry sites, the presence and degree of aortic insufficiency, and the flow pattern in the true and false lumen as well as in critical aortic branches. The latter is crucial for patient selection for transcatheter endovascular repair of type B acute and chronic aortic dissection as an alternative to open surgery.[38,39] For diagnostic purposes, the true lumen can be differentiated from the false lumen by the anatomic and functional (flow-related) features. In addition, the visualization of remnants of the dissected media as cobwebs adjacent to the outer wall of the lumen may help to identify the false lumen. The leakage of blood from the descending aorta into the periaortic space, which can appear with high signal intensity and can result in a left-sided pleural effusion, is usually better visualized on axial images. A high signal intensity of a pericardial effusion indicates a bloody component and is a sign of impending rupture of the ascending aorta into the pericardial space. A detailed anatomic map of aortic dissection must indicate the type and extension of dissection and distinguish the origin and perfusion of branch vessels from the true or false channels. In stable patients, adjunctive gradient echo sequences or phase-contrast images can be instrumental in identifying aortic insufficiency and entry or reentry sites as well as in differentiating slow flow from thrombus in the false lumen.[20,40] The third step in the diagnosis of aortic dissection and definition of its anatomic detail relies on the use of gadolinium-enhanced 3D MRA. Because 3D MRA is rapidly acquired without any need of ECG triggering and gadolinium has minimal toxicity in patients with good renal function, this technique may even be used with severely ill patients.[41] With spin echo sequences, artifacts caused by imperfect ECG gating, respiratory motion, or slow blood pool can result in intraluminal signal, simulating or obscuring an intimal flap. In gadolinium-enhanced 3D MRA, the intimal flap is easily detected, and the relationship with aortic vessels is clearly depicted. Entry and reentry sites appear as a segmental interruption of the linear intimal flap on axial or sagittal images. The analysis of MRA images should not be limited to viewing MIP images or surface-shaded display; it should also include a complete evaluation of reformatted images in all three planes to confirm or improve spin echo information and exclude artifacts. Combining the spin echo with MRA images completes the diagnosis and anatomic definition.[42] At present, CMR is one of the most accurate tools in the detection of aortic dissection. A high degree of spatial resolution and contrast and the capability for multiplanar acquisition provide excellent sensitivity and specificity at approximately 100%.[42,43]

In selecting the diagnostic modality of choice, one must begin by considering what diagnostic information needs to be obtained. First, any chosen study must confirm or refute the diagnosis of dissection. Second, the study must determine whether the dissection involves the ascending aorta (type A) or is confined to the descending aorta (type B). Third, several anatomic features of the dissection should be identified, including its extent, the sites of entry and reentry, the presence of thrombus in the false lumen, the extent of branch vessel involvement, the presence and severity of aortic insufficiency, the presence of pericardial effusion, and the presence of coronary artery involvement. It is also important to consider the accuracy of the diagnostic information obtained, as a false negative diagnosis may result in avoidable death, while a false-positive diagnosis might lead to unnecessary surgery.

According to the present information, CMR and TEE are the most sensitive modalities, with both performing better than aortography. The sensitivities of aortography, CT, and CMR are all quite high, while the specificity of TEE may be comparable only when a strict definition of a positive study is applied. Finally, availability, speed, safety, and cost should be taken into consideration when comparing various modalities. Aortography is rarely immediately available, requires transport of the patient, is a lengthy study, has the associated risks of both an invasive study and intravenous contrast, and is the most expensive. Yet it may be necessary in selected patients who are being considered for combined surgical treatment, especially those with a high likelihood of coronary artery disease or evidence of involvement of major arterial trunks arising from the aorta. CT scanning has the advantage that it is more easily obtained in less time and is noninvasive, but it is overall less accurate than the other techniques. CMR is usually less available in most hospitals, requires transportation of the patient, and is considered undesirable for unstable patients or those requiring very close monitoring. Meanwhile, TEE is readily obtained, quick to complete at the bedside, and thus ideal for unstable patients, and it is the least costly of the four imaging techniques. These options render angiography obsolete in the diagnostic workup of aortic dissection. Thus, detecting dissection of the thoracic aorta should be a noninvasive strategy using CT or CMR in hemodynamically stable patients and TEE in patients who are too unstable for transportation. Comprehensive and detailed evaluation can thus be reduced to a single noninvasive imaging modality in the evaluation of suspected aortic dissection.

While CMR may be less practical than CT and TEE to evaluate patients presenting with suspected aortic dissection, it is well suited for patients with stable chronic dissections.[31–33] The extraordinary accuracy of CMR and the optional functional images may render CMR the gold standard for defining aortic anatomy and risk of rupture in dissection patients; for surveillance of dissection, CMR has already been widely accepted regardless of medical treatment, surgical repair, or endovascular management.

MRI can in fact be used to custom design an individualized endovascular approach to aneurysms, aortic dissections, and localized aortic ulcers. With customized aortic endoprosthesis, such entities are more frequently becoming an ideal target for interventional treatment rather than surgical approaches, which have high mortality and morbidity (Fig. 39.7).[44]

Moreover, the identification of "high risk" conditions of hemodynamically stable type B dissection by virtue of flow analysis is becoming an attractive concept to select patients for elective endovascular interventions; antegrade high-velocity flow conditions in the true lumen and low-velocity retrograde flow in the false lumen can coexist, probably identifying a high-risk subset of type B aortic dissection.[45,46] Multivelocity-encoding 4D flow MRI has been proposed for short- and long-term risk stratification in chronic aortic dissection.[47]

AORTIC INTRAMURAL HEMATOMA

An important differential diagnosis of aortic dissection is intramural hematoma (IMH), which usually presents with the same clinical picture and risk profile as overt aortic dissection.[48] Tomographic modalities such as CMR may be used to identify IMH with no luminal component, which is considered an imminent precursor of aortic dissection.[49,50] With high-resolution tomographic imaging, the imaging diagnosis of IMH is now feasible, suggesting IMH as a precursor of dissection, with one-third progressing to overt dissection.[50,51] Because of these findings in vivo before death, IMH appears more likely to be a variant of dissection than a separate entity.[52,53] Typical epiphenomena of dissection such as aortic insufficiency and pericardial or pleural effusion may also occur in IMH. Spontaneous rupture of aortic vasa vasorum, especially of nutrient vessels to the media layer, has been suggested to initiate the process of aortic disintegration without an intimal tear. With a pathogenesis that explains the high rate of progression to overt aortic dissection and a prognosis and survival that are like those in aortic dissection, urgent diagnosis of IMH is important.

The diagnosis of IMH relies on the visualization of intramural blood and/or evidence of localized increased wall thickness.[54] CMR techniques, however, not only visualize the blood in the wall, but also allow an assessment of the age of the hematoma based on signal changes caused by the formation of methemoglobin (Fig. 39.8). Acute IMH (early stage) is well imaged on T2-weighted spin echo images due to high initial signal intensity of blood, whereas blood of 1 to 5 days of age has lower signal intensity on T2 images. High signal intensity within the aortic wall on T1 spin echo images suggests subacute IMH, whereas acute IMH may be determined on T1 images from the isodense appearance of blood and aortic wall.[52,55] Although TEE has an excellent sensitivity to detect aortic dissection, the definite distinction between IMH and normal findings may require a second tomographic modality such as CT or CMR, since a false-negative result (or false exclusion of IMH) is more likely to be avoided with independent morphologic information. In conclusion, as a precursor of dissection, IMH requires diagnostic attention by using high-resolution tomographic imaging; owing to its physical properties, CMR may play a prominent role not only in diagnosing IMH, but also in assessing its age and differentiating IMH from mural thrombosis; angiography certainly is not diagnostic in the setting of IMH.

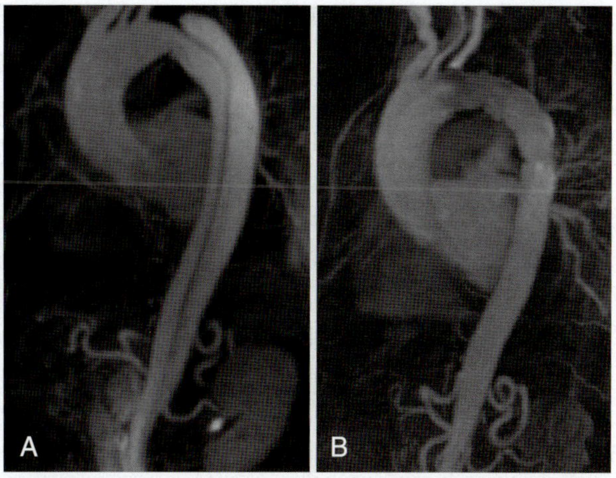

FIG. 39.7 Contrast-enhanced magnetic resonance angiography (MRA) of chronic type B dissection originating from the aortic arch region. (A) Follow-up MRA at 7 days after stent-graft placement shows a completely sealed proximal entry to the thrombosed false lumen. (B) The diameter of the true lumen is normalized, and the descending aorta is reconstructed.

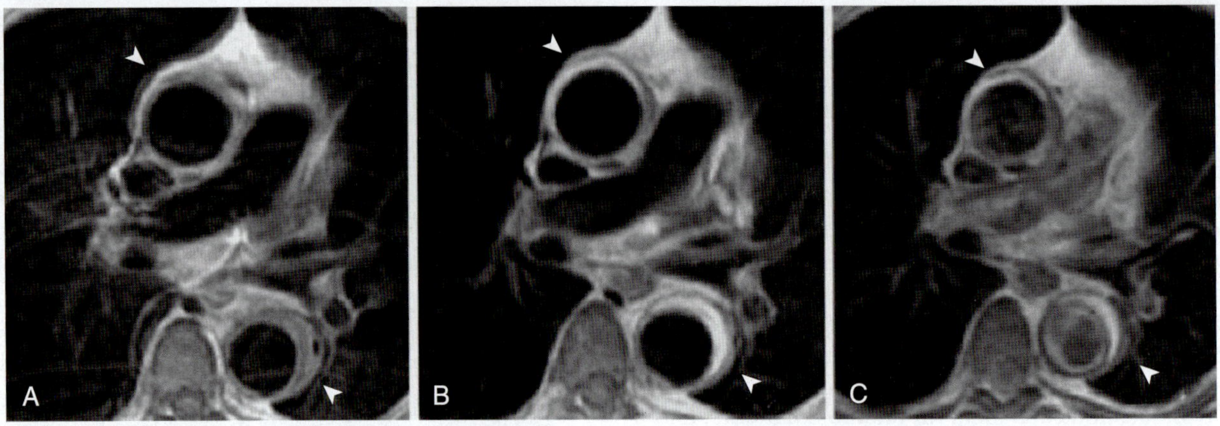

FIG. 39.8 T1-weighted spin echo axial image of intramural hematoma of the ascending and descending aorta. The abnormal wall thickening (*arrows*) presents with intermediate signal intensity in panel (A) (oxyhemoglobin, acute phase) and high signal intensity in panel (B) (*methemoglobin, subacute phase*). (C) T2-weighted spin echo image signal intensity is high in the acute phase (*recent hemorrhage*).

PENETRATING AORTIC ULCER

Ulcers occur in the presence of aortic atherosclerosis and may mimic subacute dissection or may develop without major symptoms. In contrast to IMH, aortic ulcers are characterized on angiography by focal contrast enhancement beyond the confines of the aortic lumen, but communicating with the lumen (Fig. 39.9).[55] At present, there is emerging consensus on the prognosis and outcome of aortic ulcers. Persistent pain, hemodynamic instability, or expansion of width or depth >20 mm should trigger surgical or endovascular treatment. An incidence of transmural rupture ranging from 8% to 42% has been reported in the medical literature.[56,57] Both IMH and ulcers are unrelated to intimal lacerations as in acute aortic dissection. Lacerations and IMH usually occur at points of greatest hydraulic stress (right lateral ascending aorta or adjacent to the ligamentum arteriosum), whereas penetrating ulcers are typically found in the descending or abdominal aorta. Conversely, discrete penetrating atheromatous ulcers ("giant ulcers") have been suspected as one cause of intramural bleeding. Both MRI and TEE have helped to elucidate the pathogenic background and the complex anatomic peculiarities of these important features, but accurate diagnosis of penetrating ulcers is sometimes difficult, and no test is ideal.[58] CT may demonstrate the surrounding hematoma and displaced calcifications in most cases; in addition to this, CMR can differentiate subacute intramural hematoma from chronic intraluminal thrombus. No large-scale studies of CMR and aortic ulcers are currently available, but owing to its versatility and imaging features, CMR appears best suited to characterize this form of aortic pathology as a constellation of diffuse aortic atherosclerosis, an ulceration with focal wall thickening, and missing evidence of aortic dissection.

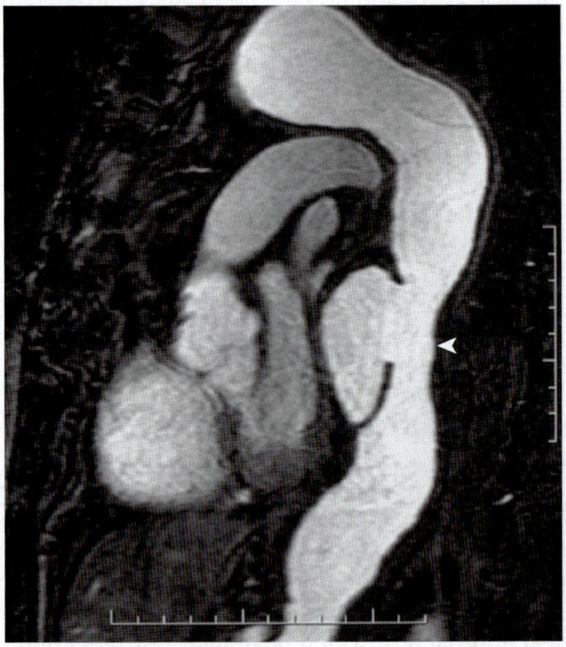

FIG. 39.9 Penetrating atherosclerotic ulcer in a 61-year-old male with high blood pressure. Sagittal oblique contrast-enhanced magnetic resonance angiography shows a diffusely aneurysmal descending aorta with a large outpouching in the medial anterior region (*arrow*), an appearance consistent with penetrating atherosclerotic ulcer. Prior studies showed development of a focal aneurysm 2 years earlier.

THORACIC AORTIC ANEURYSM

Limited dilatation of a blood vessel can either be a true aneurysm or a false aneurysm. True aneurysms involve all layers of the aortic wall and result from the degeneration of the elastin fibers within the media. A false aneurysm, or pseudoaneurysm, is not a true aneurysm but rather a contained perforation of the vessel wall with penetration of the intima and media. Pseudoaneurysms form after focal penetration of the intima and media by trauma (20% to 25% of thoracic aneurysms) or by infection (about 5% of thoracic aneurysms). Atherosclerosis may result in the formation of pseudoaneurysms if a true aneurysm ruptures but is contained by the adventitia and periaortic tissues. Pseudoaneurysms, therefore, have a narrow "neck" leading to the "aneurysm." Thoracic aortic aneurysms are common, with a recently reported incidence of 10.9 cases per 100,000 persons per year.[59] They may involve all thoracic aortic segments, requiring different therapeutic strategies with a surgical, interventional, or hybrid

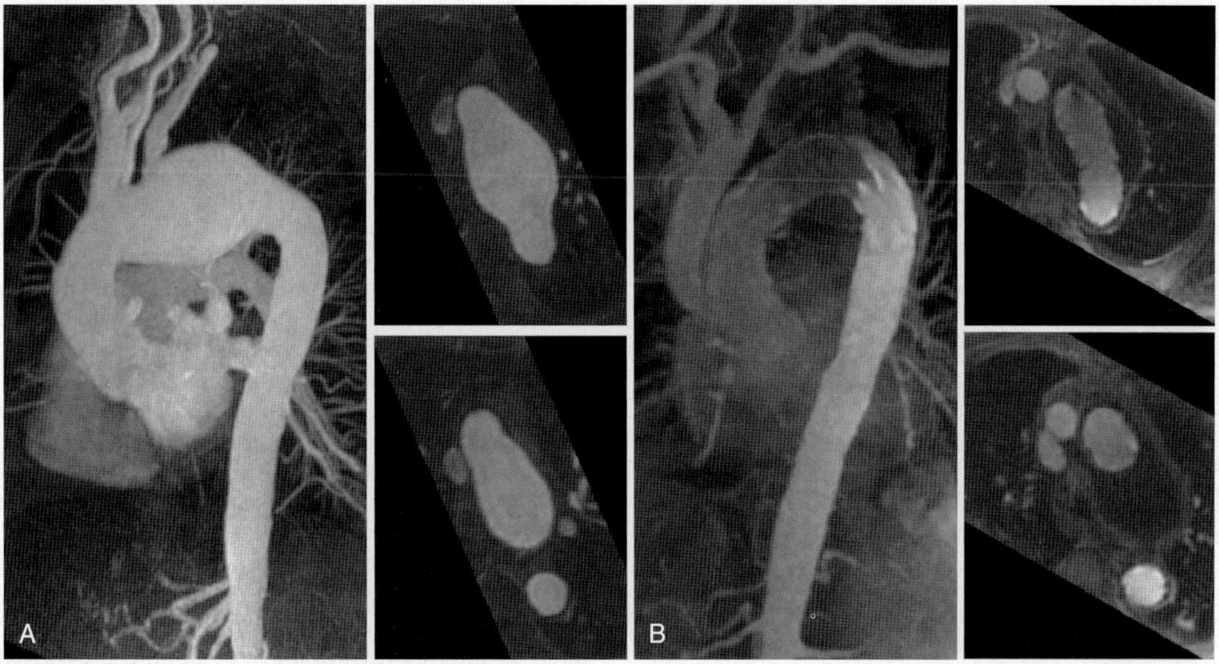

FIG. 39.10 (A) Magnetic resonance angiography images of an aortic arch aneurysm in parasagittal-oblique and axial orientation. (B) Follow-up study after a hybrid-procedure with initial head-vessel-debranching and staged endovascular stent-graft repair demonstrates perfect reconstruction of the proximal aorta.

approach (Fig. 39.10). In modern series, aneurysms of the ascending aorta occur most commonly (60%), followed by aneurysms of the descending aorta (40%), whereas aneurysms involving the arch or thoracoabdominal aorta occur less often.[60] Atherosclerotic aneurysms are usually fusiform, involving long segments of the aorta. Conversely, ascending aortic aneurysm or annuloaortic ectasia are often caused by Marfan syndrome, syphilis, or poststenotic dilatation resulting from aortic stenosis; the sinotubular junction is preserved in aortic stenosis but markedly dilated in the other entities. If isolated to the descending aorta, saccular aneurysms may be traumatic or infective, but atherosclerosis remains the leading cause. Saccular and sinus Valsalva aneurysms in the aortic root very often have associated aortic insufficiency. The clear delineation of the location, extent, and shape of an aneurysm; its relation to branch vessels and adjacent structures; and its associated complicating factors, such as rupture, periaortic hematoma or infection, hemopericardium, and aortic valve insufficiency are all of importance.

CMR is effective in the identification and characterization of thoracic aortic aneurysms as well as in the evaluation of their pathophysiologic consequences.[8,61,62] Standard spin echo sequences are helpful in the evaluation of alterations of the aortic wall and periaortic space. Periaortic hematoma and areas of high signal intensity within the thrombus may indicate instability of the aneurysm and are well depicted on spin echo images. Atherosclerotic lesions are visualized as areas of increased thickness with high signal intensity and irregular profiles. In contrast to transaxial imaging, oblique planes allow precise determination of lumen diameter. With fat suppression techniques, the outer wall of the aneurysm can easily be distinguished from periadventitial fat

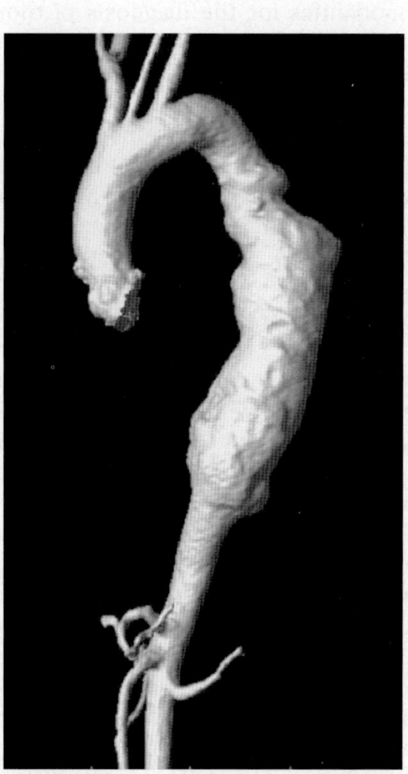

FIG. 39.11 Three-dimensional shaded surface–rendered contrast-enhanced magnetic resonance angiography depicts a large true aneurysm of the thoracic descending aorta in a 38-year-old male.

tissue. Contrast-enhanced 3D MRA can provide precise topographic information about the extent of an aneurysm and its relationship to the aortic branches (Fig. 39.11). The capability of contrast MRA to visualize the Adamkiewicz artery represents an important advance in avoiding postoperative neurologic deficit secondary to spinal cord ischemia.[63,64]

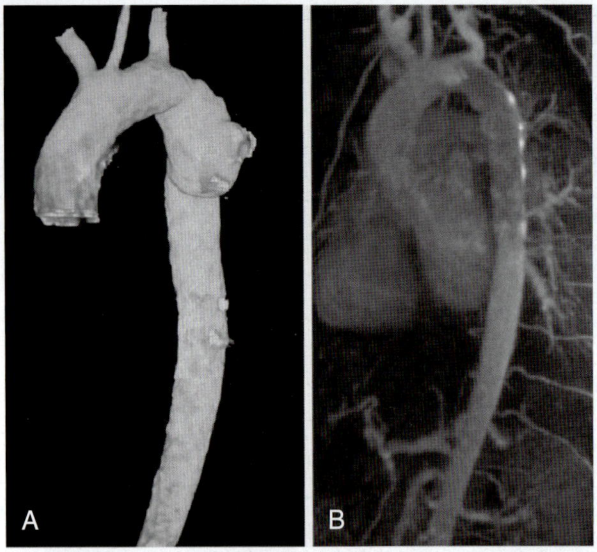

FIG. 39.12 Contrast-enhanced magnetic resonance angiography of chronic traumatic aortic lesion. (A) Partial laceration of the aortic wall results in a diverticular aneurysm (*shaded surface rendering*). (B) Discharge imaging after endovascular stent-graft repair reveals complete restitution of thoracic aortic integrity.

At present, no trials exist to compare the value of CMR and other modalities for the diagnosis of thoracic aneurysms; there is, however, consensus that CMR is accurate and versatile but most likely not as cost effective in serial studies. Although CMR promises to emerge as the standard in the diagnosis and management of thoracic aortic aneurysms, cost considerations must be evaluated before recommendation of widespread use of MRI scanning to follow stable patients with subcritical aneurysms.

TRAUMA TO THE AORTA

Aortic trauma is usually generated by deceleration of the body in serious motor vehicle crashes, pedestrian injuries, and falls from height.[65] The aortic segment that is subjected to the greatest strain by rapid deceleration forces is located just beyond the area of the isthmus aortae. In clinical series, aortic rupture occurs at this location in 90% of cases.[66,67] The traumatic lesion is a transverse tear variably extending from the intimal to adventitial layers. Intimal hemorrhage without any laceration has been described in pathologic series but was not recognized in the clinical setting before the advent of high-resolution tomographic imaging modalities. Recent reports indicate that intimal hemorrhage with and without partial intimal laceration tends to heal spontaneously. When the lesion involves intimal and medial layers, false aneurysm formation occurs. The aneurysm is fusiform in the case of a circumferential lesion, while in a partial laceration, it appears as localized diverticulum (Fig. 39.12). Periaortic hemorrhage may occur irrespective of the type of lesion. Complete rupture of the aorta, including the adventitial layer and periadventitial connective tissue, leads to immediate exsanguination. However, false aneurysm or occlusion of the side of rupture may permit temporary survival. A long examination time and difficult access to the polytraumatized patient have been the main limitations of CMR in acute aortic pathology. The development of fast CMR techniques has shortened the examination time to a few minutes; therefore, MRI can be used even in critically ill patients. The value of CMR in detecting traumatic aortic rupture in comparison to angiography and conventional CT was reported in a series of 24 consecutive patients.[68] The potential for CMR to detect the hemorrhagic component of a lesion by its high signal intensity is beneficial in traumatized patients. On spin echo images in the sagittal plane, a longitudinal visualization of the thoracic aorta makes it possible to distinguish a partial lesion from a lesion encompassing the entire aortic circumference. This discrimination is of prognostic significance because a circumferential lesion may be more likely to rupture.[68] The presence of periadventitial hematoma and/or pleural and mediastinal hemorrhagic effusion may also be considered a sign of instability. In the same sequence used to evaluate the aortic lesion, without the need of any additional time, the wide field of view of CMR provides a comprehensive evaluation of chest trauma such as lung contusion and edema and pleural effusion and rib fractures. MRA does not add any diagnostic value to spin echo CMR, and it cannot supply information on parietal lesions and hemorrhagic fluids outside the aortic vessel. Recently, the development of endovascular techniques has provided additional opportunities in the treatment of acute onset and chronic traumatic aortic disease (Fig. 39.12).[69–71]

AORTIC COARCTATION

Coarctation is a common congenital anomaly, with an incidence of 20 to 60 per 100,000 live births, and represents 5% to 8% of all congenital cardiovascular disorders. The obstructive lesion results from an abnormality in the aortic media and refers to an enfolding of the posterolateral aortic wall in the region of the ligamentum or ductus arteriosus. This is usually a discrete phenomenon that occurs just distal to the ductus and is also labeled postductal coarctation. Since it is usually asymptomatic in the neonatal period, it is also referred to as adult coarctation versus preductal or infantile coarctation, which is less common than adult coarctation and usually associated with hypoplasia of the arch. There is usually a dilation of the descending aorta distal to the coarctation. As a result of the obstruction caused by the coarctation, collateral vessels develop that increase flow into the descending aorta. Increased flow through intercostal arteries results in their dilation and notching along the inferior aspect of the ribs, which usually takes 8 to 10 years to become significant enough to be observed on a chest radiograph.

With its multiplanar image acquisition, large field of view, and dynamic quantitative flow imaging capacity, CMR appears to be the modality of choice for the evaluation of coarctation (Fig. 39.13). The left oblique sagittal view centered on the middle of the ascending and descending aortas is an ideal orientation that may also demonstrate associated aortic stenosis, left ventricular hypertrophy, and ventricular septal defects. This is important because

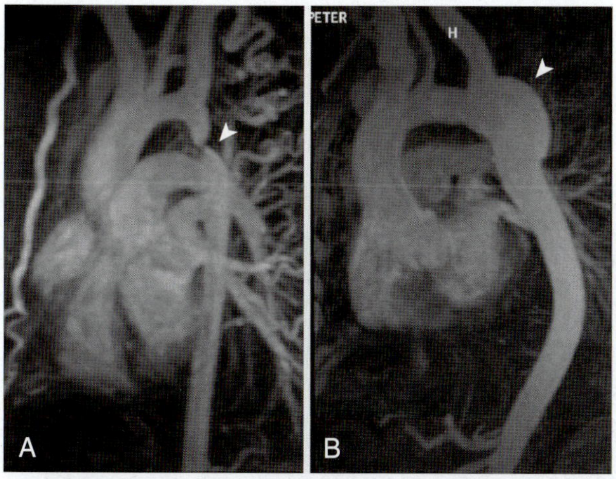

FIG. 39.13 (A) Magnetic resonance angiography of aortic coarctation depicts focal stenotic segment (*arrow*) at the isthmic zone and multiple intercostal collateral arteries joining the descending aorta. (B) Medium-sized Dacron patch aneurysm (*arrow*) diagnosed 30 years after coarctation surgery.

there is a high association of bicuspid aortic valve and ventricular septal defects with coarctation. The severity of the stenosis can be expressed as the ratio of the diameters or cross-sectional areas measured at the coarcted segment and above the diaphragm.[72] However, although the anatomic narrowing of the aorta establishes the diagnosis of coarctation, an assessment of its clinical significance depends on determining its hemodynamic effects. Cine CMR has been applied to evaluate flow turbulence across the coarctation; the severity of coarctation is quantified on the basis of the length of flow void.[73] Further functional information can be provided by CMR flow mapping, which can define the severity of the stenosis by measuring velocity jets at the level of coarctation and mean flow deceleration in the descending aorta.[74] With this technique, it is possible to predict the coarctation severity with good sensitivity and specificity (95% and 82%, respectively) compared with catheter angiography. Flow mapping is also able to quantify the flow pattern and volume of collateral flow in the descending aorta, which are other important parameters of the severity of coarctation, and this information may be crucial in the choice of surgical strategy. Collateral flow is present if distal aortic flow is greater than proximal flow, and it is possible to quantify collateral circulation by subtracting flow volume in the proximal descending aorta from that in the distal portion. The presence of collateral flow indicates a hemodynamically significant coarctation. Furthermore, a pressure gradient calculated with flow mapping CMR by use of the modified Bernoulli equation ($\Delta P = 4V^2$)[75] can be used to determine the need for surgical/endovascular repair (a pressure gradient greater than 15 mm Hg is considered an indication for intervention). However, this threshold is arbitrary; therefore, it may be more appropriate to use the measurement of collateral flow.

Several therapeutic strategies are available for the treatment of aortic coarctation, depending on the morphology of the affected aorta as well as the age and clinical condition of the patient.[76,77] Surgery for aortic coarctation is recommended at an early age because long-term results seem to be better. Recently, interventional procedures and balloon angioplasty have come into wide use and provide good results, especially in mild or moderate cases.[78,79] An accurate selection of favorable anatomy by high-resolution imaging modalities is particularly important in interventional procedure to ensure a low rate of complications and restenosis.[80] An increased risk for aneurysm formation at the site of repair has been reported after both synthetic patch aortoplasty and subclavian-flap arterioplasty (Fig. 39.13).[81,82] Moreover, restenosis, aortic dissection, and pseudoaneurysms have been reported after surgery or balloon angioplasty in around 40% of patients.[83] Therefore, routine follow-up is recommended for patients who underwent repair of an aortic coarctation, independently of surgical technique used and timing of the repair. New interventional techniques, such as endovascular stent-grafting, have currently been applied to the treatment of postsurgical patch aneurysms with excellent results, avoiding the need for further surgical intervention.[84,85]

AORTITIS

Although there are many causes of aortitis, Takayasu arteritis is the type most often studied with CMR because of the diffuse stenotic nature of the disease, which often makes vascular access difficult or impossible by catheterization.[86] In Takayasu disease, the aortic arch vessels are primarily affected, but thoracic and abdominal aorta may also be involved (Fig. 39.14). Active inflammatory disease demonstrates diffuse thickening of the aortic wall, which is typically enhanced after gadolinium administration in T1-weighted images. The chronic stage, however, is characterized by extensive perivascular fibrosis without postcontrast enhancement.[87] MRA is the preferred imaging modality for the study of branch vessel stenosis and has replaced invasive angiography, which carries a risk of pseudoaneurysm formation at the site of arterial puncture. Recently, the capability of Fludeoxyglucose F 18 (F-18 FDG) hybrid camera positron emission tomography combined with CMR to detect early stages of Takayasu aortitis has been demonstrated.[88]

INTERVENTIONAL CARDIOVASCULAR MAGNETIC RESONANCE IMAGING

CMR guidance of vascular interventional procedures offers several potential advantages over fluoroscopy-guided techniques, including image acquisition in any desired orientation, superior 3D soft tissue contrast with simultaneous visualization of the interventional device and 4D functional imaging, and absence of ionizing radiation. The feasibility of real-time, CMR-guided interventions has been demonstrated for a wide range of vascular interventional procedures in animals and patients.[89–91] In terms of endovascular aortic stent-graft placement, MRI appears to be particularly useful, as it can provide preinterventional evaluation of aortic pathology, real-time interventional image guidance,

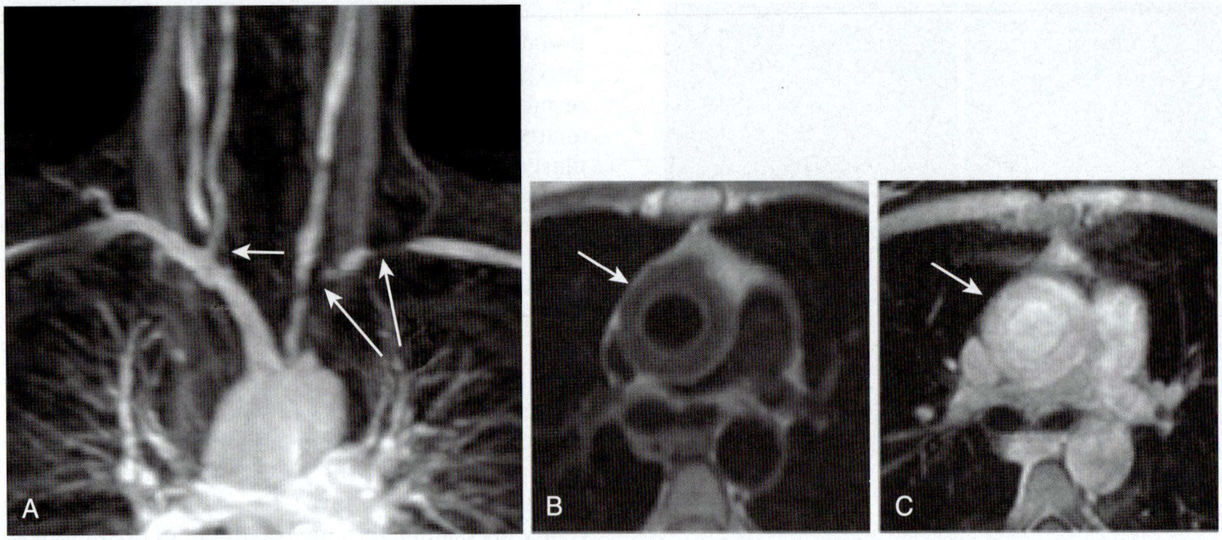

FIG. 39.14 Takayasu arteritis. (A) Coronal maximum intensity projection 3D magnetic resonance angiography shows significant stenosis of right common carotid artery at its origin (*small arrow*). The left subclavian artery has two stenotic segments (*large arrows*) with a small area of poststenotic dilatation in between. There are also some luminal irregularities of the left common carotid artery. Axial unenhanced (B) and gadolinium-enhanced (C) T1-weighted cardiovascular magnetic resonance shows wall thickening of the ascending aorta (*arrow*), which is enhanced on the gadolinium-enhanced image.

and immediate evaluation of treatment success or procedure-related complications as well as follow-up examinations.[92] Passive device tracking using material-induced susceptibility artifacts of the interventional instrument for CMR visualization requires no hardware or instrument modifications and appears to be promising in terms of potential clinical applications. However, MR-compatible instruments with satisfactory susceptibility artifacts are required, as well as CMR-compatible guidewires with adequate mechanical support. To date, the limitations of interventional CMR are long procedure times, lack of true real-time monitoring, and stent artifacts, which necessitate further modifications before they can be recommended for clinical use.[93,94] However, MRI-guided interventions are feasible and may become an important advance in the near future.

CONCLUSION

With recent advances in the understanding of aortic diseases, both power and versatility have put magnetic resonance imaging in the focus of diagnostic workup and surveillance of all aortic pathology. Technical refinements, from classic anatomic imaging, 3D gadolinium-enhanced MRA, and tissue characterization to 4D functional imaging have rendered CMR highly suitable for the assessment of acquired disease such as aortic dissection, intramural hematoma, and aneurysm, along with postoperative follow-up evaluation, with better diagnostic reliability and prognostic information than other imaging modalities; the more recently developed MR sequences allowing for blood flow measurements in the aortic lumens may provide important prognostic information beyond the classic diagnostic features. Finally, guidance of vascular interventional procedures by real-time CMR offers potential advantages over fluoroscopy-guided techniques and constitutes an interesting research tool, but has not hit the clinical arena yet.

REFERENCES

1. Hayashi K, Meaney TF, Zelch JV, et al. Aortographic analysis of aortic dissection. *Am J Roentgenol Radium Ther Nucl Med*. 1974;122(4):769–782.
2. Singh H, Fitzgerald E, Ruttley MS. Computed tomography: the investigation of choice for aortic dissection? *Br Heart J*. 1986;56(2):171–175.
3. Wilbers CR, Carrol CL, Hnilica MA. Optimal diagnostic imaging of aortic dissection. *Tex Heart Inst J*. 1990;17(4):271–278.
4. Nienaber CA, von Kodolitsch Y, Nicolas V, et al. The diagnosis of thoracic aortic dissection by noninvasive imaging procedures. *N Engl J Med*. 1993;328(1):1–9.
5. Cigarroa JE, Isselbacher EM, DeSanctis RW, et al. Diagnostic imaging in the evaluation of suspected aortic dissection: old standards and new directions. *N Engl J Med*. 1993;328(1):35–43.
6. Ballal RS, Nanda NC, Gatewood R, et al. Usefulness of transesophageal echocardiography in assessment of aortic dissection. *Circulation*. 1991;84(5):1903–1914.
7. Galvin IF, Black IW, Lee CL, et al. Transesophageal echocardiography in acute aortic transection. *Ann Thorac Surg*. 1991;51(2):310–311.
8. Russo V, Renzulli M, Buttazzi K, Fattori R. Acquired diseases of the thoracic aorta: role of MRI and MRA. *Eur Radiol*. 2006;16(4):852–865.
9. Nienaber CA, Kische S, Skriabina V, Ince H. Noninvasive imaging approaches to evaluate the patient with known or suspected aortic disease. *Circ Cardiovasc Imaging*. 2009;2(6):499–506.
10. Trimarchi S, Nienaber CA, Rampoldi V, et al. Role and results of surgery in acute type B aortic dissection: insights from the international registry of acute aortic dissection (IRAD). *Circulation*. 2006;114(1 Suppl):I357–I364.
11. Abernethy LJ. Cost effectiveness of magnetic resonance imaging. *BMJ*. 1992;304(6820):183.
12. Stemerman DH, Krinsky GA, Lee VS, et al. Thoracic aorta: rapid black-blood MR imaging with half-Fourier rapid acquisition with relaxation enhancement with or without electrocardiographic triggering. *Radiology*. 1999;213(1):185–191.
13. Powell AJ, Maier SE, Chung T, et al. Phase-velocity cine magnetic resonance imaging measurement of pulsatile blood flow in children and young adults: in vitro and in vivo validation. *Pediatr Cardiol*. 2000;21(2):104–110.
14. Bogren HG, Buonocore MH. 4D magnetic resonance velocity mapping of blood flow patterns in the aorta in young vs. elderly normal subjects. *J Magn Reson Imaging*. 1999;10(5):861–869.
15. Hopkins KD, Lehmann ED, Gosling RG. Aortic compliance measurements: a non-invasive indicator of atherosclerosis? *Lancet*. 1994;343(8911):1447.
16. Groenink M, de Roos A, Mulder BJ, et al. Biophysical properties of the normal-sized aorta in patients with Marfan syndrome: evaluation with MR flow mapping. *Radiology*. 2001;219(2):535–540.
17. Lee VS, Martin DJ, Krinsky GA, et al. Gadolinium-enhanced MR angiography: artifacts and pitfalls. *AJR Am J Roentgenol*. 2000;175(1):197–205.
18. Sodickson DK, McKenzie CA, Li W, et al. Contrast-enhanced 3D MR angiography with simultaneous acquisition of spatial harmonics: a pilot study. *Radiology*. 2000;217(1):284–289.
19. Riederer SJ, Bernstein MA, Breen JF, et al. Three-dimensional contrast-enhanced MR angiography with real-time fluoroscopic triggering: design specifications and technical reliability in 330 patient studies. *Radiology*. 2000;215(2):584–593.
20. Clough RE, Hussain T, Uribe S, et al. A new method for quantification of false lumen thrombosis in aortic dissection using magnetic resonance imaging and a blood pool contrast agent. *J Vasc Surg*. 2011:1–14.

21. Clough RE, Waltham M, Giese D, Taylor PR, Schaeffter T. A new imaging method for assessment of aortic dissection using four-dimensional phase contrast magnetic resonance imaging. *J Vasc Surg*. 2012;55(4):914–923.
22. Francois CJ, Markl M, Schiebler ML, et al. Four-dimensional, flow-sensitive magnetic resonance imaging of blood flow patterns in thoracic aortic dissections. *J Thorac Cardiovasc Surg*. 2013;145(5):1359–1366.
23. Jarral OA, Tan MKH, Salmasi MY, et al. Phase-contrast magnetic resonance imaging and computational fluid dynamics assessment of thoracic aorta blood flow: a literature review. *Eur J Cardiothorac Surg*. 2020;57:438–446.
24. Adriaans BP, Wildberger JE, Westenberg JJM, et al. Predictive imaging for thoracic aortic dissection and rupture: moving beyond diameters. *Eur Radiol*. 2019;29:6396–6404.
25. Garcia J, van der Palen RLF, Bollache E, et al. Distribution of blood flow velocity in the normal aorta: effect of age and gender. *J Magn Reson Imaging*. 2018;47:487–498.
26. Willinek WA, Hadizadeh DR, Von Falkenhausen M, et al. 4D time-resolved MR angiography with keyhole (4D-TRAK): more than 60 times accelerated MRA using a combination of CENTRA, keyhole, and SENSE at 3.0T. *J Magn Reson Imaging*. 2008;27(6):1455–1460.
27. Kauhanen SP, Hedman M, Kariniemi E, et al. Aortic dilatation associates with flow displacement and increased circumferential wall shear stress in patients without aortic stenosis: a prospective clinical study. *J Magn Reson Imaging*. 2019;50:136–145.
28. Sieren MM, Schultz V, Fujita B, et al. 4D flow CMR analysis comparing patients with anatomically shaped aortic sinus prostheses, tube prostheses and healthy subjects introducing the wall shear stress gradient: a case control study. *J Cardiovasc Magn Reson*. 2020;22:59–68.
29. Bollache E, Guzzardi DG, Sattari S, et al. Aortic valve-mediated wall shear stress is heterogeneous and predicts regional aortic elastic fiber thinning in bicuspid aortic valve-associated aortopathy. *J Thorac Cardiovasc Surg*. 2018;156:2112–2120.
30. Berhane H, Scott M, Elbaz M, et al. Fully automated 3D aortic segmentation of 4D flow MRI for heamodynamic analysis using deep learning. *Magn Reson Med*. 2020;84:2204–2218.
31. Hamid A, Gupta M, Rajiah PS, et al. The current and future role of imaging of thoracic aortic disease: a north American society for cardiovascular imaging commentary on the 2022 AHA/ACC guidelines for the diagnosis and management of aortic disease. *Int J Cardiovasc Imaging*. 2024;40:5–14.
32. Evangelista A, Sitges M, Jondeau G, et al. Multimodality imaging in thoracic aortic diseases: a clinical consensus statement from the European association of cardiovascular imaging and the European society of cardiology working group on aorta and peripheral vascular diseases. *Eur Heart J Cardiovasc Imaging*. 2023;24:65–85.
33. Czerny M, Grabenwöger M, Berger T, et al. EACTS/STS Guidelines for diagnosing and treating acute and chronic syndromes of the aortic organ. *Ann Thorac Surg*. 2024;118:5–115.
34. VIRTUE Registry Investigators. Mid-term outcomes and aortic remodelling after thoracic endovascular repair for acute, subacute, and chronic aortic dissection: the VIRTUE Registry. *Eur J Vasc Endovasc Surg*. 2014;48(4):363–371.
35. Acosta S, Blomstrand D, Gottsater A. Epidemiology and long-term prognostic factors in acute type B aortic dissection. *Ann Vasc Surg*. 2007;21(4):415–422.
36. Nienaber CA, Eagle KA. Aortic dissection: new frontiers in diagnosis and management: part II: therapeutic management and follow-up. *Circulation*. 2003;108(6):772–778.
37. Nienaber CA, Eagle KA. Aortic dissection: new frontiers in diagnosis and management: part I: from etiology to diagnostic strategies. *Circulation*. 2003;108(5):628–635.
38. Nienaber CA, Fattori R, Lund G, et al. Nonsurgical reconstruction of thoracic aortic dissection by stent-graft placement. *N Engl J Med*. 1999;340(20):1539–1545.
39. Dake MD, Kato N, Mitchell RS, et al. Endovascular stent-graft placement for the treatment of acute aortic dissection. *N Engl J Med*. 1999;340(20):1546–1552.
40. Chang JM, Friese K, Caputo GR, et al. MR measurement of blood flow in the true and false channel in chronic aortic dissection. *J Comput Assist Tomogr*. 1991;15(3):418–423.
41. Fernandez GC, Tardaguila FM, Duran D, et al. Dynamic 3-dimensional contrast-enhanced magnetic resonance angiography in acute aortic dissection. *Curr Probl Diagn Radiol*. 2002;31(4):134–145.
42. Bogaert J, Meyns B, Rademakers FE, et al. Follow-up of aortic dissection: contribution of MR angiography for evaluation of the abdominal aorta and its branches. *Eur Radiol*. 1997;7(5):695–702.
43. Sommer T, Fehske W, Holzknecht N, et al. Aortic dissection: a comparative study of diagnosis with spiral CT, multiplanar transesophageal echocardiography, and MR imaging. *Radiology*. 1996;199(2):347–352.
44. Nienaber CA, Zannetti S, Barbieri B, et al. Investigation of stent grafts in patients with type B aortic dissection: design of the INSTEAD trial—a prospective, multicenter, European randomized trial. *Am Heart J*. 2005;149(4):592–599.
45. Callaghan FM, Kozor R, Sherrah AG, et al. Use of multi-velocity encoding 4D flow MRI to improve quantification of flow patterns in the aorta. *J Magn Reson Imaging*. 2016;43:352–363.
46. Takei Y, Itatani K, Miyazaki S, et al. Four-dimensional flow magnetic resonance imaging analysis before and after thoracic endovascular aortic repair of chronic type B aortic dissection. *Interact Cardiovasc Thorac Surg*. 2019;28:413–420.
47. Trojan M, Rengier F, Kotelis D, et al. Time-resolved three-dimensional contrast-enhanced magnetic resonance angiography in patients with chronic expanding and stable aortic dissections. *Contrast Media Mol Imaging*. 2017;2017:5428914.
48. Nienaber CA, Sievers HH. Intramural hematoma in acute aortic syndrome: more than one variant of dissection? *Circulation*. 2002;106(3):284–285.
49. Nienaber CA, von Kodolitsch Y, Petersen B, et al. Intramural hemorrhage of the thoracic aorta: diagnostic and therapeutic implications. *Circulation*. 1995;92(6):1465–1472.
50. Sueyoshi E, Imada T, Sakamoto I, et al. Analysis of predictive factors for progression of type B aortic intramural hematoma with computed tomography. *J Vasc Surg*. 2002;35(6):1179–1183.
51. Evangelista A, Dominguez R, Sebastia C, et al. Long-term follow-up of aortic intramural hematoma: predictors of outcome. *Circulation*. 2003;108(5):583–589.
52. Murray JG, Manisali M, Flamm SD, et al. Intramural hematoma of the thoracic aorta: MR image findings and their prognostic implications. *Radiology*. 1997;204(2):349–355.
53. Sawhney NS, DeMaria AN, Blanchard DG. Aortic intramural hematoma: an increasingly recognized and potentially fatal entity. *Chest*. 2001;120(4):1340–1346.
54. Wolff KA, Herold CJ, Tempany CM, et al. Aortic dissection: atypical patterns seen at MR imaging. *Radiology*. 1991;181(2):489–495.
55. Kazerooni EA, Bree RL, Williams DM. Penetrating atherosclerotic ulcers of the descending thoracic aorta: evaluation with CT and distinction from aortic dissection. *Radiology*. 1992;183(3):759–765.
56. Coady MA, Rizzo JA, Elefteriades JA. Pathologic variants of thoracic aortic dissections: penetrating atherosclerotic ulcers and intramural hematomas. *Cardiol Clin*. 1999;17(4):637–657.
57. Movsowitz HD, Lampert C, Jacobs LE, et al. Penetrating atherosclerotic aortic ulcers. *Am Heart J*. 1994;128(6 Pt 1):1210–1217.
58. Hayashi H, Matsuoka Y, Sakamoto I, et al. Penetrating atherosclerotic ulcer of the aorta: imaging features and disease concept. *Radiographics*. 2000;20(4):995–1005.
59. Clouse WD, Hallett JJW, Schaff HV, et al. Improved prognosis of thoracic aortic aneurysms: a population-based study. *JAMA*. 1998;280(22):1926–1929.
60. Isselbacher EM. Thoracic and abdominal aortic aneurysms. *Circulation*. 2005;111(6):816–828.
61. Goldfarb JW, Holland AE, Heijstraten FM, et al. Cardiac synchronized gadolinium-enhanced MR angiography: preliminary experience for the evaluation of the thoracic aorta. *Magn Reson Imaging*. 2006;24(3):241–248.
62. Tatli S, Lipton MJ, Davison BD, et al. From the RSNA refresher courses: MR imaging of aortic and peripheral vascular disease. *Radiographics*. 2003;23(Spec No):S59–S78.
63. Yoshioka K, Niinuma H, Kawakami T, et al. Three-dimensional demonstration of the artery of adamkiewicz with contrast-enhanced magnetic resonance angiography. *Ann Thorac Surg*. 2005;79(5):1785–1794.
64. Yamada N, Takamiya M, Kuribayashi S, et al. MRA of the Adamkiewicz artery: a preoperative study for thoracic aortic aneurysm. *J Comput Assist Tomogr*. 2000;24(3):362–368.
65. Richens D, Kotidis K, Neale M, et al. Rupture of the aorta following road traffic accidents in the United Kingdom 1992–1999: the results of the co-operative crash injury study. *Eur J Cardiothorac Surg*. 2003;23(2):143–148.
66. Hunt JP, Baker CC, Lentz CW, et al. Thoracic aorta injuries: management and outcome of 144 patients. *J Trauma*. 1996;40(4):547–555;discussion 555–556.
67. Kodali S, Jamieson WR, Leia-Stephens M, et al. Traumatic rupture of the thoracic aorta: a 20-year review: 1969–1989. *Circulation*. 1991;84(Suppl 5):III40–III46.
68. Fattori R, Celletti F, Descovich B, et al. Evolution of post-traumatic aortic aneurysm in the subacute phase: magnetic resonance imaging follow-up as a support of the surgical timing. *Eur J Cardiothorac Surg*. 1998;13(5):582–586. discussion 586–587.
69. Rousseau H, Soula P, Perreault P, et al. Delayed treatment of traumatic rupture of the thoracic aorta with endoluminal covered stent. *Circulation*. 1999;99(4):498–504.
70. Scheinert D, Krankenberg H, Schmidt A, et al. Endoluminal stent-graft placement for acute rupture of the descending thoracic aorta. *Eur Heart J*. 2004;25(8):694–700.
71. Demers P, Miller C, Scott Mitchell R, et al. Chronic traumatic aneurysms of the descending thoracic aorta: mid-term results of endovascular repair using first and second-generation stent-grafts. *Eur J Cardiothorac Surg*. 2004;25(3):394–400.
72. Godart F, Labrot G, Devos P, et al. Coarctation of the aorta: comparison of aortic dimensions between conventional MR imaging, 3D MR angiography, and conventional angiography. *Eur Radiol*. 2002;12(8):2034–2039.
73. Simpson IA, Chung KJ, Glass RF, et al. Cine magnetic resonance imaging for evaluation of anatomy and flow relations in infants and children with coarctation of the aorta. *Circulation*. 1988;78(1):142–148.
74. Weber OM, Higgins CB. MR evaluation of cardiovascular physiology in congenital heart disease: flow and function. *J Cardiovasc Magn Reson*. 2006;8(4):607–617.
75. Mohiaddin RH, Kilner PJ, Rees S, et al. Magnetic resonance volume flow and jet velocity mapping in aortic coarctation. *J Am Coll Cardiol*. 1993;22(5):1515–1521.
76. Carr JA. The results of catheter-based therapy compared with surgical repair of adult aortic coarctation. *J Am Coll Cardiol*. 2006;47(6):1101–1107.
77. Gibbs JL. Treatment options for coarctation of the aorta. *Heart*. 2000;84(1):11–13.

78. Mullen MJ. Coarctation of the aorta in adults: do we need surgeons? *Heart.* 2003;89(1):3–5.
79. Ovaert C, McCrindle BW, Nykanen D, et al. Balloon angioplasty of native coarctation: clinical outcomes and predictors of success. *J Am Coll Cardiol.* 2000;35(4):988–996.
80. Paddon AJ, Nicholson AA, Ettles DF, et al. Long-term follow-up of percutaneous balloon angioplasty in adult aortic coarctation. *Cardiovasc Intervent Radiol.* 2000;23(5):364–367.
81. Ala-Kulju K, Jarvinen A, Maamies T, et al. Late aneurysms after patch aortoplasty for coarctation of the aorta in adults. *Thorac Cardiovasc Surg.* 1983;31(5):301–306.
82. von Kodolitsch Y, Aydin MA, Koschyk DH, et al. Predictors of aneurysmal formation after surgical correction of aortic coarctation. *J Am Coll Cardiol.* 2002;39(4):617–624.
83. Varma C, Benson LN, Butany J, et al. Aortic dissection after stent dilatation for coarctation of the aorta: a case report and literature review. *Catheter Cardiovasc Interv.* 2003;59(4):528–535.
84. Bell RE, Taylor PR, Aukett M, et al. Endoluminal repair of aneurysms associated with coarctation. *Ann Thorac Surg.* 2003;75(2):530–533.
85. Ince H, Petzsch M, Rehders T, et al. Percutaneous endovascular repair of aneurysm after previous coarctation surgery. *Circulation.* 2003;108(24):2967–2970.
86. Nastri MV, Baptista LP, Baroni RH, et al. Gadolinium-enhanced three-dimensional MR angiography of Takayasu arteritis. *Radiographics.* 2004;24(3):773–786.
87. Choe YH, Kim DK, Koh EM, et al. Takayasu arteritis: diagnosis with MR imaging and MR angiography in acute and chronic active stages. *J Magn Reson Imaging.* 1999;10(5):751–757.
88. Meller J, Grabbe E, Becker W, et al. Value of F-18 FDG hybrid camera PET and MRI in early takayasu aortitis. *Eur Radiol.* 2003;13(2):400–405.
89. Buecker A, Adam GB, Neuerburg JM, et al. Simultaneous real-time visualization of the catheter tip and vascular anatomy for MR-guided PTA of iliac arteries in an animal model. *J Magn Reson Imaging.* 2002;16(2):201–208.
90. Raval AN, Karmarkar PV, Guttman MA, et al. Real-time magnetic resonance imaging-guided endovascular recanalization of chronic total arterial occlusion in a swine model. *Circulation.* 2006;113(8):1101–1107.
91. Raman VK, Karmarkar PV, Guttman MA, et al. Real-time magnetic resonance-guided endovascular repair of experimental abdominal aortic aneurysm in swine. *J Am Coll Cardiol.* 2005;45(12):2069–2077.
92. Eggebrecht H, Kuhl H, Kaiser GM, et al. Feasibility of real-time magnetic resonance-guided stent-graft placement in a swine model of descending aortic dissection. *Eur Heart J.* 2006;27(5):613–620.
93. Eggebrecht H, Zenge M, Ladd ME, et al. In vitro evaluation of current thoracic aortic stent-grafts for real-time MR-guided placement. *J Endovasc Ther.* 2006;13(1):62–71.
94. Ladd ME, Quick HH, Debatin JF. Interventional MRA and intravascular imaging. *J Magn Reson Imaging.* 2000;12(4):534–546.

40 Pulmonary Artery Magnetic Resonance Imaging

JOHN D. GRIZZARD

INTRODUCTION

Magnetic resonance imaging (MRI) of the pulmonary arterial system has been the subject of investigation for many years. Continued advances in gradient design and software sequences have resulted in progressive improvements in angiographic image quality while also shortening acquisition times, increasing its potential applications (Fig. 40.1). High-resolution images can be obtained in most patients within a manageable breath-hold, and techniques such as time-resolved imaging allow sequential discrete assessment of the pulmonary and systemic circuits (Fig. 40.2).[1] Angiographic images can also be combined with velocity-encoded flow analysis to provide a comprehensive evaluation of pulmonary valvular and arterial stenoses; 4D flow techniques may provide information about both with one technique that does not require breath-holding. The following chapter will review some of the potential applications of MRI in the assessment of disorders affecting the pulmonary arterial system including pulmonary embolism, pulmonary artery hypertension, congenital abnormalities, and pulmonary artery tumors.

PULMONARY EMBOLISM

Pulmonary embolism is the third most common cause of cardiovascular death in the United States, exceeded only by myocardial infarction and stroke. Incidence figures vary by age, with an overall incidence of 39 to 115 per 100,000 persons/year with an increase to ~200 to 700 in patients 70 or older. Additionally, incidence rates appear to be increasing over time,[2] although that this data may be affected by increasing sensitivity of diagnostic imaging techniques.[3] Case fatality rates in the multicenter RIETE registry showed a progressive decrease in mortality over the period from 2001–2013.[4] However, while a US study showed a similar decrease over the period from 1999 to 2008, from 2008 to 2019 a slight progressive increase was found, with racial and geographic disparities noted.[5] Moreover, mortality remains significant, with an estimated 300,000 deaths per year in the United States and similar numbers in Europe.[2] Predisposing causes of venous thromboembolism are commonly present, including major trauma, surgery, lower-limb fractures, and spinal cord injury. Cancer is also known to be a predisposing factor, particularly pancreatic cancer, hematologic malignancies, lung cancer, and gastric cancer. Oral contraceptives are the most frequent risk factor in females of reproductive age.

Clinical recognition of pulmonary embolism (PE) is hampered by the protean and nonspecific nature of the symptoms it may produce. Common symptoms include chest pain (often pleuritic) and dyspnea, with syncope frequently noted in those with large pulmonary emboli. Leg swelling when present may be a clue to the diagnosis and may suggest the vessel of origin. Because of the nonspecific nature of the signs and symptoms of pulmonary embolism, imaging has assumed a prominent role in its diagnosis and management. However, the increased awareness of clinicians regarding the possible diagnosis of pulmonary embolism combined with ready access to advanced imaging techniques has led to concerns regarding potential overuse of these techniques, particularly with regard to possible unnecessary radiation exposure. Clinical prediction rules have been developed (the Wells rule, Geneva rule, and their modifications)[6–9] that aim to assess the clinical pretest probability of PE and have been shown to allow accurate triage of patients into low-probability, moderate-probability, and high-probability categories with an estimated risk of confirmed PE of <10%, 30%, and 65% respectively.[2] In addition, the D-dimer assay, a marker of the simultaneous activation of coagulation and thrombolysis, is often used to risk stratify patients. An elevated D-dimer value has low predictive power, but a normal level is strong evidence against venous thromboembolism/PE. As an example, a D-dimer of <500 ng/mL combined with a low-probability Wells score can safely exclude 34% of patients from further workup. The YEARS score combines three elements of the Wells score (*absence of* clinical evidence of deep venous thrombosis, hemoptysis, and clinical assessment that PE is more likely than alternative diagnoses) with D-dimer values of <1000 ng/mL or D-dimer <500 ng/mL and one or more clinical items and allows exclusion of 48% of patients from further imaging workup.[10] Nonetheless, a substantial number of patients will still require advanced imaging to either exclude pulmonary embolism or to assess its extent.

Initially, pulmonary angiography was the method of choice due to its high spatial and temporal resolution and was long considered the gold standard for diagnosis. However, it requires exposure to ionizing radiation, and it is invasive, requiring manipulation of a catheter through the right heart and injection of potentially nephrotoxic contrast. It is contraindicated in patients with pulmonary hypertension, which may be present in patients with a large clot burden.

Noninvasive alternatives that mitigate some of these limitations were sought and planar ventilation-perfusion

(V/Q) nuclear scintigraphic imaging was found to be a useful alternative to invasive angiography and was rapidly adopted in many centers. It has the advantage of being noninvasive and does not require nephrotoxic iodinated contrast. In addition, it conveys a lower radiation dose compared to catheter angiography. Pulmonary embolism is diagnosed when there are photon deficits on perfusion imaging in a pulmonary artery distribution with normal ventilation. Although widely used for a number of years, over time the limitations of V/Q scanning became apparent. In particular, the Prospective Investigation of Pulmonary Embolism Detection (PIOPED) study showed that the majority of those with angiographically proven pulmonary embolism did not have a high-probability scan and found that a high-probability scan had a sensitivity of only 41%.[11] If intermediate- and low-probability scans were considered positive the sensitivity improved to 98% but the specificity decreased to 10%. In the clinical setting, low- to intermediate-probability scan interpretations are frequent (approaching 50% in some studies) and the limited diagnostic utility is such that these readings are considered nondiagnostic. However, there is value in the finding of a normal V/Q scan in a patient with a low clinical suspicion of PE in whom anticoagulation may be safely avoided. Additionally, V/Q scanning remains in use in selected populations, such as those with renal insufficiency or in pregnant patients. The addition of single-photon emission computed tomography imaging has been reported to improve the diagnostic performance of scintigraphic imaging, but at present has a limited evidence base.[2]

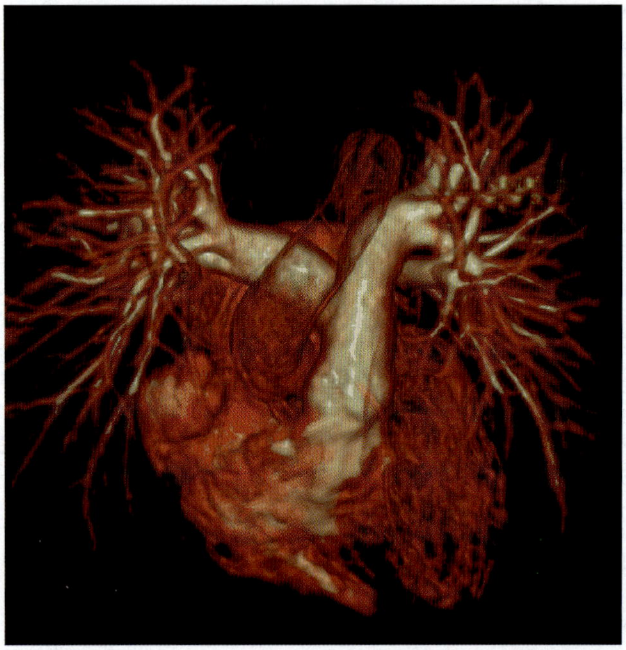

FIG. 40.1 Angled frontal view of a volume-rendered magnetic resonance (MR) angiogram demonstrating the excellent image quality possible with current MR systems.

In recent years, computed tomography pulmonary angiography (CTPA) has assumed a preeminent role in the diagnosis of pulmonary embolism. The PIOPED II trial demonstrated its diagnostic utility with a sensitivity of 83% and a specificity of 96% for the diagnosis of PE.[12] The assessment of pretest clinical probability was also shown to be important, with a negative CTPA in a patient with low clinical probability having a negative predictive value of 96%, and one with an intermediate probability a negative predictive value of 89%. Computed tomography (CT) scanners have undergone continued improvement since the PIOPED study, which mostly used 4-slice scanners, and 64 slice and higher scanners with rapid gantry rotation are now ubiquitous. Its excellent diagnostic performance has led to its recommendation as the first-line imaging test for the diagnosis of pulmonary embolism by both the European Society of Cardiology and the American College of Radiology.[2,13] Advantages of CTPA include its wide availability around the clock at most centers, its excellent accuracy, and its strong validation in prospective management outcome studies. Perhaps most importantly, it can often provide an alternative diagnosis if PE is excluded, such as aortic dissection or pneumonia. It does require exposure to ionizing radiation and iodinated contrast, decreasing

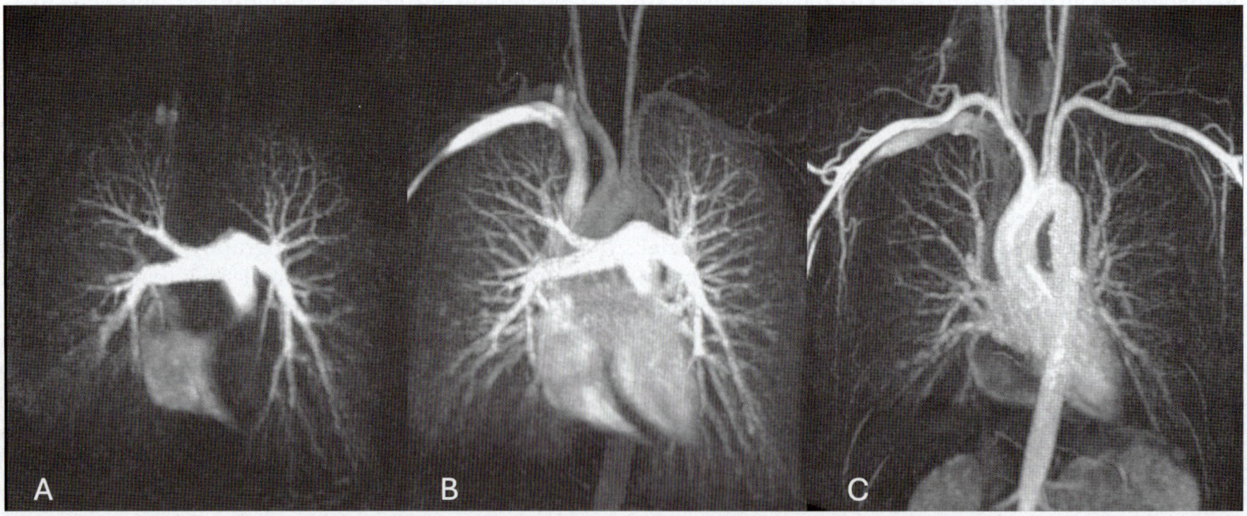

FIG. 40.2 Maximum intensity projection magnetic resonance angiographic image from a time-resolved study demonstrating early pulmonary arterial filling (A), late pulmonary artery filling (B), and systemic arterial filling (C) as discrete angiograms.

its desirability in young and/or pregnant patients or those with impaired renal function.

Magnetic resonance angiography (MRA) shares many desirable features with CT angiography in that it is noninvasive and provides a comprehensive assessment of a large volume of interest. It has advantages over CT in that it does not require ionizing radiation or potentially nephrotoxic iodinated contrast. Unfortunately, in reported studies, its sensitivity and specificity have been largely inferior to those of CTPA. Most notably, in the often-referenced PIOPED III study, MRAs were technically inadequate in 25% of patients.[14] In patients with adequate examinations, the sensitivity was 78% and the specificity was 99%. Similar results were found in the IRM-EP study, in which ~30% of scans were inconclusive.[15] A meta-analysis from 2015 evaluating the use of MRI in the diagnosis of pulmonary embolism reported that in 15 studies reviewed, 19% were technically inadequate, and that the overall sensitivity was 75% (84% for those with adequate images) and specificity was 80% (97% for those with adequate images).[16] Several studies have noted that the diagnostic accuracy of MRA decreases with decreased vessel size, with 90%+ sensitivity for large-vessel emboli and with subsegmental vessels having the lowest sensitivity. However, the importance of diagnosing isolated subsegmental pulmonary emboli is a matter of some controversy and is the subject of ongoing investigation (SAFE-SSPE study).[17]

In light of its importance in the assessment of the value of MRA for PE, further detailed evaluation of the PIOPED III data is warranted.[18] Technical factors for the MRA studies in the PIOPED III study were as follows: images were acquired with 3 mm slice thickness and a fixed field of view of 40 cm with a matrix of 384 × 288, resulting in a voxel size of 1.04 mm × 1.4 mm × 3 mm (interpolated to 1.5 mm with zero filling), which is significantly lower resolution than current techniques. In large or obese patients, the field of view was kept constant, and the matrix was reduced, further decreasing the in-plane resolution. The scan time was 14–22 seconds. Analysis of the technical quality of the PIOPED III MRA data revealed that the proportion of uninterpretable studies varied significantly by site from 11% to 51%, with poor arterial opacification responsible for 67% of uninterpretable scans and motion artifact 36%. Gadobenate dimeglumine was used for 84% of patients in a dose of 0.1 mmol/kg with an average volume of 20 mL and was administered at 2 mL/sec resulting in a nominal bolus duration of 10 seconds. Newer studies have been reported that modified these parameters with improved results. For example, given the increased relaxivity of gadobenate dimeglumine, Pressaco et al. diluted the contrast agent with saline to a total volume of 40 mL and injected it at 2.5 mL/sec, resulting in a 16 second bolus duration.[19] This longer bolus duration significantly mitigated the truncation and blurring artifacts known to occur if the contrast concentration varies during the image acquisition. Technical factors used in their MRA acquisition on a 3 T scanner resulted in a significantly higher resolution scan with a voxel size of 1.14 × 0.9 × 2.1 mm that was acquired with a parallel imaging factor of 4 resulting in a consistent 16 second scan duration. A second acquisition with similar factors but a lower flip angle was then performed, with an additional 3D volumetric interpolated breath-hold examination in the chest and abdomen/pelvis to complete the study. They reported a sensitivity of 100% and specificity of 97% for the detection of the main, lobar, and segmental arteries compared to CTPA. For subsegmental arteries the sensitivity was 75% with 100% specificity.[19] Several technical factors likely explain the improved results—the contrast bolus dilution and the longer infusion time substantially reduced truncation and "ringing" artifacts, correcting the main source of artifacts and inadequate scans in the PIOPED III study. The shorter breath-hold decreased respiratory motion artifacts, and the higher scan resolution was likely also helpful in improving image quality. Finally, the authors noted that the opacification of the vessel walls provided by delayed-phase imaging with contrast agents with blood pool properties allows improved visualization of intraluminal thrombus (Fig. 40.3). Note that in a standard pulmonary arterial magnetic resonance (MR) angiogram pulmonary emboli may be difficult to recognize if they are eccentric in location (see figure) or result in total vessel occlusion. Lastly, their use of gadobenate dimeglumine allowed delayed-phase imaging of the pelvic and thigh veins to exclude venous thrombosis. Importantly,

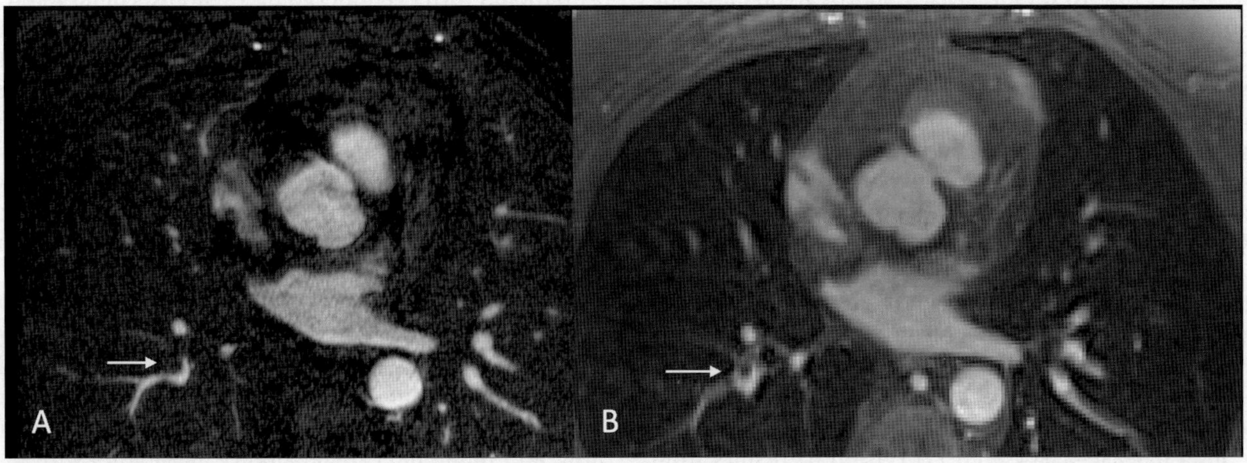

FIG. 40.3 Axial magnetic resonance angiographic image (A) demonstrating a small pulmonary embolus (*arrow*). Note how the fat-suppressed postcontrast T1 volumetric breath-hold examination image (B) demonstrates improved conspicuity of the small embolus (*arrow*) due to opacification of the vessel wall. This significantly improves the detectability of the embolus.

an outcomes study using a similar multiphase image MR acquisition (arterial and early delayed-phase angiographic images with delayed-phase, fat-suppressed T1 volumetric imaging) showed a negative predictive value of 97% at 3 months and 96% at 1 year, similar to values reported for CT.[20]

Other studies have been performed with ferumoxytol, an ultrasmall superparamagnetic iron oxide compound with T1-shortening properties that can be safely administered to renal failure patients, and which has prolonged intravascular retention, minimizing the impact of errors of bolus timing. An initial study of its use combined with ultrashort echo time (TE) imaging has provided encouraging results.[21]

In summary, while current guidelines do not support the use of MR for the evaluation of pulmonary embolism, it may still be considered in those allergic to iodinated contrast, or in young patients to avoid radiation exposure. In the future, it is likely that continued advances in the acceleration of image acquisition paired with the use of delayed imaging with improved vessel wall visualization using blood pool contrast agents will expand the indications for MRA for pulmonary embolism imaging over time.

PULMONARY HYPERTENSION

Pulmonary hypertension (PH) comprises a group of disorders that have in common persistent abnormal elevation of mean pulmonary artery pressure above 20 mm Hg and pulmonary vascular resistance >2 Woods units; previously, a cut-off of 25 mm Hg and 3 Woods units was used, but recent investigations have demonstrated that these new values correlate with the upper limits of normal and that values exceeding these levels are associated with a significant and continuous increase in mortality.[22] It is estimated that 1% of the world's population is affected, with low- and middle-income countries thought to have a disproportionate number of cases.

The World Health Organization recognizes five groups of disorders causing PH:

Group 1—pulmonary artery hypertension (rare)
Group 2—PH due to left heart disease (very common)
Group 3—PH due to lung diseases and/or hypoxia (common) (e.g., chronic obstructive pulmonary disease, interstitial lung disease)
Group 4—PH associated with pulmonary artery obstructions (usually due to chronic thromboembolic PH) (rare)
Group 5—PH with unclear and/or multifactorial mechanisms (rare)

Pulmonary artery hypertension (group 1—previously termed "primary pulmonary hypertension"), while rare, has been the subject of considerable study and is characterized by pulmonary artery remodeling and obstruction resulting in increased precapillary pulmonary vascular resistance to >2 Woods units. PH associated with left heart disease (group 2) may have isolated postcapillary PH or combined post and precapillary PH, while lung disease–associated PH (group 3) results from precapillary obstruction. Regardless of the cause of PH, all forms are characterized by conversion of the normal low-pressure/low-resistance pulmonary artery circuit into a high-pressure/high-resistance circuit. Initially, the right ventricle responds with hypertrophy, but ultimately right heart failure develops with resultant premature mortality. Clinical symptoms are nonspecific, including dyspnea on exertion and other symptoms that may be mistaken for coronary artery disease. Echocardiography, often performed for the evaluation of these nonspecific symptoms, is often the initial modality to suggest the presence of the disorder. Visualization of a jet of tricuspid regurgitation exceeding 2.8 cm/sec may provide evidence of elevated pulmonary artery pressure. A definitive diagnosis is made by right heart catheterization, which confirms the degree of PH and determines the level of elevated pulmonary vascular resistance. However, it is an invasive procedure and requires the use of ionizing radiation.

CT pulmonary angiography, while requiring ionizing radiation and iodinated contrast, can noninvasively demonstrate indirect signs of right ventricular (RV) dysfunction and elevated pulmonary artery pressures, such as RV hypertrophy and abnormal curvature of the intraventricular septum. In addition, it may provide information regarding the possible etiology of PH such as findings of lung disease (emphysema or interstitial fibrosis) or chronic thrombi in cases of chronic thromboembolic pulmonary hypertension (CTEPH).[23] However, functional assessments with CT and repetitive CT examinations are unappealing as they can result in significant radiation exposure.

Cardiovascular MR (CMR) imaging has significant advantages in the assessment and monitoring of patients with PH. Right ventricular health is the key determinant of the prognosis of patients with PH, and CMR is recognized as the reference standard for the noninvasive assessment of RV structure and function. Cine steady-state free precession (SSFP) sequences can accurately quantify RV systolic and diastolic volume and stroke volume and can measure RV mass. Two-dimensional velocity-encoded flow studies can accurately measure pulmonary artery flow. Importantly, in this era of new treatment regimens for PH, serial measurements of RV function and mass to assess treatment response can be performed accurately and without exposure to radiation or iodinated contrast.[23] This data has been shown to have prognostic significance; in a study of 91 patients with PH undergoing 12 months of targeted therapy, CMR-derived functional parameters at baseline and at 12-month follow-up reflected changes in functional status and predicted survival.[24] A recent meta-analysis of 22 studies encompassing 2000 patients confirmed that CMR measures of RV function were a strong predictor of mortality; for every 1% decrease in RV ejection fraction there was a 4.9% increase in the risk of clinical worsening as well as an increased risk of mortality over the subsequent 22 and 54 months, respectively.[25]

Multiple other parameters can be assessed with CMR that can also provide useful information regarding the pulmonary artery-right ventricular unit. Two-dimensional velocity-encoded flow studies have been shown to demonstrate reduced pulmonary artery (PA) velocities, blood flow, and pulmonary distensibility in patients with pulmonary arterial hypertension (PAH) compared to normal.[26] Heterogenous flow profiles and regions of retrograde flow in the main PA have also been observed. Other investigators have shown that prolonged mean transit time and decreased pulmonary blood flow were common in patients with PAH.[27] Late gadolinium enhancement at the RV insertion sites may be observed in patients with PH and is strongly associated with elevated PA pressures, RV dilatation and RV hypertrophy, as well as adverse outcomes in patients with PH (Fig. 40.4).[28]

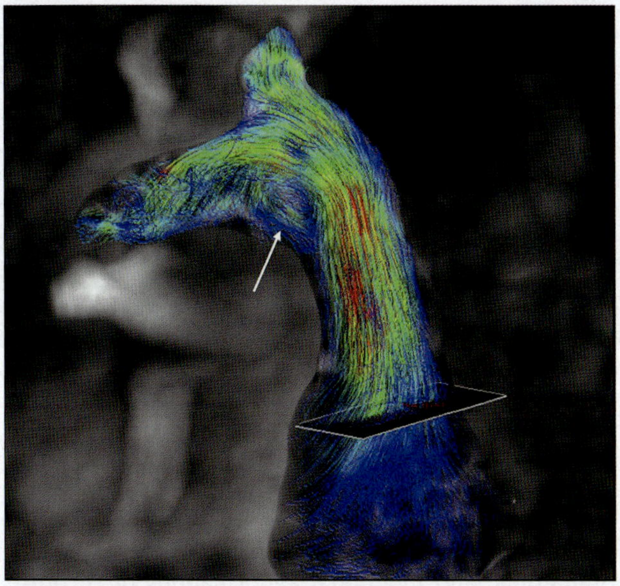

FIG. 40.4 Still-frame image from a 4D flow study through the pulmonary artery demonstrates a flow vortex (*arrow*), a finding seen on 4D flow images in patients with pulmonary hypertension. The percentage of the cardiac cycle with vortical flow has been found to correlate with the mean pulmonary artery pressure.

CMR visualization of the interventricular septum (IVS) in patients with PH demonstrates displacement from right to left with loss of the normal rightward convexity as pulmonary artery pressures rise (Fig. 40.4). As the PA systolic pressure rises to meet or exceed the left ventricular (LV) pressure the displacement of the IVS into the LV results in a decrease in cardiac output. Similarly, as the RV fails and RV diastolic pressure rises, flattening of the septum during diastole may decrease LV filling, also decreasing cardiac output. The abnormal septal dynamics are readily observable on short-axis cine imaging.[29]

CMR has also been used as a means of detecting and quantifying the degree of PH. Measured pulmonary artery diameters exceeding 30 mm correlate with elevated pressure. Recently, studies have been reported to provide accurate estimations of PA pressure using various parameters determined by CMR. One group used a composite model incorporating measurement of the interventricular septal angle, the ventricular mass index (RV mass/LV mass), and a score based on black-blood images showing slow flow in the PA. In a study of 300 patients, this model demonstrated excellent correlation with invasive mean pulmonary artery pressure measurements, with the area under the receiver operating characteristic (ROC) curve of 0.95.[30] Mean PA pressures >25 mm Hg were detected with a sensitivity of 93% and a specificity of 79% and a positive predictive value of 96%. Similar accuracy was reported for this model at a lower threshold of 20 mm Hg.[31]

An alternative means to diagnose and monitor mean PA pressure in cases of PH using the persistence of flow vortices (Fig. 40.5) in the pulmonary artery on 4D flow sequences has also been reported. Reiter et al. found that the percentage duration of the cardiac cycle with flow

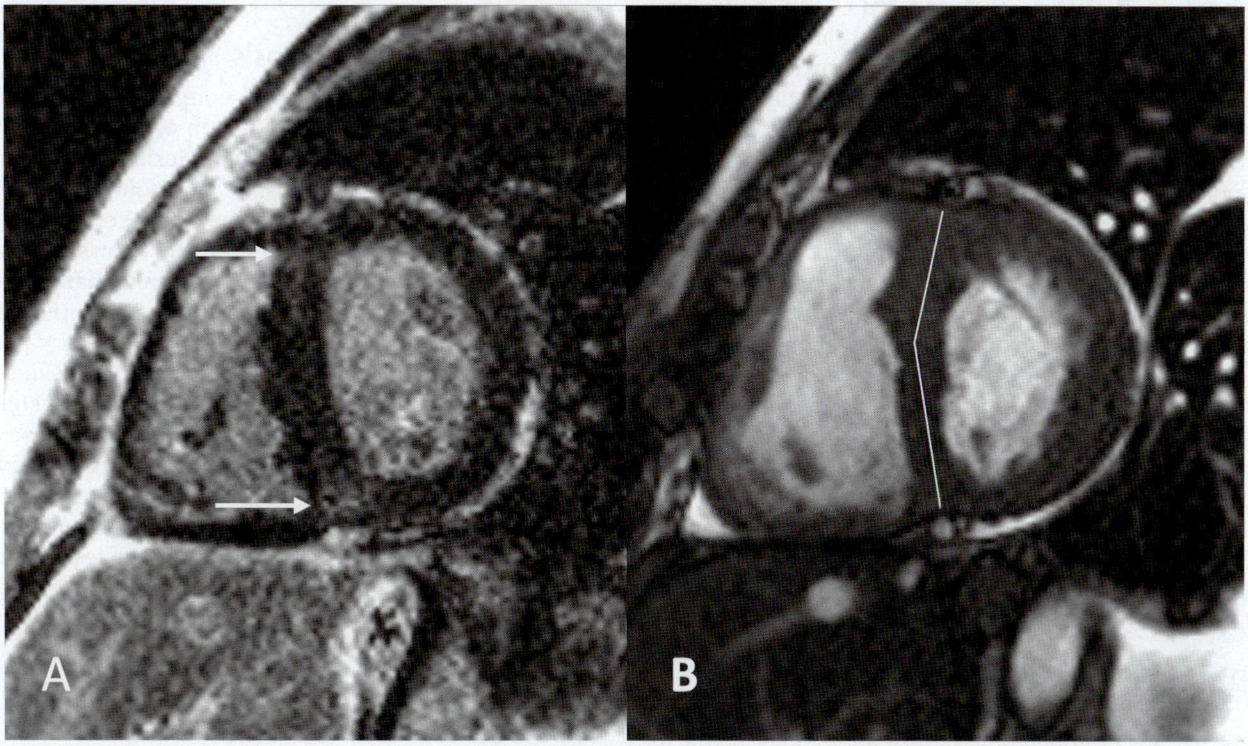

FIG. 40.5 Short-axis late gadolinium enhanced (A) image from a patient with pulmonary hypertension demonstrates abnormal enhancement of the right ventricular insertion sites upon the septum (*arrows*) as well as mild midwall septal enhancement. Short-axis cine steady-state free precession image at end systole (B) shows an abnormal angle of septal curvature (*lines*), a finding that is proportional to the mean pulmonary artery pressure.

vortices evident correlated in a linear fashion with the mean arterial pressure, with an area under the ROC curve of 0.994. A calculated cut-off value of 14.3% of the cardiac cycle showing vortical flow had a sensitivity of 97% and specificity of 96% for the diagnosis of PH.[32] The standard deviation of mean PA pressure estimations compared to invasive measurements was 3.9 mm Hg. Additional CMR techniques have been applied to assess the RV in cases of PH including T1 mapping of the RV, perfusion imaging of the RV, and strain analysis to detect subtle abnormalities of RV structure and function.[23,33] These provide information that is complementary to standard hemodynamic data and are the subject of ongoing research. These investigations, while preliminary in nature, suggest that CMR can provide comprehensive functional and hemodynamic data regarding the RV and may serve in the future as a complement to (and possibly a partial replacement for) invasive measurements.

CTEPH, although uncommon, is the largest component of group 4 noted above. Importantly, surgical intervention and/or balloon angioplasty in appropriate patients can meaningfully impact outcomes, leading to improvements in prognosis and quality of life.[34] It is characterized by the presence of chronic, organized, fibrotic clots that often result in ringlike stenoses, webs/slits, and chronic total pulmonary artery occlusions on imaging that are persistent findings noted after 3 months of therapeutic anticoagulation. In some patients it is accompanied by small-vessel arteriopathy. It is estimated that 2%–4% of cases of acute PE may develop CTEPH.[35] To facilitate early diagnosis and treatment, European Society of Cardiology guidelines currently recommend echocardiography in all patients with symptoms of CTEPH and/or predisposing factors to CTEPH. More recently, clinical prediction rules to risk-stratify patients with suspected CTEPH have been developed and allow a significant reduction in the number of patients requiring echocardiography, particularly when combined with findings noted on CTPA at the time of initial PE diagnosis.[36] However, a clear history of PE is lacking in up to 25% of patients, and imaging plays an important role in the diagnosis of CTEPH. Societal guidelines recommend the use of V/Q scanning to diagnose or exclude the disorder, with positive cases showing unmatched perfusion defects.[2] Dual-energy CT examinations may also depict areas of perfusion abnormality similar to V/Q scanning by using iodine mapping and are the subject of ongoing study. However, MR has also been reported to provide accurate information for this disorder, with one study showing that time-resolved MRA combined with noncontrast SSFP imaging had a sensitivity of 98% for proximal chronic thrombotic disease and 94% for distal disease and was superior to CTPA. In addition, perfusion images obtained using the MRA dataset had a sensitivity of 92%.[37] Larger studies confirming and extending these promising data are needed.

CONGENITAL VASCULAR DISORDERS

A wide variety of congenital abnormalities may result in abnormalities of the pulmonary artery circuit, and CMR has emerged as the most comprehensive means of assessing the anatomic and functional abnormalities often present in these disorders and following their repair. CMR's lack of ionizing radiation makes it especially appealing given the young age of the affected patients and the frequent need for repeated examinations. Selected examples are noted below.

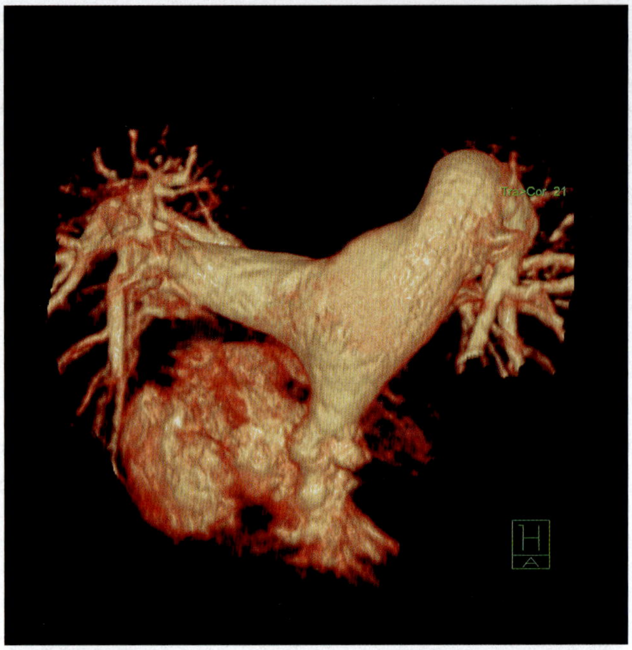

FIG. 40.6 Frontal view of a volume-rendered magnetic resonance pulmonary angiogram of a patient with uncorrected valvular pulmonary stenosis. Note that the main and left pulmonary arteries are larger than the right pulmonary artery. This classic finding is due to the jet of turbulent flow produced by the stenotic valve extending in line towards the main and left pulmonary arteries.

Valvular Pulmonic Stenosis

This makes up ~ 8% of cases of congenital heart disease cases. Most cases result from fusion of the valve leaflets, resulting in a "doming" appearance during systole, which is readily observable on SSFP cine MR sequences. Velocity-encoded flow sequences can determine the gradient in a noninvasive fashion, and MRA typically shows the classic enlargement of the main and left main pulmonary arteries, which are noticeably larger than the right PA (Fig. 40.6). This asymmetry is thought to result from the flow jet produced by the abnormal valve extending in an in-line fashion into the main and left pulmonary arteries. Poststenotic dilatation of the main PA can be extreme in some cases and can result in aneurysm formation. Balloon valvuloplasty is the preferred treatment but is frequently complicated by mild pulmonary regurgitation; significant pulmonary regurgitation requiring intervention is much less common. CMR flow and volumetric studies provide precise and reproducible data and are an excellent means of follow-up in these patients.

Tetralogy of Fallot

This is the most common cyanotic defect, accounting for 10% of cases of congenital heart disease. Relief of the right ventricular outflow tract obstruction may require augmentation of the pulmonary valve annulus with a transannular patch, which often disrupts the function of the valve with resultant pulmonary regurgitation, which may be severe. CMR flow studies can quantify the degree of regurgitation. MRA can demonstrate aneurysmal dilation of the outflow tract when present and any residual central or branch pulmonary artery stenoses, the latter of which known to occur in up to 37% of cases (Fig. 40.7). The severity of branch PA stenoses can also be quantified using velocity-encoded flow studies.

Patent Ductus Arteriosus

These lesions, representing persistence of the embryologic connection between the aorta and pulmonary artery, are occasionally detected in adulthood as incidental findings on CT or MR examinations performed for other reasons. Far less commonly they present as hemodynamically significant lesions in adults. Patent ductus arteriosus is readily detected on MR angiographic images and larger lesions may be visualized on cine SSFP imaging (Fig. 40.8). Over time, uncorrected larger lesions result in Eisenmenger's physiology with reversal of the left-to-right shunt and development of right-to-left shunting. The degree of shunting can be assessed with MR flow studies.

D-Transposition of the Great Arteries

The currently preferred repair is the arterial switch (Jatene) procedure, in which the proximal portions of the pulmonary artery and aorta are transected, and the pulmonary artery is moved anterior to the aorta (LeCompte maneuver) before anastomoses are performed. Branch PA stenosis may develop in up to 25% of patients as an early or late complication, more commonly affecting the left PA

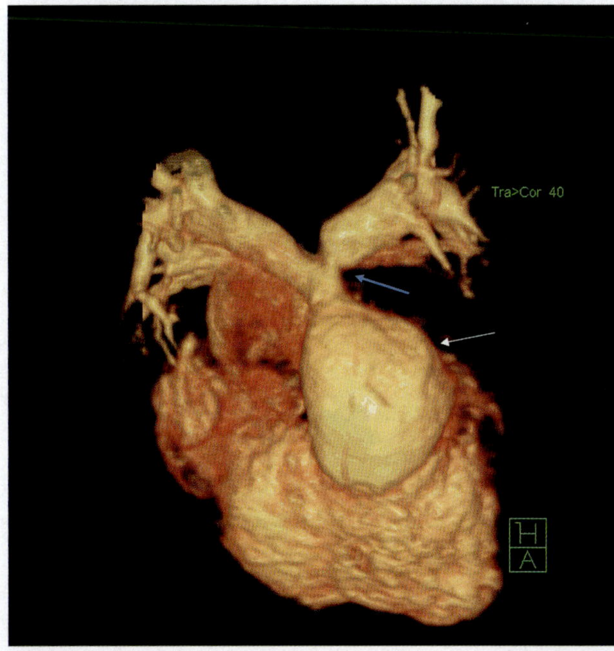

FIG. 40.7 Frontal view of a volume-rendered magnetic resonance angiogram of a patient who is status-post patch annuloplasty for repair of tetralogy of Fallot. Note the aneurysmal ballooning of the right ventricular outflow tract (*white arrow*) and the residual branch stenosis of the left pulmonary artery (*blue arrow*).

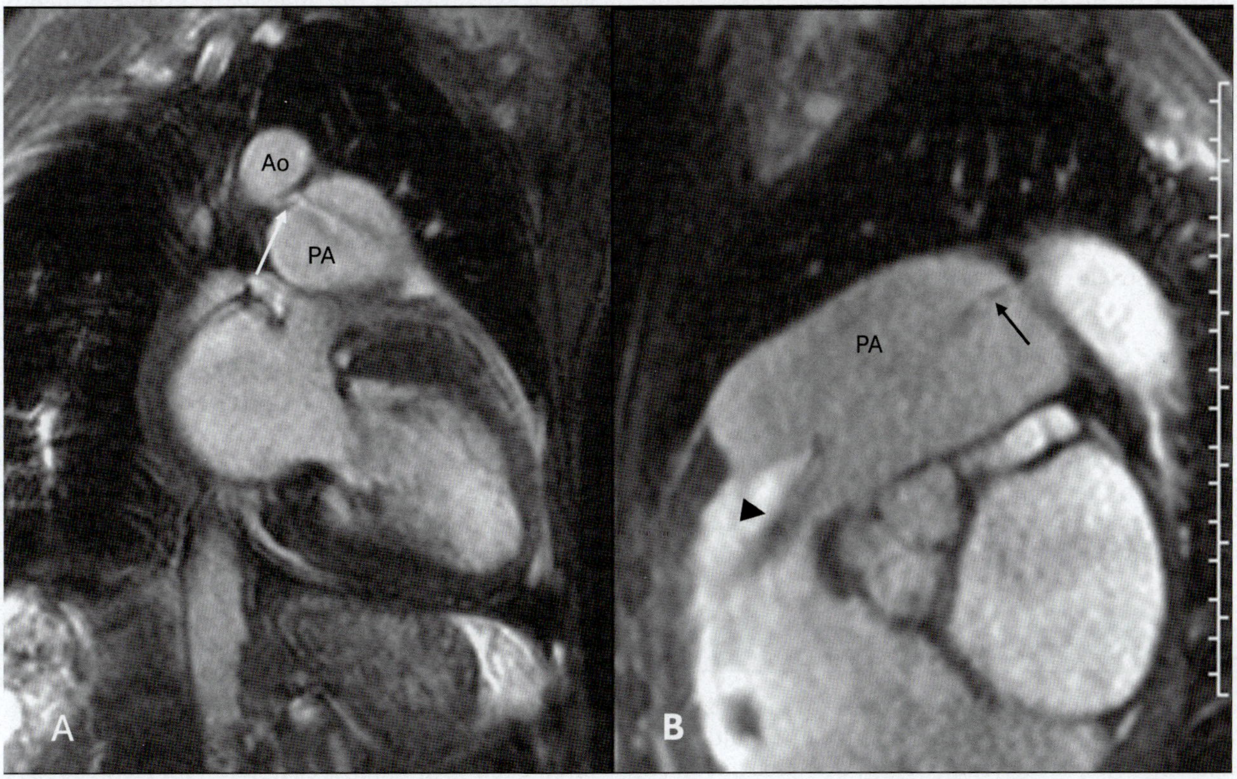

FIG. 40.8 Cine steady-state free precession two-chamber view (A) shows a patent ductus arteriosus transmitting flow from the aorta (Ao) into a dilated pulmonary artery (PA). A right ventricular outflow tract cine image (B) shows a flow jet (*black arrow*) from the aorta into the dilated pulmonary artery. This has resulted in pulmonary hypertension with dilatation of the pulmonary artery and secondary pulmonary regurgitation with a flow jet noted to extend into the right ventricle (*black arrowhead*).

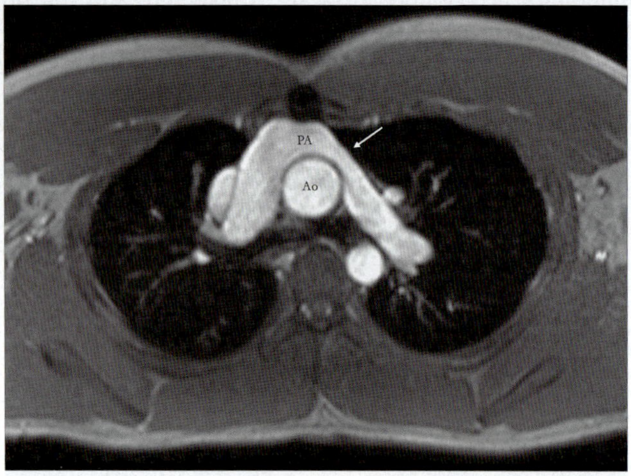

FIG. 40.9 Axial cine steady-state free precession image of a patient who had a Jatene procedure for repair of DTransposition of the great arteries. Note that the pulmonary arteries (PA) are "draped" over the ascending aorta (Ao), and that there is moderate narrowing of the proximal left pulmonary artery (*arrow*), a common complication of the repair.

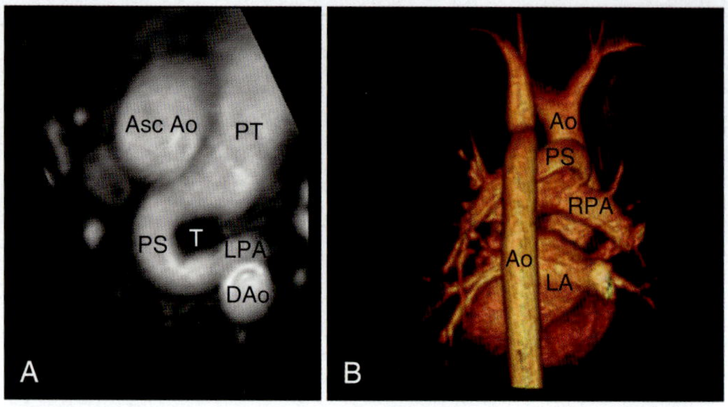

FIG. 40.10 Pulmonary artery sling. (A) Axial contrast-enhanced cardiovascular magnetic resonance reconstruction demonstrating an aberrant left pulmonary artery (*LPA*), also known as pulmonary artery sling (*PS*), coursing between the ascending aorta (*Asc Ao*) and descending aorta (*DAo*), posterior to the trachea (*T*). (B) Three-dimensional volume-rendered image of the same patients showing the PS arising from the right pulmonary artery (*RPA*) coursing posterior to the aorta (*Ao*). *LA*, left atrium; *PT*, pulmonary trunk.

(Fig. 40.9). CMR studies incorporating angiography and flow studies is an ideal technique for the follow-up of these patients.

Fontan Circuits

In these patients the pulmonary arteries are passively perfused, most often with some combination of anastomosis of the superior vena cava (SVC) to the right pulmonary artery (Glenn procedure) along with creation of a conduit connecting the inferior vena caval/right atrial flow to the PA. Pulmonary artery imaging studies in such patients are complicated by the differential opacification times of the components of the pulmonary circulation, and often necessitate multiple angiographic image acquisitions. Although CT examinations are often used, the need for complex bolus shaping and/or multiple acquisitions requiring additional radiation exposure has led to an increased interest in MR techniques. MR angiographic imaging can be performed with multiple acquisitions with a single bolus of contrast and without radiation penalty, and functional analysis of the single ventricle can be easily added to the study.

Pulmonary Artery Sling

This is an uncommon abnormality in which the left pulmonary artery originates from the posterior margin of the right pulmonary artery and passes posterior to the trachea and anterior to the esophagus. It is frequently associated with tracheomalacia, and airway abnormalities are often the means of presentation (Fig. 40.10).

PULMONARY ARTERY TUMORS

Primary pulmonary artery tumors are rare malignancies with an estimated incidence of 0.001% to 0.03%,[38] although the exact incidence is uncertain as they are often mistaken clinically and on imaging as pulmonary emboli. The majority are histologically intimal sarcomas and demonstrate extensive intraluminal growth. Clinically, they often present with dyspnea (86%), cough (73%), and chest pain (64%) and less commonly with hemoptysis (50%). Although a few series report a slight female predominance, most show an approximately equal sex distribution, with an average age of ~49 years at presentation. Notably, in a recent clinical series the tumors were initially misdiagnosed as pulmonary emboli in 95% of cases on initial CT examination.[39] Clinical differentiation may be aided by the finding of normal D-dimer levels and lower brain natriuretic peptide (BNP) levels in patients with pulmonary artery sarcomas.[40] Imaging differentiation from acute or chronic PE is often difficult on CT but is aided by the recognition of vessel expansion of the affected main and branch pulmonary arteries, with sarcomas tending to fill the vessel and have a rounded proximal edge. A "grapelike," aneurysm-like dilatation of the distal vessel involvement is seen in ~45%. The main PA is involved in 95% of cases, the right PA in 71%, and the left PA in 41%–65%. Extraluminal extension and involvement of the right ventricular outflow tract and pulmonic valve are highly suggestive of the correct diagnosis and are seen in 25%–30% of patients.[40] MRI has been reported to be very helpful when used, as high signal is characteristically seen on T2 fat-suppressed and diffusion-weighted images. Contrast enhancement of the tumor is seen on T1-weighted images, allowing accurate differentiation from thrombi[41] (Fig. 40.11). The prognosis of pulmonary artery sarcomas is unfortunately dismal, as up to 25% of patients have metastases at presentation. Life expectancy of untreated patients is ~ 2–3 months. Multimodality treatment, including surgical resection when possible, combined with chemoradiation therapy has resulted in improved survival of 24.7 months.[42]

Secondary tumor involvement of the pulmonary artery circuit most often results from direct tumor invasion by adjacent lung or mediastinal malignancies, with the primary tumor sources most often lung cancer or tumor-laden mediastinal lymph nodes. Embolic disease is most often seen with lung, breast, and stomach cancer and is a known cause of significant dyspnea and may result in PH.[43] While microemboli are most common, on occasion

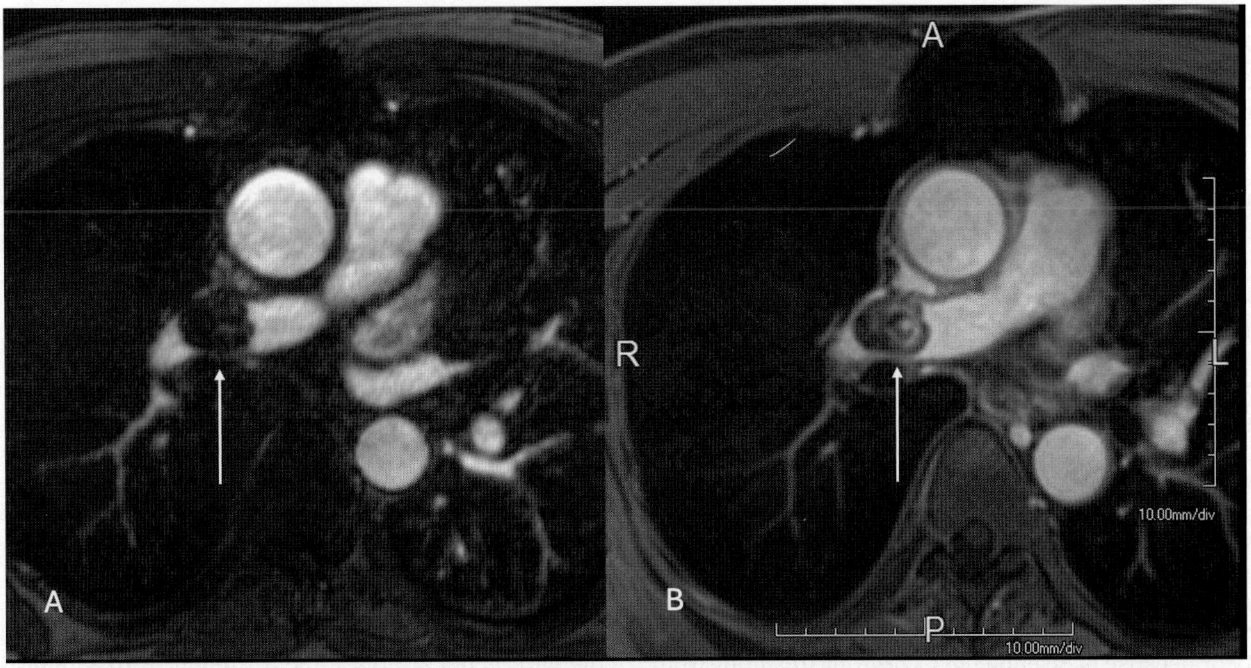

FIG. 40.11 Axial images from an arterial phase magnetic resonance angiogram (A) and delayed-phase images from a volumetric interpolated breath-hold examination (B) showing a rounded sarcoma in the right pulmonary artery (*arrows*). The lesion does not appear to enhance on immediate postcontrast images but shows avid enhancement on the delayed images (B), allowing clear differentiation from nonenhancing thrombus.

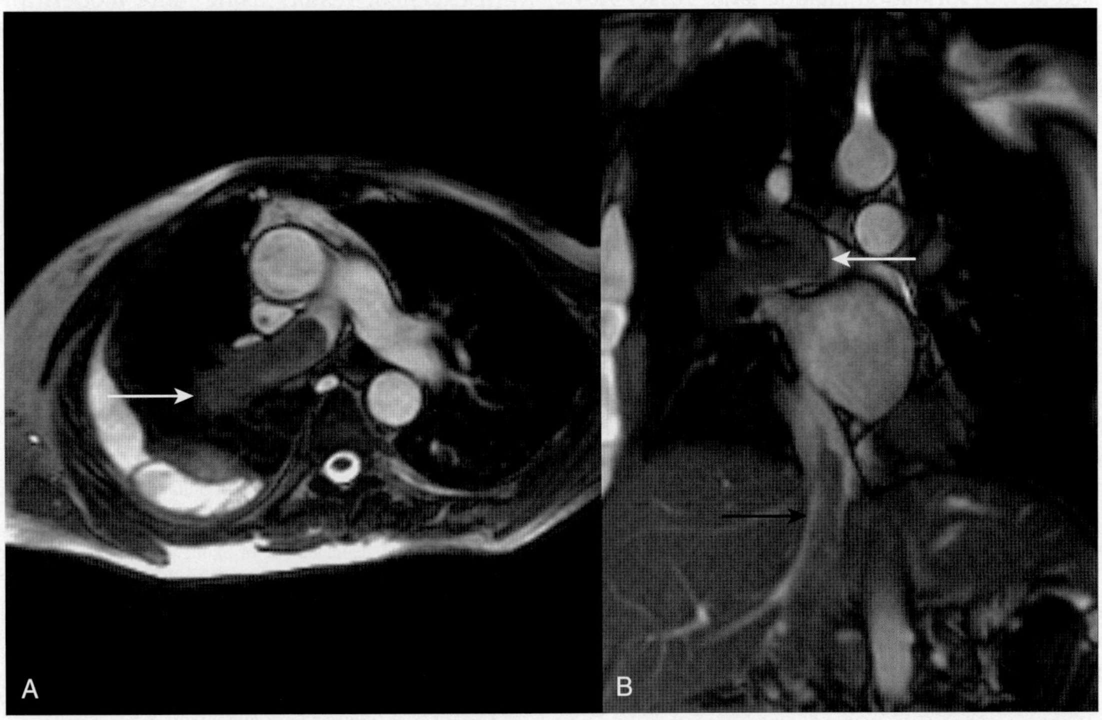

FIG. 40.12 Axial steady-state free precession (SSFP) cine image (A) demonstrates a large tumor thrombus in the right pulmonary artery (*white arrow*). Coronal SSFP image with a large field of view (B) demonstrates transvenous extension of a renal carcinoma (*black arrow*), which was the source of the tumor embolism.

large tumor emboli can occur and can mimic bland thromboembolism. Typically, such emboli occur in the setting of inferior vena caval tumor involvement, most often by renal, adrenal, or hepatocellular malignancies, which are usually evident at the time of embolism detection (Fig. 40.12).

An increasingly recognized benign tumor, papillary fibroelastoma, is known to involve the pulmonary valve in a minority of cases (8%–13%).[44] These small tumors have a "frondlike" appearance and most often occur on the aortic and mitral valve leaflets, where they can result in problematic systemic emboli. Involvement of the pulmonary valve is often clinically silent and most of the lesions are detected as incidental findings. On cine SSFP MRI, they present as small (~8 mm average size), rounded, low-signal lesions attached to the valve. On T1-weighted images, they are iso or hypointense and are hyperintense on T2-weighted images. They do not show uptake on first-pass perfusion imaging. Hyperenhancement is usually seen on late gadolinium-enhanced images but may require delayed images up to 15 to 20 minutes postcontrast. They do not usually require any specific therapy (see Chapter 35).

PULMONARY ARTERY ANEURYSMS

Pulmonary artery aneurysms (PAAs) are significantly less common than aortic aneurysms and tend to occur in a younger population. Although some authors define a PAA as one that exceeds 29 mm, most use a cut-off of 40 mm diameter. It is said that 89% involve the main PA with 11% in the pulmonary branches. Congenital abnormalities are said to constitute ~50% of cases, with shunt lesions such as patent ductus arteriosus, ventricular septal defects, and atrial septal defects most often seen, likely due to abnormal wall shear stress.[45–47] Valvular pulmonary stenosis may also result in abnormal dilatation of the main and left pulmonary arteries (see Fig. 40.6). Acquired causes including pulmonary artery hypertension, either as a primary abnormality or because of Eisenmenger syndrome resulting from a preexisting left-to-right shunt, are also associated with PAA formation (see Fig. 40.8).

Rare causes of PAA formation include large-vessel vasculitis, with Behcet syndrome being the most common vasculitis to cause PAA followed by Takayasu and giant-cell arteritis. Behcet syndrome is unique in that it involves both small and large vessels, as well as veins. It is a multisystem relapsing and remitting disorder that is thought to result from exposure of a genetically susceptible host to a wide variety of environmental triggers. The mean age at diagnosis is 30, and males and females have an equal incidence, but males tend to have more severe involvement. Oral and genital aphthous ulcers are a frequent mode of presentation, often accompanied by uveitis. Vascular involvement is seen in up to 40% of cases, with thrombophlebitis and deep venous thrombosis the most frequent manifestations. Arterial involvement is most commonly seen in the aorta and peripheral vessels, but pulmonary artery involvement when noted is highly suggestive of the diagnosis.[48] Hughes-Stovin syndrome, once thought to be a separate disorder, is now thought to be a limited form of Behcet syndrome. It is also characterized by PAA formation with a tendency of the aneurysms to rupture, but does not have the same incidence of skin and ocular involvement.[47]

Pulmonary artery pseudoaneurysms most often result from infection or trauma. Septic pulmonary emboli from right-sided endocarditis may result in a pseudoaneurysm when they lodge in a pulmonary artery branch and cause necrotizing infection that results in a loss of integrity of the vessel wall. Similar destructive changes can result from angioinvasive infectious agents as may be seen in immunocompromised patients. Traumatic pseudoaneurysms may result when Swan-Ganz catheters are placed in a peripheral pulmonary arterial branch and are subsequently inflated to a diameter that exceeds that of the vessel with resultant injury. They may also be seen following penetrating trauma.

MRA is well suited to the diagnosis and follow-up of patients with PAAs, as many are seen in young patients with congenital lesions in whom its excellent image quality can be combined with the acquisition of hemodynamic data in the same setting and without radiation.

SUMMARY

MRI has many appealing features that have generated substantial interest in its use for evaluation of the pulmonary artery circuit. MRA of the pulmonary arteries is an integral part of the evaluation of many forms of congenital heart disease and is readily combined with cine imaging and flow studies to provide a comprehensive assessment of the right ventricular-pulmonary arterial unit. It provides reproducible functional and anatomic data that is the reference standard for follow-up studies in these young patients and does so without ionizing radiation. Additionally, pulmonary artery masses—like other cardiac masses—are best characterized with MRI, which has superior soft tissue contrast relative to CT and provides comprehensive anatomic coverage not possible with echocardiography. Although prior studies have cast doubt on its efficacy in the evaluation of pulmonary embolism, some centers are performing these studies with excellent results using more modern protocols for image acquisition and contrast administration.[19,49] For selected patients such as those with contrast allergies or other concerns regarding iodinated CT contrast administration, MRA can be a useful alternative. It has been shown to be potentially useful in patients with suspected chronic thromboembolic PH, although V/Q scanning remains the first-line imaging study. Lastly, it is an important component of the evaluation and follow-up of patients with PH. Ongoing research in this area shows promising data that in addition to accurate RV functional assessments, noninvasive estimations of PA pressures may be possible using CMR.

REFERENCES

1. Kocaoglu M, Pednekar A, Fleck RJ, Dillman JR. Cardiothoracic magnetic resonance angiography. *Curr Probl Diagn Radiol.* 2024;53(1):154–165.
2. Konstantinides SV, Meyer G, Becattini C, et al. 2019 ESC guidelines for the diagnosis and management of acute pulmonary embolism developed in collaboration with the European respiratory society (ERS). *Eur Heart J.* 2020;41(4):543–603.
3. Wiener RS, Schwartz LM, Woloshin S. Time trends in pulmonary embolism in the United States: evidence of overdiagnosis. *Arch Intern Med.* 2011;171(9):831–837.
4. Jimenez D, de Miguel-Diez J, Guijarro R, et al. Trends in the management and outcomes of acute pulmonary embolism: analysis from the RIETE registry. *J Am Coll Cardiol.* 2016;67(2):162–170.
5. Martin KA, Molsberry R, Cuttica MJ, Desai KR, Schimmel DR, Khan SS. Time trends in pulmonary embolism mortality rates in the United States, 1999 to 2018. *J Am Heart Assoc.* 2020;9(17):e016784.
6. Gibson NS, Sohne M, Kruip MJ, et al. Further validation and simplification of the wells clinical decision rule in pulmonary embolism. *Thromb Haemost.* 2008;99(1):229–234.
7. Klok FA, Mos IC, Nijkeuter M, et al. Simplification of the revised Geneva score for assessing clinical probability of pulmonary embolism. *Arch Intern Med.* 2008;168(19):2131–2136.
8. Le Gal G, Righini M, Roy PM, et al. Prediction of pulmonary embolism in the emergency department: the revised Geneva score. *Ann Intern Med.* 2006;144(3):165–171.
9. Wessels JN, de Man FS, Vonk Noordegraaf A. The use of magnetic resonance imaging in pulmonary hypertension: why are we still waiting? *Eur Respir Rev.* 2020;29(156).
10. van der Hulle T, Cheung WY, Kooij S, et al. Simplified diagnostic management of suspected pulmonary embolism (the YEARS study): a prospective, multicentre, cohort study. *Lancet.* 2017;390(10091):289–297.

11. Investigators P. Value of the ventilation/perfusion scan in acute pulmonary embolism. Results of the prospective investigation of pulmonary embolism diagnosis (PIOPED). *JAMA*. 1990;263(20):2753–2759.
12. Stein PD, Fowler SE, Goodman LR, et al. Multidetector computed tomography for acute pulmonary embolism. *N Engl J Med*. 2006;354(22):2317–2327.
13. Expert Panel on Cardiac I, Kirsch J, Wu CC, et al. ACR appropriateness criteria(R) suspected pulmonary embolism: 2022 update. *J Am Coll Radiol*. 2022;19(11S):S488–S501.
14. Stein PD, Chenevert TL, Fowler SE, et al. Gadolinium-enhanced magnetic resonance angiography for pulmonary embolism: a multicenter prospective study (PIOPED III). *Ann Intern Med*. 2010;152(7):434–443.
15. Revel MP, Sanchez O, Couchon S, et al. Diagnostic accuracy of magnetic resonance imaging for an acute pulmonary embolism: results of the 'IRM-EP' study. *J Thromb Haemost*. 2012;10(5):743–750.
16. Zhou M, Hu Y, Long X, et al. Diagnostic performance of magnetic resonance imaging for acute pulmonary embolism: a systematic review and meta-analysis. *J Thromb Haemost*. 2015;13(9):1623–1634.
17. Baumgartner C, Klok FA, Carrier M, et al. Clinical surveillance vs. anticoagulation for low-risk patiEnts with isolated subsegmental pulmonary embolism: protocol for a multicentre randomised placebo-controlled non-inferiority trial (SAFE-SSPE). *BMJ Open*. 2020;10(11):e040151.
18. Sostman HD, Jablonski KA, Woodard PK, et al. Factors in the technical quality of gadolinium enhanced magnetic resonance angiography for pulmonary embolism in PIOPED III. *Int J Cardiovasc Imaging*. 2012;28(2):303–312.
19. Pressacco J, Papas K, Lambert J, et al. Magnetic resonance angiography imaging of pulmonary embolism using agents with blood pool properties as an alternative to computed tomography to avoid radiation exposure. *Eur J Radiol*. 2019;113:165–173.
20. Schiebler ML, Nagle SK, Francois CJ, et al. Effectiveness of MR angiography for the primary diagnosis of acute pulmonary embolism: clinical outcomes at 3 months and 1 year. *J Magn Reson Imaging*. 2013;38(4):914–925.
21. Knobloch G, Colgan T, Schiebler ML, et al. Comparison of gadolinium-enhanced and ferumoxytol-enhanced conventional and UTE-MRA for the depiction of the pulmonary vasculature. *Magn Reson Med*. 2019;82(5):1660–1670.
22. Johnson S, Sommer N, Cox-Flaherty K, Weissmann N, Ventetuolo CE, Maron BA. Pulmonary hypertension: a contemporary review. *Am J Respir Crit Care Med*. 2023;208(5):528–548.
23. Freed BH, Collins JD, Francois CJ, et al. MR and CT imaging for the evaluation of pulmonary hypertension. *JACC Cardiovasc Imaging*. 2016;9(6):715–732.
24. Peacock AJ, Crawley S, McLure L, et al. Changes in right ventricular function measured by cardiac magnetic resonance imaging in patients receiving pulmonary arterial hypertension-targeted therapy: the EURO-MR study. *Circ Cardiovasc Imaging*. 2014;7(1):107–114.
25. Alabed S, Shahin Y, Garg P, et al. Cardiac-MRI predicts clinical worsening and mortality in pulmonary arterial hypertension: a systematic review and meta-analysis. *JACC Cardiovasc Imaging*. 2021;14(5):931–942.
26. Ley S, Mereles D, Puderbach M, et al. Value of MR phase-contrast flow measurements for functional assessment of pulmonary arterial hypertension. *Eur Radiol*. 2007;17(7):1892–1897.
27. Ohno Y, Hatabu H, Murase K, et al. Primary pulmonary hypertension: 3D dynamic perfusion MRI for quantitative analysis of regional pulmonary perfusion. *AJR Am J Roentgenol*. 2007;188(1):48–56.
28. Sanz J, Garcia-Alvarez A, Fernandez-Friera L, et al. Right ventriculo-arterial coupling in pulmonary hypertension: a magnetic resonance study. *Heart*. 2012;98(3):238–243.
29. Dellegrottaglie S, Sanz J, Poon M, et al. Pulmonary hypertension: accuracy of detection with left ventricular septal-to-free wall curvature ratio measured at cardiac MR. *Radiology*. 2007;243(1):63–69.
30. Johns CS, Kiely DG, Rajaram S, et al. Diagnosis of pulmonary hypertension with cardiac MRI: derivation and validation of regression models. *Radiology*. 2019;290(1):61–68.
31. Whitfield AJ, Solanki R, Johns CS, Kiely D, Wild J, Swift AJ. MRI prediction of precapillary pulmonary hypertension according to the sixth world symposium on pulmonary hypertension. *Radiology*. 2020;294(2):482.
32. Reiter G, Reiter U, Kovacs G, Olschewski H, Fuchsjager M. Blood flow vortices along the main pulmonary artery measured with MR imaging for diagnosis of pulmonary hypertension. *Radiology*. 2015;275(1):71–79.
33. Broncano J, Bhalla S, Gutierrez FR, et al. Cardiac MRI in pulmonary hypertension: from magnet to bedside. *Radiographics*. 2020;40(4):982–1002.
34. Delcroix M, Lang I, Pepke-Zaba J, et al. Long-term outcome of patients with chronic thromboembolic pulmonary hypertension: results from an international prospective registry. *Circulation*. 2016;133(9):859–871.
35. Valerio L, Mavromanoli AC, Barco S, et al. Chronic thromboembolic pulmonary hypertension and impairment after pulmonary embolism: the FOCUS study. *Eur Heart J*. 2022;43(36):3387–3398.
36. Luijten D, Valerio L, Boon G, et al. Optimisation of detecting chronic thromboembolic pulmonary hypertension in acute pulmonary embolism survivors: the InShape IV study. *Eur Respir J*. 2024;64(4).
37. Rajaram S, Swift AJ, Capener D, et al. Diagnostic accuracy of contrast-enhanced MR angiography and unenhanced proton MR imaging compared with CT pulmonary angiography in chronic thromboembolic pulmonary hypertension. *Eur Radiol*. 2012;22(2):310–317.
38. Assi T, Kattan J, Rassy E, et al. A comprehensive review on the diagnosis and management of intimal sarcoma of the pulmonary artery. *Crit Rev Oncol Hematol*. 2020;147:102889.
39. Li J, Liu L, Song LX, et al. Clinical features and outcomes of pulmonary artery sarcoma. *Heart Lung Circ*. 2022;31(2):230–238.
40. Guo R, Yang H, Xi L, et al. Comparison of pulmonary artery sarcoma and pulmonary thromboembolism according to clinical and computed tomography pulmonary angiography and magnetic resonance imaging characteristics: a single-center retrospective study. *Quant Imaging Med Surg*. 2024;14(2):1686–1698.
41. Liu MX, Ma ZH, Jiang T, et al. Differential diagnosis of pulmonary artery sarcoma and central chronic pulmonary thromboembolism using CT and MR images. *Heart Lung Circ*. 2018;27(7):819–827.
42. Blackmon SH, Rice DC, Correa AM, et al. Management of primary pulmonary artery sarcomas. *Ann Thorac Surg*. 2009;87(3):977–984.
43. Roberts KE, Hamele-Bena D, Saqi A, Stein CA, Cole RP. Pulmonary tumor embolism: a review of the literature. *Am J Med*. 2003;115(3):228–232.
44. Gowda RM, Khan IA, Nair CK, Mehta NJ, Vasavada BC, Sacchi TJ. Cardiac papillary fibroelastoma: a comprehensive analysis of 725 cases. *Am Heart J*. 2003;146(3):404–410.
45. Metras D, Ouattara K, Quezzin-Coulibaly A. Aneurysm of the pulmonary artery with cystic medial necrosis and massive pulmonary valvular insufficiency. Report of two successful surgical cases. *Eur J Cardiothorac Surg*. 1987;1(2):119–124.
46. Deterling Jr RA, Clagett OT. Aneurysm of the pulmonary artery; review of the literature and report of a case. *Am Heart J*. 1947;34(4):471–499.
47. Kreibich M, Siepe M, Kroll J, Hohn R, Grohmann J, Beyersdorf F. Aneurysms of the pulmonary artery. *Circulation*. 2015;131(3):310–316.
48. Saadoun D, Bodaghi B, Cacoub P. Behcet's syndrome. *N Engl J Med*. 2024;390(7):640–651.
49. Nagle SK, Schiebler ML, Repplinger MD, et al. Contrast enhanced pulmonary magnetic resonance angiography for pulmonary embolism: building a successful program. *Eur J Radiol*. 2016;85(3):553–563.

41 Safety Monitoring and Protocols in Infants and Children

MARK A. FOGEL

INTRODUCTION

Clinical cardiac magnetic resonance (CMR) has been in use for over 35 years and has become firmly established in the evaluation of congenital heart disease (CHD) in many ways, including anatomy, physiology, ventricular function, blood flow, and tissue characterization.[1–15] In many instances, it is used as an adjunct to other imaging modalities such as echocardiography and angiography; however, in a number of areas such as vascular rings, blood flow, and ventricular volumes and mass,[16,17] it has become the "gold standard." In addition, CMR offers several advantages over other imaging modalities including its lack of ionizing radiation, which is extremely important in children who are more susceptible to neoplastic disease from DNA breakage and who have more time to manifest cancer symptomatology than adults.

In the world of CHD CMR, there are special safety considerations when it comes to successfully performing scans in infants and children as well as protocols for obtaining the diagnostic information needed to treat patients with CHD. All safety issues in adults apply to infants and children, and this chapter will focus on the additional ones. Further, basic principles of protocol procedures in adult heart disease also apply in patients with CHD, however, the nuances of anatomy and pathophysiology dictate a more individualized approach rather than strictly following a protocol. Nevertheless, there are generalized themes that can be formulated in this age range.

The first half of this chapter will discuss safety and monitoring in this age range while the second half will discuss the generalized protocol in CHD with specific types of technical challenges the imager may encounter.

SAFETY AND MONITORING

Remaining Motionless in the Magnetic Resonance Imaging Scanner: Anesthesia and Sedation

The degree of cooperation necessary for successful performance of CMR is generally greater than that of any other type of magnetic resonance imaging (MRI) examination; scans require no significant movement, repeated breath-holds at the same point of the respiratory cycle over 45–60 minutes (although there are some free breathing techniques that can be used at times), and can be lengthy. Couple this with the strange environment of the scanning room and loud banging noises, it is no wonder that both adults and children alike find this very intimidating. Therefore, the use of medication may be required. Either conscious sedation or general anesthesia is generally administered so that children who are too young to cooperate or teenagers with CHD who may not be able to cooperate for one reason or another (e.g., claustrophobia, attention deficit hyperactivity disorder) can still undergo successful CMR. With conscious sedation, patients continue to breathe throughout the scan and imaging has to be substantially altered because of this, whereas in a paralyzed, intubated, and mechanically ventilated patient under general anesthesia, the effect of "breath-holding" can be created by having the anesthesiologist temporarily suspend ventilation. This is not to say that anytime a patient undergoes general anesthesia in the CMR environment that suspending respiration should be performed, but rather that this technique is available to the CMR imager if needed. It should be noted that imaging with free breathing, whether under sedation or general anesthesia, is more physiologic than imaging with positive pressure mechanical ventilation and breath-holding and, therefore, may be more advantageous than the minor increase in image fidelity with breath-holding. For example, a single-ventricle patient after Fontan depends upon both cardiac and respiratory effects to allow for pulmonary blood flow; suspending respiration may alter the physiology artificially and therefore, although accurate for suspended respiration, the physiology is not reflective of the patient's true state. In addition, because systemic venous return changes during the respiratory cycle, imaging during suspended respiration will obtain data only in that state, while if the patient is imaged during free breathing, the loading conditions across the respiratory cycle are "averaged" into the image, which is more reflective of the patient's true physiologic state.

There is no definitive cut-off for the age range in which medication is needed to remain motionless for a successful CMR study; however, in general, most children greater than or equal to 10–12 years old can cooperate. Of course, this is just a rule of thumb, as there can be 7 year olds who are very mature and can follow directions while there are some 15 year olds who will simply not cooperate and will require pharmacology. Limited scans with reduced times may be possible with younger patients who would normally require conscious sedation or general anesthesia and may be considered; it is all in the judgment and purview of the family, physicians, and other healthcare providers caring for the patient. Preparation of the child prior to the scan is important; the involvement of child life experts or a supportive parent or other regular caregiver in the scanner room can reduce anxiety and be the difference between a scan under medication versus without medication or a successful versus an unsuccessful scan.

As the CMR environment can be a challenging one for the anesthesiologist or pediatrician/nurse sedation specialist, monitoring is extremely important; since the patient's body will be mostly within the scanner itself, direct visualization during the study is not possible without removing the patient from the bore of the magnet and removing the coil. Many centers utilize a direct video feed with cameras designed to work within the CMR environment and placed in critical positions. For example, a camera pointed down the bore of the magnet is essential along with cameras in other areas to get a good view of what is occurring in the scan room. In addition, extensive physiological monitoring of subjects using equipment specifically designed to be operated in the magnetic resonance (MR) scan room is essential for the safe conduct of the study. Pulse oximetry, limb-lead ECG, blood pressure monitoring, inspiratory and expiratory gas analysis such as end-tidal carbon dioxide, and temperature monitoring (especially in young children) should all be available and used. The monitoring systems should be available wherever the anesthesiology/sedation teams are positioned, which is generally either in the control room or scan rooms. Many facilities position the anesthetic equipment and gas tanks directly outside the scan room, with the gas lines passing through "wave guides" in the wall of the scanner room installed for just this purpose. This arrangement has two advantages: (A) there is reduced risk of inadvertently introducing non-CMR–compatible equipment into the scan room and (B) communication between the anesthesiology/sedation team and imaging teams is much easier in this setup. It should be noted, however, that this comes at the cost of increased compliance in the anesthetic circuit. If the decision is made to keep both monitoring and anesthetic equipment in the scan room, there is usually a minimum distance that this equipment must be kept from the magnet within which it may not operate correctly, may interfere with the images, and may even be attracted into the scanner bore. Careful establishment of this distance from the manufacturer is mandatory before the equipment is first introduced into the scan room. Even consideration of the use of physical restraints to prevent incursion of the equipment within such a distance, and thus avoid accidents, should be considered. Direct verbal communication between the anesthesiology/sedation teams and the imaging teams should be ongoing at all times, preferably with visual contact as well. It should be noted that if there is a code, the patient needs to be moved out of "zone 4" (the scanner room) and at a minimum, moved to zone 3 (preferably zone 2) to perform resuscitation.

Neonates and very small infants less than 6 months of age may undergo CMR successfully while sleeping using a "feed and swaddle" technique.[18–21] The patient usually is kept awake for a while prior to scanning (3–4 hours) and not fed. When the child enters the preparation area, the intravenous is inserted and the ECG leads are placed. At this point, the baby is very fussy, however, feeding the infant and subsequently swaddling with a warm blanket in a quiet and dimly lit environment prior to the study will allow the patient to fall asleep. The neonate/infant is subsequently transported to the scanner room. Vacuum-shaped support bags can also be utilized to reduce patient motion. Placing ear plugs, a hat over the head and ears, as well as blankets around the head at the time of swaddling all aid in keeping the child comfortable and asleep. Imaging sequences that allow for free breathing (e.g., using multiple excitations) must be used.

Whether to use deep sedation or anesthesia to perform CMR has been debated for many years. Consideration should be given to how long the CMR scan is likely to take, the patient's age, the flexibility of CMR scanner time, and the availability of anesthesiology staffing and/or specialized sedation teams that include nurses and pediatricians. The practice is obviously a matter for individual, institutional, and patient preferences. Anesthesia is much more predictable when it comes to onset of action and duration/depth of impaired consciousness; this is advantageous in scheduling CMR examinations and running the schedule smoothly. Deep sedation use has been associated with reduced image quality in some studies[22] but not in others,[23] and in some institutions it is far more likely to fail than anesthesia,[24] though failure rates can be reduced to close to zero by careful use of expert personnel and strict sedation regimes.[25–27] Anesthesia has been reported to be marginally safer than deep sedation in some studies[22,28] and equal in others,[23] but there is no doubt that it is more costly and invasive. There are numerous pediatric centers with many years of experience performing CMR under deep sedation with excellent safety records.[23,25,26] The end result is that both techniques are likely to remain in practice for the foreseeable future.

ANESTHESIA SAFETY FOR CHILDREN LESS THAN 3 YEARS OLD

In 2016, the Food and Drug Administration (FDA) issued a warning for children younger than 3 years of age on the safety of administering anesthesia.[29,30] The warning stated that exposure of patients in this age range to repeated or lengthy anesthesia (>3 hours) may affect the development of their brains. According to the warning, this was suggested by some animal studies that demonstrated changes in learning and behavior. There have been some retrospective human studies as well, some of which may support this in children. The warning goes on to state that, consistent with human studies, it is unlikely that a single, relatively short exposure will have an effect on children.

Suffice it to say that nearly all CMR studies performed in children require significantly less time than the 3 hours the FDA advises against. Since the warning, there have been a number of retrospective studies in humans to determine whether this is indeed an issue, and there is general agreement that there is a lack of definitive evidence in humans, since the results have been unclear. Studies in humans have demonstrated contradictory results with important limitations, most importantly, the difficulty of distinguishing the effect of anesthesia from other patient and perioperative factors (e.g., factors related to the underlying surgery or medical condition). Study limitations include being limited to one geographic area or institution, heterogeneous or unknown anesthetic drug administration, use of a variety of outcome measures with variable sensitivity for the assessment of anesthetic effects, and varied timing of the neurodevelopmental assessment of the children being exposed to anesthesia. As seems to be the general consensus, the best evidence suggests that exposure to anesthesia has limited to no association with detrimental effects on intelligence. A number of questions still remain, however, particularly regarding behavior and the effect of prolonged or multiple exposures. See references in the next 2 paragraphs.

The only randomized trial has been the General Anaesthesia compared to Spinal anaesthesia (GAS) trial which was an international, multicenter study of local versus general anesthesia (sevoflurane) with the Wechsler Preschool and Primary Scale of Intelligence Third Edition Full Scale Intelligence Score [FSIQ] at age five years.[31] Three hundred and sixty three infants, mostly male, were randomized to either group (general anesthesia of a median duration of 54 minutes) and there was no difference in the primary outcome measure. The majority of secondary behavioral and neurocognitive outcomes were also similar. Of course, there were limitations to this study, including longer periods of anesthesia, multiple exposures, and sex, as most participants were male.

There have been multiple observational studies spanning the gamut from learning disabilities,[32–34] developmental and psychiatric disorders,[35–39] academic/teacher evaluations,[40–42] neuropsychologic assessments, to parental reports of behavior,[43–46] all with mixed results. The literature is replete with these, and space limitations preclude a long treatise on this topic. The ultimate resolution of this topic is that it is so far unclear what impact, if any, this safety issue presents in infants and children. There is no definitive answer, so as always in these circumstances, clinical judgement is required.

Contrast Agents: Gadolinium and Ferumoxytol

GADOLINIUM

Gadolinium has been the contrast agent of choice in CMR for years. With administration, blood can be visualized as it traverses the cardiovascular system (dynamic imaging), high resolution two-dimensional (2D) and three-dimensional (3D) imaging can be obtained, 2D phase-contrast mapping and four-dimensional (4D) flow can be acquired with increased signal, and tissue characterization (i.e., T1 mapping with extracellular volume and viability) can occur. With literally hundreds of millions of doses administered throughout this time, the safety of this agent has been proven time and time again, with a very low hypersensitivity reaction in children on the order of a tenth of a percent.[47] Two safety issues must be considered that are rare but important to keep in mind—nephrogenic systemic fibrosis (NSF) and gadolinium retention in the brain.

Nephrogenic Systemic Fibrosis

First reported in 1997, NSF is a disorder of retention of gadolinium in the skin where it becomes thickened, fibrotic, and tethered to the underlying tissue, similar to scleroderma, with reduced range of motion and contractures. It was relatively uncommon and occurred mostly in adults in the general population, especially those with kidney disease, and was extremely rare in children.[48] Since the dosage of gadolinium was limited its use in kidney disease was restricted, a greater adherence to guidelines occurred, and safer gadolinium agents were developed, the occurrence of NSF has nearly disappeared. Although it is extremely rare, this complication should always be kept in mind.

Gadolinium Retention in the Brain

In 2015, the FDA put out a warning regarding gadolinium retention in the brain[49] and updated its warning in 2017[50] and 2022[51] to state that no harmful effects have been found but that investigations continue. This warning was in reference to those individuals who have had four or more exposures to the agent. There is no definitive evidence that gadolinium retention in the brain affects intelligence or behavior or causes any neuropsychiatric or neurodevelopmental disorder. Pathology reports of regions of the brain with gadolinium demonstrate no cellular death or other issues.

FERUMOXYTOL

This agent is an iron-based contrast material that has a high relaxivity and remains in the blood stream for an extended period of time (half-life ~12–15 hours). As it is a not a "first-pass" contrast agent, it has found utility in creating high resolution static and dynamic 3D imaging (e.g., multiphase steady-state imaging with contrast [MUSIC])[52] and increasing signal in 2D phase-contrast mapping and 4D flow. The safety of this agent was demonstrated in a large cohort of children and adults with a <1% rate of hypersensitivity reaction.[53] The practitioner should be aware that out of the millions of doses administered to chronic kidney disease patients, there were ~87 patients who had a fatal allergic reaction to the medication when given therapeutically, causing the FDA to issue a black box warning.[54] It should be noted that when given as a contrast agent, a much smaller dose is used (2–4 mg/kg/dose) and infused slower (over 15 minutes) than the therapeutic dose.

Implantable Device Safety

In CHD, it is not uncommon to have devices implanted in the cardiovascular system during cardiac catheterization, and on occasion via surgery, such as stents, patent ductus arteriosus or atrial septal defect occluder devices, coils, and abandoned leads or valves. In addition, there are noncardiovascular devices such as Harrington rods and cochlear implants that may have been placed in the patient. The practitioner should be aware of all implantable devices and either call the manufacturer or search the website to assure MRI safety at the strength of the magnet used (1.5 or 3 T). Some devices are not compatible while others may need to limit the energy deposition used.

Pacemakers present a special safety concern and are not uncommon in, for example, single-ventricle patients after Fontan, tetralogy of Fallot and endocardial cushion defects after repair, Ebstein's anomaly, and transposition of the great arteries. Originally, pacemakers were not considered safe in the MRI environment, and over the years it has been determined that CMRs can be performed safely in adults as well as children. Special protocols should be followed and the reader is referred to their institutional safety protocols or other manuscripts in the literature for a lengthier treatise.[55]

Miscellaneous Safety Issues

As with adult imaging, there are a number of other safety issues that must be looked after. External devices such are respirators that are not MRI compatible or that are MRI compatible but not necessarily MRI safe must be kept either outside zone 4 or outside the 5 Gauss line (or whatever the manufacturer's restrictions are). Noise remediation must be considered and the ears protected, even if the patient is under anesthesia. ECG lead placement must be performed in such a way as to not burn the patient.

PROTOCOLS

Although the application of CMR to CHD utilizes nearly all of the techniques discussed in the various chapters of this book, it nevertheless stands on its own as a separate discipline in the world of CMR. The multiple reasons for this can be divided into a few broad categories:

1. **Technical challenges:** Imaging children is very demanding as they require both increased spatial resolution because of their small size as well as increased temporal resolution because of their higher heart rates compared to adults. Many tradeoffs are made in CMR for adults to make imaging quicker and simpler without sacrificing diagnostic accuracy, such as obtaining spatial resolution at the cost of temporal resolution and vice versa. As many pulse sequences are made to image adult patients, the tradeoffs that can be performed in children can only be taken advantage of to a limited degree. In addition, because of the physiology of CHD, free-breathing imaging is preferred since it is more physiologic and the data obtained is more reflective of the true hemodynamic state of the patient. As the breath-holding technique is the mainstay of adult CMR, "work-arounds" have been developed to successfully image children <10 years old in this more physiologic state. Of course, under anesthesia, respiration can be suspended if all else fails, however, it should be noted that many anesthesiologists prefer giving supplemental oxygen during suspended respiration. This can clearly add to the complexity of the interpretation of data (e.g., shunts). These modifications or new approaches to CMR must be understood for children to be imaged successfully.
2. **Anatomy of CHD:** The anatomy of native CHD is very different from adult cardiology and demands a rigorous and systematic approach to make the correct diagnosis. In addition, as many of the diseases in CHD rely on surgical as well as an increasing number of catheter-based therapies, the anatomic and physiologic information extracted from the CMR examination needs to keep these approaches in mind. As a corollary, the postoperative/interventional anatomy and hemodynamics in CHD must also be familiar to the physician performing the examination to assess for the adequacy of the therapy and follow-up. For example, the connections between the major cardiac segments (atria, ventricles, and great vessels) along with venous anatomy can and are altered in many types of the diseases encountered in CHD (e.g., transposition of the great arteries). Communications are present where they should not be (e.g., ventricular septal defects), blood vessels from fetal life may still be present (e.g., patent ductus arteriosus), and some cardiac structures might not even be present or present in a markedly hypoplastic form (e.g., hypoplastic left heart syndrome). In the evaluation of CHD after surgery, conduits and baffles constructed to separate the circulations has little parallel in the adult world. As such, anatomy and morphology must be delineated by CMR in ways that are not required in adult heart disease, and the physician interpreting the study needs to be schooled in the nuances of both the pre and postoperative anatomy of CHD.
3. **Physiology:** The unique physiology of CHD is most often a result of the altered anatomy. The evaluation of shunts (e.g., ventricular septal defects) plays a critical role in the assessment of any disease entity in pediatrics and yet has a minor role in the adult world. CMR has recently become the only imaging modality to quantify aortic-to-pulmonary collateral flow development in single ventricles, again, a unique province of CHD.[56–58] The determination of ventricular function in ventricles with strange and unusual shapes (e.g., single ventricles, L-looped ventricles) are routine in the practice of CMR in children and demand unique solutions. Assessment of the postoperative/interventional physiology where the surgeon, for example, creates a systemic-to-pulmonary artery shunt or creates an anastomosis between the cava and the pulmonary artery must be dealt with. CMR in CHD and in pediatrics must be adapted to fit these needs and the physician interpreting the study needs to understand the complex physiology.

GENERALIZED PROTOCOL OF CARDIAC MAGNETIC RESONANCE FOR CONGENITAL HEART DISEASE (FIG. 41.1)

CMR for CHD is a technique that constantly requires fine tuning during an examination in general since unexpected findings turn up all the time, especially in pediatrics. Nevertheless, certain basic principles exist that can be formulated into a generalized protocol of CMR in CHD, as depicted in Fig. 41.1. The author does not claim this to be the only way to think about the process, but it is, in the author's opinion, the most efficient and complete. It should be noted that the protocol needs to be individualized to the patient and the disease process.

Anatomic Imaging (Noncontrast)

After localizers, anatomic data is acquired not only to survey the cardiovascular anatomy and make the "anatomic diagnosis," but also to act as a localizer as well for future physiologic and functional imaging. This is important in that physiologic and functional data must be interpreted in light of the prevailing anatomy. A full contiguous set

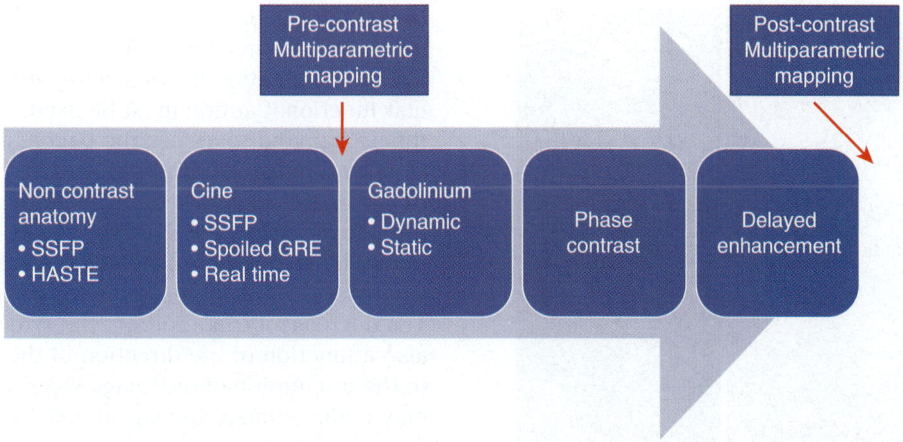

FIG. 41.1 Generalized protocol for CMR imaging of CHD. This is a generalized protocol and needs to be individualized to the patient and the specific disease. *CHD*, congenital heart disease; *CMR*, cardiac magnetic resonance; *GRE*, gradient echo; *HASTE*, half-Fourier acquisition single-shot turbo spin-echo; *SSFP*, steady-state free precession.

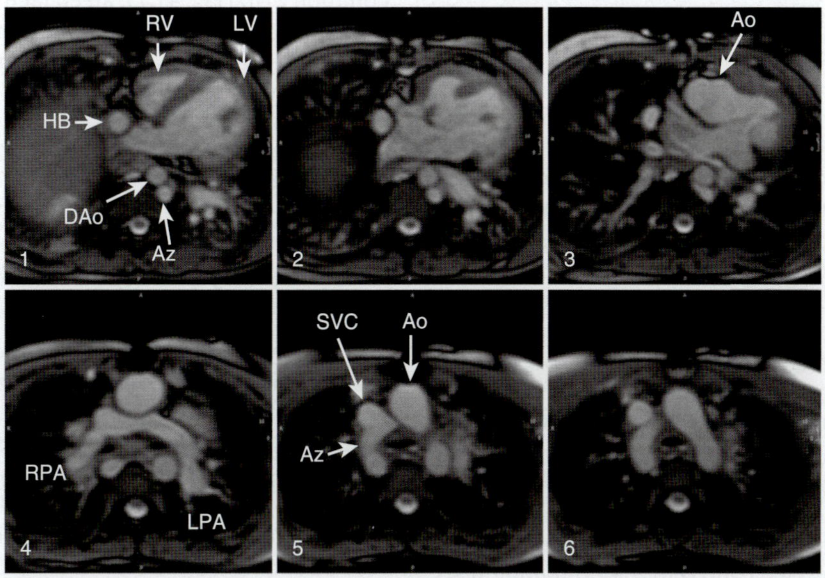

FIG. 41.2 Stack of contiguous static steady-state free precession images. This is a set of selected axial images of a patient with heterotaxy syndrome, tricuspid stenosis with pulmonary atresia {S,D,X} with a hypoplastic right ventricle, and interrupted inferior vena cava with azygous continuation to the right superior vena cave (SVC) after a Kawashima operation (SVC to pulmonary artery connection in the presence of an interrupted inferior vena cava with azygous continuation) and a hepatic baffle to the pulmonary arteries. Images progress from inferior to superior as the panels go from left to right and from top to bottom (numbers 1–6). *Ao*, aorta; *Az*, azygous vein; *DAo*, descending aorta; *HB*, hepatic baffle; *LPA*, left pulmonary artery, *LV*, left ventricle; *RPA*, right pulmonary artery; *RV*, right ventricle; *SVC*, superior vena cava.

of axial images from the diaphragm to the thoracic inlet is obtained (typically 40–50 images); the author prefers "static" steady-state free precession (SSFP) images (e.g., true-Fast Imaging with Steady state Precession [FISP]) (Fig. 41.2). This must be extended outside the thorax for special cases such as to the neck if arch anatomy is being evaluated (e.g., innominate artery branches in the neck) or if total anomalous pulmonary venous connections are suspected (e.g., connection below the diaphragm). Imaging utilizing SSFP depends upon contrast between blood and the surrounding tissue, which is enhanced by using a high flip angle, and, therefore, the practice is to allow the scanner to select the highest flip angle possible. These axial images form the basis of examining the anatomy.

One disadvantage to utilizing "static" SSFP is that turbulence may present on the image as an absence of a structure (signal loss), as in the case of the pulmonary arteries in a single-ventricle patient after a Blalock-Taussing shunt—typically, these are very difficult to visualize by this technique because the turbulence creates a major signal loss. This drawback can be compensated for by performing half Fourier acquisition single-shot turbo spin echo (HASTE) imaging, which yields a set of dark-blood images rapidly (or another type of dark-blood imaging such as 3D Sampling Perfection with Application optimized Contrasts using different flip angle Evolution [3D SPACE]—see below, although HASTE is the quickest) and is performed while multiplanar reconstruction (MPR) is being done (see below). Alternatively, a set of axial cines can be performed to visualize these structures in the hope that a phase of the cardiac cycle will demonstrate the "missing" structure.

After the axial stack above is obtained, multiplanar reformatting (MPR) can be used to a) inspect the anatomy from multiple angles and b) determine the exact slice orientation and position for any future imaging during the study.

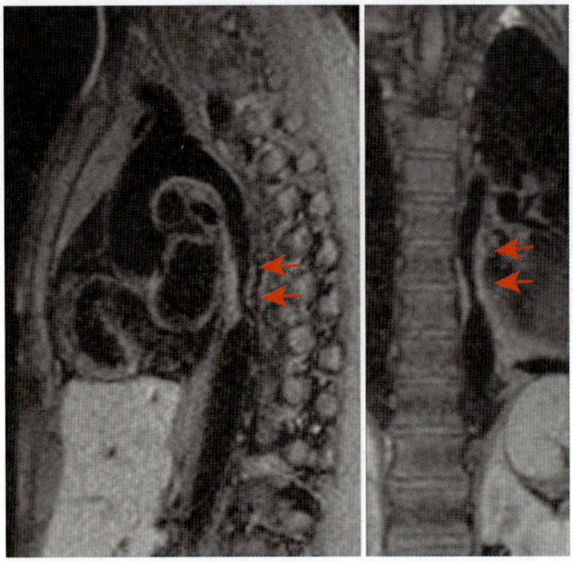

FIG. 41.3 Dark-blood imaging. Example of a 3 year old with a midthoracic long-segment aortic coarctation of the aorta (*arrows*) in the candy cane view (*left*). On the right is the coarctation in the orthogonal view to the candy cane view.

If needed, dark-blood imaging can complement the bright-blood imaging, as in instances of vascular rings to visualize the trachea, coarctation of the aorta (Fig. 41.3), or a systemic-to-pulmonary artery shunt. This type of imaging is used judiciously since it requires relatively long scanning times. A set of high-resolution double inversion recovery dark-blood images can be obtained or, if available, 3D SPACE (3D sampling perfection with application-optimized contrasts using different flip angle evolutions),[59] which can obtain a high resolution slab in 5 minutes or less.

Newer techniques such as bright-blood and black-blood phase-sensitive inversion recovery (BOOST) can be utilized to acquire a high resolution (to the submillimeter level of both bright- [Fig. 41.4] and dark-blood techniques) of anatomy without contrast agents (although it can also be utilized with contrast agents).

Function/Anatomy—Cine Cardiac Magnetic Resonance (Figs. 41.5–41.8)

Either SSFP or spoiled gradient echo (GRE) sequences are used and are tailored to the lesion under study. Cine, along with phase-contrast CMR (PCMR), are the major sequences utilized to delineate physiology (Fig. 41.4) and function (ventricular and valvar) in CMR of CHD. We nearly always determine ventricle function in CHD (Fig. 41.5). For example, in a patient with ventricular septal defect, left ventricular (LV) volume overload is determined by a stack of LV short-axis images measuring volumes, ejection fraction, and cardiac index; in the absence of valve regurgitation, the difference between left and right ventricular stroke volumes is the added volume overload. If the LV volume overload was due to aortic regurgitation (Fig. 41.4), a cine of the LV outflow tract in multiple views will be added to the short-axis stack to visualize the insufficiency jet. If there is aortic stenosis or hypertrophic cardiomyopathy, LV mass is determined.

Cine imaging can also be used to delineate the anatomy as stated in the previous section (Fig. 41.6). If coarctation of the aorta is present, for example, turbulence should be noted on cine imaging unless there are multiple collaterals, the coarctation is not severe, or there is poor ventricular function. Caution must be used, however, when using this signal void to assess the degree of stenosis (or insufficiency if imaging valves) as it must be viewed in light of CMR physics, similar to echocardiography (e.g., frame rate, angle of incidence). The size of the signal void is a function of a number of factors such as the echo time (TE, where longer TEs increase the signal void size and shorter TEs decrease it). In addition, the size of the signal void is also a function of the direction of the stenotic jet relative to the orientation of the image voxel. Finally, SSFP imaging may underestimate the signal void seen on gradient echo sequences.

Cine can also be used to visualize the anatomy of valves, typically en face, and is obtained many times during PCMR. For example, to visualize a bicuspid aortic valve, the most common CHD (Fig. 41.7), an en face view of the valve is performed by lining up the imaging plane perpendicular to the LV outflow tract in two orthogonal views at the level of the aortic annulus (or slightly above). This typically results in the equivalent of a "parasternal short axis view" by echocardiography. Either SSFP, GRE with a high flip angle (e.g., 25 degrees), or PCMR can be used. Quadracuspid and unicuspid aortic valves are shown in Fig. 41.8.

Anatomy/Physiology/Function—Contrast-Based Cardiac Magnetic Resonance

The two types of 3D gadolinium techniques for anatomy (both static [Figs. 41.4 and 41.11] and time resolved [also called "dynamic"] [Figs. 41.9 and 41.10])[60] are then performed to obtain a high-resolution, 3D data set to either view in 2D, create a volume-rendered 3D image (Figs. 41.4, 41.10 and 41.11), or generate an .stl file to be used to build a 3D-printed model or visualize in virtual reality. Time-resolved imaging such as time-resolved angiography with interleaved stochastic trajectories (TWIST) will yield multiple 3D image sets in as little as 2 seconds but is not ECG gated (Figs. 41.9 and 41.10). This type of imaging not only yields a large field of view of both anatomy and physiology but the contrast agent is also followed through the cardiovascular tree so shunts may be seen, as well as regions of perfusion and nonperfusion of lung fields, and others. The injection should be as fast as possible for a tight bolus, depending upon the IV size.

A static, high resolution ECG and navigator-based inversion recovery gradient echo (IR-GRE) technique (Figs. 41.4 and 41.11) can follow immediately after dynamic imaging to allow for submillimeter resolution and has been extremely useful in infants and children, especially for small vessels such as the coronaries (see coronary subsection below). This has to be performed within a minute or so afterwards to obtain acceptable contrast. Alternatively, if dynamic imaging is not being utilized, a "slow drip" technique can be used with the IR-GRE in which the contrast should be completely injected within approximately the first third of the sequence. Finally, important in children with high heart rates or small babies, if performing combined dynamic and static imaging, the dose must be split between the two techniques either 50/50% or 75/25%.

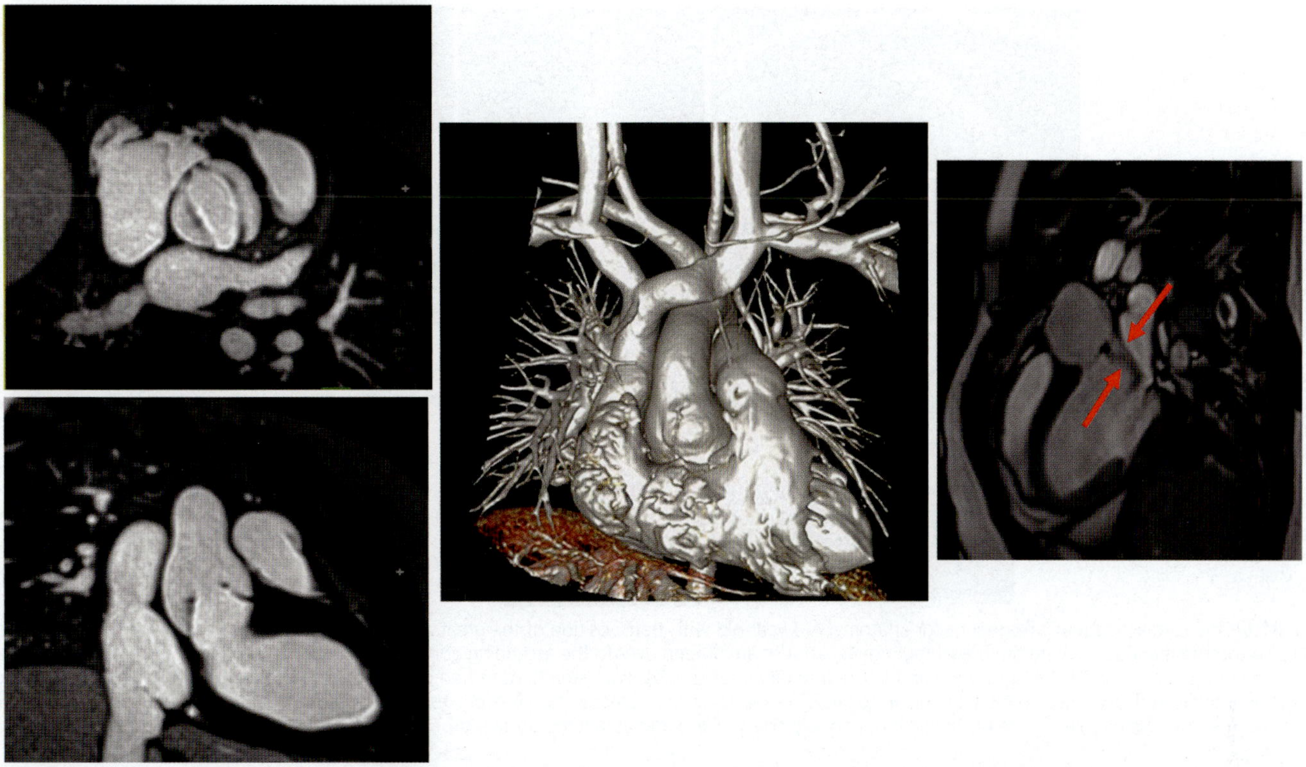

FIG. 41.4 Noncontrast bright-blood and black-blood phase-sensitive inversion recovery (BOOST). A 7 year old with aortic insufficiency and a bicuspid aortic valve (fusion right and left coronary commissures) in systole. Upper left image is an en face image of the valve while the lower left is the left ventricular outflow tract and the valve in long axis. Middle panel is a noncontrast 3D reconstruction of the heart demonstrating the dilated aortic root. The right panel is a diastolic steady-state free precession cine image of the aortic insufficiency jet hitting the mitral valve (*red arrows*).

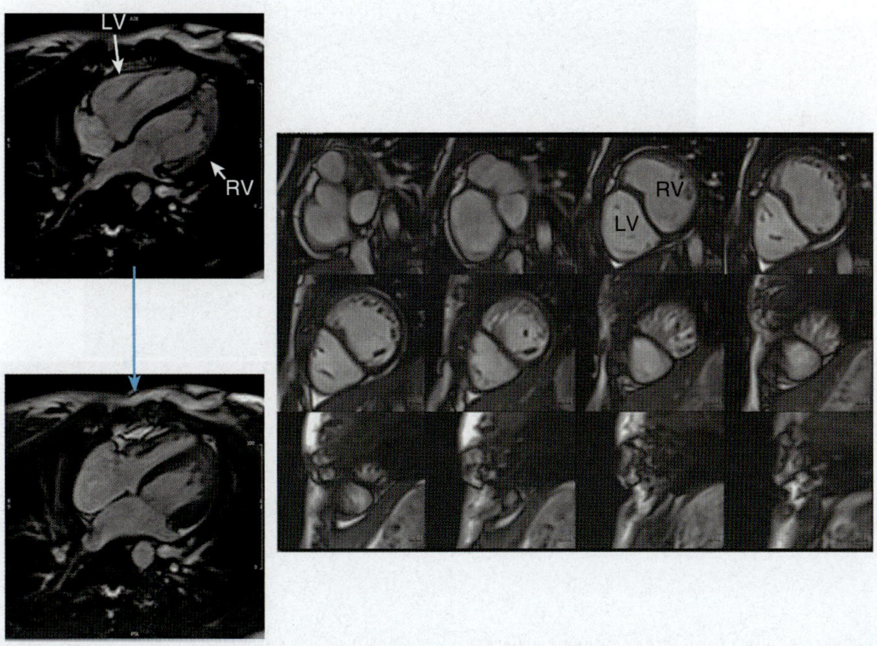

FIG. 41.5 Cine cardiac magnetic resonance for ventricular function. A 2 year old with corrected transposition of the great arteries (TGA {S,L,L} or L-TGA) demonstrating the left-sided right ventricle (*RV*) and the right-sided left ventricle (*LV*) in the four-chamber view in diastole (*upper left*) and systole (*lower left*). The panel on the right demonstrates 12 contiguous short-axis images from base to apex in diastole based on the 4-chamber view on the left.

A Special Note on Ferumoxytol-Based Imaging

As mentioned above, ferumoxytol is not a first-pass contrast agent and has a long half-life in blood. Static IR-GRE or BOOST imaging is performed with this agent or MUSIC (Fig. 41.12) if both static and 3D cine imaging is needed. For safety, it is not injected as a bolus as used with dynamic gadolinium sequence. One advantage of the long half-life is that it can be injected prior to the patient entering the scanner, and sequences using this agent may be obtained anytime in the following couple of hours afterwards. Cine SSFP cannot be used, and generally spoiled-gradient GRE

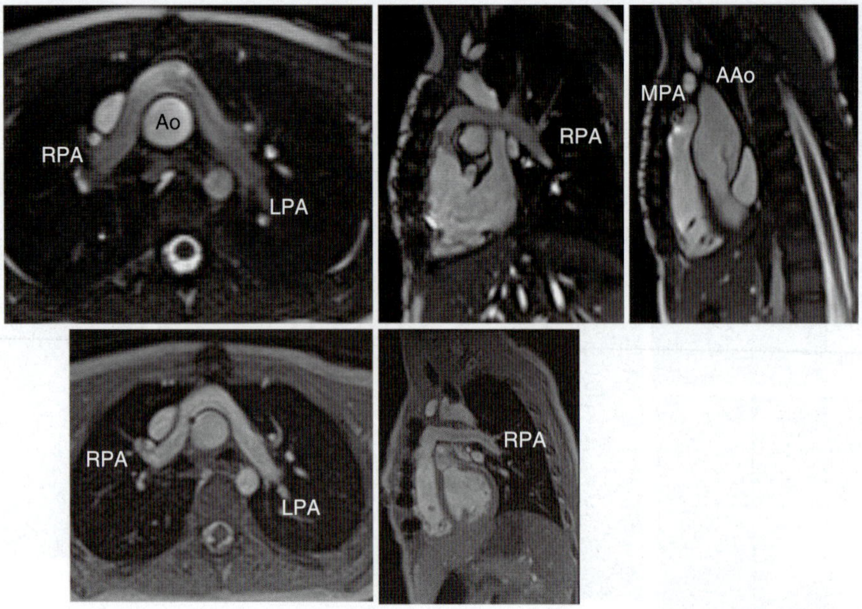

FIG. 41.6 Cine cardiac magnetic resonance for anatomy. A 4 year old with transposition of the great arteries (TGA [S,D,D]) after arterial switch operation and a LeCompte maneuver where the branch pulmonary arteries are draped over to the ascending aorta (*Ao*). The upper left and lower left image demonstrate the bifurcation view of the right (*RPA*) and left pulmonary arteries (*LPA*) with steady-state free precession and gradient echo imaging, respectively. The upper middle and lower right panels demonstrate the RPA in long axis with steady-state free precession and gradient echo imaging respectively as well. Upper right shows the parallel nature of the main pulmonary artery (*MPA*) and ascending aorta (*AAo*), which is common in this lesion.

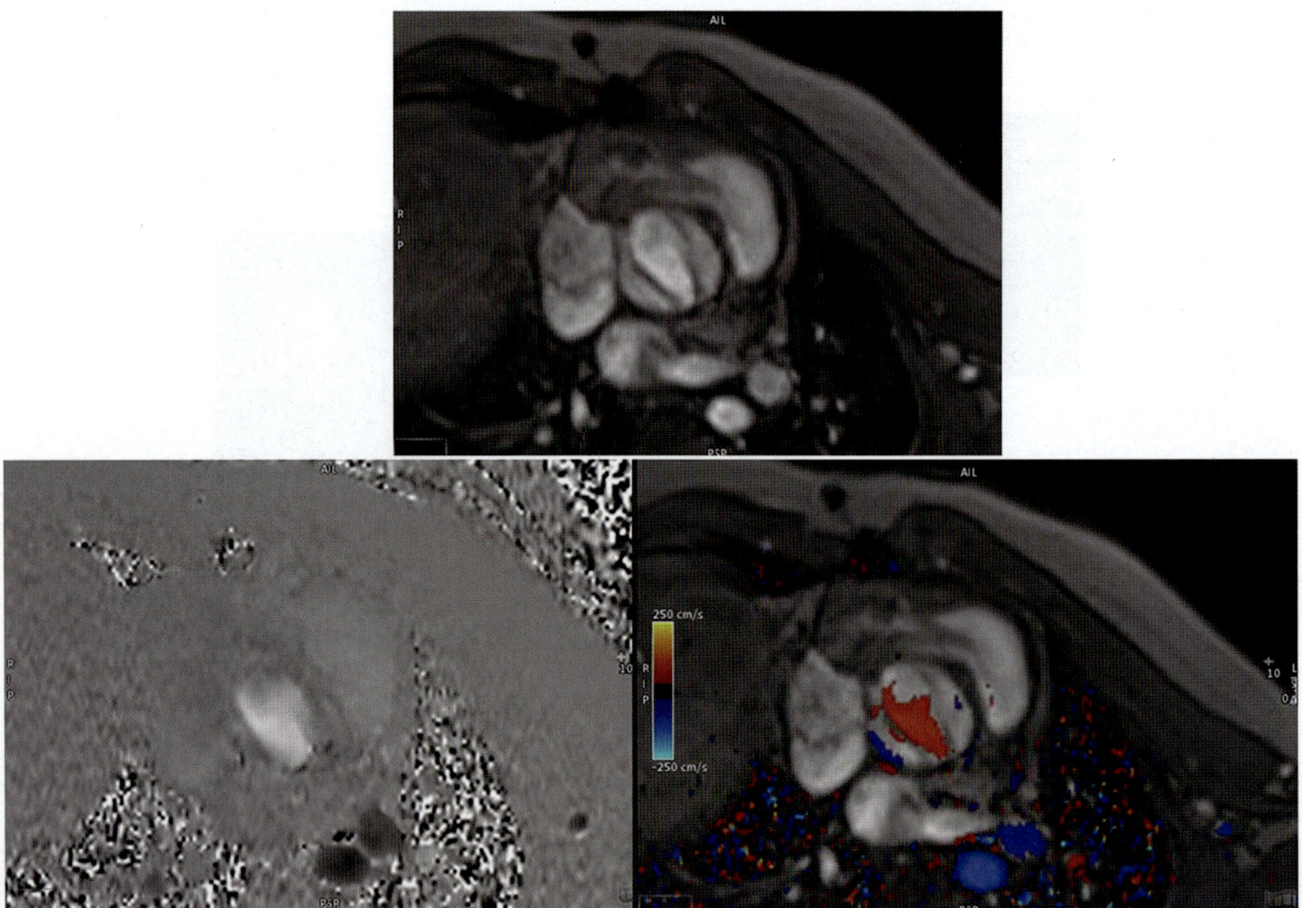

FIG. 41.7 Bicuspid aortic valve with fusion of right and left coronary commissures en face. Top panel is a spoiled gradient echo image while bottom left (*phase*) and right (*magnitude*) panels are from phase-contrast mapping with the right image color coded to outline the valve.

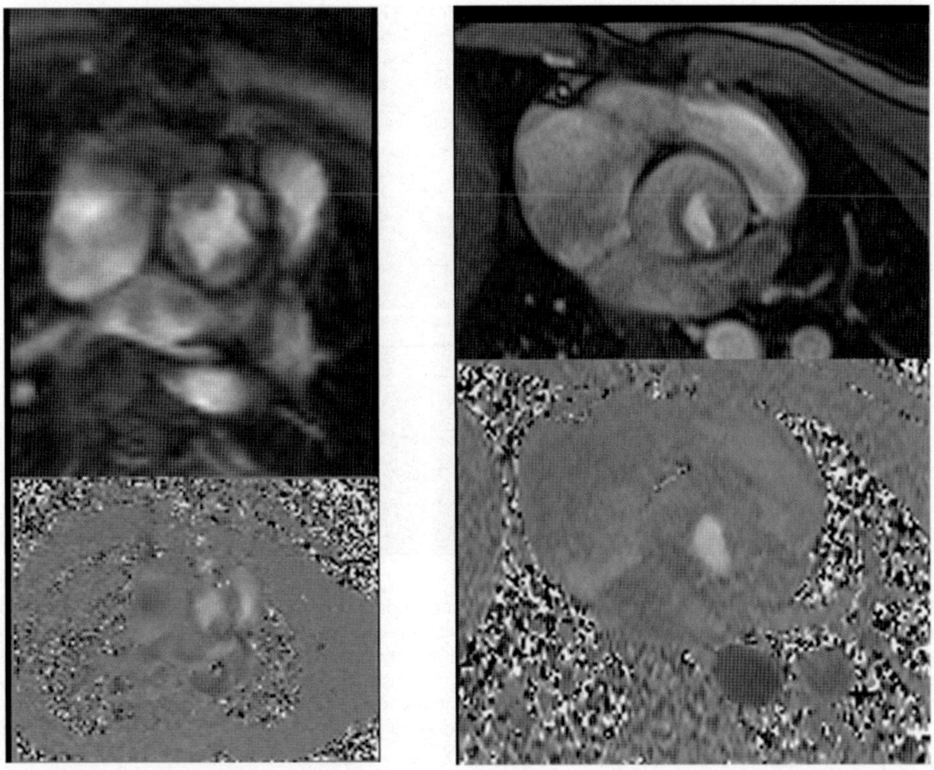

FIG. 41.8 Quadracuspid aortic valve from a 4 year old with truncus arteriosus (*left*) and a unicuspid aortic valve (only open commissure is left-non) from a 7 month old with small left-sided structures (*right*). Images are from phase-contrast magnetic resonance. Top panels are magnitude images and bottom panels are phase images.

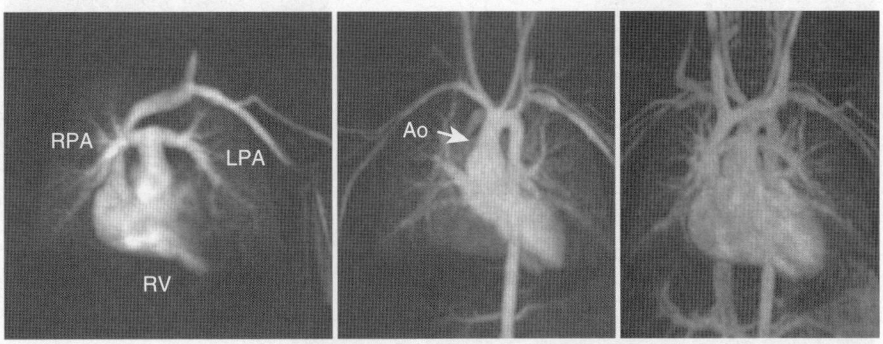

FIG. 41.9 Time-resolved gadolinium cardiac magnetic resonance. From left to right, the panels are maximum intensity projections that demonstrate the pulmonary phase, the systemic phase, and the recirculation phase of the patient in figure six with transposition of the great arteries (TGA [S,D,D]) after arterial switch operation and a LeCompte maneuver. Each maximum intensity projection is a three-dimensional image in and of itself. *Ao*, aorta; *LPA*, left pulmonary artery; *RPA*, right pulmonary artery; *RV*, right ventricle.

imaging is performed instead. If cine SSFP is needed or preferred, it should be performed prior to ferumoxytol injection and the agent infused on the table. Similarly, if tissue characterization is needed (e.g., anomalous coronaries, Fontan, tetralogy of Fallot), this should also be performed prior to ferumoxytol injection.

The MUSIC sequence is especially useful as it acquires multiple high-resolution ECG-gated phases of the cardiac cycle with respiratory navigation (Fig. 41.12). After acquisition, MPR allows for a stack of short-axis images for function, anatomy to visualize valve morphology and function, as well as other general anatomy including anatomy dependent upon dynamic imaging (e.g., LV outflow tract obstruction, LV-to-aortic pathway for two-ventricle repair in, for example, double-outlet right ventricle).

Blood Flow—Phase-Contrast Cardiac Magnetic Resonance

After gadolinium imaging, blood flow data is obtained and, similar to cine CMR, is tailored to the lesion under study. By performing PCMR after gadolinium injection, increased signal to noise is obtained in the PCMR sequences. "Through-plane retrospectively-gated" images are acquired so that flow can be measured across the entire cardiac cycle while in-plane velocity mapping can be used for measuring peak velocities and visualizing flow directionality. PCMR is extremely useful in CHD for understanding hemodynamics and physiology and is used for most cases. For example, in an atrial septal defect, through-plane PCMR is obtained across the aortic and

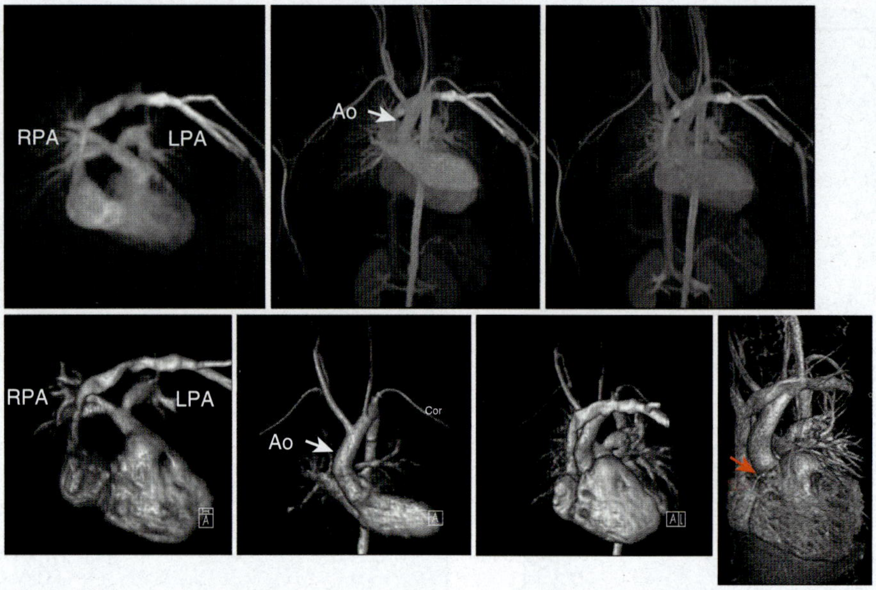

FIG. 41.10 Time-resolved gadolinium cardiac magnetic resonance and 3D volume rendering. The patient is a 7 year old with tetralogy of Fallot with pulmonary atresia and multiple aortopulmonary collaterals after unifocalization in which the aortopulmonary collaterals were brought together to form "branch pulmonary arteries." The top three panels, from left to right, are maximum intensity projections that demonstrate the pulmonary phase, the systemic phase, and the recirculation phase of a left arm injection. As each maximum intensity projection is a 3D dataset, the bottom left, second from left, and second from right panels are volume-rendered images from each of the phases in the top panels, respectively. Afterwards, a 3D inversion recovery gradient echo sequence was run with 1 mm isotropic resolution, which is shown from the anteroposterior view in the lower right panel; the right coronary is shown by the arrow. *Ao*, aorta; *LPA*, left pulmonary artery; *RPA*, right pulmonary artery.

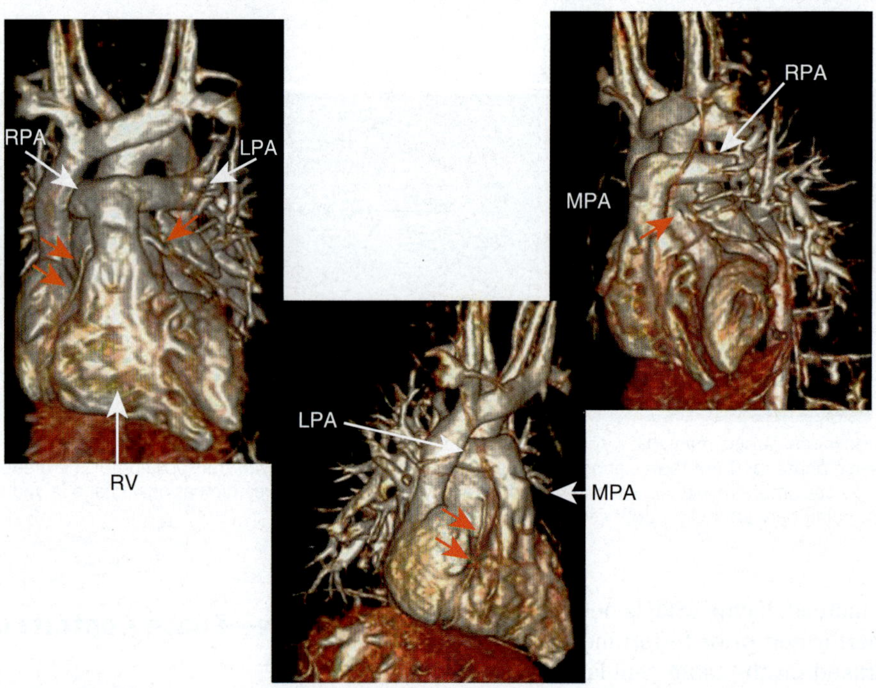

FIG. 41.11 Static three-dimensional gadolinium cardiac magnetic resonance. These are created from a 3D-inversion recovery-gradient echo imaging sequence utilizing gadofosveset trisodium of the patient in figures 6 and 7 with transposition of the great arteries (TGA [S,D,D]) after arterial switch operation and a LeCompte maneuver. The upper left panel is viewing the heart anteroposterior while the lower panel and upper right panel depict the heart rotated to further define the long axis of the left (*LPA*) and right pulmonary arteries (*RPA*), respectively. *Red arrows* point to the proximal origins of the reimplanted coronary arteries. *MPA*, Main pulmonary artery; *RV*, right ventricle.

pulmonary valves to measure the pulmonary-to-systemic flow ratio (Qp/Qs), which has been validated against oximetry.[11] As an internal check (one of the strengths of the accuracy of PCMR), flow in the branch pulmonary arteries (should equal flow across the pulmonary valve) and in the cavae (should equal flow in the aorta in the absence of aortic-to-pulmonary collaterals) are obtained. As another internal check, LV output as calculated using cine CMR (in the absence of mitral insufficiency) should equal the forward flow as measured across the aorta utilizing through-plane PCMR, and the same is true of right ventricular output.

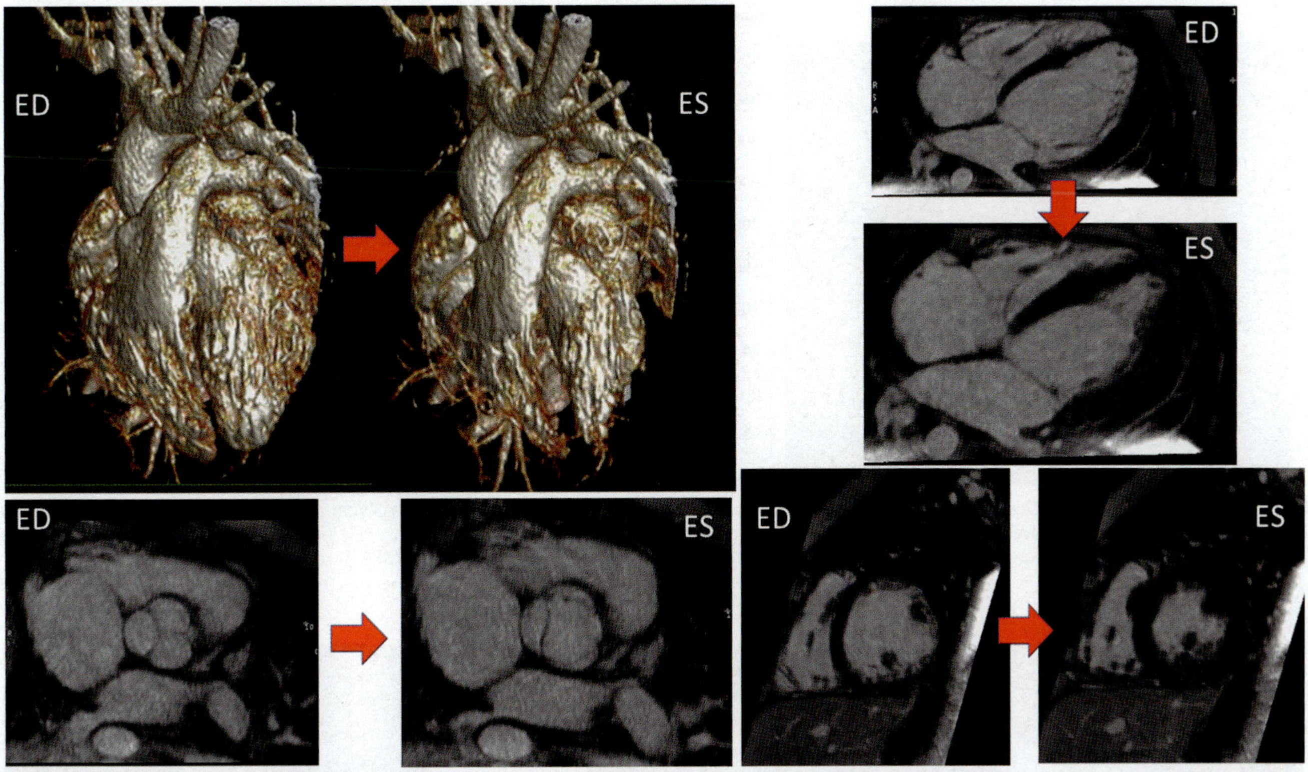

FIG. 41.12 Multiphase steady-state imaging with contrast (MUSIC). The patient is a 4 year old with moderate aortic insufficiency; MUSIC was acquired at 15 phases at a heart rate of 122 beats per minute. Top left panels are 3D images at end diastole (*ED*) and end systole (*ES*) demonstrating 3D ventricular function. Bottom left panels are 2D cuts of the 3D images at the level of the aortic valve at ED and ES. Right panels demonstrate 2D cuts of the 3D images in the 4-chamber (*top*) and short-axis views (*bottom*) at ED and ES.

PCMR alone or in conjunction with cine CMR can calculate other important parameters of function such as valve insufficiency (Fig. 41.13). For example, patients who have undergone complete common atrioventricular canal repair can sometimes manifest left atrioventricular valve insufficiency as a sequelae. To assess this quantitatively, the difference in the stroke volume of the left ventricle and the forward flow out the aorta would be the left atrioventricular valve regurgitant volume. Subtraction of net flow across the aortic valve from forward flow across the left atrioventricular valve (in the absence of any other residual shunts) can also quantify this regurgitant volume, however, it may be difficult at times to line this imaging plane exactly perpendicular to flow.

PCMR evaluation of aortic insufficiency is almost never performed directly in dilated aortas as this is fraught with inaccuracies. Instead, pulmonary artery flow or systemic venous return is subtracted from forward flow across the aortic valve[61] to yield the regurgitant volume (divided by 0.95 to account for bronchial flow).[56]

As mentioned above, PCMR can also be used to assess valve anatomy (Figs. 41.7, 41.8 and 41.13). Through-plane PCMR can outline the leaflets of valves when imaged en face (both on the phase and magnitude images) and can be successful when routine cine imaging is not.

Finally, 4D flow imaging is becoming more commonplace in CHD and the techniques and tools used are continually being developed. A full treatment of 4D flow in CHD is beyond the scope of this chapter, however, 4D flow of a Fontan patient as well as one with normal anatomy for comparison are shown in Fig. 41.14.

Tissue Characterization/Multiparametric Mapping (Figs. 41.13 and 41.14)

There are a number of different techniques utilized in CHD that are helpful to characterize myocardial tissue.

- *Delayed-enhancement (DE) imaging* (Fig. 41.15): DE imaging (viability), a gadolinium-based technique first described in the mid-1980s,[62] can achieve signal intensity differences between normal and infarcted myocardium of up to 500%.[63] It is not just the province of adult heart disease.[64–66] Children with congenital abnormalities of the coronaries (e.g., anomalous left coronary artery from the pulmonary artery), those who have had surgical manipulation of the coronaries (e.g., transposition of the great arteries after an arterial switch procedure or Ross procedure), those who have had specific or acquired inflammatory diseases (e.g., Kawasaki disease), as well as those who have cardiac tumors (see below) can all benefit from DE assessment. In addition, in general, hearts that have undergone surgical reconstruction are candidates for DE imaging to assess for myocardial scar tissue in both the substance of the myocardium as well as areas that were reconstructed such as the infundibulum and pulmonary annulus in a patient after transannular patch repair of tetralogy of Fallot or the ventricle of a patient who had a Sano shunt placed (Fig. 41.15).
- *T1 mapping* (Fig. 41.15): The ability to quantify the T1 of the myocardium, both before and after contrast administration, has enabled the ability to determine diffuse fibrosis within the heart with a disproportionate

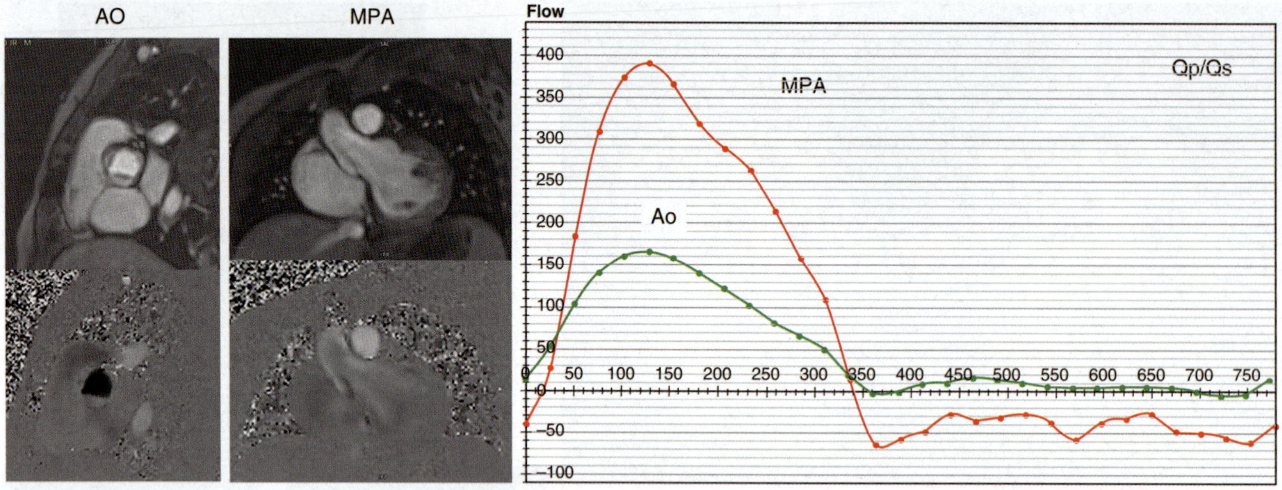

FIG. 41.13 Two-dimensional phase-contrast cardiac magnetic resonance (PCMR). These images are from a 3 year old with a large atrial septal defect and pulmonary insufficiency. Aortic valve (*Ao*) PCMR magnitude (*top*) and phase (*bottom*) images are on the left while main pulmonary artery (*MPA*) magnitude (*top*) and phase (*bottom*) images are in the middle. Flow-time graph is on the right with Ao in *green* and MPA in *red*.

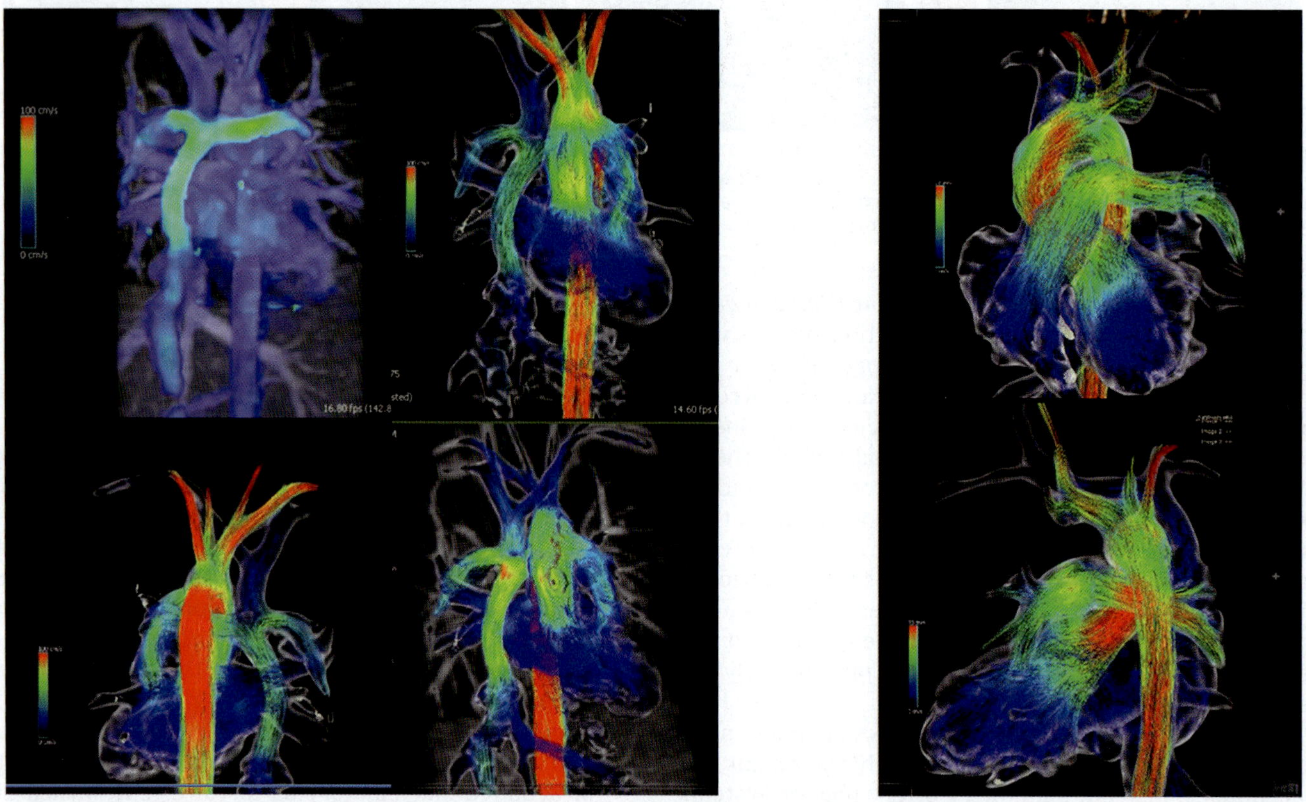

FIG. 41.14 Four-dimensional (4D) Flow. The four panels on the left are 4D flow images of an 8 year old after Fontan with speed display in the upper left and velocity vectors displayed anteriorly in the right panels and posteriorly in the lower left panel. The two panels on the right demonstrate 4D flow in a patient with normal anatomy anteriorly (*top*) and posteriorly (*bottom*).

amount of collagen. This may be quantified by native T1 times and extracellular volume calculations. There is emerging evidence to suggest that this may be of value clinically in CHD and in the pediatric age group. For example, in tetralogy of Fallot, the left and right ventricular T1 mapping values are different than normal individuals[67] and may be prognostic of exercise performance and adverse events.[68]

- *Myocardial iron*: The T2 star technique is utilized to assess myocardial iron and hematologists use this in conjunction with other parameters such as liver and blood iron to adjust chelation therapy. This applies to children with thalassemia, sickle cell disease, and other hematologic disorders of red blood cell destruction.
- *Myocarditis*: Although there is a paucity of data in the pediatric age group for the CMR assessment of myocarditis, it is not an uncommon diagnosis to entertain in an adolescent with chest pain and elevated troponins. Similar to the adult assessment, the Lake Louise criteria are used, including T2 imaging (edema), T1 mapping, and DE.

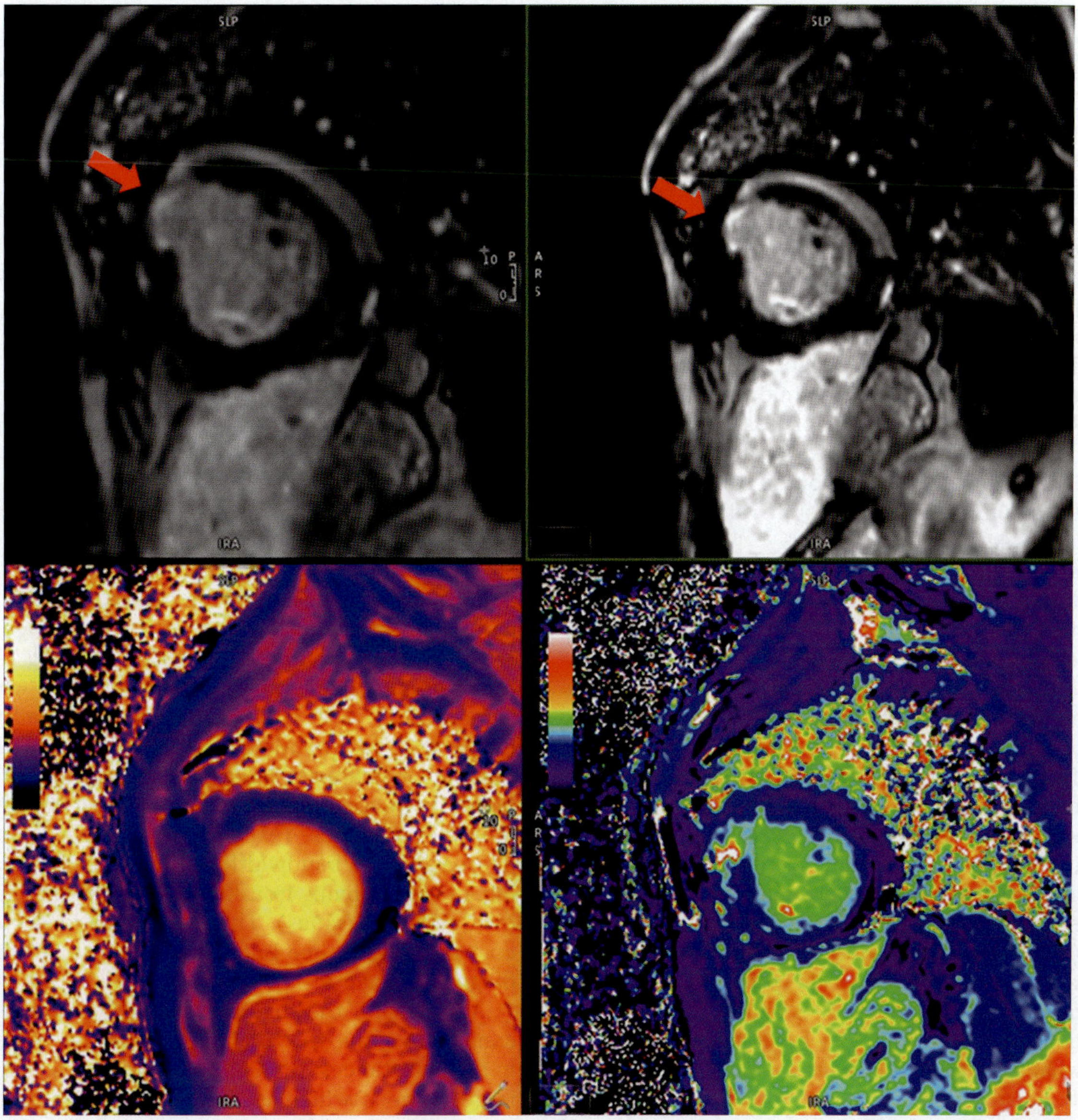

FIG. 41.15 Tissue characterization. Patient is a 3 year old with hypoplastic left heart syndrome after Sano shunt and bidirectional Glenn reconstruction. Top images are magnitude- (*left*) and phase-sensitive (*right*) delayed-enhancement images at the Sano shunt insertion into the right ventricle demonstrating scar (*arrows*). Lower panels are T1 mapping (*left*) and an extracellular volume map (*right*) of the same patient.

Other Important Techniques Utilized in Congenital Heart Disease

There are special techniques that do not fall into this generalized protocol which may be inserted at different points, depending on the lesion.

- *Perfusion* (Fig. 41.14): The same patient populations who are candidates for DE imaging are also candidates for perfusion imaging, which, similar to DE, is not only a consideration for adults with heart disease but also for patients with CHD.[64] It is gadolinium based and is typically imaged with either an MRI-compatible exercise ergometer, regadenoson stress imaging (400 mcg/dose for patients >40 kg body weight or 8 mcg/kg/dose for patients ≤40 kg) followed by theophylline reversal (50 mg for patients > 40 kg body weight or 0.25 mg/kg/dose for patients ≤40 kg), or with dobutamine stress.[69] In CHD, utilizing exercise or regadenoson stress is more common. All techniques utilize rest imaging after stress as well as DE.
- *Real-time cine imaging and PCMR*: real-time cine imaging, techniques that acquire single-shot images at a temporal resolution of ~30–40 milliseconds and can be utilized in exercise CMR (see below), in patients with arrhythmias or in those who have a problem remaining motionless in the scanner. In addition, real-time cine can be performed interactively by utilizing a "real-time window" and three other localizer windows controlled with a cursor and sweeping the ventricle to assess ventricular function or finding small atrial and ventricular septal defects. These sweeps can be used to survey the cardiovascular anatomy in conjunction with the static SSFP imaging.

Real-time PCMR acquires single-shot flow images and can have a similar temporal resolution to real-time cine images. This also may be utilized for exercise CMR, patients with arrhythmias, or simply to speed up the examination.

It is becoming more common for real-time cine and PCMR to utilize compressed sensing technologies and/or artificial intelligence/deep learning techniques. Other techniques use low-resolution real-time cine over an extended period of time and then "bin" the images with the recorded EGC.[70]

- *Coronary artery imaging*[66,71,72] (Fig. 41.11): Using T2-prepared SSFP imaging combined with the navigator technique,[71] the IR-GRE technique mentioned in the contrast section above, or BOOST imaging, coronary evaluation is indicated in a variety of CHDs, similar to those who obtain DE imaging In children with fast heart rates (RR intervals of 500 msec or less), minimizing the motion of the coronary arteries by acquiring lines of k-space at the quiescent phase of the cardiac cycle may require obtaining data at end systole rather than mid to late diastole like in adults.
- *Exercise CMR*: With the advent of MRI-compatible ergometers, the patient can exercise in the MRI environment with subsequent imaging of function and flow, generally with "real-time" techniques. This is useful in children with chest pain in whom perfusion at exercise can be assessed, in those with hypertrophic cardiomyopathy with poor echocardiographic windows to visualize the LV outflow tract, and in adolescents with poor exercise performance to assess ventricular function. For example, it was discovered that poor exercise performance of single-ventricle patients after Fontan was related to increased power loss in the systemic venous pathway in this manner.[73]
- *Tumor/mass characterization*[74,75]: Although relatively rare, cardiac tumors/masses do occur in pediatrics. Many cardiac tumors and masses can be differentiated from each other not only by where they occur in the heart, what symptoms they cause, and at what age they occur, but also by their tissue characteristics on CMR. For example, a fibroma will accumulate gadolinium and be signal intense on DE imaging and T1-weighted images after gadolinium administration, whereas lipomas will be signal intense on T1-weighted images and become signal poor after fat saturation. Tumor characterization procedures by CMR are a protocol in themselves and typically include SSFP imaging, T1- and T2-weighted sequences, T1 images with fat saturation, GRE imaging, myocardial tagging, perfusion (e.g., for hemangiomas), DE imaging, T1-weighted images after gadolinium administration, and a TI scout. If time permits, functional imaging can be used to assess for effects of the tumor such as obstruction to flow and decreased cardiac output.
- *Arrhythmogenic right ventricular cardiomyopathy*: This disease is the replacement of myocardium by fatty or fibrofatty tissue and imaging fulfills only one of the criteria set forth.[76,77] CMR has been successfully utilized in adults for this disease, however, in pediatrics, there is question as to how useful it truly is.[78] The findings by CMR in adults with arrhythmogenic right ventricular dysplasia vary from study to study.[79] Findings to look for in children are regional wall motion abnormalities of the right ventricle (and LV), ventricular dilation, decreased ejection fraction, dyskinetic bulges or dyskinesia of RV wall motion, and the accordion sign. The protocol includes cine for ventricular function, phase-encoded velocity mapping, and DE.[80]

TECHNICAL CONSIDERATIONS IN PEDIATRIC CARDIAC MAGNETIC RESONANCE

Because of the demands of high spatial and temporal resolution in infants and children along with the inability to breath-hold, alternative means are needed to allow the CMR sequences designed for adults to work. Strategies have been created to successfully image these youngsters and have been employed to various degrees for many years.

Spatial and Temporal Resolution

Small voxels needed to image infants and small children can be problematic because of the poor signal-to-noise ratio (SNR). By employing parallel imaging techniques, this becomes even worse. Simply imaging without consideration for SNR will result in a poor-quality, "grainy" image that will nondiagnostic. To increase the SNR, a number of strategies have been employed, either in isolation or in combination, such as using contrast agents, multiple averages (excitations), phase oversampling, decreasing the bandwidth, forgoing using parallel imaging, or even moving from 1.5 to 3 T (which comes with its own separate issues). These modifications come at the cost of imaging time but are worth it to get high-quality diagnostic images.

At times, for the smallest voxels, even these strategies cannot be employed to affect SNR to the degree needed. In these instances, the CMR imager must be satisfied with larger voxels, which is done by decreasing the matrix size—typically, when imaging an adult, a base matrix (in the frequency-encoding direction) of 256 or 192 is used, which can be decreased in varying steps to as low as 128 which can yield diagnostic images well in the range of fields of view of ~200 mm or less, yielding pixels of 1.5–2 mm or less depending upon the field of view used. Slice thicknesses generally do not go below 2.5 to 3 mm because of SNR considerations. Note that gadolinium/ferumoxytol images, however, because of the T1 shortening from the contrast agent, can achieve submillimeter isotropic resolution.

When imaging small children, small fields of view are needed, but at certain settings sequences are written that do not allow for the fields of view to go down very low (e.g., 200 mm or less in a 3 kg baby). Similarly, slice thicknesses need to be smaller than when imaging the adult, and because of SNR considerations the matrix size needs to be smaller at times, but at certain settings sequences are written that do not allow for these manipulations. When that occurs, the imager must find combinations by trial and error of changing bandwidths, repetition time (TR), matrix, segments of k-space ("views"), field of view, and slice thickness to allow for optimal imaging for the size of the patient. Each manufacturer has their own idiosyncrasies which make it prohibitive to list all the combinations here. By relaxing some parameters (e.g., longer TR, increasing the segments), other parameters may be allowed to be optimized to image the smaller patients (e.g., smaller field of view).

As heart rates can be very high in infants (not uncommonly 140–170 beats per minute), a successful CMR scan in this age group needs to accommodate this. As a rule of thumb, 15–20 phases of the cardiac cycle should be used under an RR interval of 500 msec, 20–25 phases should be obtained from 500–750 msec, and 25–30 phases should be used for >750 msec. To be able to obtain this kind of temporal resolution at fast heart rates, the TR needs to be low, and to do this, in general, the number of segments need to be as low as possible. If the TR and the number of segments are not low enough, in retrospectively gated imaging, the walls of the heart will appear blurry and with a double or triple shadow while in prospectively triggered imaging, the heart motion will look stilted and jerky. Adequate temporal resolution can be obtained at fast heart rates with three segments at a minimum. Various compressed sensing techniques may be used.

In retrospective-gating types of sequences, it is important to understand that the MR scanner is acquiring data continuously and recording the ECG tracing. After all the lines of k-space are acquired, the computer then "bins" each line of k-space to the closest phase of the cardiac cycle it is calculating, interpolating the data as it is performing the "bin." It is, therefore, important to be cognizant of the fact that the number of calculated phases should not exceed twice the measured phases (essentially the RR interval [msec]/TR [msec] where TR is the line TR x lines of k-space obtained) as there should be two measured points between each interpolated point to obtain robust data. The formula used is:

$$2\,x\,\text{RR interval (msec)} / \text{number of calculated phases} = \text{TR (msec)}$$

where TR is defined as the line TR x lines of k-space obtained. This is especially important in velocity mapping for accurate data to be obtained.

At times, it is advantageous to utilize "single-shot" imaging in children because of respiratory motion or arrhythmia, where all the lines of k-space are acquired in one heartbeat. A typical "single-shot" imaging sequence is the HASTE sequence mentioned above, but other sequences such as static SSFP and cine SSFP can be performed in "single-shot" mode. If the heart rate is too fast, it may be advantageous to obtain the image over two heartbeats (i.e., imaged at the end of 2 heartbeats - 2 × RR interval) instead of one and this should be considered in imaging sequences such as HASTE, double inversion dark-blood imaging, or viability imaging if the heart cannot be successfully imaged in one heartbeat.

When performing tissue characterization with fast heart rates, it is imperative that the spins in the tissue are allowed to relax prior to the next excitation. In these instances, the RR interval set in the acquisition window may be purposely doubled or even tripled and the acquisition of data occur at the end of the last heartbeat. This technique has indeed saved many scans in the past from failure albeit at the cost of doubling or tripling the time involved.

Inability of Pediatric Patients to Breath-Hold

As mentioned, to perform CMR in patients who cannot hold their breath, general anesthesia may be used so the anesthesiologist can do the breath-holding for the patient. That being said, deep sedation has been successfully utilized for many years without untoward effects and allowed patients to free-breath during the CMR examination. The advantage to deep sedation and free breathing is of course the less invasive nature of this approach and imaging in "normal" day-to-day physiology.

Imaging the patient who is allowed to free breathe utilizes:

a) Multiple excitations to "average out" the respiratory motion. Typically, three excitations are needed to obtain good image quality (which also increases SNR), although at times, four to five excitations may be needed for the vigorous breather.
b) Navigator-based techniques to monitor diaphragmatic motion
c) Navigator techniques to monitor heart motion such as SIMBA[81] or iNav
d) "Real-time" or single-shot techniques
e) Specialized motion correction (MOCO) algorithms may be used

In addition to these strategies, placing a saturation band over the chest wall can also aid in minimizing any respiratory artifact that does occur. These are the most common strategies to allow high-quality images to be created, albeit at the cost of a little extra time, which is not prohibitive. It is true that breath-holding will yield much crisper images, however, the marginal benefit in many instances is not worth the cost as the above strategies for free breathing yield diagnostic information.

Contrast-Based Techniques

The above applies to all types of imaging, but the gadolinium-based techniques have a couple of additional considerations.

a) Infants and children generally have quick circulatory times. When performing dynamic imaging, this should be kept in mind for temporal resolution. As always, there is a tradeoff in CMR and increasing temporal resolution generally comes at the cost of spatial resolution. This should be balanced depending upon the disease state and the information needed. For example, assessing shunts, continuity of vessels, and lung perfusion may require higher temporal resolution while anatomy such as searching for vessels not visualized by echocardiography will require more spatial resolution.
b) When performing solely "static" imaging such as DE, using the "tracking" or "Combined Application to Reduce Exposure (CARE)" bolus technique allows for the imager to ensure the contrast agent has entered the circulation (as opposed to an injector malfunction, infiltrated IV, or broken stopcock) before imaging. Once again, it should be noted that children will have a quick circulatory time and the imager should not be caught off guard when this occurs, missing the first pass gadolinium in the process.

c) For viability imaging, as mentioned above, two or more RR intervals may be needed to allow the tissue to relax enough for the next excitation.
d) When performing the "slow-drip" 3D inversion recovery technique (as well as other contrast-based techniques), even at a "double dose," the dosage may be a small amount (e.g., 2–3 cc). In this particular case, the contrast is diluted (1:1 or greater) for better overall image quality.
e) The perfusion technique obtains images at a single slice position at different time points in the cardiac cycle after a delay. With heart rates in infants and children so high, it may only be possible to fit two slices (or rarely one slice with really high heart rates) within an RR interval. If this occurs, the imager can perform the sequence over 2 RR intervals without degradation of diagnostic quality and obtain more slices (3–4) during the scan.

A TASTE OF THE FUTURE

With the many advances in CMR, the future holds great promise for CHD with work in the area of interventional CMR (e.g., balloon valvuloplasty, stent placement), molecular imaging, tissue and blood characterization techniques (e.g., T1 rho),[82] diffuse fibrosis, oxygen content, as well as continued development of 4D flow imaging, 5D imaging, and "real-time" flow assessment.

CONCLUSION

CMR of CHD in infants and children is a unique field unto itself in the world of CMR for many reasons. The imager needs to understand the anatomy, physiology, and function of native CHD as well as the treatments (surgical and catheter based) to perform the examination correctly in addition to tackling the myriad technical issues associated with imaging in pediatrics. With both hardware and software advances in the field, CMR will only become more important in CHD in the years to come.

REFERENCES

1. Didier D, Higgins CB, Fisher M, Osakai L, Silverman NH, Cheitlin MD. Congenital heart disease: gated magnetic resonance imaging in 72 patients. *Radiology*. 1986;158:227–235.
2. Adams R, Fellows KE, Fogel MA, Weinberg PM. Anatomic delineation of congenital heart disease with 3D magnetic resonance imaging. Proceedings SPIE-medical imaging. *Physiol Funct Multidimens Images*. 1994;2168:184–194.
3. Fogel MA, Ramaciotti C, Hubbard AM, Weinberg PW. Magnetic resonance and echocardiographic imaging of pulmonary artery size throughout stages of fontan reconstruction. *Circulation*. 1994;90:2927–2936.
4. Fogel MA, Weinberg PM, Gupta KB, et al. Mechanics of the single left ventricle: a study in ventricular-ventricular interaction II. *Circulation*. 1998;98:330–338.
5. Fogel MA, Weinberg PM, Rychik J, et al. Caval contribution to flow in the branch pulmonary arteries of fontan patients using a novel application of magnetic resonance presaturation pulse. *Circulation*. 1999;99:1215–1221.
6. Fogel MA, Weinberg PM, Hubbard A, Haselgrove J. Diastolic biomechanics in normal infants utilizing MRI tissue tagging. *Circulation*. 2000;102:218–224.
7. Eyskens B, Reybrouck T, Bagaert J, et al. Homograft insertion for pulmonary regurgitation after repair of tetralogy of Fallot improves cardiorespiratory exercise performance. *Am J Cardiol*. 2000;85:221–225.
8. Niezen RA, Helgbing WA, van der Wall EE, van der Geest RJ, Rebergen SA, de Roos A. Biventricular systolic function and mass studied with MRI imaging in children with pulmonary regurgitation after repair for tetralogy of Fallot. *Radiology*. 1996;201:135–140.
9. Rebergen SA, Chin JGJ, Ottenkamp J, van der Wall EE, de Roos A. Pulmonary regurgitation in the late postoperative follow-up of tetralogy of fallot. Volumetric quantification by MR velocity mapping. *Circulation*. 1993;88:2257–2266.
10. Rebergen SA, Ottenkamp J, van der Wall EE, Chin JDJ, de Roos A. Postoperative pulmonary flow dynamics after Fontan surgery: assessment with nuclear magnetic resonance velocity mapping. *J Am Coll Cardiol*. 1993;21:123–131.
11. Beerbaum P, Korperich H, Barth P, Esdorn H, Gieseke J, Meyer H. Noninvasive quantification of left-to-right shunt in pediatric patients. Phase-contrast cine magnetic resonance imaging compared with invasive oxymetry. *Circulation*. 2001;10:2476–2482.
12. Fogel MA, Weinberg PM, Chin AJ, Fellows KE, Hoffman EA. Late ventricular geometry and performance changes of functional single ventricle throughout staged Fontan reconstruction assessed by magnetic resonance imaging. *J Am Coll Cardiol*. 1996;28(1):212–221.
13. Fogel MA, Weinberg PM, Fellows KE, Hoffman EA. A study in ventricular - ventricular interaction: single right ventricles compared with systemic right ventricles in a dual chambered circulation. *Circulation*. 1995;92(2):219–230.
14. Fogel MA, Gupta KB, Weinberg PW, Hoffman EA. Regional wall motion and strain analysis across stages of Fontan reconstruction by magnetic resonance tagging. *Am J Physiol*. 1995;269 (Heart and Circulatory Physiology 38):H1132–H1152.
15. Fogel MA, Weinberg PM, Hoydu A, et al. The nature of flow in the systemic venous pathway in Fontan patients utilizing magnetic resonance blood tagging. *J Thorac Cardiovasc Surg*. 1997;114:1032–1041.
16. Mor-Avi V, Sugeng L, Weinert L, et al. Fast measurement of LV mass with real-time 3-dimensional echocardiography: comparison with MRI. *Circulation*. 2004;110:1814–1818.
17. Bu L, Munns S, Zhang H, et al. Rapid full volume data acquisition by real-time 3-dimensional echocardiography for assessment of LV indexes in children: a validation study compared with MRI. *J Am Soc Echocardiogr*. 2005;18:299–305.
18. Fogel MA, Pawlowski TW, Harris MA, et al. Comparison and usefulness of cardiac magnetic resonance versus computed tomography in infants six months of age or younger with aortic arch anomalies without deep sedation or anesthesia. *Am J Cardiol*. 2011;108:120–125.
19. Shariat M, Mertens L, Seed M, et al. Utility of feed-and-sleep cardiovascular magnetic resonance in young infants with complex cardiovascular disease. *Pediatr Cardiol*. 2015;36:809–812.
20. Srinivasan R, Faerber JA, DeCost G, et al. Right ventricular strain is associated with increased length of stay after tetralogy of fallot repair. *J Cardiovasc Imaging*. 2022;30(1):50–58.
21. DiLorenzo M, Goldmuntz E, Nicolson SC, Fogel MA, Mercer-Rosa L. Early postoperative remodeling following repair of tetralogy of fallot utilizing unsedated cardiac magnetic resonance: a pilot study. *Cardiol Young*. 2018;28(5):697–701.
22. Malviya S, Voepel-Lewis T, Eldevik OP, Rockwell DT, Wong JH, Tait AR. Sedation and general anaesthesia in children undergoing MRI and CT: adverse events and outcomes. *Br J Aneasth*. 2000;84:743–748.
23. Fogel MA, Weinberg P, Parave E, Harris C, Montenegro L, Concepcion M. Safety and efficacy of deep sedation in infants, children and adolescents undergoing cardiac magnetic resonance. *J Pediatr*. 2008;152:534–539.
24. Malviya S, Voepel-Lewis T, Tait AR. Adverse events and risk factors associated with the sedation of children by nonanesthesiologists. *Anesth Analg*. 1997;85:1207–1213.
25. Bluemke DA, Breiter SN. Sedation procedures in MR imaging: safety, effectiveness, and nursing effect on examinations. *Radiology*. 2000;216:645–652.
26. Vade A, Sukhani R, Dolenga M, Habisohn-Schuck C. Choral hydrate sedation of children undergoing CT and MR imaging: safety as judged by American academy of pediatrics guidelines. *Am J Roentgenol*. 1995;165:905–909.
27. Shepherd JK, Hall-Craggs MA, Finn JP, Bingham RM. Sedation in children scanned with high-field magnetic resonance: experience at the hospital for sick children, great ormond street. *Br J Radiol*. 1990;63:794–797.
28. Lawson GR. Sedation of children for magnetic resonance imaging. *Arch Dis Child*. 2000;82:150–154.
29. https://www.fda.gov/drugs/drug-safety-and-availability/fda-drug-safety-communication-fda-review-results-new-warnings-about-using-general-anesthetics-and (accessed Oct 14, 2024).
30. https://www.fda.gov/drugs/drug-safety-and-availability/fda-drug-safety-communication-fda-approves-label-changes-use-general-anesthetic-and-sedation-drugs (accessed Oct 14, 2024).
31. McCann ME, de Graaff JC, Dorris L, et al. Neurodevelopmental outcome at 5 years of age after general anaesthesia or awake-regional anaesthesia in infancy (GAS): an international, multicentre, randomised, controlled equivalence trial. *Lancet*. 2019;393(10172):664.
32. Wilder RT, Flick RP, Sprung J, et al. Early exposure to anesthesia and learning disabilities in a population-based birth cohort. *Anesthesiology*. 2009;110:796.
33. Hu D, Flick RP, Zaccariello MJ, et al. Association between exposure of young children to procedures requiring general anesthesia and learning and behavioral outcomes in a population-based birth cohort. *Anesthesiology*. 2017;127:227.
34. Flick RP, Katusic SK, Colligan RC, et al. Cognitive and behavioral outcomes after early exposure to anesthesia and surgery. *Pediatrics*. 2011;128:e1053.
35. DiMaggio C, Sun LS, Kakavouli A, et al. A retrospective cohort study of the association of anesthesia and hernia repair surgery with behavioral and developmental disorders in young children. *J Neurosurg Anesthesiol*. 2009;21:286.

36. Shi Y, Dykhoff HJ, Guevara LRH, et al. Moderators of the association between attention-deficit/hyperactivity disorder and exposure to anaesthesia and surgery in children. *Br J Anaesth*. 2021;127:722.
37. Ing C, Ma X, Sun M, et al. Exposure to surgery and anesthesia in early childhood and subsequent use of attention deficit hyperactivity disorder medications. *Anesth Analg*. 2020;131:723.
38. Sprung J, Flick RP, Katusic SK, et al. Attention-deficit/hyperactivity disorder after early exposure to procedures requiring general anesthesia. *Mayo Clin Proc*. 2012;87:120.
39. DiMaggio C, Sun LS, Li G. Early childhood exposure to anesthesia and risk of developmental and behavioral disorders in a sibling birth cohort. *Anesth Analg*. 2011;113:1143.
40. O'Leary JD, Janus M, Duku E, et al. Influence of surgical procedures and general anesthesia on child development before primary school entry among matched sibling pairs. *JAMA Pediatr*. 2019;173:29.
41. O'Leary JD, Janus M, Duku E, et al. A population-based study evaluating the association between surgery in early life and child development at primary school entry. *Anesthesiology*. 2016;125:272.
42. Graham MR, Brownell M, Chateau DG, et al. Neurodevelopmental assessment in kindergarten in children exposed to general anesthesia before the age of 4 years: a retrospective matched cohort study. *Anesthesiology*. 2016;125:667.
43. Sun LS, Li G, Miller TL, et al. Association between a single general anesthesia exposure before age 36 months and neurocognitive outcomes in later childhood. *JAMA*. 2016;315:2312.
44. Ing C, DiMaggio C, Whitehouse A, et al. Long-term differences in language and cognitive function after childhood exposure to anesthesia. *Pediatrics*. 2012;130:e476.
45. Bong CL, Ho D, Allen JC, et al. Early neurodevelopmental outcomes following exposure to general anesthesia in infancy: Egain, a prospective cohort study. *J Neurosurg Anesthesiol*. 2023;35:394.
46. Walkden GJ, Gill H, Davies NM, et al. Early childhood general anesthesia and neurodevelopmental outcomes in the avon longitudinal study of parents and children birth cohort. *Anesthesiology*. 2020;133:1007.
47. McDonald JS, Larson NB, Kolbe AB, et al. Acute reactions to gadolinium-based contrast agents in a pediatric cohort: a retrospective study of 16,237 injections. *AJR Am J Roentgenol*. 2021;216(5):1363–1369.
48. Nardone B, Saddleton E, Laumann AE, et al. Pediatric nephrogenic systemic fibrosis is rarely reported: a RADAR report. *Pediatr Radiol*. 2014;44(2):173–180.
49. https://www.fda.gov/drugs/drug-safety-and-availability/fda-drug-safety-communication-fda-evaluating-risk-brain-deposits-repeated-use-gadolinium-based (accessed Oct 14, 2024).
50. https://www.fda.gov/drugs/drug-safety-and-availability/fda-drug-safety-communication-fda-identifies-no-harmful-effects-date-brain-retention-gadolinium (accessed Oct 14, 2024).
51. www.fda.gov/drugs/fda-drug-safety-podcasts/fda-drug-safety-podcast-fda-identifies-no-harmful-effects-date-brain-retention-gadolinium-based#:~:text=On%20May%2022%2C%202017%2C%20FDA,not%20warranted%20at%20this%20time. (accessed Oct 14, 2024).
52. Nguyen KL, Han F, Zhou Z, et al. 4D MUSIC CMR: value-based imaging of neonates and infants with congenital heart disease. *J Cardiovasc Magn Reson*. 2017;19(1):40.
53. Nguyen KL, Yoshida T, Kathuria-Prakash N, et al. Multicenter safety and practice for off-label diagnostic use of ferumoxytol in MRI. *Radiology*. 2019;293(3):554–564.
54. https://www.fda.gov/drugs/drug-safety-and-availability/fda-drug-safety-communication-fda-strengthens-warnings-and-changes-prescribing-instructions-decrease (accessed Oct 14, 2024).
55. De Leon-Benedetti LS, Ramirez-Suarez KI, Otero HJ, et al. How we do it: cardiac implantable devices are not a contraindication to MRI: time for a paradigm shift. *Pediatr Radiol*. 2024;54(6):863–875.
56. Whitehead KK, Gillespie MJ, Harris MA, Fogel MA, Rome JJ. Noninvasive quantification of systemic to pulmonary collateral flow: a major source of inefficiency in patients with superior cavopulmonary connections. *Circ Cardiovasc Imaging*. 2009;2:405–411.
57. Glatz AC, Rome JJ, Small AJ, et al. Systemic-to-pulmonary collateral flow, as measured by cardiac magnetic resonance imaging, is associated with acute post-fontan clinical outcomes. *Circ Cardiovasc Imaging*. 2012;5:218–225.
58. Grosse-Wortmann L, Al-Otay A, Yoo SJ. Aortopulmonary collaterals after bidirectional cavopulmonary connection or fontan completion: quantification with MRI. *Circulation: Cardiovasc Imaging*. 2009;2:219–225.
59. Edelman RR, Chien D, Kim D. Fast selective black blood MR imaging. *Radiology*. 1991;181:655–660.
60. Finn JP, Baskaran V, Carr JC, et al. Low-dose contrast-enhanced three-dimensional MR angiography with subsecond temporal resolution—initial results. *Radiology*. 2002;224:896–904.
61. Iwamoto Y, Inage A, Tomlinson G, et al. Direct measurement of aortic regurgitation with phase-contrast magnetic resonance is inaccurate: proposal of an alternative method of quantification. *Pediatr Radiol*. 2014;44(11):1358–1369.
62. McNamara MT, Tscholakoff D, Revel D, et al. Differentiation of reversible and irreversible myocardial injury by MR imaging with and without gadolinium-DTPA. *Radiology*. 1986;158:765–769.
63. Simonetti OP, Kim RJ, Fieno DS, et al. An improved MRI technique for the visualization of myocardial injury. *Radiology*. 2001;218:215–223.
64. Prakash A, Powell AJ, Krishnamurthy R, Geva T. Magnetic resonance imaging evaluation of myocardial perfusion and viability in congenital and acquired pediatric heart disease. *Am J Cardiol*. 2004;93:657–661.
65. Harris MA, Ghods S, Weinberg PM, Fogel MA. Magnetic resonance delayed enhancement for detection of fibrous tissue in postoperative pediatric patients with various forms of congenital heart disease. *J Cardiovasc Mag Reson*. 2005;7:157.
66. Taylor AM, Dymarkowski S, Hamaekers P, et al. MR coronary angiography and late-enhancement myocardial MR in children who underwent arterial switch surgery for transposition of great arteries. *Radiology*. 2005;234:542–547.
67. Kozak MF1, Redington A, Yoo SJ, Seed M, Greiser A, Grosse-Wortmann L. Diffuse myocardial fibrosis following tetralogy of fallot repair: a T1 mapping cardiac magnetic resonance study. *Pediatr Radiol*. 2014;44(4):403–409.
68. Broberg C, Huang J, Hogberg I, et al. Diffuse LV myocardial fibrosis and its clinical associations in adults with repaired tetralogy of fallot. *J Am Coll Cardiol Img*. 2016;9(1):86–87.
69. Paetsch I, Jahnke C, Wahl A, et al. Comparison of dobutamine stress magnetic resonance, adenosine stress magnetic resonance, and adenosine stress magnetic resonance perfusion. *Circulation*. 2004;110:835–842.
70. Xue H, Kellman P, Larocca G, Arai AE, Hansen MS. High spatial and temporal resolution retrospective cine cardiovascular magnetic resonance from shortened free breathing real-time acquisitions. *J Cardiovasc Magn Reson*. 2013;15(1):102.
71. Kim WY, Danias PG, Stuber M, et al. Coronary magnetic resonance angiography for the detection of coronary stenoses. *NEJM*. 2001;345:1863–1869.
72. Tangcharoen T, Hegde S, Bell A, et al. Feasibility of whole-heart, steady-state free precession magnetic resonance coronary angiography (MRCA) in infants and children with congenital heart disease. *J Soc Cardiovasc Magn Resonan – Abstr 11th annu SCMR Sci Sess*. 2008:80–81 (abstract 219).
73. Khiabani RH, Whitehead KK, Han D, et al. Exercise capacity in single ventricle patients after fontan correlates with hemodynamic energy loss in TCPC. *Heart*. 2015;101(2):139–143. PMID: 25184826.
74. Beroukhim RS, Prakash A, Buechel ER, et al. Characterization of cardiac tumors in children by cardiovascular magnetic resonance imaging: a multicenter experience. *J Am Coll Cardiol*. 2011;58(10):1044–1054.
75. Beroukhim RS, Ghelani S, Ashwath R, et al. Accuracy of cardiac magnetic resonance imaging in diagnosing pediatric cardiac masses: a multicenter study. *JACC Cardiovasc Imaging*. 2022;15(8):1391–1405.
76. Corrado D, van Tintelen PJ, McKenna WJ, et al. Arrhythmogenic right ventricular cardiomyopathy: evaluation of the current diagnostic criteria and differential diagnosis. *Eur Heart J*. 2020;41:1414–1429.
77. Graziano F, Zorzi A, Cipriani A, et al. The 2020 "Padua criteria" for diagnosis and phenotype characterization of arrhythmogenic cardiomyopathy in clinical practice. *J Clin Med*. 2022;11(1):279.
78. Fogel MA, Weinberg PM, Rhodes L. Usefulness of magnetic resonance imaging for the diagnosis of right ventricular dysplasia in children. *Am J Cardiol*. 2006;97(8):1232–1237.
79. Midiri M, Finazzo M, Brancato M, et al. Arrhythmogenic right ventricular dysplasia: MR features. *Eur Radiol*. 1997;7:307–312.
80. Tandri H, Saranathan M, Rodriguez ER, et al. Noninvasive detection of myocardial fibrosis in arrhythmogenic right ventricular cardiomyopathy using delayed-enhancement magnetic resonance imaging. *J Am Coll Cardiol*. 2005;45(1):98–103.
81. Roy CW, Di Sopra L, Whitehead KK, et al. Free-running cardiac and respiratory motion-resolved 5D whole-heart coronary mr angiography in pediatric cardiac patients using ferumoxytol. *J Cardiovasc Mag Reson*. 2022;24:39.
82. Bustin A, Witschey WRT, van Heeswijk RB, et al. Magnetic resonance myocardial T1ρ mapping. *J Cardiovasc Magn Reson*. 2023;25:34.

42 Pediatric and Congenital Heart Disease

M. JAY CAMPBELL, ANDREW J. POWELL, AND ANNE MARIE VALENTE

ABBREVIATIONS

3D three-dimensional
4D four-dimensonal
ASD atrial septal defect
BSA body surface area
CC-TGA congenitally corrected transposition of the great arteries
CHD congenital heart disease
CMR cardiovascular magnetic resonance
ECG electrocardiogram
LGE late gadolinium enhancement
MRA magnetic resonance angiography
PAPVC partially anomalous pulmonary venous connections
Qp/Qs pulmonary-to-systemic flow
SSFP steady-state free precession
TGA Transposition of the great arteries
TOF tetralogy of Fallot
VSD ventricular septal defect

INTRODUCTION

Congenital heart disease (CHD) is the most common birth defect, occurring in 8/1000 live births.[1] The majority of children born with CHD are now living well into adulthood; consequently, the number of adults with CHD has grown significantly.[2] For young patients with CHD, echocardiography is the first-line imaging modality. Cardiac magnetic resonance imaging (CMR) and cardiac computed tomography are superior in imaging extracardiac structures. CMR also has a unique ability to quantify ventricular size and systolic function, which is particularly important in many patients with CHD.[3] Improvements in hardware and the development of new highly efficient imaging techniques have allowed for sufficient spatial and temporal resolution to comprehensively evaluate cardiac anatomy and function in pediatric patients despite their small body size and rapid heart rate. Although echocardiography provides the necessary diagnostic information for most patients in this age group, CMR offers an important alternative in several circumstances: (1) when transthoracic echocardiography fails to provide the required diagnostic information, (2) when clinical assessment and diagnostic tests are inconsistent, (3) as an alternative to diagnostic cardiac catheterization with its associated higher risk and cost, and (4) to obtain diagnostic information for which it offers unique advantages (e.g., flow measurements, myocardial assessment).

This chapter reviews the anatomy, clinical management, and CMR evaluation of selective CHD and pediatric conditions. For each, we will present goals of the CMR protocol with the acknowledgement that there is considerable anatomic variability and individualization of protocols is required. Knowledge of the patient's anatomy, history of interventions, and prior imaging is critical to focus the protocol so that the essential information is obtained within a reasonable amount of time, as many of these patients will undergo serial examinations. Patient preparation, sedation, and monitoring strategies for children undergoing CMR are discussed in Chapter 41.

PRINCIPLES OF CARDIAC MAGNETIC RESONANCE EVALUATION IN CONGENITAL HEART DISEASE

Preexamination planning is crucial given the wide array of imaging sequences available and the often complex nature of the clinical, anatomic, and functional issues in patients with CHD. It is essential to perform a careful review of the patient's medical history, including details of all cardiovascular surgical procedures, interventional catheterizations, previous diagnostic test results, and current clinical status. As with echocardiography and cardiac catheterization, CMR examination of CHD is a dynamic diagnostic procedure that is optimally performed with continuous review and interpretation of the data by the supervising physician. Unexpected findings or suboptimal image quality often require adjustment of the examination protocol, imaging planes, techniques, and sequence parameters. Reliance on standardized protocols and postexamination review alone in these patients may result in incomplete or even erroneous interpretation.

One of the strengths of CMR is the ability to accurately and precisely measure ventricular and vascular structures. Care must be taken, however, when determining whether these measurements fall within the normal range, as adjustment for variation in body size remains challenging. Simply dividing by body surface area (BSA) is inadequate for most parameters, particularly in children and unusually large or small adults.[4] Several authors have shown that linear dimensions (e.g., ascending aorta diameter) are best adjusted to the square root of BSA, area measurements to BSA, and volumetric measurements to BSA raised to the 1.3–1.4 power.[5,6] Thus, for example, one cannot simply apply to children a normative range for ventricular volume indexed to BSA that was derived in adults. CMR-based normative data from children are available, though they are often limited by a smaller than ideal sample size, particularly in the youngest age range.[7–15] Furthermore, it is essential to apply the same measurement technique (e.g., whether to include papillary muscles or myocardial trabeculations in the blood pool) as that which was used to derive the normative data.

ATRIAL SEPTAL DEFECTS AND OTHER INTERATRIAL COMMUNICATIONS

Anatomically, five different defects can result in an interatrial shunt (Fig. 42.1): (1) A patent foramen ovale is bordered on the left by septum primum and by the superior limbic band of the fossa ovalis (septum secundum) on the right. A patent foramen ovale is seen in almost all newborns and often closes over the first several months of life. (2) A secundum atrial septal defect (ASD) (Fig. 42.2) is the most common cause of an atrial level shunt after patent foramen ovale. Usually, the defect is due to deficiency of the septum primum, but rarely, it results from a deficiency of the septum secundum. (3) A primum ASD is a variant of incomplete common atrioventricular canal and almost always associated with a cleft anterior mitral valve leaflet. Any associated defect within the fossa ovalis (e.g., secundum ASD) is regarded as a separate abnormality. (4) A sinus venosus defect results from deficiency of the sinus venosus septum, which separates the pulmonary veins from the systemic veins and the sinus venosus portion of the right atrium (Fig. 42.3). Most commonly, a sinus venosus defect is between the right upper pulmonary vein and the cardiac end of the superior vena cava. Rarely, the defect involves the right lower and/or middle pulmonary veins and the inferior aspect of the right atrium near its junction with the inferior vena cava. From an anatomic standpoint, a sinus venosus defect is not an ASD because it does not allow direct communication between the left and right atria. Instead, the interatrial flow travels between the left atrium, one or more of the pulmonary veins, the sinus venosus septal defect, the superior (or inferior) vena cava, and the right atrium. The defect usually allows pulmonary vein flow to drain to the right atrium through the defect as well. Patients with sinus venosus defects may have additional accessory right upper pulmonary veins connecting to the superior vena cava or azygous vein. (5) A coronary sinus septal defect is a rare type of interatrial communication in which the septum between the coronary sinus and the left atrium is either partially or completely unroofed, allowing the right and left atria to communicate through the defect and the coronary sinus orifice. This may be accompanied by a persistent left superior vena cava that drains to the coronary sinus, unless the coronary sinus is completely unroofed, in which case the left superior vena

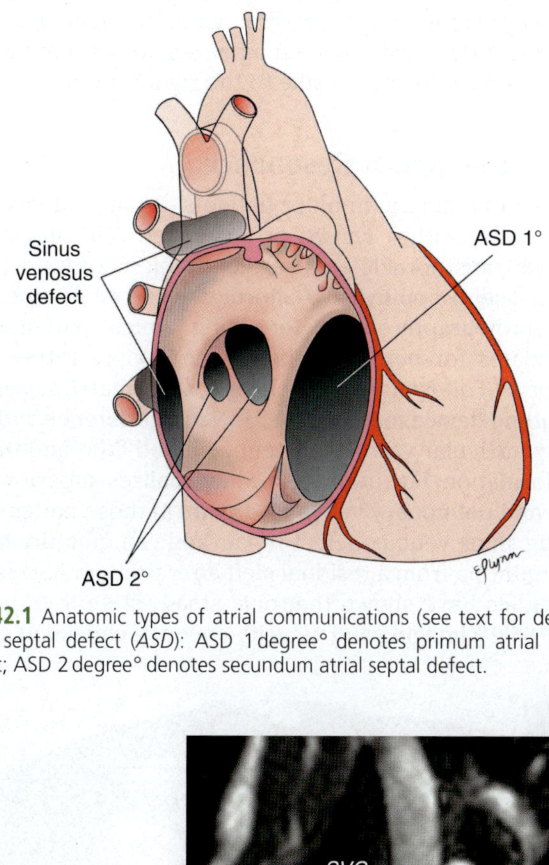

FIG. 42.1 Anatomic types of atrial communications (see text for details). Atrial septal defect (*ASD*): ASD 1degree° denotes primum atrial septal defect; ASD 2degree° denotes secundum atrial septal defect.

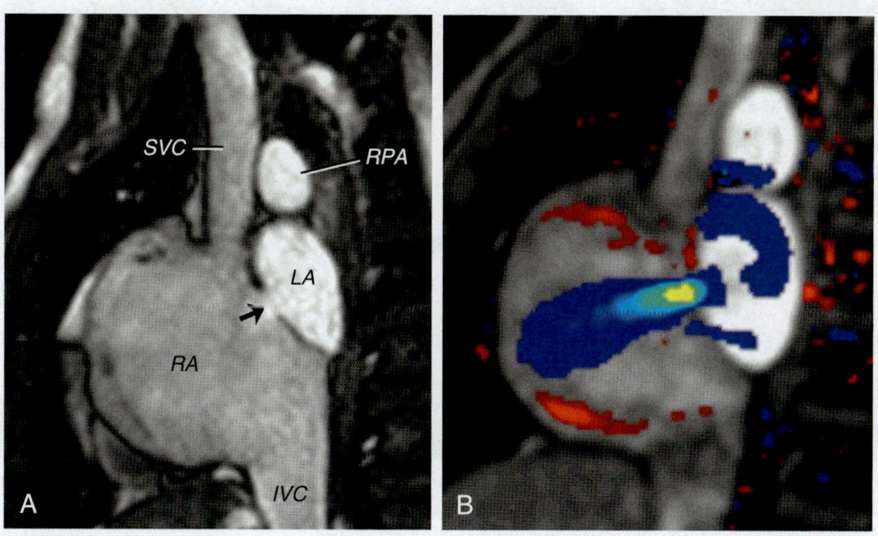

FIG. 42.2 Secundum atrial septal defect. (A) Oblique steady-state free precession cine showing a centrally located defect (*arrow*). (B) Color-coded, velocity-encoded cine showing flow from the left atrium (*LA*) to the right atrium (*RA*) through the defect. *IVC*, inferior vena cava; *RPA*, right pulmonary artery; *SVC*, superior vena cava. (From Geva T, Powell AJ. Magnetic resonance imaging. In: Allen HD, Shaddy RE, Penny DJ, Feltes TF, Cetta F, eds. *Moss and Adams' Heart Disease in Infants, Children, and Adolescents.* 9th ed. Philadelphia: Wolters Kluwer; 2016:373–412.)

cava drains to the left atrium. The coexistence of a coronary sinus septal defect and persistent left superior vena cava is termed Raghib syndrome and results in cyanosis.[16]

Regardless of the specific anatomic type, the amount of shunting through an interatrial communication is determined by the defect size and relative compliance of the right and left ventricles. Over the first few months of life, left ventricular compliance typically rises, leading to an increasing left-to-right shunt. During adulthood, right ventricular compliance normally decreases, further augmenting the left-to-right flow. Shunt flow through the right heart and lungs leads to dilation of the right atrium, right ventricle, pulmonary arteries, and pulmonary veins. Up to 5%–10% of patients with a significant left-to-right shunt may develop pulmonary vascular disease by adulthood, leading to pulmonary hypertension. Adults with unrepaired atrial level defects are also at risk for exercise intolerance, atrial arrhythmias, and paradoxical emboli.

In general, current practice is to refer patients for interatrial defect closure if the patient is symptomatic or the defect results in a significant left-to-right shunt. Evidence for the latter including right ventricular dilation, flattening of the ventricular septum in diastole (caused by elevated right ventricular diastolic pressure from the volume load), and a pulmonary-to-systemic flow (Q_p/Q_s) ratio ≥1.5. All these defect types can be closed surgically with a very low mortality and morbidity in centers with expertise. Many secundum ASDs can be closed by percutaneous transcatheter devices. Device closure requires that the defect is of an appropriate size and has adequate rims for anchoring the device.[17] Attempted device placement in a patient with inadequate rims can result in a failed attempt, device embolization, or erosion into the aorta. Secundum ASDs may be closed surgically (either closed primarily or with a patch). For primum ASDs, the defect is closed with a patch and, in most cases, the associated mitral valve cleft is partially closed with a suture. Sinus venosus septal defects can often be closed by placing a patch to reconstruct the missing portion of the sinus venosus septum, thereby eliminating interatrial and right pulmonary vein-to-right atrial flow ("single patch repair"). A second patch may be placed anteriorly on the superior vena cava to enlarge it ("two patch repair"). In some cases, especially when a right upper pulmonary vein drains relatively high to the superior vena cava, the superior vena cava is transected superior to the anomalous veins and the distal caval end anastomosed to the right atrial appendage (Warden procedure). The sinus venosus defect is then closed in such a way that the proximal superior vena cava and anomalous veins drain to the left atrium. Short-term outcomes for all three techniques are excellent, but caval or pulmonary venous obstruction may develop over time. Rarely, sinus venous defects in older patients may be amenable to percutaneous device closure. For a coronary sinus septal defect, the os of the coronary sinus is usually patched closed. If a left superior vena cava is present, it is redirected to the right atrial side either through ligation when an adequate left innominate vein is present or via a baffle to the right atrium.

Cardiac Magnetic Resonance

CMR can be helpful in older patients, usually adolescents and adults, with a known or suspected ASD and inconclusive transthoracic echocardiographic findings. CMR is also a useful noninvasive alternative to transesophageal echocardiography for determining which patients are candidates for percutaneous device closure rather than surgery.[18] Following device closure, CMR may be useful in excluding device malposition, device interference with the atrioventricular valves and venous blood flow, and thrombus formation. Furthermore, CMR visualizes superior vena cava and pulmonary vein obstruction in those patients following sinus venous defect repair and can quantify mitral regurgitation from a residual cleft after primum ASD repair.

Studies have shown that cine steady-state free precession (SSFP) imaging and velocity-encoded cine imaging are

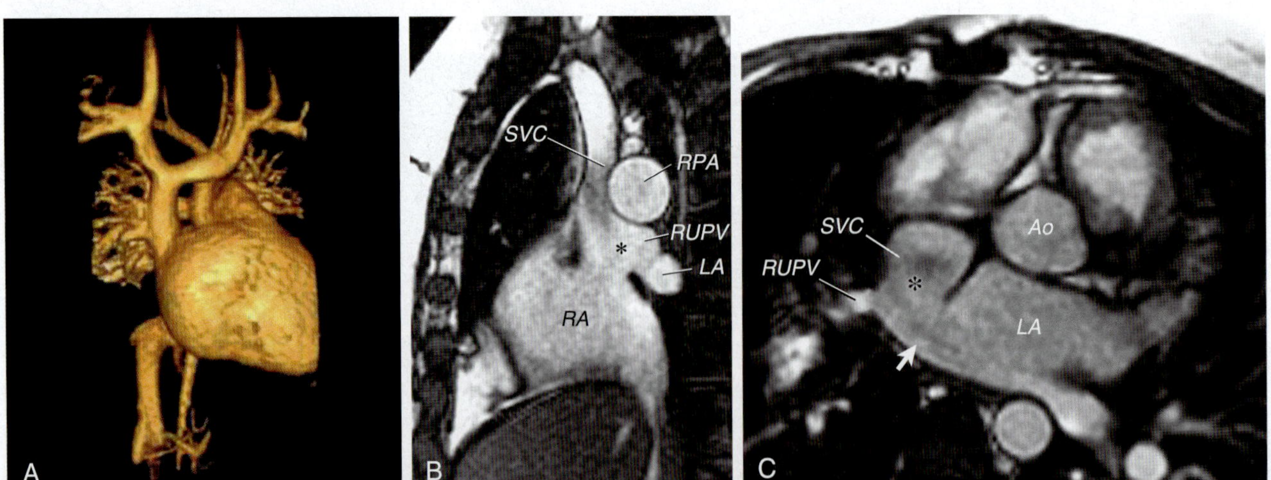

FIG. 42.3 Sinus venosus atrial septal defect. (A) Volume-rendered, contrast-enhanced, three-dimensional magnetic resonance angiography showing several pulmonary veins from the right upper lobe draining into the superior vena cava. (B) Steady-state free precession (SSFP) cine in the sagittal plane showing the defect *(*)* between the right upper pulmonary vein *(RUPV)* and the superior vena cava *(SVC)*. (C) Cine SSFP in the axial plane showing the defect *(*)* between the RUPV and SVC. The *arrow* points to the left atrial orifice of the RUPV. A left-to-right shunt results from the drainage of the RUPV to the SVC and from left atrial blood entering the right atrium through the orifice of the RUPV (*arrow*) and the unroofed wall between the RUPV and the SVC *(*)*. *Ao*, ascending aorta; *LA*, left atrium. (From Valente AM, Sena L, Powell A, Del Nido P, Geva T. Cardiac MRI evaluation of sinus venosus defects: comparison to surgical findings. *Pediatr Cardiol* 2007; 28:51–56.)

able to accurately identify ASD size, shape, proximity to adjacent structures, and associated findings (e.g., anomalous pulmonary venous return).[18–22] Similarly, CMR is useful for diagnosis and preoperative planning in patients with sinus venosus defects.[23,24] Moreover, multiple reports have demonstrated that calculation of the Q_p/Q_s ratio by measuring flow in the main pulmonary artery (Q_p) and ascending aorta (Q_s) agrees closely with catheterization-based oximetry measurements of Q_p/Q_s.[25–27]

In the absence of significant valve regurgitation or an additional shunt, the Q_p/Q_s ratio can also be derived from the right (Q_p) and left (Q_s) ventricular stroke volumes measured from the short-axis cine stack of the ventricles. In clinical practice, it is recommended to measure the Q_p/Q_s ratio by both of these methods and check the data for consistency. In addition, review of the ventricular short-axis cine images also allows one to make a qualitative estimate of right ventricular systolic pressure based on the configuration of the ventricular septum. The septal geometry is concave toward the right ventricle when the right ventricle-to-left ventricle pressure ratio is low and assumes a flat configuration, or even a concave shape toward the left ventricle, as the right ventricle-to-left ventricle pressure ratio increases. Interpretation of the septal configuration may be confounded by factors such as dyssynchronous contraction, conduction delay (e.g., right or left bundle branch block and preexcitation), and a high left ventricular pressure.

The goals of the CMR examination include (1) delineating ASD number, location, size, and rim length; (2) evaluating pulmonary venous return; (3) estimating the right ventricular pressure based on septal configuration; (4) measuring the Q_p/Q_s ratio; and (5) quantifying ventricular volumes, mass, and function. These goals can be achieved by the following protocol:[28]

- Cine SSFP: stack of contiguous thin slices in an axial (sinus venosus defect) or four-chamber plane (secundum ASD) to span the atrial septum and cardiac ends of the vena cavae
- Cine SSFP: stack of contiguous thin slices in an oblique sagittal plane perpendicular to the atrial septum to span the atrial septum and cardiac ends of the vena cavae (Fig. 42.4)
- Velocity-encoded cine: one to three contiguous slices positioned parallel to the atrial septum with through-plane velocity encoding to obtain an *en-face* view of the defect (Fig. 42.4)
- Velocity-encoded cine: stack of contiguous thin slices in a four-chamber and/or oblique sagittal plane to span the atrial septum and with velocity encoding in the direction of ASD flow to visualize the ASD (Fig. 42.2(B))
- Cine SSFP: ventricular long-axis planes and a ventricular short-axis stack from base to apex for quantitative assessment of ventricular dimensions and ejection fraction
- Contrast-enhanced three-dimensional (3D) magnetic resonance angiography (MRA) and/or ECG and respiratory navigator-gated 3D whole-heart angiography of the thorax to confirm the pulmonary venous anatomy
- Blood flow measurements: ascending aorta (Q_s) and main pulmonary artery (Q_p); optional, superior vena cava and descending aorta at the diaphragm (Q_s), and left and right pulmonary arteries (Q_p)

PARTIALLY ANOMALOUS PULMONARY VENOUS CONNECTIONS

In partially anomalous pulmonary venous connections (PAPVCs), one or more (but not all) of the pulmonary veins connect to a systemic vein. PAPVCs may be seen in isolation or as a component in complex congenital heart lesions, particularly heterotaxy syndrome with polysplenia. Common anomalous pulmonary vein connection sites are the left innominate vein, the right superior vena cava, the azygous vein, and the inferior vena cava. Anomalous connection of some or all of the right pulmonary veins to

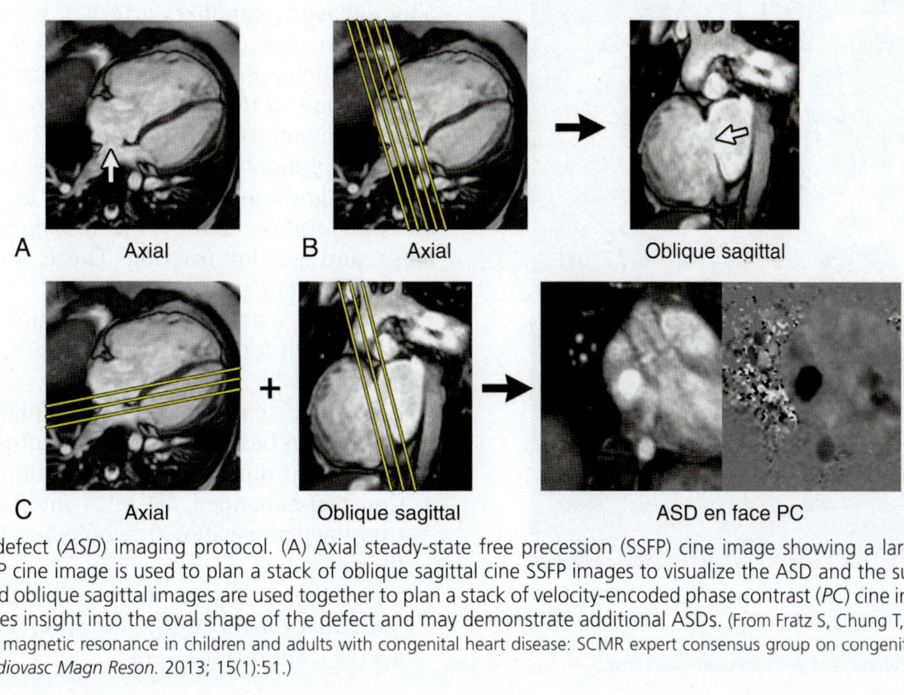

FIG. 42.4 Atrial septal defect (*ASD*) imaging protocol. (A) Axial steady-state free precession (SSFP) cine image showing a large secundum ASD *(white arrow)*. (B) The axial SSFP cine image is used to plan a stack of oblique sagittal cine SSFP images to visualize the ASD and the superior and inferior defect margins. (C) The axial and oblique sagittal images are used together to plan a stack of velocity-encoded phase contrast (*PC*) cine images to visualize the ASD flow en face. This provides insight into the oval shape of the defect and may demonstrate additional ASDs. (From Fratz S, Chung T, Greil GF et al. Guidelines and protocols for cardiovascular magnetic resonance in children and adults with congenital heart disease: SCMR expert consensus group on congenital heart disease. *J Cardiovasc Magn Reson : Off J Soc Cardiovasc Magn Reson*. 2013; 15(1):51.)

the inferior vena cava is termed "scimitar syndrome" (Fig. 42.5). The name is derived from the curvilinear shadow in the right lung on chest radiography caused by the anomalous vein as it descends toward the right hemidiaphragm, which resembles a scimitar, or Turkish sword. Other abnormalities commonly seen in scimitar syndrome include hypoplasia of the right lung and pulmonary artery, secondary dextrocardia, and anomalous systemic arterial collateral vessels, usually from the descending aorta to the right lung.

PAPVC results in a left-to-right shunt as blood draining from the lungs returns to the lungs via the systemic veins and right heart without passing through the systemic arterial circulation. This physiology leads to increased pulmonary blood flow and resembles that of an ASD and other pretricuspid valve shunts. The magnitude of the shunt is determined by the number and size of the involved veins, the site of their connections, the pulmonary vascular resistance, the size of their vascular bed, and the presence of associated defects. Dilation is commonly seen in the systemic veins downstream of the anomalous pulmonary vein insertion site, the right atrium and ventricle, and the pulmonary arteries. Young patients are usually asymptomatic, but dyspnea on exertion becomes increasingly common in the third and fourth decades of life. Development of pulmonary hypertension is rare. Patients may come to attention after auscultation of a pulmonary flow murmur or when diagnostic imaging is performed for another indication. Evidence of right ventricular volume overload with no apparent intracardiac shunt should prompt a search for PAPVC. The presentation of scimitar syndrome varies widely depending on the severity of the associated abnormalities. Infants may be critically ill with respiratory compromise whereas adults may have minimal symptoms.

A single small anomalous pulmonary vein is associated with a modest left-to-right shunt and does not usually require intervention.[29] In those with much or all of the left pulmonary veins returning to the left innominate vein, the connecting vertical vein is usually large and long enough to detach from the innominate vein and anastomose to the left atrium. For veins connecting to the superior vena cava, a baffle within the superior vena cava and across the atrial septum can be constructed to channel the pulmonary venous return to the left atrium similar to sinus venosus defect repair. Alternatively, the superior vena cava can be transected superior to the anomalous veins and the caval end anastomosed to the right atrial appendage (Warden procedure). A baffle across the atrial septum is then created to direct the pulmonary venous flow in the cardiac end of the superior vena cava to the left atrium. Pulmonary veins entering the inferior vena cava can either be baffled through the right atrium to the left atrium or directly anastomosed to the left atrium. The most common postoperative complications seen in patients with PAPVC correction are obstruction and residual defects in the surgically created pathways. CMR examinations following PAPVC repair should include tailored cine SSFP imaging planes to visualize the pulmonary venous connection to the left atrium to assess for obstruction and defects along the surgically created pulmonary venous drainage pathway.

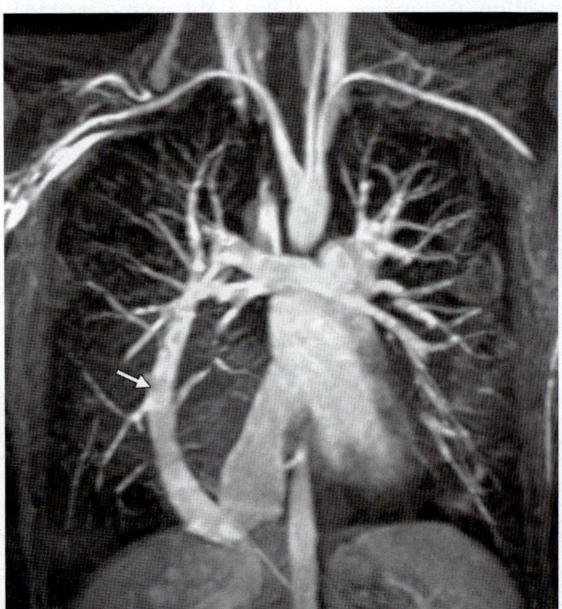

FIG. 42.5 Partially anomalous pulmonary venous connection. Contrast-enhanced three-dimensional magnetic resonance angiogram showing drainage of the right upper pulmonary vein (*arrow*) to the inferior vena cava-right atrial junction in a patient with scimitar syndrome.

Cardiac Magnetic Resonance

Several studies have demonstrated that CMR angiography techniques for PAPVC have a high level of agreement with surgical inspection and x-ray angiography and are more accurate than transthoracic and transesophageal echocardiography.[30–34] In addition to defining anatomy, the size of the shunt can be calculated directly by measuring blood flow in the main pulmonary artery (Q_p) and the ascending aorta (Q_s). In some cases, it may also be possible to measure the flow in the anomalously draining vein itself. In the absence of significant valvular insufficiency, the ventricular stoke volume differential should be equal to the shunt size and thus serve as a useful check. For cases in which there is a hypoplastic pulmonary artery or pulmonary venous pathway obstruction, it is also important to measure blood flow in the branch pulmonary arteries to assess differential flow.

The goals of the CMR examination include (1) delineating pulmonary venous drainage, (2) measuring the Q_p/Q_s ratio and pulmonary artery flow distribution, (3) estimating the right ventricular pressure by evaluating the septal configuration, and (4) calculating ventricular volumes, mass, and ejection fraction. These goals can be achieved by the following protocol:

- Cine SSFP: axial stack from the midliver to the top of the aortic arch for thoracic and upper abdominal vascular anatomy
- Cine SSFP: ventricular long-axis planes and a short-axis stack from base to apex for quantitative assessment of ventricular dimensions and ejection fraction
- Contrast-enhanced 3D MRA and/or ECG and respiratory navigator-gated 3D whole-heart angiography of the thorax
- Blood flow measurements: ascending aorta (Q_s), main pulmonary artery (Q_p), left and right pulmonary arteries (Q_p), anomalous vein

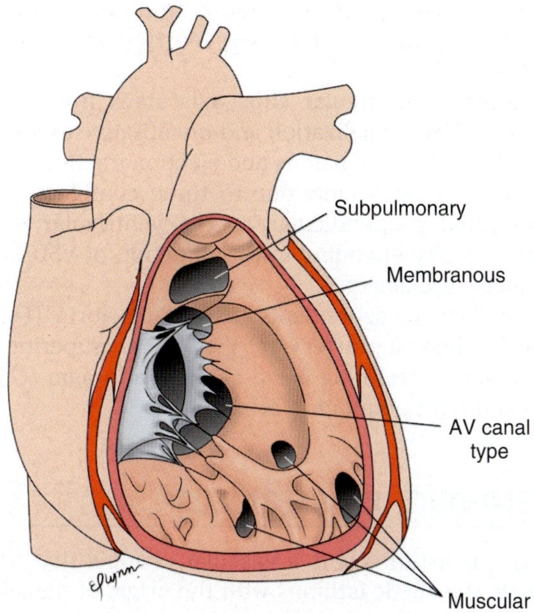

FIG. 42.6 Anatomic types of ventricular septal defects (see text for details). *AV*, Atrioventricular.

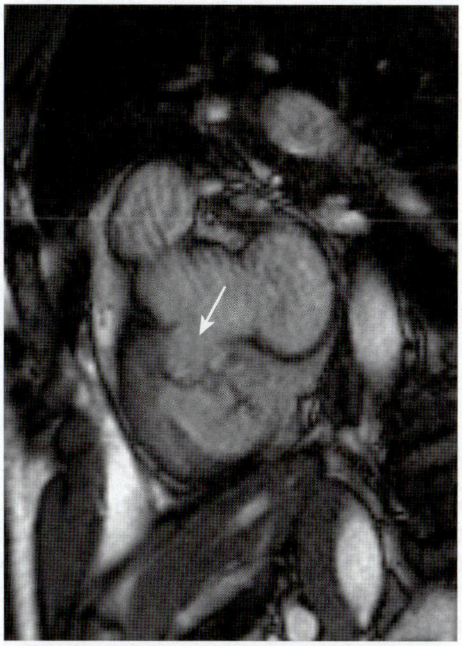

FIG. 42.7 Steady-state free precession cine image illustrating a patient with a large conoventricular ventricular septal defect (*arrow*) partially covered by tricuspid valve tissue.

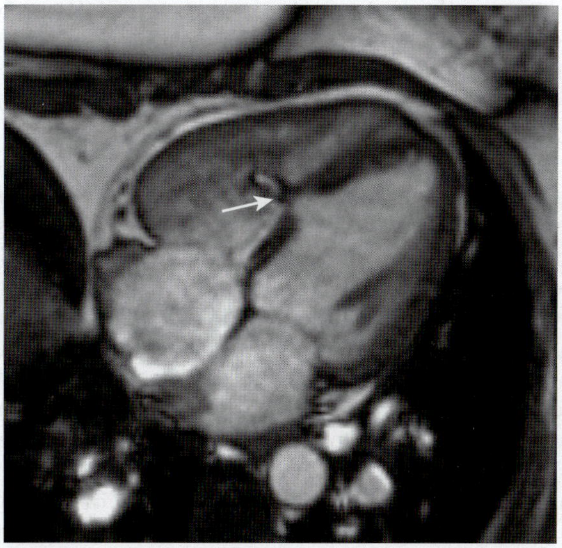

FIG. 42.8 Steady-state free precession cine four-chamber image illustrating a small midmuscular ventricular septal defect *(arrow)*.

VENTRICULAR SEPTAL DEFECTS

A ventricular septal defect (VSD) is a communication between the right and left ventricles through an opening in the ventricular septum. Several VSD anatomic classification systems exist. Fig. 42.6 shows one such system modified from Van Praagh et al., which includes the following: (1) defects at the junction between the conal septum and the muscular septum bordering the membranous septum (referred to as membranous defects) or associated with malalignment of the conal septum (conoventricular defects) (Fig. 42.7), (2) defects in the muscular septum (called muscular or trabecular defects) (Fig. 42.8), (3) defects in the inlet septum (known as atrioventricular canal-type or inlet defects), and 4) defects in the outlet septum (variably called outlet, doubly committed subarterial, subpulmonary, conal septal, or supracristal defects).[35]

The natural history of a VSD relates to the size and location of the defect. Defects in the membranous or muscular septum often become smaller over time and may spontaneously close. In contrast, malalignment conoventricular defects, outlet septum defects, and atrioventricular canal-type defects are usually large and remain so. Consequently, such patients often undergo surgical closure in infancy. Venturi effects associated with VSDs in the membranous or outlet septum may cause aortic valve leaflets (usually the right coronary leaflet) to prolapse through the defect. Although the leaflet prolapse typically reduces the effective orifice size of the defect, it may also lead to aortic insufficiency. VSDs, particularly those associated with turbulent flow jets, also predispose patients to the development of endocarditis.

Symptoms are predominantly determined by the size of the shunt through the VSD which, in turn, is related to the defect size and the relative resistances of the pulmonary and systemic vascular beds. In most situations, pulmonary resistance is lower than systemic resistance, and there is a left-to-right shunt. The resulting increased blood flow to the lungs and left heart may lead to dilation of the pulmonary arteries, pulmonary veins, left atrium, and left ventricle. Since most of the shunt flow passes through the VSD into the right ventricle in systole, right ventricular dilation is usually not present. If the shunt is small and the patient is asymptomatic, an intervention to close the defect is not warranted. When the shunt is large, symptoms from pulmonary overcirculation (e.g., tachypnea, diaphoresis, poor feeding, and slow weight gain) may develop in the first few months of life. If the defect is unlikely to become small over time or if these symptoms cannot be managed medically, surgical closure in infancy is recommended. Untreated, patients with VSDs and large left-to-right shunts may develop irreversible pulmonary hypertension from elevated pulmonary vascular resistance. In such cases, the flow through the defect will become increasingly right to left, resulting in cyanosis (Eisenmenger syndrome).

A surgical approach is by far the most common technique used to close VSDs and carries a low mortality risk, even when performed in the first few months of life. Typically, the surgeon works through the tricuspid valve and applies a patch to cover the defect. In selected patients, such as those with apical defects, a limited right ventriculotomy may be required for effective closure. Experience with transcatheter delivery of occlusion devices is growing, and this approach may be appropriate in selected circumstances.

Cardiac Magnetic Resonance

Transthoracic echocardiography is the primary diagnostic imaging modality in patients with suspected or known VSDs, and is usually adequate. Occasionally, in larger patients acoustic windows may be insufficient and CMR is indicated to define the defect size and location as well as identify associated conditions such as aortic valve prolapse. CMR may also be of use when the hemodynamic burden of a defect is uncertain by providing reliable quantitative data on the Q_p/Q_s ratio and ventricular dimensions and function. Moreover, CMR has been shown to be an important, noninvasive test in the diagnosis and management of defects in the outlet septum when echocardiographic assessment of this region is inadequate.[36]

VSD location and size can be demonstrated by cine gradient echo or spin echo sequences.[37,38] Very small defects may be difficult to resolve; however, the associated turbulent flow can be made conspicuous on gradient echo sequences provided the echo time is long enough to allow for sufficient spin dephasing (Fig. 42.8). It is useful to assess the ventricular septum using stacks of images oriented in at least two planes. The four-chamber plane provides base-to-apex localization whereas the short-axis plane shows the location in the superior-to-inferior axis (Figs. 42.7 and 42.8). Also, as described in the section on ASDs above, the ventricular septal configuration can be used to estimate right ventricular systolic pressure. Finally, quantification of the VSD shunt should be performed by calculating the Q_p/Q_s ratio. This can be accomplished by measuring the net blood flow in the main pulmonary artery (Q_p) and the ascending aorta (Q_s) using velocity-encoded cine CMR.[26,39] Alternatively, in the absence of significant valve regurgitation or other shunts, the ventricular stroke volume data can be used. The Q_p/Q_s ratio is equal to the left ventricular stroke volume divided by the right ventricular stroke volume. In practice, both approaches are recommended and the two results should be compared for consistency.

The goals of the CMR examination include (1) delineating VSD number, location, and size; (2) measuring the Q_p/Q_s ratio; (3) estimating right ventricular pressure by evaluating the septal configuration; (4) calculating ventricular volumes, mass, and ejection fraction; and (5) quantifying aortic valve regurgitation, if significant. These goals can be achieved by the following protocol:

- Cine SSFP: stack of contiguous thin slices in a four-chamber plane to span the ventricular septum for VSD visualization
- Cine SSFP: ventricular short-axis stack from base to apex for VSD visualization and quantitative assessment of ventricular dimensions and ejection fraction
- Velocity-encoded cine: one to three contiguous slices positioned perpendicular to the ventricular septum with velocity encoding in the direction of VSD flow to visualize the defect
- Blood flow measurements: ascending aorta (Q_s) and main pulmonary artery (Q_p); optional, superior vena cava and descending aorta at the diaphragm (Q_s) and left and right pulmonary arteries (Q_p)

PATENT DUCTUS ARTERIOSUS

The ductus arteriosus is a vascular channel that usually connects the aortic isthmus with the origin of the left pulmonary artery (Fig. 42.9). During fetal life, the ductus arteriosus allows the majority of the right ventricular output to bypass the lungs by carrying blood flow to the descending aorta. Normally, the ductus arteriosus closes shortly after birth. A persistent patent ductus arteriosus (PDA) is common in premature infants and is associated with increased morbidity. In full-term infants and children, the clinical course and sequelae of an isolated PDA are usually related to ductal size and direction of flow. In the absence of elevated pulmonary vascular resistance, isolated PDAs have left-to-right flow, leading to increased pulmonary flow and a volume load on the left heart. Larger PDAs cause a significant left-to-right shunt and, if untreated, lead to pulmonary overcirculation, respiratory distress, growth failure, and, eventually, pulmonary vascular disease. Smaller PDAs pose little hemodynamic burden but place the patient at risk for infective endarteritis; the benefit of closure in older children or adults is debated.[40] When indicated, PDA closure can be accomplished either surgically or in the catheterization laboratory using occluding devices.

Cardiac Magnetic Resonance

CMR is seldom requested primarily for assessment of an isolated PDA as this usually presents in childhood and is a straight-forward echocardiographic diagnosis. In several types of complex congenital heart disease, evaluation of the ductus arteriosus is an important element of the examination. For example, in patients with tetralogy of Fallot and pulmonary atresia, the ductus arteriosus may persist and be a significant source of pulmonary blood supply. PDAs can be visualized using a gadolinium-enhanced 3D MRA or electrocardiogram (ECG) and respiratory navigator-gated 3D whole-heart angiography of the thorax.[41] Cine CMR is also useful in detecting PDAs, particularly those that are small with turbulent flow. As with VSD jets, a longer echo time will allow more time for spin dephasing and make the turbulent flow more conspicuous. Blood flow measurements are useful to quantify the Q_p/Q_s ratio. Note that with a PDA and no other shunting lesions, systemic flow (Q_s) is equal to the main pulmonary artery flow and pulmonary flow (Q_p) is equal to ascending

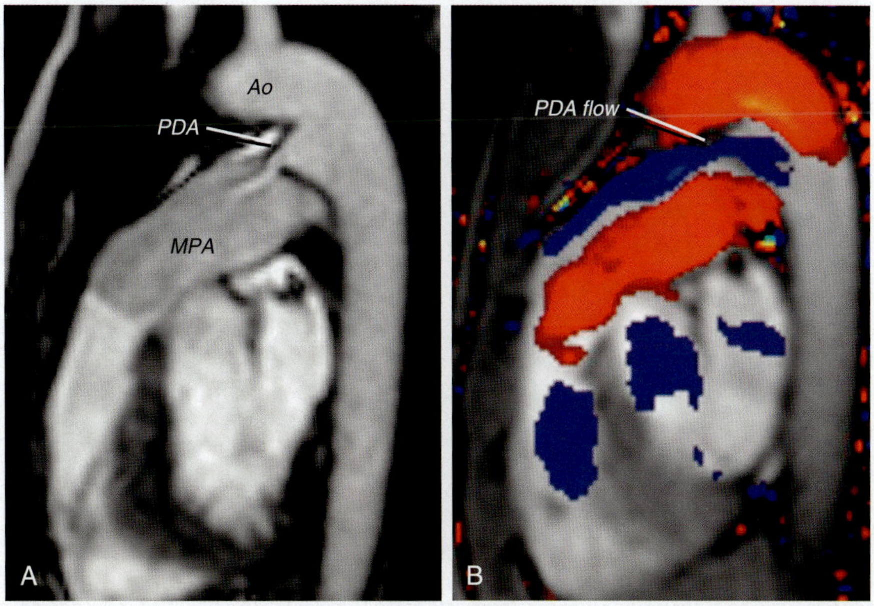

FIG. 42.9 Patent ductus arteriosus (*PDA*). (A) Steady-state free precession cine image in an oblique sagittal plane showing a small patent ductus arteriosus. (B) Color-coded, velocity-encoded cine showing left-to-right flow through the PDA. *Ao*, aorta; *MPA*, main pulmonary artery. (From Geva T, Powell AJ. Magnetic resonance imaging. In: Allen HD, Shaddy RE, Penny DJ, Feltes FT, Cetta F, eds. *Moss and Adams' Heart Disease in Infants, Children, and Adolescents*. 9th ed. Philadelphia: Wolters Kluwer; 2016:373–412.)

aorta flow. It is also helpful to measure ventricular volumes and function and assess right ventricular pressure by evaluating ventricular septal position in systole.

The goals of the CMR examination include (1) delineating the PDA size, (2) measuring the Q_p/Q_s ratio, (3) assessing the direction of PDA flow, (4) estimating the right ventricular pressure by evaluating the septal configuration, and (5) calculating ventricular volumes, mass, and ejection fraction. These goals can be achieved by the following protocol:

- Cine SSFP: stack of contiguous thin slices in an oblique sagittal plane positioned between the transverse aortic arch and the left pulmonary artery for PDA visualization (Fig. 42.9(A))
- Velocity-encoded cine: in the same location as above with velocity encoding in the direction of PDA flow to visualize the defect and direction of flow (Fig. 42.9(B))
- Contrast-enhanced 3D MRA and/or ECG and respiratory navigator-gated whole-heart angiography of the thorax
- Cine SSFP: ventricular short-axis stack from base to apex for quantitative assessment of ventricular dimensions and ejection fraction
- Blood flow measurements: ascending aorta (Q_p) and main pulmonary artery (Q_s); optional, superior vena cava and descending aorta at the diaphragm (Q_s) and left and right pulmonary arteries distal to the PDA (Q_p). *Note that the Q_p is the amount of blood that is from the lungs and, therefore, includes the contribution of flow from the ductus.

COARCTATION OF THE AORTA

Coarctation of the aorta is a discrete narrowing most commonly located just distal to the left subclavian artery at the ductus arteriosus insertion site (Figs. 42.10 and 42.11). Hypoplasia and elongation of the distal transverse arch is a frequent association. Coarctation may be present alone or in combination with other heart lesions including a bicuspid aortic valve, subvalvar and valvar aortic stenosis, mitral valve abnormality, ASD, VSD, persistent PDA, and conotruncal anomaly. Coarctation is a diffuse vascular abnormality and is associated with aortic aneurysm, cerebral aneurysms, and endothelial dysfunction. Awareness of these abnormalities is important as the entire aorta and cerebral vessels should be imaged in these patients.

Infants often present with symptoms of heart failure and systemic hypoperfusion as the ductus arteriosus closes; if untreated, they may progress to shock or death. Older children and adults typically present with difficult to control systemic hypertension and diminished lower extremity pulses or arm-leg blood pressure discrepancy. Note that there may be little upper-to-lower extremity blood pressure differential even with important aortic obstruction when there is a significant collateral circulation bypassing the obstruction. Even in asymptomatic patients, relief of the aortic obstruction is indicated for hemodynamically significant lesions because of the high rate of late complications, including congestive heart failure, systemic hypertension, premature coronary artery disease, ruptured aortic or cerebral aneurysms, stroke, aortic dissection, infective endarteritis, and premature death.[42]

Therapeutic options for coarctation include surgical repair and percutaneous balloon angioplasty and stent placement. Currently, resection of the coarctation with an end-to-end anastomosis and augmentation of the transverse arch, if needed, is the most widely practiced surgical repair and has the lowest incidence of recurrent obstruction. The subclavian flap procedure was performed in the early surgical experience and involved transecting the left subclavian artery and placing it over

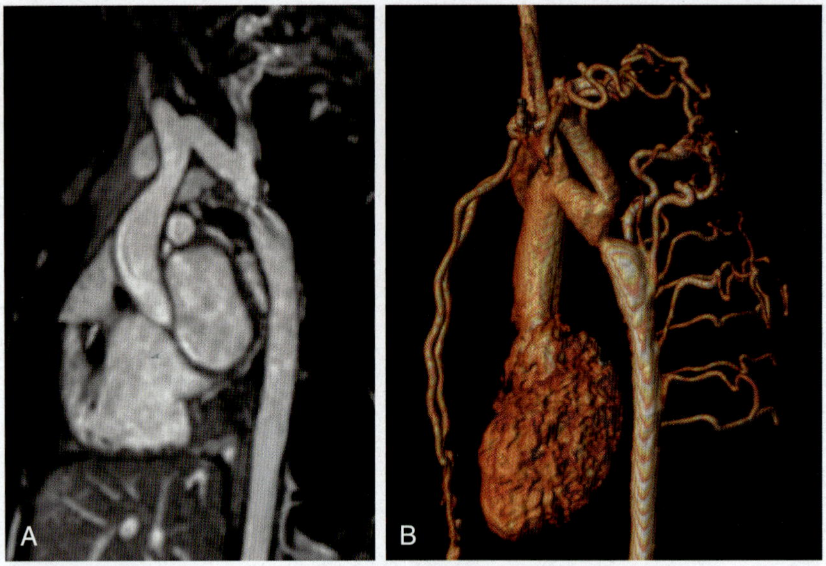

FIG. 42.10 Aortic coarctation. (A) Electrocardiogram and respiratory navigator-gated three-dimensional (3D) steady-state free precession oblique sagittal reformat showing severe discrete narrowing at the aortic isthmus with an associated turbulent flow jet. (B) Volume-rendered, contrast-enhanced 3D magnetic resonance angiography revealing several tortuous collateral vessels and dilated internal mammary arteries.

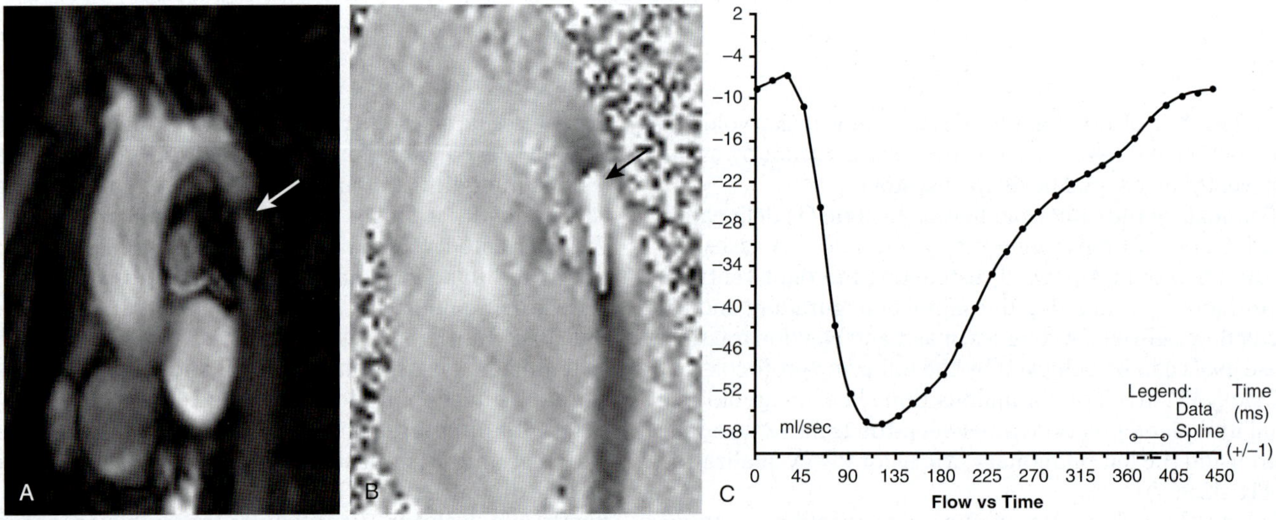

FIG. 42.11 (A) Steady-state free precession cine long-axis image showing coarctation of the aorta (*arrow*) with dephasing of flow distal to the area of coarctation. (B) Velocity-encoded, phase-contrast, in-plane image at the same position as (A) illustrating flow acceleration across the coarctation of the aorta (*arrow*). (C) Flow analysis of velocity-encoded phase contrast through plane image at the level of the diaphragm denoting decreased amplitude and forward flow in diastole characteristic of proximal obstruction.

the narrowed portion of the descending aorta. Patients who have undergone this procedure will no longer have the left subclavian artery attached to the transverse arch. Some patients with complex CoA (coarctation of the aorta) have undergone interposition graft repairs, and those with Dacron material are particularly susceptible to aneurysm formation. Coarctation of the aorta in infants is treated surgically in the majority of centers because of the lower risk of residual obstruction, recurrence, and technique-related complications compared with percutaneous interventions.[43] In the event of recurrent coarctation following surgical repair, balloon angioplasty with or without stent placement is often the preferred approach. Coarctation in older children or adults is increasingly being treated primarily by percutaneous interventions. Regardless of the initial treatment, subsequent surveillance for restenosis, aneurysm formation, and dissection is warranted.[44]

Cardiac Magnetic Resonance

In young children, transthoracic echocardiography may be the only diagnostic imaging needed, however, CMR provides high-quality anatomic imaging of the aortic arch in its entirety (Fig. 42.10), assessment of the hemodynamic severity of the obstruction, and quantitative evaluation of left ventricular mass and function. In a retrospective study of 84 adult patients following intervention for coarctation of the aorta, Therrien et al. showed that the combination of clinical assessment and CMR on every patient was more cost effective for detecting complications than combinations that relied on echocardiography or chest radiography as imaging modalities.[45] Other studies have shown the utility of CMR in infants and children with coarctation and other anomalies of the aortic arch.[46–48] Computed tomography (CT) can also provide excellent anatomic imaging of the aorta but has the disadvantage of ionizing radiation exposure, making it a less attractive modality for serial follow-up.

With regard to aortic anatomy, careful attention should be given to the transverse aortic arch and isthmus, brachiocephalic vessels, collateral vessels that may bypass the obstruction, and possible aneurysms or dissections at the repair sites. Regions of vessel narrowing should ideally be measured in cross-section as elliptical lesions are common. If a coarctation of the aorta is present, its diameter, length, and distance to neighboring vessels should be reported since they may influence decisions regarding percutaneous intervention. Given the association of a bicuspid aortic valve with coarctation, the aortic valve morphology should be noted as well as the dimensions of the aortic root and ascending aorta, as they may be dilated.

Blood velocity and flow measurements with CMR have been used to gain insight into the functional significance of an obstruction. One approach has been to assess the flow pattern in the descending aorta distal to the coarctation, preferably at the level of the diaphragm (Fig. 42.11(C)). Characteristics suggestive of a hemodynamically significant coarctation include decreased peak flow, decreased time-averaged flow, delayed onset of descending aorta flow compared with the onset of flow in the ascending aorta, decreased acceleration rate, and prolonged deceleration with increased antegrade diastolic flow.[49–52] Another approach to assessing coarctation severity is to measure the peak coarctation jet velocity and estimate a pressure gradient using the modified Bernoulli equation.[53–56] Note, however, that such measurements may be technically difficult in a long, tortuous coarctation segment and that the pressure estimates may not be indicative of anatomic severity because of collateral flow. Finally, CMR has been used to quantify collateral flow entering the descending aorta distal to the obstruction via retrograde flow from the intercostal arteries or vessels arising off the aortic arch and arch branches.[50,57–59] With this technique, proximal flow is measured just proximal or distal to the site of obstruction, and distal flow in the descending aorta at the level of the diaphragm. A greater distal-to-proximal flow ratio is seen with increased collateral flow and suggests more severe obstruction. If little collateral flow is found, the surgeon may elect to perform left heart bypass to the descending aorta during the repair to reduce the risk of spinal cord ischemic injury when correction requires interruption of aortic flow.

CMR evaluation of a coarctation should also include calculation of left ventricular dimensions, ejection fraction, mass, and mass-to-volume ratio. This data is clinically relevant because hypertension is often present and may lead to ventricular hypertrophy and dysfunction.[60]

The goals of the CMR examination include (1) assessing the aortic arch anatomy and degree of obstruction; (2) calculating ventricular volumes, mass, and ejection fraction; and (3) evaluating aortic valve morphology and function. These goals can be achieved by the following protocol.[28]

- Cine SSFP: stack of contiguous thin slices in an oblique sagittal plane oriented in long axis (parallel) to the aortic arch for evaluation of arch anatomy
- Black-blood spin echo (optional): stack of contiguous thin slices in an oblique sagittal plane oriented in long axis (parallel) to the aortic arch for evaluation of arch anatomy. This is particularly valuable following endovascular stent placement because there is less metallic susceptibility artifact than with cine sequences.
- Cine SSFP: ventricular long-axis planes and a short-axis stack from base to apex for quantitative assessment of ventricular size, mass, and ejection fraction
- Contrast-enhanced 3D MRA and/or ECG and respiratory navigator-gated 3D SSFP imaging of the thorax (Fig. 42.10)
- Blood flow measurements: ascending aorta, main pulmonary artery, descending aorta at the level of the diaphragm for assessment of the descending aorta flow profile (Fig. 42.11(C)) and aortic valve function.
- Blood flow measurements (optional): just distal to the coarctation in long axis and cross-section for measurement of the peak velocity and/or quantitation of collateral flow

Four-dimensional velocity mapping is an emerging technique for showing turbulence at the CoA and characterizing altered aortic velocity profiles, providing insight into which patients may be at higher risk for aortic wall complications, such as dissection.

TETRALOGY OF FALLOT

Tetralogy of Fallot (TOF) is the most common type of cyanotic congenital heart disease.[61] Although TOF involves several anatomic components, the anomaly is thought to result from a single developmental anomaly: underdevelopment of the subpulmonary infundibulum (conus).[62] The resulting pathology is notable for anterior, superior, and leftward deviation of the infundibular (conal) septum causing subpulmonary stenosis; pulmonary valve stenosis from annular hypoplasia, thickened leaflets, and abnormal commissures; a large conoventricular septal defect; and overriding aortic valve above the ventricular septum. The degree of right ventricular outflow obstruction varies from mild to complete obstruction (i.e., TOF with pulmonary atresia). The mediastinal pulmonary arteries are often small and may even be discontinuous or absent. In patients with pulmonary atresia or absent branch pulmonary arteries, pulmonary blood flow comes from a patent ductus arteriosus and/or collateral vessels arising from the aorta and its branches. Approximately 5%–6% of patients with TOF have a major coronary artery crossing the anterior aspect of the right ventricular outflow tract.[63] Most commonly, it is the left anterior descending coronary artery that arises from the right coronary artery and traverses the infundibular free wall to reach the anterior interventricular groove. Preoperative identification of a major coronary artery crossing the right ventricular outflow tract is important to avoid inadvertent damage to the coronary artery during surgical relief of right ventricular outflow tract obstruction. Additionally, approximately 25% of patients with TOF have a right aortic arch.

Although the clinical presentation and course of patients with TOF varies, most patients develop cyanosis during the first year of life. In the current era, the majority of patients undergo surgical repair in infancy or childhood, although older adults may have first undergone a palliative shunt (Blalock-Taussig-Thomas, Waterston, or Potts shunt) as a young child and then undergone a complete repair at an older age. A typical repair includes patch closure of the VSD and right ventricular outflow tract obstruction relief using a combination of resection of obstructive muscle bundles and an overlay patch. When the pulmonary valve annulus is moderately or severely hypoplastic, the right ventricular outflow tract patch is extended across the pulmonary valve annulus into the main pulmonary artery, destroying the valve mechanism and leading to pulmonary regurgitation. In patients with TOF and pulmonary atresia, or when a major coronary artery crosses the right ventricular outflow tract, a conduit—either a homograft or a prosthetic tube—is placed between the right ventricular outflow tract and the pulmonary arteries.

Patients undergoing surgical repair of TOF as young children have excellent short-term survival.[64] However, they experience significant morbidity and mortality related to biventricular dysfunction and arrhythmia in their adult years.[65–67] These sequelae are believed to be at least in part related to chronic pulmonary regurgitation caused by efforts to relieve pulmonary valve stenosis with the initial TOF repair. Thus, pulmonary valve replacement is often performed in later life.[68,69] Other common concerns in repaired TOF patients include right ventricular outflow tract or pulmonary arterial obstruction, tricuspid regurgitation, and residual ASDs and VSDs.

Cardiac Magnetic Resonance

PREOPERATIVE

For most infants, echocardiography provides all of the necessary diagnostic information for surgical repair; however, when the pulmonary arteries are hypoplastic and aortopulmonary collateral vessels are suspected, other modalities are often needed to adequately delineate these structures. Contrast-enhanced MRA is well-suited for this task. Compared with conventional x-ray angiography, MRA has been shown to be highly accurate in depicting all sources of pulmonary blood supply in patients with complex pulmonary stenosis or atresia, including infants with multiple small aortopulmonary collaterals.[32,41]

POSTOPERATIVE

CMR provides a comprehensive imaging assessment of postoperative TOF patients and its use is recommended by a number of expert guideline statements.[70–73] Accurate quantification of right ventricle (RV) size, function, and mass is particularly important in repaired TOF patients, as RV dilatation, dysfunction, and hypertrophy are associated with adverse outcomes in this group.[74,75] Pulmonary regurgitation is the most common sequelae of TOF repair and is often associated with RV dilation (Fig. 42.12(A, B)), predisposing to RV dysfunction, arrhythmias, and death. Phase-contrast sequences assess antegrade and retrograde flow across the main pulmonary artery (Fig. 42.13), and studies demonstrate this to be a highly reproducible technique for quantifying pulmonary regurgitation volume.[76] Pulmonary regurgitation fraction is calculated as retrograde flow volume divided

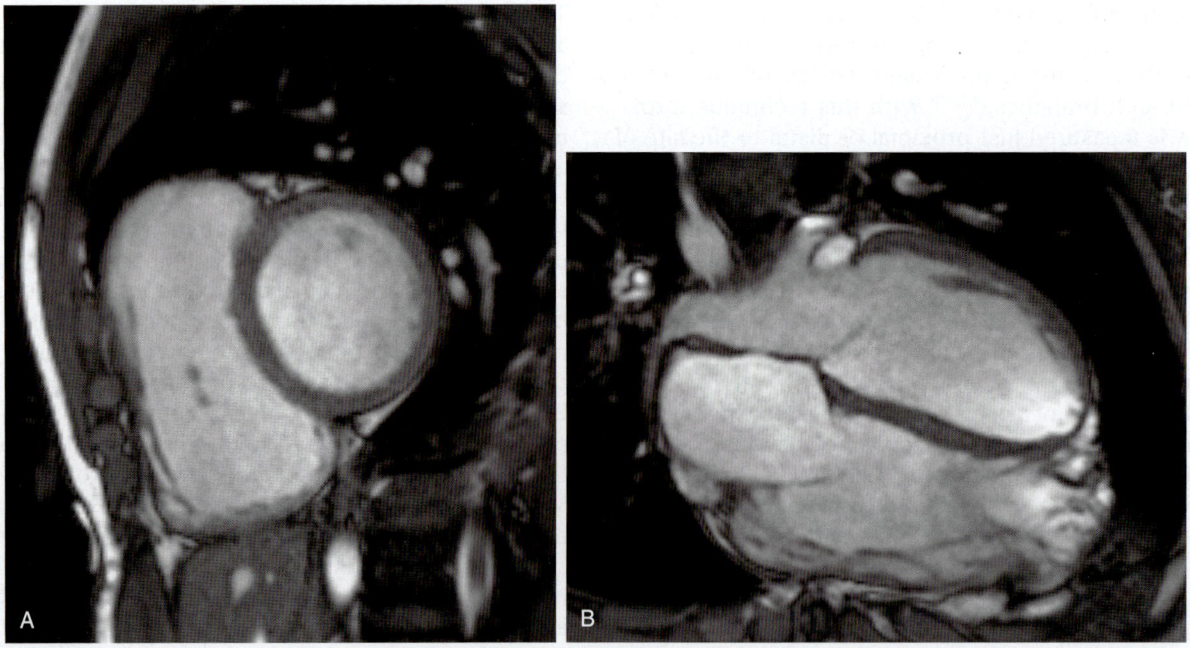

FIG. 42.12 Short-axis (A) and four-chamber (B) steady-state free precession cine images illustrating right ventricular dilation.

by antegrade flow volume, and in our laboratory a PR (pulmonary regurgitation) fraction greater than 40% is considered severe. CMR is useful for determining the geometry of the right ventricular outflow tract (RVOT) (Fig. 42.14(A, B)) and identifying potential candidates for percutaneous pulmonary valve placement. Delineation of the coronary artery course is essential prior to any RVOT intervention, as an anomalous coronary artery coursing across the RVOT (5%–6%) may complicate both surgical and transcatheter pulmonic valve implantation.

There are several mechanisms that lead to tricuspid regurgitation (TR) in repaired TOF patients, including annular dilation, structural valve abnormalities, or as a consequence of valve disruption during prior TOF repair.[77] CMR allows for quantification of TR, and significant TR should be considered in surgical plans at the time of pulmonary valve replacement (PVR).

Ascending aortic dilation is common in adults with repaired TOF; however, aortic dissection is exceedingly rare. In fact, up to 25% of adults with repaired TOF have an aortic root diameter >4 cm, however, only 2.3% have an aortic diameter >5 cm.[78] Some patients develop progressive dilation of the aortic root that can lead to significant aortic regurgitation.[79]

In an effort to improve risk stratification, a growing number of studies have linked CMR data to adverse outcomes. The International Multicenter TOF Registry (INDICATOR) cohort demonstrated that right ventricular hypertrophy and decreased left and right ventricular ejection fraction measured by CMR are associated with death or sustained ventricular tachycardia.[80] Focal fibrosis as identified by late gadolinium enhancement (LGE) is common after TOF repair (Fig. 42.15), and a greater extent of right ventricular involvement is associated with older age, worse symptoms, exercise intolerance, right ventricular dysfunction, and clinical arrhythmia.[81] The utility of diffuse fibrosis assessment using T1 measurement techniques is now being explored.[82,83]

The goals of the CMR examination include (1) quantitative assessment of biventricular volume, mass, stroke volume, and ejection fraction; (2) imaging the right ventricular outflow tract, pulmonary arteries, aorta, and aortopulmonary collaterals; (3) quantification of pulmonary regurgitation, tricuspid regurgitation, cardiac output, and the Q_p/Q_s ratio; and (4) assessment of myocardial fibrosis. These objectives can be achieved with the following protocol.[28]

- Cine SSFP: ventricular long-axis planes and a short-axis stack from base to apex for quantitative assessment of ventricular size, mass, and ejection fraction
- Cine SSFP: stack parallel to the right ventricular outflow tract
- Cine SSFP: axial plane to image the branch pulmonary arteries
- Contrast-enhanced 3D MRA and/or ECG and respiratory navigator-gated 3D SSFP imaging of the thorax

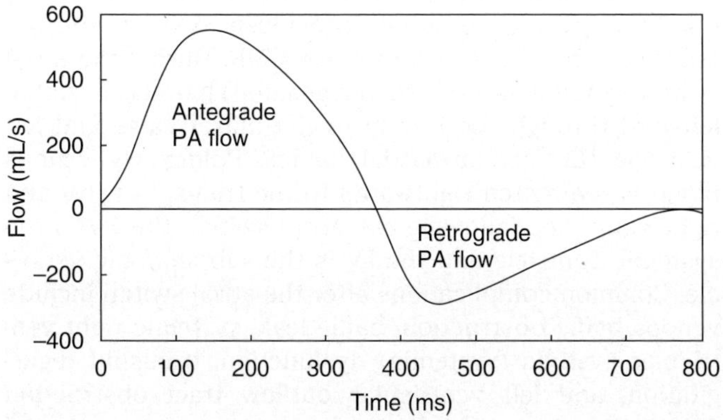

FIG. 42.13 Flow analysis of velocity-encoded phase contrast thru-plane image at the level of the right ventricular outflow tract. Reversal of flow in diastole as a result of pulmonary regurgitation is seen. *PA*, pulmonary artery.

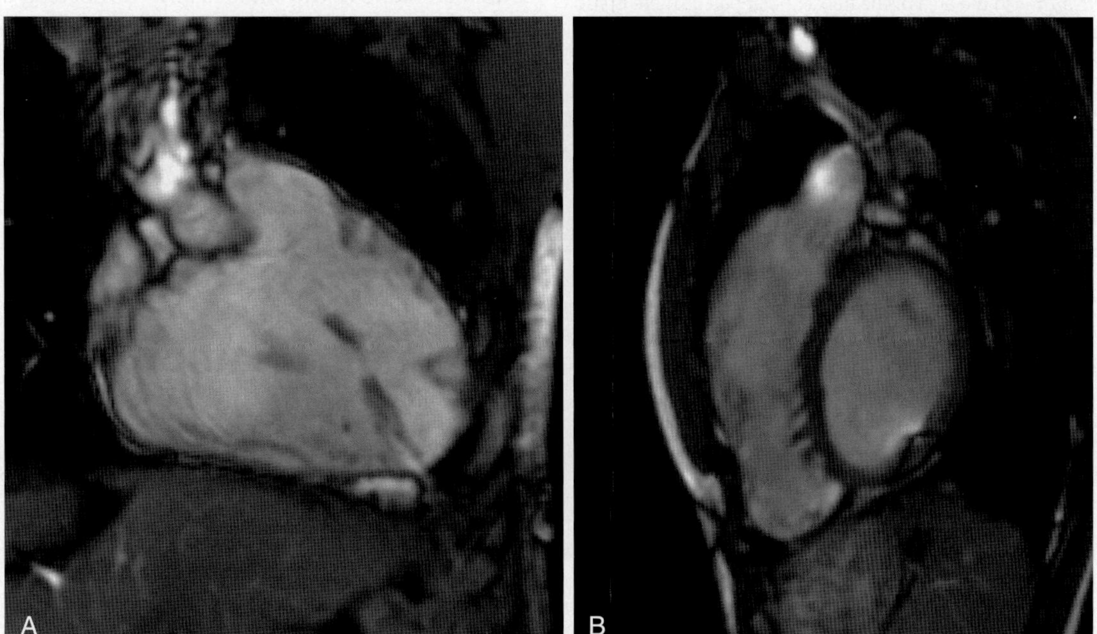

FIG. 42.14 Steady-state free precession cine image long-axis views visualizing the right ventricular outflow tract in coronal (A) and sagittal (B) views.

- Blood flow measurements: main and branch pulmonary arteries, ascending aorta, and atrioventricular (AV) valves
- LGE: ventricular long- and short-axis planes

TRANSPOSITION OF THE GREAT ARTERIES

Transposition of the great arteries (TGA) is defined as discordant alignments between the ventricles and the great arteries; the aorta arises from the right ventricle and the pulmonary artery arises from the left ventricle. The most common type of TGA and the focus of the subsequent discussion is viscero-atrial situs solitus (S), ventricular D-loop (D), and dextro malposition of the aortic valve relative to the pulmonary valve (D). This anatomical arrangement can be summarized as (S,D,D) TGA. Associated cardiac anomalies with their approximate prevalence include VSDs in 45% of patients, coarctation or interrupted aortic arch in 12%, pulmonary stenosis in 5%, right ventricular hypoplasia in 4%, and juxtaposition of the atrial appendages in 2%.[84] The principal physiological abnormality is that desaturated systemic venous blood flows to the right atrium, right ventricle, and aorta, and oxygenated pulmonary venous blood flows to the left atrium and left ventricle and then back to the lungs. These parallel systemic and pulmonary circulations result in profound hypoxemia. Consequently, survival depends on the presence of an ASD, VSD, and/or PDA that allows mixing of blood between the systemic and pulmonary circulations.

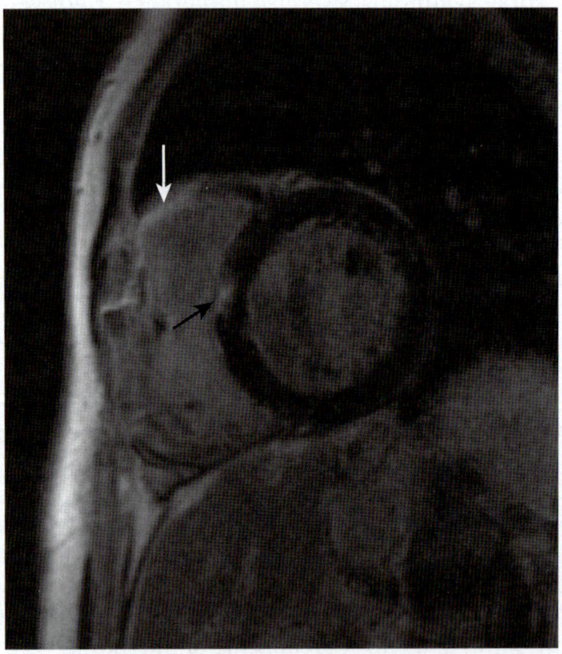

FIG. 42.15 Late gadolinium enhancement image in a patient with repaired tetralogy of Fallot. There is hyperenhancement in the right ventricular outflow tract (*white arrow*) in the area of the transannular patch. There is also septal hyperenhancement (*black arrow*).

For several decades beginning in the late 1950s, the atrial switch procedure was used to treat D-loop TGA and is often described by the eponymous Mustard or Senning procedures (Fig. 42.16).[85,86] Even though the atrial switch has been largely abandoned (see below), there is a large population of adults previously treated with the atrial switch who are referred for CMR. During the atrial switch, systemic venous (deoxygenated) blood is rerouted leftward through the atrium to the mitral valve and left ventricle (LV) by intraatrial baffles. Pulmonary venous blood is redirected rightwards to the tricuspid valve and right ventricle. Following the atrial switch, the RV is the systemic ventricle and the LV is the subpulmonic ventricle. Common complications after the atrial switch include venous baffle obstruction, baffle leak, systemic right ventricular systolic (systemic) dysfunction, tricuspid regurgitation, and left ventricular outflow tract obstruction (pulmonary stenosis).[87–89]

In the 1990s, the arterial switch operation (ASO) succeeded the atrial switch as the preferred treatment for D-loop TGA (Fig. 42.17). In the ASO, the great arteries are transected above the sinuses and the aorta is brought posteriorly to align with the LV while the pulmonary arteries

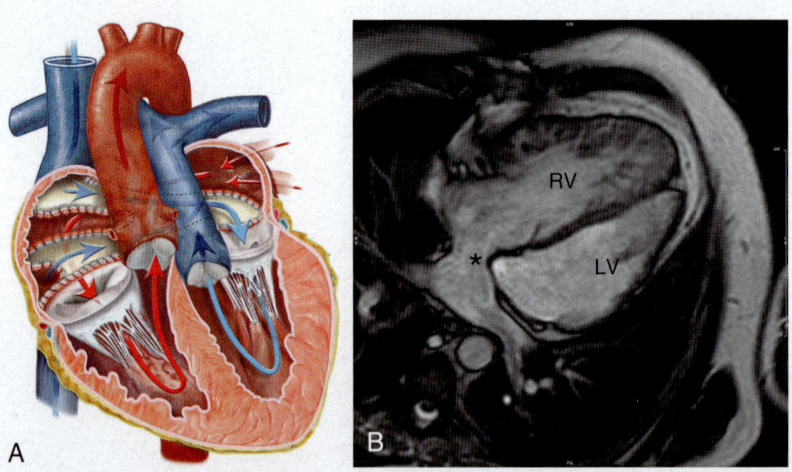

FIG. 42.16 (A) The atrial switch operation (Mustard or Senning) for D-loop transposition of the great arteries. The atrial switch procedure uses intraatrial baffles to redirect systemic venous return to the subpulmonic left ventricle and pulmonary venous return to the systemic right ventricle. (B) Steady-state free precession cine four-chamber image. Note the thin-walled subpulmonic ventricle and hypertrophied systemic right ventricle. The * indicates the pulmonary venous pathway. *LV*, Left ventricle; *RV*, right ventricle. (From Krieger EVDJ. Transposition of the Great Arteries. In: CM O, ed. *Practice of Clinical Echocardiography.* 5th ed. Philadelphia: Elsevier Saunders; 2017.)

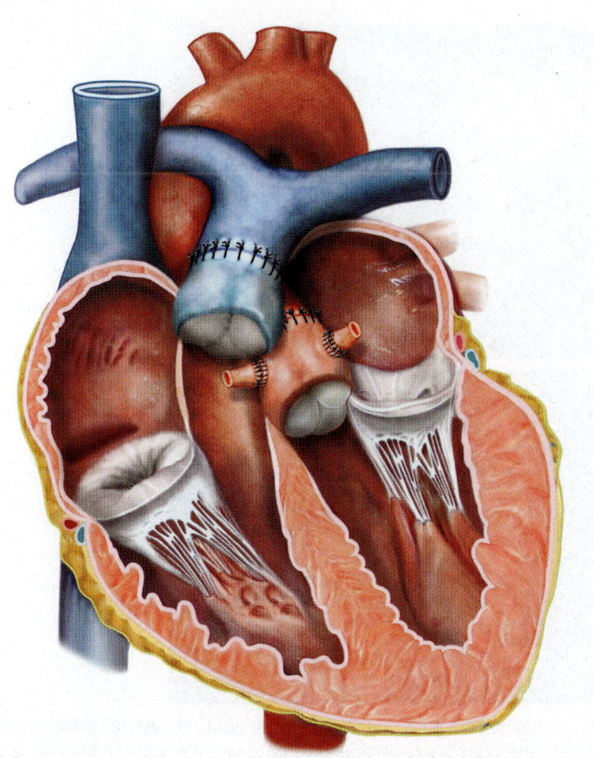

FIG. 42.17 The arterial switch procedure. This provides for a systemic left ventricle and a subpulmonic right ventricle but requires a neonatal coronary transfer. (From Krieger EVDJ. Transposition of the Great Arteries. In: CM O, ed. *Practice of Clinical Echocardiography.* 5th ed. Philadelphia: Elsevier Saunders; 2017.)

are brought anteriorly where they straddle the aorta to come into alignment with the RV. A coronary artery translocation is performed. Late complications after the ASO include neoaortic dilation and regurgitation, supravalvar pulmonic stenosis, branch pulmonary artery stenosis, and coronary artery obstruction.[90–92]

The Rastelli operation is performed on those with a VSD and pulmonic stenosis. In the Rastelli operation, a VSD patch is fashioned to baffle oxygenated blood across the VSD to the anterior aorta. The pulmonic artery is oversewn and an RV-to-pulmonary artery conduit is inserted. Late complications include dysfunction of the right ventricle-to-pulmonary artery conduit, residual VSD, and left ventricular outflow tract obstruction.[93]

Cardiac Magnetic Resonance

POSTOPERATIVE ATRIAL SWITCH OPERATION

CMR has a central role in the noninvasive imaging surveillance of patients who have undergone an atrial switch operation. Assessment of the systemic right ventricle, a key concern in this patient group, can be difficult by echocardiography because of its substernal position and complex shape. CMR, however, routinely provides complete tomographic imaging of the right ventricle, which allows for accurate and reproducible measurements of volume, mass, and ejection fraction.[94,95] CMR is also useful for evaluating the systemic and pulmonary venous baffle pathways for obstruction and leaks.[96,97] The physiologic impact of baffle leaks can be gauged by measuring blood flow in the main pulmonary artery and ascending aorta to calculate the Q_p/Q_s ratio. Note, however, that a Q_p/Q_s ratio close to 1 can be seen even in large baffle leaks when there is bidirectional flow; thus, anatomic imaging information and systemic oxygen saturation must also be considered.

Studies in patients who have undergone an atrial switch operation have found right ventricular LGE indicative of focal myocardial fibrosis, though the reported prevalence of this finding varies.[98–101] In cross-sectional studies, the presence and extent of LGE have been associated with greater age, RV dysfunction, reduced peak oxygen uptake, electrophysiological parameters, arrhythmia, and adverse clinical events. The value of LGE comes from a longitudinal study of 55 subjects who underwent the atrial switch, and right ventricular LGE was independently associated with a composite endpoint primarily composed of atrial tachyarrhythmia.[100]

The goals of the CMR evaluation include (1) quantitative assessment of the systemic right ventricular volume, mass, and ejection fraction; (2) imaging of the systemic and pulmonary venous pathways for obstruction and baffle leaks; (3) quantitation of tricuspid valve regurgitation; (4) evaluation of the left and right ventricular outflow tracts for obstruction, and (5) assessment of myocardial fibrosis. These goals can be achieved with the following protocol.[28]

- Cine SSFP: axial stack from the midliver through the top of the aortic arch for dynamic imaging of the venous pathways, atrioventricular valve regurgitation, and the great arteries
- Cine SSFP: oblique planes to image the superior and inferior limbs of the systemic venous pathway in long axis (Fig. 42.18)
- Cine SSFP: ventricular long-axis planes to assess ventricular function and the outflow tracts
- Cine SSFP: ventricular short-axis stack from base to apex for quantitative assessment of ventricular size, mass, and ejection fraction
- Contrast-enhanced 3D MRA and/or ECG and respiratory navigator-gated 3D whole-heart angiography of the chest
- Blood flow measurements: main pulmonary artery, ascending aorta, tricuspid valve, and mitral valve
- LGE: ventricular long- and short-axis planes

POSTOPERATIVE ARTERIAL SWITCH OPERATION

Studies have shown that detection of pulmonary artery stenosis in ASO patients by CMR is accurate and superior to the information obtained by echocardiography (Fig. 42.19).[102–104] CMR can also provide high-resolution imaging of the proximal coronary arteries and define their relationship to the surrounding structures such as the aorta and main pulmonary artery.[105–107] The largest report consisted of 84 CMR examinations and yielded diagnostic image quality of the proximal coronary arteries in 95% and showed stenosis in 11% of patients.[107] There are two principal CMR techniques to diagnose inducible myocardial ischemia: (1) evaluation for perfusion defects using vasodilator stress agents (e.g., adenosine or dipyridamole) and (2) evaluation of wall motion, most commonly using dobutamine stress. In addition, the LGE technique is highly sensitive for detecting myocardial infarction

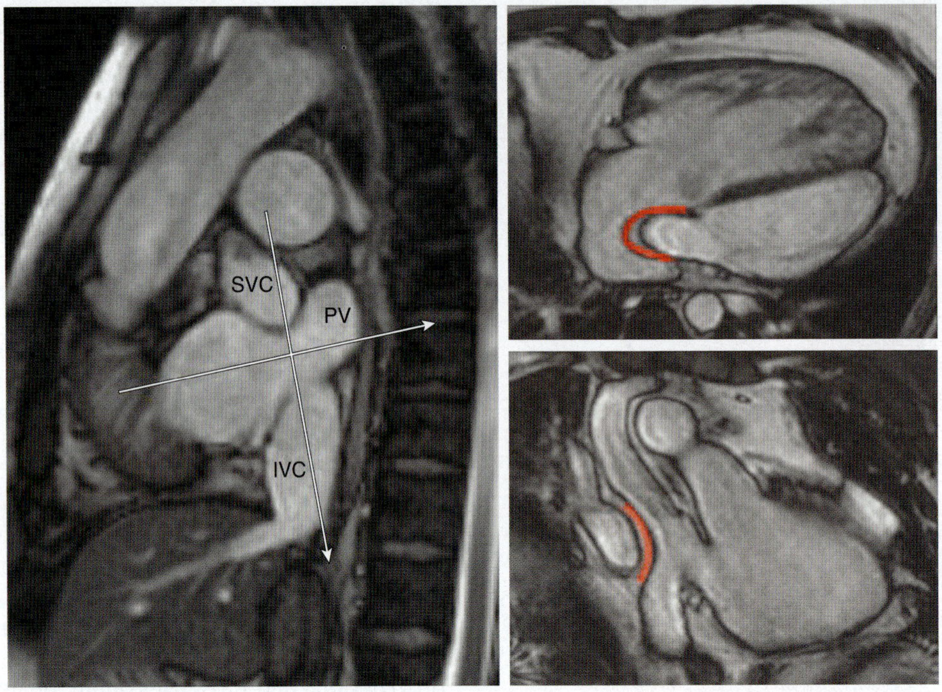

FIG. 42.18 An approach to the initial plane selection for cardiovascular magnetic resonance of a Mustard/Senning patient. In sagittal projections, the superior vena cava (*SVC*) and inferior vena cava (*IVC*) are identified at the point where the pulmonary venous (*PV*) pathway transects them. Using these landmarks provides horizontal and vertical long-axis views (*smaller panels at right*) that can be used for additional imaging, starting with a short-axis scout stack. *Red* denotes the location of the baffle. (From Broberg CS. Cardiac magnetic resonance imaging of the patient with an atrial switch palliation for transposition of the great arteries. *Prog Pediat Cardiol*. 2014; 38:49–55.)

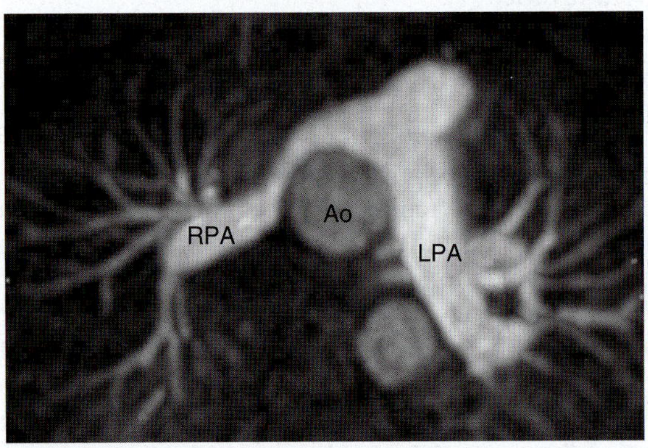

FIG. 42.19 Axial contrast-enhanced magnetic resonance angiogram demonstrating the relationship of the pulmonary arteries and ascending aorta after an arterial switch operation with LeCompte maneuver. Branch pulmonary artery stenosis often occurs, where the pulmonary arteries are draped over the ascending aorta. Quantifying differential pulmonary blood flow provides information to the hemodynamic significance of narrowing. *Ao*, Aorta; *LPA*, left pulmonary artery; *RPA*, right pulmonary artery.

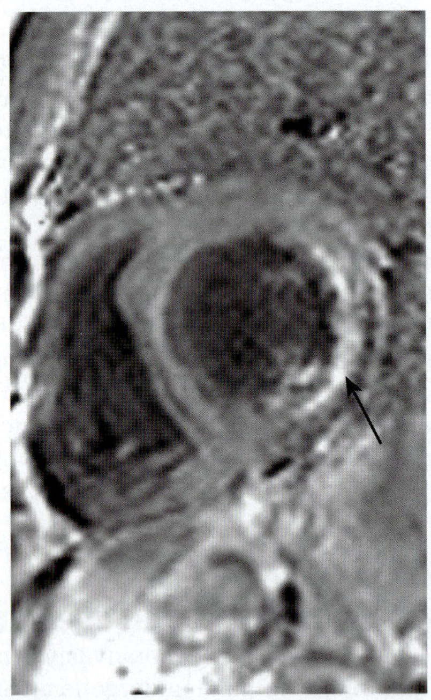

FIG. 42.20 Black-blood late gadolinium enhancement image illustrating a subendocardial infarction in the lateral wall (*arrow*) in a patient with D-loop transposition of the great arteries and history of the arterial switch procedure.

and focal fibrosis (Fig. 42.20). In two reports describing a total of 55 asymptomatic subjects with prior ASO, no defects were detected with stress perfusion CMR.[106,108] Moreover, the LGE technique has identified prior myocardial infarction in only a small proportion of patients after ASO.[106,108,109] Thus, based on these studies, both CMR stress imaging and LGE appear to have a low positive yield in asymptomatic ASO patients. Larger studies that include symptomatic patients and have longer-term follow-up are needed to better define the indications and prognostic value of these CMR techniques.

The goals of the CMR evaluation include (1) quantitative assessment of biventricular size and function; (2) imaging the left and right ventricular outflow tracts for obstruction; (3) imaging the aorta, main pulmonary artery, and branch pulmonary arteries for obstruction; (4) measurement of aortic root size; (5) quantitation of aortic and pulmonary valve regurgitation; (6) identification of residual atrial and ventricular septal defects and calculation of the Q_p/Q_s ratio; and (7) description of the proximal coronary origins, course, and degree of obstruction. These goals can be achieved with the following protocol:[28]

- Cine SSFP: ventricular long-axis planes and a short-axis stack from base to apex for quantitative assessment of ventricular dimensions and ejection fraction
- Cine SSFP: stack parallel to the right ventricular outflow tract to assess for right ventricular outflow tract, pulmonary valve, and main pulmonary artery (MPA) obstruction
- Cine SSFP: axial stack to assess for branch pulmonary artery obstruction
- Cine SSFP: stack in short axis to the aortic root to assess the degree of dilation and visualize any regurgitation jet
- Cine SSFP: ascending aorta long-axis plane to assess for obstruction
- Contrast-enhanced 3D MRA
- ECG and respiratory navigator-gated 3D whole-heart angiography of the coronary arteries
- Blood flow measurements: main and branch pulmonary arteries, ascending aorta

If there is a concern for inducible myocardial ischemia, a vasodilator or dobutamine stress protocol and myocardial LGE imaging should be considered.

CONGENITALLY CORRECTED TRANSPOSITION OF THE GREAT ARTERIES

Congenitally corrected transposition of the great arteries (CC-TGA) (or L-looped TGA) is characterized by atrioventricular discordance and ventriculoarterial discordance (Fig. 42.21). Systemic venous blood returns to the morphologic right atrium which then empties through the mitral valve into the morphologic left ventricle. The morphologic left ventricle is connected to the pulmonary arteries and ejects into the pulmonary circulation. Pulmonary venous blood flow then returns to the morphologic left atrium which then empties, via the tricuspid valve, into the morphologic right ventricle. The morphologic right ventricle is attached to the aorta and systemic circulation. Commonly associated problems include VSD, Ebstein anomaly of the tricuspid valve, subpulmonary stenosis, and heart block. Given that systemic venous return is ultimately directed to the pulmonary arteries and pulmonary venous return to the aorta, patients with CC-TGA (in the absence of other anomalies) have normal oxygen saturations. As children, these patients are often asymptomatic unless significant associated anomalies exist. It is not unusual for some patients with this diagnosis to be diagnosed in adulthood.

The main late complications for patients diagnosed with CC-TGA are systemic ventricular (morphologic right ventricle) and atrioventricular (tricuspid) valve failure. The morphologic right ventricle is intended to be a subpulmonary ventricle subject to low afterload and the tricuspid valve is also intended to prevent regurgitation from a low-pressure ventricle into the atrium. Long-term exposure to systemic pressure in CC-TGA can ultimately lead to systemic right ventricular and tricuspid valve failure.[110–112] These complications most often manifest in the fifth and sixth decades of life.[111,113] At the time these complications

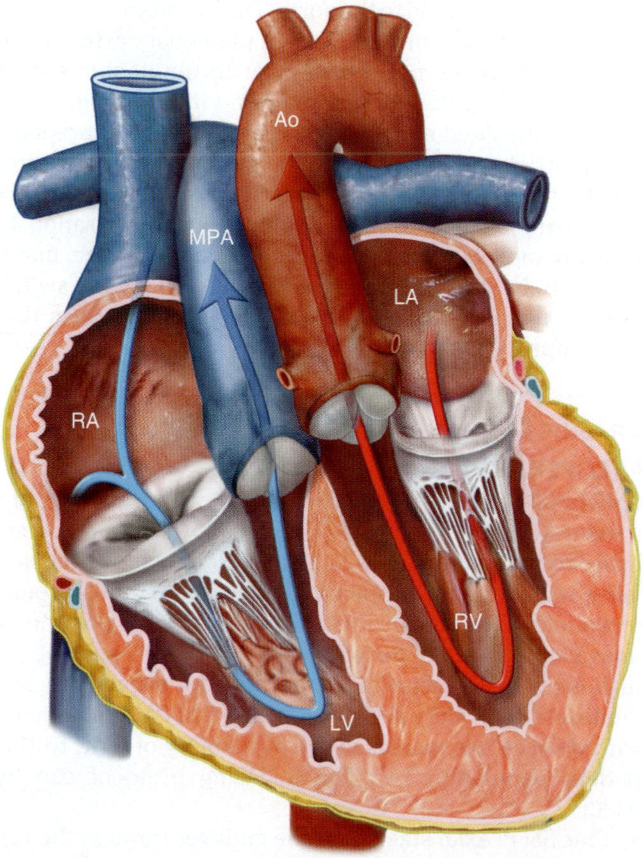

FIG. 42.21 Congenitally corrected transposition of the great arteries (L-looped transposition). In this rare acyanotic congenital heart defect there is ventricular inversion and transposed great arteries. The right ventricle (*RV*) pumps oxygenated blood to the aorta (*Ao*), while the left ventricle (*LV*) pumps deoxygenated blood to the pulmonary artery. *LA*, left atrium; *MPA*, main pulmonary artery; *RA*, right atrium. (From Krieger EVDJ. Transposition of the Great Arteries. In: CM O, ed. *Practice of Clinical Echocardiography.* 5th ed. Philadelphia: Elsevier Saunders; 2017.)

develop, therapeutic surgical options are limited. Those with isolated ventricular failure can be placed on medical therapy but may ultimately require cardiac transplantation.[111] Patients with significant tricuspid valve regurgitation can undergo tricuspid valve repair, which can result in an improvement in outcomes.[114,115] Worsening tricuspid valve regurgitation is correlated with worsening clinical outcomes.[110,116] The AV node and His bundles are abnormally located and complete heart block occurs at a rate of approximately 2% per year.[112]

Surgical repairs in childhood can be performed to prevent late complications. In patients with associated lesions such as VSD or tricuspid valve regurgitation, this could include VSD patch closure and/or tricuspid valve repair. This can be referred to as a "physiologic repair."[117] These types of repairs still result in a systemic morphologic right ventricle, and outcomes are limited.[118,119] To establish the morphologic left ventricle as the systemic ventricle, a double switch operation can be performed.[120–123] This is also known as an "anatomic repair." This combines an atrial switch operation with an arterial switch or Rastelli operation. This operation reroutes systemic venous return to the left-sided, morphologic right ventricle that is now connected to the pulmonary arteries and the pulmonary venous return to the right-sided morphologic left ventricle that is now connected to the aorta. This results in a systemic morphologic left ventricle. Often, a pulmonary artery band operation must be performed prior to the double switch operation.[124] A pulmonary artery band increases afterload for the right-sided morphologic left ventricle and prepares this ventricle to ultimately be the systemic ventricle after the double switch operation.[124] CMR is recommended after pulmonary band and before double switch operation to measure morphologic left ventricular chamber size, mass, and systolic function.[125] Outcomes from the double switch operation are mixed, with initial high mortality rates that have improved with time.[125–130]

Cardiac Magnetic Resonance

PREOPERATIVE

CMR is an essential imaging modality for the evaluation of a patient with unrepaired CC-TGA.[131] It allows for a thorough anatomic evaluation as well as quantification of tricuspid valve regurgitation, subpulmonary stenosis, and systemic morphologic right ventricle function. CMR was previously unavailable to many patients with CC-TGA because of the high incidence of heart block and need for pacemaker. The demonstrated safety and expanded use of CMR in patients with devices has increased the availability of CMR to this patient population.[132,133] The following protocol can be used:[28]

- Cine SSFP: axial stack from the midliver through the top of the aortic arch
- Cine SSFP: oblique planes to image tricuspid valve function
- Cine SSFP: ventricular long-axis planes and a short-axis stack from base to apex for quantitative assessment of ventricular size, mass, and ejection fraction
- Contrast-enhanced 3D MRA and/or ECG and respiratory navigator-gated whole-heart angiography imaging of the thorax
- Blood flow measurements: ascending aorta, main pulmonary artery, tricuspid valve
- LGE: ventricular long- and short-axis planes

Patients with unrepaired CC-TGA have been documented to have evidence of fibrosis in the systemic morphologic right ventricle as well as the left ventricle.[117,134,135] These abnormalities have been associated with increased risk of arrhythmia and reduced ventricular function.[117,134,135] Late gadolinium enhancement and T1 mapping imaging should be considered in all patients with CC-TGA.

POSTOPERATIVE AFTER DOUBLE SWITCH OPERATION

CMR is an essential imaging modality for the patient after a double switch operation. Complications of the double switch operation include those of both the atrial and arterial switch operations.

- Cine SSFP: axial stack from the midliver through the top of the aortic arch
- Cine SSFP: oblique planes to image tricuspid valve function and to assess atrial baffles
- Cine SSFP: ventricular long-axis planes and a short-axis stack from base to apex for quantitative assessment of ventricular size, mass, and ejection fraction
- Contrast-enhanced 3D MRA and/or ECG and respiratory navigator-gated 3D whole-heart angiography of the thorax
- Blood flow measurements: ascending aorta, main pulmonary artery, tricuspid valve, mitral valve, main pulmonary artery, branch pulmonary arteries
- LGE: ventricular long- and short-axis planes

EBSTEIN ANOMALY

The Ebstein anomaly is a malformation of the tricuspid valve and RV, which encompass a large spectrum of disease severity. There is failure of delamination of the septal and posterior tricuspid valve leaflets from the myocardium resulting in apical displacement of the tricuspid valve ($\geq$0.8 cm/m^2 relative to the anterior mitral leaflet insertion site).[136] The portion of the RV proximal to the functional tricuspid valve becomes “atrialized.” The anterior leaflet of the tricuspid valve is large and redundant, and often has fenestrations and tethering attachments to the free wall of the right ventricle. The posterior leaflet is often dysplastic and apically displaced.

The etiology of the Ebstein anomaly is not known; however, in rare cases, genetic factors such as mutations in the transcription factor NKX2.5,10p13-p14 deletion, or 1p34.3-p36.11 deletion have been described.[137,138] The most severe cases of Ebstein anomaly result in fetal hydrops and fetal demise. Patients with Ebstein anomaly often develop progressive right heart failure and exercise intolerance. However, some with mild forms of this disease can be asymptomatic into adulthood.

When possible, the surgical intervention for Ebstein anomaly involves tricuspid valve repair. In the current era, the repair generally involves a right atrium (RA) reduction, plication of the atrialized RV, and a tricuspid valve repair involving the creation of a monocusp tricuspid valve using the redundant anterior tricuspid valve leaflet with a posterior annuloplasty (cone procedure).[139]

In patients who are unsuitable for tricuspid valve repair, a bioprosthetic tricuspid valve replacement is generally performed. Evaluation of the patient after Ebstein repair involves assessing the degree of residual tricuspid regurgitation or stenosis and assessing the RA size and RV size and function. The right coronary artery lies in close proximity to the repaired tricuspid valve annulus site, and it is important to assess for evidence of LGE following surgery for Ebstein anomaly.

The goals of the CMR examination include (1) assessing tricuspid valve anatomy and regurgitant fraction; (2) calculating right ventricular volumes, mass, and ejection fraction; (3) calculating right atrial area and volume, and (4) evaluating for associated anomalies, including atrial septal defects, RVOT obstruction, and myocardial noncompaction. These goals can be achieved by the following protocol:

- Cine SSFP: axial stack from the midliver through the top of the aortic arch for dynamic imaging of the pulmonary arteries and atrioventricular valve regurgitation
- Cine SSFP: oblique planes to image tricuspid valve inflow orientation

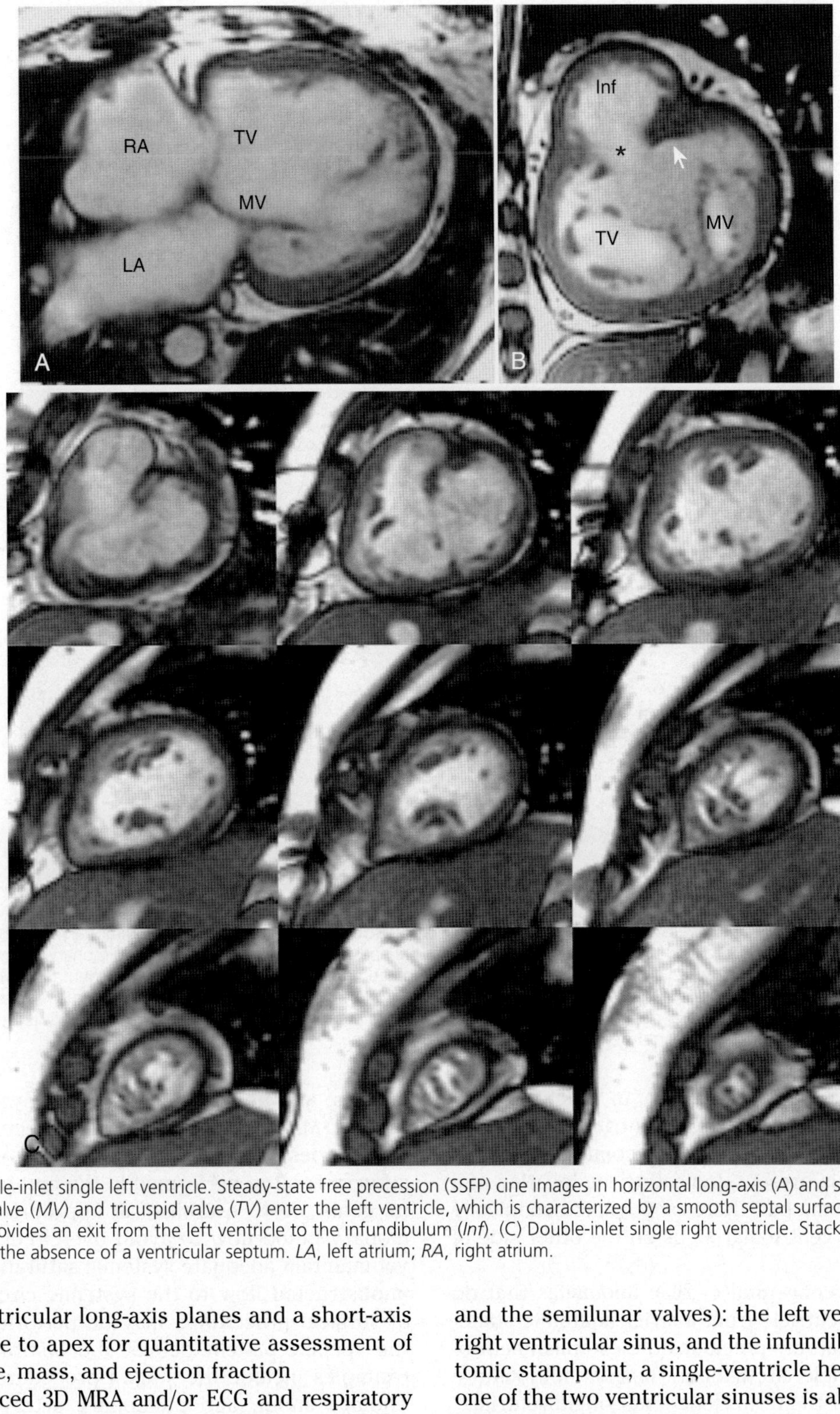

FIG. 42.22 (A,B) Double-inlet single left ventricle. Steady-state free precession (SSFP) cine images in horizontal long-axis (A) and short-axis (B) planes. Note that both the mitral valve (*MV*) and tricuspid valve (*TV*) enter the left ventricle, which is characterized by a smooth septal surface (*arrow*). The bulboventricular foramen (*) provides an exit from the left ventricle to the infundibulum (*Inf*). (C) Double-inlet single right ventricle. Stack of SSFP cine images in a short-axis plane. Note the absence of a ventricular septum. *LA*, left atrium; *RA*, right atrium.

- Cine SSFP: ventricular long-axis planes and a short-axis stack from base to apex for quantitative assessment of ventricular size, mass, and ejection fraction
- Contrast-enhanced 3D MRA and/or ECG and respiratory navigator-gated 3D whole-heart angiography of the thorax
- Blood flow measurements: ascending aorta, main pulmonary artery, tricuspid valve, mitral valve
- LGE: ventricular long- and short-axis planes

SINGLE VENTRICLE

The normal human heart is composed of three chambers at the ventricular level (between the atrioventricular valves and the semilunar valves): the left ventricular sinus, the right ventricular sinus, and the infundibulum. From an anatomic standpoint, a single-ventricle heart is present when one of the two ventricular sinuses is absent. The infundibulum is always present and has a variety of names such as infundibular outlet chamber, rudimentary or hypoplastic right ventricle, and rudimentary chamber. There are two types of single ventricles:

1. Single left ventricle (Fig. 42.22(A,B)), in which there is an absence of the right ventricular sinus and the presence of a left ventricle and an infundibulum. The communication between the left ventricle and the infundibulum is termed the bulboventricular foramen.

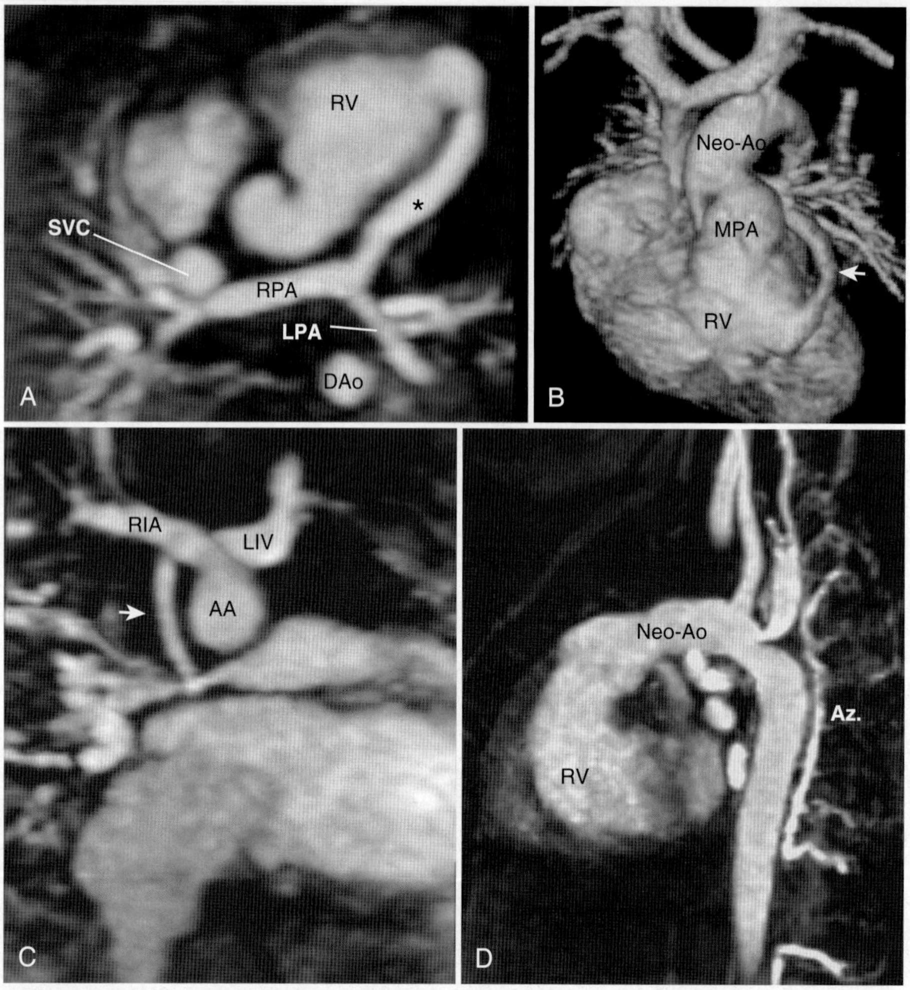

FIG. 42.23 Contrast-enhanced three-dimensional magnetic resonance angiography in infants before bidirectional Glenn shunt. (A) Subvolume maximum intensity projection (MIP) in an oblique transverse plane showing a conduit (*) from the right ventricle (*RV*) to the pulmonary arteries. (B) Three-dimensional volume rendering in the same patient showing the conduit (*arrow*) as well as the anastomosis between the main pulmonary artery and the reconstructed neo-aorta (*Neo-Ao*). (C) Oblique coronal subvolume MIP in a patient with a modified right Blalock-Taussig shunt. The shunt (*arrow*) extends from the right innominate artery (*RIA*) to the right pulmonary artery, and there is pulmonary artery stenosis at the insertion site. (D) Oblique sagittal subvolume MIP showing a reconstructed *Neo-Ao. AA,* ascending aorta; *Az.*, azygous vein; *DAo*, descending aorta; *LIV*, left innominate vein; *LPA*, left pulmonary artery; *MPA*, main pulmonary artery; *RPA*, right pulmonary artery; *SVC*, superior vena cava.

2. Single right ventricle (Fig. 42.22(C)), in which the ventricular mass consists of the right ventricular sinus and the infundibulum, together forming a common chamber. The septal band is present, indicating the location of a ventricular septum, but there is no macroscopically recognizable left ventricular sinus on the other side of the septum.

There are other congenital cardiac anomalies that do not have a single ventricle from a strict anatomic standpoint but whose anatomy precludes the establishment of a normal two-ventricle circulation. These conditions are often grouped under the term "functional single ventricle" or "functional univentricular hearts" and are managed similarly to single-ventricle hearts. Examples include tricuspid atresia, mitral atresia, severely unbalanced common atrioventricular canal defect, and hypoplastic left heart syndrome.

Single-ventricle physiology is characterized by complete mixing of the systemic and pulmonary venous return flows. The proportion of the ventricular output distributed to the pulmonary versus systemic circulations is determined by the relative resistance to flow in the two circuits, and heavily influences the systemic oxygen saturation. Management is typically directed toward a series of surgeries culminating in the Fontan operation. The first surgery is often performed in the first week or two of life. Its goals are to establish an appropriate amount of pulmonary blood flow to avoid overcirculation to the lungs yet maintain adequate systemic saturation and to provide unobstructed flow to the systemic circulation. A variety of surgical procedures may be performed depending on the specific patient details and institutional preference. Examples include the stage I procedure, Blalock-Taussig-Thomas shunt, and pulmonary artery band placement (Fig. 42.23). The next surgery is typically a superior cavopulmonary anastomosis (bidirectional Glenn) operation, performed at 4–6 months of age. As a result of this procedure, the superior vena cava supplies pulmonary flow and the inferior vena cava blood skips the lungs and is directed to the ventricle and then out to the systemic circulation. The third and often final surgery is the Fontan operation, performed between 18 months and 3 years of age. With this procedure, inferior vena cava blood is also directed to the pulmonary arteries. Thus, the systemic and pulmonary

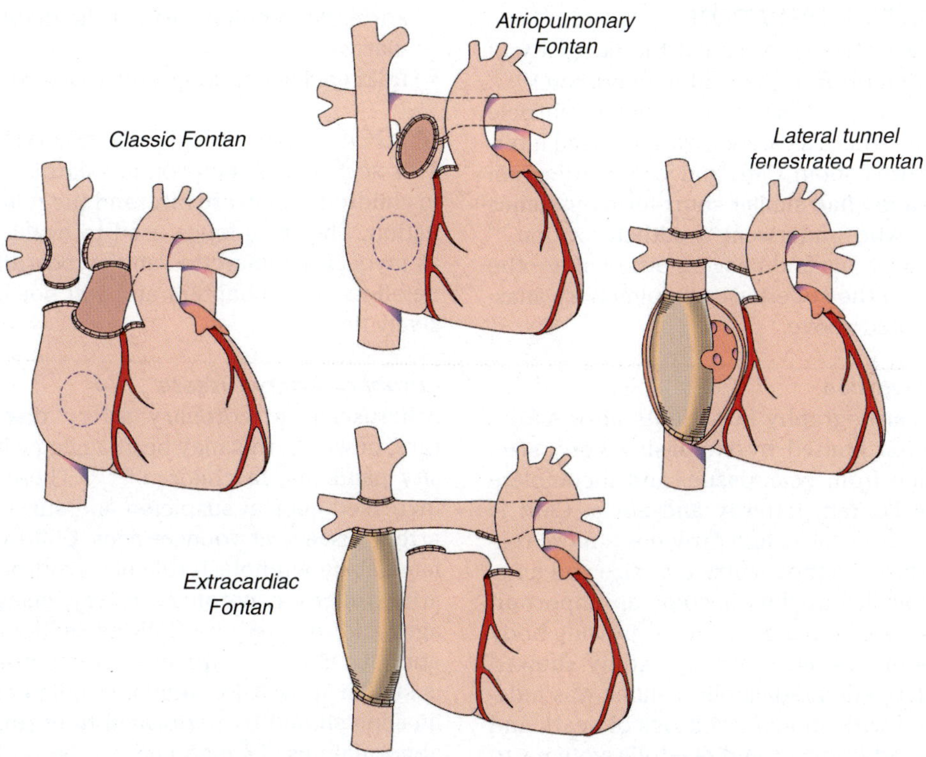

FIG. 42.24 Diagram of four variations of the Fontan operation.

circulations are separated with inferior and superior vena cava flow passively draining to the lungs and pulmonary venous return actively pumped by the single ventricle out to the body. This largely eliminates hypoxemia. Since it was first described in 1971,[140] the Fontan operation has undergone multiple modifications (Fig. 42.24), including direct anastomosis of the right atrial appendage to the main pulmonary artery (called an atriopulmonary anastomosis), a right atrium-to-right ventricle conduit, a lateral tunnel between the inferior vena cava and the undersurface of the ipsilateral branch pulmonary artery, fenestration of the lateral tunnel baffle, and an extracardiac conduit between the inferior vena cava and the ipsilateral branch pulmonary artery.

With refinement of patient selection criteria, medical therapy, and surgical techniques, the results of this staged surgical management approach to single-ventricle heart disease have improved. Nevertheless, this patient population continues to be at risk for complications including ventricular systolic and diastolic dysfunction; valve regurgitation; aortic arch, Fontan pathway, and pulmonary artery obstruction; pulmonary vein compression; thromboembolism; protein-losing enteropathy; plastic bronchitis; hepatic and renal dysfunction; arrhythmias; and premature death. Such adverse developments are usually poorly tolerated; thus, prompt detection with diagnostic imaging is an important element in caring for these patients.

Cardiac Magnetic Resonance

PRIOR TO THE FIRST OPERATION

CMR is seldom requested prior to the first palliative operation because echocardiography usually provides all of the necessary diagnostic information.

Prior to the Superior Cavopulmonary Anastomosis Operation

Traditionally, the superior cavopulmonary anastomosis operation is preceded by cardiac catheterization for assessment and planning. However, in a prospective randomized clinical trial, CMR was shown to be a safe, effective, and less costly alternative to routine catheterization in selected patients.[141,142]

The goals of the CMR examination include (1) measuring ventricular mass, volume, and function; (2) quantifying significant valve regurgitation; (3) evaluating the pulmonary arteries, pulmonary veins, atrial septum, and aortic arch for obstruction; and (4) assessing aortopulmonary and venovenous collateral vessels.[143,144] These goals can be achieved by the following protocol:

- Cine SSFP: axial stack from the midliver through the top of the aortic arch for dynamic imaging of the heart and vasculature
- Cine SSFP: ventricular long-axis planes and a ventricular short-axis stack from base to apex for quantitative assessment of ventricular dimensions and ejection fraction
- Cine SSFP: aortic arch long-axis plane
- Fast (turbo) spin echo with blood suppression (optional): axial plane to image the branch pulmonary arteries and aortic arch in long axis
- Contrast-enhanced 3D MRA and/or ECG and respiratory navigator-gated 3D whole-heart angiography of the chest (Fig. 42.23)
- Blood flow measurements: main and branch pulmonary arteries, ascending aorta, descending aorta at the diaphragm; superior vena cava, inferior vena cava, pulmonary veins, and atrioventricular valves
- LGE: ventricular long- and short-axis planes

PRIOR TO THE FONTAN OPERATION

Several reports have critically examined the necessity of cardiac catheterization prior to the Fontan operation.[145–147] One retrospective study showed that single-ventricle patients who did not require a catheterization-based intervention and had a pre-Fontan CMR and echocardiogram but not a catheterization had similar short-term outcomes compared to those who underwent a catheterization.[148] The CMR examination goals and imaging protocol are the same as those prior to the superior cavopulmonary anastomosis operation noted above.

After the Fontan Operation

The utility of echocardiography in patients after a Fontan operation is often limited by increasing body size, acoustic interference from scar tissue, and incomplete visualization of the Fontan pathway and aorta. CMR is not subject to these drawbacks and provides a more reliable quantitative assessment of ventricular size and function[149] and blood flow. It has thus become an important clinical tool in these fragile patients with a growing body of research to support its use.[70,72,150] One study showed that a larger CMR-derived end-diastolic volume was independently associated with an increased risk of death and transplant, and the addition of end-diastolic volume to clinical variables led to improved risk stratification for transplant-free survival.[151] In another report, LGE was seen in 28% of Fontan patients, and a greater extent of LGE was associated with lower ejection fraction, increased end-diastolic volume, increased mass, and a higher frequency of nonsustained ventricular tachycardia.[152] Studies using CMR blood flow measurements have also revealed new information about the importance of aortopulmonary collateral vessels,[143,144,153–157] energy losses in the Fontan connection,[150,158,159] and the value of computational fluid dynamics in surgical planning.[160]

The goals of the CMR examination include (1) assessing the systemic veins, Fontan baffle, and pulmonary arteries for obstruction and thrombus; (2) detecting Fontan baffle fenestrations or leaks; (3) evaluating the pulmonary veins for compression; (4) quantifying ventricular volumes, mass, and function; (5) detecting ventricular outflow tract obstruction; (6) quantifying significant valve regurgitation; (7) imaging the aorta for obstruction or aneurysm; and (8) assessing aortopulmonary and venovenous collateral vessels. These goals can be achieved by the following protocol:[28]

- Cine SSFP: axial stack from the midliver through the top of the aortic arch for dynamic imaging of the heart and vasculature
- Cine SSFP: ventricular long-axis planes and a ventricular short-axis stack from base to apex for quantitative assessment of ventricular dimensions and ejection fraction
- Cine SSFP: aortic arch long-axis plane
- Contrast-enhanced 3D MRA
- ECG and respiratory navigator-gated 3D whole-heart angiography of the thorax
- Blood flow measurements: superior vena cava, Fontan baffle above and below any fenestration or baffle leak, branch pulmonary arteries, pulmonary veins, ascending aorta, descending aorta at the diaphragm, atrioventricular valves
- LGE: ventricular long- and short-axis planes

MYOCARDIAL DISEASE IN PEDIATRICS

This section will focus on myocardial diseases that occur in children, which are rare, and the role of CMR in this evaluation. The techniques used to evaluate conditions such as myocardial infarction and myocarditis are described in detail in other chapters and will not be discussed extensively here.

Coronary Artery Disease

Atherosclerotic coronary artery disease in children is rare; however, this may be changing with the ongoing obesity pandemic in children.[161–165] There will be a need for increased clinical suspicion and surveillance of coronary artery disease at younger ages. Children with a history of familial hypercholesterolemia syndromes are at risk for atherosclerotic coronary artery disease at very young ages and may require CMR evaluation.[166] The CMR evaluation for children with suspected coronary artery disease is similar to that for adults. Detailed SSFP cine short-axis imaging should be performed to evaluate for wall motion abnormalities. T2 mapping can be performed to evaluate for peri-infarct edema and has been proposed as a method to determine ischemic area at risk, although there are limitations to this evaluation, and one study has shown this method to be unreliable.[167] T1 mapping can also be performed to detect fibrosis associated with chronic infarction; however, this method has limitations such as the presence of fat within the infarct that complicates the sensitivity of the test.[168] LGE imaging, bright- and dark-blood methods, should be performed to evaluate for myocardial infarction.[169,170] Dark-blood LGE has been shown to be superior for the evaluation of subendocardial infarction.[171] Bright-blood LGE can be superior for midmyocardial hyperenhancement. Stress CMR imaging in children can also be performed to evaluate patients at risk for ischemia. Dobutamine stress imaging can be used to accentuate wall motion abnormalities.[172,173] Adenosine and/or regadenoson stress perfusion can also be used in children and are sensitive in the detection of coronary artery stenosis.[174–176]

Congenital anomalies of the coronary arteries such as anomalous origin from the pulmonary arteries and from the contralateral sinus of Valsalva place the patient at risk for myocardial infarction. Children with anomalous origin of the left (ALCAPA) or right coronary artery (ARCAPA) from the pulmonary artery most often present at several months of age when pulmonary artery resistance has decreased and there is "steal" of coronary flow into the low-pressure pulmonary arteries. The reduced coronary blood flow leads to myocardial ischemia and infarction with resulting ventricular dysfunction and mitral regurgitation. Occasionally, children will develop sufficient collaterals within the coronary system such that acute ischemia and infarction do not occur in infancy. These patients can present at older ages, and this is known as Bland-White-Garland syndrome.[177–180] CMR, using ECG and respiratory navigator-gated 3D whole-heart angiography, can be used in patients with suspected ALCAPA or

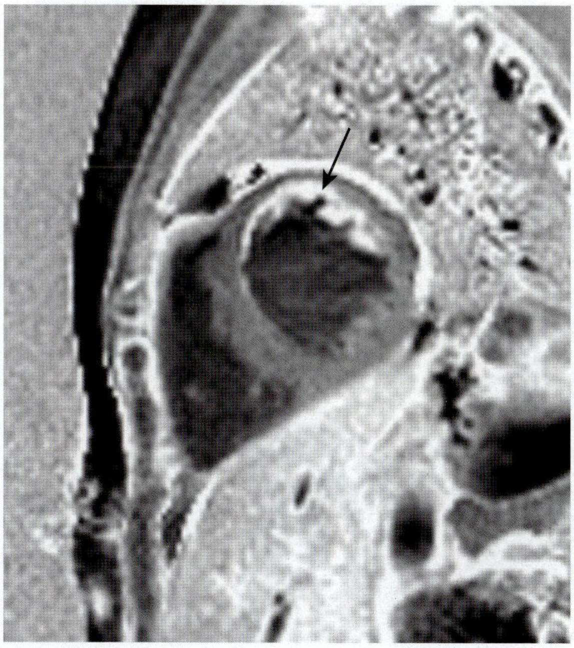

FIG. 42.25 Black-blood late gadolinium enhancement short-axis image of a patient with a history of anomalous origin of the left coronary artery. A subendocardial myocardial infarction (*arrow*) is noted.

ARCAPA to define coronary artery anatomy. This can be a challenge in infants given the limited spatial resolution of CMR angiography. CT, echocardiography, or invasive angiography may better define the coronary artery anatomy. LGE can provide a quantitative assessment of infarct burden, which can serve as a baseline for future comparison (Fig. 42.25).[181,182] ALCAPA and ARCAPA patients should undergo surgical translocation of the anomalous coronary artery onto the aorta. Often, with improved coronary perfusion, wall motion and global systolic function will improve.[179] Postrepair stenosis is a possible postoperative complication. The CMR evaluation of a patient following repair should evaluate for changes in ventricular function via SSFP cine imaging, changes in infarct burden via LGE, and for inducible ischemia using cine angiography and stress imaging.[173,179,181,183,184]

Patients with anomalous origin of the left coronary artery from the right sinus of Valsalva can be at risk for ischemia, infarction, and sudden death.[185,186] The left coronary artery most often has an interarterial course between the aorta and main pulmonary artery. Many of these patients are asymptomatic and the initial presentation can be chest pain, infarction, and sudden death.[186,187] The risk of ischemia is such that patients with this diagnosis should undergo surgical repair with either unroofing or reimplantation of the coronary artery to the correct sinus of Valsalva. Patients with anomalous origin of the right coronary artery from the left sinus of Valsalva with an interarterial course also have a risk of ischemia and sudden death, although they are thought to have significantly less risk of sudden death than those with anomalous origin of the left coronary artery.[188,189] Management of patients with this diagnosis, including exercise restrictions and surgical reimplantation, is more challenging because the risk of sudden death is felt to be very low and there are also risks of a sedentary lifestyle and/or surgery.[188]

The CMR assessment of patients with anomalous coronary arteries should include SSFP cine imaging to evaluate for wall motion abnormalities, LGE and T1 mapping to detect prior infarction, and angiography to visualize the proximal coronary arteries. Stress imaging can be used as a mechanism of risk stratification.[185,190] A positive stress test should lead to exercise restrictions and surgical correction. On the other hand, a negative test is not predictive of a risk-free outcome and must be interpreted with caution. Some anatomical features such as a "slit-like" orifice and intramural course have been proposed as risk factors for ischemia and sudden death; however, data supporting these conclusions is limited and anecdotal. Surgical repair of an anomalous coronary artery most often consists of unroofing or reimplantation of the anomalous coronary artery so that it arises from the correct sinus of Valsalva. Postoperative coronary artery occlusion is a possibility and patients with a history of repair can be evaluated by CMR for coronary artery origin stenosis, wall motion abnormalities, infarcts detected by LGE, and stress imaging abnormalities.

Patients with small- and medium-sized vessel vasculitis such as Kawasaki disease (KD) and multisystem inflammatory syndrome of children (MIS-C) associated with COVID-19 can develop coronary artery aneurysms, thrombi, stenosis, and rupture.[191–193] These coronary artery abnormalities can place the patient at risk for myocardial ischemia and infarction. In patients with a history of coronary artery aneurysms, CMR should be considered.[194,195] This evaluation should include SSFP cine imaging, LGE, and angiography to visualize the coronary arteries.[195] Direct visualization of the coronary arteries and aneurysms by angiography has been previously described, but imaging by CMR is often not as sensitive as CT.[196,197] CMR evaluation could also include stress imaging, which has been shown to be sensitive for the detection of coronary artery stenosis in KD.[198] Patients with KD and MIS-C can also develop myocarditis (discussed below).[199]

Heart Transplant Recipients

The field of pediatric heart transplantation has continued to develop, with improved patient outcomes.[200–203] Pediatric heart transplant recipients are at risk for rejection and coronary vasculopathy. Historically, cardiac catheterization and endomyocardial biopsy have been the "gold standard" for screening and diagnosing rejection.[203–205] The utility of this is questionable because of the potential for sampling error. Despite this, patients continue to undergo invasive routine surveillance, in large part due to the absence of a noninvasive alternative. CMR, given its ability to assess the myocardium using LGE, myocardial strain, and T1 and T2 mapping, could provide such an alternative (Fig. 42.26).[203,206] The results from initial studies investigating the use of parametric mapping for the detection of acute rejection are mixed. In adult patients, some studies have shown promise with elevated T2 and ECV (extracellular volume) levels being associated with acute rejection.[207–210] Other studies have not been able to replicate this result.[211] Results of pediatric studies designed to investigate the utility of parametric mapping in detecting acute rejection and coronary vasculopathy are similarly mixed,

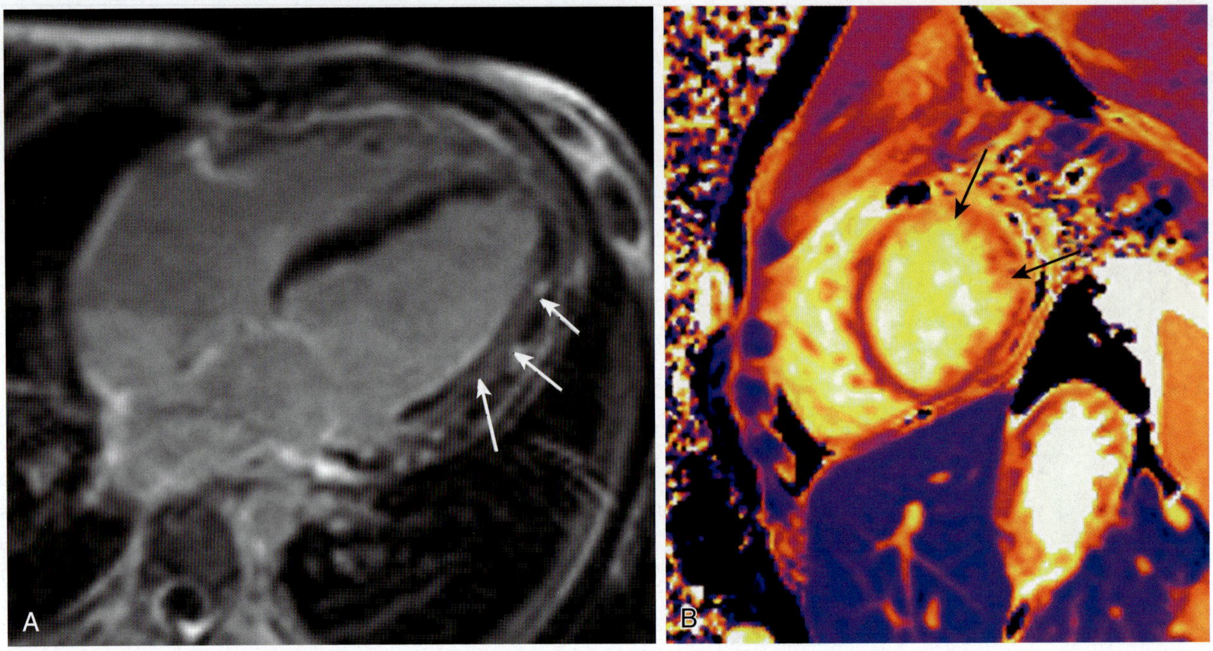

FIG. 42.26 A. Late gadolinium enhancement long-axis image illustrating patchy midmyocardial hyperenhancement in the left ventricle lateral wall. B. T1 map in a short-axis plane in the same patient (A) illustrating elevated T1 values in the lateral wall.

with some positive[203,212–215] and some negative[216] results. Pediatric studies have also demonstrated that abnormalities of myocardial strain as detected by CMR may be able to detect acute rejection and coronary vasculopathy.[203,206] LGE in heart transplant patients has been associated with poor clinical outcomes in adults.[217] Adenosine stress CMR could be beneficial in identifying coronary artery vasculopathy, and recent studies have demonstrated the safety of adenosine and regadenoson for this purpose in adult and pediatric heart transplant recipients.[218–221] In summary, CMR holds promise as a noninvasive test for the detection of acute rejection and coronary artery vasculopathy in pediatric heart transplant recipients; however, experience is limited and CMR is not used clinically for this purpose in most institutions. In a multicenter study of 59 children who underwent heart transplantation, global circumferential strain was worse in acute rejection and cardiac allograft vasculopathy compared to healthy patients. ECV, native T1, and T2 *z*-scores were elevated in patients with acute rejection.[203]

Cardiomyopathies

The first phenotypic manifestations of dilated, restrictive, and hypertrophic cardiomyopathies often begin in childhood. Early detection is important, but it is also vital to differentiate abnormal findings from normal phenotypic variations. The fact that young, well-conditioned athletes can have increased cardiac size (athlete's heart) can further complicate this assessment.[222,223] CMR, with its combined ability to evaluate morphology, hemodynamics, ventricular function, and myocardial health, is ideally positioned to perform this evaluation.

Hypertrophic cardiomyopathy (HCM) is the leading cause of sudden death in the young.[186,189,224] CMR is an excellent imaging modality to evaluate the phenotypic findings of HCM. Patients are often directed to CMR after abnormalities are noted on other screening tests, such as left ventricular hypertrophy on ECG or echocardiogram, family history of HCM or sudden unexplained death, an abnormal genetic finding, an abnormal physical examination finding, or concerning symptoms such as exercise-induced chest pain, palpitations, or syncope. SSFP cine imaging allows for assessment of ventricular wall thickness, mass, chamber sizes, and systolic function. It also allows for the identification of systolic anterior motion of the mitral valve and left ventricular apical aneurysms. SSFP cine long-axis views and velocity-encoded phase-contrast imaging can also allow for the characterization and quantification of left ventricular outflow tract obstruction. A velocity-encoded, phase-contrast, in-phase image of the left ventricular outflow tract may be helpful in identifying the location of obstruction. T1 mapping should be performed and can demonstrate diffuse myocardial fibrosis.[225] LGE can reveal areas of hyperenhancement and patients typically have midwall hyperenhancement in hypertrophied areas (Fig. 42.27(A)).[226] The presence of hyperenhancement in a pattern typical for HCM when seen in a young patient with left ventricular hypertrophy greatly increases the likelihood of a diagnosis of HCM, and the finding of hyperenhancement has been associated with worse clinical outcomes.[227,228] Adenosine stress perfusion CMR can also be performed and microvascular perfusion defects can be noted (Fig. 42.27(B)). The prognostic value of this finding is uncertain; however, perfusion defects are never a normal finding and would support a diagnosis of HCM in a patient with a borderline phenotype.[174]

CMR should also be considered in patients with dilated and restrictive cardiomyopathies. In adult patients, LGE, stress CMR, and T1/T2 mapping can help differentiate between ischemic and nonischemic cardiomyopathies. In children, most cardiomyopathies are nonischemic with the exception of congenital coronary anomalies (discussed above). CMR can identify abnormalities of T1/T2 and LGE in these patients. Some genetic abnormalities are

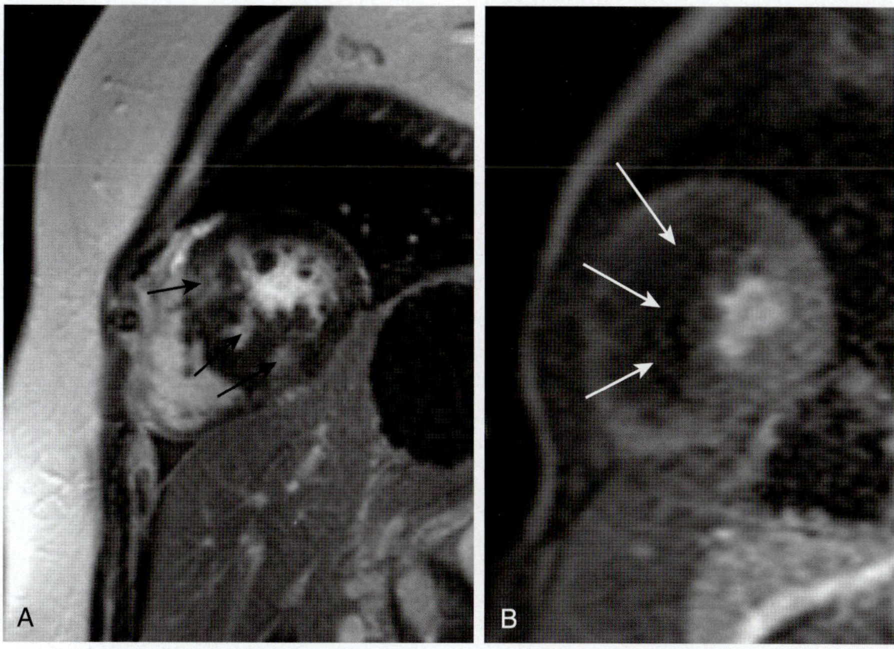

FIG. 42.27 (A) Late gadolinium enhancement short-axis image of a patient with hypertrophic cardiomyopathy. There is patchy midmyocardial hyperenhancement of the septal wall (*arrows*). (B) Adenosine stress cardiac magnetic resonance image of a patient with hypertrophic cardiomyopathy. There is a large perfusion defect in the septal wall (*arrow*).

associated with characteristic CMR findings. Patients with neuromuscular genetic disorders such as Duchenne muscular dystrophy (DMD) are one such population. Patients with DMD can have a characteristic LGE pattern of epicardial hyperenhancement predominantly in the LV anterolateral, inferolateral, and inferior segments (Fig. 42.28).[229] Patients with Fabry disease characteristically have low T1 values in affected areas.[230] Strain measurements from CMR images can also be performed in these patients to detect early subclinical disease. One population who can particularly benefit from this is cardio-oncology patients.[231,232] Cardiac toxicity associated with anthracycline agents is well described. Cardiac imaging, including CMR, should be used to detect disease at early stages so that chemotherapy can be adjusted, if needed. Strain and parametric mapping have been demonstrated to be beneficial in this regard.

Arrhythmogenic cardiomyopathy (ACM) is a myocardial disease that involves fatty infiltration of the myocardium, ventricular arrhythmias, and sudden death.[233,234] This condition is often caused by genetic defects in desmosomes and can present in childhood.[235] The most recent diagnostic criteria include CMR findings and incorporate both right and left ventricular subtypes.[236,237] The CMR evaluation of ACM is described thoroughly in another chapter. This diagnosis should be suspected in patients being evaluated for unexplained syncope, aborted sudden death, arrhythmia, family history of sudden death, or concern for ventricular enlargement and/or dysfunction. CMR evaluation should include detailed SSFP cine images of the ventricles with careful attention to regional wall motion abnormalities and ejection fraction. The right and left ventricles should be evaluated for wall motion abnormalities and aneurysms. SSFP cine images can be performed in phase and out of phase to attenuate the appearance of fatty infiltration.[238] T2-weighted images can also be obtained

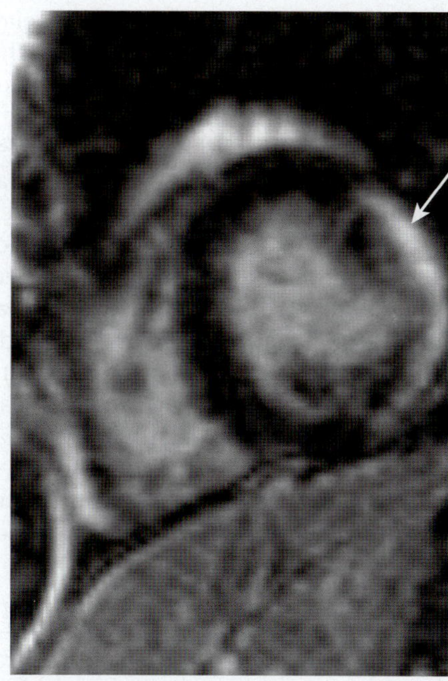

FIG. 42.28 Late gadolinium enhancement short-axis image illustrating epicardial hyperenhancement (*arrow*) in the lateral wall of a patient with Duchenne muscular dystrophy.

with and without fat saturation to facilitate the detection of fatty infiltration. Parametric mapping and LGE should also be acquired to assist in the visualization of fatty infiltrates or other areas of abnormal myocardium. Patients with desmoplakin mutations are particularly likely to have left ventricular findings and often present with a myocarditis-type clinical picture.[239]

Myocarditis and Pericarditis

Myocarditis is defined as inflammation of the myocardium. The most common etiology is viral; however, bacterial, fungal, other inflammatory conditions, drugs, and immunizations are also causes of myocarditis. The gold standard for diagnosis is endomyocardial biopsy, with the presence of lymphocytic infiltrates being diagnostic. Over the last 2 decades, CMR, as a result of its tissue characterization capabilities, has emerged as a noninvasive alternative. The CMR community has established CMR diagnostic criteria for myocarditis in the Lake Louise and modified Lake Louise guidelines.[240,241] Elevated cardiac enzymes are a hallmark of myocardial damage and occur with myocarditis. In young patients with elevated cardiac enzymes, myocarditis is a much more likely cause than atherosclerotic coronary artery disease. Because of this, CMR can be considered as a first-line test in young patients with elevated cardiac enzymes and a history consistent with myocarditis. This approach allows many young patients to avoid unnecessary invasive coronary angiography. Patients with inflammatory conditions such as KD and multisystem inflammatory syndrome in children and adults (MIS-C and MIS-A) can also have myocarditis, which can be a predominant cardiac feature of these syndromes.[191,192,199,242] Recently, cases of myocarditis were noted following vaccination with mRNA vaccines for the COVID-19 virus.[243] These cases occurred predominantly in teenage and young adult males.[244,245] The COVID-19 pandemic, through direct viral infections, MIS-C/MIS-A, and vaccine-associated myocarditis, has increased our knowledge of the pathogenesis of myocarditis and increased the diagnostic role of CMR.

The CMR evaluation of myocarditis should include stacks of SSFP cine images in short-axis, axial, and ventricular long-axis planes. Careful attention should be paid to the presence of wall motion abnormalities and atrioventricular valve regurgitation. T1 mapping should be performed to assess for inflammation and fibrosis. T2-weighted images and T2 mapping are used to evaluate for myocardial edema. The presence of significant edema can be an indicator of acute inflammation. Delayed-enhancement imaging is also helpful in evaluating for intracardiac thrombus (early gadolinium enhancement) and for myocardial inflammation and necrosis (LGE). The typical LGE patterns for myocarditis are midmyocardial and/or epicardial hyperenhancement, as opposed to the subendocardial pattern associated with myocardial ischemia (Fig. 42.29).

CMR can also evaluate for pericardial disease. Patients with pericarditis will have hyperenhancement of the pericardium on LGE. Constrictive pericarditis is characterized by a thickened pericardium. Evaluation for constrictive physiology should include real-time imaging in a short-axis plane at the level of the ventricles while the patient is free breathing. Patients with constrictive physiology will have dyskinetic ventricular septal wall motion with respiration. Pericardial effusions will also be apparent on CMR imaging. Indicators of cardiac tamponade such as right atrial and ventricular collapse can also be seen. Pericardial tumors and cysts can occur but are rare in children.

Cardiac Mass

Cardiac masses in children are rare and most often benign. Histologic diagnosis is the "gold standard'; however, CMR, given its tissue characterization capabilities, is an excellent noninvasive alternative. Studies have assessed the typical CMR characteristics of pediatric cardiac masses and, from this data, diagnostic tools have been developed.[246,247] The most common pediatric masses are rhabdomyomas and fibromas.[246,247] Rhabdomyomas are associated with tuberous sclerosis and often spontaneously regress. Recent developments have demonstrated the utility of mTOR inhibitors in accelerating regression of rhabdomyomas.[248] Indications to surgically remove a cardiac mass in children include hemodynamically significant ventricular inflow or outflow obstruction, reduced ventricular function, refractory arrhythmias, unexplained syncope or arrested sudden death, and unsure diagnosis with concern for malignancy. The CMR evaluation of cardiac masses should include SSFP cine imaging in multiple imaging planes, T1-weighted images and mapping, T2-weighted images with and without fat saturation to evaluate for lipomas, perfusion imaging to evaluate for vascular tumors, early gadolinium enhancement to assess for thrombi, and LGE. ECG and respiratory-gated whole-heart angiography to evaluate the coronary artery courses may also be needed if a coronary artery is surrounded by the cardiac mass.

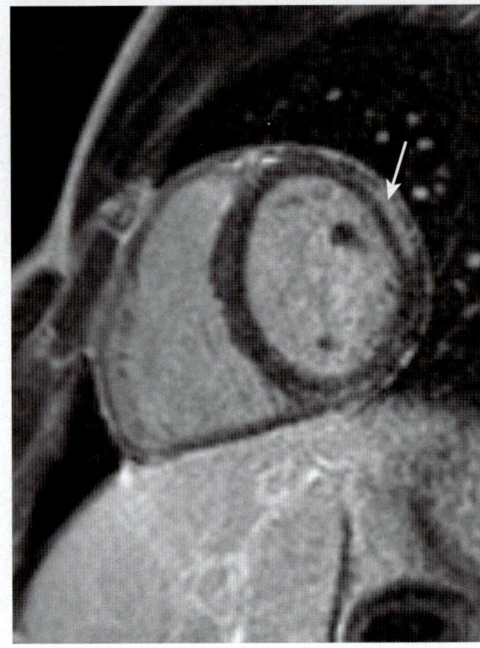

FIG. 42.29 Late gadolinium enhancement short-axis image of a patient with myocarditis. There is midmyocardial hyperenhancement of the lateral wall (*arrow*).

In conclusion, an increasing number of people with CHD are undergoing CMR imaging. Knowledge of the congenital heart anatomy, prior surgical interventions, and incorporation of an imaging protocol for each individual patient is crucial to perform a successful CMR examination. The information provided by CMR may identify prognostic information regarding future risk for adverse outcomes in this unique set of patients.

REFERENCES

1. L B. Epidemiology and prevention of congenital heart defects, United States. In: Allen H, ed. *Moss and Adams Heart Disease in Infants, Children, and Adolescents*. 1. 7th ed. Lippincott & Wilkins; 2016:524–545.
2. Marelli AJ, Ionescu-Ittu R, Mackie AS, Guo L, Dendukuri N, Kaouache M. Lifetime prevalence of congenital heart disease in the general population from 2000 to 2010. *Circulation*. 2014;130(9):749–756.

3. Sechtem U, Pflugfelder P, Higgins CB. Quantification of cardiac function by conventional and cine magnetic resonance imaging. *Cardiovasc Interventional Radiol*. 1987;10(6):365–373.
4. Dewey FE, Rosenthal D, Murphy Jr DJ, Froelicher VF, Ashley EA. Does size matter? Clinical applications of scaling cardiac size and function for body size. *Circulation*. 2008;117(17):2279–2287.
5. Sluysmans T, Colan SD. Theoretical and empirical derivation of cardiovascular allometric relationships in children. *J App Physiol*. 2005;99(2):445–457.
6. Cantinotti M, Scalese M, Molinaro S, Murzi B, Passino C. Limitations of current echocardiographic nomograms for left ventricular, valvular, and arterial dimensions in children: a critical review. *J Am Soc Echocardiogr: Off Pub Am Soc Echocardiogr*. 2012;25(2):142–152.
7. Voges I, Jerosch-Herold M, Hedderich J, et al. Normal values of aortic dimensions, distensibility, and pulse wave velocity in children and young adults: a cross-sectional study. *J Cardiovas Magn Reso: Off J Soc Cardiovas Magn Reson*. 2012;14(1):77.
8. Buechel EV, Kaiser T, Jackson C, Schmitz A, Kellenberger CJ. Normal right- and left ventricular volumes and myocardial mass in children measured by steady state free precession cardiovascular magnetic resonance. *J Cardiovas Magn Reson: Off J Soc Cardiovas Magn Reson*. 2009;11(1):19.
9. Robbers-Visser D, Boersma E, Helbing WA. Normal biventricular function, volumes, and mass in children aged 8 to 17 years. *J Magn Reson Imaging: JMRI*. 2009;29(3):552–559.
10. Sarikouch S, Peters B, Gutberlet M, et al. Sex-specific pediatric percentiles for ventricular size and mass as reference values for cardiac MRI: assessment by steady-state free-precession and phase-contrast MRI flow. *Circ Cardiovasc Imaging*. 2010;3(1):65–76.
11. Alfakih K, Plein S, Thiele H, Jones T, Ridgway JP, Sivananthan MU. Normal human left and right ventricular dimensions for MRI as assessed by turbo gradient echo and steady-state free precession imaging sequences. *J Magn Reson Imaging: JMRI*. 2003;17(3):323–329.
12. Hudsmith LE, Petersen SE, Francis JM, Robson MD, Neubauer S. Normal human left and right ventricular and left atrial dimensions using steady state free precession magnetic resonance imaging. *J Cardiovas Magn Reson: Off J Soc Cardiovas Magn Reson*. 2005;7(5):775–782.
13. Kaiser T, Kellenberger CJ, Albisetti M, Bergsträsser E, Valsangiacomo Buechel ER. Normal values for aortic diameters in children and adolescents-assessment in vivo by contrast-enhanced CMR-angiography. *J Cardiovas Magn Reson: Off J Soc Cardiovas Magn Reson*. 2008;10(1):56.
14. Kawel-Boehm N, Maceira A, Valsangiacomo-Buechel ER, et al. Normal values for cardiovascular magnetic resonance in adults and children. *J Cardiovas Magn Reson: Off J Soc Cardiovas Magn Reson*. 2015;17(1):29.
15. Sarikouch S, Koerperich H, Boethig D, et al. Reference values for atrial size and function in children and young adults by cardiac MR: a study of the German competence network congenital heart defects. *J Magn Reson Imaging: JMRI*. 2011;33(5):1028–1039.
16. Raghib G, Ruttenberg HD, Anderson RC, Amplatz K, Adams Jr P, Edwards JE. Termination of left superior vena cava in left atrium, atrial septal defect, and absence of coronary SINUS; a developmental complex. *Circulation*. 1965;31:906–918.
17. Muroke V, Jalanko M, Haukka J, Sinisalo J. Cause-specific mortality of patients with atrial septal defect and up to 50 Years of follow-up. *J Am Heart Assoc*. 2023;12(2):e027635.
18. Durongpisitkul K, Tang NL, Soongswang J, Laohaprasitiporn D, Nanal A. Predictors of successful transcatheter closure of atrial septal defect by cardiac magnetic resonance imaging. *Pediatr Cardiol*. 2004;25(2):124–130.
19. Beerbaum P, Körperich H, Esdorn H, et al. Atrial septal defects in pediatric patients: noninvasive sizing with cardiovascular MR imaging. *Radiology*. 2003;228(2):361–369.
20. Piaw CS, Kiam OT, Rapaee A, et al. Use of non-invasive phase contrast magnetic resonance imaging for estimation of atrial septal defect size and morphology: a comparison with transesophageal echo. *Cardiovasc Interventional Radiol*. 2006;29(2):230–234.
21. Teo KS, Disney PJ, Dundon BK, et al. Assessment of atrial septal defects in adults comparing cardiovascular magnetic resonance with transoesophageal echocardiography. *J Cardiovasc Magn Reson: Off J Soc Cardiovasc Magn Reson*. 2010;12(1):44.
22. Thomson LE, Crowley AL, Heitner JF, et al. Direct en face imaging of secundum atrial septal defects by velocity-encoded cardiovascular magnetic resonance in patients evaluated for possible transcatheter closure. *Circ Cardiovasc Imaging*. 2008;1(1):31–40.
23. Valente AM, Sena L, Powell AJ, Del Nido PJ, Geva T. Cardiac magnetic resonance imaging evaluation of sinus venosus defects: comparison to surgical findings. *Pediatr Cardiol*. 2007;28(1):51–56.
24. Prompona M, Muehling O, Naebauer M, Schoenberg SO, Reiser M, Huber A. MRI for detection of anomalous pulmonary venous drainage in patients with sinus venosus atrial septal defects. *Int J Cardiovas Imaging*. 2011;27(3):403–412.
25. Powell AJ, Tsai-Goodman B, Prakash A, Greil GF, Geva T. Comparison between phase-velocity cine magnetic resonance imaging and invasive oximetry for quantification of atrial shunts. *Am J Cardiol*. 2003;91(12):1523–1525. a1529.
26. Beerbaum P, Körperich H, Barth P, Esdorn H, Gieseke J, Meyer H. Noninvasive quantification of left-to-right shunt in pediatric patients: phase-contrast cine magnetic resonance imaging compared with invasive oximetry. *Circulation*. 2001;103(20):2476–2482.
27. Hundley WG, Li HF, Lange RA, et al. Assessment of left-to-right intracardiac shunting by velocity-encoded, phase-difference magnetic resonance imaging. A comparison with oximetric and indicator dilution techniques. *Circulation*. 1995;91(12):2955–2960.
28. Fratz S, Chung T, Greil GF, et al. Guidelines and protocols for cardiovascular magnetic resonance in children and adults with congenital heart disease: SCMR expert consensus group on congenital heart disease. *J Cardiovasc Magn Reson: Off J Soc Cardiovasc Magn Reson*. 2013;15(1):51.
29. Dyme JL, Prakash A, Printz BF, Kaur A, Parness IA, Nielsen JC. Physiology of isolated anomalous pulmonary venous connection of a single pulmonary vein as determined by cardiac magnetic resonance imaging. *Am J Cardiol*. 2006;98(1):107–110.
30. Riesenkampff EM, Schmitt B, Schnackenburg B, et al. Partial anomalous pulmonary venous drainage in young pediatric patients: the role of magnetic resonance imaging. *Pediatr Cardiol*. 2009;30(4):458–464.
31. Greil GF, Powell AJ, Gildein HP, Geva T. Gadolinium-enhanced three-dimensional magnetic resonance angiography of pulmonary and systemic venous anomalies. *J Am Coll Cardiol*. 2002;39(2):335–341.
32. Prasad SK, Soukias N, Hornung T, et al. Role of magnetic resonance angiography in the diagnosis of major aortopulmonary collateral arteries and partial anomalous pulmonary venous drainage. *Circulation*. 2004;109(2):207–214.
33. Ferrari VA, Scott CH, Holland GA, Axel L, Sutton MS. Ultrafast three-dimensional contrast-enhanced magnetic resonance angiography and imaging in the diagnosis of partial anomalous pulmonary venous drainage. *J Am Coll Cardiol*. 2001;37(4):1120–1128.
34. Vyas HV, Greenberg SB, Krishnamurthy R. MR imaging and CT evaluation of congenital pulmonary vein abnormalities in neonates and infants. *Radiographics : Rev Pub Radiol Soc N Am, Inc*. 2012;32(1):87–98.
35. Van Praagh R, Geva T, Kreutzer J. Ventricular septal defects: how shall we describe, name and classify them? *J Am Coll Cardiol*. 1989;14(5):1298–1299.
36. Bremerich J, Reddy GP, Higgins CB. MRI of supracristal ventricular septal defects. *J Comput Ass Tomogr*. 1999;23(1):13–15.
37. Lowell DG, Turner DA, Smith SM, et al. The detection of atrial and ventricular septal defects with electrocardiographically synchronized magnetic resonance imaging. *Circulation*. 1986;73(1):89–94.
38. Baker EJ, Ayton V, Smith MA, et al. Magnetic resonance imaging at a high field strength of ventricular septal defects in infants. *Br Heart J*. 1989;62(4):305–310.
39. Mohiaddin RH, Underwood R, Romeira L, et al. Comparison between cine magnetic resonance velocity mapping and first-pass radionuclide angiocardiography for quantitating intracardiac shunts. *Am J Cardiol*. 1995;75(7):529–532.
40. Fortescue EB, Lock JE, Galvin T, McElhinney DB. To close or not to close: the very small patent ductus arteriosus. *Congenit Heart Dis*. 2010;5(4):354–365.
41. Geva T, Greil GF, Marshall AC, Landzberg M, Powell AJ. Gadolinium-enhanced 3-dimensional magnetic resonance angiography of pulmonary blood supply in patients with complex pulmonary stenosis or atresia: comparison with x-ray angiography. *Circulation*. 2002;106(4):473–478.
42. Campbell M. Natural history of coarctation of the aorta. *Br Heart J*. 1970;32(5):633–640.
43. Rao PS, Jureidini SB, Balfour IC, Singh GK, Chen SC. Severe aortic coarctation in infants less than 3 months: successful palliation by balloon angioplasty. *J Invasive Cardiol*. 2003;15(4):202–208.
44. Chen SS, Dimopoulos K, Alonso-Gonzalez R, et al. Prevalence and prognostic implication of restenosis or dilatation at the aortic coarctation repair site assessed by cardiovascular MRI in adult patients late after coarctation repair. *Int J Cardiol*. 2014;173(2):209–215.
45. Therrien J, Thorne SA, Wright A, Kilner PJ, Somerville J. Repaired coarctation: a "cost-effective" approach to identify complications in adults. *J Am Coll Cardiol*. 2000;35(4):997–1002.
46. Simpson IA, Chung KJ, Glass RF, Sahn DJ, Sherman FS, Hesselink J. Cine magnetic resonance imaging for evaluation of anatomy and flow relations in infants and children with coarctation of the aorta. *Circulation*. 1988;78(1):142–148.
47. Mendelsohn AM, Banerjee A, Donnelly LF, Schwartz DC. Is echocardiography or magnetic resonance imaging superior for precoarctation angioplasty evaluation? *Catheter Cardiovasc Diagn*. 1997;42(1):26–30.
48. Didier D, Saint-Martin C, Lapierre C, et al. Coarctation of the aorta: pre and postoperative evaluation with MRI and MR angiography; correlation with echocardiography and surgery. *Int J Cardiovasc Imaging*. 2006;22(3–4):457–475.
49. Muzzarelli S, Ordovas KG, Hope MD, Meadows JJ, Higgins CB, Meadows AK. Diagnostic value of the flow profile in the distal descending aorta by phase-contrast magnetic resonance for predicting severe coarctation of the aorta. *J Magn Reson Imaging: JMRI*. 2011;33(6):1440–1446.
50. Steffens JC, Bourne MW, Sakuma H, O'Sullivan M, Higgins CB. Quantification of collateral blood flow in coarctation of the aorta by velocity encoded cine magnetic resonance imaging. *Circulation*. 1994;90(2):937–943.
51. Nielsen JC, Powell AJ, Gauvreau K, Marcus EN, Prakash A, Geva T. Magnetic resonance imaging predictors of coarctation severity. *Circulation*. 2005;111(5):622–628.
52. Muzzarelli S, Meadows AK, Ordovas KG, et al. Prediction of hemodynamic severity of coarctation by magnetic resonance imaging. *Am J Cardiol*. 2011;108(9):1335–1340.
53. Mohiaddin RH, Kilner PJ, Rees S, Longmore DB. Magnetic resonance volume flow and jet velocity mapping in aortic coarctation. *J Am Coll Cardiol*. 1993;22(5):1515–1521.

54. Oshinski JN, Parks WJ, Markou CP, et al. Improved measurement of pressure gradients in aortic coarctation by magnetic resonance imaging. *J Am Coll Cardiol*. 1996;28(7):1818–1826.
55. Rengier F, Delles M, Eichhorn J, et al. Noninvasive pressure difference mapping derived from 4D flow MRI in patients with unrepaired and repaired aortic coarctation. *Cardiovasc Diagn Ther*. 2014;4(2):97–103.
56. Riesenkampff E, Fernandes JF, Meier S, et al. Pressure fields by flow-sensitive, 4D, velocity-encoded CMR in patients with aortic coarctation. *JACC Cardiovasc Imaging*. 2014;7(9):920–926.
57. Araoz PA, Reddy GP, Tarnoff H, Roge CL, Higgins CB. MR findings of collateral circulation are more accurate measures of hemodynamic significance than arm-leg blood pressure gradient after repair of coarctation of the aorta. *J Magn Reson Imaging: JMRI*. 2003;17(2):177–183.
58. Holmqvist C, Ståhlberg F, Hanséus K, et al. Collateral flow in coarctation of the aorta with magnetic resonance velocity mapping: correlation to morphological imaging of collateral vessels. *J Magn Reson Imaging: JMRI*. 2002;15(1):39–46.
59. Julsrud PR, Breen JF, Felmlee JP, Warnes CA, Connolly HM, Schaff HV. Coarctation of the aorta: collateral flow assessment with phase-contrast MR angiography. *AJR Am J Roentgenol*. 1997;169(6):1735–1742.
60. Krieger EV, Clair M, Opotowsky AR, et al. Correlation of exercise response in repaired coarctation of the aorta to left ventricular mass and geometry. *Am J Cardiol*. 2013;111(3):406–411.
61. Hoffman JI, Kaplan S. The incidence of congenital heart disease. *J Am Coll Cardiol*. 2002;39(12):1890–1900.
62. Van Praagh R, Van Praagh S, Nebesar RA, Muster AJ, Sinha SN, Paul MH. Tetralogy of Fallot: underdevelopment of the pulmonary infundibulum and its sequelae. *Am J Cardiol*. 1970;26(1):25–33.
63. Need LR, Powell AJ, del Nido P, Geva T. Coronary echocardiography in tetralogy of fallot: diagnostic accuracy, resource utilization and surgical implications over 13 years. *J Am Coll Cardiol*. 2000;36(4):1371–1377.
64. Ishigami S, Ye XT, Buratto E, Ivanov Y, Chowdhuri KR, Fulkoski N, Robertson T, Davies B, Brizard CP, Konstantinov IE. Long-term outcomes of tetralogy of Fallot repair: A 30-year experience with 960 patients. *J Thorac Cardiovasc Surg*. 2024;167(1):289–302.e11. https://doi.org/10.1016/j.jtcvs.2023.04.015. Epub 2023 May 9. PMID: 37169063.
65. Bacha EA, Scheule AM, Zurakowski D, et al. Long-term results after early primary repair of tetralogy of Fallot. *J Thorac Cardiovasc Surg*. 2001;122(1):154–161.
66. Nollert G, Fischlein T, Bouterwek S, Böhmer C, Klinner W, Reichart B. Long-term survival in patients with repair of tetralogy of Fallot: 36-year follow-up of 490 survivors of the first year after surgical repair. *J Am Coll Cardiol*. 1997;30(5):1374–1383.
67. Cuypers JA, Menting ME, Konings EE, et al. Unnatural history of tetralogy of Fallot: prospective follow-up of 40 years after surgical correction. *Circulation*. 2014;130(22):1944–1953.
68. Ferraz Cavalcanti PE, Sá MP, Santos CA, et al. Pulmonary valve replacement after operative repair of tetralogy of Fallot: meta-analysis and meta-regression of 3,118 patients from 48 studies. *J Am Coll Cardiol*. 2013;62(23):2227–2243.
69. O'Byrne ML, Glatz AC, Mercer-Rosa L, et al. Trends in pulmonary valve replacement in children and adults with tetralogy of fallot. *Am J Cardiol*. 2015;115(1):118–124.
70. Valsangiacomo Buechel ER, Grosse-Wortmann L, Fratz S, et al. Indications for cardiovascular magnetic resonance in children with congenital and acquired heart disease: an expert consensus paper of the Imaging Working Group of the AEPC and the Cardiovascular Magnetic Resonance Section of the EACVI. *Cardiol Young*. 2015;25(5):819–838.
71. Valente AM, Cook S, Festa P, et al. Multimodality imaging guidelines for patients with repaired tetralogy of fallot: a report from the AmericanSsociety of echocardiography: developed in collaboration with the Society for cardiovascular magnetic resonance and the Society for pediatric Radiology. *J Am Soc Echocardiog: Off Pub Am Soc Echocardiogr*. 2014;27(2):111–141.
72. Kilner PJ, Geva T, Kaemmerer H, Trindade PT, Schwitter J, Webb GD. Recommendations for cardiovascular magnetic resonance in adults with congenital heart disease from the respective working groups of the European Society of Cardiology. *Eur Heart J*. 2010;31(7):794–805.
73. Silversides CK, Kiess M, Beauchesne L, et al. Canadian Cardiovascular Society 2009 Consensus Conference on the management of adults with congenital heart disease: outflow tract obstruction, coarctation of the aorta, tetralogy of Fallot, Ebstein anomaly and Marfan's syndrome. *Can J Cardiol*. 2010;26(3):e80–e97.
74. Geva T, Mulder B, Gauvreau K, et al. Preoperative predictors of death and sustained ventricular tachycardia after pulmonary valve replacement in patients with repaired tetralogy of fallot enrolled in the INDICATOR cohort. *Circulation*. 2018;138(19):2106–2115.
75. Majeed A, Geva T, Sleeper LA, et al. Cardiac MRI predictors of good long-term outcomes in patients with repaired TOF. *Am Heart J*. 2022;245:70–77.
76. Wald RM, Redington AN, Pereira A, et al. Refining the assessment of pulmonary regurgitation in adults after tetralogy of Fallot repair: should we be measuring regurgitant fraction or regurgitant volume? *Eur Heart J*. 2009;30(3):356–361.
77. DeZorzi C, Marenco A, Valente AM. Tricuspid Regurgitation in Patients with Tetralogy of Fallot. *J Clin Med*. 2023;12(7):2470. https://doi.org/10.3390/jcm12072470. PMID: 37048554; PMCID: PMC10095308.
78. Mongeon FP, Gurvitz MZ, Broberg CS, et al. Aortic root dilatation in adults with surgically repaired tetralogy of fallot: a multicenter cross-sectional study. *Circulation*. 2013;127(2):172–179.
79. Niwa K. Aortic root dilatation in tetralogy of Fallot long-term after repair-histology of the aorta in tetralogy of Fallot: evidence of intrinsic aortopathy. *Int J Cardiol*. 2005;103(2):117–119.
80. Valente AM, Gauvreau K, Assenza GE, et al. Contemporary predictors of death and sustained ventricular tachycardia in patients with repaired tetralogy of Fallot enrolled in the INDICATOR cohort. *Heart*. 2014;100(3):247–253.
81. Babu-Narayan SV, Kilner PJ, Li W, et al. Ventricular fibrosis suggested by cardiovascular magnetic resonance in adults with repaired tetralogy of fallot and its relationship to adverse markers of clinical outcome. *Circulation*. 2006;113(3):405–413.
82. Chen CA, Dusenbery SM, Valente AM, Powell AJ, Geva T. Myocardial ECV fraction assessed by CMR is associated with type of hemodynamic load and arrhythmia in repaired tetralogy of fallot. *JACC Cardiovasc Imaging*. 2016;9(1):1–10.
83. Broberg CS, Huang J, Hogberg I, et al. Diffuse LV myocardial fibrosis and its clinical associations in adults with repaired tetralogy of fallot. *JACC Cardiovasc Imaging*. 2016;9(1):86–87.
84. Blume ED, Altmann K, Mayer JE, Colan SD, Gauvreau K, Geva T. Evolution of risk factors influencing early mortality of the arterial switch operation. *J Am Coll Cardiol*. 1999;33(6):1702–1709.
85. Senning A. Surgical correction of transposition of the great vessels. *Surgery*. 1959;45(6):966–980.
86. Mustard WT. Successful two-stage correction of transposition of the great vessels. *Surgery*. 1964;55:469–472.
87. Roubertie F, Thambo JB, Bretonneau A, et al. Late outcome of 132 Senning procedures after 20 years of follow-up. *Ann Thorac Surg*. 2011;92(6):2206–2213; discussion 2213-2204.
88. Moons P, Gewillig M, Sluysmans T, et al. Long term outcome up to 30 years after the Mustard or Senning operation: a nationwide multicentre study in Belgium. *Heart*. 2004;90(3):307–313.
89. Krieger EVDJ. Transposition of the great arteries. In: CM O, ed. *Practice of Clinical Echocardiography*. 5th ed. Elsevier Saunders; 2017.
90. Villafañe J, Lantin-Hermoso MR, Bhatt AB, et al. D-transposition of the great arteries: the current era of the arterial switch operation. *J Am Coll Cardiol*. 2014;64(5):498–511.
91. van der Bom T, van der Palen RL, Bouma BJ, et al. Persistent neo-aortic growth during adulthood in patients after an arterial switch operation. *Heart*. 2014;100(17):1360–1365.
92. Fricke TA, d'Udekem Y, Richardson M, et al. Outcomes of the arterial switch operation for transposition of the great arteries: 25 years of experience. *Ann Thorac Surg*. 2012;94(1):139–145.
93. Kreutzer C, De Vive J, Oppido G, et al. Twenty-five-year experience with rastelli repair for transposition of the great arteries. *J Thorac Cardiovasc Surg*. 2000;120(2):211–223.
94. Lorenz CH, Walker ES, Graham Jr TP, Powers TA. Right ventricular performance and mass by use of cine MRI late after atrial repair of transposition of the great arteries. *Circulation*. 1995;92(9 Suppl):Ii233–Ii239.
95. Mooij CF, de Wit CJ, Graham DA, Powell AJ, Geva T. Reproducibility of MRI measurements of right ventricular size and function in patients with normal and dilated ventricles. *Journal of Magnetic Resonance Imaging : JMRI*. 2008;28(1):67–73.
96. Groenink M, Mulder BJ, van der Wall EE. Value of magnetic resonance imaging in functional assessment of baffle obstruction after the Mustard procedure. *J Cardiovasc Magn Reson: Off J Soc Cardiovasc Magn Reson*. 1999;1(1):49–51.
97. Johansson B, Babu-Narayan SV, Kilner PJ, Cannell TM, Mohiaddin RH. 3-dimensional time-resolved contrast-enhanced magnetic resonance angiography for evaluation late after the mustard operation for transposition. *Cardiol Young*. 2010;20(1):1–7.
98. Babu-Narayan SV, Goktekin O, Moon JC, et al. Late gadolinium enhancement cardiovascular magnetic resonance of the systemic right ventricle in adults with previous atrial redirection surgery for transposition of the great arteries. *Circulation*. 2005;111(16):2091–2098.
99. Fratz S, Hauser M, Bengel FM, et al. Myocardial scars determined by delayed-enhancement magnetic resonance imaging and positron emission tomography are not common in right ventricles with systemic function in long-term follow up. *Heart*. 2006;92(11):1673–1677.
100. Rydman R, Gatzoulis MA, Ho SY, et al. Systemic right ventricular fibrosis detected by cardiovascular magnetic resonance is associated with clinical outcome, mainly new-onset atrial arrhythmia, in patients after atrial redirection surgery for transposition of the great arteries. *Circ Cardiovasc Imaging*. 2015;8(5).
101. Preim U, Hoffmann J, Lehmkuhl L, et al. Systemic right ventricles rarely show myocardial scars in cardiac magnetic resonance delayed-enhancement imaging. *Clin Res Cardiol: Off J German Cardiac Soc*. 2013;102(5):337–344.
102. Beek FJ, Beekman RP, Dillon EH, et al. MRI of the pulmonary artery after arterial switch operation for transposition of the great arteries. *Pediatr Radiol*. 1993;23(5):335–340.
103. Weiss F, Habermann CR, Lilje C, et al. [MRI of pulmonary arteries in follow-up after arterial-switch-operation (ASO) for transposition of great arteries (d-TGA)]. *RoFo: Fortschritte auf dem Gebiete der Rontgenstrahlen und der Nuklearmedizin*. 2005;177(6):849–855.
104. Gutberlet M, Boeckel T, Hosten N, et al. Arterial switch procedure for D-transposition of the great arteries: quantitative midterm evaluation of hemodynamic changes with cine MR imaging and phase-shift velocity mapping-initial experience. *Radiology*. 2000;214(2):467–475.

105. Taylor AM, Thorne SA, Rubens MB, et al. Coronary artery imaging in grown up congenital heart disease: complementary role of magnetic resonance and x-ray coronary angiography. *Circulation*. 2000;101(14):1670–1678.
106. Tobler D, Motwani M, Wald RM, et al. Evaluation of a comprehensive cardiovascular magnetic resonance protocol in young adults late after the arterial switch operation for d-transposition of the great arteries. *J Cardiovasc Magn Reson: Off J Soc Cardiovasc Magn Reson*. 2014;16(1):98.
107. Marín Rodríguez C, Lancharro Zapata Á, Rodríguez Ogando A, et al. [Quality of 3D magnetic resonance imaging of coronary arteries in patients with D-transposition of the great arteries after the Jatene switch procedure]. *Radiologia*. 2015;57(4):326–332.
108. Manso B, Castellote A, Dos L, Casaldáliga J. Myocardial perfusion magnetic resonance imaging for detecting coronary function anomalies in asymptomatic paediatric patients with a previous arterial switch operation for the transposition of great arteries. *Cardiol Young*. 2010;20(4):410–417.
109. Taylor AM, Dymarkowski S, Hamaekers P, et al. MR coronary angiography and late-enhancement myocardial MR in children who underwent arterial switch surgery for transposition of great arteries. *Radiology*. 2005;234(2):542–547.
110. Prieto LR, Hordof AJ, Secic M, Rosenbaum MS, Gersony WM. Progressive tricuspid valve disease in patients with congenitally corrected transposition of the great arteries. *Circulation*. 1998;98(10):997–1005.
111. Beauchesne LM, Warnes CA, Connolly HM, Ammash NM, Tajik AJ, Danielson GK. Outcome of the unoperated adult who presents with congenitally corrected transposition of the great arteries. *J Am Coll Cardiol*. 2002;40(2):285–290.
112. Graham Jr TP, Bernard YD, Mellen BG, et al. Long-term outcome in congenitally corrected transposition of the great arteries: a multi-institutional study. *J Am Coll Cardiol*. 2000;36(1):255–261.
113. van Dissel AC, Opotowsky AR, Burchill LJ, et al. End-stage heart failure in congenitally corrected transposition of the great arteries: a multicentre study. *Eur Heart J*. 2023;44(34):3278–3291.
114. Emani SM, Del Nido PJ. Systemic atrioventricular valve regurgitation in corrected transposition of the great arteries: where are we? *J Am Coll Cardiol*. 2023;82(23):2209–2211.
115. Abdelrehim AA, Stephens EH, Miranda WR, et al. Systemic atrioventricular valve surgery in patients with congenitally corrected transposition of the great vessels. *J Am Coll Cardiol*. 2023;82(23):2197–2208.
116. Connelly MS, Liu PP, Williams WG, Webb GD, Robertson P, McLaughlin PR. Congenitally corrected transposition of the great arteries in the adult: functional status and complications. *J Am Coll Cardiol*. 1996;27(5):1238–1243.
117. Wilson HC, Lu JC, Yu S, et al. Ventricular function in physiologically repaired and unrepaired congenitally corrected transposition of the great arteries. *Am J Cardiol*. 2022;165:95–100.
118. Hraska V, Duncan BW, Mayer Jr JE, Freed M, del Nido PJ, Jonas RA. Long-term outcome of surgically treated patients with corrected transposition of the great arteries. *J Thorac Cardiovasc Surg*. 2005;129(1):182–191.
119. Yeh Jr T, Connelly MS, Coles JG, et al. Atrioventricular discordance: results of repair in 127 patients. *J Thorac Cardiovasc Surg*. 1999;117(6):1190–1203.
120. Yamagishi M, Imai Y, Hoshino S, et al. [Surgical correction of atrioventricular discordance-results and follow-up]. *[Zasshi] [Journal] Nihon Kyobu Geka Gakkai*. 1992;40(8):1167–1176.
121. Yagihara T, Kishimoto H, Isobe F, et al. Double switch operation in cardiac anomalies with atrioventricular and ventriculoarterial discordance. *J Thorac Cardiovasc Surg*. 1994;107(2):351–358.
122. Devaney EJ, Charpie JR, Ohye RG, Bove EL. Combined arterial switch and Senning operation for congenitally corrected transposition of the great arteries: patient selection and intermediate results. *J Thorac Cardiovasc Surgy*. 2003;125(3):500–507.
123. Ilbawi MN, DeLeon SY, Backer CL, et al. An alternative approach to the surgical management of physiologically corrected transposition with ventricular septal defect and pulmonary stenosis or atresia. *J Thorac Cardiovasc Surg*. 1990;100(3):410–415.
124. Winlaw DS, McGuirk SP, Balmer C, et al. Intention-to-treat analysis of pulmonary artery banding in conditions with a morphological right ventricle in the systemic circulation with a view to anatomic biventricular repair. *Circulation*. 2005;111(4):405–411.
125. Marathe SP, Chávez M, Schulz A, et al. Contemporary outcomes of the double switch operation for congenitally corrected transposition of the great arteries. *J Thorac Cardiovasc Surg*. 2022;164(6):1980–1990.
126. Duncan BW, Mee RBB, Mesia CI, et al. Results of the double switch operation for congenitally corrected transposition of the great arteries. *Eur J Cardiothorac Surg*. 2003;24(1):11–20.
127. Murtuza B, Barron DJ, Stumper O, et al. Anatomic repair for congenitally corrected transposition of the great arteries: a single-institution 19-year experience. *J Thorac Cardiovasc Surg*. 2011;142(6):1348–1357.
128. Sharma R, Talwar S, Marwah A, et al. Anatomic repair for congenitally corrected transposition of the great arteries. *J Thorac Cardiovasc Surg*. 2009;137(2):404–412.e404.
129. Gaies MG, Goldberg CS, Ohye RG, Devaney EJ, Hirsch JC, Bove EL. Early and intermediate outcome after anatomic repair of congenitally corrected transposition of the great arteries. *Ann Thorac Surg*. 2009;88(6):1952–1960.
130. Hraška V, Mattes A, Haun C, et al. Functional outcome of anatomic correction of corrected transposition of the great arteries. *Eur J Cardiothorac Surg*. 2011;40(5):1227–1234.
131. Gurvitz M, Krieger EV, Fuller S, et al. 2025 ACC/AHA/HRS/ISACHD/SCAI Guideline for the Management of Adults With Congenital Heart Disease: A Report of the American College of Cardiology/American Heart Association Joint Committee on Clinical Practice Guidelines. *J Am Coll Cardiol*. 2026;87(7):822–976. https://doi.org/10.1016/j.jacc.2025.09.006. Epub 2025 Dec 18. PMID: 41411480.
132. Al-Wakeel N, O h-Ici D, Schmitt KR, et al. Cardiac MRI in patients with complex CHD following primary or secondary implantation of MRI-conditional pacemaker system. *Cardiol Young*. 2016;26(2):306–314.
133. Vuorinen AM, Paakkanen R, Karvonen J, et al. Magnetic resonance imaging safety in patients with abandoned or functioning epicardial pacing leads. *Eur Radiol*. 2022;32(6):3830–3838.
134. Giardini A, Lovato L, Donti A, et al. Relation between right ventricular structural alterations and markers of adverse clinical outcome in adults with systemic right ventricle and either congenital complete (after Senning operation) or congenitally corrected transposition of the great arteries. *Am J Cardiol*. 2006;98(9):1277–1282.
135. Al-Wakeel-Marquard N, Ferreira da Silva T, Berger F, Kuehne T, Messroghli DR. Myocardial extracellular volume is a non-invasive tissue marker of heart failure in patients with transposition of the great arteries and systemic right ventricle. *Front Pediatr*. 2022;10:949078.
136. Edwards WD. Embryology and pathologic features of Ebstein's anomaly. *Progr Pediatr Cardiol*. 1993;2(1):5–15.
137. Benson DW, Silberbach GM, Kavanaugh-McHugh A, et al. Mutations in the cardiac transcription factor NKX2.5 affect diverse cardiac developmental pathways. *J Clin Investig*. 1999;104(11):1567–1573.
138. Yang H, Lee CL, Young DC, Shortliffe M, Yu W, Wright JR. A rare case of interstitial del(1)(p34.3p36.11) diagnosed prenatally. *Fetal Pediatr Pathol*. 2004;23(4):251–255.
139. da Silva JP, Baumgratz JF, da Fonseca L, et al. The cone reconstruction of the tricuspid valve in Ebstein's anomaly. The operation: early and midterm results. *J Thorac Cardiovasc Surg*. 2007;133(1):215–223.
140. Fontan F, Baudet E. Surgical repair of tricuspid atresia. *Thorax*. 1971;26(3):240–248.
141. Brown DW, Gauvreau K, Powell AJ, et al. Cardiac magnetic resonance versus routine cardiac catheterization before bidirectional glenn anastomosis in infants with functional single ventricle: a prospective randomized trial. *Circulation*. 2007;116(23):2718–2725.
142. Brown DW, Gauvreau K, Powell AJ, et al. Cardiac magnetic resonance versus routine cardiac catheterization before bidirectional Glenn anastomosis: long-term follow-up of a prospective randomized trial. *J Thorac Cardiovasc Surg*. 2013;146(5):1172–1178.
143. Grosse-Wortmann L, Al-Otay A, Yoo SJ. Aortopulmonary collaterals after bidirectional cavopulmonary connection or Fontan completion: quantification with MRI. *Circ Cardiovasc Imaging*. 2009;2(3):219–225.
144. Whitehead KK, Gillespie MJ, Harris MA, Fogel MA, Rome JJ. Noninvasive quantification of systemic-to-pulmonary collateral flow: a major source of inefficiency in patients with superior cavopulmonary connections. *Circ Cardiovasc Imaging*. 2009;2(5):405–411.
145. Prakash A, Khan MA, Hardy R, Torres AJ, Chen JM, Gersony WM. A new diagnostic algorithm for assessment of patients with single ventricle before a Fontan operation. *J Thorac Cardiovasc Surg*. 2009;138(4):917–923.
146. Ro PS, Rychik J, Cohen MS, Mahle WT, Rome JJ. Diagnostic assessment before Fontan operation in patients with bidirectional cavopulmonary anastomosis: are noninvasive methods sufficient? *J Am Coll Cardiol*. 2004;44(1):184–187.
147. Banka P, McElhinney DB, Bacha EA, et al. What is the clinical utility of routine cardiac catheterization before a Fontan operation? *Pediatr Cardiol*. 2010;31(7):977–985.
148. Fogel MA, Pawlowski TW, Whitehead KK, et al. Cardiac magnetic resonance and the need for routine cardiac catheterization in single ventricle patients prior to Fontan: a comparison of 3 groups: pre-Fontan CMR versus cath evaluation. *J Am Coll Cardiol*. 2012;60(12):1094–1102.
149. Margossian R, Schwartz ML, Prakash A, et al. Comparison of echocardiographic and cardiac magnetic resonance imaging measurements of functional single ventricular volumes, mass, and ejection fraction (from the Pediatric Heart Network Fontan Cross-Sectional Study). *Am J Cardiol*. 2009;104(3):419–428.
150. Hjortdal VE, Emmertsen K, Stenbøg E, et al. Effects of exercise and respiration on blood flow in total cavopulmonary connection: a real-time magnetic resonance flow study. *Circulation*. 2003;108(10):1227–1231.
151. Rathod RH, Prakash A, Kim YY, et al. Cardiac magnetic resonance parameters predict transplantation-free survival in patients with fontan circulation. *Circ Cardiovasc Imaging*. 2014;7(3):502–509.
152. Rathod RH, Prakash A, Powell AJ, Geva T. Myocardial fibrosis identified by cardiac magnetic resonance late gadolinium enhancement is associated with adverse ventricular mechanics and ventricular tachycardia late after Fontan operation. *J Am Coll Cardiol*. 2010;55(16):1721–1728.
153. Grosse-Wortmann L, Drolet C, Dragulescu A, et al. Aortopulmonary collateral flow volume affects early postoperative outcome after Fontan completion: a multimodality study. *J Thorac Cardiovasc Surg*. 2012;144(6):1329–1336.
154. Glatz AC, Harrison N, Small AJ, et al. Factors associated with systemic to pulmonary arterial collateral flow in single ventricle patients with superior cavopulmonary connections. *Heart*. 2015;101(22):1813–1818.

155. Whitehead KK, Harris MA, Glatz AC, et al. Status of systemic to pulmonary arterial collateral flow after the fontan procedure. *Am J Cardiol.* 2015;115(12):1739–1745.
156. Odenwald T, Quail MA, Giardini A, et al. Systemic to pulmonary collateral blood flow influences early outcomes following the total cavopulmonary connection. *Heart.* 2012;98(12):934–940.
157. Prakash A, Rathod RH, Powell AJ, McElhinney DB, Banka P, Geva T. Relation of systemic-to-pulmonary artery collateral flow in single ventricle physiology to palliative stage and clinical status. *Am J Cardiol.* 2012;109(7):1038–1045.
158. Khiabani RH, Whitehead KK, Han D, et al. Exercise capacity in single-ventricle patients after Fontan correlates with haemodynamic energy loss in TCPC. *Heart.* 2015;101(2):139–143.
159. Be'eri E, Maier SE, Landzberg MJ, Chung T, Geva T. In vivo evaluation of Fontan pathway flow dynamics by multidimensional phase-velocity magnetic resonance imaging. *Circulation.* 1998;98(25):2873–2882.
160. Haggerty CM, Kanter KR, Restrepo M, et al. Simulating hemodynamics of the Fontan Y-graft based on patient-specific in vivo connections. *J Thorac Cardiovasc Surg.* 2013;145(3):663–670.
161. Di Cesare M, Sorić M, Bovet P, et al. The epidemiological burden of obesity in childhood: a worldwide epidemic requiring urgent action. *BMC Med.* 2019;17:1–20.
162. Ng M, Fleming T, Robinson M, et al. Global, regional, and national prevalence of overweight and obesity in children and adults during 1980-2013: a systematic analysis for the Global Burden of Disease Study 2013. *Lancet (London, England).* 2014;384(9945):766–781.
163. Ajala O, Mold F, Boughton C, Cooke D, Whyte M. Childhood predictors of cardiovascular disease in adulthood. A systematic review and meta-analysis. *Obe Rev : Off J Int Assoc Study Obes.* 2017;18(9):1061–1070.
164. Baker JL, Olsen LW, Sørensen TI. Childhood body-mass index and the risk of coronary heart disease in adulthood. *N Engl J Med.* 2007;357(23):2329–2337.
165. Umer A, Kelley GA, Cottrell LE, Giacobbi Jr P, Innes KE, Lilly CL. Childhood obesity and adult cardiovascular disease risk factors: a systematic review with meta-analysis. *BMC Public Health.* 2017;17(1):683.
166. Santos RD, Gidding SS, Hegele RA, et al. Defining severe familial hypercholesterolaemia and the implications for clinical management: a consensus statement from the International Atherosclerosis Society Severe Familial Hypercholesterolemia Panel. *Lancet Diabetes Endocrinol.* 2016;4(10):850–861.
167. Kim HW, Van Assche L, Jennings RB, et al. Relationship of T2-weighted MRI myocardial Hyperintensity and the ischemic area-at-risk. *Circ Res.* 2015;117(3):254–265.
168. Kaolawanich Y, Azevedo CF, Kim HW, et al. Native T1 mapping for the diagnosis of myocardial fibrosis in patients with chronic myocardial infarction. *JACC Cardiovasc Imaging.* 2022;15(12):2069–2079.
169. Kim RJ, Chen EL, Lima JA, Judd RM. Myocardial Gd-DTPA kinetics determine MRI contrast enhancement and reflect the extent and severity of myocardial injury after acute reperfused infarction. *Circulation.* 1996;94(12):3318–3326.
170. Kim RJ, Fieno DS, Parrish TB, et al. Relationship of MRI delayed contrast enhancement to irreversible injury, infarct age, and contractile function. *Circulation.* 1999;100(19):1992–2002.
171. Kim HW, Rehwald WG, Jenista ER, et al. Dark-blood delayed enhancement cardiac magnetic resonance of myocardial infarction. *JACC Cardiovasc Imaging.* 2018;11(12):1758–1769.
172. Strigl S, Beroukhim R, Valente AM, et al. Feasibility of dobutamine stress cardiovascular magnetic resonance imaging in children. *J Magn Reson Imaging: JMRI.* 2009;29(2):313–319.
173. Stagnaro N, Moscatelli S, Cheli M, Bondanza S, Marasini M, Trocchio G. Dobutamine stress cardiac MRI in pediatric patients with suspected coronary artery disease. *Pediatr Cardiol.* 2023;44(2):451–462.
174. Campbell MJ, Barker P, Hayes B, Kim RJ. CMR adenosine stress perfusion in pediatrics and congenital heart disease: effects on clinical decision making and outcomes. *J Cardiovasc Magn Reson.* 2012;14(1):1–2.
175. Campbell MJ, Barker PC, Bailliard F, Kim RJ. Evaluation of coronary artery disease in congenital heart disease and pediatrics utilizing adenosine stress perfusion. *J Cardiovasc Magn Reson.* 2011;13:1–2.
176. Noel CV, Krishnamurthy R, Masand P, et al. Myocardial stress perfusion MRI: experience in pediatric and young-adult patients following arterial switch operation utilizing regadenoson. *Pediatr Cardiol.* 2018;39(6):1249–1257.
177. Lee AC, Foster E, Yeghiazarians Y. Anomalous origin of the left coronary artery from the pulmonary artery: a case series and brief review. *Congenit Heart Dis.* 2006;1(3):111–115.
178. Ramana RK, Varga P, Leya F. Late presentation of an anomalous origin of the left coronary artery from the pulmonary artery: case report and review. *J Invasive Cardiol.* 2008;20(10):564–566.
179. Straka N, Gauvreau K, Huang Y, et al. Analysis of Perioperative and long-term outcomes among presentations of anomalous left coronary artery from the pulmonary artery diagnosed beyond infancy versus during infancy. *Pediatr Cardiol.* 2023.
180. Berre LL, Baruteau AE, Fraisse A, et al. Anomalous origin of the left coronary artery from the pulmonary artery presenting in adulthood: a French nationwide retrospective study. *Sem Thorac Cardiovasc Surg.* 2017.
181. Latus H, Gummel K, Rupp S, et al. Cardiovascular magnetic resonance assessment of ventricular function and myocardial scarring before and early after repair of anomalous left coronary artery from the pulmonary artery. *J Cardiovasc Magn Reson: Off J Soc Cardiovasc Magn Reson.* 2014;16(1):3.
182. Browne LP, Kearney D, Taylor MD, et al. ALCAPA: the role of myocardial viability studies in determining prognosis. *Pediatr Radiol.* 2010;40(2):163–167.
183. Schmitt B, Bauer S, Kutty S, et al. Myocardial perfusion, scarring, and function in anomalous left coronary artery from the pulmonary artery syndrome: a long-term analysis using magnetic resonance imaging. *Ann Thorac Surg.* 2014;98(4):1425–1436.
184. Secinaro A, Ntsinjana H, Tann O, et al. Cardiovascular magnetic resonance findings in repaired anomalous left coronary artery to pulmonary artery connection (ALCAPA). *J Cardiovasc Magn Reson: Off J Soc Cardiovasc Magn Reson.* 2011;13(1):27.
185. Doan TT, Wilkes JK, Reaves O'Neal DL, et al. Clinical presentation and medium-term outcomes of children with anomalous aortic origin of the left coronary artery: high-risk features beyond Interarterial course. *Circ Cardiovasc Interven.* 2023;16(5):e012635.
186. Maron BJ, Doerer JJ, Haas TS, Tierney DM, Mueller FO. Sudden deaths in young competitive athletes: analysis of 1866 deaths in the United States, 1980–2006. *Circulation.* 2009;119(8):1085–1092.
187. Basso C, Maron BJ, Corrado D, Thiene G. Clinical profile of congenital coronary artery anomalies with origin from the wrong aortic sinus leading to sudden death in young competitive athletes. *J Am Coll Cardiol.* 2000;35(6):1493–1501.
188. Brothers JA, Frommelt MA, Jaquiss RDB, Myerburg RJ, Fraser Jr CD, Tweddell JS. Expert consensus guidelines: anomalous aortic origin of a coronary artery. *J Thorac Cardiovasc Surg.* 2017;153(6):1440–1457.
189. Maron BJ, Shirani J, Poliac LC, Mathenge R, Roberts WC, Mueller FO. Sudden death in young competitive athletes: clinical, demographic, and pathological profiles. *JAMA.* 1996;276(3):199–204.
190. Doan TT, Molossi S, Sachdeva S, et al. Dobutamine stress cardiac MRI is safe and feasible in pediatric patients with anomalous aortic origin of a coronary artery (AAOCA). *Int J Cardiol.* 2021;334:42–48.
191. Cannon L, Campbell MJ, Wu EY. Multisystemic inflammatory syndrome in children and kawasaki disease: parallels in pathogenesis and treatment. *Curr Allergy Asthma Rep.* 2023;23(6):341–350.
192. Wu EY, Campbell MJ. Cardiac manifestations of multisystem inflammatory syndrome in children (MIS-C) following COVID-19. *Curr Cardiol Rep.* 2021;23(11):168.
193. McCrindle BW, Rowley AH, Newburger JW, et al. Diagnosis, treatment, and long-term management of kawasaki disease: a Scientific statement for health professionals from the American heart association. *Circulation.* 2017;135(17):e927–e999.
194. Crean A, Benson L, Shah A, Han K, Lesser J, McCrindle BW. Imaging the delayed complications of childhood Kawasaki disease. *F1000Research.* 2022;11:147.
195. Dorfman AL, Geva T, Samyn MM, et al. SCMR expert consensus statement for cardiovascular magnetic resonance of acquired and non-structural pediatric heart disease. *J Cardiovasc Magn Reson : Off J Soc Cardiovasc Magn Reson.* 2022;24(1):44.
196. Greil GF, Stuber M, Botnar RM, et al. Coronary magnetic resonance angiography in adolescents and young adults with kawasaki disease. *Circulation.* 2002;105(8):908–911.
197. van Stijn D, Planken N, Kuipers I, Kuijpers T. CT angiography or cardiac MRI for detection of coronary artery aneurysms in kawasaki disease. *Front Pediatr.* 2021;9:630462.
198. Campbell MJ, Barker P, Li J, Abstract O. 55: utility of adenosine cardiac stress MRI to evaluate ischemia in patients with kawasaki disease. *Circulation.* 2015;131(suppl l_2):AO55.
199. Dove ML, Jaggi P, Kelleman M, et al. Multisystem inflammatory syndrome in children: survey of protocols for early hospital evaluation and management. *J Pediatr.* 2021;229:33–40.
200. Rossano JW, Singh TP, Cherikh WS, et al. The International thoracic organ transplant Registry of the International Society for heart and lung transplantation: twenty-second pediatric heart transplantation report–2019; focus theme: donor and recipient size match. *J Heart Lung Transplant.* 2019;38(10):1028–1041.
201. Singh TP, Cherikh WS, Hsich E, et al. The International thoracic organ transplant Registry of the International Society for heart and lung transplantation: Twenty-fourth pediatric heart transplantation report—2021; focus on recipient characteristics. *J Heart Lung Transplant.* 2021;40(10):1050–1059.
202. Singh TP, Hsich E, Cherikh WS, et al. The International thoracic organ transplant Registry of the International Society for heart and lung transplantation: 23rd pediatric heart transplantation report—2020; focus on deceased donor characteristics. *J Heart Lung Transplant.* 2020;39(10):1028–1037.
203. Kikano S, Lee S, Dodd D, et al. Cardiac magnetic resonance assessment of acute rejection and cardiac allograft vasculopathy in pediatric heart transplant. *J Heart Lung Transplant.* 2023;43(5):745–754.
204. Nandi D, Chin C, Schumacher KR, et al. Surveillance for cardiac allograft vasculopathy: practice variations among 50 pediatric heart transplant centers. *J Heart Lung Transplant.* 2020;39(11):1260–1269.
205. Godown J, Harris MT, Burger J, Dodd DA. Variation in the use of surveillance endomyocardial biopsy among pediatric heart transplant centers over time. *Pediatr Transplant.* 2015;19(6):612–617.
206. Grotenhuis HB, Nyns ECA, Kantor PF, et al. Abnormal myocardial contractility after pediatric heart transplantation by cardiac MRI. *Pediatr Cardiol.* 2017;38(6):1198–1205.
207. Dolan RS, Rahsepar AA, Blaisdell J, et al. Multiparametric cardiac magnetic resonance imaging can detect acute cardiac allograft rejection

after heart transplantation. *JACC: Cardiovasc Imaging*. 2019;12(8 Part 2):1632–1641.
208. Imran M, Wang L, McCrohon J, et al. Native T1 mapping in the diagnosis of cardiac allograft rejection: a prospective histologically validated study. *JACC: Cardiovasc Imaging*. 2019;12(8 Part 2):1618–1628.
209. Vermes E, PantalΩon C, Auvet A, et al. Cardiovascular magnetic resonance in heart transplant patients: diagnostic value of quantitative tissue markers: T2 mapping and extracellular volume fraction, for acute rejection diagnosis. *J Cardiovasc Magn Reson*. 2018;20(1):59.
210. Anthony C, Imran M, Pouliopoulos J, et al. Cardiovascular magnetic resonance for rejection surveillance after cardiac transplantation. *Circulation*. 2022;145(25):1811–1824.
211. Miller CA, Naish JH, Shaw SM, et al. Multiparametric cardiovascular magnetic resonance surveillance of acute cardiac allograft rejection and characterisation of transplantation-associated myocardial injury: a pilot study. *J Cardiovasc Magn Reson*. 2014;16:1–11.
212. Richmann DP, Gurijala N, Mandell JG, et al. Native T1 mapping detects both acute clinical rejection and graft dysfunction in pediatric heart transplant patients. *J Cardiovasc Magn Reson*. 2022;24(1):51.
213. Soslow JH, Godown J, Bearl DW, et al. Cardiac magnetic resonance imaging noninvasively detects rejection in pediatric heart transplant recipients. *Circulation: Cardiovascular Imaging*. 2022;15(4):e013456.
214. Soslow JH, Samyn MM. Multi-modal imaging of the pediatric heart transplant recipient. *Transl Pediatr*. 2019;8(4):322.
215. Sethi N, Doshi A, Doshi T, et al. Quantitative cardiac magnetic resonance T2 imaging offers ability to non-invasively predict acute allograft rejection in children. *Cardiol Young*. 2020;30(6):852–859.
216. Greenway SC, Dallaire F, Kantor PF, et al. Magnetic resonance imaging of the transplanted pediatric heart as a potential predictor of rejection. *W J Transplant*. 2016;6(4):751.
217. Pedrotti P, Vittori C, Facchetti R, et al. Prognostic impact of late gadolinium enhancement in the risk stratification of heart transplant patients. *Eur Heart J Cardiovasc Imaging*. 2017;18(2):130–137.
218. Kazmirczak F, Nijjar PS, Zhang L, et al. Safety and prognostic value of regadenoson stress cardiovascular magnetic resonance imaging in heart transplant recipients. *J Cardiovasc Magn Reson: Off J Soc Cardiovasc Magn Reson*. 2019;21(1):9.
219. Patel SG, Husain N, Rigsby CK, Robinson JD. Safety and efficacy of regadenoson for pediatric stress perfusion cardiac MRI with quantification of myocardial blood flow. *Children (Basel, Switzerland)*. 2022;9(9):1332.
220. Jiménez-Jaso JM, Ezponda A, Sáenz-Diez JM, Caballeros M, Rábago G, Bastarrika G. Cardiac magnetic resonance imaging myocardial perfusion reserve index in heart transplant patients. *Radiologia*. 2020;62(6):493–501.
221. Erbel C, Mukhammadaminova N, Gleissner CA, et al. Myocardial perfusion reserve and strain-encoded CMR for evaluation of cardiac allograft Microvasculopathy. *JACC Cardiovasc Imaging*. 2016;9(3):255–266.
222. Luijkx T, Velthuis BK, Prakken NH, et al. Impact of revised Task Force Criteria: distinguishing the athlete's heart from ARVC/D using cardiac magnetic resonance imaging. *Eur J Prevent Cardiol*. 2012;19(4):885–891.
223. Franzen E, Mangold S, Erz G, et al. Comparison of morphological and functional adaptations of the heart in highly trained triathletes and long-distance runners using cardiac magnetic resonance imaging. *Heart Vessels*. 2013;28(5):626–631.
224. Maron BJ, Haas TS, Ahluwalia A, Murphy CJ, Garberich RF. Demographics and epidemiology of sudden deaths in young competitive athletes: from the United States National Registry. *Am J Med*. 2016;129(11):1170–1177.
225. Hussain T, Dragulescu A, Benson L, et al. Quantification and significance of diffuse myocardial fibrosis and diastolic dysfunction in childhood hypertrophic cardiomyopathy. *Pediatr Cardiol*. 2015;36(5):970–978.
226. Axelsson Raja A, Farhad H, Valente AM, et al. Prevalence and progression of late gadolinium enhancement in children and adolescents with hypertrophic cardiomyopathy. *Circulation*. 2018;138(8):782–792.
227. Petryka-Mazurkiewicz J, Ziolkowska L, Kowalczyk-Domagala M, et al. LGE for risk stratification in primary prevention in children with HCM. *JACC Cardiovasc Imaging*. 2020;13(12):2684–2686.
228. Ali LA, Marrone C, Martins DS, et al. Prognostic factors in hypertrophic cardiomyopathy in children: an MRI based study. *Int J Cardiol*. 2022;364:141–147.
229. Silva MC, Meira ZM, Gurgel Giannetti J, et al. Myocardial delayed enhancement by magnetic resonance imaging in patients with muscular dystrophy. *J Am Coll Cardiol*. 2007;49(18):1874–1879.
230. Thompson RB, Chow K, Khan A, et al. T_1 mapping with cardiovascular MRI is highly sensitive for Fabry disease independent of hypertrophy and sex. *Circ Cardiovasc Imaging*. 2013;6(5):637–645.
231. Mertens L, Singh G, Armenian S, et al. Multimodality imaging for cardiac surveillance of cancer treatment in children: recommendations from the American Society of Echocardiography. *J Am Soc Echocardiogr: Off Pub Am Soc Echocardiogr*. 2023;36(12):1227–1253.
232. Toro-Salazar OH, Ferranti J, Lorenzoni R, et al. Feasibility of echocardiographic techniques to detect subclinical cancer therapeutics-related cardiac dysfunction among high-dose patients when compared with cardiac magnetic resonance imaging. *J Am Soc Echocardiogr: Off Pub Am Soc Echocardiogr*. 2016;29(2):119–131.
233. Thiene G, Nava A, Corrado D, Rossi L, Pennelli N. Right ventricular cardiomyopathy and sudden death in young people. *N Engl J Med*. 1988;318(3):129–133.
234. Corrado D, Basso C, Thiene G. Arrhythmogenic right ventricular cardiomyopathy: diagnosis, prognosis, and treatment. *Heart*. 2000;83(5):588.
235. Corrado D, Link MS, Calkins H. Arrhythmogenic right ventricular cardiomyopathy. *N Engl J Med*. 2017;376(1):61–72.
236. Corrado D, Anastasakis A, Basso C, et al. Proposed diagnostic criteria for arrhythmogenic cardiomyopathy: European Task Force consensus report. *Int J Cardiol*. 2024;395:131447.
237. Corrado D, Marra MP, Zorzi A, et al. Diagnosis of arrhythmogenic cardiomyopathy: the Padua criteria. *Int J Cardiol*. 2020;319:106–114.
238. Azevedo CF, Jenista ER, Kaolawanich Y, et al. Assessment of myocardial lipomatous metaplasia using an optimized out-of-phase cine steady-state free-precession sequence: Validation and clinical implementation. *NMR Biomed*. 2022;35(10):e4777.
239. Piriou N, Marteau L, Kyndt F, et al. Familial screening in case of acute myocarditis reveals inherited arrhythmogenic left ventricular cardiomyopathies. *ESC Heart Failure*. 2020;7(4):1520–1533.
240. Friedrich MG, Sechtem U, Schulz-Menger J, et al. Cardiovascular magnetic resonance in myocarditis: a JACC White Paper. *J Am Coll Cardiol*. 2009;53(17):1475–1487.
241. Ferreira VM, Schulz-Menger J, Holmvang G, et al. Cardiovascular magnetic resonance in nonischemic myocardial inflammation: expert recommendations. *J Am Coll Cardiol*. 2018;72(24):3158–3176.
242. La Vecchia G, Del Buono MG, Bonaventura A, et al. Cardiac involvement in patients with multisystem inflammatory syndrome in adults. *J Am Heart Assoc*. 2024:e032143.
243. Kim HW, Jenista ER, Wendell DC, et al. Patients with acute myocarditis following mRNA COVID-19 vaccination. *JAMA Cardioly*. 2021;6(10):1196–1201.
244. Oster ME, Shay DK, Su JR, et al. Myocarditis cases reported after mRNA-based COVID-19 vaccination in the US from December 2020 to August 2021. *JAMA*. 2022;327(4):331–340.
245. Truong DT, Dionne A, Muniz JC, et al. Clinically suspected myocarditis temporally related to COVID-19 vaccination in adolescents and young adults: suspected myocarditis after COVID-19 vaccination. *Circulation*. 2022;145(5):345–356.
246. Beroukhim RS, Ghelani S, Ashwath R, et al. Accuracy of cardiac magnetic resonance imaging in diagnosing pediatric cardiac masses: a multicenter study. *JACC Cardiovasc Imaging*. 2022;15(8):1391–1405.
247. Beroukhim RS, Prakash A, Buechel ER, et al. Characterization of cardiac tumors in children by cardiovascular magnetic resonance imaging: a multicenter experience. *J Am Coll Cardiol*. 2011;58(10):1044–1054.
248. Aw F, Goyer I, Raboisson MJ, Boutin C, Major P, Dahdah N. Accelerated cardiac rhabdomyoma regression with Everolimus in infants with tuberous sclerosis complex. *Pediatr Cardiol*. 2017;38(2):394–400.

APPENDIX A

Cardiac Magnetic Resonance Screening Form: Duke Cardiovascular Magnetic Resonance Center

M2326
Rev. 8/15

Duke Medicine

PATIENT MRI SAFETY SCREENING

Place Patient Label Here

Place Patient Label Here

☐ Duke University Hospital ☐ Duke Raleigh Hospital

☐ Duke Regional Hospital ☐ Davis Ambulatory Surgery Center

☐ Other ______________________ (Please specify)

Please list all surgeries and year performed:

____

____

____

WARNING: Certain implants, devices, or objects may be hazardous to you and/or may interfere with the MR procedure (i.e., MRI, MR angiography, functional MRI, MR spectroscopy). Do not enter the MR system room or MR environment if you have any questions or concerns regarding an implant, device, or object. Consult the MRI Staff, Radiologist or Physician BEFORE entering the MR system room. The MR system magnet is ALWAYS on.

Please indicate if you have any of the following:

☐ Yes ☐ No Aneurysm clip(s)
☐ Yes ☐ No Cardiac pacemaker
☐ Yes ☐ No Implanted cardioverter defibrillator (ICD)
☐ Yes ☐ No Electronic implant or device
☐ Yes ☐ No Magnetically-activated implant or device
☐ Yes ☐ No Neurostimulation system
☐ Yes ☐ No Spinal cord stimulator
☐ Yes ☐ No Internal electrodes or wires
☐ Yes ☐ No Bone growth/bone fusion stimulator
☐ Yes ☐ No Cochlear, eye or other ear implant
☐ Yes ☐ No Insulin or other infusion pump
☐ Yes ☐ No Implanted drug infusion device
☐ Yes ☐ No Any type of prostheses (eye, penile, etc.)
☐ Yes ☐ No Heart valve prosthesis
☐ Yes ☐ No Eyelid spring or wire
☐ Yes ☐ No Artificial or prosthetic limb
☐ Yes ☐ No Metallic stent, filter or coil
☐ Yes ☐ No Shunt (spinal or intraventricular)
☐ Yes ☐ No Vascular access port and/or catheter
☐ Yes ☐ No Radiation seeds or implants
☐ Yes ☐ No Swan-Ganz or thermodilution catheter
☐ Yes ☐ No Medication patch (Nicotine, Nitroglycerine)
☐ Yes ☐ No Any metallic fragment or foreign body
☐ Yes ☐ No Wire mesh implant
☐ Yes ☐ No Tissue expander (e.g., breast)
☐ Yes ☐ No Surgical staples, clips or metallic sutures
☐ Yes ☐ No Joint replacement (hip, knee, etc.)
☐ Yes ☐ No Bone/joint pin, screw, nail, wire, plate, etc.
☐ Yes ☐ No IUD, diaphragm or pessary
☐ Yes ☐ No Dentures or partial plates
☐ Yes ☐ No Tattoo or permanent makeup
☐ Yes ☐ No Body piercing jewelry
☐ Yes ☐ No Hearing aid
☐ Yes ☐ No Other implant ______________
☐ Yes ☐ No Breathing problem or motion disorder
☐ Yes ☐ No Claustrophobia
☐ Yes ☐ No Any chance of pregnancy?

IMPORTANT INSTRUCTIONS

Before entering the MR environment or MR system room, you must remove all metallic objects including hearing aids, dentures, partial plates, keys, beeper, cell phone, eyeglasses, hair pins, barrettes, jewelry, body piercing jewelry, watch, safety pins, paperclips, money clip, credit cards, bank cards, magnetic strip cards, coins, pens pocket knife, nail clipper, tools, clothing with metal fasteners & clothing with metallic threads.

Please consult the MRI Technologist, Radiologist, Physician or MRI Staff if you have any questions or concerns BEFORE you enter the MR system room.

NOTE: You may be advised to wear earplugs or other hearing protection during the MR procedure to prevent possible problems or hazards related to acoustic noise.

M2326

I attest that the above information is correct to the best of my knowledge. I read and understand the contents of this form and had the opportunity to ask questions regarding the information on this form and regarding the MR procedure that I am about to undergo.

Signature of Person Completing Form: ______________________ **Date:** ____/____/____ **Time:** ________

Form Completed By: ☐ Patient ☐ Relative ☐ Nurse

______________________ Print name ______________________ Relationship to Patient

Form Information Reviewed By: ______________________ Print name ______________________ Signature

☐ MRI Technologist ☐ Nurse ☐ Radiologist/Physician ☐ Other______________ Date: ____/____/____ Time: ______

Page 1 of 2

M2326
Rev. 8/15

Duke Medicine **PATIENT MRI SAFETY SCREENING**	Name MAN/History Number (Inpatient) Account Number Birthdate (DRM Clinics and PDC)

Initials	Safety Check
	Confirmed correct patient through: 1) full name; and 2) date of birth or medical record number
	Confirmed body part being scanned and laterality
	Confirmed patient MRI screening is complete
	Confirmed only MRI conditional/safe equipment is being used
	Confirmed all staff compliance with zone IV conditionality

Technologist: (Print Name) ______________________

Signature: ______________________ Date: __________ Time: ________

*The technologist signing this form indicates that all criteria have been met as per the Duke Medicine MRI Safety Pause Policy.

For DRAH and DRH Only: Patient History

1) Reason for exam (per patient's explanation): ______________________

2) Have you ever had an MRI on the body part being studied? Yes/No Patient weight ____________

If yes: Date: __________ Location of study: ______________________

3) Have you ever had surgery on the body part being studied? Yes / No

If yes: Date __________ Procedure: ______________________

4) How long has this been a problem? ______________________

5) Personal history of cancer? Yes / No Typo ______________________

Date of diagnosis ____________ Last Chemo date ____________ Last Radiation date ____________

6) Additional information: ______________________

Technologist: (Print Name) ______________________

Signature: ______________________ Date: __________ Time: __________

Page 2 of 2

APPENDIX B

Cardiac Magnetic Resonance Pulse Sequence Parameters and Protocols at Duke Cardiovascular Magnetic Resonance Center

Abbreviations
GRAPPA Generalized Autocalibrating Partially Parallel Acquisition
GRE Gradient Recalled Echo
Hz/px Hertz/pixel
SSFP Steady-state Free Precession
TE Echo Time
TR Repetition Time
TI Inversion Time

1.5 T:

SSFP cine imaging

Readout type: SSFP
TE/TR/flip angle: 1.09 ms/2.73 ms/60 degrees
Matrix size: 256 × 200
Acceleration: GRAPPA: 2, phase partial Fourier: 7/8, asymmetric echo: strong
Slice thickness: 6 mm, interslice spacing: 4 mm
Bandwidth: 1085 Hz/Px
Temporal resolution: <40 ms

Segmented delayed enhancement imaging:

Readout type: GRE
TE/TR/flip angle: 3.38 ms/8.8 ms/25 degrees
Matrix size: 256 × 195
Acceleration: GRAPPA: none, phase partial Fourier: none, asymmetric echo: weak
Slice thickness: 7 mm, interslice spacing: 3 mm
Bandwidth: 130 Hz/Px
Temporal resolution: <180 ms
Inversion time: set to null normal myocardium (~300 ms)

Single-shot delayed enhancement imaging:

Readout type: SSFP
TE/TR/flip angle: 1.24 ms/3.06 ms/80 degrees
Matrix size: 208 × 150
Acceleration: GRAPPA: 2, phase partial Fourier: 7/8, asymmetric echo: weak
Slice thickness: 8 mm, interslice spacing: 0 mm
Bandwidth: 601 Hz/Px
Temporal resolution: <200 ms
Inversion time: 600 ms (thrombus; long TI), ~300 ms (TI to null normal myocardium)

Phase-contrast imaging:

Readout type: GRE
TE/TR/flip angle: 2.72 ms/4.94 ms/20 degrees
Matrix size: 256 × 192
Acceleration: GRAPPA: 2, phase partial Fourier: none, asymmetric echo: strong
Slice thickness: 7 mm
Bandwidth: 444 Hz/Px
Temporal resolution <40 ms

Contrast-enhanced MR angiography

Readout type: 3D GRE
TE/TR/flip angle: 1.07 ms/3.18 ms/23 degrees
Matrix size: 288 × 248 × 190
Acceleration: GRAPPA: phase: 2; slice: 2, phase partial Fourier: none, slice partial Fourier: 6/8, asymmetric echo: allowed
Slice thickness: 1.6 mm
Bandwidth: 390 Hz/Px
Temporal resolution: heart rate–dependent

Perfusion:

Readout type: GRE
TE/TR/flip angle: 1.18 ms/2.67 ms/15 degrees
Matrix size: 208 × 131
Acceleration: GRAPPA: 2, phase partial Fourier: 7/8, asymmetric echo: weak
Slice thickness: 9 mm, gap: dependent on heart size
Bandwidth: 586 Hz/Px
Temporal resolution: 160.7 ms

3.0 T:

SSFP cine imaging

Readout type: SSFP
TE/TR/flip angle: 1.39 ms/3.21 ms/50 degrees
Matrix size: 240 × 163
Acceleration: GRAPPA: 3, phase partial Fourier: 7/8, asymmetric echo: weak
Slice thickness: 6 mm, interslice spacing: 4 mm
Bandwidth: 1157 Hz/Px
Temporal resolution: <40 ms

Segmented delayed enhancement imaging:

Readout type: GRE
TE/TR/flip angle: 2.43 ms/3.34 ms/ 35 degrees
Matrix size: 256 × 204
Acceleration: GRAPPA: 2, phase partial Fourier: none, asymmetric echo: none
Slice thickness: 7 mm, interslice spacing: 3 mm
Bandwidth: 930 Hz/Px
Temporal resolution: <180 ms
Inversion time: set to null normal myocardium (~400 ms)

Single-shot delayed enhancement imaging:

Readout type: SSFP
TE/TR/flip angle: 1.17 ms/2.78 ms/ 45 degrees

Matrix size: 256 × 184
Acceleration: GRAPPA: 2, phase partial Fourier: 7/8, asymmetric echo: weak
Slice thickness: 7 mm, interslice spacing: 0 mm
Bandwidth: 977 Hz/Px
Temporal resolution: <200 ms
Inversion time: 875 ms (thrombus; longTI), ~400 ms (TI to null normal myocardium)

Phase-contrast imaging:

Readout type: GRE
TE/TR/flip angle: 2.57 ms/4.53 ms/ 15 degrees
Matrix size: 256 × 187
Acceleration: GRAPPA: 2, phase partial Fourier: none, asymmetric echo: strong
Slice thickness: 8 mm
Bandwidth: 574 Hz/Px
Temporal resolution <40 ms

Contrast-enhanced MR angiography

Readout type: 3D GRE
TE/TR/flip angle: 1.22 ms/3.86 ms/ 20 degrees
Matrix size: 320 × 224 × 234
Acceleration: GRAPPA: phase: 2; slice: 2, phase partial Fourier: none, slice partial Fourier: 6/8, asymmetric echo: allowed
Slice thickness: 1.5 mm
Bandwidth: 290 Hz/Px
Temporal resolution: heart rate–dependent

Perfusion:

Readout type: GRE
TE/TR/flip angle: 1.79 ms/3.31 ms/ 12 degrees
Matrix size: 256 × 172
Acceleration: GRAPPA: 3, phase partial Fourier: 6/8, asymmetric echo: off
Slice thickness: 8 mm, gap: dependent on heart size
Bandwidth: 610 Hz/Px
Temporal resolution: 140 ms

APPENDIX C

Cardiac Magnetic Resonance Acronyms Used by Various Vendors

SEQUENCE TYPE	SIEMENS	GE	PHILIPS	HITACHI	CANNON (TOSHIBA)
SPIN ECHO	**SE**	**SE**	**SE**	**SE**	**SE**
Fast spin echo	Turbo SE (TSE)	FSE (fast SE)	Turbo SE (TSE)	FSE (fast SE)	FSE (fast SE)
Number of echoes in TSE	Turbo factor	Echo train length (ETL)	Turbo factor	Echo factor	Echo train length (ETL)
Multispin echo	Multi echo/MS	SE	Multi SE	SE	Multi echo
Fast spin echo with variable flip angle	SPACE	CUBE	VISTA	isoFSE	3D MV/OX
Fast spin echo with 90-degree flip-back pulse	RESTORE	FRFSE	DRIVE	Driven equilibrium FSE	T2 plus FSE
Ultrafast spin echo (echo planar fast spin echo)	HASTE	SS-FSE	Single shot TSE	Sigle shot FSE	FASE/SuperFASE
Fat/Water Imaging Techniques					
Chemical shift fat saturation	Fat-Sat	Fat sat/chem sat	SPIR	SINC, H–SINC	MSOFT
Combined chemical shift and inversion recovery	SPIR	SPECIAL/SSRF	SPIR		
Combined chemical shift and adiabatic inversion recovery	SPAIR	ASPIR	SPAIR		SPAIR
DIXON fat/water separation for TSE	DIXON TSE	IDEAL	mDIXON XD, mDIXON TSE	fatSep	
DIXON water/fat separation for 3D GRE	DIXON VIBE	LAVA-flex	mDIXON		WFS
Water excitation	WE	SSRF	ProSet	WE	PASTA
Preparation Modules					
Inversion recovery	IR	IR	IR	IR	IR
Fast inversion recovery	Turbo IR/TIRM	FSE-IR	IR TSE	FIR	Fast IR
Short T1 inversion recovery	STIR	STIR	STIR	STIR	STIR
Long tau inversion recovery	FLAIR/TURBO FLAIR	FLAIR/FAST FLAIR	FLAIR/FLAIR TSE	FLAIR/fast FLAIR	FLAIR/fast FLAIR
True inversion recovery (phase-sensitive inversion recovery)	True IR/PSIR	T1 FLAIR/PSIR	Real IR/PSIR	T1 FLAIR/PSIR	PSIR
Imaging Readouts					
Gradient recall echo	GRE	GRE	FFE	GE	Field echo (FE)
Spoiled gradient echo	FLASH	SPGR	T1-FFE	RSSG	T1-FFE/RF spoiled FE
ULTRAFAST GRADIENT ECHO	TurboFLASH, VIBE	Fast GRE/fast SPGR, VIBRANT/FAME/LAVA	T1-TFE, T2-TFE, THRIVE, eTHRIVE	RGE, SARGE	Fast FE, RADIANCE/ QUICK 3D
Ultrafast 3D gradient echo	MP-RAGE	3D FGRE, 3D fast SPGR	TFE/3D T1-TFE	MP-RAGE	
Ultrafast gradient echo with magnetization preparation	T1/T2 TurboFLASH	IR-prepared, DE-SPGR, BRAVO	IR TFE		Fast FE
T1-weighted gradient echo with fat suppression	VIBE	LAVA, LAVA XV, LAVA FLEX, FAME	IR TFE	TIGRE	QUICK 3D
Coherent gradient echo	FISP	GRASS	FFE	Reshaped SARGE	FE
Coherent gradient echo with echo refocusing	PSIF	SSFP	T2-FFE	Time-resolved SARGE	SSFP
Balanced gradient echo	TrueFISP	FIESTA	Balanced FFE (BFFE)/BTFE	BASG	True SSFP
Coherent balanced gradient echo with dual excitation	CISS	FIESTA-C		PBSG	

SEQUENCE TYPE	SIEMENS	GE	PHILIPS	HITACHI	CANNON (TOSHIBA)
Echo planar	EPI	EPI	EPI	EPI	EPI
Gradient recall echo plus spin echo (hybrid echo)	TGSE		GRASSE		Hybrid EPI
Spoiled gradient echo using combined multiple free induction decays	MEDIC	MERGE	M-FFE		
Spin echo black blood (cardiac)	Dark-blood prepared TSE, HASTE	Double IR FSE with blood suppression	Black-blood prepulse		
Spin echo fat-suppressed black blood (cardiac)	TIRM	Double IR FSE with fat suppression	Black-blood prepulse with SPIR or SPAIR		
Single shot black blood	HASTE	Single-shot FSE (SS-FSE)	Single-shot TSE (SSH-TSE), ultrafast spin echo (UFSE)	Single-shot fast SE	Fast advanced SE (FASE)
Magnetic Resonance Angiography					
Time-of-flight MR angiography	TOF	TOF	Inflow MRA		
Fluoroscopic triggering sequence	Care bolus	Fluoro trigger	Bolus TRAK	FLUTE	VISUAL PREP
Time-resolved contrast-enhanced MR angiography with k-space manipulation	TWIST	TRICKS	4D-TRAK		
Contrast-enhanced MR angiography	CE-MRA	CE-MRA	CE angio	CE-MRA	CE-MRA
Noncontrast angiography (inflow balanced SSFP with inversion recovery saturation)	NATIVE TrueFISP	Inhance Inflow IR (IFIR)	TRANCE/B-TRANCE	VASC-ASL	Time-SLIP
Contrast-enhanced MR angiography with moving table (bolus-chase)	TimCT	SmartStep	MobiTrak, MobiFlex		
Real-time interactive scan	CARE	iDRIVE	Interactive		
Susceptibility-weighted imaging	SWI	SWAN	Venous BOLD		
Acceleration Techniques					
Parallel imaging technique	iPAT	ASSET	SENSE		RAPID
Parallel imaging	mSENSE	SENSE	SENSE	SENSE	SENSE
Parallel imaging with k-space-based algorithm	GRAPPA	ARC			
Compressed sensing	CS	HyperSense	Compressed SENSE		Compressed SPEEDER
Advanced Imaging Acronyms					
T1/T2/T2* mapping	MyoMaps	StarMap (T2*), CartiGram (T2)	T1 mapping, StarQuant	T2* relax map	
Phase-contrast (velocity) imaging	Phase contrast (PC)	Phase contrast (PC)	Phase contrast (PC)	Phase contrast (PC)	Phase shift (PS)
Diffusion-weighted imaging	DWI	DWI	DWI	DWI	DWI
Apparent diffusion coefficient map	ADC	ADC	ADC	ADC	ADC
Diffusion tensor imaging	Multidirectional diffusion imaging (MDDI), DTI	DTI	DTI	DTI	DTI
DTI tractography	DTI tractography	FiberTrak	FiberTrak	DTT (diffusion tensor tractography)	DTI tractography
High-resolution diffusion imaging	RESOLVE	PROPELLER DWI	DWI with segmented EPI	FASE DWI	RADAR DWI
Flow compensation with gradient moment nulling	GMR/FlowComp	FlowComp	FlowComp, FLAG	GR	FC
Motion correction with radial blades	BLADE	PROPELLER	MultiVane	RADAR	JET

SEQUENCE TYPE	SIEMENS	GE	PHILIPS	HITACHI	CANNON (TOSHIBA)
Sequence Parameters					
Repetition time	TR	TR	TR	TR	TR
Echo time	TE	TE	TE	TE	TE
Inversion time	TI	TI	TI	TI	TI
Interecho spacing (TSE/EPI)	Echo spacing	Echo spacing	Echo spacing	Interecho time (IET)	Echo spacing
Averages	Averages	NEX	NSA	NSA	NAQ
Scan measurement time	Acquisition time (TA)	Acquisition time	Acquisition time	Scan time	Acquisition time
Shifting slices off-center	Off-center shift	Off-center FoV	Off-center FoV	Off-center FoV	Phase & frequency shift
Distance between slices	Distance factor (as % of slice thickness)	GAP	GAP	Slice interval	GAP
Simultaneous excitation	Simultaneous excitation	POMP (phase offset multiplanar)	Multislice	Dual slice	QuadScan
RF excitation pulse in gradient echo	Flip angle	Flip angle	Flip angle	Flip angle	Flip angle
Bandwidth	Bandwidth (Hz/px)	Receive bandwidth (kHz)	Fat/water shift (pixel)	Bandwidth	Bandwidth
Half-Fourier imaging	Half-Fourier, phase partial Fourier	Half NEX, fractional NEX	Half scan	Half scan	AFI
Partial echo	Asymmetric echo	Asymmetric echo	Partial echo	Half echo	Matched bandwidth
Phase oversampling	Phase oversampling	No phase wrap	Fold-over suppression	Antiwrap	Phase wrap suppression
Segmented K-space	Lines/segments	Views per segment	Views/segments	Segments	Segments
Scan synchronization with ECG	ECG triggered	Cardiac gated/triggered	ECG triggered/ VCG	ECG triggered	Cardiac gated
Delay after R-wave	Trigger delay (TD)	Trigger delay (TD)	Trigger delay (TD)	Delay time	Trigger delay (TD)
Respiratory gating	Respiratory gated	Respiratory comp	Trigger PEAR	MAR	Respiratory gated
Multichannel RF coil sensitivity normalization	Prescan normalize	PURE	CLEAR	NATURAL	
Centric K-space filling	Central elliptical	Elliptic centric	CENTRA	P	

Index

Note: Page numbers followed by *f* indicate figures and *t* indicate tables.

B

N

Q

R

S

T

U

V